Recommended Dietary Allowances (RDA), 1980[a]

Age (years)	Weight (kg)	Weight (lbs)	Height (cm)	Height (in)	Protein (g)	Vitamin A (RE)	Vitamin D (µg)	Vitamin E (mg)	Vitamin C (mg)	Thiamin (mg)	Riboflavin (mg)	Niacin (mg equiv.)	Vitamin B₆ (mg)	Folacin (µg)	Vitamin B₁₂ (µg)	Calcium (mg)	Phosphorus (mg)	Magnesium (mg)	Iron (mg)	Zinc (mg)	Iodine (µg)
Infants																					
0.0-0.5	6	13	60	24	kg × 2.2	420	10	3	35	0.3	0.4	6	0.3	30	0.5	360	240	50	10	3	40
0.5-1.0	9	20	71	28	kg × 2.0	400	10	4	35	0.5	0.6	8	0.6	45	1.5	540	360	70	15	5	50
Children																					
1-3	13	29	90	35	23	400	10	5	45	0.7	0.8	9	0.9	100	2.0	800	800	150	15	10	70
4-6	20	44	112	44	30	500	10	6	45	0.9	1.0	11	1.3	200	2.5	800	800	200	10	10	90
7-10	28	62	132	52	34	700	10	7	45	1.2	1.4	16	1.6	300	3.0	800	800	250	10	10	120
Males																					
11-14	45	99	157	62	45	1,000	10	8	50	1.4	1.6	18	1.8	400	3.0	1,200	1,200	350	18	15	150
15-18	66	145	176	69	56	1,000	10	10	60	1.4	1.7	18	2.0	400	3.0	1,200	1,200	400	18	15	150
19-22	70	154	177	70	56	1,000	7.5	10	60	1.5	1.7	19	2.2	400	3.0	800	800	350	10	15	150
23-50	70	154	178	70	56	1,000	5	10	60	1.4	1.6	18	2.2	400	3.0	800	800	350	10	15	150
51+	70	154	178	70	56	1,000	5	10	60	1.2	1.4	16	2.2	400	3.0	800	800	350	10	15	150
Females																					
11-14	46	101	157	62	46	800	10	8	50	1.1	1.3	15	1.8	400	3.0	1,200	1,200	300	18	15	150
15-18	55	120	163	64	46	800	10	8	60	1.1	1.3	14	2.0	400	3.0	1,200	1,200	300	18	15	150
19-22	55	120	163	64	44	800	7.5	8	60	1.1	1.3	14	2.0	400	3.0	800	800	300	18	15	150
23-50	55	120	163	64	44	800	5	8	60	1.0	1.2	13	2.0	400	3.0	800	800	300	18	15	150
51+	55	120	163	64	44	800	5	8	60	1.0	1.2	13	2.0	400	3.0	800	800	300	10	15	150
Pregnant					+30	+200	+5	+2	+20	+0.4	+0.3	+2	+0.6	+400	+1.0	+400	+400	+150	[b]	+5	+25
Lactating					+20	+400	+5	+3	+40	+0.5	+0.5	+5	+0.5	+100	+1.0	+400	+400	+150	[b]	+10	+50

[a] The allowances are intended to provide for individual variations among most normal, healthy people in the United States under usual environmental stresses. They were designed for the maintenance of good nutrition. Diets should be based on a variety of common foods in order to provide other nutrients for which human requirements have been less well defined. See the text for a more detailed discussion of the RDA and of nutrients not tabulated.

[b] Supplemental iron is recommended.

The Committee on RDA has published a separate table showing energy allowances in ranges for each age-sex group and another table for vitamins and minerals not previously covered by the recommendations. These tables appear in Appendix I. The FDA has published a special table of selected RDA values for use on food labels: these, the U.S. RDA, appear on the inside back cover.

Reproduced from *Recommended Dietary Allowances,* 9th ed. (1980), with the permission of the National Academy of Sciences, Washington, D.C.

Understanding Normal and Clinical Nutrition

Second Edition

Eleanor Noss Whitney

Corinne Balog Cataldo

Sharon Rady Rolfes

West Publishing Company
St. Paul   New York
Los Angeles   San Francisco

Copyediting Mary Berry, Naples Editing Service
Composition Carlisle Graphics; Appendixes by K. F. Merrill Co.
Text Design Design Office, Bruce Kortebein, Leigh McLellan
Text Illustrations Chapters 1–16 by Kidd & Company
Cartoons Chapters 17–27 by Kirk Barron
Diagrams Chapters 17–27 by Asterick Group
Cover Image Photomicrograph of Vitamin B$_6$ Tore Johnson of Woodfin Camp and Associates
Cover Design David Farr, Imagesmythe, Inc.

Photo Credits

Chapter Openings
1, 51, 89, 133, 167, 203, 239, 289, 371, 407, 437, 491, 529, 549 From D. W. Fawcett, *The Cell*, 2nd ed. (Philadelphia: Saunders, 1981); color by Kidd & Company; **17** Woodfin Camp & Associates, Tore Johnson; **341, 605, 649, 677, 717, 737, 759, 789, 809, 835** Sandra Silvers, electron microscopist at Florida State University Electron Microscope Facility, color by Kidd & Company; **575** © Joel Gordon 1984; **697** B. F. King, Univ. of California School of Medicine/BPS.

Text
5, 27, 36, 40, 41, 69, 72, 75, 78 Ray Stanyard; **46** Drawing by Donald Reilly; © 1971 The New Yorker Magazine, Inc.; **79** © 1977 King Feature Syndicate, Inc.; **90** © Tony Duffy, Woodfin Camp & Associates; **92, 108, 109, 110, 111, 113** Ray Stanyard; **124** (A and B) Reproduced by permission. Original material provided by Abel L. Robertson, M.D. Ph.D., University of Illinois at Chicago, Dept. of Pathology, College of Medicine, Chicago, IL 60612, © *Scientific American* 236 (1977): 75. Reprinted by permission of Scientific American, Inc.; **136** Human hemoglobin

model constructed by Dr. Makio Murayama, NIH, Bethesda, Maryland (scaled to ½ inch to angstrom). Atomic coordinates were supplied for the model by Dr. Max F. Perutz, Cambridge, England; **145** Ray Stanyard; **152** (margin) Wide World Photos, reprinted with permission; **152** (bottom) Courtesy of Dr. Robert S. Goodhard, M.D.; **157, 158, 162** Ray Stanyard; **179** Courtesy of Dr. Susumu Ito; **224** © Karen Eberhardt/Jeroboam, Inc.; **241, 242, 264** Ray Stanyard; **295** © *Nutrition Today*, C. Butterworth and G. Blackburn, Hospital Nutrition and How to Assess the Nutritional Status of a Patient. Nutrition Today Teaching Aid Number 18 (Nutrition Today: Annapolis, MD), 1975; **300** Courtesy of Dr. Samuel Dreizen, D.D.S., M.D.; **301** © *Nutrition Today*, H. Sandstead, J. Carter, and W. Darby, Nutritional Deficiencies, Nutrition Today Teaching Aid Number 5 (Nutrition Today: Annapolis, MD), 1975; **306, 311** Ray Stanyard; **317** © *Nutrition Today*, H. Sandstead, J. Carter, and W. Darby, Nutritional Deficiencies, Nutrition Today Teaching Aid Number 5 (Nutrition Today: Annapolis, MD), 1975; **317** From C. Conn, *The Specialities in General Practice*, 2nd ed. (Philadelphia: Saunders, 1957); **320** Ray Stanyard; **322** Anthony Vannelli; **324** (top) Bernard Pierre Wolfe/FPG International; (bottom) Courtesy of the Upjohn Company; **325** Ray Stanyard; **347** David J. Farr; **348** © *Nutrition Today*, H. Sandstead, J. Carter, and W. Darby, Nutritional Deficiencies, Nutrition Today Teaching Aid Number 5 (Nutrition Today: Annapolis, MD), 1975; **354** Ray Stanyard; **356** Courtesy of Parke-Davis & Company; **372** Anthony Vannelli; **389** (A) Courtesy of Gjon Mill; (B) © *Nutrition Today*; (C) Adapted from Why Should Adults Drink Milk? (Tallahassee, Fla.: Nutrition Company, 1983); **393, 400** Ray Stanyard; **409** Courtesy of Dr. M. F. Perutz; **411** © Michael Abbey, Science Source/Photo Researchers; **423** Reproduced with permission of *Nutrition Today*,

magazine, P.O. Box 1829, Annapolis, MD 21404, March 1968; **427** Ray Stanyard; **429** Courtesy of FAO; **433** Courtesy of H. Kaplan and V.P. Rabbach; **456, 457** Ray Stanyard; **493** (L) Photo copyright © Camera, M.D. Studios, 1973. All rights reserved; (R) Photo copyright © Camera M.D. Studios, 1977. All rights reserved; **497** Woodfin Camp & Associates, © William Hubbell; **499** Photos courtesy of Ann Pytkowicz Streissguth, University of Washington. Reprinted by permission from the CIBA Foundation; **502** Woodfin Camp & Associates, © William Hubbell; **513, 515**, Anthony Vannelli; **516** Courtesy of H. Kaplan and V.P. Rabbach; **526** Woodfin Camp & Associates, © Lawrence Manning; **532, 533, 540** Anthony Vannelli; **542** © Donald Dietz, 1980, Stock, Boston; **550** Anthony Vannelli; **559** Woodfin Camp & Associates, © Burk Uzzle 1983; **568** Woodfin Camp & Associates, © Michal Heron 1981; **571** Woodfin Camp & Associates, © Jeff Lowenthal 1985; **572** Woodfin Camp & Associates, © Sylvia Johnson, 1984; **581** Billy E. Barnes/FPG International; **582** Susan Leavines/Photo Researchers, Inc.; **588, 597** Stephen McBrady/InfoEdit; **606** Woodfin Camp & Associates, © Michal Heron; **616** Woodfin Camp & Associates, © Alon Reininger; **625** Illustration courtesy of Ross Laboratories; **638** Stephen McBrady/InfoEdit **646** Photograph courtesy of Cornmed, Inc.; **650** Biomedical Communications/Photo Researchers, Inc., **652** L & M Photo/FPG International; **667, 668** Anthony Vannelli; **681** Hans Halberstadt/Photo Researchers, Inc.; **699, 719** Anthony Vannelli; **731** Reproduced with permission of *Nutrition Today* Magazine, P.O. Box 1829, Annapolis, Maryland 21404, September 1968; **734** Anthony Vannelli; **766** Biophoto Associates/Photo Researchers, Inc.; **768** Dennis Hallinan/FPG International; **772** Anthony Vannelli; **791** Ray Stanyard; **796** (top) Stephen McBrady/InfoEdit; **796** (bottom), **798** Anthony Vannelli.

Library of Congress Cataloging-in-Publication Data

Whitney, Eleanor Noss.
    Understanding normal and clinical nutrition.

    Includes bibliographical references and index.
    1. Nutrition.   2. Diet in disease.   3. Nutrition disorders.   I. Cataldo, Corinne Balog.   II. Rolfes, Sharon Rady.   III. Title.
[DNLM: 1. Diet Therapy   2. Nutrition.
QU 145 W618ua]
QP141.W458   1987   612'.3   87-6139
ISBN 0-314-24245-7
1st Reprint—1987

To Kara, Russ, and Lynn, whose astonishing strides in new realms bring me joy. And to my parents, Edith and Henry Noss, who delight me by continuing to learn and grow.

Ellie

To the memory of my sister and friend, Keesy, whose words of encouragement, happiness for my happiness, and love made the good times better and the bad times less ominous. I miss your presence, your voice, and your laughter dearly. But you live in my heart and thoughts and I hear you often in the part of me that is you.

Corkie

To Tom, Lyle, and Marni, whose love and laughter brighten my life. To Mom and Dad, who nourish me with affection and encouragement to pursue my dreams. And to Ellie, who gave me an understanding of nutrition, and the opportunity to share it with others.

Sharon

About the Authors

Eleanor Noss Whitney, Ph.D., R.D., received her B.A. in Biology from Radcliffe College in 1960 and her Ph.D. in Biology from Washington University, St. Louis, in 1970. Formerly on the faculty at the Florida State University, she now devotes full time to research, writing, and consulting in nutrition and health. She is president of Nutrition and Health Associates, a nutrition information resource center in Tallahassee, Florida. Her previous publications include articles in *Science*, the *Journal of Nutrition, Genetics,* and other journals, and the textbooks *Understanding Nutrition, Nutrition: Concepts and Controversies,* and *Nutrition and Diet Therapy.*

Corinne Balog Cataldo, M.M. Sc., R.D., L.D., received her B.S. in Community Health Nutrition from Georgia State University in 1976 and her M.M. Sc. in Clinical Dietetics from Emory University in 1979. She has worked as a nutrition counselor in private practice in Atlanta, as a clinical dietitian and metabolic support nutritionist at Georgia Baptist Medical Center in Atlanta, and as a faculty member and dietetic internship director at Emory University. She has made numerous presentations, and in addition to this book, she has published a tube feeding manual and the book *Nutrition and Diet Therapy.*

Sharon Rady Rolfes, M.S., R.D., received her B.S. in Psychology and Criminology in 1974 and her M.S. in Nutrition and Food Science in 1982 at the Florida State University. She serves on the board of directors of Nutrition and Health Associates, an information resource center in Tallahassee, Florida. Her publications include several *Nutrition Clinics* on topics such as cancer, heart disease, vegetarian diet planning, and hypoglycemia. As a contributing editor of the monthly newsletter, *Healthline,* she has written articles on bulimia, cancer, fish oils and heart disease, and fasting. She prepared the *Instructor's Manual* and *Student Study Guide* that accompany *Understanding Nutrition, Nutrition: Concepts and Controversies,* and *Understanding Normal and Clinical Nutrition* and is currently co-authoring a nutrition textbook entitled *Maternal and Child Nutrition.*

Contents in Brief

continued

Contents

4   The Lipids: Fats, Oils, Phospholipids, and Sterols   89

5   Protein: Amino Acids   133

6   Digestion, Absorption, and Transport   167

7   Metabolism: Nutrient Transformations and Interactions   203

8   Energy Balance and Weight Control   239

9   The Water-Soluble Vitamins: B Vitamins and Vitamin C   289

10   The Fat-Soluble Vitamins: A, D, E, and K   341

11   Water and the Major Minerals   371

12   The Trace Minerals   407

19   Nutrition and Drug Therapy   649

20   Nutrition and Stress: Surgery, Infection, and Burns   677

21   Disorders of the Upper GI Tract   697

22   Disorders of Intestines   717

23 Disorders of the Liver, Exocrine Pancreas, and Gallbladder 737

24 Diabetes and Hypoglycemia 759

25 Disorders of the Heart and Blood Vessels 789

Appendixes

Preface

When we wrote the first edition of *Understanding Normal and Clinical Nutrition* our goal was to provide an up-to-date and accurate textbook that included both normal and clinical nutrition. We wanted the book to hold the reader's attention—to provide more than just facts. We also wanted readers to understand how the facts apply to people and to everyday life. Our goals for this second edition of the book are basically unchanged. However, the book has been revised substantially to reflect the many changes that have taken place in the field of nutrition since the first book was written.

Among new and substantially revised subject matter are many sections of the chapters, and many of the highlights. Chapter 1 has been expanded to two chapters, so that it can accommodate information on food labels and the U.S. RDA in close proximity to the RDA. New discussions appear in the first twelve chapters on the glycemic effect of foods, protein quality, stress and nutrition, common digestive problems, the assessment and treatment of obesity, B vitamin roles and interactions, toxicity of micronutrients, fluid and electrolyte balance and imbalance, acid-base balance, water balance, blood pressure regulation, calcium and osteoporosis, milk substitutes, calcium supplements, iron supplements and contamination iron, marginal iron deficiency, behavioral effects of iron deficiency, and many other subjects. Chapter 13 on foods and food safety is new: it brings together information on food additives, pesticide residues in foods, engineered and convenience foods, natural food toxicants, food contaminants, and food poisoning. Chapter 14 contains a new section comparing human milk with other milks and infant formula.

The clinical chapters are substantially revised and include new or expanded sections on preventing protein-kcalorie malnutrition, encouraging the adult and child who is ill to eat, current recommendations for the administration of tube feedings, special considerations in feeding infants and children by tube or intravenous feeding, and additional information on the administration of medications through feeding tubes. The discussion on disorders of the gastrointestinal system has been revised and divded into two chapters to ease reading and to include additional current information. Chapter 24 now incorporates the new diabetic exchange list system and has additional information on diabetes during pregnancy and special considerations for the child with diabetes. Chapter 25 includes the latest recommendations of the American Heart Association on the treatment of hyperlipidemias and contains information on many new studies that have surfaced during the past few years.

At the ends of the chapters on normal nutrition are self-study sections, permitting students to analyze their own diets; the needed forms are all in Appendix K. In the chapters on clinical nutrition, you will find many new case studies and sample menus. In addition, many of the chapters throughout the book have new figures, tables, and study questions.

Many of the highlights are also new, delving into such fascinating topics as natural foods, nutrition and cancer, vegetarianism, nutrition and the brain, nutrition and fitness, controversial uses of vitamin B_6, nutrition and premenstrual syndrome (PMS), cancer and the Delaney Clause, nutrition and children's behavior, uses of computers in nutrition, ethical issues in clinical nutrition, and the roles of diet in the prevention and treatment of kidney disorders. Especially notable is Highlight 8, which gives an expanded treatment of anorexia nervosa and bulimia, commensurate in extent and depth with students' interest in these eating disorders. Highlight 18B provides a significantly revised discussion of home enteral and parenteral nutrition programs, and Highlight 19 on nutrition and the immune system includes information on acquired immune deficiency syndrome (AIDS).

The appendixes are also all revised, and we are pleased to present several new ones. Appendix A provides background on the endocrine and nervous sytems, complementing B and C on basic chemistry, chemical structures, and metabolic pathways. Appendix D assists the student with routine nutrition calculations. Appendix F offers our recommendations on nutrition books and journals. Appendix G contains the elegant, revised Food Exchange System first presented at the American Dietetic Association's annual meeting in October, 1986 (and the chapters incorporate the new system). Most pleasing to us is that Appendix H contains a new nutrient data base assembled by ESHA Research, Inc. of Salem, Oregon: it presents the composition of over 1,000 foods with respect to 19 nurients, including for the first time dietary fiber, magnesium, phosphorus, and vitamin B_6. This appendix also includes sodium, potassium, cholesterol, and the fatty-acid breakdown of foods, eliminating the necessity of presenting this information in separate appendixes. Appendix L is also new; it contains the composition of commercially-made enteral formulas and feeding modules.

The concept of nutrient density has received greater emphasis in this edition than in previous editions. It's an old term, now, but its applications are still new and surprising. Tables throughout the chapters on vitamins and minerals present the nutrient contents of foods in two ways: the left side of each table does it the old way (ranked by nutrient per serving); the right side does it the new way—ranked by nutrient per 100 kcalories of the food. This puts foods into a new perspective, and together with the color photographs of foods rich in various nutrients, helps the reader to appreciate the value of certain foods— especially vegetables—more realistically than ever before. The impact is heightened by a presentation that begins by contrasting two meals in Chapter 2, discusses those two meals in chapter after chapter in the first half of the book, and culminates with a synthesis in Chapter 13.

As before, one of the main missions of the book is to assist the reader who wants not only to learn nutrition "facts," but also to become a discriminating consumer of newly emerging nutrition information. "How can I decide what to believe?" the reader wants to know. In the first half of the book, portions of each chapter—the digressions—and most of the Highlights are devoted to construction of a sieve through which readers can filter new nutrition claims and separate the valid ones from the rest. In the clinical chapters, the digressions are designed to show the human element amid the "facts" about treating various disorders with a diet. Digressions ask the reader to stop and think about the implications to clients of the recommendations presented in the chapters. The book continues to deliver the message that there is no absolute certainty, even in science's most logical theories, and that human critical thinking and judgment must always be applied in assessing nutrition claims or providing advice to clients.

> The digressions are set off with color like this; if they prove too distracting you can skip them and possibly come back to them later. But they contain a theme that runs throughout the book.

We have tried to keep the number of footnotes to a minimum. Many statements that appeared in the previous edition with footnotes now appear without them, but every statement is backed by evidence and the authors will supply references on request. Also, as before, we have retained our informal, conversational writing style, hoping this will make the reader's study of nutrition as enjoyable as possible. It is a fascinating subject; we hope our enthusiasm for it comes through on every page.

Eleanor N. Whitney
Corinne B. Cataldo
Sharon R. Rolfes
February, 1987

Acknowledgments

The first sixteen chapters of this book discuss normal nutrition as presented also in the separate textbook *Understanding Nutrition*, by Eleanor N. Whitney, Eva May Nunnelly Hamilton, and Marie A. Boyle. We appreciate the spirit of that book as originally conceived by May Hamilton, and the contributions made by Marie Boyle to the third and fourth editions.

We have been assisted and supported by the finest group of associates any authors could ask for. We are especially grateful to Annette Franklin for her cheerful and careful attention to round after round of word processing; to Jeannie Weingarth for her enthusiastic and efficient assistance with a multitude of production details; to Betty and Bob Geltz for their meticulous and monumental effort in assembling the new food composition appendix; to Sandra Silvers for her beautiful electron micrographs; to Sharon Rady Rolfes and Jana R. Kicklighter for the high-quality Instructor's Manual and Student Study Guide that accompany this book; to Stan Winter for sharing his creative ideas and criticism; to Linda DeBruyne for her efficient production of the index; to Paul Sharpe for his patient work on the food tables; to Linda Patton for her skilled library detective work; to Dee Dee Celander, Danny Johnson, and Joe Antonacci for their artistic creations; to Louise March for her artistry with page makeup; to Phyllis Mueller for her smooth coordination of reviews; and to our editors Pete Marshall, Becky Tollerson, and Sharon Walrath for their powerful support activities. We also thank our many reviewers, whose contributions have enhanced the quality and accuracy of the information this book presents. A special thank you to our families for their encouragement and support in helping us complete this project.

Reviewers of *Understanding Normal and Clinical Nutrition*, 2e

Kathryn Anderson
Florida State University

Yvonne Bronner
Howard University

Kara Caldwell
California State Polytechnic University–San Luis Obispo

Patricia Carey
Miami Dade Community College

Wen Chiu
Shoreline Community College

Dorothy Coltrin
DeAnza College

Christine Condit
Appalachian State University

Connie Ellif
Lamar University

Pam Fletcher
Albequerque Technical Vocational Institute

Gayle Gess
Fullerton College

Nancy Green
Florida State University

Mary Jane Hamilton
Del Mar College

Margaret Hedley
University of Guelph

Maren Hegsted
Louisiana State University

Elaine Johnson
City College of San Francisco

Mary Kelso
Antelope Valley College

Margaret Kessel
Ohio State University

Kathleen M. Koehler
University of New Mexico

Barbara Kurtz
North Central Michigan Community College

Betty Kutter
Evergreen State College

Carolyn Lara-Braud
University of Iowa

Louise Little
University of Delaware

Elaine Long
Boise State University

Anne McLaughlin
Indiana University

Rose Martin
Scottsdale Community College

Sharleen Matter
University of Louisville

Stella Miller
Mt. San Antonio College

Connie Mobley
Incarnate Word College

Karen Mondrone
William Paterson College

Peggy Morrison
Pensacola Junior College

James T. Mullen
Somerset Community College

Maria Museler
Suffolk Community College

Ellen S. Parham
Northern Illinois University

Janice R. Peach
Western Washington University

Irvin P. Plitzuweit
Rochester Community College

Mary Jane Reumann
University of Alabama–Huntsville

Gerald Robinson
University of South Florida

Betty Schaffner
Baldwin-Wallace College

Robin Sesan
University of Delaware

Rose Ann Shorey-Kutschke
University of Texas–Austin

Mary Sirotnik
Mac Nursing Education Center

Harry Sitren
University of Florida

Samuel C. Smith
University of New Hampshire

Joanne Spaide
University of Northern Iowa

Janet White
Rochester Institute of Technology

Carol Whitlock
Rochester Institute of Technology

Stan Winter
Golden West College

Nutrition and Health

1

Contents

The body's cells are highly sensitive and energetic, and require many nutrients to sustain their activities. Shown here are three white blood cells—the body's defenders against disease.

You are a collection of molecules that move. All these moving parts are arranged in complexity and order—cells, tissues, and organs. The arrangement is constant, but its parts are continually being replaced by processes using nutrients, and using energy derived from nutrients. Your skin, which seems to have covered you without changing from when you were born, is not the same skin that covered you seven years ago; it is made entirely of new cells. The fat beneath your skin is not the same fat that was there a year ago. Your oldest red blood cell is only 120 days old, and the entire lining of your digestive tract is renewed every three days. To maintain your "self," you must continually replenish the energy you burn and replace the pieces you lose.

To put together a human being from the purified chemical ingredients, supposing it could be done, would be an expensive proposition, because we contain such a gold mine of molecular information in such highly organized form. The protein hemoglobin of the red blood cells costs several dollars a gram; the hormone insulin, close to $50 a gram. A whimsical calculation estimates the value of the chemical constituents of a single human body at over $6,000,000—before computing the cost of assembly, preservation, and maintenance. As fanciful as this calculation may be, it illustrates that "we are, at the molecular level, the most information-dense structures around, surpassing computers by many orders of magnitude."[1]

All the pieces you are made of have come from your food. You are made entirely of what you have eaten. Amazingly, though, you can eat foods entirely different from those someone else eats and still construct a normal human body from the nutrients in them. The secret is in the genetic code you inherited from your parents—which gives the instructions for raw materials to be assembled into the structures of your body. As long as the nutrients you need are all there in sufficient amounts, your genetic blueprint and assembly machinery will ensure that you are constructed according to plan and working as you should. The science of nutrition is the study of how this takes place—the study of the nutrients in foods and the body's handling of those nutrients.

The Nutrients

science of nutrition: the study of nutrients and of their ingestion, digestion, absorption, transport, metabolism, interaction, storage, and excretion. A broader definition includes the study of the environment and of human behavior as it relates to these processes.

nutrient: a substance obtained from food and used in the body to promote growth, maintenance, and/or repair. The **essential nutrients** are those the body cannot make for itself in sufficient quantity to meet physiological need, and so has to obtain from food.

food: nutritive material taken into the body for the maintenance of life and the growth and repair of tissues (**nutritive:** containing nutrients).

The six classes of nutrients are carbohydrate, fat, protein, vitamins, minerals, and water.

Almost any food you eat is composed of dozens or even hundreds of different kinds of materials—atoms and molecules, tinier by far than the smallest things that can be seen with the most powerful microscope. The complete chemical analysis of a food such as spinach shows that it is composed mostly of water (95 percent) and that most of the solid materials are organic compounds: carbohydrate, fat, and protein. If you could remove these materials, you would find a tiny residue of minerals, vitamins, and other items. Water, carbohydrate, fat, protein, vitamins, and some of the minerals are nutrients. Some of the other materials are not.

A complete chemical analysis of the body would show that it is made of similar materials. A healthy 150-pound person's body contains about 90 pounds of water and about 30 pounds of fat. The other 30 pounds are mostly protein and carbohydrate, related organic compounds made from them, and the major minerals of the bones: calcium and phosphorus. Vitamins, other minerals, and incidental extras constitute a fraction of a pound. Thus the human body, like spinach, is composed largely of nutrients (see Figure 1-1).

Atoms, molecules, and compounds: Appendix B summarizes basic chemistry facts and provides definitions.

FIGURE 1-1

Foods and the human body are made of the same classes of chemicals. (Vitamins and other constituents are not shown, because the amounts are too small to be seen on a graph this size.)

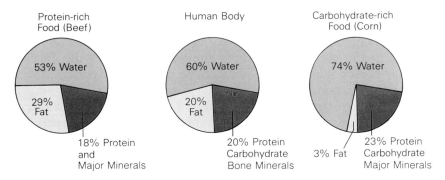

Protein-rich Food (Beef): 53% Water, 29% Fat, 18% Protein and Major Minerals

Human Body: 60% Water, 20% Fat, 20% Protein Carbohydrate Bone Minerals

Carbohydrate-rich Food (Corn): 74% Water, 3% Fat, 23% Protein Carbohydrate Major Minerals

GEE, I BETTER GO BACK TO AISLE 6 AND GET 40 MORE MILLIGRAMS OF IRON.

When we buy foods, we are really buying nutrients.

(This book is devoted mostly to the nutrients, but you should be aware that other constituents are found in foods and in your body—alcohols, organic acids, pigments, intentional and incidental additives, and others. Some are beneficial, some are of no recognized positive value to human beings, and some are harmful. Later sections of the book focus on some of these constituents and their significance.)

If you burn a food such as spinach in air, it "disappears." The water evaporates, and all the organic compounds are oxidized to gas (carbon dioxide) and water vapor, leaving only a residue of ash (minerals). This leads us to a definition of the word *organic*.

An organic compound is one that contains carbon atoms. The first organic compounds known were natural products synthesized by plants or animals; indeed, it used to be thought that only living things contributed organic compounds to our world. The term has since been expanded to include all carbon compounds, whatever their origin. Actually, in a sense, all organic compounds are produced by living things. Some of them, like petroleum (which comes from the remains of microorganisms, plants, and animals that grew in prehistoric times), began and ended their lives millions of years ago. Others are produced

Constituents other than nutrients, such as additives, toxicants, and contaminants, are treated in Chapter 13.

organic: containing carbon or, more strictly, containing carbon and hydrogen or carbon-carbon bonds. This definition excludes coal (which has no defined bonds) and a few carbon-containing compounds which contain only a single carbon and no hydrogen such as carbon dioxide (CO_2), calcium carbonate ($CaCO_3$), magnesium carbonate ($MgCO_3$), and sodium cyanide ($NaCN$). See also p. 46

Labels on food products sometimes claim that the products are "organic," implying that they are therefore somehow superior. By our definition, any carbon compound is organic—even a synthetic vitamin preparation from the laboratory of a pharmaceutical company. Is there any reason to believe that "organic" or "natural" foods or nutrient preparations sold in "health food" stores are superior to grocery store foods or synthetic vitamins? Highlight 2 investigates this question.

The organic nutrients are carbohydrate, fat, protein, and vitamins. The first three yield energy for human use.

oxidation: a reaction in which electrons are removed from a molecule (see Appendix B). Often, this occurs when a molecule reacts with oxygen; hence the name. Oxidation reactions usually result in the release of energy. In chemical oxidation of nutrients, the energy released is largely chemical and mechanical; in oxidative combustion (burning), the energy released is mostly heat and light energy.

Metabolism, the set of processes by which nutrients are rearranged into body structures or broken down to yield energy, is defined and described in Chapter 7.

The energy nutrients—that is, the nutrients that break down to yield energy the body can use—are carbohydrate, fat, and protein.

calorie: a unit in which energy is measured. Technically, a calorie is the amount of heat necessary to raise the temperature of a gram of water one degree Celsius. Food energy is measured in **kilocalories** (thousands of calories), abbreviated **kcalories** or **kcal**. A capitalized version is also sometimes used: **Calories**. Most people, even nutritionists, speak of these units simply as calories, but on paper they should be prefaced by a *k*. (The pronunciation of *kcalories* ignores the *k*, but some people when speaking pronounce it "KAY-calories" or "KAY-cal.") We will use *kcalories* and *kcal* throughout this book.
1 gram carbohydrate = 4 kcalories.
1 gram protein = 4 kcalories.
1 gram fat = 9 kcalories.

1 gram alcohol = 7 kcalories.

by plants and animals alive today. Still others come from laboratories where chemists (who are also living things) produce them in the test tube.

In any case, four of the six classes of nutrients (carbohydrate, fat, protein, and vitamins) are organic, while the other two (minerals and water) are inorganic. On being oxidized during metabolism, three of these four (carbohydrate, fat, and protein) provide energy the body can use. In contrast, minerals and water are inorganic and do not yield energy in the human body.

The Energy Nutrients

You can metabolize all four classes of organic nutrients, but derive energy from only three. These three are the energy nutrients. They are vital to life, for without continual replenishment of the energy you spend daily, you would soon die. When oxidized in the body, the energy nutrients break down; that is, their carbon and hydrogen atoms (and others) come apart and are combined with oxygen, yielding carbon dioxide and water, waste materials that must be excreted. As they break down, they release energy. Some of this energy is released as heat, some is transferred into other compounds (including fat) that compose the structures of your body cells, and some is used as fuel for your activities.

The amount of energy the energy nutrients release can be measured in calories (or more properly, kilocalories or kcalories), which are familiar to everyone as a measure of food energy and of the energy the body spends in large quantities during heavy exercise. People think of "kcalories" as a constituent of foods, but strictly speaking, they are not; they are a *measure* of the energy in foods. Thus to speak of the kcalories in an apple or a cookie is technically incorrect, just as to speak of the inches in a person is incorrect. It is correct to speak of the *energy* in a food (and of the *height* of a person), and that is what this book will do.* A gram of carbohydrate contains 4 kcalories; a gram of protein also contains 4; and a gram of fat contains 9 kcalories. The energy content of a food thus depends on how much carbohydrate, fat, and protein it contains. If you don't use these nutrients immediately after you eat them, your body rearranges them (and the energy they contain) into storage compounds such as body fat, and puts them away for use between meals and overnight. If more are consumed than are used, no matter from which of the three energy nutrients, this can lead to overweight. Too much meat (a protein-rich food) is just as fattening as too many potatoes (a carbohydrate-rich food).

One other substance contributes kcalories: alcohol. Alcohol is not called a nutrient, because it doesn't promote growth, maintenance, or repair in the body. Still, people do consume it, and it shares several characteristics with the energy nutrients. Like them, it is metabolized in the body to yield energy (7 kcalories per gram). When taken in excess of energy need, alcohol, too, is converted to body fat and stored. But when alcohol contributes a substantial portion of the energy in a person's diet, it is harmful. It is especially dangerous during preg-

---

* Food energy can also be measured in kilojoules (kJ). A kilojoule is the amount of energy expended when a kilogram is moved one meter by a force of one newton. (It is thus a measure of work energy, whereas the kcalorie is a measure of heat energy. Both are metric measures.)

One kcal equals 4.2 kilojoules. The kilojoule is now the international unit of energy. The United States and Canada will slowly be switching over to it in the next decades, but it is not in popular use yet. This book does not use the kilojoule.

For Canadians: 1 gram carbohydrate = 17 kilojoule; 1 gram protein = 17 kilojoule; and 1 gram fat = 37 kilojoule. 1 gram alcohol (discussed next) = 29 kilojoule.

nancy, because it can cause irreversible retardation and deformity in the developing fetus. (Highlight 7B is devoted to alcohol and nutrition.)

Practically all foods contain mixtures of all three energy nutrients, although they are sometimes classified by the predominant nutrient. Thus it is not correct to speak of meat as a protein or of bread as a carbohydrate; they are *foods* rich in these nutrients. A protein-rich food like beef actually contains a lot of fat as well as protein; a carbohydrate-rich food like corn also contains fat and protein (recall Figure 1-1). Only a few foods are exceptions to this rule, the common ones being sugar (which is pure carbohydrate) and oil (which is almost pure fat).

The body's use (metabolism) of the energy nutrients can be summarized, simply as follows. First, food protein, fat, and carbohydrate are broken down to simpler compounds. The process yields energy, and fragments of the original materials. Then, the fragments may be:

- Used to build new compounds (contributing to fat, muscle, or other tissues), or
- Excreted as waste materials.

The energy may:

- Help build new compounds (and some energy may be stored in them).
- Help move the body (do work).
- Escape as heat.

The energy nutrients are (by molecular standards) tremendous in size. A single molecule of carbohydrate may be composed of 300 sugar (glucose) units, each containing 24 atoms, for a total of some 7,000 atoms. Fats and proteins are similar in size. Only if they are oxidized for fuel do they diminish in size to tiny molecules of carbon dioxide and water (three atoms each). When this occurs, they release tremendous quantities of energy for your use.

Furthermore, you eat (by molecular standards) tremendous quantities of the three energy nutrients. Some people eat 100 grams or more a day of each. If you could purify the carbohydrate, fat, and protein in your daily diet, they

The damage caused by alcohol to the developing fetus is known as *fetal alcohol syndrome*. See Chapter 14.

A huge molecule, composed of hundreds or thousands of atoms, is a **macromolecule**. A molecule of water, by contrast, is composed of only three atoms: 2 H (hydrogen) and 1 O (oxygen).

Carbohydrate, fat, and protein: people eat 50 to 200 grams per day of each.

A Note about Grams

Most people don't think of foods in terms of grams. It's easy to learn to do so, though, and a good idea for those who plan to work with foods in the future. A standard portion (a half cup) of most vegetables or a half cup of milk or juice has a volume of about 125 milliliters and weighs roughly 100 grams. A teaspoon of any dry powder such as sugar, salt, or flour weighs (very roughly) 5 grams. For accurate conversion factors, look on the inside back cover.

100 g Peas.

100 g Juice.

5 g Salt.

Normal (half-cup) vegetable servings are about 125 ml (100 g if weighed). A half-cup of juice or milk is also about 125 ml and weighs about 100g. One teaspoon of any dry powder is about 5 g.

TABLE 1–1

The Vitamins[a]

The Fat-Soluble Vitamins
  Vitamin A
  Vitamin D
  Vitamin E
  Vitamin K
The Water-Soluble Vitamins
  B vitamins
    Thiamin
    Riboflavin
    Niacin
    Vitamin B_6
    Vitamin B_{12}
    Folacin
    Biotin
    Pantothenic acid
  Vitamin C

[a]The names given here for the vitamins are those agreed on by the American Institute of Nutrition and other scientific societies and published in Nomenclature policy: Generic descriptors and trivial names for vitamins and related compounds, *Journal of Nutrition* 112 (1982): 7–14.

Vitamins are small, organic molecules.

Vitamins yield no energy.

vitamin: an organic, essential nutrient required in minute amounts.
vita = life
amine = containing nitrogen (the first vitamins discovered were amines)

The water-soluble vitamins are the B vitamins and vitamin C. The fat-soluble vitamins are vitamins A, D, E, and K.

Minerals are small, inorganic molecules.

Minerals yield no energy.

would fill two or three measuring cups each. The foods they come in weigh much more and occupy much more volume. A hundred grams of food may contain only 10 or 50 grams of energy nutrients, the rest being water, fiber, and other non-kcaloric materials.

The vitamins, the next class of nutrients, differ profoundly from the first three classes in almost every way: in their size and shape, in the roles they play, and in the amounts you consume. Perhaps the only characteristics they share with the first three classes of nutrients are that they are vital to life, they are organic, and they are available in food.

The Vitamins

The vitamins are organic compounds generally much smaller than the energy nutrients. The body may break them down but cannot extract usable energy from them; their role is rather to serve as helpers, making possible the processes by which the other nutrients are digested, absorbed, and metabolized to body compounds or excreted. There are 13 different vitamins, each with its own special roles to play (see Table 1-1).

That vitamins are organic has several consequences. For one thing, they are destructible. They can be broken down, oxidized, and altered in shape. They must therefore be handled with care. The body makes special provisions to absorb and transport them, providing many of them with custom-made protein carriers. A vitamin may be useful in one form here and another there, so special metabolic equipment is provided that can subtly alter the characteristics of a vitamin to allow it to perform a particular task.

The destructibility of vitamins also has implications for food handlers and cooks. You are well-advised, when working with food, to keep in mind that excessive acid, alkali, air, heat, or light can destroy vitamins.

The vitamins are divided into two classes: some are soluble in water (the B vitamins and vitamin C), and others in fat (vitamins A, D, E, and K). This fact has many implications for the kinds of foods that contain them and the ways the body absorbs, transports, stores, and excretes them. The vitamins are the subjects of Chapters 9 and 10.

The Minerals

Minerals are inorganic elements, smaller than vitamins and they occur in even simpler forms. Sodium, for example, can exist as a single charged atom (an ion), tiny in comparison with starch, which may be composed of thousands of atoms. Some minerals may be put together into orderly arrays in such structures as bones and teeth—but only with the help of the body's lively metabolic machinery, which itself is composed of protein and assisted by vitamins and some minerals. When minerals are withdrawn from bone and excreted, they yield no energy. When they float about in the fluids of the body, they give the fluids certain characteristics, but they are not metabolized—arranged and rearranged—in the complicated ways or to the same extent as the energy nutrients are. You consume small amounts of minerals daily, roughly similar to the amounts of vitamins in your diet. Of the dozens of minerals found in nature, 21 are essential in human nutrition (see Table 1-2). Others are important to nutrition, not because they are nutrients, but because they displace the mineral nutrients in the body, causing deranged body functions—a problem discussed in Chapters 12 and 13.

The minerals are elements, whereas the other nutrients are all compounds (see Appendix B for the definition of an *element*.) This means the minerals cannot lose their identity; they exist "forever." When you cook a food containing vitamins and minerals, the elements that make up the vitamins can undergo rearrangement, and so the vitamins can lose their chemical identity; the minerals, however, remain unchanged. Because they are indestructible, minerals in foods need not be handled with the very special care that vitamins need. They can be bound by substances that make them difficult to absorb, though, so if they are scarce in your diet, you have to choose food sources of them with care. And you do need to make sure not to soak them out of food or throw them away in cooking water. Chapters 11 and 12 are devoted to the minerals.

Water

Water, indispensable and abundant, forms the major part of every body tissue. It is often ignored—because, like air, it is everywhere and we take it for granted. Water is inorganic, being composed of two atoms of hydrogen to every one of oxygen (H_2O). The amounts you must consume relative to the other nutrients are enormous: two to three liters (about two to three quarts) a day. That's 2,000 to 3,000 grams, whereas you eat only 50 or so grams of protein each day, and perhaps 100 or so grams of carbohydrate. Of course, you need not drink water as such in these quantities; it comes abundantly in foods and beverages.

Water provides the medium in which nearly all the body's activities are conducted. It participates in many metabolic reactions, and supplies the medium for transporting vital materials to cells and waste products away from them.

In addition to the obvious dietary source—water itself—virtually all foods contain water. In addition, water is generated from the energy nutrients in foods (recall that the carbon and hydrogen in these nutrients combine with oxygen during metabolism to yield carbon dioxide and water). Daily water intake from these three sources normally balances perfectly with daily water losses. Water is further discussed in Chapter 11, but is mentioned in every chapter. If you watch for it, you cannot help but be impressed by its participation in all life processes.

Assessment of Nutrition Status

What happens when people don't get enough of the nutrients? They get sick, one way or another, and they exhibit symptoms. Assessment techniques were first developed to detect nutrient deficiencies, but both undernutrition and overnutrition can be assessed.

Undernutrition

The mineral iron can be used to illustrate the stages in the development of an overt nutrient deficiency. The overt, or outside, symptoms of an iron deficiency are pallor, weakness, tiredness, apathy, and headaches. These symptoms are the outward manifestations of an internal state of the blood—anemia—in which

---

TABLE 1–2

The Minerals

The Major Minerals
  Calcium
  Phosphorus
  Potassium
  Sodium
  Chloride
  Magnesium
  Sulfur
The Trace Minerals
  Iron
  Iodine
  Zinc
  Chromium
  Selenium
  Fluoride
  Cobalt
  Molybdenum
  Copper
  Manganese
  Vanadium
  Tin
  Silicon
  Nickel

Water is inorganic.

Water yields no energy.

undernutrition: underconsumption of energy or nutrients.
overnutrition: overconsumption of energy or nutrients.
Both undernutrition and overnutrition are forms of **malnutrition**, which also includes an imbalance of nutrient intakes.
mal = bad

overt (oh-VERT): out in the open. A condition can be **covert** (KOH-vert), or hidden, but when it has become obvious, it is said to be overt.
ouvrire = to open
co + operire = to hide thoroughly

there is too little of the iron-containing protein hemoglobin to carry oxygen to the cells and enable them to get energy.

The appearance of an overt iron deficiency is the last of a long sequence of events, as shown in Figure 1-2. First, too litte iron gets into the body—either because there is not enough iron in the person's food (a primary deficiency) or because the person's body cannot absorb enough of the iron taken in or use it normally (a secondary deficiency). The body then begins to use up its own stores of iron, so there is a period of declining stores. At this point, the deficiency might be said to exist already, but it shows no outward signs yet, and the person hasn't started to feel bad. Finally, the stores are used up, and the body can't make enough hemoglobin to fill the developing, new red blood cells. At this point, the number of red blood cells declines, the new cells made are smaller than normal and pale, and every part of the body feels the effects of an oxygen lack. Weakness, fatigue, pallor, and headaches ensue.

A **primary deficiency** is a nutrient deficiency caused by inadequate dietary intake of a nutrient. A **secondary deficiency** is caused by something other than diet, such as a disease condition that reduces absorption, increases excretion, or causes destruction of the nutrient. Either of these can be a **subclinical deficiency**—that is, a deficiency in the early stages, before the outward signs have appeared.

FIGURE 1-2

Stages in the development of a nutrient deficiency. Notice that attention to diet can prevent problems at the earliest possible time.

Source: Adapted from H. H. Sandstead and W. N. Pearson, Clinical evaluation of nutrition status, in *Modern Nutrition in Health and Disease*, ed. R. S. Goodhart and M. E. Shils (Philadelphia: Lea and Febiger, 1973), p. 585.

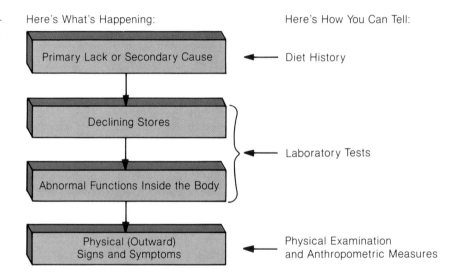

Here's What's Happening:

Primary Lack or Secondary Cause

Declining Stores

Abnormal Functions Inside the Body

Physical (Outward) Signs and Symptoms

Here's How You Can Tell:

Diet History

Laboratory Tests

Physical Examination and Anthropometric Measures

Figure 1-2 shows how to get at the problem of deficiencies before the end stage is reached. One way a deficiency can be deduced early is by obtaining information about the person's diet. For example, a careful recording can be made of all the foods the person eats over a period of time (say, three days or a week), with special attention to portion sizes. The foods are looked up in a table of food composition like Appendix H in this book, which shows the amounts of nutrients in each food. Then the nutrient intakes are compared with recommended intakes. This kind of study is recommended for you, the reader, in the exercises at the ends of the chapters. To interpret them correctly, you have to be aware that the Appendix H values are not absolute (different oranges vary in vitamin C content, for example), and that the values presented assume that reasonable care was taken in the preparation of foods (for example, they weren't so seriously overcooked that vitamins were lost). You are assumed to be healthy, to be taking no medications that interfere with your body's use of nutrients, and to absorb and use the nutrients normally. You also have to know that the standard of comparison (usually the RDA, or Recommended Dietary Allowance, or the Canadian RNI—see Chapter 2) provides only a guideline for

Methods Used in Nutrition Assessment
Data on Diet (history, recall, diary)
Physical Examination
Laboratory Tests
Anthropometric Measures

how much of a nutrient you might choose to try to consume, because people's needs vary.

A second nutrition assessment technique is a physical examination that looks for clues to poor nutrition status. Every part of the body that can be inspected can offer such clues: the hair, eyes, skin, posture, tongue, fingernails, and others. Evidence pointing to deficiencies, imbalances, and toxicity states can be detected this way.

A third way to detect a developing deficiency, imbalance, or toxicity state is to take samples of body tissues (like blood or urine) and study them in the laboratory for the effects of these abnormal states. If body changes are already occurring but are not yet obvious, such laboratory tests may reveal them. In the case of iron, for example, many tests can detect declining stores; other tests reveal iron overload.

A fourth technique that may reveal nutrient deficiencies or other nutrition problems (although it is not useful for iron) is the taking of anthropometric measures such as height, weight, and limb circumferences (*anthropos* means "person"; *metric* means "measuring"). These measures alert the clinician to such serious problems as growth failure in children and wasting or swelling of body tissue in adults, which may reflect severe nutrient or kcalorie deficiencies or imbalances. Many more details of nutrition assessment techniques are offered in later chapters and in Appendix E.

One way nutrition status is assessed is by comparing people's heights and weights with standards.

Overnutrition

Overnutrition and imbalances of some nutrients may be assessed, using anthropometric tests. Height, weight, and fatfold measures can help to indicate excessive body fatness (see Chapter 8). In addition, blood tests showing abnormal concentrations of fat-carrying compounds can indicate overnutrition or unbalanced nutrition with respect to fat and protein intakes. Also, as mentioned, clinical and lab evidence can provide clues pointing to overdoses of vitamins and minerals.

In reading further, you may want to keep these examples of nutrition assessment in mind. They illustrate several principles. For one thing, internal changes precede outward signs of deficiencies or excesses. As a corollary, we do not have to wait for the signs of sickness to appear before taking corrective measures. Tests can reveal problems in the early stages or confirm that nutrient stores are adequate. These principles underlie several later chapters about the vitamins and minerals.

How Well Do We Eat?

Assessment techniques like those just enumerated have been used in surveys taken at intervals over the last six decades to investigate people's nutritional health in the United States and Canada. One of the first of those surveys, taken before World War II, revealed that about a third of our population appeared to be poorly fed. During the next three decades, many further surveys confirmed this impression. Then in the 1970s, malnutrition in both nations attracted additional attention, due to the findings of two major surveys. In the United States, the Ten-State (National Nutrition) Survey pinpointed nutritional deficiencies among all segments of the population, especially among the poor. A simultaneous survey in Canada (Nutrition Canada) produced similar findings. More recently, two additional U.S. Surveys (the Health and Nutrition Examination Survey, or HANES, and the Nationwide Food Consumption Survey) have extended the findings.

The details of these surveys are presented in Chapter 13, but the highlights are worth presenting in this introductory chapter, because they reveal the reality that people can and do suffer from many kinds of malnutrition on the domestic scene. Few severe deficiencies are apparent, but subclinical iron deficiency and some overt anemia are widespread. Protein deficiencies are seen here and there, particularly among poor pregnant and lactating women. Intakes of many nutrients have been impossible to study in depth to date, due to lack of knowledge about their presence in foods or lack of techniques for accurately assessing their presence in the body, but problems are suspected with respect to folacin, vitamin B_6, magnesium, and zinc.

Overnutrition is also a widespread problem. Obesity occurs with various frequencies across all socioeconomic and cultural groups. Inactivity—a low energy output—contributes to obesity, and to dieting people's inability to eat enough food to supply the nutrients they need. Fat intakes are high, and are associated with cardiovascular disease and cancer. Sugar intakes are high, and are related to dental decay. Salt intakes are high, and contribute to high blood pressure. Calcium intakes, especially in women, are not high enough to support maintenance of a healthy skeleton into the later years. The dietary guidelines presented in the next chapter are aimed at remedying these shortcomings.

At the same time, in many ways, our nations are among the best nourished in the world. Simple starvation and severe protein undernutrition are relatively rare, here, and are appallingly common in much of the rest of the world. It can be argued that where undernutrition does occur, it is more a problem of people's not knowing what foods to choose, or where to go for help, than of the true unavailability of food to them. Our food supply is comparatively (some say remarkably) safe. The additives used in foods are effective in controlling food poisoning and spoilage, and the regulations that govern their use are comprehensive and well enforced. Accidental contamination episodes occur, but monitoring procedures catch them promptly, permitting appropriate public health measures to be taken. (Chapter 13 discusses the safety of foods in detail.)

The many surveys recently conducted have yielded enough information so that it is possible to ask the research questions, "What food consumption patterns do people actually follow?"[2] and "Which of these food patterns are found in the groups with the best nutrition status?"[3] From the answers to these questions, more specific guidelines may develop, tailored to people's specific nutrient needs and based on the patterns they already follow. The "average" man, for example, would be advised to eat more vegetables, fruits, beans, and nuts; more whole-grain cereal, pasta, and other grain products; less meat, fish, and poultry; and fewer eggs.

Meanwhile, what can you do about your own nutrition status? Even after you know what nutrients you need and what foods supply them, you still have

Food does not become nutrition until it passes the lips. Ronald M. Deutsch to work out a way to combine those foods into a healthful eating plan, and tailor that eating plan to your individual or family lifestyle. How can you integrate all that you know into a way of life in which meals yield up all the benefits you want from them: social enjoyment, sensory pleasure, ease of preparation, economy, *and* good health?

Eating is not, after all, just a matter of delivering nutrients to the body. Nor do people choose foods solely for their nutrient contributions. Food choices are irrational, to a great extent, and they resist change. Before undertaking diet planning, the planner must understand the dynamics of food choices, because people will alter their eating habits only if their preferences are honored.

Why Do We Eat As We Do?

Among the reasons why you choose the foods you eat today may be any of the following:

- Personal preference (you like them).
- Habit or tradition (they are familiar; you always eat them).
- Social pressure (they are offered; you feel you can't refuse them).
- Availability (there are no others to choose from).
- Convenience (you are too rushed to prepare anything else).
- Economy (they are within your means).
- Nutritional value (you think they are good for you).

Of these seven possible reasons, only one has to do with nutrition directly. Even people who pride themselves on eating nutritious foods will admit that the other six factors also influence their food choices. No matter how nutritious a meal is, it cannot benefit a person's health until it is eaten.

Why do we like certain foods? One reason, of course, is our preferences for certain tastes. Two of these preferences are widely shared: the tastes for sugar and salt. We also like foods with which we have happy associations—those we eat in the midst of a warm family gathering on traditional holidays, those given to us as children by someone who loved us, or those eaten by people whom we admire. By the same token, we can attach an intense and unalterable dislike to foods that we ate when we were sick, or that were forced on us when we weren't hungry, or that are eaten by people we don't respect. Your parents may have taught you to like and dislike certain foods for reasons of their own, like these, without even being aware of the reasons.

Social pressure is another powerful influence on food behavior. How can you refuse when your friends are going out for pizza and beer (or ice cream or doughnuts)? Such pressure operates in all circles and across cultural lines. An almost necessary element of etiquette and politeness is to accept food or drink being shared by a group or being offered by a host; you are not a member of the social gathering until you do.

The influence of availability, convenience, and economy on our food selections is clear. You cannot eat foods if they are not available, if you cannot prepare

People choose foods—and also avoid them—for many different reasons.

Your parents may have taught you to dislike certain foods.

Record What You Eat

Our purpose in providing these exercises is to encourage you to study your own diet. Your reaction to them may be that they are both good news and bad news. The bad news is that they will slow you down, and filling out all the forms is tedious. Like your checkbook, they have to be done carefully, with frequent checking of arithmetic and tidy handwriting, so that they will be accurate and meaningful.

The good news, however, may well outweigh the drawbacks. Most students who do these activities with thoughtful attention report that unlike income tax returns they are intriguing, informative, and often reassuring. They are also rewarding—in direct proportion to your honesty.

In this first exercise you are to make a record of your typical food intake; in the next one, you will analyze it for the nutrients it contains. You are undertaking this analysis before you have learned very much about the nutrients, but there's an advantage in that: having the results in front of you as you read will make the reading more meaningful. As you learn about each nutrient and ask yourself how much of it you consume, you will already have the answer in front of you, ready for interpretation and action.

Use three copies of Form 1 (Appendix K) and record on them all the foods you eat for a three-day period. If, like most people, you eat differently on weekdays than on weekends, then to get a true average you should probably record for two weekdays and one weekend day. Better still, make seven copies of Form 1 and record your food intakes for a week.

As you record each food, make careful note of the amount. Estimate the amount to the nearest ounce, quarter cup, tablespoon, or other common measure. In guessing at the sizes of meat portions, it helps to know that a piece of meat the size of the palm of your hand weighs about 3 or 4 ounces. If you are unable to estimate serving sizes in cups, tablespoons, or teaspoons, try measuring out servings the size of a cup, tablespoon, and teaspoon onto a plate or into a bowl to see how they look. It also helps to know that a slice of cheese (such as sliced American cheese) or a 1 1/2-inch cube of cheese weighs about 1 ounce.

You may have to break down mixed dishes to their ingredients. However, many mixed dishes, including soups, are listed in Appendix H. Other mixtures are simple to analyze. A ham and cheese sandwich, for example, can be listed as 2 slices of bread, 1 tablespoon of mayonnaise, 2 ounces of ham, 1 ounce of cheese, and so on. If you can't discover all the ingredients, estimate the amounts of only the major ones, like the beef, tomatoes, and potatoes in a beef-vegetable soup.

You will, of course, make errors in estimating amounts. In calculations of this kind, errors of up to 20 percent are expected and tolerated. Still, you will have a rough approximation that will enable you to compare your nutrient intakes with the recommended ones.

Do not record any nutrient supplements you take. It will be interesting to discover whether your food choices alone deliver the nutrients you need. If they don't, you'll know better after analyzing your diet what supplement to choose.

them, or if you cannot afford them. Although these factors influence everyone's food choices, the nutritional value of food has become an important consideration for many consumers today. They are interested in selecting foods that will provide the nutrients they need to achieve optimal health. The next chapter shows how to go about doing this.

Study Questions

1. What is a nutrient? Name the nutrients found in foods and discuss their significance to the human body.

2. What happens when people don't get enough of the nutrients? How are nutrient deficiencies and excesses detected?

3. Summarize the findings of the major nutrition surveys.

4. Why do people eat certain foods and avoid others?

Notes

1. H. J. Morowitz, The high cost of being human, *The New York Times,* 11 February 1976.

2. F. J. Cronin and coauthors, Characterizing food usage by demographic variables, *Journal of the American Dietetic Association* 81 (1982): 661-673.

3. H. S. Schwerin and coauthors, Food eating patterns and health—A reexamination of the Ten-State and HANES I surveys, *American Journal of Clinical Nutrition* 34 (1981): 568-580.

The Wisdom of the Body

Anyone interested in nutrition needs not only to study nutrients and foods, but also to acquire an understanding of the human body as well. The interactions among foods, nutrients, and the body are not as simple as one might expect. Every consumer needs this information, and people in the health professions especially need it so that they can advise their clients on matters of nutrition. Many false claims in advertising are based on misunderstandings of how the body works; you will be at a great advantage in the world of mass media if you can see through the misinformation.

This highlight introduces the principle of homeostasis, which underlies wise nutrition judgment and competent diet advice. In everyday terms, this principle means that the body operates according to its own regulatory systems, and handles nutrients according to its own laws. Most misguided nutrition behavior neglects this principle.

A few examples will illustrate misguided nutrition behavior, based on incorrect assumptions about the way the body works. Unfortunately, many people engage in these practices; they are not at all uncommon. The end of this highlight reveals a more correct view of each situation.

■ A person with a low blood sugar level decides to eat a sugary snack. The blood sugar rises briefly in response, but soon falls back to below the level it started from. Sugar is a poor choice, because it evokes an insulin surge and a return to an even lower blood sugar level, as Chapter 3 explains in more detail. The person's

mistake? To think that a simple move like eating sugar would raise the blood sugar level; to forget that eating sugar is followed by an adjustment, made as the body returns to its preset level. The principle at work is homeostasis—the maintenance of constancy.

■ A middle-aged woman has read that women's bones lose calcium after the menopause. She decides to take calcium supplements. Her body, however, decides how much calcium to absorb. If her bones are not used often (if she doesn't exercise), or if a number of other conditions are not met, the body's decision may be to excrete the extra calcium she is eating. The money she spends on calcium supplements is wasted. (Chapter 11 discusses osteoporosis prevention.)

■ A young man wants big muscles and he knows that muscles and meat are both high in protein. He eats large quantities of meat and also supplements his diet with protein powders, but his body doesn't deposit this protein in his muscles. Instead, it converts it to fuel and either oxidizes it or stores it as fat— the last thing the young man wants. What he doesn't know is that his body's rules, not his will, determine the fate of the protein he ingests. The body will build muscle only in response to muscle work, not to diet. (See Highlight 7A for more on nutrition, fitness, and sports.)

■ An ulcer patient experiences pain at mealtimes and fears that his foods are irritating his stomach lining. He adopts a strict, bland diet and eliminates all brightly colored, strongly flavored, coarse-textured

foods. Unfortunately, this necessitates excluding most of the foods he likes, as well as foods containing nutrients and fiber that he needs. Then he begins to dread mealtimes and ironically, his pain gets worse. His mistake? To think that the foods were irritating his stomach, when in fact his stomach was irritating itself by secreting too much acid in response to stress. His body has its own set point for acid secretion—too high, and not primarily caused by diet.

■ A dieter wants to lose weight as rapidly as possible, so she chooses to fast. She knows that fasting will induce degradation of her body's protein tissue as well as of its fat, so she decides to allow herself a daily drink made from a commercial high-protein powder to "spare" her body's protein. However, her body does not respond as she has planned. Her fat loss is no more, and may be less, than if she had eaten more kcalories;[1] she does lose weight but it is mostly lean tissue; and she also feels quite ill. Her mistake? To forget that her body would respond to this diet by altering its internal balances. (Chapter 7 offers more on fasting metabolism.)

■ A man whose father has heart disease learns that the lesions of his father's atherosclerosis (see Highlight 4B) are plaques in the arteries, made largely of cholesterol. He decides to stop eating all high-cholesterol foods, including eggs, shellfish, and others that he likes and enjoys. However, the buildup of cholesterol in his own arteries proceeds unchecked. He doesn't realize that his body is synthesizing cholesterol in response to its own controls.

- A woman notices that she tends to accumulate fluid during the week before her menstrual period every month. She therefore cuts down on her fluid intake at that time, thinking that if she gives her body less water, it will swell less. To her dismay, it swells more, obeying some mysterious rules of its own.
- A college student notices that he has been getting sick more easily lately and is more sensitive to various kinds of environmental influences. He thinks that foods may be causing the trouble and he adopts a monotonous and bizarre diet in order to "purify" his body. However, he begins to feel worse rather than better. What he doesn't know is that an adequate, varied, and balanced diet is the most important nutrition factor that prevents people from getting ill.

In every one of these cases the body is behaving as it typically does, but its owner is misinterpreting that behavior. In every case the effect of the nutrient input is feeble or nonexistent in comparison with the powerful controls exerted by the body itself. Here—briefly—is what is happening in each case. What is important to learn is not the individual facts (those are the subjects of chapters throughout the book), but the common thread that runs through all of them viewed together:

- The person with low blood sugar needs a diagnosis, for low blood sugar is not a disease; it is a symptom that can signify many different diseases, each of which demands a different treatment.[2] For one of these diseases, some dietary measures will help control the blood sugar level, but simply trying to push sugar into the blood will not help. The person needs to eat in such a way as to elicit the desired response from the body: to enhance secretion of the hormones that raise the blood glucose level.*

- The woman who fears bone loss is entirely right. A woman's bones do lose calcium—sometimes great amounts of it—after the menopause. This can create major problems in later life, but the woman can't reverse the process simply by pushing calcium into her body. The hormones of menopause are a powerful factor influencing bone maintenance; the bone-building activity stimulated by exercise also has an important effect; and the hormone-like vitamin D is indispensable for the absorption of calcium. The woman may need more calcium, indeed, but only a naive, misinformed, or malpracticing health professional would recommend that she just take calcium supplements. She needs to undertake a multifaceted approach—to create the circumstances that promote bone building, rather than bone breakdown, by her body (see Chapter 11).

- When the young man who wants bigger muscles eats meat, he is indeed providing the material they are made of, but this is having no effect. In fact, he almost certainly had enough building material for muscles in his diet before he made the change. He needs to set in motion the muscle-building activity that occurs in response to exercise. He needs an adequate, not a high-protein, diet; then he needs to work out, in order to build muscle.

- As for the ulcer patient, he has yielded to the widely held belief that foods are the cause of stomach irritation. Foods can irritate, it is true; almost everyone can identify particular foods that "disagree with" him or her. But a far more powerful factor in ulcer causation is the individual's particular nervous and hormonal system, which responds to stress with enhanced stomach acid secretion. To avoid eating particular foods may be adding a burden to an already heavy load. Except for coffee, alcohol, and possibly meat extracts and pepper, no specific foods deserve black marks in the ulcer patient's book. An understanding of the real dynamics of ulcer causation permits the sufferer to take more effective measures (see Chapter 6).

- The dieter has been deceived, as have thousands of others, by some complicated but logical-sounding reasoning in a book by someone with an impressive title. Diet frauds like this are among the most successful of all nutrition profiteering schemes, and they are hard to see through because they are based on sophisticated-sounding descriptions of the body's metabolic processes. The public knows too little physiology to see through the distortion. Nurses, doctors, and even dietitians are more often and more easily tricked by these subtle persuasions than they would like to believe. Because quick-weight-loss diets cause serious health harm to people who follow them, there is

---

*The appropriate strategy is based on eating protein foods to stimulate glucagon secretion, and avoiding simple sugars to prevent oversecretion of insulin. See Chapter 3.

This is an exciting time to be studying nutrition, precisely because so much is being learned about the body's control systems. The more that is learned, the more effective diet advice can become. But because authorities are still in the process of learning how the body responds to different diet therapies, their conclusions have to be revised from time to time. Even advice from authorities can change, and it is important to keep up to date.

heavy emphasis on their metabolic effects in Chapters 7 and 8.

- About the man who fears heart disease: Many people believe that cutting out dietary cholesterol will be enough to reduce inside-the-body cholesterol. Actually, the body makes cholesterol not from the cholesterol a person eats, but from other compounds eaten, according to the body's own rules and in response to other factors in that person's lifestyle—for example, exercise habits. A long and complex sequence of events leads to the depositing of cholesterol in someone's arteries. The body's internal chemical and hormonal balances have much more to do with the narrowing of arteries than the eating of cholesterol does.

- What makes the body retain fluid and swell before menstruation is a series of events that readies it for pregnancy. If fertilization doesn't occur, the fluid is excreted at the same time as the menstrual blood is lost. The woman who tries to restrict her fluid intake at this time makes her body's task more difficult, but doesn't prevent this important process from occurring. The body will obey the rule that fluid must accumulate prior to menstruation. The woman who restricts her water intake may not only hinder water excretion, but make her swelling worse.

- For the college student: It's not so much what you are exposed to that determines whether you get ill but rather how well you can resist disease-causing organisms. The degree to which a person resists illness is dependent on the strength of the body's immune system. The immune system is composed of various organs whose function is to defend the body against foreign invaders such as bacteria and viruses. Every vitamin and mineral is involved in making the structures and supporting the functions of the cells

that fight infection and disease. Research in the last five years on the influence of nutrition on immunity has revealed much new and remarkable information. For example, physicians are learning that their patients' nutritional preparedness before a hospital admission is a key factor in how long they stay sick or how fast they get well.

All of these examples show mistaken uses of diet tactics. Choosing to eat a certain food or to follow a certain kind of diet in the hope of having a special effect on the body is a hit-or-miss process. In all these cases, the people described mistakenly thought of nutrients as medicines. However, nutrients do not work as drugs might, to cure an illness. Nutrients delivered from foods work with one another under the body's directions. The nourished, healthy body best keeps itself well. The well body—the body that best resists disease, lives the longest, and enjoys the highest quality of life in the later years—is a body that receives all of the nutrients necessary for optimum living. This kind of thinking is an example of the attitude of preventive nutrition, which supports people's well-being before they get sick. Nutrition as a preventive strategy is discussed throughout this book.

In every case, however, diet is relevant. For each problem, researchers have learned what to do about diet by first studying the body's internal regulation and control systems. Then they design experiments to learn the effects that changes in diet will have, not only on the body's end products (like muscle, fluids, or bones), but also on its regulatory systems (the hormones, enzymes, and nervous system). Managing these regulatory systems is the only way to get at the end products.

As described here, the human body is a homeostatic system that is regulated by a complex set of controls. An airport is a comparable system. Should you want to shift a single small plane onto a different runway, you might try to position yourself in its path and wave your arms wildly to persuade the pilot to change course in response. If you use your head, however, you will seek to discover where and how the commands are given. You will get into the control tower and work from there. Much of the rest of this book delves into the body's control systems.

Note: Appendix A presents the basic details of how cells work, and of the body's hormonal and nervous regulatory systems.

NOTES
1. M. F. Ball, J. J. Canary, and L. H. Kyle, Comparative effects of caloric restriction and total starvation on body composition in obesity, *Annals of Internal Medicine* 67 (1967): 60–67.
2. *Hypoglycemia and Nonhypoglycemia*, a monograph available from Stickley Publishing Co., 210 Washington Square, Philadelphia, PA 19106.

Miniglossary

homeostasis (HOME-ee-oh-STAY-sis): the maintenance of relatively constant internal conditions in body systems by corrective responses to forces that, unopposed, would cause unacceptably large changes in those conditions. A homeostatic system is not static. It is constantly changing, but within tolerable limits.
homeo = the same
stasis = staying
immune system: the body's system of defense against foreign materials.
immunity: the body's ability to recognize and eliminate foreign materials.

Recommended Nutrient Intakes and Diet Planning Guides

2

Contents

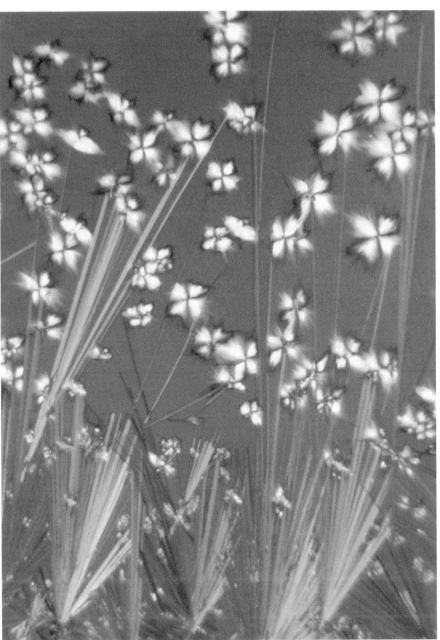

The nutrients themselves are beautiful when viewed in crystalline form under the microscope. These are crystals of the B vitamin pantothenic acid.

mong the most important questions asked by nutrition scientists are how much of each nutrient the body needs and how we can make sure it gets enough. This chapter shows how nutrition experts arrive at recommended nutrient intakes and how diets can be planned to deliver them.

Recommended Nutrient Intakes

Many countries have developed nutrient standards. Those of the United States (the Recommended Dietary Allowances, or RDA) and Canada (the Recommended Nutrient Intakes, or RNI) are examples. The RDA are presented on the inside front cover of this book, and the Canadian recommendations, in Appendix I.

The RDA have been much misunderstood. They are not recommendations for individuals, but are intended as guidelines to aid in the evaluation and planning of diets for groups of people. The following facts will help put the RDA in perspective:

- They are published by the government, but the committee that determines them is composed of highly qualified scientists selected by the National Academy of Sciences.
- They are based on available scientific evidence to the greatest extent possible. The committee reviews them about every five years in the light of new findings and revises them if necessary.
- They are recommendations, not requirements, and certainly not minimum requirements. They include a substantial margin of safety. Individuals whose needs are higher than the average are included within the RDA.
- They are for healthy persons only. Medical problems alter nutrient needs.

The Setting of the Nutrient RDA

It is important to understand how the RDA and other such recommendations are set. A theoretical discussion based on the way the Committee on RDA made its recommendation for protein will illustrate the limitations and qualifications you must keep in mind when dealing with the RDA.

Suppose we were the Committee on RDA and we had the task of setting an RDA for nutrient X (any nutrient). Ideally, our first step would be to try to find out how much of that nutrient each person needs. We would review and select the most valid studies of deficiency states, of the body's nutrient stores and their depletion, and of many other relevant factors. We could also measure the body's intake and excretion of nutrient X (in the case of nutrients that aren't changed before they are excreted) and find out how much of an intake is required to achieve balance (this is called a balance study). For each individual subject, we could determine a *requirement* for nutrient X. Below the requirement, that person would slip into negative balance, or experience declining stores.

RDA tables—inside *front* cover.
RDA: Recommended Dietary Allowances. The RDA are daily recommended intakes of nutrients intended to provide for individual variations among most normal, healthy people in the United States under usual environmental stresses. RDA are set for:

- Energy—a range.
- Vitamins—A, D, E, C, folacin, niacin, riboflavin, thiamin, B_6, and B_{12}.
- Minerals—calcium, phosphorus, iodine, iron, magnesium, and zinc.

The RDA committee has also set tentative lower and upper limits for nutrients about which less is known. These are termed "Estimated Safe and Adequate Intakes":

- Vitamins—K, biotin, and pantothenic acid.
- Minerals—sodium, potassium, chloride, copper, manganese, fluoride, chromium, selenium, and molybdenum.

The RDA are different from the U.S. RDA, used on labels. See next section. U.S. RDA—inside *back* cover.

balance study: a laboratory study in which a person is fed a controlled diet and the intake and excretion of a nutrient are measured. Balance studies are valid only for nutrients like calcium that don't change while they are in the body.

requirement: the amount of a nutrient that will just prevent the development of specific deficiency signs; distinguished from the RDA, which is a recommended allowance that includes a safety factor to provide for individual variability.

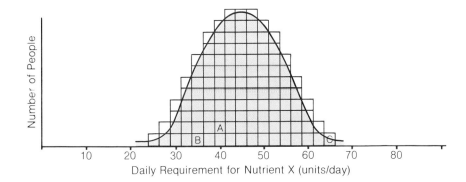

FIGURE 2-1

Different individuals have different requirements. Each square represents a person. A, B, and C are Mr. A, Ms. B, and Mr. C. The next figure shows how a recommended intake (RDA) is superimposed on these data.

We would find that different individuals have different requirements. Mr. A might need 40 units of the nutrient each day to maintain balance; Ms. B might need 35; Mr. C, 65. If we looked at enough individuals, we might find that their requirements fell into an even distribution—that most were near the midpoint, and only a few were at the extremes. Figure 2–1 depicts this situation.

Then we would have to decide what intake to recommend for everybody; that is, we would have to set the RDA. Should we set it at the mean (shown in Figure 2–1 at 45 units)? This is the average requirement for nutrient X; it is the closest to everyone's need. But if people took us literally and consumed exactly this amount of nutrient X each day, half of the population would develop deficiencies, Mr. C among them.

Perhaps we should set the RDA for nutrient X at or above the extreme—say, at 70 units a day—so that everyone would be covered. (Actually, we didn't study everyone, so we would have to worry that some individual we didn't happen to test would have a still higher requirement.) This might be a good idea in theory, but what if nutrient X is expensive or scarce? A person like Ms. B, who needs only 35 units a day, would then try to consume twice that, an unnecessary strain on her pocketbook. Or she might overeat as a consequence, or overemphasize foods containing nutrient X to the exclusion of foods containing other valuable nutrients.

The choice we would finally make, with some reservations, would be to set the RDA at a reasonably high point so that the bulk of the population would be covered. In this example, a reasonable choice might be to set it at the point where nearly everyone's needs are covered—say, at 63 units (see Figure 2–2). The point can be chosen mathematically so that it covers 98 or 99 percent of the population. By moving the RDA further toward the extreme, we would pick up very few additional people but inflate the recommendation as it applies to most people (including Mr. A and Ms. B).

It is this kind of choice that the committee members make in setting the RDA for nutrients. They set it well above the mean requirement as best they can determine it from the available information. (Actually, they don't usually have enough data to be sure that the population's requirements are evenly distributed for every nutrient under consideration.) Relatively few people's requirements, then, are not covered by the RDA.

If you have followed this line of reasoning, you will see why the RDA cannot be used as the perfect guide for nutrient intakes by any individual. Remember, you can't know exactly what your own personal requirements may be. Moreover,

Nutrient Needs

Naive View

Accurate View

The RDA are not minimum amounts but represent the approximate midpoints of ranges within which nutrient intakes probably should fall. Nutrient intakes above or below these ranges might be equally harmful.

the Committee on RDA makes several assumptions that don't apply to all real situations. It assumes, among other things, that you are eating a generally adequate diet including protein of good quality and that you are consuming adequate kcalories and nutrients. It assumes that you store and cook your foods with reasonable care and that large amounts of nutrients aren't lost in these processes. When you use the RDA for yourself and compare your nutrient intakes with them, you should keep two principles in mind:

- They are not absolute requirements. *R* stands for *recommended*, not for *required*. They are allowances, and they are generous. Even so, they do not necessarily cover every individual for every nutrient. In planning your own diet, it is probably wise to aim for average intakes, over time, of close to 100 percent of the RDA.
- Beyond a certain point, though, it is unwise to consume large amounts of any nutrient. It is naive to think of the RDA as minimum amounts. A more accurate view is to see your nutrient needs as falling within a range, with danger zones both below and above it. The 1980 recommendations reflect this consideration especially clearly in the tables that state recommended intakes in terms of "safe and adequate" ranges. As a general guide, average intakes should not exceed two times the RDA for most nutrients.

It is also important to remember that the RDA and other such recommendations are for the maintenance, not the restoration, of health. Under the stress of illness or malnutrition, a person may require a much higher intake of certain nutrients. Separate recommendations are made for therapeutic diets; for use after surgery, burns, or fractures; or in the treatment of other illnesses.

With the understanding that they are approximate, flexible, and generous, we can use the RDA as a yardstick, not to assess the adequacy of individual diets, but to measure the adequacy of diets in groups of people—for example, all the children in a certain school or all the families in a certain county. The RDA have been used as a standard in many surveys to evaluate people's nutrition status.

The RDA for Energy (kCalories)

In setting allowances for energy intakes, the Committee on RDA took a different approach than for the nutrients. Its members had reasoned that it would be sensible to set generous allowances for protein, vitamins, and minerals. They felt that small amounts of a *nutrient* in excess of the minimum required to maintain freedom from deficiency symptoms would be less harmful than small deficits. However, *energy* intakes either above or below need are undesirable, because obesity is as unhealthy as underweight. The Committee on RDA therefore set the energy RDA at the mean—halfway between the lowest and highest needs of the individuals it studied. Figure 2–2 illustrates the difference between the nutrient and energy RDA set by the committee. As the figure shows, most people's energy needs fall close to the mean, but few fit the mean exactly. The latest version of the RDA energy table provides a wide range of suggested energy intakes surrounding the mean for each age-sex group, showing how variable individual people's needs may be (see Appendix I). The best way to determine what your energy requirement may be is to monitor your food energy intake over a period of time during which your activities are typical and your weight remains constant.

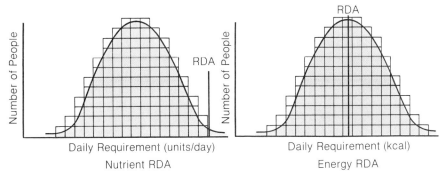

FIGURE 2-2

The nutrient RDA and the energy RDA. The nutrient RDA are set so that only a few people's requirements will exceed them. The energy RDA are set so that half the population's requirements will fall below and half above them.

No RDA is set for carbohydrate or fat. The assumption is that you will first use a certain minimum number of kcalories for the protein you specifically need, and then will use the remaining kcalories for carbohydrate, fat, and possibly alcohol (according to your personal preference) to meet your energy RDA.

Other Recommendations

As mentioned, different nations and international groups have published different sets of standards similar to the RDA. The Canadian equivalent to the RDA is the Recommended Nutrient Intakes for Canadians (RNI, of which summary examples are shown in Appendix I). The Canadian recommendations differ from the RDA in some respects, partly because of differences in interpretation of the data they were derived from and partly because conditions in Canada differ somewhat from those in the United States. Some of the differences between the two sets of recommendations will be explained as the nutrients are discussed in the coming chapters.

Among the most widely used recommendations are a set developed by two international groups: the Food and Agriculture Organization (FAO) and the World Health Organization (WHO). The FAO/WHO recommendations are considered sufficient for the maintenance of health in "nearly all people."[1] They are sometimes higher, but usually lower, than the RDA, not because the RDA are wrong, but because different judgment factors apply to each. FAO/WHO, for example, assumed a protein quality lower than that commonly available in the United States, and so recommended a higher intake of protein. The United States sets its calcium recommendation higher to keep it in balance with the higher phosphorus and protein intakes of its people. Nevertheless, the various recommending agencies have arrived at figures that are all within the same range.

The U.S. RDA and Food Labels

The term *U.S. RDA* appears on food labels and so deserves an explanation. A food label would be most meaningful if it expressed the food's nutrient contents as a percentage of your need, but of course it can't do that. The makers of the label don't know who you are: a 10-year-old boy, a 70-year-old woman, or a

U.S. RDA table—inside back cover.

pregnant teenage girl. Even if they did, they wouldn't know your particular requirements. To standardize labels, four sets of U.S. RDA were developed for different groups of people—infants, children, adults, and pregnant and lactating women. The most commonly used of these is the U.S. RDA for adults, and this is the one referred to here. The idea behind the U.S. RDA for adults was to develop a single set of standards for a sort of generalized adult human being whose nutrient needs are high—as high as people's needs generally go. So if you read on a label that a serving of cereal provides 10 percent of the U.S. RDA of a nutrient, you can be sure that it will also provide at least a tenth of *your* RDA for that nutrient. Your nutrient needs, in other words, are covered by the U.S. RDA.

The U.S. RDA are a set of figures chosen by the Food and Drug Administration (the FDA, which is responsible for nutrition labeling). They are about equal to the highest numbers for each nutrient that you can find in the RDA table. For most nutrients, the U.S. RDA are the same as the RDA for an adult man. But for iron, the woman's RDA is greater than the man's (see inside front cover), so the woman's RDA is used. The table on the inside *back* cover shows the U.S. RDA that are used on labels that make nutrition claims and gives further details about them.

The person who wants to read food labels intelligently needs to know some additional facts about the labeling laws. First of all, according to law, every food label must state:

- The common name of the product.
- The name and address of the manufacturer, packer, or distributor.
- The net contents in terms of weight, measure, or count.

Then, unless the food has a standard of identity (explained later), the label must list:

- The ingredients, in descending order of predominance by weight.

This information has to be prominently displayed, and must be expressed in ordinary words. That's all there is to the required label—but if you know how to read the front and side of a package, you're already a step ahead of the naive buyer. This is particularly true in regard to the ingredient list. Whatever is listed first is the ingredient that predominates, by weight. Consider the following ingredient lists:

- An orange powder that contains "sugar, citric acid, orange flavor . . ." versus a juice can that contains "water, tomato concentrate, concentrated juices of carrots, celery . . ."
- A cereal that contains "puffed milled corn, sugar, corn syrup, molasses, salt . . ." versus one that contains "100 percent rolled oats."
- A canned fruit that contains nothing but "apples, water."

If you read the label, you know what you're getting, and what the main ingredient is. Figure 2–3 demonstrates the reading of a label.

Labels often tell you more than the minimum, however. If a nutrient is added to a food (for example, vitamin C to a breakfast drink), or if an advertising claim is made (for example, that a food is a good source of vitamin A), then the package must provide an information panel that complies *fully* with the nutrition labeling requirements. Without a complete information panel, nutrition claims could deceive the consumer.

Several types of claims may not be made on labels:

1. That a food is effective as a treatment for a disease.
2. That a balanced diet of ordinary foods cannot supply adequate amounts of nutrients (excepting the iron requirements of infants, children, and pregnant or lactating women).
3. That the soil on which food is grown may be responsible for deficiencies in quality.
4. That storage, transportation, processing, or cooking of a food may be responsible for deficiencies in its quality.
5. That a food has particular dietary qualities when such qualities have not been shown to be significant in human nutrition.
6. That a natural vitamin is superior to a synthetic vitamin.

Labels making nutrition claims.

The nutrition labeling section of the law then states that, if any nutrition information or claim is made on the label of a food package, it must conform to the following format under the heading "Nutrition Information":

■ Serving or portion size.
■ Servings or portions per container.
■ Food energy (in kcalories) per serving.
■ Protein (grams) per serving.
■ Carbohydrate (grams) per serving.
■ Fat (grams) per serving.
■ Protein, vitamins, and minerals as percentages of the U.S. RDA. (No claim may be made that a food is a significant source of a nutrient unless it provides at least 10 percent of the U.S. RDA of that nutrient in a serving.)

The side panel of the box of cooked cereal shown in Figure 2–3 provides all this information.

With this understanding of the U.S. RDA, you can extract a lot of information from a nutrition label. The percentage of U.S. RDA tells you generally what amounts of nutrients are in the package, and if you want to know exactly how many units of a nutrient are in a serving, you can do a simple calculation. Suppose a serving provides 25 percent of the U.S. RDA for vitamin A, for example. Turn to the U.S. RDA table, find out that the U.S. RDA is 1,000 RE, and figure that 25 percent of that is 250 RE. For the nutrients included in the RDA tables, then, all the information is there that most consumers might want.

If it delivers 25 percent of the U.S. RDA for a nutrient, then it delivers at least 25 percent of *your* RDA for that nutrient.

Labeling laws also specify just what labels may say about a food's energy and sodium contents (see Figure 2–3). Furthermore, wherever additives are listed on labels, their functions must be stated.

The information just presented helps you with ordinary foods labeled "fish" or "beans," and with foods that present information panels like breakfast cereals. But what about foods that simply say "TV dinner" or "macaroni and cheese"? The FDA has devised nutritional quality guidelines for the nutrient contents of many kinds of convenience foods: frozen dinners; breakfast cereals; vitamin C-fortified beverages; and main dishes such as pizza or macaroni and cheese. If a

FIGURE 2-3

How to read a food label.

The ingredient list on the front or side panel names the ingredients in order of predominance by weight. Significance to you, the consumer: what appears first is present in the largest quantity. Only products with standards of identity (recipes defined by law) have no ingredient list.

The label may also state information about sodium and kcalories: see Miniglossary of Terms on Food Labels.

The front of the package must always tell you the product name, the name and address of the company, and the weight or measure; and it may list the ingredients.

product complies with the nutritional quality guidelines, it may carry on its label the statement that it "provides nutrients in amounts appropriate for this class of food as determined by the U.S. government."*

What if the label says nothing more than a name, such as *mayonnaise*? For some items the law provides standards of identity and excuses manufacturers

---

*For example, frozen dinners must contain one or more sources of protein from meat, poultry, fish, cheese, or eggs, and these must make up at least 70 percent of the total protein; they must include one or more vegetables or vegetable mixtures other than potatoes, rice, or cereal-based products; and they must have a certain minimum nutrient level for each 100 kcalories.

The nutrition information panel tells you the nutrients in a serving.

The serving size may or may not be the same as the amount you eat. Check the servings per container to get an idea if it is.

FIGURE 2–3 (continued)

Nutrition Information (per serving)
Serving Size = 1 C
Servings Per Container = 24

	Cereal	Cereal + Butter, Milk, Water, Salt
Calories	140	280
Protein (g)	4	6
Total carbohydrates (g)	30	32
Simple sugars (g)	25	27
Complex carbohydrates	5	5
Fat (g)	0	14
Sodium	460 mg	975 mg

The nutrient contents are listed in the food as served (after cooking, in this example).

The kcalorie-bearing ingredients are given in grams (units of weight). This is especially meaningful with respect to protein, because you need 40 to 80 g a day, depending on your size and other factors. Protein is also given in percentage of U.S. RDA in the list below.

Sodium is listed in milligrams. About 1,000 to 3,000 mg/day is considered a safe intake, but the average U.S. citizen consumes 5,000 to 7,000 mg/day. A teaspoon of salt contains nearly 2,000 mg sodium.

The carbohydrate breakdown tells you how much simple sugar and how much starch is in the product. A fat breakdown may also be listed, including saturated fat, polyunsaturated fat, and cholesterol.

Percentage of U.S. Recommended Daily Allowances (U.S. RDA)

Protein	4	8
Vitamin A	2	10
Vitamin C	80	80
Thiamin	10	15
Riboflavin	2	8
Niacin	10	10
Calcium	2	4
Iron	4	4

Protein, vitamins, and minerals are given in percentages of U.S. RDA (see inside back cover). Significance to you, the consumer: if it meets 10% of the U.S. RDA, it almost undoubtedly meets at least 10% of your daily needs.

*Prepared according to recipe on back of package.

from the requirement of listing ingredients. Standards of identity exist for such foods as bread and mayonnaise—common foods that at one time were often prepared at home, so that the basic recipe was understood by almost everyone. Certain ingredients must be present in a specific percentage before the food may use the standard name.*

*Any product like mayonnaise, for example, may use that name on the label only if it contains 65 percent by weight of vegetable oil, either vinegar or lemon juice, and egg yolk. The FDA does not have the authority to require that ingredients be listed for these foods, but it urges manufacturers to give the consumer more detailed information, and many manufacturers do so voluntarily.

Miniglossary of Terms on Food Labels

Sodium terms:

- sodium free: less than 5 mg/serving.
- very low sodium: 35 mg or less per serving.
- low sodium: 140 mg or less per serving.
- reduced sodium: processed to reduce the usual level of sodium by 75%.
- unsalted: processed without the normally used salt (may still contain sodium present in the food originally).*

Energy terms:

- low in kcalories: no more than 40 kcalories per serving or 0.9 kcal per gram.
- reduced-calorie food: a food at least a third lower in kcalories than the food it most closely resembles.

Weight terms:

- gram: a unit of weight. Teaspoons of food often weigh about 5 grams; servings are often about 100 grams; see p. 5.
- milligram (mg): 1/1,000 of a gram.
- microgram: 1/1,000 of a milligram (1 millionth of a gram).

*R. W. Miller, Food labels to tell more about sodium, *FDA Consumer*, July–August 1984, pp. 30–31.

A Wheat Plant

A food that is used daily, so that it contributes a significant percentage of the kcalories in the diet, can be called a **staple** food. Examples are milk, bread, and potatoes, for most people in the United States. It is important that all foods you eat contribute nutrients, but it is especially important that staple foods do.

Another class of foods that concerns consumers is made up of foods developed in imitation of, and as substitutes for, familiar foods. With the new food technology, many imitation food products on the market may be superior to traditional foods; so it is misleading to the consumer to imply that they are inferior. For this reason, the law requires that the word *imitation* be used on the label only if the product is "a substitute for and resembles another food but is nutritionally inferior to the food imitated. . . . Nutritional inferiority is defined as a reduction in the content of an essential vitamin or mineral or of protein that amounts to 10 percent or more of the U.S. RDA."

Three other terms are commonly used to describe grain foods: *refined, enriched,* and *whole grain*. Grain has to have its inedible external coat (the husk, or chaff) removed before it is used for food. Except for the chaff, however, the whole grain is edible, and for nutrition's sake, the bran and the germ should be retained in the milling process. In extensive milling, however, *all* the rough parts are removed, including the bran and the germ; all that is left is the starchy endosperm. A light, delicious flour can be made from the endosperm, and this refined flour is popular for baking. But it is so lacking in nutrients that it causes deficiencies when it displaces other, more nutritious foods from the diet.

During the 1930s in the United States, a survey revealed that people were actually suffering from nutrient deficiencies due to the replacement of whole-

TABLE 2-1

Nutrients in One-Pound Loaves of Bread

Type of Bread	Iron (mg)	Thiamin (mg)	Riboflavin (mg)	Niacin (mg)
Whole wheat	13.6	1.36	0.45	12.7
Italian (unenriched)	3.2	0.41	0.27	3.6
Italian (enriched)	10.0	1.32	0.91	11.8

Learn to like the hearty flavor of whole grains.

grain products with refined products. The nutrients known at the time to be affected were the mineral iron and the B vitamins thiamin, riboflavin, and niacin. The Enrichment Act of 1942 required that these lost nutrients be returned to flour. Thus, in enriched bread, iron and the vitamins thiamin and niacin have been restored to the levels found in whole wheat; riboflavin is added to a higher level. This doesn't make a single slice of bread "rich" in these nutrients, but people who eat several or many slices of bread a day obtain significantly more of them than they would from plain, refined white bread. Table 2–1 compares the nutrient contents of several breads.

Enrichment doesn't remedy all the deficits created by the refinement of grain. Since the Enrichment Act, better research tools have shown that other nutrients besides the classic four are lost when grains are refined. Evidence is piling up that fiber needs are not being met as fiber is refined out of bread, cereal, and other foods. Trace mineral deficiencies are also being discovered. Therefore, although the enrichment of wheat and other cereal products restores four of the lost nutrients, increasing evidence suggests that we should return to the use of some whole-grain products in order to restore fiber and trace minerals to our diets. Whole-grain items are preferred over enriched products, because they contain more magnesium, zinc, folacin, and vitamin B_6. If you eat bread every day, you would be well advised to learn to like the hearty flavor of whole-grain bread.

Fortified is another term that you often see on labels. A fortified food is like an enriched food in that nutrients have been added to it, but a fortified food is different in that the nutrients added may or may not have been there in the original product. Examples are:

- Milk, to which vitamins A and D may be added.
- Soy milk, to which calcium and vitamin B_{12} are added.
- Salt, to which iodine is added.
- A sweetened drink, to which vitamin C is added.

As mentioned earlier, fortified foods may appear to be nutritious because of all the nutrients listed on their labels, but they may not contain the several dozen other nutrients that natural, whole foods have. To know whether a food is really nutritious, you have to know more than just what's on the label.

Among the most highly fortified of all foods on the market today are breakfast cereals, some of which have every vitamin and mineral of the U.S. RDA tables added to them. When a food has nutrients added in amounts greater than 50 percent above the U.S. RDA, it has to be labeled as a *supplement*, the same term as is used to describe a vitamin-mineral pill or powder. Thus some breakfast cereals (those made from refined flour and described as supplements on their

refined food: a food from which the coarse parts have been removed. Specifically, with respect to grains, a product from which the bran, germ, and chaff have been removed, leaving only the endosperm.

whole grain: a grain that retains much of the material of its outside layers (except the chaff); one that has not been refined.

enriched food: a food to which nutrients have been added. Specifically, in the case of refined bread or cereal, four nutrients have been added: thiamin, niacin, and iron in amounts approximately equivalent to those originally present in the whole grain; and riboflavin in about twice the amount originally present.

fortified: a term referring to the addition of nutrients to a food, often not originally present, and often added in amounts greater than might be found there naturally. The term *enriched* sometimes also has this meaning, but also has the special meaning previously given.

Fortified foods.

supplement: as used on labels, a term that means that nutrients have been added in amounts greater than 50% above the U.S. RDA.

Some cereals are described as vitamin-mineral supplements on their labels.

Diet-planning principles are ABCMV—adequacy, balance, kcalorie control, moderation, and variety.

Iron deficiency causes fatigue.

labels) are more like pills disguised as cereal than like whole grains. They are nutritious—with respect to the nutrients added—but they may not contain the full spectrum of nutrients that an unrefined whole food (or better, a mixture of such foods) might have.

Diet Planning Guides

Knowing the individual nutrients and their recommended intakes, you can now ask how the available foods can be juggled to create a diet that supplies all the needed nutrients in the appropriate amounts for good health. The principle is simple enough: just select a variety of foods that present the nutrients you need. But in practice, how does this work out? It is helpful to think in terms of adequacy, balance, kcalorie control, moderation, and variety. We named adequacy first here, for alphabetical order, but let's begin by discussing dietary balance.

The minerals calcium and iron illustrate the importance of dietary balance. Iron is one of the essential nutrients. You can only get it into your body by eating foods that contain it. If you miss out on these foods you can develop iron-deficiency anemia. You feel weak, tired, and unenthusiastic; may have frequent headaches; and can do very little muscular work without disabling fatigue. If you make the needed correction and add iron-rich foods to your diet, you soon feel more energetic.

Some foods are rich in iron; others are notoriously poor. Meats, fish, poultry, and legumes are in the iron-rich category, and an easy way to obtain the needed iron is to include these foods in your diet regularly. Most food group plans recommend two or more servings a day.

Calcium is another essential nutrient. A diet lacking calcium causes poor bone development during the growing years and a gradual bone loss in adults that can totally cripple a person in later life. The foods just named (meats and meat alternates) are poor sources of calcium; you can get enough of this nutrient only by making frequent use of milk and milk products or carefully selected milk substitutes. Most food group plans recommend two or more cups of milk or the equivalent every day for adults and more for growing children, teenagers, and older women or women who are either pregnant or breastfeeding their babies.

Most foods that are rich in iron are poor in calcium, and vice versa. In fact, milk (except breast milk) and milk products are so low in iron that the overuse of these foods, by displacing iron-rich foods from the diet, can actually cause iron-deficiency anemia. And yet no one could accuse milk of being a nutrient-poor food. It is the single most nutritious food for infants and can be an important calcium-contributor in the diet of people of all ages.

This discussion illustrates the need for dietary balance. Use enough—but not too many—meat or meat alternates for iron; use enough—but not too many—milk and milk products for calcium. Save some space for other foods needed for other nutrients.

Iron and calcium are only two of some 40–odd essential nutrients, and meat and milk are their most outstanding food sources in most people's diets. Yet there are other nutrients that are not abundant in either milk or meat; to obtain these nutrients, you have to eat vegetables, fruits, grains, or other foods. The task of designing an adequate, balanced diet therefore requires some skill.

Several approaches are possible. We will discuss here the three diet-planning guides most widely used by nutrition-conscious people today: food group plans, dietary guidelines, and exchange patterns. Each has its strengths and weaknesses, and these are compared in Table 2–2. (The table shows, as you can see, that exchange systems probably best combine the virtues of the other systems with a minimum of pitfalls.) The person who understands and appreciates all three is in the best position to design an optimal diet.

Food Group Plans

One of the most familiar ways of grouping foods in the United States fits the major foods into four groups, as shown in Table 2–3. Each of the four groups contains foods that are similar in origin and nutrient content. The nutrients named in the table are representative of all the nutrients. The assumption is that once you have adequate amounts of these, you'll probably have enough of the

When iron is restored, energy returns.

An **adequate** diet is one that provides all the essential nutrients and kcalories necessary to maintain health and body weight. Ideally, a diet will be more than just adequate; it will be **optimal**, providing an assortment and balance of nutrients and kcalories that maintain appropriate body weight and the best possible state of health.

TABLE 2-2

Diet-Planning Guidelines Compared

Guideline	Emphasis	Helps Avoid	Pitfalls
Four Food Group Plan: eat two meat, two milk, four vegetable/fruit, four grain each day	Adequacy	Undernutrition	Overnutrition, imbalance, because only gives minimum number of servings and no serving sizes.
Dietary guidelines: limit fat, sugar, salt; increase complex carbohydrate and fiber intake; eat more whole foods	kCalorie control, moderation	Overnutrition	Undernutrition, imbalance, because does not provide minimum numbers of servings in each of several food groups supplying different nutrients.
Exchange pattern: follow a pattern (example: Four Food Group Plan), but select foods primarily from exchange lists	Adequacy, kcalorie control, control of fat intake, variety	Overnutrition, undernutrition, imbalance	

TABLE 2-3

The Four Food Group Plan

Food Group	Sample Foods	Main Nutrient Contributions
Meat and meat alternates	Beef, pork, lamb, fish, poultry, eggs, nuts, legumes	Protein, iron, riboflavin, niacin, zinc, vitamin B_{12},[a] thiamin
Milk and milk products	Milk, buttermilk, yogurt, cheese, cottage cheese, soy milk, ice cream	Calcium, protein, riboflavin, zinc, vitamin, B_{12},[a] thiamin
Fruits and vegetables	All fruits and vegetables	Vitamin A, vitamin C,[b] thiamin, additional iron and riboflavin, fiber, folacin
Grains (bread and cereal products)	All whole-grain[c] and enriched flours and products	Additional amounts of niacin, iron, thiamin,[d] zinc in whole grains; fiber

As described here, this could be either the U.S. or Canadian plan.

[a]Vitamin B_{12} is contributed only by the animal food members of this group.

[b]Dark green and deep orange vegetables are especially reliable vitamin A sources; other fruits and vegetables are not. For vitamin C, citrus fruits, green leafy vegetables, and selected other fruits and vegetables are superior sources. See Chapters 9 and 10 for more details.

[c]Whole grains include wheat, oats, rice, barley, millet, rye, and bulgur.

[d]One serving is not a significant source of any of these nutrients, but the recommended four or more servings contribute significant quantities to the diet. This group also contributes most of the complex carbohydrate of the diet. Whole-grain products are highly recommended in place of refined enriched products.

other two dozen or so essential nutrients as well, because they occur in the same groups of foods. This is not an entirely safe assumption; as mentioned, when fortified foods are involved, some eight or ten nutrients may be listed on the label, making the food appear nutritious, but they may be the only nutrients present. Still, with the precaution that primarily whole foods be used, the Four Food Group Plan provides a suitable foundation for diet planning.

The Four Food Group Plan specifies that a certain quantity of food must be consumed from each group. For the adult, the number of servings recommended is two, two, four, and four (see Table 2–4).

TABLE 2-4

Servings in the Four Food Group Plan

Food Group	Servings (Adult)	Food Item	Serving Size
Meat and meat alternates	2	Cheese (cheddar, cottage, processed)	2 oz
		Cooked lean meat, poultry, or fish	2 oz
		Dried beans or peas	1 c
		Eggs	2
		Lunch meats	2 oz
		Nuts	½ c
		Peanut butter	4 tbsp
		Sunflower seeds	½ c
		Tofu	1 c
		Tuna fish	2 oz

TABLE 2-4

(continued)

Food Group	Servings (Adult)	Food Item	Serving Size
Milk and milk products	2	Cheese	1 to 1½ oz
		Cottage cheese[a]	1½ to 2 c
		Ice cream[a]	1¾ c
		Milk	1 c
		Pudding or custard	1 c
		Yogurt	1 c
Fruits and vegetables	4[b]	Most vegetables and fruits, including canned:	½ c
		Sources of Vitamin A:	
		apricot	
		broccoli[c]	
		cantaloupe[c]	
		carrots	
		greens	
		spinach	
		sweet potato[c]	
		Sources of Vitamin C:	
		cabbage	
		grapefruit	
		green pepper	
		orange	
		potato	
		strawberries	
		tomato	
		Apple, banana, orange, pear, potato, tomato	1 medium
		Cantaloupe	¼ medium
		Chili peppers	¼ c
		Corn	1 medium
		Grapefruit	½ medium
		Green pepper	½ medium
		Lettuce/salad greens	1c
		Vegetable/fruit juices	½ c
		Vegetable-base soups	1 c
Grains (bread and cereal products)	4[d]	Bagel	½ (3-in)
		Biscuit	1 (2-in)
		Bread	1 slice
		Bun (hamburger/hotdog)	½ bun
		Crackers	6
		Dinner roll	1 oz roll
		Dry cereal	1 oz
		English muffin	½ muffin
		Pasta	½ c (cooked)
		Pancake	1 (4-in)
		Pita pocket bread	½ (6-in)
		Rice, oatmeal, grits	½ c (cooked)
		Tortilla	1 (7-in)

[a]The amount of a nutritional serving is much larger than an average serving.

[b]One should be rich in vitamin C; at least one every other day should be rich in vitamin A.

[c]Good sources of both vitamins A and C.

[d]Enriched or whole-grain products only.

The seeds of legumes are high in protein.

The roots of legumes "fix" nitrogen, contributing to the soil more nitrogen than the plants take out.

Legumes have long been scorned by the middle class as "beans" or "the poor man's meat," but they are now coming into their own as an inexpensive, health-promoting, land-sparing, nutritious food. From them are made food products that are used in many kinds of cooking: Orientals' bean curd (tofu) and soy sauce, Americans' peanut butter and baked beans, vegetarians' bean sprouts, and Mexicans' bean paste, among others.

Many terms describe vegetarian foodways. **Ovovegetarians** eat eggs; **lactovegetarians** use milk; "pure" vegetarians, or **vegans** (VEJ-ans, VEG-ans), use neither animal flesh nor any animal products.

Many foods don't fit into any of the four food groups. Consider butter, margarine, cream, sour cream, salad dressing, mayonnaise, jam, jelly, broth, coffee, tea, alcoholic beverages, synthetic products, and others. These items are grouped together into a miscellaneous category. Some of them do contribute some nutrients to the day's intake. However, either they are not foods, their nutrient content is not significant in enough of the nutrients characteristic of a food group, or their nutrient content has been greatly diluted by fat, sugar, or water.

The Four Food Group Plan appears quite rigid, but it can be used with great flexibility once its intent is understood. For example, cheese can be substituted for milk because it supplies protein, calcium, and riboflavin in about the same amounts. Legumes and nuts are alternative choices for meats. The plan can be adapted to casseroles and other mixed dishes, as well as to different national and cultural cuisines.

The Four Food Group Plan has been much criticized. Of people who follow it, many overconsume kcalories, especially kcalories from fat. Critics say that half of the food classes identified (two of the four groups) are animal products, milk and meat, which leads many people to think that half of the foods they consume should be milk and meat. (Actually, though, the plan recommends *two* milk items, *two* meat items, and *eight* food items from the plant food groups.) Also, a person can follow all the Plan's rules and still fail to meet the day's needs for some nutrients—especially vitamin B_6, vitamin E, iron, magnesium, and zinc. If the Plan is modified to include generous servings of legumes as well as meat, these problems are somewhat relieved, but at the cost of adding more kcalories than most people think they can afford to consume. Actually the full Four Food Group Plan plus 1−1/2 cups of cooked legumes a day can add up to fewer than 2,000 kcalories, but when abundant, hidden sugar and fat are present along with the nutritious foods, it may seem as if the foods have made the kcalories excessive. They haven't; it's the sugar and fat, but these are hard to give up.

Some people choose to exclude certain foods or food classes from their diets for religious, philosophical, cultural, or other reasons. Some exclude red meat only, while eating poultry and fish. Some eat only fish among these foods. Some exclude all animal flesh, but eat products produced by animals such as eggs, cheese, and milk. Some are "pure" vegetarians, eating plant foods only, and some go to the extreme of eating only fruit, not vegetables or grains. Each of these foodways presents a challenge to the planner—that of obtaining the needed nutrients from fewer foods or food groups.

The person who excludes meat and poultry has a nutritionally similar food to rely on—fish. But the person who eats no animal flesh, not even fish, needs an alternative source of iron, zinc, and some of the vitamins offered by meat; the liberal use of legumes is recommended. The person who uses only plant foods has to plan still more knowledgeably. For example, one nutrient, vitamin B_{12}, is found *only* in animal foods, so this person has to take a vitamin B_{12} supplement or use vitamin B_{12}-fortified soy milk or similar products daily. (As for people who attempt to eat fruit only, there is no way that such people can maintain their health for very long.) There is much more the vegetarian needs to learn, and later chapters offer more information. Table 2−5 presents a foundation for diet planning without meat.

Dietary Guidelines

One way to plan diets is to emphasize adequacy—getting enough. Another way, which can seem to conflict with the first, is to emphasize fat and kcalorie control—not getting too much. The Four Food Group Plan was designed primarily with adequacy in mind, as it originated during the 1940s, a time of dawning awareness of the prevalence of undernutrition in the population. The guidelines we are about to discuss originated from a new awareness, largely during the mid-1960s, that overnutrition was contributing to the illnesses many people suffer from today: heart disease, cancer, diabetes, liver disease, and others. These diseases are aggravated by excess intake of fat, salt, sugar, and even protein. Government authorities are now as much concerned about protecting people from consuming too much of these substances as they once were about deficient intakes. In the last decade, the governments of several of the developed countries have published recommendations that their people reduce their intakes of fat, salt, and sugar and turn back toward the more whole-food-based diets of their predecessors.

Among the new sets of recommendations have been the *Nutrition Recommendations for Canadians* (1977); the *Dietary Goals for the United States* (1977); and the *Dietary Guidelines for Americans* (1980). These sets of guidelines differ somewhat from each other, but there is more agreement than disagreement. The emphasis in all of them is on prevention of overnutrition and disease.

Nutrition scientists are of divergent opinions about advising the public on diet. Some feel justified in offering very concrete advice; others feel that no advice can reasonably be given at all. The two points of view might be characterized as the preventive approach and the medical approach. The first of these positions emphasizes everyone's health, and if it errs, it does so on the side of urging more people to make more changes than may be necessary. The object is to help prevent anyone's developing disease from any preventable diet-related cause. Proponents believe that since we can't predict just which individuals may be susceptible to dietary factors related to diseases, we should offer the same advice to all. The second position represents the more conservative, traditional approach. It emphasizes cure rather than prevention, and the physician rather than the health promoter as the agent.

The *Dietary Goals* and other guidelines offered to the public represent a compromise between the two extremes, not a consensus of all scientists. They are tentative, and they are offered here not because they represent the absolute truth on diet, but because students of nutrition need to know what they are.

The first U.S. *Dietary Goals* were seven in number.[2] One of them had to do with energy (kcalorie) consumption; two, with carbohydrate; three, with fat and cholesterol; and one, with salt. The recommended changes in diet are illustrated in Figure 2–4, which shows that the most dramatic change recommended was that we should increase our consumption of complex carbohydrate. Chapter 3 presents the reasons for this and the message, surprising to many consumers, that carbohydrate is not "bad," but "good," for you.

An objection to the *Dietary Goals* was that they had come out under the auspices of a political body—a powerful Senate committee—rather than a group of scientists. In 1979, after much discussion and disagreement, two departments of the government produced the *Dietary Guidelines for Americans,* which included

TABLE 2-5

Four Food Group Plan without Meat

- 2 servings of milk or milk products (or soy milk fortified with vitamin B_{12})
- 2 servings of protein-rich foods (include 2 c legumes daily to help meet iron requirements for women; count 4 tbsp peanut butter as 1 serving)
- 4 servings of whole-grain foods
- 4 servings of fruits and vegetables (include 1 c dark greens to help meet iron requirements for women)

Source: Adapted from *Vegetarian Food Choices* (Gainesville: Shands Teaching Hospital and Clinics, Food and Nutrition Service, University of Florida, 1976).

FIGURE 2-4

The U.S. Dietary Goals.

Source: U.S. Senate, Select Committee on Nutrition and Human Needs, *Dietary Goals for the United States,* 2nd ed. (Washington, D.C.: Government Printing Office, 1977).

Current Diet

Fat, 42% of kCalories

Protein, 12%

Complex Carbohydrate, 22%

Sugar, 24%

Recommended Diet

Fat, 30% of kCalories

Protein, 12%

Complex Carbohydrate, 48%

Sugar, 10%

seven guidelines similar to the *Dietary Goals,* but less specific and less controversial (see box on page 35).

The publication of these two sets of recommendations—the *Dietary Goals* and the *Dietary Guidelines*—so close together in time reveals the nation's intense interest in nutrition, and especially its concern about overnutrition. The United States is not alone in being concerned about its citizens' ways of eating. Many other nations have studied the same issues and have presented their people with similar sets of recommendations. The Canadian government's recommendations are shown here for comparison; you can see that many of the concerns are the same (see box on page 37).

To demonstrate the differences between the "standard American" way of eating and the "dietary goals" way, we've contrasted two day's meals in Figure 2–5, slightly exaggerated to make a point. One day, labeled "Preferred Choices," contains abundant plant foods, nonfat milk, modest amounts of fish and cheese, and no prepared or processed foods. The other day, labeled "Poor Choices," heavily emphasizes meat, eggs, and fats, and includes a fast-food lunch. Both days' foods add up to between 1,800 and 1,860 kcalories, but the preferred choices offer more than twice the bulk of the poor choices with only 24 percent of the kcalories from fat. The poor choices supply a whopping 48 percent of the kcalories from fat.

Real people eat both ways. Those who eat the abundant vegetable way are astonished that others can eat so much meat and fat. Those who eat the meat-and-potatoes way wonder how anyone could consume such a large bulk of food. Neither party lacks for protein; both get a sweet dessert, but the "preferred choices" person does much better in terms of vitamins, minerals, and fat than does the "poor choices" person. A compromise between the two styles might be the reasonable alternative for many people or at least a good starting point. But you can clearly see several things: You can eat a lot of fat without consuming much bulk of food. You can eat a large amount of food without having to consume too much food energy. In fact, for purposes of this demonstration, we had to add butter and sugar to the "preferred choice" meals to bring the kcalories up to 1,800, because to add vegetables would have made the meals too high in

Dietary Guidelines for Americans/Suggestions for Food Choices

1. *Eat a variety of foods daily*. Include these foods every day: fruits and vegetables; whole-grain and enriched breads and cereals and other products made from grains; milk and milk products; meats, fish, poultry, and eggs; and dried peas and beans.

2. *Maintain desirable weight*. Increase physical activity; control overeating by eating slowly, taking smaller portions, and avoiding "seconds"; eat fewer fatty foods and sweets and less sugar, drink fewer alcoholic beverages, and eat more foods that are low in calories and high in nutrients.

3. *Avoid too much fat, saturated fat, and cholesterol*. Choose low-fat protein sources such as lean meats, fish, poultry, and dry peas and beans; use eggs and organ meats in moderation; limit intake of fats on and in foods; trim fats from meats; broil, bake, or boil—don't fry; limit breaded and deep-fried foods; read food labels for fat contents.

4. *Eat foods with adequate starch and fiber*. Substitute starchy foods for foods high in fats and sugars; select whole-grain breads and cereal, fruits and vegetables, and dried beans and peas, to increase fiber and starch intake.

5. *Avoid too much sugar*. Use less sugar, syrup, and honey; reduce concentrated sweets like candy, soft drinks, cookies, and the like; select fresh fruits or fruits canned in light syrup or their own juices; read food labels—sucrose, glucose, dextrose, maltose, lactose, fructose, syrups, and honey are all sugars; eat sugar less often to reduce dental caries.

6. *Avoid too much sodium*. Learn to enjoy the flavors of unsalted foods; flavor foods with herbs, spices, and lemon juice; reduce salt in cooking; add little or no salt at the table; limit salty foods like potato chips, pretzels, salted nuts, popcorn, condiments (soy sauce, steak sauce, and garlic salt), some cheeses, pickled foods and cured meats, and some canned vegetables and soups; read food labels for sodium or salt contents, especially in processed and snack foods; use lower-sodium products when available.

7. *If you drink alcoholic beverages, do so in moderation*. For individuals who drink, limit all alcoholic beverages (including wine, beer, liquors, and so on) to one or two drinks per day. "One drink" means 12 ounces of beer, 3 ounces of wine, or 1 1/2 ounces of distilled spirits. Pregnant women should refrain from the use of alcohol. If you drink, do not drive.

Source: U.S. Department of Agriculture, U.S. Department of Health and Human Services, *Nutrition and Your Health, Dietary Guidelines for Americans*, 2nd ed. (Washington, D.C.: Government Printing Office, 1985).

protein. You can afford a sweet treat in a nutritious diet, and you can eat it without guilt. You can even enjoy a fast food meal now and then, too. Much of the art of balancing the diet, as the later chapters will continue to demonstrate, is a matter of learning appropriate frequencies with which to eat various foods.

FIGURE 2-5

Preferred choices versus poor choices. The contrast is slightly exaggerated to make a point.

Preferred Choices
1,809 kCalories
18% of kCalories from Protein
24% of kCalories from Fat
57% of kCalories from Carbohydrate

1 c Coffee
1 c Oatmeal
¼ c Raisins
½ c Nonfat Milk
½ Grapefruit

1 c Cooked Brown Rice   ⅔ c Strawberries
2 c Mixed Vegetables   1 c Nonfat Milk
2 oz Cheddar Cheese   2 Packets Sugar
2 Pats Butter

3 oz Broiled Fish   2 Pats Butter
½ c Green Beans   ½ c Peas
½ c Carrots   1 c Nonfat Milk

¼ Cantaloupe
1 Brownie

Poor Choices
1,860 kCalories
18% of kCalories from Protein
48% of kCalories from Fat
34% of kCalories from Carbohydrate

½ c Orange Juice   1 c Coffee
2 Scrambled Eggs   1 Packet Sugar
2 Slices Raisin Bread   1 tbsp Cream
2 Pats Butter

Fast Food Hamburger
Fast Food Small French Fries

6 oz Steak   1 tbsp Blue Cheese Dressing
½ Baked Potato   1 tbsp Sour Cream
¼ Head Lettuce   2 Pats butter

1 Brownie

Nutrition Recommendations for Canadians

1. Consume a nutritionally adequate diet, as outlined in Canada's Food Guide.
2. Reduce kcalories from fat to 35 percent of total kcalories. Include a source of polyunsaturated fatty acid (linoleic acid) in the diet.
3. Consume a diet that emphasizes whole-grain products and fruits and vegetables and minimizes alcohol, salt, and refined sugars.
4. Prevent and control obesity through reducing excess consumption of kcalories and increasing physical activity. Take precautions that no deficiency of vitamins and minerals occurs when total kcalories are reduced.

Source: Adapted from J. L. Beare-Rogers, Dietary goals and recommendations in Canada, *Journal of the Canadian Dietetic Association* 41 (1984): 325–329; edited for consistency with this book's style.

Nutrient Density

So far we have offered the Four Food Group Plan as a means of achieving dietary adequacy, and the *Dietary Guidelines* as a means of preventing overnutrition. Yet the Four Food Group Plan fails to prevent overeating, while the *Dietary Guidelines* stress negatives. A positive guide to good nutrition and moderate energy intake is still lacking.

Part of the secret to eating well without overeating is to select the foods within each group that deliver the most nutrients at the lowest kcalorie cost. Take foods containing iron, for example: a 3–ounce portion of either sirloin steak or sardines provides 2.6 milligrams of iron; but the beef contains 240 kcalories and the sardines, only 175 kcalories.* Both are nutritious, but based on the amount of iron they offer for a given kcalorie amount, the sardines have higher nutrient density than the beef. This way of evaluating foods is based on the concept of nutrient density.

The concept of nutrient density can help the health-conscious consumer make informed choices. The food industry has enthusiastically endorsed the selling of the nutritional *adequacy* concept. The dairy people proclaim, "Drink milk—it's good for you." The meat people boast that meat is rich in protein and iron, as indeed it is. But aware consumers realize that whole milk and meat can also contribute many fat kcalories, and they use those that are lowest in fat, thereby obtaining more nutrients for the kcalories. This book offers many tables of foods showing their density (nutrients per kcalorie) in later chapters, to assist readers in buying nutrients for a low kcalorie cost.

Exchange Patterns

Systems have long existed that are useful to the consumer who wants to eat well and control kcalories at the same time. These are known as exchange systems. Appendix G gives complete details of the U.S. and Canadian exchange systems.

nutrient density: a characteristic of a food. A nutrient-dense food provides a high quantity (relative to need) of one or (preferably) several essential nutrients, with a small quantity (relative to need) of kcalories.

Nutrient density helps with the third principle of diet planning mentioned earlier—kcalorie control. It also helps you to be moderate in your use of sugar and salt and still obtain an adequate diet.

All the kcalories from protein and lactose—280 mg calcium, 180 RE vitamin A, 0.4 mg riboflavin, and more.

All the kcalories from sucrose—insignificant nutrients.

An example of nutrient density.

---

* These figures were taken from items 605 and 585 in Appendix H.

If honey and wheat germ would enter a contest for the title of "nutritious food," the wheat germ would win, hands down. Chapter 3 offers more about honey.

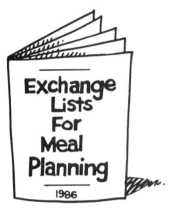

The exchange lists were originally developed for people with diabetes. They proved so useful, however, that they are now in general use for diet planning. Weight Watchers, a well-known organization that helps people control their weight while eating a nutritious diet, bases its eating plans on the exchange system. (Other kinds of exchange systems also exist—for example, those based on the sodium content of foods.)

Another case in point is honey, a much-beloved sweetener, and one often advertised as being more nutritious than sugar. Honey does provide a few B vitamins and trace minerals in very small amounts, in contrast to white sugar, which does not supply them at all. But to say that honey is actually nutritious is to mislead the consumer. On the other hand, wheat germ, a favorite item among nutrition-conscious people, provides abundant B vitamins, iron, and other nutrients relative to its kcalorie content. If the two should enter a contest for the title of "nutritious food," the wheat germ would win, hands down.

The person who learns to use an exchange system can gain mastery over dietary balance, and especially kcalorie intake. Unlike the Four Food Group Plan, which sorts foods by their protein, vitamin, and mineral contents, the exchange system pays special attention to kcalories; proportions of carbohydrate, fat, and protein; and portion sizes. All the food portions in a list have approximately the same number of kcalories and the same amounts of energy nutrients (protein, fat, and carbohydrate).

There are six lists of foods in the exchange system, and each has a typical member—with portion size specified—that you can remember it by. Each food has an associated number of kcalories—which is not exact, but is an average number of kcalories for the group. The lists and their typical representatives are:

- Starch/Bread—1 slice bread (80 kcalories).
- Meat/Meat Alternates—1 ounce lean meat or nonfat-milk cheese (55 kcalories).
- Vegetable—½ cup carrots (25 kcalories).
- Fruit—½ small banana (60 kcalories).
- Milk—1 cup nonfat milk (90 kcalories).
- Fat—1 teaspoon butter (45 kcalories).

Table 2–6 shows the protein, fat, and carbohydrate values that pertain to each list, and Figure 2–6 shows the foods that belong together in this system. Notice that cheese is classed as a meat in this system, because its protein and fat contents are similar to those of meat. In the Four Food Group Plan, cheese is classed with milk because of its calcium content, and in Canada's Food Group System it is permitted to serve either role but not both at any one time. Foods are not always where you might first expect them to be in the exchange system, because they are grouped according to their energy nutrient contents rather than by their outward appearances. Corn is not a "vegetable," for example; it is listed with breads as a "starchy vegetable." Similarly, olives are not a "vegetable"; they are "fats," and so is bacon. These groupings permit you to see resemblances among foods that are significant to nutrition.

The user of the exchange system is encouraged to think of nonfat milk as milk and of whole milk as milk with added fat. The vegetable list includes only low-kcalorie vegetables, so a half cup of any of them will provide about 25 kcalories. The fruit list specifies "no added sugar or sugar syrup"—not necessarily to forbid you to eat fruits with sugar, but help you keep track of sugar consumption. Portion sizes are adjusted so that fruit portions are equal in kcalories. One small banana counts as two fruits. But a piece of cherry pie is *not* a fruit. It *includes* a fruit if it contains ten large cherries, but it also

TABLE 2-6

The Six Exchange Lists

List	Portion Size	Carbohydrate (g)	Protein (g)	Fat (g)	Energy (kcal)
Starch/Bread[a]	1 slice	15	3	trace	80
Meat[b]	1 oz				
Lean		—	7	3	55
Medium-Fat		—	7	5	75
High-Fat		—	7	8	100
Vegetable[c]	½ c	5	2	—	25
Fruit	1 portion	15	—	—	60
Milk	1 c				
Nonfat		12	8	trace	90
Low-fat		12	8	5	120
Whole		12	8	8	150
Fat	1 tsp	—	—	5	45

This is the U.S. exchange system. The complete details, and those of the Canadian system, are shown in Appendix G.

[a]This list includes starchy vegetables such as lima beans and corn, as well as cereal, bread, pasta, and other grain products. For portion sizes see Appendix G.

[b]This list includes cheese and peanut butter as well as meat.

[c]This list includes low kcalorie vegetables only.

Energy Values of Carbohydrate, Fat, and Protein

If you know the number of grams of carbohydrate, fat, and protein in a food, you can derive the number of kcalories. Simply multiply the carbohydrate grams times 4, the fat grams times 9, and the protein grams times 4, and add them all together.

The energy values for the exchange list items were derived this way. For example, a slice of bread contains 15 grams of carbohydrate (that's 60 kcalories) and 3 grams of protein (that's another 12 kcalories), or 72 kcalories, plus a trace of fat—rounded off to 80 kcalories for ease in calculating. A half cup of vegetables (not including starchy vegetables) contains 5 grams of carbohydrate (20 kcalories) and 2 grams of protein (8 more) and has been rounded *down* to 25 kcalories. This slight understatement of the energy value of vegetables is probably intended to encourage people to use them in abundance. At 25 kcalories a half cup, you could eat *4 cups* of vegetables for less than the kcalorie cost of a single 3–ounce hamburger patty—which is 3 medium-fat meat exchanges. The contrast between the two sets of meals in Figure 2–5 illustrated that a person who eats large quantities of vegetables is unlikely to consume as many kcalories as a person who eats servings of fatty meat that many people think of as reasonable.

1 g carbohydrate = 4 kcal.

1 g fat = 9 kcal.

1 g protein = 4 kcal.

---

includes bread and fat exchanges, and added sugar. (Thus it might be counted as one fruit, two bread, and three fat, with three teaspoons added sugar.) The starch/bread list also clearly specifies portion sizes and makes clear which grain products contain added fat. Lima beans, potatoes, and other starchy vegetables are listed with the breads, not the vegetables, because they are similar to breads in kcalorie and carbohydrate content.

FIGURE 2–6

The exchange system

Starch/Breads
1 slice bread is like:
¾ c ready-to-eat cereal
⅓ c cooked beans
½ c corn
1 small (3 oz) potato
(1 bread = 15 g carbohydrate, 3 g protein, trace of fat, and 80 kcal.)

Milks
1 c nonfat milk is like:
1 c nonfat yogurt, plain
1 c nonfat buttermilk
½ c evaporated nonfat milk
(1 milk = 12 g carbohydrate, 8 g protein, trace of fat, and 90 kcal.)

Vegetables
½ c carrots is like:
½ c greens
½ c brussels sprouts
½ c beets
(1 vegetable = 5 g carbohydrate, 2 g protein, and 25 kcal.)

Fruits
½ small banana is like:
1 small apple
½ grapefruit
½ c orange juice
(1 fruit = 15 g carbohydrate and 60 kcal.)

Meats (Lean)

1 oz lean meat is like:

1 oz chicken meat without the skin

1 oz any fish

¼ c canned tuna

1 oz low-fat cheese[a]

(1 lean meat = 7 g protein, 3 g fat, and 55 kcal.)

(One 3-oz portion of meat, (such as a hamburger patty) = 3 meat exchanges. One meat exchange = ⅓ of a 3-oz hamburger patty.)

[a] Cheeses are grouped with milk in food group plans because of their calcium content but with meats in this system because, like meat, they contribute kcalories from protein and fat and have negligible carbohydrate content.

Meats (Medium Fat)

1 oz medium-fat meat is like 1 oz lean meat in protein content, but has 5 g fat (2 g more fat than lean meat).

Examples:

1 oz pork loin

1 egg

¼ cup creamed cottage cheese[a]

(1 medium-fat meat = 7 g protein, 5 g fat, and about 75 kcal.)

Meats (High Fat)

1 oz high-fat meat is like 1 oz lean meat in protein content but is estimated to have an **extra "1 fat"**—that is, to have the 3 g fat of a lean meat and 5 g additional fat. Examples:

1 oz country-style ham

1 oz cheddar cheese[a]

1 small hotdog (frankfurter)[b]

(1 high-fat meat = 7 g protein, 8 g fat, and 100 kcal.)

[b]The frankfurter counts as one high-fat meat exchange plus one fat exchange.

Legumes

Legumes are an odd kind of plant food. They are like meats because they are rich in protein and iron, but many are lower in fat than meat. Besides, they contain a lot of starch. They can be treated as:

1 c legumes = 1 lean meat + 2 starch.

(1 c legumes = 30 g carbohydrate, 13 g protein, 3 + g fat, and 215 kcal.)

Legumes can also be considered similar to breads in being rich in complex carbohydrate, and the additional protein can be ignored. However, this treatment underestimates their kcalorie value, especially that of the higher-fat legumes such as peanuts.

Whatever you do with legumes on paper, however, use them often in cooking. You will learn many more reasons why they are an inexpensive, nutritious, high-quality, and health-promoting food.

Fats

1 tsp butter is like:

1 tsp margarine

1 tsp any oil

1 tbsp salad dressing

1 strip crisp bacon

5 large olives

10 whole Virginia peanuts

(1 fat = 5 g fat and 45 kcal.)

Peanut Butter

Peanut butter is like a meat in terms of its protein content. It is estimated as:

1 tbsp peanut butter = 1 high-fat meat (1 tbsp peanut butter = 7 g protein, 8 g fat, and 100 kcalories.)

(Don't stop reading now, and don't swear off peanut butter, necessarily. You'll need to read about the polyunsaturated character of its fat in Chapter 4, and the B-vitamin contributions it makes in Chapter 9, before deciding how much of a place it should have in your diet.)

Perhaps most important of all, meats and cheeses are separated into three categories—lean, medium fat, and high fat— and the fat list, by including items like bacon and avocadoes, alerts the user to foods that are unexpectedly high in fat kcalories. A warning: meat list items are exchanged ounce for ounce, not serving for serving. That is, an "exchange" or unit of meat is only one ounce, whereas a serving is usually three or more ounces, or several exchanges. This book reminds you of that whenever you need to know it, to ease your use of the system.

If you are a diet planner who wants to choose foods that contain all the nutrients you need, you may find both the food group plan and the exchange system useful. The food group plan promotes adequacy and balance, helping you to avoid overemphasis on any one class of food. The exchange system provides the lists from which to make your food selections; by following it, you can employ moderation and control kcalories without effort.

Only one additional principle is necessary to successful diet planning: variety. It is generally agreed that people should not eat the same foods day after day (except for staples, of course). Variety permits you to take advantage of the fact that some foods are better sources of some nutrients than other foods are. Also, a monotonous diet may deliver unwanted amounts of undesirable food constituents, such as contaminants (see Chapter 13). Each food's ingredients are diluted by the bulk of all the other foods eaten and even further diluted if several days are skipped before it is eaten again.

The principle of variety being referred to here could also be called the principle of **dilution**.

The demonstration in Table 2−7 shows that when you use the Four Food Group Plan as a pattern and the exchange system as a guide for choosing the items to eat, you can get by with surprisingly few kcalories. All 12 recommended items can total about 1,000 kcalories while providing adequacy for most of the major nutrients. An average adult would still have more than 1,000 kcalories to spend. A wise choice would be to invest many of those additional kcalories in additional fruits, vegetables, and whole-grain foods, or in large servings of

TABLE 2-7

Diet Planning with Exchange Pattern

Pattern from Four Food Group Plan	Selections Made Using the Exchange System	Example	Energy Cost (kcal)
Milk—2 c	Milk list—select 2 exchanges	2 c nonfat milk	180
Meat—2 servings (2 to 3 oz each)	Meat list—select 6 exchanges[a]	6 oz lean meat	330
Fruits and vegetables—4 servings	Fruit and vegetable lists— select 4 exchanges	2 vegetable exchanges; 2 fruit exchanges	50 120
Grains (breads and cereals)—4 servings	starch/bread— select 4 exchanges	2 bread exchanges 2 starchy vegetable exchanges	320
Total			1,000

[a]In the Four Food Group Plan, 1 serving is 2 to 3 oz. In the exchange system, 1 exchange is 1 oz.

legumes or nuts in place of or in addition to some of the meat. (Two 3/4–cup portions of legumes at about 160 kcalories each would add less than 400 kcalories to the total and still leave some room to spare.) Some of the extra kcalories could be spent adding more starch-containing foods like starchy vegetables or snacks like unbuttered popcorn. Others could be invested in occasional sweet desserts; some butter, margarine, or oil; or even alcohol. If these additions were made, they would be made by choice rather than through the unintentional use of high-kcalorie foods to begin with. Adequacy and balance would be achieved, not necessarily at each meal, but within each day.

At the same time, you can exercise to "earn" additional kcalories. Clearly, the person interested in good health, fitness, and weight control will not just diet, and not just eat an adequate diet, but combine diet and exercise into a daily pattern that supports optimal health.

With judicious selections, the diet can meet the need for all the nutrients and provide some luxury items as well. The final plan might be like that outlined in Table 2–8 (one of many possible examples). The planner then could achieve variety by selecting different foods each day from the exchange lists.

Diet planners use different patterns of exchanges for different kcalorie levels. A person eating 3,000 kcalories per day could use considerably more bread exchanges, for example, than a person eating 1,500 kcalories per day. Table 2–9 shows diet plans for different kcalorie intakes.

TABLE 2-8

A Sample Diet Plan

Exchanges	Energy (kcal)[a]
7 starch/bread	560
6 medium-fat meat	450
2 vegetable	50
3 fruit	180
2 nonfat milk	180
4 fat	180
	1,600

[a]This diet derives about 20% of its kcalories from protein, about 30% from fat, and nearly 50% from carbohydrate.

TABLE 2-9

Diet Patterns for Different kCalorie Levels[a]

Exchanges	Energy Level (kcal)					
	1,000	1,200	1,500	1,800	2,000	2,200
Starch/Bread	3	4	6	8	10	11
Meat	4	5	5	5	6	6
Vegetable	2	3	4	4	4	6
Fruit	3	3	4	5	5	5
Milk	2	2	2	2	2	2
Fat	3	4	5	7	7	8

[a]These patterns of exchanges supply about 30% of the kcalories as fat, in accordance with the view that a moderate fat intake is desirable.

Study Questions

1. What factors are considered in setting nutrient intake recommendations?
2. What is the difference between the RDA and U.S. RDA?
3. What information is required on food labels? What claims may not be made on labels?
4. Describe the diet planning guides and how they are used. What are each of their strengths and weaknesses?

Notes

1. FAO Nutrition Meetings, *Requirements of Vitamin A, Thiamine, Riboflavin, and Niacin,* report series 41 (Rome: Food and Agriculture Organization, 1967).
2. U.S. Senate, Select Committee on Nutrition and Human Needs, *Dietary Goals for the United States,* 2nd ed. (Washington, D.C.: Government Printing Office, 1977).

This Self-Study takes up where the last one left off, and directs you to calculate your nutrient intakes for the three-day period in which you wrote down what foods you ate.

1. Using Appendix H, calculate for each day your total intakes of kcalories, protein, fat, fatty acids, carbohydrate, fiber, and all of the nutrients listed in Appendix H. If the foods you have eaten are not included in the appendix, read the label on the package or use your ingenuity to guess their composition, using the most similar food you can find as a guide.

Be careful in recording the nutrient amounts in odd-size portions. For example, if you used a quarter-cup of milk, then you will have to record a fourth of the amount of every nutrient listed for a cup of milk. And note the units in which the nutrients are measured:

- Energy is measured in kcalories as explained on p. 4
- Protein, fat, fatty acids, and carbohydrate are measured in grams (g).
- Calcium, iron, zinc, thiamin, riboflavin, niacin, vitamin C (ascorbic acid), and cholesterol are measured in milligrams (mg)—thousandths of a gram (0.001 g). Folacin is measured in micrograms (mcg or μg)—thousandths of a milligram or millionths of a gram (0.001 mg or 0.000001 g). Thus "800 mg calcium" is the same as "0.8 g calcium," and

Calculate Your Nutrient Intakes

"400 μg folacin" is the same as "0.4 mg folacin." Be sure to convert all calcium amounts to milligrams and all folacin amounts to micrograms before calculating.

- Vitamin A can be measured in international units (IU) or retinol equivalents (RE); 1 RE equals 3 IU of vitamin A from animal foods or 10 IU of vitamin A from plant foods. Appendix H lists vitamin A in RE to ease comparison with the RDA, which is also in RE. (For more details, see Chapter 10.) If you eat a packaged food whose label lists vitamin A in IU, be sure to convert to RE before calculating.

If you eat a packaged food whose label lists nutrient amounts as "percent of U.S. RDA," use the table on the inside back cover to convert to grams, milligrams, micrograms, or RE. Suppose a food portion contains "25 percent of the U.S. RDA of iron," for example. The table shows that the U.S. RDA for iron is 18 milligrams. The food portion therefore contributes a fourth of 18 milligrams, or 4.5 milligrams of iron.

2. Now total the amount of each nutrient you've consumed for each day, and transfer your totals to Form 2 in

Appendix K. Form 2 provides a convenient means of deriving and keeping on record an average intake for each nutrient.

3. As a final step, transfer your average intakes to Form 3 for future reference. For comparison, enter the intakes recommended for a person of your age and sex, using either the RDA (on the inside front cover) or the Canadian RNI (in Appendix I), whichever you prefer. Note that no recommendations are made for intakes of fat or carbohydrate. Guidelines for these nutrients and for others, like cholesterol and fiber, will be presented and discussed later. Succeeding Self-Studies will guide you in focusing on each of the nutrients provided by your diet.

Suspend judgment about the adequacy of your diet for the moment. You have much to learn about your individuality, the nutrients, and the recommendations before you can reach any reasonable conclusions.

4. What percentage of the kcalories you consumed comes from protein, fat, and carbohydrate? (Use Form 4 to calculate.) Is your diet in line with the U.S. *Dietary Goals* in this respect? Remember, the *Dietary Goals* are not commandments; not everyone agrees with them.

5. You can get an indication of whether your diet is balanced by using the Food Group Plan Scorecard (Form 5—one copy for each day). How does your diet score by these criteria?

Natural Foods

Chapter 2 talked a lot about foods, but didn't say what kind of foods to buy. Some people say that, to be healthy, one must eat only "health" foods or "natural" foods—that grocery store foods are no good. They seem quite confident of the rightness of their convictions. Others, who aren't sure exactly what the advantages of natural foods may be, still feel vaguely comforted when served them. Still others aggressively combat the natural-food enthusiasts, insisting that grocery store foods are fine—the best in the world—and that there's no reason to fear them.

What exactly are natural foods? The popular definition is unclear, and there is no legal definition, but let's assume for the moment that most people who use the term mean unprocessed, unsprayed, additive-free foods that have been fertilized with "organic," rather than "chemical," fertilizer. Are such foods better than the ordinary foods most people buy and eat? In brief, here are the arguments:

- Grocery store foods are inferior because they are processed; they lack nutrients. Natural foods are unprocessed, wholesome, and nutritious.
- Grocery store foods have been sprayed with insecticides; they are poisonous. Natural foods are unsprayed and clean.
- Grocery store foods are full of pollutants and environmental contaminants. Natural foods are unpolluted and pure.
- Grocery store foods have chemicals added to them—additives and preservatives. Natural foods are additive-free.
- Grocery store foods have been grown on poor soil, and probably lack nutrients. Natural foods are grown on natural, usually "organic," fertilizer; they are healthier and more nutritious.

Who's right? Whom should we believe? How can we tell? All of these issues will receive detailed treatment later, but it seems appropriate to highlight them here, define the terms, and lay out the principal lines of argument.

Processed versus Unprocessed Foods

A processed food is, literally, any food subjected to a process such as alteration of texture, mixing with additives, or cooking. Some processed foods are more nutrient-dense, and some less, than their unprocessed counterparts. Foods such as potato chips are heavily processed; they have been subjected to extensive heat treatment, alteration of form, and addition of fat and salt; and they have lost nutrients and gained kcalories along the way. Fortified pasteurized nonfat milk is also a processed food, but in contrast to potato chips, it has been minimally heat-treated, has gained nutrients, and has lost kcalories. Potato chips are nutritionally inferior to potatoes, then, but fortified nonfat milk is nutritionally superior to whole milk for people whose energy intakes limit their nutrient intakes. Evidently it's not whether a food is processed or unprocessed, but *how* it is processed, that determines its nutritional value.

Sprayed versus Pesticide-free Foods

Part of modern agriculture is the extensive use of pesticides to control pests that otherwise might diminish or destroy crops. However, what is poisonous to insects is usually poisonous to human beings as well, and people rightly fear that when they eat foods that were sprayed in the fields, they are ingesting poisons.

If all grocery store foods were permeated with poisons and all natural foods were free of them, then the choice would be obvious: buy natural foods. Two important qualifications bear on this choice, though.

First, anything, even water, can be toxic if you consume enough of it. Whether a food has been exposed to pesticides at some time in the past is not the right question to ask about that food's effect on your health. The question to ask is how much residue remains in the food at the time you eat it, in relation to the threshold at which harm might occur. If a food has been sprayed and the poison has since evaporated, or changed into a nontoxic compound, or been diluted below the point at which it can do any harm, then the food may not be inferior to an unsprayed food; it may even be nutritionally superior, because it has not been weakened by attacks of pests.

Second, even though natural foods sold in special stores claim not to have been sprayed, testing shows they sometimes contain pesticide residues in the same amounts as grocery store foods. Where these residues come from is not clear; perhaps in some cases farmers secretly spray them, and perhaps in other cases pesticides drift onto farms that are not directly using them themselves. The question is not what's on the label, then; the question is what's really in the food. Foods labeled "natural," "organic," or "health food" may not be superior to ordinary grocery store foods in this sense.

Pesticides are not the only contaminants natural-food buyers are concerned about. Contamination of the environment is a serious problem these days, and part of Chapter 13 is devoted to discussing this subject in detail.

Foods with or without Chemicals

An advantage often claimed by natural or health foods is that they contain no added chemicals. To say this is to imply that chemicals aren't natural. A moment's thought will reveal the fallacy: *all* foods are made of chemicals, whether or not anything is added to them. All *bodies* are made of chemicals; even water is a chemical. This being the case, what is intrinsically wrong with adding chemicals to foods? Is it that they are added—that they were not there originally?

Additives are used in foods for many purposes—for example, to help preserve them, to stabilize their texture, to enhance their color or flavor, or to improve their nutritional quality. As with pesticides, discussed earlier, the question is not whether an additive is present in a food, but whether that additive is harmful to health at any level, and if so, whether it is present above or below that harmful level.

People who oppose the use of additives argue that we don't always know what hazards they may present, that some are known to be harmful, and that to be on the safe side it is best not to use them in foods at all. People who favor the use of additives say they confer more advantages than disadvantages on foods. "Natural foods spoil," they say, "don't taste good, and don't look good. Give me the best

today's food industry can produce—additives to make my food palatable, protect it against infestation of pests, enhance its flavor and color, and keep it safe." The argument is developed further later, but for the moment, the question still remains as to what is most nutritious. The question whether additives are present or not has no bearing on the *nutritive* value of foods (except for nutrient additives, of course).

Chemically versus Organically Fertilized Foods

Some foods are grown with "chemical" fertilizers, others with "organic" fertilizers. What is the difference, and is one better than the other?

Before we go any further we had better define some terms. The term *organic* has two meanings. One meaning was made popular by J. I. Rodale, a Pennsylvania editor whose magazine *Prevention* has enjoyed a wide readership for several decades among people interested in health. According to Rodale, an organic food is a food fertilized with natural organic matter such as manure rather than chemical fertilizers, grown without application of pesticides, and processed without the use of food additives. However, as defined by chemists, the term *organic* merely means containing organic compounds, or molecules with carbon atoms in them, as defined in Chapter 1. By this definition, all foods are organic. Your body can't tell whether the nutrients it receives come from an "organic" food or any other food.

When you read the word *organic* on a food label, it usually conveys the Rodale meaning: free of chemical fertilizers, pesticides, and additives. The word *natural* has similar connotations but means, more generally, foods altered as little as possible from their original farm-grown state. *Health foods* encompass both organic and natural foods. They include ordinary foods that

"Remember, now, the stuff is organic for those that want organic."

Organic foods are not necessarily pesticide-free.

have been subjected to less processing than usual (such as whole-grain flours) and some special foods such as brewer's yeast, yogurt, wheat germ, and herb teas. The latter items are supposed to have special power to promote health. None of these words has any legal meaning, and the Food and Drug Administration (FDA) has taken no position on the use of these terms on food labels, so they may express different intents when used on different labels.[1]

The same analysis as before applies to the use of the word *chemical*. All fertilizers are made of chemicals—so the question is not whether they are organic ("natural") or chemical; it is what chemicals they contain. A plant grown without the chemicals it needs (its essential nutrients, in a sense) can't grow well; a good fertilizer is one that meets the plant's chemical needs. In one set of circumstances, an organic fertilizer may do this best; in another, a chemical fertilizer may. And incidentally: *all* fertilizers, whatever the names on the bags they come in, have to break down to their inorganic constituents before plants can use them anyway.

Still, organic fertilizers, which are made of manure, rotted vegetable matter, and other compost, offer two advantages unique to them. One is their texture, which is coarse and

Fertilizer conveys nutrients to plants just as food does to people.

fibrous and conveys desirable structural and drainage characteristics—a quality called *tilth*—to the soil with which they are mixed. Plants may grow better in soil with these characteristics.

The other advantage of organic fertilizers has to do with ecology, not with nutrition. The materials of compost are manure and garbage (vegetable matter, rotted and consumed by growing plants). If they are not used as fertilizer, they often wind up in the rivers and lakes where they pollute the water, or they have to be burned, and so pollute the air. If used as fertilizer, they are recycled the natural way; they are broken down during use to water and carbon dioxide, which disappear back into the waterways and air as if they had never been there at all. The tradition of organic farming is beneficial in this sense.

Foods carrying the labels *organic*, *health*, and *natural* thus have no proven nutritional advantage over conventional, comparable grocery store foods. They are often considerably more expensive; they are often fraudulently advertised; and their use—especially that of herbal preparations—may be risky, because they are not well regulated or inspected. Organic foods are not different chemically from their conventional counterparts, and often are not even pesticide-free.

Does all this mean there is *no* advantage to natural foods? No, but a more useful distinction than that between natural and grocery store foods

might be that between whole foods and partitioned foods, described next.

High-Nutrient-Density Foods versus Nutrient-Empty Foods

Generally speaking, the more a food resembles the original, farm-grown product, the more nutritious it is likely to be. During processing, nutrients are lost, and often nutrient-empty additions like sugar, salt, and fat are made. A potato contains 20 milligrams of vitamin C; the same number of kcalories in french fries contains only about 7 milligrams; and the same number of kcalories in potato chips contains only 2 milligrams of vitamin C. (By this standard, it isn't really fair to call potato chips "natural" even if they are organically grown.) A glass of nonfat milk contains 302 milligrams of calcium; a glass of chocolate milk with more kcalories contains 280 milligrams, and a cup of ice cream with still more kcalories contains only 176 milligrams. And so forth. Regardless of where these products were purchased—whether at the health-food store or at the grocery store—there is something to be said for buying the potato and the milk. They don't have to be *labeled* natural; they only have to *be* natural.

Something funny about health-food stores is that they ignore the nutrient density principle being applied here. Among their most popular items are candy bars loaded with sugar and fat.

A potato—even a grocery store potato—is more nutritious than potato chips—even "natural" potato chips. It doesn't have to be *labeled* natural; it *is* natural.

Because the candy bars are made from sources labeled "natural," like fruit sugar, honey, and carob beans, rather than from cane sugar and chocolate, they are advertised as superior sources of nutrients. They are still candy, though—low in nutrients, high in kcalories. A bunch of broccoli from the grocery store would be much more nutritious.

When you want to choose nutritious foods, a useful guideline is to choose whole, natural foods. But you don't have to do this all the time. Not every potato product you use must be recognizably potato. A principle that helps with making food choices is to ask, "What am I using this food for?" or "How big a part of my diet is this food?" Most important are the nutrient densities of the foods you use as staples (see p. 26). If bread, for example, is one of your staple foods, then whole-grain bread is certainly a better choice than refined, white bread. In the same way, the less often or less heavily you use a food, the less its quality matters. An example is candy bars. If you eat them only on picnics and you picnic only once a year, they'll hardly detract from your nutrition on a year-round basis. But if you are eating nothing but candy bars for breakfast and lunch every day, then they are a staple item in your diet, and a very poor choice indeed. You can no doubt think of many other examples of beneficial versus harmful uses of food items.

Some choices, of course, may be neither beneficial nor harmful, but neutral. An example is the hearty loaf of whole-grain bread available at the local organic foods store. You may know that the same nutrients are available at a lower price in the supermarket, but the organic bread is simply delicious. You opt for the bread for a good reason: you like it. But if you don't have the money or the personal taste that justifies choices like this, no matter. It is perfectly possible to obtain all the wholesome, nutritious foods you need for a balanced and adequate diet by making educated choices in the grocery store.

Healthful Foods and the Wellness Concept

We just said you can construct an adequate and balanced diet from ordinary, grocery store foods. What if you want more than mere adequacy? What if you want an *optimal* diet? Health-conscious consumers have been buying special, high-priced health foods out of fear for years; they want to be as healthy as they can possibly be. Their thinking goes something like this:

- People can eat all four food groups and still be malnourished. They need to eat the best foods in all four food groups.
- If people have no deficiency symptoms, that doesn't mean they have the best possible diet. Besides the obvious deficiency symptoms, there can be subtle ones that we sometimes fail to see.
- It isn't enough to simply "eat the RDA" of nutrients. People vary, and some have one or more nutrient needs greater than the RDA. Besides, the RDA were designed for healthy people, and not everyone is perfectly healthy.
- It isn't enough to simply eat *more* than the RDA of all known nutrients. There may be still other nutrients; there's fiber; and there are combinations of nutrients that work together.

Given all these axioms, it seems important indeed not to simply scrape by, eating ordinary foods that fit the four food group pattern. It's desirable to do better than that—the best we possibly can do.

Chapter 2 presented the Four Food Group Plan, stating that with knowledgeable choices, it provided a good start toward dietary adequacy. Let's begin with that plan, then, and attempt to make it do more than offer mere adequacy. How can we get from an adequate diet to the optimal diet? At first glance, there seems to be two possibilities: take nutrient supplements, or eat extraordinarily nutritious foods.

Vitamin-Mineral Supplements

The choice to take supplements is a choice many people make. In fact, the people who care most about their nutrition are most likely to make this choice. Some take a single, once-daily type of multivitamin-mineral supplement; others gulp down a whole arsenal of pills, powders, and potions purchased individually from the pharmacy or health-food store, intended to meet every ordinary and extraordinary health need they think they have or may develop.

The whole phenomenon of supplement taking is fascinating to anyone interested in human nature, and the questions of whether and when supplements are needed are obviously important to anyone interested in nutrition. Highlight 10 explores these subjects in detail, but we'd better offer the punchline here: supplements are probably not a wise choice except when people really cannot get the nutrients they need from food. This fact will be demonstrated over and over again throughout the book. Among the points that support it are:

- All nutrients are toxic in excess.
- People vary in their tolerances for excess nutrients; no one knows how much is too much for a given individual.
- The body is designed to handle foods, not supplements.
- No one knows just what nutrients are needed in just what amounts; no one knows how to formulate the ideal supplement.
- No two people have exactly the same nutrient needs anyway, and no one can know just what his or her own nutrient needs are.
- People have to eat foods for energy, anyway. The foods they eat will either deliver nutrients or will be empty-kcalorie foods—loaded with sugar, fat, or both.

This brings us to the choice of trying to develop an optimal diet from foods, which is just what the natural-food users are attempting to do. But which foods?

Whole Foods versus Partitioned Foods

Two-thirds of the foods consumed in the U.S. diet are foods completely or almost completely empty of nutrients: sugar, fat, alcohol, and refined flour.[2] These are partitioned foods—that is, they are composed of *parts* of the plant and animal tissues we need to eat to obtain our nutrients. They are former whole foods that have been peeled, separated, refined, purified, sweetened, enriched, dried, and then packed in cellophane bags, cardboard boxes, and tin cans. Anyone who eats a diet composed largely of these foods— especially the most highly refined of them—is bound to be malnourished.[3]

The other one-third of the foods in the U.S. diet are relatively whole foods—whole in the sense of being unaltered from their original farm-grown state. These are the foods that contribute our nutrients. They are also, in a sense, "natural"—although labels bearing that word are no guarantee that foods are, as they should be, whole.

Figure H2–1 shows four sets of foods. It makes both of the distinctions we've been discussing here: natural versus grocery store foods, and whole versus partitioned foods. Examples in each category of food might be:

- *Whole, natural food*: apples labeled "natural."
- *Whole, grocery store food*: apples.
- *Partitioned, natural food*: apple jelly labeled "natural."
- *Partitioned, grocery store food*: apple jelly.

It's easy to see that two sets of foods are likely to be more nutritious than the other two sets. The nutritious foods are the whole foods—whether labeled

FIGURE H2-1

Distinctions among types of foods. The foods to the left of the vertical line which are whole are the nutritious ones. The horizontal line which distinguishes "natural" from grocery store foods is meaningless.

	Whole Foods	Partitioned Foods
"Natural" Foods		
Grocery Store Foods		

"natural" or not. The less nutritious foods are the partitioned foods—even if labeled "natural."

Food Choices

The implications of this discussion for food choices should now be clear: for an optimally nutritious diet, choose whole foods to the greatest extent possible. Being realistic, few of us have the resources to milk cows and churn butter; feed chickens and collect their eggs; plant, harvest, and can tomatoes; or grind wheat for the flour needed to bake our bread. But we do have a choice at the grocery store. We can select whole foods or partitioned foods, or any of the many foods that fall on the continuum in between. This continuum is apparent within each of the four food groups:

- Whole grain bread > refined white bread > sugared doughnuts.
- Milk > fruit-flavored yogurt > canned chocolate pudding.
- Corn on the cob > canned creamed corn > caramel popcorn.
- Baked ham > deviled ham > fried pork rind.

It would be wise to select foods from the whole foods end of the continuum in your efforts to reach the optimum end of the nutrition continuum.

We have concluded that *adequate* nutrition is not necessarily *optimal* nutrition. The nutrition continuum ranges from deficiency, through adequacy, and on to optimum paralleling the food continuum that ranges from partitioned foods to whole foods:

- Optimal > adequate > deficient.
- Whole foods > partitioned foods.

For a guarantee of meeting all your nutrient needs, because you don't know exactly what they are, you have to aim for the RDA. But the way to do this is not by taking more than twice the RDA, and not by taking vitamin supplements. A variety of whole foods from nature's bountiful array will best satisfy your nutrient requirements, and probably bring the greatest personal satisfaction as well.

Miniglossary

health food: a misleading term used on labels, usually of organic or natural foods, to imply unusual power to promote health. This term has no legal definition.

natural food: a food that has been altered as little as possible from the original farm-grown state. As used on labels, this term may misleadingly imply unusual power to promote health. It has not been legally defined.

organic: the chemist's definition is given on page 000. There is also a popular definition: a food or nutrient produced without the use of chemical fertilizers, pesticides, or additives. As used on labels, this term may misleadingly imply unusual power to promote health. It has not been legally defined.

Note: Although there is no legal definition of the word natural as used on food labels, the National Advertising Division of the Council of Better Business Bureaus has voluntarily adopted some guidelines. They are logical, but they permit use of the word under conditions that might surprise consumers. Foods that can, under these guidelines, be labeled "natural" include ice cream, carbonated beverages, chewing gum, syrup, flavored drink mixes, pan spray coating, and purified fructose—even though they contain added refined sugar, added salt, added fat, or no nutrients at all.[4]

Notes
1. M. Stephenson, The confusing world of health foods, *FDA Consumer,* July-August 1978, pp. 18-22.
2. Parts of this discussion are adapted from L. K. DeBruyne and S. R. Rolfes, *Optimal Nutrition versus the RDA: How Wide a Gap Between?* This monograph is available from Stickley Publishing Co., 210 Washington Square, Philadelphia, PA 19106.
3. D. R. Davis, Nutrition in the United States: Much room for improvement, *Journal of Applied Nutrition* 35 (1983): 17-29.
4. Food cases involving "natural" claims, *NAD Case Report* (a newsletter from the Council of Better Business Bureaus, 845 Third Ave., New York, NY 10022), October 1984.

The Carbohydrates: Sugar, Starch, and Fiber

3

Contents

Within a single cell lie hundreds of coils of membranes enfolding materials the cell makes and uses. Shown here is part of a liver cell. The clusters of dark beads are glycogen—the form in which the cell stores carbohydrate energy.

carbohydrate: a compound composed of carbon, hydrogen, and oxygen, arranged as monosaccharides or multiples of monosaccharides.
carbo = carbon (C)
hydrate = water (H_2O)

complex carbohydrates: the polysaccharides (starch, glycogen, and some fibers).

simple carbohydrates: the monosaccharides (glucose, fructose, and galactose) and the disaccharides (sucrose, lactose, and maltose); also called the sugars.

monosaccharide (mon-oh-SACK-uh-ride): a carbohydrate of the general formula $C_nH_{2n}O_n$; *n* maybe any number, but the monosaccharides important in nutrition are all hexoses (*n* = 6) with the formula $C_6H_{12}O_6$.
mono = one
saccharide, ose = sugar
hex = six

disaccharide: a pair of monosaccharides bonded together.
di = two

polysaccharide: many monosaccharides bonded together.
poly = many

Glucose, a simple sugar, is the principal carbohydrate in mammalian blood (see also p. 58). It is often called blood sugar.

For the chief exception to this rule, ketosis, see Chapter 7.

homeostasis: see Highlight 1.

A **milligram (mg)** is 1/1,000 of a gram; a **milliliter (ml)** is 1/1,000 of a liter. Blood concentrations of many substances are measured in milligrams per 100 milliliters (mg/100 ml).
milli = 1,000.

When someone speaks of *carbohydrate*, what comes to mind? People correctly associate the word with sugars and starches, but most fibers are also carbohydrates. People think of carbohydrates as "fattening," but they aren't—unless, of course, you eat too much of them. Their primary role in human nutrition is to supply an indispensable commodity—energy—and they are preferred over the other available energy nutrients for this purpose. Their second role is to spare protein from being used for energy, so that it can do the work it is uniquely suited for. Carbohydrates appear in virtually all plant foods and in only one food taken from animals—namely, milk.

All carbohydrates are composed of simple sugars. They come in three main sizes: sugars with a single ring like glucose (see p. 58); sugars made from pairs of the single ring carbohydrates (for example, two glucose molecules bonded together); and large molecules which are long chains of the single ring carbohydrates (for example, 3,000 or so glucose molecules linked together). The chemist's terms for these three types of carbohydrates are monosaccharides, disaccharides, and polysaccharides. The monosaccharides and disaccharides are also known as the simple carbohydrates; store-bought white sugar is a disaccharide. The polysaccharides include starch, glycogen, and most types of fibers, and are also known as the complex carbohydrates. The body almost invariably converts carbohydrates, whatever form they come in, to its own energy currency, "blood sugar," properly termed glucose.

The Constancy of the Blood Glucose Level

A certain amount of glucose in your blood is indispensable to your feeling of well-being. If your blood glucose concentration falls below normal, you may become tired, hungry, and shaky; if it goes above normal, you may become sleepy. If either extreme is pushed far enough, you go into a coma. Optimal functioning is only possible when blood glucose is within a certain range of values.

Every body cell depends on glucose to a greater or lesser extent. Ordinarily the cells of your brain and nervous system depend *solely* on this sugar for their energy. The brain cells are continually active, even while you're asleep, so they are continually drawing on the supply of glucose in the fluid surrounding them. To maintain the supply, a steady stream of blood moves past these cells, replenishing the glucose as the cells use it up.

What do you have to do, to maintain a normal blood glucose level? Your body does it for you, as part of its job of maintaining homeostasis, but you can help by attending to your eating habits, as we shall show in a moment.

When you wake up in the morning, your blood probably contains between 70 and 120 milligrams of glucose in each 100 milliliters of blood. This range, which is known as the fasting blood glucose concentration, is normal and is accompanied by a feeling of alertness and well-being (provided that nothing else is wrong, of course—that you don't have the flu, for example). If you don't eat, the blood glucose level gradually falls as the cells all over your body keep drawing on the diminishing supply. At 60 or 65 milligrams per 100 milliliters, the low end of the normal range, a feeling of hunger is often experienced. The normal response to this sensation is to eat; then the blood glucose level rises again.

It is important that the blood glucose level not rise too high, and the body works to prevent this. The first organ to respond to raised blood glucose is the pancreas, which detects the excess and puts out a hormonal message about it; then liver and muscle cells receive the message, remove the glucose from the blood, and store it as glycogen.

Special cells of the pancreas are sensitive to the blood glucose concentration.* When it rises, they respond by secreting more of the hormone insulin into the blood. As the circulating insulin bathes the body's other cells, many respond by taking up glucose from the blood. Most of the cells can only use the glucose for energy right away, but the liver and muscle cells have the ability to store it for later use: they assemble the small glucose units into long branching chains characteristic of glycogen. The liver cells also take the glucose apart and convert it to a different compound, fat, for export to other body cells. The fat cells can pick up this ready-made fat the liver cells have sent to them or can make fat from glucose themselves (see Figure 3–1).

After you have eaten, then, your blood glucose concentration returns to normal and any excess glucose is put in storage as glycogen and fat. During the

Chapter 6 describes the functions of the pancreas and liver. Their places in the digestive system are shown in Figure 6–1 in that chapter. For the workings of the cells, see Appendix A.

glycogen (GLIGH-co-gen): a storage form of glucose in liver and muscle cells.
glyco = glucose
gen = gives rise to

A **hormone** is a chemical messenger. Hormones are secreted in response to altered conditions by a variety of glands in the body. Each hormone affects one or more specific target tissues or organs and elicits specific responses to restore normal conditions. Appendix A provides more information about hormones.

insulin (IN-suh-lin): a hormone secreted by the pancreas in response to (among other things) increased blood glucose concentration.

FIGURE 3–1

Regulation of blood glucose concentration.
1. High blood glucose stimulates the pancreas to release insulin.
2. Insulin stimulates the uptake of glucose into cells. Liver and muscle cells store the glucose as glycogen.
3. Liver cells also convert it into fat and release it. The fat cells pick up the fat and store it.
4. Later, low blood glucose stimulates the pancreas to release glucagon into the bloodstream.
5. Glucagon stimulates liver cells to break down glycogen and release glucose into the blood.

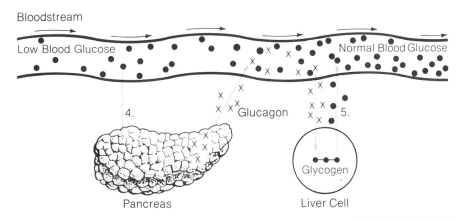

*These special cells are the **beta** (BAY-tuh) **cells;** one of several types of cells in the pancreas. The beta cells secrete insulin in response to increased blood glucose concentration.

glucagon (GLOO-ka-gon): a hormone that elicits release of glucose from storage. Glucagon is produced by the alpha cells of the pancreas.

epinephrine (EP-ih-NEF-rin): one of the stress hormones, so called because it is secreted (from the adrenal glands, which lie on top of the kidneys) whenever emergency action is called for; it readies body systems for fast action and mobilizes fuel to support that action. Epinephrine used to be called **adrenaline** (a-DREN-a-lin).
epi = on top of
nephron = kidney

hours that follow, before you eat again, a hormone that opposes insulin's action—glucagon—works to bring glucose back out of storage as needed. Thus the stored liver glycogen (but not the muscle glycogen* or fat) can keep replenishing the blood glucose as the brain and other body cells keep drawing on it to meet their energy needs.

Another hormone that elicits release of glucose from the liver cells is the famous "fight-or-flight" hormone, epinephrine. Epinephrine is produced quickly when you are under stress, ensuring that all your body cells have energy fuel in emergencies.

Muscle glycogen, too, can be dismantled to glucose, but this glucose is used primarily within the muscle cells themselves, where it serves as an important fuel for muscle action. Long-distance runners know that adequate stores of muscle glycogen can make a crucial difference in their endurance toward the end of a race. Before an event, the athlete is well advised to eat meals high in carbohydrate (see Highlight 7).

The maintenance of a normal blood glucose level thus depends ordinarily on two processes. When the level gets too low, it can be replenished quickly either from liver glycogen stores or from food. When the level gets too high, insulin is secreted to siphon the excess into storage.

The way you eat can help your body keep a happy medium between the extremes. Two guidelines apply. First, when you are hungry, you should eat without waiting until you are famished. Second, when you do eat, you should eat a balanced meal, including some protein and fat as well as complex carbohydrate. The fat slows down the digestion and absorption of carbohydrate, so that it trickles gradually into the blood, providing a steady, ongoing supply. The protein elicits the secretion of glucagon, whose effects are generally opposite to those of insulin, and this damps insulin's effect.

In some people, blood glucose regulation fails for one reason or another. Two groups of conditions are especially common: the hypoglycemias, and several kinds of diabetes. Both are surrounded by many myths and misconceptions, including much misguided advice on diet, so both are worth a moment's attention here.

Hypoglycemia

hypoglycemia (HIGH-po-gligh-SEEM-ee-uh): a too-low blood glucose concentration. Hypoglycemia may arise briefly in any normal person or can be a symptom of a number of disease conditions.
hypo = too little
glyce = glucose
emia = in the blood

Strictly speaking, the term *hypoglycemia* simply means "low blood glucose." It refers to a symptom, not to a disease. More accurately still, it refers to a lab test

---

*Normally, only glycogen from the liver, not from muscle, can return glucose units to the blood; muscle cells only use them internally. Muscle cells can restore blood glucose level indirectly, however: when they are oxidizing glucose for energy, they can release a breakdown product, lactic acid, into the blood, and the liver can pick this up and reconvert it to glucose. This is the so-called Cori cycle. For more about lactic acid, see Highlight 7.

result (blood glucose below a certain value), and it may or may not have symptoms associated with it. When low blood glucose does precipitate symptoms, however, they can be upsetting.

The symptoms most people associate with hypoglycemia are similar to those of an anxiety attack: weakness, rapid heartbeat, sweating, anxiety, hunger, and trembling. This is not surprising, since they are caused by the "emergency hormone," epinephrine. Most people, after eating, experience a rise in their blood glucose level, followed by a gradual decline, during which time the hormone insulin dominates the scene and is promoting fuel storage—the physiologic condition characteristic of the "fed state." Then they shift gently into the reverse condition, as the opposing hormones glucagon and epinephrine assume dominance and promote the release of fuels from storage—the "fasting state." Throughout, blood glucose remains in the normal range, and for most people, the transition is not noticeable.

In some, however, the transition is stressful because of the associated effects of epinephrine. The condition in which hypoglycemia (low blood glucose) with symptoms arises several hours after a meal and causes distress has been named reactive hypoglycemia, and it has attracted a lot of attention and misguided advice.

A different situation—and a different kind of hypoglycemia—exists in a person who has symptoms while well advanced into the fasting state. A person may have fasted for 8 to 14 hours (for example, overnight), so that all available stored glucose is used up. The body should then be compensating by producing glucose from body protein; but if blood glucose continues to fall without this compensation, the nerve cells are seriously deprived. The symptoms of fasting hypoglycemia are different from those of reactive hypoglycemia: headache, mental dullness, fatigue, confusion, amnesia, and even seizures and unconsciousness.

Both kinds of hypoglycemia can have a multitude of causes, from tumors of the pancreas through abnormalities and diseases of the intestinal tract, the liver, the muscles, and the brain. No one treatment is appropriate for all these conditions, and it is crucial for a person with hypoglycemia to get an accurate diagnosis from a medical professional qualified and experienced in working with hormone abnormalities. Still, many quacks "diagnose" hypoglycemia on the basis of their "clients'" verbal reports alone, and "prescribe" all sorts of "remedies" for it with transparently thin rationale. People also "diagnose" themselves, so commonly that physicians have identified a special category for their condition: *non*hypoglycemia.[1]

The problem of dealing with supposed hypoglycemia is further complicated, in that the same symptoms can arise from a multitude of other causes that don't even have anything to do with low blood glucose. For example, anything that reduces the flow of blood to the brain feels the same as glucose deprivation, because it cuts off the brain's energy supply. Poor circulation, as from heart and artery disease; poor lung function; dehydration, which lowers the blood volume; depression, which slows the metabolism; and other conditions have the same effect. Eating a large meal makes you sleepy, partly because the brain synthesizes compounds that favor sleep and partly because the blood is routed temporarily to the digestive tract to pick up nutrients, so that less blood flows to the brain. Neither has anything to do with the blood glucose level. Some people can even bring on symptoms by simply eating a large dose of simple sugar. The sugar attracts large volumes of water from the bloodstream into the intestine, lowering

reactive hypoglycemia: hypoglycemia experienced simultaneously with epinephrine-release symptoms four to five hours after a meal.

fasting hypoglycemia: hypoglycemia found after 8 to 14 hours of fasting.

nonhypoglycemia: a term used when persons think they have hypoglycemia but don't.

the blood volume and causing a temporary reduction in the blood supply to the brain. And plain anxiety, of course, evokes epinephrine-release symptoms indistinguishable from those of reactive hypoglycemia.

Hypoglycemia can be identified by directly testing the blood glucose concentration. The finding that a person has reactive hypoglycemia requires three simultaneous observations: (1) low blood glucose and (2) the simultaneous presence of symptoms (3) four to six hours after a meal or after a dose of glucose. (Remember, though, that if a low blood glucose level is found, this does not constitute a diagnosis—it only says the level is low, not why it is low.) Traditionally, reactive hypoglycemia is identified by performing a glucose tolerance test—measuring the blood glucose level at intervals for several hours after the fasting subject consumes a large dose of simple sugar. This test has been criticized, though, because people don't normally fast and then consume simple sugar. A new way of testing is now preferred by many: permit the subjects to eat as usual; have them record their mealtimes and foods eaten, as well as symptoms experienced; and have them also take periodic fingerpricks of blood to be tested for glucose. The simultaneous appearance of symptoms with low glucose under these conditions reflects problems clients may experience in normal life—problems that need to be dealt with.[2]

To discuss the problems of diagnosis further would be inappropriate in a book about normal nutrition, but we are now in a position to understand better how the way you eat can affect your feeling of well-being. Two findings about hypoglycemia are relevant:

- People with *normal* glucose regulation can develop the symptoms of reactive hypoglycemia if they take a large dose of simple sugar after three days of following a low-carbohydrate diet.[3]
- People who appear to have reactive hypoglycemia by traditional testing, properly performed, do not have it after mixed meals—only after a simple sugar load.[4]

These findings suggest that the way you eat can certainly affect how you feel. Even if you are prone to hypoglycemia, you can probably avoid it by eating normal mixed meals rather than sugar snacks. And even if you are *not* prone to hypoglycemia, you can wreak havoc with your system by depriving it of carbohydrate and then dumping in a large dose all at once! (We will say more against low-carbohydrate diets later, but this section is about blood glucose regulation.) Eat regularly, then; eat balanced meals; and some problems may clear right up.

The exact carbohydrate-containing food you eat may have an effect on your blood glucose, too. Under "The Carbohydrates in Foods" later in this chapter, we discuss the *glycemic effect of foods*.

Diabetes

Diabetes is a disease, most probably hereditary, characterized either by a deficiency of insulin in the circulating blood or by a surplus of ineffective insulin. Either the pancreas becomes unable to synthesize insulin (Type I diabetes) or the cells become unable to respond to the insulin that is present (Type II). In either case, blood glucose rises too high when the person with diabetes eats foods or drinks beverages containing carbohydrate.

When the blood glucose rises too high, and insulin fails to bring it back down to normal, the body brings a second control mechanism into play. The kidneys, through which blood flows each time it passes through the lower body,

diabetes (DYE-uh-BEET-eez): a disorder of blood glucose regulation usually caused by insufficiency or relative ineffectiveness of insulin. Diabetes takes two main forms.

Type I diabetes, or **insulin-dependent diabetes mellitus (IDDM)** is the more rare (about 20% of cases). Persons with IDDM are usually thin, usually contract the disease suddenly and early in life, and cannot synthesize insulin at all. IDDM used to be called **juvenile-onset diabetes,** but some cases arise in adulthood.

serve as a filter to allow unwanted materials to leave the blood and funnel them into the urinary bladder for excretion. Blood glucose levels above about 170 milligrams per 100 milliliters trigger a compensatory action of the kidneys that causes the excess glucose to spill into the urine.

An early symptom of diabetes is excessive hunger (perhaps glucose is slow to get into brain cells when insulin is lacking, so the brain doesn't know that the person has eaten). Another symptom is excessive thirst, because the kidneys excrete water to get rid of the excess blood glucose. The person with diabetes who learns to use nutrition knowledge to manage the disease may be able to live a nearly normal life in spite of this defect in carbohydrate metabolism. The exchange system, useful to many people for balancing their diets, was originally developed to assist people with diabetes. We will talk to the person with diabetes at intervals throughout this book. The end of this chapter has some additional information for people with diabetes. See pp. 80–81.

Type II diabetes, or **non-insulin-dependent diabetes mellitus (NIDDM)** is the more common (80% of cases). Persons with NIDDM are usually obese and usually contract the disease gradually and later in life. While they can synthesize insulin, their insulin is ineffective. NIDDM used to be called **adult-onset diabetes**.

A too-high blood glucose level is **hyperglycemia**. Glucose in the urine is **glycosuria** (GLIGH-cose-YOUR-ee-uh).

The Chemist's View of Carbohydrates

One way to understand things is in terms of the next smaller units of which they are made. An understanding of how energy is contained in glucose molecules and how it is released when these molecules are metabolized in the body will provide the basis for understanding how the body needs and uses its energy nutrients.

Chemical Symbols

Chemists describe a glucose molecule as a compound composed of 6 carbon atoms, 12 hydrogen atoms, and 6 oxygen atoms. These atoms are symbolized by the letters C, H, and O. The chemical formula for glucose is thus $C_6H_{12}O_6$.

Each type of atom has a characteristic amount of energy available for forming chemical bonds with other atoms. A carbon atom can form four such bonds; a nitrogen atom, three; an oxygen atom, two; and a hydrogen atom, only one. Chemists represent the bonds as lines between the letters that represent the atoms (see Figure 3–2).

Atoms are put together to form molecules in ways that satisfy the bonding requirements of each atom. The structure of ethyl alcohol, the active ingredient of alcoholic beverages, is shown in Figure 3–2 as an example. You can see that the bonding requirements of each atom are met. The two carbons each have

Compound, chemical formula: Appendix B presents basic chemistry.

A. Each atom has a characteristic number of bonds it can form with other atoms.

B. Ethyl alcohol, a simple molecule showing bonding.

FIGURE 3–2

Atoms and their bonds.
The four main types of atoms found in nutrients are hydrogen, oxygen, nitrogen, and carbon. (Nitrogen doesn't appear in glucose, but is important in protein and B vitamins; see Chapters 5 and 9.)

FIGURE 3–3

Chemical structure of glucose.
On paper, it has to be drawn flat, but in nature the 5 carbons and oxygen are roughly in a plane, with the darkened bonds extending out of the paper toward you. The atoms attached to the ring carbons extend above and below it.

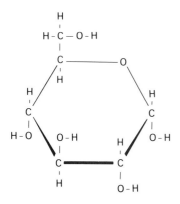

Chemical reaction: see Appendix B.

 condensation: a chemical reaction in which two reactants combine to yield a larger product.

four bonds represented by lines, the oxygen has two, and each hydrogen has one bond connecting it to other atoms. In any drawing of a chemical structure these conditions must be met, not because a fussy scientist made them up, but because they are what nature demands.

Glucose is a larger and more complicated molecule than ethyl alcohol, but it obeys the same rules—as do all chemical compounds. The complete structure of a glucose molecule is shown in Figure 3–3. Again, each carbon atom has four bonds; each oxygen, two bonds; and each hydrogen, one bond.

The diagram of a glucose molecule shows all the relationships between the parts and proves simple on examination. Since you will be viewing other complex structures (not necessarily to memorize them, but rather to understand certain things about them), let us adopt a simpler way to depict them. In the drawings of Figure 3–4, the letters C that represent carbon atoms in the ring have been left out. Also left out are the letters H, for the hydrogens attached to these carbons. You can easily reconstruct the complete structure, with all its details, from such a picture, just by filling in the missing carbons and hydrogens. Put a C for carbon wherever lines intersect and an H for hydrogen at the end of each single line.

Next, we'll examine how these units are put together and taken apart in the continuous flow of matter and energy through living things.

Making and Breaking Pairs: Chemical Reactions

When a disaccharide is formed from two monosaccharides, a chemical reaction known as a condensation reaction takes place (see Figure 3–5). In a condensation reaction, two molecules are linked together. First, some atoms are removed (since all the atoms in glucose had their bonding needs met). A hydrogen atom is removed from one monosaccharide and an oxygen-hydrogen (OH) group is removed from the other, creating a molecule of water, and leaving the two originally separate molecules linked together by a single O.

When a disaccharide is taken apart to form two monosaccharides, as during digestion in the body, a molecule of water is also broken apart to obtain the H and OH needed to complete the separated structures. This reaction is called a

FIGURE 3–4

Simplified diagrams of glucose.

A. The carbons at the corners are not shown and the atoms on the flagpole carbon are written as a partial formula, CH_2OH.

B. The letters H circled in (A) are now not shown, but lines still extend upward or downward from the ring to show where they belong. This is the traditional chemical shorthand used for carbohydrates.

C. Another way to look at glucose is to notice that its six carbon atoms are all connected.

FIGURE 3–5

Condensation.

A. Water is being removed from two glucoses.

B. The disaccharide maltose, with a new bond between the two glucose pieces, is the product.

FIGURE 3–6

Hydrolysis.

A. The dissaccharide maltose.

B. Two glucose units.

hydrolysis reaction (Figure 3–6). It is by condensation and hydrolysis reactions that all of the carbohydrates are put together and taken apart.

In living systems, condensation and hydrolysis reactions almost always require enzymes to facilitate them. Enzymes are discussed in Chapter 5, but for the moment, let us adopt a simple definition. An enzyme is a giant protein molecule that provides a surface on which other molecules react with one another. Since the making and breaking of chemical bonds is required for growth, maintenance, and change in all living creatures, the enzymes that facilitate these reactions are indispensable to life.

But enough about chemical bonds. You know now that glucose is the predominant energy source for all the body's cells, and you can appreciate the importance of having a constant energy supply if you are to feel well. So let's return to the more familiar term, *sugars,* and consider where they come from and what they do for you. Table 3–1 shows the six sugars most important in nutrition and symbolizes them simply as circles, triangles, squares, and combinations of these.

hydrolysis (high-DROL-ih-sis): a chemical reaction in which a major reactant is split into two products, with the addition of H to one and OH to the other (from water).
hydro = water
lysis = breaking

An enzyme is not a hormone. Enzymes facilitate specific chemical reactions; hormones act as master controllers, often regulating enzymes. Enzymes are discussed in Chapter 5.

TABLE 3–1

The Major Sugars

Monosaccharides	Disaccharides
Glucose ●	Maltose ●—●
Fructose ▲	Sucrose ●—▲
Galactose ■	Lactose ●—■
(found only as part of lactose)	

The Single Sugars: Monosaccharides

Practically all your energy comes from the food you eat—about half from carbohydrate and half from protein and fat. In fact, one of the principal roles of carbohydrate in the diet is to supply energy in the form of blood glucose. Starch is the most significant contributor of glucose to people's diets, but any of the sugars can be converted to glucose. Six common sugars are found in foods—glucose, fructose, galactose, sucrose, lactose, and maltose. A number of other sugars are familiar to the users of special dietary products, notably the sugar alcohols—maltitol, mannitol, sorbitol, and xylitol.

Glucose

Glucose is not as sweet tasting as sucrose; a pinch of the purified sugar on your tongue gives only a mild sweet flavor. Glucose, like most monosaccharides, is absorbed rapidly into the bloodstream from the intestines, but is unique in that it can be absorbed to some extent through the lining of the mouth. Thus if a person with diabetes has become unconscious with extreme hypoglycemia (for example, from an overdose of insulin), a quick way to supply the needed blood glucose is to tip the head to one side and drip a water solution of glucose into the cheek pocket. The glucose will be absorbed directly into the bloodstream.

Fructose

If you have ever sampled pure, powdered fructose, you will not be surprised to learn that it is the sweetest of the sugars. Curiously, fructose has exactly the same chemical formula as glucose—$C_6H_{12}O_6$—but its structure is different (see Figure 3–7). The different arrangements of the atoms in these two sugars stimulate the taste buds on your tongue in different ways.

Fructose can be absorbed through the intestinal wall directly into the bloodstream. When the blood circulates past the liver, the fructose is taken up into the liver cells, where enzymes rearrange the C, H, and O atoms to make compounds indistinguishable from those derived from glucose, and sometimes to make glucose itself. Fructose and glucose are not used in exactly the same ways in the body. Fructose has no need of insulin's help to get into cells, so it has

glucose: a monosaccharide; sometimes known as blood sugar, sometimes as grape sugar. Nearly all plant foods contain glucose.

 = Glucose

fructose: a monosaccharide; sometimes known as fruit sugar or **levulose**. Most plants contain fructose; it is especially abundant in fruits and saps.
fruct = fruit

▲ = Fructose

FIGURE 3–7

Two monosaccharides: glucose and fructose.
Can you see the similarities? If you learned the rules in Figure 3–4, you will be able to "see" 6 carbons (numbered), 12 hydrogens, and 6 oxygens in both these compounds.

Glucose   Fructose

some advantages as a sweetener for use by people with diabetes. Counterbalancing this advantage is fructose's somewhat greater tendency to be converted to fat rather than to glycogen—a tendency that contributes to high levels of fat in the blood. For purposes of the discussions of metabolism in this book, though, glucose and fructose are handled in essentially the same way and are treated as being metabolically identical. The differences are only differences in degree.

Food chemists have studied sweet-tasting substances, such as fructose, and have identified the exact arrangement of the atoms that stimulates the sweet-taste receptors in the tongue. All sweet-tasting substances share this structure, including the artificial sweeteners saccharin, cyclamate, and aspartame (Chapter 13 deals with these).

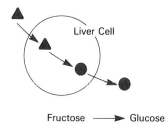

The liver cell converts fructose to gluclose and releases it. (Sometimes fructose breaks down to intermediates, which are used for other purposes.)

Galactose

Glucose and fructose are the only monosaccharides of importance in foods. A third, galactose, is seldom found free in nature but occurs as part of the disaccharide lactose. Like glucose and fructose, galactose is a hexose with the formula $C_6H_{12}O_6$. It is shown in Figure 3–8 beside a molecule of glucose for comparison.

galactose: a monosaccharide; part of the disaccharide lactose.

■ = Galactose

The Double Sugars: Disaccharides

The other three common sugars are disaccharides—pairs of monosaccharides linked together. Glucose is found in all three; the second member of the pair is either fructose, galactose, or another glucose.

Sucrose

Sucrose, or table sugar, is the most familiar of the three disaccharides. Sugar cane and sugar beets are two sources from which it is purified and granulated to various extents to provide the brown, white, and powdered sugars available in the supermarket. Because the fructose part is in an accessible position, sucrose is very sweet, and it accounts for some of the sweetness of sweet fruits. It is the principal energy-nutrient ingredient of carbonated beverages, candy, frostings, and other concentrated sweets.

sucrose: a disaccharide composed of glucose and fructose; commonly known as table sugar, beet sugar, or cane sugar. Actually, sucrose occurs in many fruits and some vegetables and grains.
sucro = sugar

 = Sucrose

FIGURE 3–8

Two monosaccharides: glucose and galactose.

Glucose

Galactose

Digestion of sucrose

1 tsp = 22 kcal.   1 tsp = 16 kcal.

1 tsp = 2 kcal
with vitamins,
minerals,
and fiber.

la =gu+ga

lactose: a disaccharide composed of glucose and galactose; commonly known as milk sugar.
lact = milk

 = Lactose

When you eat a food containing sucrose, enzymes in your digestive tract hydrolyze the sucrose to yield glucose and fructose. These monosaccharides are absorbed, and the fructose may be converted to glucose in the liver. (Alternatively, the fructose may be broken down to smaller compounds identical to those derived from glucose.) Thus one molecule of sucrose can ultimately yield two of glucose.

You can see from this description that it ultimately makes no difference whether you eat these monosaccharides hitched together as table sugar or already broken apart. In either case they will end up as monosaccharides in the body. People who think that the "natural sugar" honey is chemically different from purified table sugar fail to understand this point.

It so happens that honey, like table sugar, contains glucose and fructose. The only difference is that in table sugar they are hitched together, and in honey some of them are not. Like table sugar, honey is concentrated to the point where it contains very few impurities, even such desirable ones as vitamins and minerals. In fact, being a liquid, honey is more dense than its crystalline sister and so contains more kcalories per spoon. Table 3–2 shows that honey is not significantly more nutritious than sugar.

To say that honey is no more nutritious than sugar, however, is not to say that there are no differences among sugar sources. Consider a piece of fruit, like an orange. From the fruit you could receive the same monosaccharides and the same kcalories as from sugar or honey. But the packaging is different. The fruit's sugars are diluted in a large volume of water that contains valuable trace minerals and vitamins, and the flesh and skin of the fruit are supported by fibers that also offer health value.

From these two comparisons you can see that the really significant difference between sugar sources is not between "natural" and "purified" sugar but between concentrated sweets and the dilute, naturally occurring sugars that sweeten nutritious foods. You can suspect an exaggerated nutrition claim when you hear the assertion that a product is more nutritious because it contains honey.

Lactose

Lactose is the principal carbohydrate of milk, making up about 5 percent of its weight. A human baby is born with the digestive enzymes necessary to hydrolyze lactose into its two monosaccharide parts, glucose and galactose, so that they can be absorbed. The galactose is then converted to glucose in the liver, so each molecule of lactose eventually yields two molecules of glucose to supply energy for the baby's growth and activity. Babies can digest lactose at birth, but they don't develop the ability to digest starch until they are several months old. This is one of the many reasons why breast milk and formula are such good foods

TABLE 3–2

Sample Nutrients in Sugars and Other Foods The indicated portion of any of these foods would provide 100 kcalories. Notice what nutrients the eater receives along with those 100 kcalories.

Food	Size of 100-kCal Portion	Percentage of U.S. RDA[a]				
		Protein	Calcium	Iron	Vitamin A	Thiamin
Milk, low fat	¾ c	17	26	—	3	5
Kidney beans	½ c	12	4	13	< 1	9
Watermelon	4-by-8-inch wedge	3	3	12	50	9
Bread, whole wheat	1½ slices	7	4	7	—	9
Sugar, white	2 tbsp	0	0	0	0	0
Molasses, blackstrap	2 tbsp	0	27	35	0	3
Cola beverage	1 c	0	0	0	0	0
Honey, strained or extracted	1½ tbsp	—	< 1	1	0	—

[a] Percentages are rounded to nearest whole number. A dash means the percentage has not been determined and is not significant. The U.S. RDA are recommended adult intakes (see Chapter 2 and inside back cover).

for babies; they provide simple, easily digested carbohydrate supplying the right amount of energy.

Many individuals lose the ability to digest lactose and become lactose intolerant. If the lactose in the intestine is not rapidly hydrolyzed and absorbed, then numerous small sugar molecules remain in the intestine undigested, attract water, and cause fullness, discomfort, cramping, nausea, and diarrhea. The lactose also becomes food for intestinal bacteria, which multiply and produce irritating acid and gas, making the person sicker.

Lactose intolerance becomes more common as people grow older. It is the rule, not the exception, in the majority of the world's people: Native American, Asian, African, Mediterranean, and Middle Eastern peoples. It can also appear temporarily in anyone who is ill, making the person unable to tolerate milk for a while. Lactose intolerance is not the same as the commonly observed milk allergy, which is caused by an immune reaction to the protein in milk.

People who can't or won't drink milk, for whatever reason, urgently need to find another food source of the calcium and riboflavin it provides in abundance. Chapter 11 offers help with finding milk substitutes.

Maltose

The third disaccharide is found at only one stage in the life of a plant. When the seed is formed, it is packed with starch—glucose units strung together in long arrays—to be used as fuel for the germination process. When the seed begins to sprout, an enzyme cleaves the bonds between pairs of glucose units, making maltose. Another enzyme then splits the maltose units into glucose units, and other enzymes degrade these still further, releasing energy for the sprouting of the plant's shoot and root. Then the plant's leaves reach for the sun, whose light offers additional energy for growth.

As you might predict, when you eat or drink a food source of maltose, your digestive enzymes hydrolyze the maltose into two glucose units, which are then absorbed into the blood. Thus maltose, like the other disaccharides, contributes glucose to the body.

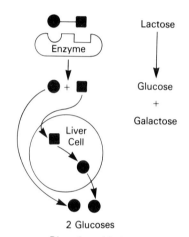

Lactose

Glucose
+
Galactose

2 Glucoses

Digestion of lactose.

lactose intolerance: inherited or acquired inability to digest lactose, due to failure to produce the enzyme lactase. Lactose intolerance is discussed in detail with calcium in Chapter 11.

ma = gu + gu

maltose: a disaccharide composed of two glucose units; sometimes known as malt sugar.

●━━● = Maltose

Digestion of maltose.

In summary, then, the major simple carbohydrates, or sugars, are those shown earlier in Table 3–1. Glucose, fructose, maltose, and sucrose are from plants; lactose and its component galactose, from milk.

Health Effects of Sugars

The sugars are all quite similar in their effects on health. Anything true of sucrose is probably true of the other sugars as well. Many accusations have been made against sucrose:

- *It's unnatural.* It isn't a nutrient; it's an additive, and so it's dangerous. (This is largely unfounded.)
- *It causes malnutrition.* (This is well supported.)
- *It causes obesity.* (It depends, as we'll show in a moment.)
- *It causes diabetes (Type II).* (This is not well supported.)
- *It causes high blood lipid levels and cardiovascular disease.* (This is not well supported.)
- *It causes tooth decay.* (This is confirmed.)

With respect to the first accusation, it is true that sugar is new in our environment. Our cave ancestors did not have a source of pure, refined sucrose, and we are not biologically adapted to cope with large quantities of it. We do require carbohydrates in our diet, but not from sugar as such. In the United States, sugar consumption was only about 20 pounds per person per year in 1820, but had reached over 100 pounds per person per year in the 1970s. In Canada it is now between 85 and 100 pounds per person per year. By now, over a third of the kcalories in our diet come from sugars and visible fats, and sugar is today's leading additive. Our consumption of it is thus not voluntary; of the 100-plus pounds that we eat in a year, 70-some pounds are already added to foods during processing.

Sugar is not a poison, however; sucrose is just glucose plus fructose hitched together, in no way toxic to the system. It's not dangerous—at least not in the sense that true poisons are dangerous. It can even substitute adequately for starch in some roles. It can be beneficial to a child with kidney disease, for example. The feeding of children with kidney disease presents problems. They need protein to grow, but their kidneys can handle only a limited amount of the nitrogen waste from protein. Furthermore, these children often lack appetite. They'll accept sugary treats, and the kcalories permit them to use the protein they receive for growth rather than for energy. Protein used for growth produces a minimum of waste nitrogen for the kidneys to handle. The sugar, then, spares the protein. Nutritionists therefore offer Popsicles and hard candies freely to children with kidney disease, knowing it will help their growth. In such a situation, sugar provides a source of valuable needed energy.

As for the second accusation, it is partly true. Sugar can displace needed nutrients from the diet. Starch usually comes in foods with other nutrients, but sugar contains no other nutrients—no protein, vitamins, or minerals—and so can be termed an empty-kcalorie food. If you have 200 kcalories to "spend" on something, and you spend them on sugar, you get nothing of value for your outlay. If you spend your 200 kcalories on three slices of whole wheat bread instead, you get 14 percent of the protein, 18 percent of the thiamin, and 12 percent of the niacin recommended for a day, as well as comparable amounts

empty-kcalorie food: a popular term used to denote foods that contribute kcalories but are relatively empty of the nutrients protein, vitamins, and minerals. The most notorious empty-kcalorie foods are sugar, fat, and alcohol.

of many other nutrients (Table 3–2). Whether you can afford to eat sugar, then, depends on how many kcalories you have to spend altogether.

It is theoretically possible, with careful food selection, to obtain all the needed nutrients within an allowance of about 1,500 kcalories—but this is not easy for most people. (The Four Food Group Plan with legumes added to it as suggested on p. 32 requires ingesting about 2,200 kcalories.) A teenage boy needs as many as 4,000 kcalories to get all the energy he needs; if he eats some very nutritious foods, then perhaps the "empty kcalories" of cola beverages are an acceptable addition to his diet. On the other hand, many teenage girls eat only 1,200 kcalories or even less, so they can't afford any but the most nutrient-dense foods. Sugar can clearly cause malnutrition, then—not by any positive action of its own, but by displacing nutrients that prevent malnutrition. The appropriate attitude to take is not that sugar is "bad" and that we must avoid it, but that nutritious foods must come first. If the nutritious foods end up crowding sugar out of the diet, that is fine.

The third accusation, that sugar causes obesity, can be answered as follows. Excess energy from any food source, even protein, is stored in body fat. Evidence from population studies shows that in many countries obesity rises as sugar consumption increases. But sugar cannot be singled out as the sole cause. In populations studied, increases in sugar intake are often simultaneous with declines in physical activity and with increases in fat and total kcalorie intakes. Obesity occurs sometimes where sugar intake is low, though, and in some instances, fat people eat less sugar than thin people. Sugar doesn't cause obesity by itself, then, and obesity can occur without it.

On diabetes, the evidence is conflicting and interesting. In vast areas of the world, as the diet has changed in the direction of increased sugar consumption, a profound increase—by as much as tenfold—in the incidence of Type II diabetes has occurred. (This is true for the Japanese, Israelis, Africans, Native Americans, Inuits, Polynesians, and Micronesians.) Yet in other populations, no relation has been found between sugar intake and diabetes. Wherever starch is a major part of the diet, diabetes is rare, but this may not be an effect of the starch itself, but of the nutrients, such as trace minerals and fiber, that accompany it in foods. Wherever obesity is rare, diabetes is also rare, suggesting that sugar alone is, in any case, not enough to cause the disease.

In animals, however, diets very high in sugar can cause a diabetes-like disease even if the animals do not become obese. The fairest conclusion is that obesity is a major factor in the causation of adult onset (Type II) diabetes, but that sugar has not been proven innocent as a special factor.

One of the earliest symptoms of diabetes is excessive hunger. As the common form of diabetes (Type II) develops, the person typically first becomes hungry and then becomes obese; finally, symptoms of diabetes appear. Thus sugar may contribute not to diabetes, but to the obesity that brings the disease into the open. Obesity then aggravates the situation by causing resistance to insulin. In fact, in this type of diabetes there is too much, rather than too little, insulin in the blood, but the tissues fail to respond to it. Both weight control and avoidance of sugar are therefore recommended for people who are susceptible to, or who have, diabetes.

Does sugar raise blood lipid levels and cause cardiovascular disease? No simple answer is available. The blood lipid of greatest interest in connection with cardiovascular disease is cholesterol, and it is discussed in the next chapter,

Some of the effects sugar is thought to have on behavior probably come about indirectly, by way of poor nutrition. See Highlight 14.

The study of populations, **epidemiology** (ep-uh-deem-ee-OLL-uh-gee), involves collecting and interpreting data on the incidence and distribution of diseases. Epidemiology often can demonstrate a correlation between two variables, but cannot prove a cause.

correlation: the simultaneous increase or decrease of two variables.

variable: a factor that may vary (increase or decrease). One variable may depend on another; for example, the height of the average child depends partly on his age. One variable may be independent of another; for example, the intelligence of a child is independent of her height.

which shows that dietary fat is by far the most influential factor affecting the blood cholesterol level. Another blood lipid, not conclusively linked with heart disease, is triglycerides (also discussed in Chapter 4); moderate amounts of sugar may raise blood triglyceride levels in a special subgroup of the population—"carbohydrate-sensitive" individuals. As many as one in five adults may fall in this category. Sugar in the amounts usually consumed seems to have no discrete influence on lipid levels in most people, however. Deaths from heart disease correlate most closely with high blood cholesterol levels, next most closely with obesity, and only loosely with sugar intake; a moderate amount of sugar (5 to 10 percent of total kcalories) has not been shown to affect the disease process.

Does sugar cause dental caries? Here the evidence is strongly positive. Dental caries are actually caused by the acid by-product of bacterial growth in the mouth. Bacteria thrive on carbohydrate, and so it is logical to implicate sugar as the cause of cavities. However, any carbohydrate-containing food, including bread, bananas, or milk, as well as sugar—can support bacterial growth. Equally important is the length of time the food stays in the mouth, and this depends on how soon you brush your teeth after eating and how sticky the food is. Because the damage sugar does is related to both the amount and the stickiness of the sugar, it has been suggested that food labels express their sugar contents in terms of both. Rather than stating simply how much sugar is in a food, the label should state how much dental decay the food causes under defined test conditions. By such a measure, a sticky, sugary food like raisins or granola would be seen to be more caries causing than an easily rinsed-off sugary food like a sweetened beverage.

Sugar can be eaten and then removed from tooth surfaces soon enough to prevent decay, however. A rule of thumb is that bacterial action is maximal within the first 20 minutes after the mouth bacteria have had access to carbohydrate. If immediate brushing is not possible, milk or water drunk with a meal will help wash some of the carbohydrate off the teeth.

Alternatively, you can remove the bacteria themselves by flossing. It takes 24 hours for a large enough clump of bacteria to accumulate on a tooth to produce caries-causing acid, so once-a-day flossing may effectively prevent formation of caries, regardless of the carbohydrate content of the diet. And some people may *never* get cavities, because they have inherited resistance to them. In this matter, as in the others, sugar may not be the extreme villain that some have made it out to be. Still, if sugar is guilty of any of the six accusations listed at the start, it is guilty of contributing to tooth decay.

In summary, there is no reason to believe that the moderate consumption of sugar (5 to 10 percent of kcalories) is in any way dangerous to the normal, healthy human being. Clearly, however, it may be associated with other factors that are harmful: obesity, the displacement of needed nutrients and fiber, and dental decay. If on these grounds you conclude that sugar is indeed to be avoided, it is important to recognize that all kcaloric sweeteners—including fructose, honey, and the rest—are no better.

You have to know, too, that only about a third of the sugar you eat is added to foods by you. The average North American eats at least 100 pounds of sugar a year, and two-thirds of this is hidden in common products to which it has been added by manufacturers. Much of it is not as sucrose but as high-fructose corn syrup (HFCS), the chief sweetening agent used by the food industry today.

A statement of the amount of dental decay a food would produce would be a **cariogenicity** (CARE-ee-oh-jen-ISS-it-ee) **index** for the food.

A normal tooth. Bacteria tend to collect in areas where tooth and tooth or tooth and gum are in contact. Given carbohydrate, they multiply, adhere more firmly, and produce acid, which eats into tooth enamel.

This raises the problem of how food labels should declare their sugar contents. Consumers want, and are entitled to, this information, but food producers are concerned that the labels not put them at an unfair disadvantage; so the exact requirements for labeling still have to be worked out. What should be called "sugar," for example: all monosaccharides and disaccharides, including those found naturally in the food? Or all added sugars, including honey, corn syrup, and the like? Or only added sucrose? How should sugar contents be listed? If given in grams per serving, then the amount of sugar in a cola beverage will be seen to be more than that in a serving of sugar-coated cereal; but if sugar is stated as a percentage, then the amount in the cereal will appear very high, because it isn't diluted by water. These questions have not been resolved, so you can't tell how much sugar is in the products you buy unless the manufacturer has listed the amount voluntarily.

The presence of sugar does have to be revealed in the ingredient list, however, and if sugar is the first ingredient named there, you know it's the predominant substance in the product. A ploy used to avoid revealing this is to list sugar's different forms separately—for example, "corn starch, sucrose, corn syrup," and so on. This way, even though sugar is the main ingredient, it doesn't appear first on the label. But your acquaintance with the terminology presented in this chapter should enable you to see through this ploy and recognize sugar in all its forms.

Sugar is concealed in many common products.

Source: Adapted from Too much sugar, Consumer Reports, March 1978, pp. 137, 139.

Alternative Sweeteners

For people who want to avoid or cut down on their use of the sugars just described, two sets of alternatives are available. One set is the sugar alcohols and other energy-yielding sweeteners; the other is the artificial sweeteners, which contain virtually no kcalories. The sugar alcohols are true sugars and are discussed here; the artificial sweeteners are sugar substitutes and are discussed under "Additives" in Chapter 13.

The sugar alcohols are familiar to people who use special dietary products. Among them are mannitol, sorbitol, xylitol, and maltitol. These carbohydrates are either absorbed more slowly or metabolized to glucose more slowly than most of the other sugars and so may be suitable for use by people who can't handle large amounts of glucose efficiently and so must restrict their intake of ordinary sweets, which provide glucose from the glucose portion of sucrose. They also can't be metabolized as rapidly as sugar by ordinary mouth bacteria, so they don't contribute as much to tooth decay.

Mannitol is the least satisfactory of the alternative sweeteners just named. It is considerably less sweet than sucrose, so sizable amounts have to be used when it is substituted for sucrose. Because it lingers unabsorbed in the intestine for a long time, it is available to intestinal bacteria for their energy. As they consume the mannitol, they multiply, they attract water, and they produce irritating waste, which causes diarrhea. Mannitol is therefore not much used as an alternative sweetener.

Sorbitol has been popular as a sweetener for sugar-free gums and candies, but it, too, has drawbacks. It is only half as sweet as sucrose, so sorbitol with twice as many kcalories has to be used to deliver a given amount of sweetness. Also, like mannitol, it causes diarrhea. Advantages are that it is absorbed very slowly, so it has little or no effect on blood glucose; and little or no insulin is needed to make it available to the body's cells. Thus people with diabetes, who have ineffective insulin or who have to take insulin, may benefit from using small amounts of sorbitol. Its threshold for causing diarrhea is higher than mannitol's, so of the two, sorbitol is preferred.

Xylitol has also been popular, especially in chewing gums, because it has been reported to help prevent dental caries. (It not only doesn't support caries-producing bacteria; it actually inhibits their growth.[5]) Like all the sugar alcohols, it has as many kcalories per gram as sucrose, but it is as sweet as fructose, so that less can be used. Xylitol occurs in foods, and some xylitol is produced in the body during normal metabolic processes; so it is not a foreign substance. Xylitol is widely used in many Western European countries and in Canada; however, reports that it may cause tumors in animals have led to the voluntary curtailing of its use by U.S. food producers.

Maltitol has a sweetness equal to about 90 percent that of sucrose. It is used in some carbonated beverages and canned fruits, and in Japanese bakery products and other sweets intended not to cause tooth decay. At first thought not to be absorbed from the gastrointestinal tract, maltitol was recommended for use in food products for dieters and people with diabetes. This claim is doubtful, however; the sugar probably does have kcalorie value. The manufacture of maltitol from maltose is expensive and limits its use; using maltose directly costs less.

The person who wishes to cut kcalories should be aware that the sugar alcohols *do* contain kcalories—just as many per gram as sucrose. In spite of this fact, products that contain them are labeled "sugar-free." The reason they are suitable for people who must limit their intakes of ordinary sweets is because the body handles them differently, not because they are kcalorie-free. The person who is limiting kcalories must limit sugar alcohols just as carefully as sugars.

Another sweetener of possible usefulness to people with abnormal carbohydrate metabolism is fructose, already discussed. It is one and a half times as sweet as sucrose when tasted in a simple solution, and it neither requires nor stimulates insulin secretion. Thus it has been advocated, in amounts up to 75 grams per day (about 12 teaspoons), as an alternative sweetener for use by people with diabetes and hypoglycemia.[6] Many authorities oppose the use of fructose by people with diabetes, however, because it may tend to increase their already high blood lipid levels.[7] In any case, because fructose, like sucrose, contains 4 kcalories per gram, it still contributes kcalories and so its usefulness as a weight-loss aid is limited. Still, it is so sweet that a small dose will do the job that a larger dose of sucrose would do.

The Complex Carbohydrates: Polysaccharides

While the sugars contain three monosaccharides in different combinations, the polysaccharides are composed almost entirely of only one—glucose. The differences between them have to do with the ways glucose is condensed into the large molecules of starch, glycogen, and cellulose.

Starch

As the chemist sees it, starch is a long, straight or branched chain of hundreds of glucose units connected together. These units would have to be magnified more than 10 million times to appear at the size shown on this page. However, as molecules go, starches are rather large. A single starch molecule may contain 3,000 or more glucose units linked together. These giant molecules are packed side by side in the rice grain or potato tuber—as many as a million in a cubic inch of food.

In the plant, starch serves a function similar to that served by the glycogen in the body. It is a storage form of glucose needed for the plant's first growth. (When you eat the plant, of course, you get the glucose to use for your own purposes.)

All starchy foods are in fact plant foods. Grains are the richest food source. Many human societies have a staple grain from which 50 to 80 percent of their people's food energy is derived—rice in the Orient; wheat in Canada, the United States, and Europe; corn in much of Central and South America; and millet, rye, barley, and oats elsewhere.

A second important source of starch is the legume (bean and pea) family, including peanuts and such dry beans found in the supermarket as butter beans, kidney beans, "baked" beans, black-eyed peas (cowpeas), chickpeas (garbanzo beans), and soybeans. These legumes are not only rich in starch but also contain a significant amount of protein. A third major source of starch is the tubers, such as the potato, yam, and cassava of many non-Western societies.

When you eat any of these foods, enzymes in your mouth and intestine hydrolyze the starch molecules to yield glucose units, which are absorbed across the intestinal wall into the blood. One to four hours after a meal, all the starch has been digested and is circulating to the cells as glucose.

Glycogen

Glycogen is not found in plants and is stored in animal meats only to a limited extent. It is not, therefore, of importance as a nutrient, although it performs an important role in the body, as already described. Glycogen is more complex and more highly branched than starch; its structure permits rapid breakdown. When the hormonal message "Break down glycogen" arrives at a liver or muscle cell, enzymes can attack all the branches simultaneously, producing a surge of energy for emergency action. The drawing at the start of this chapter shows part of a single liver cell, in which a multitude of glycogen packages await such a call.

● = Glucose

Portion of a starch molecule.

starch: a plant polysaccharide composed of glucose and digestible by humans. For structures, see Appendix C.

Different kinds of grains

Starch can be broken down to shorter chains of glucose units known as **dextrins**. The word sometimes appears on food labels, because dextrins can be used as thickening agents in foods.

glycogen (GLIGH-co-gen): an animal polysaccharide composed of glucose, manufactured and stored in liver and muscle. For structure, see Appendix C.

Cellulose

cellulose (CELL-you-loce): a plant polysaccharide composed of glucose and indigestible by humans.

The third polysaccharide of importance in nutrition is cellulose. Cellulose, like starch, is found abundantly in plants and is composed of glucose units connected in long, branching chains. However, the bonds holding its glucose units together are not digestible by human enzymes; only bacterial enzymes can digest them. Cellulose is not, therefore, of much significance as an energy source for human beings, but is of great importance as one of the food fibers, to which the next section is devoted.

Health Effects of Complex Carbohydrates

The dietary goals and guidelines offered to the public by various agencies in the United States and Canada all agree that it would do no harm, and that it might do some good, for people to reduce their intakes of concentrated sweets and increase their intakes of foods containing complex carbohydrates. This advice is based on two distinctions. First, not all sugars need to be restricted; those in ordinary foods such as fruits, vegetables, and milk are excepted. *Concentrated* sweets, relatively empty of nutrients and high in kcalories, are the ones singled out for avoidance. Second, the concentrated sweets are to be replaced, not just with complex carbohydrates, but with *foods* containing carbohydrates. In a word, the trade is between relatively pure sugar on the one hand and complex whole foods on the other. Many people have failed to understand this distinction and have thought that they should avoid fruits or try to ingest more pure starch, but neither of these courses is recommended.

Typical consumers derive close to 25 percent of their kcalories from sugar, and about 25 percent from complex carbohydrates. The recommendation is that they reduce their sugar intake to the point where it represents 10 percent or less of their kcalories, and increase their complex carbohydrate energy to about 50 percent of the total. Total carbohydrate intake would increase, then, even though sugar intake would decline. The major additions to the diet would be foods containing starch and fiber—vegetables, grains, legumes, and fruits.

The health benefits to be expected from such a change would be many. Before enumerating them, though, let us hasten to say that it is difficult to sort out just what dietary factors might contribute to each health benefit. A diet lower in pure sugars and higher in foods containing complex carbohydrates would almost certainly be lower in fat, lower in kcalories, and higher in fiber as well. The constellation of all these factors working together might be expected to bring about, or contribute to, lower rates of obesity, cardiovascular disease, diabetes, cancer, malnutrition, and tooth decay.

Starch and fiber almost invariably appear together in foods (except refined foods), so it is especially hard to separate their effects. The next section, "The Fibers," shows what health effects are especially closely associated with fibers, and the section on "The Carbohydrates in Foods" shows the effects of foods that contain both starch and fiber on blood glucose regulation.

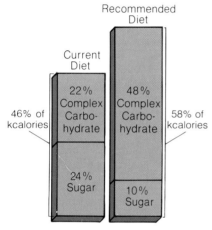

Dietary Goals: Carbohydrate

Dietary goals: carbohydrate.
While total carbohydrate in the diet is supposed to increase, sugar as a percentage of the carbohydrate and as a percentage of the total diet is supposed to decrease, making a major increase in the amount of complex carbohydrate—starch and fiber.

The Fibers

Plant foods contain many fibers, predominantly as constituents of their cell walls. These fibers, especially the polysaccharide ones, are important in the human diet. Cellulose has already been mentioned; other fibers are pectins, hemicelluloses, lignins, gums, and mucilages. Those of particular interest are the ones found in foods and not digested by the body—dietary fiber.

Although cellulose and other fibers are not attacked by human enzymes, some fibers, notably hemicellulose, can be digested by bacteria in the human digestive tract, and can yield some absorbable products. Food fibers are therefore not totally kcalorie-free, although their energy contribution can, practically speaking, be considered negligible.[8]

Health Effects of Fiber

Based on the experience of researchers in Africa, the "fiber hypothesis" suggests that consumption of unrefined, high-fiber, carbohydrate foods protects against many Western diseases. Rural Africans naturally consume a diet very high in fiber and show a low incidence of many chronic conditions. Some researchers, however, stress that it may be the higher Western intake of salt, sugar, and animal fat rather than the absence of fibrous foods that should be credited for this advantage.

Fiber may also play a role in weight control. According to the fiber hypothesis, obesity is not seen in those parts of the world where people eat large amounts of fiber. Foods high in fiber tend to be low in fat and simple sugars. High-fiber breads have fewer kcalories per pound than refined breads. High-fiber foods, because of their water-holding capacity, satisfy hunger readily. Many of the diet aids on the market today are composed of bulk-inducing fibers such as methylcellulose.

Indeed, producers of some diet aids base the success of their products on the ability of certain fibers to provide bulk and satiety. If you wish to apply this principle in adopting a low-kcalorie diet, you may be relieved to learn that you do not need to spend extra money on these diet aids. Selecting fresh fruits, vegetables, legumes, and other high-fiber foods would represent both an economic and a nutritious means of adding bulk to your diet.

fiber: a loose term denoting the substances in plant food that are not digested by human digestive enzymes. The terms *crude fiber* and *dietary fiber* are more precise.

crude fiber (CF): the residue of plant food remaining after extraction with dilute acid followed by dilute alkali in a laboratory procedure; that is, the fiber that remains in food after a harsh chemical digestive procedure.

dietary fiber (DF): the residue of plant food resistant to hydrolysis by human digestive enzymes; that is, the fiber that remains from food after digestion in the body.
1 g crude fiber ~ 2–3 g dietary fiber.

pectin and **hemicellulose:** polysaccharide fibers found in plant foods.

lignin: a carbohydrate-like fiber that occurs in plant foods.

gums, mucilages: other fibers.

available carbohydrate: another term for starch and the sugars, the carbohydrates made available to the body by human digestive enzymes (in contrast to the fibers, which are **unavailable carbohydrates**).

A fiber that yields kcalories by way of bacterial digestion is a **digestible,** but not **available,** carbohydrate. In the body such a fiber *would* normally be digested, because there are always abundant bacteria in the normal, healthy human digestive tract.

We are advised to increase our intakes of complex carbohydrates and fiber.

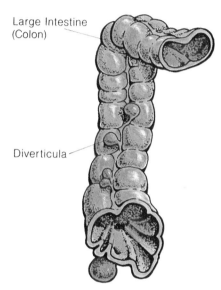

Large Intestine (Colon)

Diverticula

The outpocketings of intestinal linings that balloon through the weakened intestinal wall muscles are known as **diverticula**.

diverticulosis (DYE-ver-tic-you-LOH-sis): the condition of having outpocketings of weakened areas of the intestinal wall (like blowouts in a tire). The danger of diverticulosis is that it can give rise to **diverticulitis** (-EYE-tis), in which the pockets become infected or inflamed and may rupture. About one in every six people in Western countries develops diverticulosis in middle or later life.

divertir = to turn side
osis = disease
itis = infection or inflammation

Some fibers in the GI tract function like a sponge, holding water, binding minerals, and binding acidic materials such as the bile salts used by the body to prepare fat for digestion. Dietary fibers exercise the intestinal muscles so that they retain their health and tone. The major impact of dietary fiber is on the colon, the last part of the GI tract, where colon cancer and diverticular disease can arise; but the addition of fibrous foods to the diet increases the bulk of food all along the intestine.

Food fibers are thought to be beneficial with respect to the following:

- *Weight control.* A diet high in fibrous foods promotes satiety and can promote weight loss, if those foods displace concentrated fats and sweets.
- *Constipation and diarrhea.* Some fibers attract water into the digestive tract, thus softening the stools. Some form gels, helping to solidify watery stools. By the one mechanism, they help relieve constipation, and by the other, they help relieve diarrhea.
- *Hemorrhoids.* Softer stools ease elimination for the rectal muscles and reduce the pressure in the lower bowel, creating less likelihood that rectal veins will swell.
- *Appendicitis.* Fiber helps prevent compaction of the intestinal contents, which could obstruct the appendix and permit bacteria to invade and infect it.
- *Diverticulosis.* Fiber exercises the muscles of the digestive tract so that they retain their health and tone and resist bulging out into the pouches characteristic of diverticulosis.
- *Colon cancer.* Some fibers speed up the passage of food materials through the digestive tract, thus shortening the "transit time" and helping to prevent exposure of the tissue to cancer-causing agents in food. Some fibers bind bile (described in Chapter 4) and carry it out of the body; this is also thought to reduce cancer risk.
- *Blood lipids and cardiovascular disease.* Fiber binds lipids such as bile and cholesterol and carries them out of the body with the feces so that the blood lipid concentrations are lowered, and possibly the risk of heart and artery disease as a consequence.
- *Blood glucose and insulin modulation.* Monosaccharides absorbed from some complex carbohydrates, in the presence of fiber, produce a moderate insulin response and a more even rise in blood glucose. Insulin levels are high in obesity, cardiovascular disease, and diabetes (Type II), so this effect of fiber may be beneficial in terms of all three diseases.
- *Diabetes control.* Thanks to its effects on blood glucose, fiber helps to manage diabetes. Persons with mild cases of diabetes, given high-fiber diets, have been able to reduce their insulin doses.

Different Fibers, Different Effects

Not all the fibers have similar effects. For example, wheat bran, which is composed mostly of cellulose, has no cholesterol-lowering effect, whereas oat bran and the fiber of apples (pectin) do lower blood cholesterol. On the other hand, wheat bran seems to be one of the most effective stool-softening fibers, especially if larger particle sizes are used. Fibers that form gels in water (pectin and guar) prolong the time of transit of materials through the intestine, whereas insoluble fibers (cellulose) tend to reduce the time. Table 3–3 shows the effects of different kinds of fiber.

TABLE 3–3

Effects of Different Kinds of Fiber

Condition and Effects of Fiber	Fiber Type		
	Cellulose, Hemicellulose (From fruits, vegetables, legumes, wheat bran, oat bran, and other cereal brans, nuts and seeds, whole grain flours)	Gums, Pectins, (From fruits, vegetables, seeds, legumes, oats, barley)	Lignin (From whole grains, seeds, woody parts of vegetables)
Obesity—displaces kcalories (gel forming)?	Yes	Yes	No
Constipation/ hemorrhoids— effect on stool bulk, ease of passage	Reduces pressure, softens stools[a]	None	Make stools move faster
Cancer—increases bile acid excretion?	No[b]	Yes	Yes
Diabetes and other disorders of blood glucose regulation— improves glucose tolerance?	Yes[c]	Yes—Some help control blood sugar in diabetes	—
Cardiovascular disease—lowers blood cholesterol?	No—except oat bran lowers it	Yes	Yes
kCalorie intake— how completely digested?	60 to 95% digested	Mostly digested	Not digested
Blocks mineral absorption?	Yes	No	Yes

[a]Wheat bran improves both constipation and diarrhea. M. S. Mathur, H. Ram, and V. S. Chadda, Effect of bran on intestinal transit time in normal Indians and in intestinal amoebiasis, *American Journal of Proctology Gastroenterology and Colon and Rectal Surgery,* November–December 1978, pp. 30–32, 34.

[b]Wheat bran binds bile acids in vitro but does *not* affect bile acid excretion in man. M. A. Eastwood and R. M. Kay, An hypothesis for the action of dietary fiber along the gastrointestinal tract, *American Journal of Clinical Nutrition* 32 (1979): 364–367.

[c]Wheat bran improves glucose tolerance; pectins do not. J. W. Anderson and W.-J. L. Chen, Plant fiber: Carbohydrate and lipid metabolism, *American Journal of Clinical Nutrition* 32 (1979): 346–363.

Hazards of Too Much Fiber

Most clinical reports are concerned with the influence of the *lack* of fiber in the diet on health and disease. The questions of whether *excessive* fiber might be harmful, and what the ideal range of fiber intakes may be, remain to be answered.

A person who eats bulky foods, and who has only a small capacity, may not be able to take in enough food energy or nutrients. Vegetarian children are especially vulnerable to this problem. People who have marginal or inadequate intakes of the vitamins and trace minerals—including elderly people, people on low-kcalorie diets, and children—may also be likely to develop nutrient deficiencies on high-fiber diets.

Maximum absorption of iron occurs early during digestion. Due to the faster transit of high-fiber foods, there may be little opportunity for absorption of iron and other nutrients from them. People given *purified* fiber under experimental conditions are seen to excrete more minerals in their feces than otherwise—including calcium, potassium, zinc, and others. Whether mineral losses are significant on ordinary high-fiber *foods* is not known. Clearly, though, fiber is like all the nutrients in that "more" is only "better" up to a point. Too much is no better for you than too little. Also, purified fiber is not as beneficial as the fiber of foods; the purified version is empty of nutrients, while the food version is loaded with them.

A compound not classed as a fiber but often found with it in foods is phytic acid. On a high-fiber diet, losses of minerals may occur if they become bound to phytic acid. Most of the phytic acid in our diet comes from seeds such as the cereal grains. (The role of phytate in the plant seed may be to store these ions and hold them in plant tissue during germination.)

phytate (FYE-tate) **(phytic acid):** a nonnutrient component of plant seeds. Phytic acid occurs in the husks of grains, legumes, and seeds and is capable of binding ions such as zinc, iron, calcium, magnesium, and copper in insoluble complexes in the intestine.

The Carbohydrates in Foods

You need some carbohydrate daily as a source of glucose. If you don't eat carbohydrate, your body devours its own protein to generate glucose—and it needs its protein for other vital purposes. The "protein-sparing effect" of carbohydrate is important and will come up again (Chapters 5 and 7). How much carbohydrate is enough?

Recommended Carbohydrate Intake

Most authorities agree that you need considerably more than 50 grams—probably more than 100 grams—of carbohydrate a day.[9] To be safe, you should probably aim for at least 125 grams; and 300 grams might be an ideal intake for many people. At 4 kcalories per gram, that would be 1,200 kcalories from carbohydrate.

The *Dietary Goals* state an intake of available carbohydrate (starch and sugar) that might be ideal to support long-term health: 55 to 60 percent of total kcalories. A person consuming 1,500 kcalories a day should therefore have 825 to 900 kcalories of carbohydrate, or about 200 to 225 grams. A person consuming 3,000 kcalories a day should have twice that, or 400 to 450 grams. Most of this would be starch, with its accompanying fiber; some would be the naturally occurring sugars of fruits, vegetables, and milk; only 10 percent or less would be concentrated sugar. Fiber isn't counted in computing energy from carbohydrate; we don't know enough yet about its energy contributions, but they are probably not large in comparison with those from starch and sugar. Fiber intakes are discussed separately, below.

The recommended intakes of 200 to 500 grams or so of carbohydrate a day are very generous in comparison with the minimum amount of carbohydrate necessary to spare protein, which has been estimated at 50 to 100 grams a day.[10] They are even more generous in comparison with the "less than 60 grams" recommended by most low-carbohydrate diets.

The exchange system described in Chapter 2 provides a convenient way to estimate the amount of carbohydrate in your lunchbox or on your dinner plate. In exchange systems, foods are sorted into lists in such a way that the carbohydrate contents of foods on any one list are similar. To use such a system, all you need to know is the carbohydrate value for the list and the members of that list with their portion sizes (see Figure 3–9).

We are beginning to build a case against the low-carbohydrate diet that will culminate in Chapter 7.

FIGURE 3–9

Foods containing carbohydrate. Four of the six food lists contain carbohydrate, so you need only know four values and learn a value for concentrated sugar (which is not on the exchange lists).

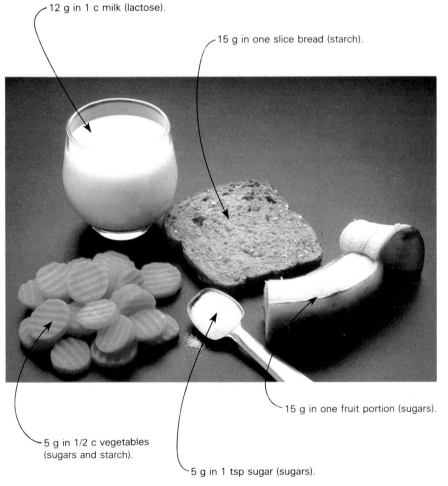

12 g in 1 c milk (lactose).

15 g in one slice bread (starch).

5 g in 1/2 c vegetables (sugars and starch).

5 g in 1 tsp sugar (sugars).

15 g in one fruit portion (sugars).

1 c nonfat milk (or any other portion of food in the milk list) provides 12 g carbohydrate as lactose, a naturally occurring sugar. Cheeses have negligible carbohydrate and so are not included with milk in this system. (See Appendix G for Canadian values, which are different.)

1 slice of bread (or any other portion of food on the starch/bread list) provides 15 g carbohydrate, mostly in the form of starch. All grain foods, such as cereal and pasta, and such starchy vegetables as corn, lima beans, and potatoes are included on this list.

1 portion of fruit (portion sizes are shown on the fruit list) provides 15 g carbohydrate, mostly as the naturally occurring sugars glucose, fructose, and sucrose.

1/2 c carrots (or any other portion of food on the vegetable list) provides 5 g carbohydrate, partly as the naturally occurring sugars fructose, glucose, and sucrose, and partly as starch. Starchy vegetables (those whose carbohydrate is predominantly starch) are not included on this list. (See Appendix G.)

1 tsp white sugar provides 4 g carbohydrate as sucrose, which for most purposes can be rounded off to 5 g. The other concentrated sweets provide sucrose, fructose, glucose, and other hexoses, or mixtures of these.

Sugar Intake

Exchange systems do not include sugary foods like candy, jam, and soft drinks, because they are not considered desirable in diet plans. But people do consume them, and they certainly contain carbohydrate. To estimate an accurate total of the carbohydrate you consume, you may need a "sugar list," and we have invented one for the purpose. Among the concentrated sweets treated as equivalent to 1 teaspoon of white sugar are:

- 1 teaspoon brown sugar.
- 1 teaspoon candy.
- 1 teaspoon corn sweeteners.
- 1 teaspoon corn syrup.
- 1 teaspoon honey.
- 1 teaspoon jam.
- 1 teaspoon jelly.
- 1 teaspoon maple sugar.
- 1 teaspoon maple syrup.
- 1 teaspoon molasses.

These sugars can all be assumed to provide about 20 kcalories per teaspoon. Some are closer to 10 kcalories (for example, 16 kcalories for sucrose), while some are over 20 (22 kcalories for honey); so an average figure of 20 kcalories is an acceptable rough approximation. For a person who uses catsup (ketchup) liberally, it may help to remember that 1 tablespoon of catsup supplies about 1 teaspoon of sugar.

1 tbsp catsup = 1 tsp sugar.

Finally, while we're still on the subject of sugar, you need to recognize its many aliases. The accompanying Miniglossary presents the multitude of names that denote sugar on food labels.

All the foods containing carbohydrate have now been identified in five categories. Some practice with estimating portion sizes and a familiarity with the gram amounts give you a command of the total carbohydrate content of any diet. The example given in Figure 3–10 demonstrates the system's usefulness.

This kind of calculation provides only an estimate, but is close enough for most purposes. A more accurate way to determine the carbohydrate composition of foods is to refer to Appendix H, which lists individual foods. Adding the individual carbohydrate amounts found in Appendix H yields 259 grams of carbohydrate for the meals shown in Figure 3–10.

It takes only one or two calculations of this kind to give you a feel for the carbohydrate content of your diet. Once you are aware of the major carbohy-

The difference between an estimate and the amount obtained by a more accurate calculation may be disconcerting. Rough estimates are often more valuable than close calculations, however, because of the time saved and because often only a ballpark figure is needed. In this example, we know that an intake of 50 grams of carbohydrate is far below the recommended minimum of 125 grams, but 255 and 269 grams are both comfortably above it and in the same range. The difference between them becomes insignificant from this perspective.

Most estimates of the nutrient contents of foods are rough but serviceable approximations. If we refer to a "90-kcalorie potato," you should understand this to mean "90 plus or minus about 20 percent," which makes it not significantly different from a 100-kcalorie potato. In general, for most purposes, a variation of about 20 percent is expected and is considered perfectly reasonable.

Miniglossary of a Few Representative kCaloric Sweeteners

brown sugar: sugar crystals contained in molasses syrup with natural flavor and color; 91 to 96% pure sucrose. (Some refiners add syrup to refined white sugar to make brown sugar.)

confectioners' sugar: finely powdered sucrose; 99.9% pure.

corn sweeteners: corn syrup and sugars derived from corn.

corn syrup: a syrup produced by the action of enzymes on cornstarch, containing mostly glucose. See also *high-fructose corn syrup*.

dextrose: glucose (an older name).

fructose, galactose, glucose: already defined (pp. 60–61).

granulated sugar: crystalline sucrose; 99.9% pure.

high-fructose corn syrup (**HFCS**): the predominant sweetener used in processed foods today. HFCS is mostly fructose; glucose makes up the balance.

honey: sugar formed from nectar (mostly sucrose) gathered by bees. An enzyme splits the sucrose into glucose and fructose. Composition and flavor vary, but honey always contains a mixture of sucrose, fructose, and glucose.

invert sugar: a mixture of glucose and fructose formed by the splitting of sucrose in a chemical process. Sold only in liquid form, sweeter than sucrose, invert sugar is used as an additive to help preserve food freshness and prevent shrinkage.

lactose: already defined (p. 62).

levulose: fructose (an older name).

maltitol, mannitol, sorbitol, xylitol: sugar alcohols, which can be derived from fruits or commercially produced from dextrose; absorbed more slowly and metabolized differently than other sugars in the human body, and not readily utilized by ordinary mouth bacteria.

maltose: already defined (p. 63).

maple sugar: a sugar (mostly sucrose) purified from concentrated sap of the sugar maple tree. Maple sugar is expensive compared with other sweeteners.

molasses: a thick brown syrup, left over from sugar cane juice during sugar refining. It retains residual sugar and other by-products and a few minerals; blackstrap molasses contains significant amounts of calcium and iron—the iron from the machinery used to process it.

raw sugar: the first crop of crystals harvested during sugar processing. Raw sugar cannot be sold in the United States because it contains too much filth (dirt, insect fragments, and the like). Sugar sold as "raw sugar" domestically has actually gone through about half of the refining steps.

sucrose: already defined (p. 61).

turbinado (ter-bih-NOD-oh) **sugar**: raw (brown) sugar from which the filth has been washed; legal to sell in the United States.

white sugar: pure sucrose, produced by dissolving, concentrating, and recrystallizing raw sugar.

FIGURE 3–10

How to estimate carbohydrate intake. A dietitian, looking at the foods in the figure, might estimate the cup of oatmeal as "2 grains," because a 1-grain portion is 1/2 cup of any cooked cereal. She would figure the quarter cup of raisins as "2 fruits," because 2 tablespoons of raisins is a fruit exchange. The ways she would view each food portion as exchanges are shown. The novice would have to become familiar with the exchange system before this technique would save time, but a few practice sessions are enough to make it easy to estimate carbohydrate grams quite closely. The actual carbohydrate grams (from Appendix H) are shown at the right; totals for the day differ by less than 2% from estimates.

		Carbohydrate Grams	
		Estimated	Actual
Breakfast			
1 c oatmeal = 2 grain portions	=	30	25
¼ c raisins = 2 fruit portions	=	30	29
½ c nonfat milk = ½ milk portion	=	6	6
½ grapefruit = 1 fruit portion	=	15	9
		81	69
Lunch			
1 c cooked rice = 2 grain portions	=	30	50
2 c mixed vegetables might be figured as follows:			
1 c vegetables = 2 vegetable portions	=	10	
and			48
1 c starchy vegetables (lima beans, peas, and corn) = 2 starchy vegetables	=	30	
2 oz cheddar cheese = 2 meat portions	=	0	1
1¼ c fresh strawberries = about 1 fruit portion	=	15	13
1 c nonfat milk = 1 milk portion	=	12	12
2 pats butter = 2 fat portions	=	0	0
2 packets sugar	=	10	12
		107	136
Dinner			
3 oz broiled fish = 3 meat portions	=	0	0
½ c green beans = 1 vegetable portion	=	5	4
½ c cooked carrots = 1 vegetable portion	=	5	6
½ c cooked peas = 1 starchy vegetable	=	15	11
2 pats butter = 2 fat portions	=	0	0
1 c nonfat milk = 1 milk portion	=	12	12
		37	33
Snack			
⅓ cantaloupe = 1 fruit portion	=	15	15
1 brownie = 1 grain portion	=	15	16
		30	31
Day's Total:	=	255	269

drate-contributing foods you eat, you can return to thinking simply in terms of the foods, developing a sense of how much of each is enough.

Fiber Intake

The amounts of dietary fiber in food are hard to estimate. Chemists can analyze food for crude fiber content in the laboratory by digesting it with acids and bases, but if you eat the same food, subjecting it to the action of your own enzymes, the undigested residue will be greater, because the body's enzymes are less harsh than the laboratory treatment. What we really need to know is the dietary fiber content of foods, but how can we measure it? One imprecise and unpleasant procedure involves collecting all the stools excreted over a 24–hour period and then drying and weighing them.

Still, with all the uncertainties, it is probably true to say that about 20 to 30 grams of dietary fiber daily is a desirable intake. The diet can supply that amount, given ample choices of whole foods, as Table 3–4 demonstrates. However, it involves eating such quantities of fruits, vegetables, legumes, and grains

TABLE 3–4

Foods to Provide 25 Grams Dietary Fiber per Day

Fruits: about 2 g of fiber per serving; use four or more per day.

Apple, 1 small	Orange, 1 small
Banana, 1 small	Peach, 1 medium
Strawberries, ½ c	Pear, ½ small
Cherries, 10 large	Plums, 2 small

Grains and Cereals: about 2 g of fiber per serving; use four or more per day.

Whole-wheat bread, 1 slice	All Bran, 1 tbsp
Rye bread, 1 slice	Cornflakes, ⅔ c
Cracked wheat bread, 1 slice	Oatmeal, dry, 3 tbsp
Shredded Wheat, ½ biscuit	Wheat bran, 1 tsp
Grape-Nuts, 3 tbsp	Puffed Wheat, 1½ cups
Barley, ½ c	

Vegetables: about 2 g of fiber per serving; use 4 or more per day. These values are for cooked portions.

Broccoli, ½ stalk	Lettuce, raw, 2 c
Brussels sprouts, 4	Green beans, ½ c
Carrots, ⅓ c	Potato, 2-inch diameter
Celery, 1 c	Tomato, raw, 1 medium
Corn on the cob, 2-inch piece	

Legumes: about 8 g of fiber per portion.

Garbanzo beans, ½ c	Baked beans, canned, ½ c
Kidney beans, ½ c	

Miscellaneous: about 1 g of fiber per portion.

Peanut butter, 2½ tsp	Pickle, 1 large
Peanuts, 10 nuts	Strawberry jam, 5 tbsp
Walnuts, ¼ c	

Source: Adapted from Recommendations for a high-fiber diet, *Nutrition and the MD*, July 1981, in turn adapted from D.A.T. Southgate and coauthors, A guide to calculating intakes of dietary fiber, *Journal of Human Nutrition* 30 (1976): 303–313.

that little room is left for meats and dairy products—a way of eating to which some people could find it hard to adjust. (Appendix H offers dietary fiber contents of additional foods.)

Glycemic Effect of Foods

The glycemic effect of a food is the effect that food has on a person's blood glucose and insulin response—how fast and how high the blood glucose rises, and how quickly the body responds by bringing it back to normal. Most people have had the impression that simple sugars produce a major surge in blood glucose while complex carbohydrates produce a flatter response curve—but now we know that the case is not so simple. The effects of different foods on blood glucose apparently depend on many factors:

- The digestibility of the starch in the food.
- Interactions of the starch with the protein in the food.
- The amounts and kinds of fat, sugar, and fiber in the food.
- The presence of other constituents, such as molecules that bind starch.
- The form of the food (dry, paste, or liquid; coarsely or finely ground; how thoroughly cooked; and so forth).

All these factors working together produce the food's glycemic effect, and it is not always what a person might expect. Ice cream, for example, produces less of a response than potatoes.

The glycemic effect of a food is important to people with abnormalities of blood glucose regulation, notably diabetes or hypoglycemia. Such people are wise to avoid foods producing too great a rise, and too sudden a fall, in blood glucose. For their use, researchers are attempting to produce a "glycemic index" that would rank foods according to their effects on blood glucose. A sample of such an index is shown in Table 3–5.

Does the glycemic index signify that people with diabetes should eat ice cream in preference to potatoes? No—although if sweet desserts have a place in their diet, then ice cream may be a better choice than several other foods in that category. They should remember, though, that foods have to be evaluated on many bases, of which the glycemic index is only one. Ice cream is high in sugar, sodium, fat, and kcalories; its nutrient density is low. The fiber of potatoes may have beneficial health effects that ice cream, lacking fiber, doesn't offer.

TABLE 3–5

Glycemic Index (A Sampling) The flatter the blood glucose curve in response to a food, the lower the glycemic index.

Fructose	20	Bread (white)	69
Milk (whole)	34	Potatoes (new)	70
Ice cream	36	Cornflakes	80
Orange juice	46	Carrots	92
Spaghetti (white)	50	Parsnips	97
Yam	51	Glucose	100

Source: D. J. A. Jenkins and coauthors, Glycemic Index of Foods, *Diabetologia* 23 (1982): 477, as adapted by P. A. Crapo, The relationship between food and blood sugar, *Nutrition and the MD*, July 1984.

Food choices should be made in the context of the total diet and of the needs of the individual.[11]

It was once believed that the person with diabetes could exchange any food containing available carbohydrate for any other with the same amount of carbohydrate. Now, however, it is clear that a half cup of rice is not necessarily the same as a small potato or a slice of bread, even though they are on the same exchange list. Nor are the following pairs of items the same:

- A slice of white bread versus a slice of whole-grain bread.
- A mashed potato versus a baked potato with the skin.
- A portion of apple juice versus an apple.

The second member of each pair creates less demand for insulin and is thus preferable in the diet of the person with diabetes who is attempting to control the disease without artificial means. This should remind you of the discussion at the end of Highlight 2: whole foods are preferable in each case.

Of all the foods that have been studied, the ones with the lowest glycemic indexes appear to be legumes, especially lentils. In fact, lentils taken for breakfast have a moderating effect on blood glucose that extends even through lunch.[12] Further study of how this effect arises should bring fascinating insights into the ways in which foods and the body interact.

This chapter began by showing you how important a constant blood glucose level is for the functioning of the brain and the body's other tissues. Then it went on to demonstrate how the body can derive glucose from all foods containing starches and sugars. Now it has shown which foods those are. Armed with this information, you can explode some of the myths perpetrated by advertisers of carbohydrate-containing foods and beverages. Sugar is "quick energy"—so when you need quick energy, you should reach for a candy bar and a cola beverage, right? Wrong. The best pick-me-ups are not concentrated sugars. True, sugars offer energy, but you now can see that any food containing carbohydrate can offer that to you. How about a delicious peanut butter and banana sandwich; a tall, cool glass of milk; and a fresh, juicy orange for your pick-me-up?

Study Questions

1. How is blood glucose maintained? What happens when it gets too high or too low?
2. What happens in a condensation reaction? In a hydrolysis reaction?
3. What three monosaccharides are important in nutrition? Where are they found?
4. What three disaccharides are important in nutrition? What are their component monosaccharides? Where are they found?
5. What are sugar alcohols?
6. What are differences between simple and complex carbohydrates?
7. What are the health effects of fiber?
8. What are the dietary goals regarding carbohydrate intake?
9. Explain the glycemic effect and give some contrasting examples.

Examine Your Carbohydrate Intake

Having read Chapter 3, you are in a position to study your carbohydrate intake. From the forms you filled out earlier, answer the following questions:

1. How many grams of carbohydrate do you consume in a day?
2. How many kcalories does this represent? (Remember, 1 gram of carbohydrate contributes 4 kcalories.)
3. It is estimated that you should have 125 grams or more of carbohydrate in a day. How does your intake compare with this minimum?
4. What percentage of your total kcalories is contributed by carbohydrate (carbohydrate kcalories divided by total kcalories times 100)?
5. How does this figure compare with the dietary goal that states that 60 percent of the kcalories in your diet should come from carbohydrate? (Note: If you are on a diet to lose weight, then this goal does not apply to you. See the exercises in Self-Study 8: Diet Planning.)
6. Another dietary goal is that no more than 10 percent of total kcalories should come from refined and other processed sugars and foods high in such sugars. To assess your intake against this standard, sort the carbohydrate-containing food items you ate into three groups:
- Foods containing complex carbohydrate (foods found on the bread and vegetable exchange lists).
- Nutritious foods containing simple carbohydrate (foods on the milk and fruit lists).
- Foods containing mostly concentrated simple carbohydrate (sugar, honey, molasses, syrup, jam, jelly, candy, cakes, doughnuts, sweet rolls, cola beverages, and so on).

How many grams of carbohydrate did you consume in each of these three categories? How many kcalories (grams times 4)? What percentage of your total kcalories comes from concentrated sugars? From other simple carbohydrates? Does your concentrated sugar intake fall within the recommended maximum of 10 percent of total kcalories?

7. Estimate how many pounds of sugar (concentrated simple carbohydrate) you eat in a year (1 pound = 454 grams). How does your yearly sugar intake compare with the estimated U.S. average of about 125 pounds per person per year?
8. You may be interested in computing fiber intake as well. Use Appendix H to compute the amount of fiber you consume. Then compare your fiber intake with the recommendation of 25 grams dietary fiber per day.

Notes

1. J. Yager and R. T. Young, Non-hypoglycemia is an epidemic condition, *New England Journal of Medicine* 291 (1974): 907–908.
2. E. N. Whitney and S. R. Rolfes, *Hypoglycemia and Nonhypoglycemia* (a monograph available from Stickley Publishing Co., 210 Washington Square, Philadelphia, PA 19106).
3. M. A. Permutt, J. Delmez, and W. Stenson, Effects of carbohydrate restriction on the hypoglycemia phase of the glucose tolerance test, *Journal of Clinical and Endocrinological Metabolism* 43 (1976): 1088–1093.
4. R. W. Buss and coauthors, Mixed meal tolerance test and reactive hypoglycemia, *Hormone and Metabolic Research* 14 (1982): 281–283.
5. Xylitol as a sucrose substitute: Relation to dental caries, *Nutrition Reviews* 39 (1981): 368–371.
6. P. A. Crapo and J. M. Olefsky, Fructose: Its characteristics, physiology, and metabolism, *Nutrition Today,* July–August 1980, pp. 10–15.
7. Both fructose and sucrose are thought to have adverse effects on blood lipids in at least 20 percent of the population. Nutritionists say reevaluation of sucrose "appears to be warranted," *Food Chemical News,* 21 February 1983, pp. 1–3.
8. W. D. Holloway, C. Tasman-Jones, and S. P. Lee, Digestion of certain fractions of dietary fiber in humans, *American Journal of Clinical Nutrition* 31 (1978): 927–930.
9. For example, *Recommended Dietary Allowances,* 9th ed. (Washington, D.C.: National Academy of Sciences, 1980), p. 33.
10. *Recommended Dietary Allowances,* 1980, p. 33.
11. P. A. Crapo, The relationship between food and blood sugar, *Nutrition and the MD,* July 1984.
12. D. J. A. Jenkins and coauthors, Slow release dietary carbohydrate improves second meal tolerance, *American Journal of Clinical Nutrition* 35 (1982): 1339–1346.

HIGHLIGHT THREE

Sugar: Why So Powerful?

Scene: your place. Time of day: afternoon or evening. You are doing nothing in particular, when suddenly you feel like eating something sweet. You resist, but the feeling gnaws at you. With guilt fluttering in your conscience, you head for the cookie jar, telling yourself, "Just one. Maybe two. Not more than three. Or four." But you already have calculated about how many cookies are in the jar. . . . A few minutes later, the jar is empty, your stomach is full, and you are in a daze.

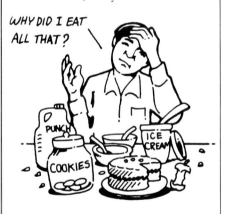

"Why did I do that?" you wonder. "What's wrong with me?"

Not all people see themselves in this description, but many more do than you might think—probably the majority of people in our society. We all have a complex and intense relationship with our food that no one completely understands. Many factors are involved, from the body's purely chemical interaction with food to the emotional involvement of the self with food and the consciousness of its social meaning. One factor is the tiny entity, the sugar molecule itself, that provides the sweet taste we all find so attractive.

The Sweet Taste

We all love sweets, from the very first time we taste them. The taste for sweetness is innate—as the photos of Figure H3–1 testify—and the reward for eating sweet foods is immediate pleasure. As a result, we quickly learn what to eat to obtain the same pleasure again. If you happen to be hungry

when you eat sweets, you experience a second reward shortly after the first—the satisfaction of your hunger. Behaviorists call these rewards *positive reinforcers:* they tend to make you repeat the behavior to obtain them again. The reward of sweetness, which comes so soon after the behavior, makes sugar an *immediate reinforcer,* and the intensity of the pleasure makes it a *supernormal reinforcer.* The later satisfaction of hunger is sugar's *postingestive effect,* another positive reinforcer. The attractiveness of sugar is therefore very great. In fact, it possesses some of the same characteristics that addictive drugs do: opiates, too, are immediate, supernormal, positive reinforcers.

Sugar has another characteristic that gives it a powerful punch: it packs much more energy into a small volume than most foods do. It might take you ten bites and fifty chews to eat a 60–kcalorie apple; but 60 kcalories of a sugar cookie might go down your gullet in only three bites and nine

FIGURE H3–1

The innate preference for sugar. This newborn baby is resting (A), and tasting distilled water (B), sugar (C), something sour (D), and something bitter (E).

(A)   (B)   (C)   (D)   (E)

Source: Taste-induced facial expressions of neonate infants from the studies of J. E. Steiner, in *Taste and Development: The Genesis of Sweet Preference,* ed. J. M. Weiffenbach, HHS publication no. NIH 77-1068 (Bethesda, Md.: U.S. Department of Health and Human Services, 1977), pp. 173–189, with permission of the author.

chews. Thus if you start eating sugary foods when you are very hungry, you can easily overeat before your stomach and sugar-laden blood have the chance to inform you that you've had enough. Of course, then you are too full for a nutritious meal. If out of guilt you postpone your next meal, you may let yourself get into the same position again—starved, and wolfing down high-kcalorie sweet foods.

The Case for Sugar as an Addictive Drug

A member of the board of Overeaters Anonymous, who calls herself a "recovered sucroholic," says she is convinced that refined sugar can be as addictive as alcohol:

> Many of us use sugar like a drug. It is our lover, friend, comforter, and when stress comes into our lives we reach for it automatically. Giving it up is terribly difficult; many people go through withdrawal and get the shakes. For some of us, complete abstinence is the only way out. We cannot be social sugar eaters just the way other people cannot be social drinkers.[1]

Another person who calls himself an "addict" is William Dufty, the author of the bestseller *Sugar Blues*.[2] Dufty describes how he kicked the sugar habit:

> I threw out everything that had sugar in it, cereals and canned fruit, soups and bread. . . . In about forty-eight hours, I was in total agony, overcome with nausea, with a crashing migraine. . . . I had it very rough for about twenty-four hours, but the morning after was a revelation. I went to sleep with exhaustion, sweating and tremors. I woke up feeling reborn.[3]

According to *Sugar Blues,* if you allow yourself to get "hooked" on sugar, your

addiction can lead to physical and mental ruin. The front cover describes sugar as "the killer in your diet," while the back cover states, "Like opium, morphine and heroin, sugar is an addictive, destructive drug."

Is sugar an addictive drug? Can it lead to total destruction? Can it kill? Some intricate reasoning from experiments with animals sheds some needed light on the question. Figure H3–2 provides the details. The outcome of the experiments was that animals can appear addicted to sugar under certain artificial circumstances; but when allowed access to normal food, they will not eat too much sugar. On a poor (low-protein) diet, however, their reliance on sugar becomes excessive. *Addiction,* then, is too strong a term to use for their relationship to sugar, but they certainly could be said to indulge in sugar *abuse*.

Can the same be said of people? Are they sugar abusers, or are they addicts? We should tell you right away that we have no final answer to this question, but can perhaps shed a little light on it. People's behavior seems more complex than animals' behavior, partly because people are conscious of what they do. They not only respond to stimuli (such as a sweet taste); they know they are responding. They think about it—and what they think may influence how they respond the next time.

You may have noticed the intensity of the feelings expressed by the two people quoted here. They shared a belief system; they *knew* they were addicted. Question: which comes first—the behavior or the belief? Some think the belief causes the behavior, and an interesting experiment provides evidence that supports the idea. The subjects were people who thought they were addicted to sugar, and who were therefore abstaining from its use. They believed that if they were to allow themselves to indulge at all, they would begin eating out of control; they would go on a binge. When made to believe they had overindulged, they did indeed proceed to overindulge some more; it was not what they actually ate, but what they believed they had eaten, that determined their subsequent behavior.[4]

This finding suggests that addiction may be a characteristic of the person, rather than of the substance. Some researchers who subscribe to this view have defined addiction, not as we have done in our Miniglossary, but largely in psychological terms. They state that loss of control is a feature of all addictive behaviors and that "low self-regard is a crucial factor." Addictive people may differ biochemically from others, but the changes are self-induced.[5]

That addictive behavior may be a characteristic of the person, rather than of the substance, is supported by abundant additional research. People who tend to overeat compulsively resemble alcohol addicts on psychological tests—even if they don't

Miniglossary

addiction: a compulsive physiological need for a habit-forming drug such as alcohol or heroin. To express the conviction that some people are addicted to carbohydrate, particularly sugar, the terms **carboholic** and **sucroholic** are in popular use.

positive reinforcer: a reward that serves to increase the probability that a behavior will be repeated. Example: the sweet taste of sugar rewards, or reinforces, the behavior of eating sweet things. Because the sweet taste is immediate and intense, sugar's sweet taste is termed an **immediate, supernormal, positive reinforcer**.

postingestive effect: an effect that occurs after eating. Sugar's postingestive effect is the raising of the blood glucose level.

FIGURE H3–2

Effects of sugar on animals: Addiction or abuse?

A. One experiment seemed to imply that rats could become addicted to sugar and could kill themselves eating it, even when good food was available to them. This kind of experiment has been widely misinterpreted to signify that if sugar is available to human beings, they will destroy themselves with it, as if it were a drug. What has been overlooked is the feeding schedule on which the rats were maintained. They were allowed access to food for only an hour a day and starved the other 23 hours. During the hour, they were given a choice between nutritious food and pure sugar (in water). They chose the pure sugar every time, and starved themselves to death. Subsequent experiments showed that it wasn't just the sweet taste, but also the postingestive effects of the sugar that reinforced the rats' choice. In other words, when they were starving, the rats consistently made the choice that most promptly gave them the feeling that their hunger was being relieved. Sugar is quickly absorbed and detected by the nervous system, so it wins the race.

B. Maintaining animals on such a schedule and allowing them to eat only when they are starving is different from allowing them free access at all times to a diet presenting a choice between sugary and more nutritious foods. With free access and free choice between sugar and other foods, rats eat enough nutritious food to stay healthy and grow, although they also eat considerable sugar. Thus, sugar alone doesn't kill rats. Rather, it is sugar administered on a weird schedule to starving rats that has this effect.

C. An unnatural schedule can even induce a rat to overuse a harmless substance like water. An underfed rat, given access to food only 3 hours a day and made to press a lever for it, will drink about half his body weight in water during that 3–hour period, even though he has plenty of water for the other 21 hours as well. The experimenter who discovered this behavior in rats named it "water abuse." On returning to a normal schedule, the rats drank water normally again.

Alcohol abuse can be made to appear in rats by a similar manipulation of feeding time (rats normally refuse to become even interested in alcohol, much less abusers of it). After consuming large amounts of alcohol under these artificial conditions for many days, the rats are "hooked" (addicted). They then react differently to alcohol. Even when returned to a normal schedule, they continue to drink alcohol as long as they have access to it.

A rat that is hooked on alcohol by the weird-schedule technique and then given the choice between alcohol and a sugar solution (still on the weird schedule) will gradually shift preference to the sugar solution. This experiment has been widely misinterpreted to mean that "sugar is even more addicting than alcohol," but sugar addiction is not what is seen here. It is sugar-preference-on-a-weird-schedule. In the words of the experimenter, "It takes unusual environmental arrangements for [water and sugar] to be abused and to become hazards to health, while ethanol and other agents with addiction liability produce their effects much more directly. . . . Further, addictive agents are viewed as instituting biochemical changes in the central nervous system which, functioning in a vicious circle, maintain a craving for the particular agent." Sugar preference in animals to the point of extreme self-harm does not persist when they are back on a normal schedule. Sweet abuse, then, is not addiction.

drink alcohol.[6] In fact, people with all sorts of addictions—to alcohol, tobacco, heroin, other drugs, and food—have much in common.[7]

Additional evidence on food addiction comes from work with antidepressant drugs. Of the 20 million or so persons in the United States who are obese, about half are compulsive eaters—and some of these people can be helped by antidepressant medication.[8] This suggests that in at least some cases, compulsive eating (a sign of addiction) may be a specific medical disorder.[9]

This being the case, can all compulsive eating—of sugar or any other food—be cured by simply prescribing antidepressant medication? It's not that simple, as Highlight 8 (on the eating disorders anorexia nervosa and bulimia) shows, and research suggests two alternative answers. Drugs help some people, as we've mentioned, but at the same time, bulimia is by definition a disease of *dieters*. It is always characterized by periods of severe food restriction—and this restriction often precedes binge episodes.[10] A very effective treatment of bulimia involves no drugs at all but diet—adequate diet. Bulimic subjects taught to eat nutrient-dense foods at regular intervals, and to eat no less than 1,400 kcalories a day, have been able to lose weight and recover from their addictive behavior without the help of drugs.[11] This suggests that sugar loses much of its attractive power when people are well nourished and not hungry.

Besides sugar's being attractive as a physical reinforcer, especially for hungry people, it offers psychological rewards as well. The next section suggests that the child who wants to rebel against authority can use sugar eating as one means of doing so.

Sugar Eating and Puritanism

The sociologist Margaret Mead first observed that the people of our culture take a puritanical attitude toward food. She wrote these three paragraphs in 1943, but what she describes is still true today:

People feel that they ought to eat correctly, or, less abstractly ("it's wrong to eat too much sweet stuff"), that, in fact, foods that are good for you are not good to eat, and foods that are good to eat are not good for you. So ingrained is this attitude that it may come as a surprise to learn that in many cultures there is no such contrast, that the foods which are thought to make people strong and well are also exclusively the foods which they like to eat, which they boast of eating, and without which they would be most unhappy. . . .

In the average home, the right food and the wrong food are both placed on the table; the child is rewarded for eating the "right" food and so taught that the right food is undesirable—for parents do not reward children for doing pleasant things. At the same time children are punished by having the "wrong" food taken away from them; here again the lesson is taught to the child that the delicious is an indulgence—for which one is punished or with which one can be rewarded. A dichotomy is set up in the child's mind between those foods which are approved and regarded by adults as undelicious and those foods which are disapproved but recognized as delightful. A permanent conflict situation is established which will pursue that child through his life— each nutritionally desirable choice is made with a sigh or rejected with a sense of guilt; each choice made in terms of sheer pleasure is either accepted with guilt or rejected with a sense of puritanical self-righteousness. Every meal becomes an experience in which an individual must decide between doing right or enjoying himself. Furthermore, as

doing right is closely associated with parental supervision, a secondary association is made linking autonomy, adulthood and masculinity with eating what one likes instead of what mother approved of.

This situation is an eternally self-defeating one, for as long as materials for making the wrong food choice are as accessible as those for making the right, many individuals will make the wrong choice, fairly often . . . we will never have a population which eats, unquestioningly, food based on the best nutritional science which we have. For each generation it has to be done all over again. The mother who has, with a great moral effort, learned to drink milk herself, does not merely place a pitcherful of milk on the table and let her children follow her example as she pours it out— although this is the simple method— but she, because of the conflict within her own personality, will argue, threaten, cajole, bribe and punish her children to make them "drink their milk."[12]

The puritanically raised child who decides to break the rules is likely to think in these terms: "This is for you, Mother [the spinach], and this is for me [ice cream]." Part of the pleasure of eating the ice cream comes from the feeling of getting away with eating a forbidden food.

Combine this reward with the others already mentioned and you have an impressive combination. First, there is the pleasure of rebelling itself; then, the immediate, intense pleasure of the sweet taste; then, especially if the person is hungry (perhaps dieting), the intense postingestive satisfaction.

All established, long-lived human societies have developed customary modes of eating that assign a limited place to sugary foods and do not allow them to push aside nutritious foods. In our culture, we refuse to let ourselves or our children eat sugary foods close to mealtimes; we save them for dessert. But our customary ways of eating family meals are breaking down, and many individuals develop their own eating patterns without models to follow. The results are often unsatisfactory, and sometimes sugary foods assume a far-too-large place in the diet. Some people turn to sugar so often, and with such damaging results, that they feel it is a truly addictive substance.

For your health's sake, then, it is important not to eat sugar's empty kcalories when your body's need is for nutritious food, but to save sugary foods for after the meal, when hunger has been satisfied, food has provided much of the desired pleasure, and a moderate dose of sugar's sweetness can just serve to top it off.

Rabbit said, "Honey or condensed milk with your bread?" [Pooh] was so excited that he said, "Both," and then, so as not to seem greedy, he added, "But don't bother about the bread, please."

A. A. Milne, *Winnie the Pooh*

NOTES
1. J. Pekkanen and M. Falco, Sweet and sour, *Atlantic Monthly*, July 1975, as quoted in *The Great American Nutrition Hassle* (Palo Alto, Calif.: Mayfield, 1978), pp. 252–259.
2. W. Dufty, *Sugar Blues* (New York: Warner Books, 1975).
3. Dufty, 1975, pp. 22–23.
4. J. Wardle and H. Beinart, Binge eating: A theoretical review, *British Journal of Clinical Psychology* 20 (1983): 97–109.
5. H. Milkman and S. Sunderwirth, The chemistry of craving, *Psychology Today*, October 1983, pp. 36–44.
6. J. B. Lauer and coauthors, Psychosocial aspects of extremely obese women joining a diet group, *International Journal of Obesity* 3 (1979): 153–167.
7. P. K. Levison, D. R. Gerstein, and D. R. Maloff, eds., *Commonalities in Substance Abuse and Habitual Behavior* (Lexington, Mass.: Lexington Books, 1983); abstract 83-1409 cited in *Alcohol Awareness Service* (National Institute on Alcohol Abuse and Alcoholism), December 1983, p. 28.
8. Bet you can't eat just one, *Science News*, 31 March 1979, p. 201.
9. E. Ely, Rx for bulimia, *Harvard Magazine*, November–December 1983, pp. 53–64.
10. Wardle and Beinart, 1983.
11. S. Dalvit-McPhillips, A dietary approach to bulimia treatment, *Physiology and Behavior* 33 (1984): 769–775.
12. M. Mead, Dietary patterns and food habits, *Journal of the American Dietetic Association* 19 (1943): 1–5.

The Lipids: Fats, Oils, Phospholipids, and Sterols

4

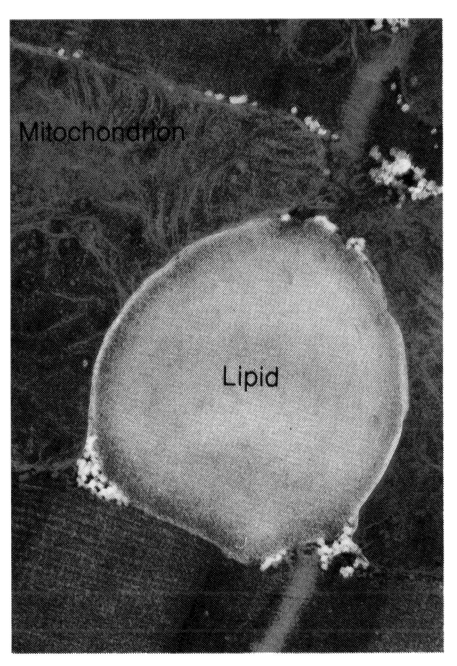

Mitochondrion

Lipid

Muscle cells derive their energy from both fat and carbohydrate. Here, a lipid droplet nestles close to a muscle fiber (bottom), while a mitochondrion snuggles up to the droplet and gathers energy from it.

Much of the cell's metabolic activity takes place inside the mitochondria. Millions of enzymes are mounted on their internal membranes, in the order in which the enzymes perform their reactions.

Most people think that the less fat you have on your body, and the less you eat, the better. This is not true. Like all the nutrients, fat is beneficial in appropriate quantities—and it is harmful to ingest either too much or too little of it. It is true, though, that in our society of abundance, we are more likely to encounter too much fat than too little.

When we speak of fat, we are actually speaking of a subset of the class of compounds known as lipids. The lipids include triglycerides (fats and oils), phospholipids, and sterols. Triglycerides predominate in quantity, both in foods and in the body, but the other compounds are also important to nutrition.

The Lipids:
triglycerides (fats and oils)
phospholipids (example: lecithin)
sterols (example: cholesterol)

Lipids in the Body and in Foods

Lipids in the body provide many services you would be hard put to do without. They are part of every cell, conferring on cell membranes an ability to convey fat-soluble substances, including vitamins and hormones, in and out of cells. Special cells also contain large stores of triglycerides, specifically to meet the body's moment to moment needs for energy; it is these cells that people refer to when they speak of their body fat. A layer of this fat tissue beneath the skin, being a poor conductor of heat, insulates the body from extremes of temperature. A pad of hard fat beneath each kidney protects it from being jarred and damaged, even during a motorcycle ride on a bumpy road. The soft fat in the breasts of a woman protects her mammary glands from heat and cold and cushions them against shock. The fat that lies embedded in the muscle tissue shares with muscle glycogen the task of providing energy when the muscles are active.

An uninterrupted flow of energy is so vital to life that in a pinch, any other function is sacrificed to maintain it. To go totally without an energy supply, even for a few minutes, would be to die. The urgency of the need for energy has ensured, over the course of evolution, that all creatures have built-in reserves to protect themselves from ever being deprived of it. Chapter 3 described one provision against this sort of emergency—the stores of glycogen in the liver that can return glucose to the blood whenever the supply runs short.

However, the liver cells can store only a limited amount of energy as glycogen; once this is depleted, the body must receive new food or start degrading body protein to continue making glucose. Unlike the liver, the body's fat mass has a virtually unlimited storage capacity, and fat supplies two-thirds of the body's ongoing energy need. During a prolonged period of food deprivation, fat stores may make an even greater contribution to energy needs.

A person who fasts (drinking only water to flush out metabolic wastes) will rapidly oxidize body fat. A pound of body fat provides 3,500 kcalories;* so you might think a fasting person who expended 2,000 kcalories a day could

Fat cells are often called **adipose** (ADD-ih-poce) **cells**.

Body fat provides much of the energy these muscles use.

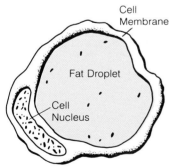

Within the fat cell, lipid is stored in a globule. This globule can enlarge indefinitely, and the fat cell membrane will grow to accommodate its swollen contents.

1 lb body fat = 3,500 kcal.

---

*The reader who knows that 1 pound = 454 grams, and that 1 gram fat = 9 kcalories, may wonder why a pound of body fat doesn't equal 9 x 454 kcalories. The reason is that body fat contains some cell water and other materials; it's not quite pure fat.

lose close to half a pound of body fat each day. Actually, the person has to obtain some energy from lean tissue, because of the brain's need for glucose, which fat can't supply; so he can't lose fat this rapidly, even if he eats nothing. Still, in conditions of enforced starvation—say, during a siege or a famine—the fatter person survives longer because of this energy reserve.

If you happen to be acquainted with a polar bear, you may be aware that the same thing is true for him. As he lumbers about on his iceberg, great masses of fat ripple beneath his thick fur coat. During the long winter hours when he sleeps, he oxidizes that fat, extracting tens of thousands of kcalories from it to maintain his body temperature and to fuel other metabolic processes. Come spring, he is a hundred or more pounds thinner than when he went to sleep.

Polar bears, like people, oxidize their body fat while they're not eating.

Although fat provides energy in a fast, it cannot provide it in the form of glucose, the substance needed for energy by the brain and nerves. After a long period of glucose deprivation, brain and nerve cells develop the ability to derive about half of their energy from a special form of fat known as ketones, but they still require glucose as well. With the available glycogen long gone, they demand this glucose from the only alternative source—protein. And since no protein is coming in from food, the only supply is in the muscles and other lean tissues of the body. These tissues give up their protein and atrophy, bringing on weakness, loss of function, and ultimately—when half the body protein has been used up—death. Death from loss of lean body tissue will occur even in a fat person who fasts too long.

ketones (KEE-tones): a condensation product of fat metabolism produced when carbohydrate is not available (see Chapter 7).

lean tissues: tissues of the body that are not predominantly fat. Muscle, blood, and organs such as the liver, brain, and intestines are examples of lean tissues.

atrophy (ATT-ro-fee): to waste away.
a = without
trophy = growth

For more about the dangers of fasting, see Chapter 7.

To sum up the roles of body fat, it helps maintain the structure and health of all cells, protects body organs from temperature extremes and mechanical shock, and provides a continuous fuel supply, helping to keep the body's lean tissue from being depleted. It is oxidized for energy by many body tissues, and when it is being used in the absence of glucose, it forms ketones that can meet about half of the energy needs of the brain and nervous system. Protein released from wasting muscle and other lean tissue provides the other half.

Not only is fat important in the body; it is also important in foods. Many of the compounds that give foods their flavor and aroma are found in fats and oils; they are fat soluble. Four vitamins—A, D, E, and K—are also soluble in fat. Whenever a fatty liquid and a watery liquid separate, the fat-soluble compounds go along with the fat, and the water-soluble compounds with the water. When the fat is removed from a food, therefore, many of the fat-soluble compounds are also removed. Significant among these are flavors and vitamins.

Fat solubility. Oil and water separate; fat-soluble compounds stay dissolved in the oil and water-soluble compounds, in the water.

Fat also lends palatability to foods, by carrying both flavor and aroma. It is the fat that makes the delicious aromas associated with bacon, ham, hamburger, and other meats, as well as onions being fried, french fries, and stir-fried Chinese vegetables. The attractiveness of fat is responsible for the popularity of fast foods, which, critics say, are too palatable for our own good. Fat also adds satiety to foods—another reason why fast foods are so popular.

Fat also carries the fat-soluble vitamins. Milk, when skimmed, loses all its vitamins A and D. To provide nonfat milk with the desired amounts of these nutrients, vitamins A and D are added to it; hence the "vitamin A and D fortified" label you see on nonfat milk. (Vitamin D is also added to whole milk, because its natural vitamin D level is low.)

An additional feature is lost when fat is removed: kcalories. A medium pork chop with the fat trimmed to within a half inch of the lean contains 275 kcalories; with the fat trimmed off completely, it contains 165 kcalories. A small baked

palatability: pleasing taste. The *palate* (PAL-ut) is the roof of the mouth, against which the tongue presses foods when tasting them.

satiety (sat-EYE-uh-tee): the feeling of satisfaction and fullness that food brings.
sate = to fill

Pork chop with a half inch of fat (275 kcal).

Potato with 1 tbsp butter and 1 tbsp sour cream (260 kcal).

Whole milk, 1 c (150 kcal).

Pork chop with fat trimmed off (165 kcal).

Plain potato (130 kcal).

Nonfat milk, 1 c (90 kcal).

Remember, fat is a more concentrated energy source than the other energy nutrients: 1 g carbohydrate or protein = 4 kcal, but 1 g fat = 9 kcal.

potato with butter and sour cream (1 tablespoon each) has 260 kcalories; plain, it has 130.* So it goes. The single most effective step you can take to reduce the energy value of a food is to eat it without the fat.

The Chemist's View of Fats

"Your blood lipid profile looks fine." If a doctor says this, the patient may be reassured. Most of us are aware nowadays that there is a close relationship between the fats in the blood and the health of the heart. A closer look at the fats will lay the foundation for an understanding of this relationship.

When we speak of fats, we are usually speaking of triglycerides. The triglycerides predominate in the diet, and the following section focuses on them.

The lipids in foods are 95% fats and oils (that is, triglycerides) and 5% other lipids (phospholipids and sterols).

```
        H
        |
   H-C—O-H
        |
   H-C—O-H
        |
   H-C—O-H
        |
        H
     Glycerol
```

glycerol (GLISS-er-ol): an organic alcohol composed of a three-carbon chain with an alcohol group attached to each carbon. An alcohol group is a reactive -OH group.
ol = alcohol

The Triglycerides

To understand the fats and the beneficial and harmful effects they have on your body, you must understand their molecular structure. Triglycerides come in many sizes and several varieties, but they all share a common structure; all have a "backbone" of glycerol to which three fatty acids are attached. All glycerol molecules are alike, but the fatty acids may vary in two ways: length of the carbon chain and degree of saturation.

*These figures were taken from items 622, 623, 159, 80, and 899 in Appendix H.

A fatty acid is an organic acid consisting of a chain of six or more carbon atoms with hydrogens attached and with an acid group (COOH) at one end. The organic acid shown in Figure 4–1 is acetic acid, the compound that gives vinegar its sour taste. This is the simplest such acid; the "chain" is only two carbon atoms long. A longer acid chain may have four, six, eight, or more carbon atoms (naturally occurring fatty acids mostly come in even numbers). Common in dairy products are fatty acids that are six to ten carbons long. Butyric acid, found in butter, is a four-carbon fatty acid. Fatty acids that predominate in meats and fish are 14 or more carbon atoms long.

To illustrate the characteristics of these fatty acids, let us look at the 18–carbon ones (two special ones among them deserve attention anyway). Stearic acid is the simplest of the 18–carbon fatty acids (see Figure 4–2):

FIGURE 4–2

Stearic acid (an 18–carbon fatty acid).

A. The structure with all details.

B. A simpler way to depict the same structure. Each "corner" on the zigzag line represents a carbon atom with two attached hydrogens.

C. Still more simply, the lines representing bonds to the hydrogens can be left out. If you count the "corners," you will see that this still represents an 18–carbon fatty acid. This is the way fatty acids will be represented in many of the following diagrams.

When three stearic acids attach to a glycerol molecule, the resulting structure is a triglyceride (see Figure 4–3).

The triglyceride shown in Figure 4–3 is a saturated fat, because the fatty acids are saturated fatty acids. They are loaded, or saturated, with all the hydrogen (H) atoms they can carry. If some Hs were to be removed, the result would be an unsaturated, or even a polyunsaturated, fat. The distinction between these kinds of fats is of interest because of their health implications. Everyone should probably control their total fat intake, but people threatened with heart trouble may be told to reduce their intake of saturated fats in particular, while people whose families show a susceptibility to cancer may be told to avoid polyunsaturated fats as well (see Highlight 4A).

FIGURE 4–1

Acetic acid (a two-carbon organic acid).

acid: a compound that tends to ionize in water solution, releasing H^+ ions. The more H^+ ions that are free in the water, the stronger the acid (see Appendix B).

acid group: the COOH group of an organic acid, which can also be represented this way:

fatty acid: an organic compound made up of a carbon chain with hydrogens attached and an acid group at one end.

triglyceride (try-GLISS-er-ride): a compound composed of carbon, hydrogen, and oxygen arranged as a molecule of glycerol with three fatty acids attached to it. Triglycerides are also called **triacylglycerols** (try-ay-seel-GLISS-er-ols).
tri = three
glyceride = a compound of glycerol
acyl = a carbon chain

saturated fatty acid: a fatty acid carrying the maximum possible number of hydrogen atoms—for example, stearic acid. A **saturated fat** is composed of triglycerides in which all or virtually all of the fatty acids are saturated.

fat: a mixture of triglycerides.

FIGURE 4–3

Formation of a fat (triglyceride): three fatty acids attached to glycerol.

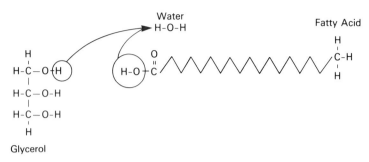

A. The first fatty acid approaches the glycerol, a condensation reaction occurs (water is eliminated), and a bond is formed between an O on the glycerol and the C at the acid end of the fatty acid.

B. Two more fatty acids can be attached to the glycerol by the same means, resulting in a triglyceride. This is tristearin (all three fatty acids are stearic acid). Most triglycerides are mixed.

Most vegetable oils are rich in polyunsaturated fats, triglycerides in which the fatty acids are carrying less than their full load of hydrogens. Consider stearic acid once more: if we remove two hydrogens from the middle of the carbon chain, we are left with a compound like that in Figure 4–4:

FIGURE 4–4

A fatty acid lacking two hydrogens—an impossible structure, since two of the carbons have only three bonds each.

Such a compound cannot exist in nature. But an extra bond can be formed between the two carbons to satisfy nature's requirement that every carbon must have four bonds connecting it to other atoms. There is then a "double bond" between them (see Figure 4–5). (The same situation exists in the acid group at the end of the chain, where an O is double-bonded to the terminal C. That carbon has its full four bonds, and the oxygen meets its requirement of having two.) The resulting structure is an unsaturated (in this case, *mono*unsaturated) fatty acid, oleic acid, which is found abundantly in the triglycerides of olive oil. The heart patient may be encouraged to use olive oil in place of butter because of its unsaturated character.

monounsaturated fatty acid: a fatty acid that lacks two hydrogen atoms and has one double bond between carbons—for example, oleic acid.

Simplified diagram (the actual shape is bent at the double bond):

Note: Rotation can occur around single bonds. These molecules, although we draw them straight, are constantly twisting and bending. At any given moment, they may be coiled, horseshoe-shaped, or straight.

FIGURE 4–5

Oleic acid (an 18–carbon fatty acid). Because it has one point of unsaturation, oleic acid is monounsaturated.

The heart patient is also advised to eat *poly*unsaturated fats in place of saturated fats; they, too, seem to reduce the risk of heart and artery disease. A polyunsaturated fat contains triglycerides in which the fatty acids have two or more points of unsaturation. An example is linoleic acid, which lacks four hydrogens and has two double bonds, as shown in Figure 4–6. Linoleic acid is found in the triglycerides of most vegetable oils—corn oil, safflower oil, soybean oil, and the like. It is the most common of the polyunsaturated fatty acids (PUFAs) in foods, and one of the most important. In fact, it is one of the special fatty acids we promised you earlier; it has a section of its own later in this chapter.

To increase your intake of polyunsaturated fats and reduce your intake of saturated fats is to increase your **P:S ratio**. For how to calculate the P:S ratio, see Appendix D.

polyunsaturated fatty acid (PUFA): a fatty acid that lacks four or more hydrogen atoms and has two or more double bonds between carbons—for example, linoleic acid (two double bonds) and linolenic acid (three double bonds). Thus a **polyunsaturated fat** is composed of triglycerides containing a high percentage of PUFAs.

FIGURE 4–6

Linoleic acid (an 18–carbon fatty acid). Its two points of unsaturation make it polyunsaturated. Linoleic acid is one of the essential fatty acids.

Simplified diagram (the actual shape is bent at the double bond):

Having looked at three of the most common fatty acids in foods, you can probably anticipate what the others look like. The fourth member of the family of 18–carbon fatty acids is linolenic acid, which has three double bonds. A similar series of 20–carbon fatty acids exists, as well as a series of 22–carbon fatty acids. These are the long-chain fatty acids. In smaller amounts, medium-chain (10 to 14 C) and short-chain (6 to 8 C) fatty acids are also present in foods.

To sum up what has been said to this point, the fats and oils are mostly (95 percent) triglycerides: glycerol backbones with fatty acids attached. Those that are fully loaded with hydrogens are the saturated fats; those that have double bonds are unsaturated and polyunsaturated fats. To complete the picture, it only remains to say that a fat or oil may contain any combination of fatty acids. A mixed triglyceride, one that contains more than one type of fatty acid, is shown in Figure 4–7. The vast majority of triglycerides are mixed.

Note: Linoleic acid (18 C, two double bonds) should not be confused with linolenic acid (18 C, three double bonds). The shorthand way of describing these two fatty acids is 18:2 and 18:3. For the fatty acid series, names, and structures, see Appendix C.

FIGURE 4–7

A mixed triglyceride typical of those found in foods. The fat in a food is a mixture of many different mixed triglycerides. (The shape of the fatty acids is shown straight for ease of viewing.)

The **essential fatty acids** are linoleic, linolenic, and arachidonic acids. See Appendix C for their structures.

Reddening and irritation of the skin are symptoms known as **dermatitis** (derm-a-TIGHT-us).
derma = skin
itis = infection or inflammation

arachidonic (a-RACK-ih-DON-ic) **acid**: a 20–carbon polyunsaturated fatty acid. Arachidonic acid is an **omega-6** fatty acid, meaning that its first double bond is six carbons away from its methyl end. (The methyl end is the other end from the acid end; a methyl group is CH_3.)

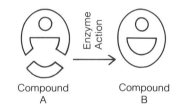

Compound A is the **precursor** of compound B. Linoleic acid is the precursor of arachidonic acid.

Acetic acid, or acetyl CoA, is formed from glucose or other compounds see Chapter 7.

Foods containing linoleic acid: meats, fish, poultry, vegetables, and vegetable oils.

EFA: the essential fatty acids. Don't confuse these with EPA, to be mentioned later.

The Essential Fatty Acids

Linoleic acid is an essential nutrient (see p. 2 for a definition of *essential nutrient*). When linoleic acid is missing from the diet, the skin reddens and becomes irritated, infections and dehydration become likely, and the liver develops abnormalities. In infants, growth failure also occurs. Adding linoleic acid back to the diet clears up these symptoms. It turns out that what the body cells need is arachidonic acid (20 C, four double bonds), and that the body can make this compound if linoleic acid is supplied in the diet. Linolenic acid cannot be synthesized from linoleic acid, and so is also essential.

The body's cells are equipped with many enzymes that can convert one compound to another. To make body fat or oil— triglycerides—all the enzymes need is a usable food source containing the atoms that triglycerides are composed of: carbon, hydrogen, and oxygen. Glucose does perfectly well. In fact, given an excess of blood glucose (and a filled glycogen storage space), this is precisely what some enzymes use. They cleave the glucose to make the 2–carbon compound acetic acid, and then combine many acetic acid molecules, with the appropriate alterations, to make long-chain fatty acids. (This is why most fatty acid carbon chains come in even numbers.) But the cells do not possess an enzyme that can arrange the double-bonding of linoleic acid, so linoleic acid must be supplied in the foods we eat. It almost inevitably is present in any diet that contains fat and/or vegetable oils, because all meats, fish, poultry, and vegetables contain it (see Table 4–2, later in this chapter). For those who wish to compare their estimated intakes with a standard, the recommendation of 3 percent of kcalories from linoleic acid has been made. A 2,000–kcalorie diet would thus contribute 60 kcalories from this fatty acid, or (at 9 kcalories per gram) about 6 1/2 grams.*

Linoleic acid, arachidonic acid, and linolenic acid together are known as "the essential fatty acids," sometimes abbreviated EFA. Nearly all diets supply enough EFA to meet the requirement. Deficiencies are usually seen only in infants fed a formula that lacks EFA and in hospital patients who have been fed

---

*Any diet that provides 25 to 50 percent of its energy in the form of fat is likely to contribute 5 to 10 percent of its energy as linoleic acid—much more than the recommended 3 percent, and sufficient linolenic acid as well. The U.S. food supply probably offers about 23 grams a day of linoleic acid to each person, on the average. Food and Nutrition Board, Committee on Recommended Allowances, *Recommended Dietary Allowances*, 9th ed. (Washington, D.C.: National Academy of Sciences, 1980), pp. 34–35.

The relief of a skin rash by linoleic acid might suggest to the unwary observer that all skin rashes indicate a deficiency of this nutrient. Not so! More than a hundred body compounds besides linoleic acid are needed to ensure the health of the skin, including other oils, vitamins, minerals, and hormones. A deficiency of any of these or an imbalance among them can cause a rash. The lack of some compound might be at fault, but the compound might also be present in excess, or might be mishandled by the skin cells. Bacterial and viral infections, allergies, physical agents such as radiation, and chemical irritants also cause rashes. There can even be a psychosomatic cause, as when excessive nervous activity in the brain generates a hormone imbalance that affects the skin. For these reasons, when you notice a symptom such as a rash, you can only know that a problem exists; you have no clue as to the cause.

In dealing with nutrition, it is important to remember the distinction being made here—the distinction between a symptom and a disease. A symptom can be alleviated (soothing oils can be applied to irritated skin to make it feel better, for example), but until you have diagnosed the disease, you cannot achieve a cure. The rule for nutritional deficiency symptoms is that if a certain nutrient clears up the symptom, then a deficiency of that nutrient *may* have been the cause. (To be certain, you would have to remove the nutrient and see the symptom reappear, then reintroduce the nutrient and see the symptom disappear; and you would have to do the experiment "blind." See Highlight 9B).

The field of nutrition is littered with misunderstandings about the interpretations of symptoms. People may think that if you are going bald, you need pantothenic acid; that if you have wrinkles, you need vitamin C; that if your hair is turning gray, you need zinc; and (yes) that if you have a skin rash, you need linoleic acid. None of these statements is true; in fact, they are all preposterous. When someone tries to persuade you of any such relationships between symptoms and nutrients, beware. Chances are, the person either doesn't see the distinction himself, or is intentionally trying to deceive you. What you need is not a nutrient, but a correct diagnosis.

The same fallacious reasoning sometimes links *foods* with symptoms. Some people think that for prevention of colds, you need to eat oranges; for health of the digestive tract, yogurt; for protection against heart attacks, fish; for sexual potency, oysters; for weight loss, grapefruits; for physical strength, beefsteak; for good eyesight, carrots; to keep the doctor away, apples; and (yes) for health of the skin, safflower oil. Actually, of course, these foods are not essential at all, although the *nutrients* in them may be, and the foods may be good sources of those nutrients. In any case, to avoid a deficiency of EFA, all you need is to eat an ordinary mixed diet; it will inevitably include some oils containing polyunsaturated fat.

The distinction between foods and nutrients has been emphasized once before (p. 48). The implication that any specific food has magical, miraculous, or curative powers is false.

When you notice a symptom, you can't be sure of the cause. Many different conditions can cause the same symptom.

psychosomatic: a term applied to any condition of the body that originates in the mind.
psyche = mind, soul
soma = body

For the effects of fish oils on the heart, see Highlight 4B.

For the polyunsaturated fat content of vegetable oils and other foods, see Appendix H.

through a vein for prolonged periods a formula that provides no EFA. Even in an otherwise totally fat-free diet, only two teaspoons of corn oil (which is 50 percent EFA) would be sufficient to supply the needed amount of EFA for an adult.

The Prostaglandins

Linoleic acid and its relatives are the precursors of prostaglandins—hormonelike compounds—in many body organs, and the prostaglandins have a multitude of diverse effects. Only recently discovered, many do not have names like other hormones (insulin and epinephrine, for example), but are designated by letters and numbers: E_1, E_2, and so forth. One prostaglandin dilates and/or constricts blood vessels. Another alters transmission of nerve impulses. Still another modulates the body tissues' responses to other hormones. Others act on the kidney, affecting its water excretion. Another, in breast milk, helps to protect the infant's digestive tract against injury. About 100 different prostaglandins are known to be produced in the body.

One prostaglandin that does have a name is of special interest in relation to nutrition and heart disease. It is thromboxane; it is made from the 20–carbon polyunsaturated fatty acid arachidonic acid; and it promotes blood clotting. Clotting is necessary to prevent excessive blood loss from wounds, of course, but it is also to blame for heart attacks and strokes. Within the intact circulatory system, even when there are no wounds, blood clots constantly form and dissolve. If the balance between these two processes favors clotting, then the clots may grow too large, lodge in arteries, and cut off vital circulation. Whatever reduces thromboxane production reduces the rate of clot formation—with the disadvantage that a person may bleed more easily when wounded, but with the offsetting advantage that the risk of heart attack and stroke will be reduced.

The connection of all this to nutrition is through fish. In recent years, many observations have led to the conclusion that the oils from fish—fatty fish in particular—contain fatty acids that displace thromboxane production. People who eat large amounts of fish have lower blood cholesterol and triglyceride levels, reduced thromboxane and clot-forming rates, and, thereby, a reduced risk of heart attacks.

Processed Fat

Ever since researchers first began to realize that saturated fats were linked to heart disease and that polyunsaturated fats might not be, advertisers have been proclaiming their oils and margarines as "high in polyunsaturates." Indeed, margarines made from vegetable oils, and plant foods such as peanut butter, do contain unsaturated fatty acids, and this is why they spread and melt more easily than foods that contain saturated fats.

Unfortunately, however, although you may gain something in health from polyunsaturated fats, you lose something in keeping quality. The more double bonds there are in a fatty acid, the more easily oxygen can destroy it. When oxygen attacks the double bond, a chain reaction occurs, yielding a variety of products that smell bad; the product has spoiled. (Other types of spoilage, due to microbial growth, can occur, too.) In general, unsaturated fatty acids are less stable than their saturated counterparts.

prostaglandins: hormonelike compounds produced in the body from the essential fatty acids; so named because the first one to be discovered was found in association with the prostate gland.

A 20–carbon fatty acid similar to linolenic acid, from which some of the prostaglandins are made. Notice the similarity of this structure to linolenic acid.

Prostaglandin E_1

Prostaglandin F_{13}

Two of the prostaglandins.

thromboxane (throm-BOX-ane): a prostaglandin that promotes blood clotting; made from arachidonic acid.

One fatty acid especially important in this regard is **eicosapentenoic** (EYE-coss-a-PEN-te-NO-ic) **acid** (**EPA** for short). EPA is an **omega-3** fatty acid; its first double bond is three carbons away from its methyl end.

Marketers of fat-containing products have three alternative ways of dealing with the problem of spoilage—none perfect. They may keep their products tightly sealed away from oxygen and under refrigeration—an expensive storage system. The consumer then has to do the same, and most people prefer not to buy products that spoil readily. Marketers may also protect their products by adding preservatives such as antioxidants, but additives are unpopular with some consumers. Finally, manufacturers may increase the products' stability by processing the fat (hardening or hydrogenating it). Figure 4–8 shows hydrogens being added at a double bond to hydrogenate fat.

Hydrogenation makes fat more solid, which is often desirable. Margarine made from vegetable oils is solid at room temperature because the oils have been partially hydrogenated, and this makes it easy to work with. Hydrogenation, however, diminishes the margarine's polyunsaturated fat content and possibly, therefore, its health value. Moreover, new evidence suggests that there may be other concerns about hydrogenated oils.

If a vegetable oil is fully hydrogenated—that is, if hydrogen is added at all its double bonds—it becomes indistinguishable from a saturated fat of the same length. If, however, the oil is partially hydrogenated, then a change takes place at some of the double bonds where hydrogen was *not* added. For one thing, some of the double bonds migrate along the molecule to positions not normally found in nature, and often they wind up near the acid group and change its reactivity. For another thing, their configuration changes from *cis* to *trans* (see Figure 4–9). One effect of this change is to create a more solid product, but double bonds are still left in the fatty acids, so the manufacturer can still say the product is unsaturated or polyunsaturated. But *trans*-fatty acids are not made by the body's cells, and they are rare in foods. It is not clear that our bodies are equipped to deal with large quantities of *trans*-fatty acids; the presence of these unusual molecules in our cells and tissues may create problems. As yet, this issue is poorly understood.

Some researchers believe that the presence of *trans*-fatty acids in processed fat may make consumers of that fat prone to develop certain kinds of cancer. However, so many dietary factors are implicated in cancer causation that it is hard to sort them all out or to decide which are significant and which are not. Undoubtedly, your total fat consumption has much more bearing on your susceptibility to cancer than does your consumption of *trans*-fatty acids. Highlight 4A puts together the many factors that relate diet to cancer.

For some questions and answers about additives, and for some special notes on BHA and BHT, see Chapter 13.

hydrogenation (high-dro-gen-AY-shun): a chemical process by which hydrogens are added to unsaturated or polyunsaturated fats to reduce the number of double bonds, making them more saturated (solid) and more resistant to oxidation.

cis (sis): same side.

trans: opposite sides.

FIGURE 4–8

Hydrogenation. Hydrogen is added at the double bond, yielding a saturated fatty acid.

Monounsaturated Fatty Acid

Hydrogenation

(Metal Catalyst Required)

Saturated Fatty Acid

FIGURE 4–9

Formation of a *trans*-fatty acid. The starting material was the same as in Figure 4–8, but this fatty acid, instead of adding hydrogens, was converted from the *cis* to *trans* form. Almost all unsaturated fatty acids occur in nature in the *cis* form; that is, the carbon chains adjacent to the double bond stick out on the same side of the molecule. During partial hydrogenation, the double bonds that do not add hydrogens are broken and re-formed into the more stable *trans* position, which has the carbon chains across from each other, where they are less crowded.

This kind of change in shape occurs at double bonds which, like a pair of sticks between two Tinker Toy wheels, can't rotate. (A single bond, like a single stick between the two wheels, allows rotation of the wheels.)

Cis-fatty acids are generally liquids, whereas *trans*-fatty acids, like saturated fatty acids, are generally solids. There are concerns that *trans*-fatty acids incorporated into cell membranes in place of *cis*-fatty acids may change the properties of the membranes.

A. A *cis*-fatty acid. The carbon chains are on the same side of the double bond.

B. A *trans*-fatty acid. The carbon chains are on opposite sides of the double bond.

One way to determine the degree of unsaturation of a fat is to perform a chemical test using iodine to obtain the "iodine number." The higher the iodine number, the greater the degree of unsaturation. Common oils, with their iodine numbers, are:
- Safflower oil, about 140.
- Most other vegetable oils, about 110 to 120.
- Soft margarines, about 90.
- Olive oil, about 75.
- Hard margarines, about 70.
- Butter, about 25 to 40.
- Coconut and palm "oil," about 10 to 15.

While the evidence on processed fats is still being collected, consumers can, if they wish, apply the principle of dilution already referred to in Chapter 2. Rather than margarine, for example, you can mix warm butter with vegetable oil in equal amounts, producing a spread that is cheaper than butter, spreads well, has the same degree of polyunsaturation as margarine but more linoleic acid, and contains fewer *trans*-fatty acids. As for peanut butter, it is possible to find unhydrogenated varieties on the shelf. The peanut mash and the oil may separate in these products, but you can stir them back together before using them or pour off the oil for a product lower in kcalories.

Ultimately, if fat processors wish to produce margarines free of *trans*-fatty acids, they can use an alternative process that hydrogenates double bonds without producing the *cis-trans* shift. This process is a little more expensive and technically more difficult than the one presently in use, so it has not yet been employed on a wide scale.

Fat Digestion

Water-fearing substances are known to chemists as **hydrophobic** or **lipophilic**.
hydro = water
phobia = fear
lipo = lipid
phile = friend

The body has a problem in digesting and using fats—how to get at them. Substances that are soluble in fat are called water fearing, and among these substances are, of course, the fats themselves. Fats are neutral; they carry no net charge. In any compartment of the digestive tract they tend to work their way upwards, separating themselves as far as possible from the watery digestive juices. Water molecules, although they too have no net charge, are polar; that is, they have a positive side and a negative side. Enzymes have positively and negatively charged groups on their surfaces, and so they mix comfortably with the ions in water—they are water loving. What the body needs to help mix fats and water together is a substance that is friendly with both water-fearing and water-loving substances. The bile acids and phospholipids meet that need.

Water-loving substances are **hydrophilic**.

FIGURE 4-10

Emulsification of fat by bile. Detergents work the same way (they are also emulsifiers), which is why they are so effective in removing grease spots from clothes. Molecule by molecule, the grease is dissolved out of the spot and suspended in the water, where it can be rinsed away. You can guess where the manufacturers of "detergents with enzymes" got their idea.

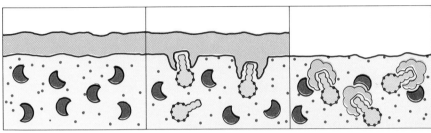

A. Fats and water separate; enzymes are in water and can't get at the fat.

B. Bile (emulsifier) has affinity for fats and for water, so it can bring them together.

C. Emulsified fat. The enzymes now have access to the fat, which is mixed in the water solution.

Water

Fat

Enzyme

Emulsifier

Manufactured from cholesterol by the liver and stored in the gallbladder until needed, the bile acids are released into the intestine whenever fat arrives there. Each molecule of bile acid has at one end an ionized group that is attracted to water and at the other end a fatty acid chain that has an affinity for fat. Molecules of bile acid surround fat droplets and draw parts of them into the surrounding solution, where they can meet enzymes. The process is known as emulsification (see Figure 4-10).

Now, after all of this preparation, the enzymes can get at the triglycerides. The enzymes digest each triglyceride by removing one, then the other, of its outer fatty acids, leaving a monoglyceride. (Rarely, they remove all three of them, leaving a molecule of glycerol.) As with the carbohydrates, the digestive process requires a molecule of water, as shown in Figure 4-11. Finally, the

bile: a compound made from cholesterol, composed of a lipophilic portion and a hydrophilic portion. Bile is not an enzyme, but an emulsifier; it comes in both salt and acid form and is referred to as "bile salts" or "bile acids." For our purposes, no distinction need be made between these.

emulsify (ee-MULL-sih-fye): to disperse and stabilize fat droplets in a watery solution. Bile is one emulsifier; lecithin and other phospholipids are others (see later).

Bile is manufactured by the liver, stored in the gallbladder, and released into the small intestine when fat is present there.

FIGURE 4-11

Digestion (hydrolysis) of a fat (triglyceride).

Bonds Break

Triglyceride

Monoglyceride + 2 Fatty Acids

A. The triglyceride and two molecules of water are split, and the pieces combine to give two fatty acids and a monoglyceride.

B. These products may pass into the intestinal cells, but sometimes the monoglyceride is split with another molecule of water to give a third fatty acid and glycerol. Absorbed into intestinal cells: fatty acids, monoglycerides, and glycerol.

These complexes are the **micelles** (MY-cells). Each contains about 20 fatty acids and/or monoglycerides. They are so small that they can fit between the tiny, hairlike microvilli of a single intestinal cell (emulsified fat particles are 100 times larger in diameter and contain tens of thousands of molecules).

monoglycerides and fatty acids form tiny spherical complexes with the bile acids and pass into the cells of the intestinal wall.

The products of lipid digestion are then rearranged and released inside the intestinal cell for transport through the body. Some of the larger ones are packaged in phospholipids and protein for this purpose. The protein-wrapped packages, called lipoproteins, are the subject of intensive research as laboratory sleuths seek to detect their structure and their relationships to heart and artery disease. The lipoproteins appear again later in this chapter.

The Phospholipids: Lecithin

The preceding pages have been devoted to one of the three classes of lipids, the triglycerides. The other two classes, the phospholipids and sterols, make up only 5 percent of the lipids in the diet, but they are nonetheless interesting and important. Among the phospholipids, the best known is lecithin (actually, there are several lecithins).

phospholipid: a compound similar to a triglyceride, but having choline or another phosphorus-containing acid in place of one of the fatty acids.

Choline: see also Chapter 9.

Like the triglycerides, the lecithins and some other phospholipids have a backbone of glycerol; they are different from the triglycerides because they have only two fatty acids attached to them. In place of the third fatty acid is a phosphate group to which is attached a molecule of choline or a similar compound containing nitrogen (N) atoms. A diagram of a lecithin molecule is shown below; other lecithin molecules differ in the nature of the attached fatty acids.

One of the lecithins. Others have other fatty acids at the upper two positions. (The plus charge on the N is balanced by a negative ion—usually chloride.)

From 2 Fatty Acids / From Choline / From Phosphate / From Glycerol

lecithin (LESS-uh-thin): one of the phospholipids; a compound of glycerol to which are attached two fatty acids, a phosphate group, and a choline molecule.

Lecithins and other phospholipids are important constituents of cell membranes. They also act as emulsifying agents, helping to keep other fats in solution in the blood and body fluids. The structure of lecithin reveals how the phospholipids can do this; the choline part of the molecule is water soluble, while the fatty acid part is fat soluble.

Food chemists take advantage of lecithin's properties and use it as an emulsifier in foods. When you read on a food label that lecithin is present, as on a chocolate bar, that's probably why it's there.

Lecithin periodically receives noisy attention in the popular press, being credited with great good deeds. You may hear that it is a major constituent of cell membranes (true), that the functioning of all cells depends on the integrity of their membranes (true), and that you must therefore purchase bottles of lecithin and give yourself daily doses (false). You might as well believe that in order to grow healthy hair or to maintain the brain you must eat hair or brains! The enzyme lecithinase in the intestine takes most of the lecithin apart before it passes into the body fluids anyway, so not much of the lecithin you eat reaches the body tissues intact. The lecithin you need for building cell membranes and for other functions is made from scratch by the liver. In other words, the lecithins are not needed in the diet; they are not essential nutrients. Furthermore, although once thought to be harmless, large doses of lecithin have now been seen to cause gastrointestinal upsets, sweating, salivation, and loss of appetite.[1] Perhaps these symptoms are beneficial, because they serve to warn people to stop self-dosing with lecithin.

Many body compounds carry on remarkable, important functions that are exciting to read about, especially when they first make the headlines. Often hucksters immediately seize on these new discoveries by bottling preparations of these compounds and selling them, on the reasoning that "This does wonderful things for you; you must not allow yourself to become deficient in it." That might be so, but then, no one seems to become deficient in lecithin. The body makes it for itself—and the same can be said for hundreds of other miraculous compounds. Before buying bottles of lecithin or any other wonder substance, ask yourself, "Do I really need this? What is the evidence that my body is likely to be deficient?"

It is wise not to self-prescribe doses of this compound.

The Sterols: Cholesterol

sterol: a compound composed of C, H, and O atoms arranged in rings like those of cholesterol, with any of a variety of side chains attached.

A student observing the chemical structure of cholesterol for the first time once remarked, "Would you believe pentamethyl hydroxy chicken wire?" He was not far wrong; chemists do create horrendous names. According to them, cholesterol is a member of the cyclopentanoperhydrophenanthrene family, whose particular designation is 3-hydroxy-5,6-cholestene. Never mind. It is not necessary to memorize a structure as complex as this one. But once having viewed it, you can say, "I have seen the structure of cholesterol."

Cholesterol is not at all an unusual type of molecule. There are dozens of similar ones in the body; all are interesting and important. Among them are the bile acids, the sex hormones (such as testosterone), the adrenal hormones (such as cortisone), and vitamin D.

Cholesterol

cholesterol: one of the sterols.

All the carbons in cholesterol come from acetyl CoA (see Chapter 7), which in turn can be derived from many other body compounds, glucose and fatty acids among them.

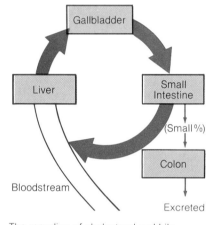

The recycling of cholesterol and bile through the intestine and liver is known as the **enterohepatic circulation** of bile.
enteron = intestine
hepat = liver

Like the lecithins, cholesterol is needed metabolically, but is not an essential nutrient. Your liver is manufacturing it now, as you read, at the rate of perhaps 5 times 10^{16} (50,000,000,000,000,000) molecules per second. The raw materials that the liver uses to make cholesterol can all be taken from glucose, amino acids, or fatty acids. (Another way of saying the same thing is that cholesterol can be made from carbohydrate, protein, or fat.)

After manufacture, cholesterol either leaves the liver or is transformed into related compounds like the hormones just mentioned. The cholesterol that leaves the liver has four possible destinations:

1. It may be made into bile and move through the gallbladder into the intestine, then be recycled back to the liver.
2. It may be made into bile, move into the intestine, and then be excreted in the feces.
3. It may be incorporated into the body's cell membranes.
4. It may wind up accumulating in arteries and causing artery disease.

The first possibility is that some of the cholesterol the liver makes becomes part of the bile salts, and these are released into the intestine to emulsify fat. After doing their job, most are reabsorbed from the intestine. The cholesterol is thus recycled.

The second possibility is that, once out in the intestine, some of the bile salts can be trapped by certain kinds of dietary fibers (notably pectin and gums), which carry them out of the body with the feces. The excretion of bile salts reduces the total amount of cholesterol remaining in the body.

The third possibility is that cholesterol leaves the liver by way of the bloodstream, packaged with other lipids for transport to the body tissues. These packages are the lipoproteins. The blood carries them through all the arteries, and any tissue can extract lipids from them; some cells take them up whole. More than nine-tenths of all the body's cholesterol is located in the cells, where it forms part of the multitude of external and internal membranes that make up the cells' structure and perform their work.[2]

The fourth possibility is that, on its way into the cells from the bloodstream, cholesterol will be deposited in the artery walls. It is deposits of cholesterol in arteries that create disease conditions leading to heart attacks and strokes. To understand how cholesterol is connected with heart disease, it is necessary to learn about the lipoproteins.

People have for some years been buying purified fiber to sprinkle onto their foods, in the hope of improving their health. But the purified fiber they buy most often is wheat bran, the type with the least cholesterol-lowering effect. Fibers better at lowering blood cholesterol include pectin and gums—found in greater abundance in fruits, vegetables, and legumes, rather than grains.

The lesson seems to be that foods, not purified nutrients or other food components, are likely to offer the greatest benefits to those who seek good health—and not so much any particular foods as a variety of foods. You may recall that other nutrition knowledge points in the same direction.

Transport of Lipids: Lipoproteins

Within the circulatory system, lipids always travel from place to place wrapped in hydrophilic coats, as lipoproteins. Lipoproteins are very much in the news these days. In fact, when doctors measure a person's blood lipid profile, they are interested not only in the types of lipid they find, such as triglycerides and cholesterol, but also in the types of proteins in their coats. Newly absorbed lipids leaving the intestinal cells are mostly packaged in large lipoproteins known as chylomicrons. Lipids that have been made or processed in the liver are released in the form of lipoproteins known as very-low-density lipoproteins (VLDL). After VLDL have deposited their triglyceride loads and undergone other changes, they become low-density-lipoproteins (LDL). The liver and intestine also make small lipoproteins known as high-density lipoproteins (HDL). HDL function in the metabolism of the other lipoproteins and in so-called "reverse transport" of cholesterol from cells back to liver.

In the scientist's laboratory, the lipoproteins are distinguished by their size and density. (The scientist layers the blood below a thick fluid in a test tube and spins the tube in a centrifuge so that the most buoyant particles, chylomicrons, will rise to the top.) But the distinction of greatest interest for the rest of us, because it has implications for the health of the heart and blood vessels, is the distinction between the HDL and the LDL. High LDL concentrations are associated with a high risk of heart attack; and high HDL, with a low risk.

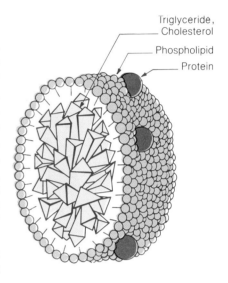

A lipoprotein.

Source: Adapted from D. Kritchevsky, An update on lipids, lipoproteins and fat metabolism, in *The Medicine Called Nutrition*, Medical Education (Meded) Programs, Ltd. (Englewood Cliffs, N.J.: Best Foods, 1979), p. 61.

Chylomicrons: From the Intestinal Cells

To help you picture the four types of lipoproteins, Figure 4–12 depicts their relative size and composition. The lipids you eat are in the form of water-insoluble triglycerides, cholesterol, and phospholipids, with the triglycerides predominating (making up about 95 percent of dietary lipid). They may be partly disassembled during digestion, but once inside an intestinal cell, these lipids are mostly reassembled. The cell then allows them to form a cluster, and a number of protein molecules then dot the surface of this aggregate, or chylomicron. In this ingenious configuration, the fat can be released from the intestinal cell and can travel through the circulatory system.

Chylomicrons are large, buoyant particles that float to the top of a sample of blood in a test tube. This floating layer of fat does not appear if blood is drawn 14 hours after a meal, for after this period of time or less, the body's cells have picked up the triglycerides, and the liver cells have disposed of the remnants.

Cells all over the body remove fat from the chylomicrons as they pass by, so the chylomicrons get smaller and smaller until, at the end of 14 hours or less, there is little left of them but protein remnants, with a few odds and ends of fat. The liver cells are programmed to recognize and remove these remnants from the blood; they have special protein receptors on their membranes for the purpose. Once they have gathered in the chylomicron remnants, they dismantle them.

chylomicron (kye-lo-MY-cron): the lipoprotein formed in the intestinal wall cells following digestion and absorption of fat. Released from these cells, chylomicrons transport ingested fats to all cells of the body, which remove the ones they need, leaving chylomicron remnants to be picked up by the liver cells. The liver cells dismantle the chylomicron remnants and construct other lipoproteins for further transport.

FIGURE 4–12

The lipoproteins. A chylomicron. The density of these particles is very, very low because they contain so little protein and so much triglyceride. You can see how the laboratory report that a person has "high blood triglycerides" might easily reflect a high concentration of chylomicrons in the blood.

HDL. These particles are denser than the others because they contain such a high percentage of protein.

VLDL and LDL. Compare these particles with the chylomicrons and HDL. Note that "high blood cholesterol" might easily reflect a high LDL concentration.

Meanwhile, the liver cells are busy making other kinds of lipids (as well as other compounds) to be shipped out to the body's cells for storage or use. These lipids they package in the VLDL.

VLDL and LDL: From the Liver

The liver cells have the task of metabolizing many compounds for the body's use. They pick up fatty acids arriving in the blood and use them to make cholesterol, other fatty acids, and other compounds. (At the same time, if they have quantities of carbohydrates, proteins, or alcohol to deal with, the liver cells may be making lipids from some of these.) Ultimately, some of the trigylcerides

VLDL: very-low-density lipoprotein. This type of lipoprotein is made by liver cells (and, to some extent, by intestinal cells). Previously called pre-beta- (pre-BAY-tuh) lipoprotein.

the liver cells manufacture will need to be used or stored in other parts of the body. To send them there, the liver packages them with proteins, cholesterol, and phospholipids, and ships them out as VLDL.

The VLDL made by the liver carry all three classes of lipids—triglycerides, phospholipids, and cholesterol. The LDL contain few triglycerides but are about half cholesterol. These particles circulate throughout the body, making their contents available to all the cells—muscle, including the heart muscle; adipose tissue; the mammary glands; and others. The body cells can select lipids from these particles to build new membranes, to make hormones or other compounds, or to store for later use. Both VLDL and LDL are much smaller than the chylomicrons, but the VLDL are still large enough to give the blood a milky appearance if there are enough of them.

Storage and Release of Body Fat

The presence of lipids in the bloodstream provides an opportunity for the body's adipose cells to take up and store some fat. They have a special enzyme on their surfaces—lipoprotein lipase—that can seize triglycerides from passing lipoproteins, hydrolyze them, and pass their parts (glycerol and fatty acids) into the cells' interiors. Inside, the cells have other enzymes that reassemble the parts into triglycerides again, so that they can't escape. Fat storage always takes place after meals when fatty acids and lipoproteins, with their cargo of triglycerides and cholesterol, are abundant.

The opposite process, fat breakdown and release, takes place whenever the body is in a fasting state. An enzyme (hormone-sensitive lipase) inside the adipose cells awaits the signal to break down triglycerides, and does so whenever fuel is needed by the body's other cells. The adipose cells release the breakdown products, glycerol and fatty acids, directly into the blood, so that they become available for uptake by any cells that need them.

HDL: From the Body Cells

When triglycerides are being released from fat cells, cholesterol and phospholipids may also be returned to the blood. The packages in which unused cholesterol is found are the HDL. It is believed that one of their functions is to return cholesterol to the liver for recycling or disposal.

Atherosclerosis and the Lipoproteins

Atherosclerosis is one of two major disease conditions leading to the heart attacks and strokes that kill the majority of adults in our country today. (The other is high blood pressure, discussed in Chapter 11.) One of the major contributors to atherosclerosis is high LDL cholesterol; LDL are the most atherogenic lipoproteins. As Highlight 4B makes clear, prudence dictates that those of us who are susceptible to heart and artery disease should take all possible means of lowering LDL cholesterol.

The HDL also carry cholesterol, but usually, raised HDL concentrations relative to LDL represent more active cholesterol, a lower risk of developing atherosclerosis, and a lower risk of heart attack. It is clearly not useful simply

LDL: low-density lipoprotein. This type of lipoprotein is derived from VLDL as cells remove triglycerides from them. Previously named beta- (BAY-tuh) lipoprotein.

lipoprotein lipase: an enzyme mounted on the surface of fat cells (and other cells) that hydrolyzes triglycerides passing by in the bloodstream, and directs their parts into the cells where they can be reassembled for storage.

hormone-sensitive lipase: an enzyme inside adipose cells that responds to the body's need for fuel by hydrolyzing triglycerides so that their parts (glycerol and fatty acids) will escape into the general circulation and thus become available to all other cells as fuel.

The signal to which this enzyme responds is the hormone glucagon, which opposes insulin (see Chapter 3).

HDL: high-density lipoprotein. These lipoproteins seem to transport cholesterol back to the liver from peripheral cells. An alternative name is alpha-lipoprotein.

High blood cholesterol:
For people in their 20s: 220 mg/100 ml.
For people in their 30s: 240 mg/100 ml.
For people over 40: 260 mg/100 ml.
Optimal blood cholesterol level for people of all ages: 180 mg/100 ml or less.

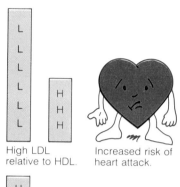

High LDL
relative to HDL.

Increased risk of
heart attack.

High HDL
relative to LDL.

Decreased risk of
heart attack.

How to control blood cholesterol level:
• Control your weight.
• Eat less saturated fat.
• Eat more water-soluble fiber.
• Exercise intensely and frequently.
See Highlight 4B.

Some foods to enjoy on a prudent diet.

to measure the total amount of cholesterol in the blood; it is necessary to know whether the cholesterol is being carried in LDL or HDL.

Some people have abnormal lipid profiles (high in chylomicrons, VLDL, or LDL) for genetic reasons, but some may have them due to such poor health habits as overeating, overconsumption of fat, or underactivity. To normalize their blood lipid profiles, these people may need to take such measures as eating less fat, increasing consumption of water-soluble fiber, losing weight, and increasing their activity levels. Activities particularly effective in raising HDL concentrations are frequent, intensive, and sustained physical activities—and these may help to reverse degenerative disease processes such as atherosclerosis, also.

An approach to preventive diet is to adopt the diet (formerly called the Prudent Diet) developed by the American Heart Association (see Table 4–1). This diet achieves a total fat intake of 30 percent of kcalories, with 10 percent coming from each type of fat (saturated, monounsaturated, and polyunsaturated), as well as a cholesterol intake below 300 milligrams per day. The menus of Figure 4–14 fit this description (see p. 110).

A dietary approach to the prevention and therapy of cardiovascular disease that people often ask about is the Pritikin Diet. Its creator, the late Dr. Nathan Pritikin, designed two diets, one for the prevention of atherosclerosis, and the other, a stricter one, for its reversal. His strict diet allows only 10 percent of kcalories from fat, for example, versus the American Heart Association's 30 percent and the 50 percent many people actually consume. Foods high in fats and sugars, as well as caffeine and alcohol, are forbidden. Dr. Pritikin also recommended vigorous daily activity, pushing the heart rate to 70 or 80 percent of its capacity for half an hour or more twice a day. Some former heart patients swear by his regimen, but authorities are cautious. The diet may be extreme. It may not be necessary to restrict fat so severely, or even at all, to obtain the benefits. But the kinds of dietary changes Pritikin recommended are in the right direction and are more likely to help than to hurt the person wishing to avoid heart trouble. Certainly the exercise is beneficial.

The Fats in Foods

Overconsumption of fat is thought to contribute to people's susceptibility to cancer; fat and cholesterol may both contribute to heart and artery disease. It makes sense to limit your intake of fat, and possibly of cholesterol, too. It is on this reasoning that many current guidelines are based. The *Dietary Guidelines for Americans*, for example, suggest that you avoid excess fat, saturated fat, and cholesterol.

This advice may be sound, but it isn't being followed, according to research on people's food habits. Food disappearance studies and diet surveys have both produced the same finding: people today are eating about 40 to 50 percent of their kcalories as fat—more than at the turn of the century, and certainly more than they need. Those who wish to reduce and alter their dietary fat intakes need to know where the fats are found in foods. Let's consider, first, the total fat in foods; then the poly-mono-saturated nature of that fat; and, finally, the accompanying cholesterol.

The exchange system presented in Chapter 2 provides a useful means of learning how much fat is present in foods. Three of the six lists in the exchange system—the milk list, the meat list, and the fat list—include foods containing appreciable amounts of fat:

- Items on the milk list contain protein, carbohydrate, and fat.
- Items on the meat list contain protein and fat (legumes contain carbohydrate as well).
- Items on the fat list contain fat only.

Figure 4–13 shows the lists that contain fat, with their portion sizes. Figure 4–14 shows how the exchange system can be used to estimate the amount of fat in a meal or in a day's meals.

The listing of milk's three fat levels emphasizes the importance of being aware of the fat content of milk. Users of the exchange system learn to think of nonfat milk as milk, and of low-fat and whole milk as milk with added fat.

A person studying the meat list for the first time may be surprised to note how many fat kcalories are in meats and some of their relatives. An ounce of lean meat supplies about half of its energy from fat: (28 protein kcalories and 27 fat kcalories). An ounce of high-fat meat supplies 72 percent of its energy from fat (28 protein kcalories and 72 fat kcalories). Two tablespoons of peanut butter supply 72 percent of their energy from fat (56 protein kcalories and 144 fat kcalories)! Thus many meats, which are often thought of as protein foods, actually contain more fat energy than protein energy, and excess consumption of meat often accounts for the excess weight meat eaters tend to gain.

TABLE 4–1

The American Heart Association Diet (formerly the Prudent Diet)

To control the amount and kind of fat you eat:
- Limit your intake of meat, seafood and poultry to no more than 5 to 7 ounces per day.
- Use chicken or turkey (without skin) or fish in most of your main meals
- Choose lean cuts of meat, trim all the fat you can see, and throw away the fat that cooks out of the meat.
- Substitute meatless or "low-meat" main dishes for regular entrees.
- Use no more than a total of 5 to 8 teaspoons of fats and oils per day for cooking, baking, and salads.
- Use low-fat dairy products.

To control your intake of cholesterol-rich foods:
- Use no more than two egg yolks a week, including those used in cooking.
- Limit your use of shrimp, lobster, sardines, and organ meats.

Source: The American Heart Association Diet, *An Eating Plan for Healthy Americans*, a booklet available (1985) from The American Heart Association National Center, 7320 Greenville Avenue, Dallas, TX 75231. Used with permission.

FIGURE 4–13

Foods containing fat.

8 g in 1 c whole milk.
3 g in 1 oz lean meat.
5 g in 1 pat butter or margarine.

Milk list
1 c nonfat milk contains	trace of fat
1 c 2% milk contains	5
1 c whole milk contains	8

Meat list
1 oz lean meat contains	3 g fat
1 oz medium-fat meat contains	5
1 oz high-fat meat contains	8
1 tbsp peanut butter contains	8

Fat list
1 tsp butter or margarine (or any other serving of food on the fat list) contributes	5 g fat

FIGURE 4–14

How to estimate fat intake. The values presented in Figure 4–13 provide a way to estimate the amount of fat eaten at a meal or in a day. Two reminders are needed. First, fat is often hidden in cooked vegetables; as a rule of thumb, vegetables served with butter or margarine can be assumed to contain one teaspoon (one exchange) of fat per half-cup serving. Second, meats and milks come in low-, medium-, and high-fat categories; be sure not to forget to count the fat in meats and milks.

Using the values of Figure 4–13, let's estimate the amounts of fat in the meals shown here. (These are the same meals used as examples in Chapters 2 and 3.) The cereal and fruit can be assumed to contain no fat; so the only foods to inspect are the meats, grains/starchy vegetables, vegetables, and milks.

The small amounts of fat in the "actual" column come from natural oils in the foods listed. As you can see, they don't affect the totals enough to be worth much attention. On the other hand, the amounts of fat in meats (even low-fat meats, as in this example) and cheeses, and the fat the person adds at mealtime (for example, the 2 pats of butter used at dinner), make a considerable difference. These meals are very low in fat and fit the American Heart Association's Prudent Diet guidelines. The exchange system overestimates actual fat in these meals by 2 percent.

		Fat Grams	
		Estimated	Actual
Breakfast			
1 c oatmeal = 2 grain portions	=	trace	2
¼ c raisins = 2 fruit portions	=	0	0
½ c nonfat milk = ½ milk portion	=	trace	0
½ grapefruit = 1 fruit portion	=	0	0
		trace	2
Lunch			
1 c cooked rice = 2 grain portions	=	trace	1
2 c mixed vegetables might be estimated to have 2 tsp fat in them, but this particular person added seasonings only (no fat)	=	0	1
2 oz cheddar cheese = 2 high-fat meat portions	=	16	19
⅔ c fresh strawberries = about 1 fruit portion	=	0	0
1 c nonfat milk = 1 milk portion	=	trace	0
2 pats butter = 2 fat portions	=	10	8
2 packets sugar	=	0	0
		26	29
Dinner			
3 oz broiled fish = 3 lean meat portions	=	9	6
½ c green beans = 1 vegetable portion	=	0	0
½ c cooked carrots = 1 vegetable portion	=	0	0
½ c cooked peas = 1 starchy vegetable	=	0	0
2 pats butter = 2 fat portions	=	10	8
1 c nonfat milk = 1 milk portion	=	trace	0
		19	14
Snack			
¼ cantaloupe = 1 fruit portion	=	0	0
1 brownie = 1 grain portion + 1 fat portion	=	5	4
		5	4
Day's Total =		50	49

Note that the unit by which meat is measured in this system is a single ounce. To use the system, you need to be aware of the number of ounces in typical servings. An egg, in this system, is equivalent to 1 ounce of meat. A hamburger is usually 3 or 4 ounces. A dinner steak may be 6 or 8 ounces or even larger.

As for the members of the fat list, everyone knows that butter, margarine, and oil belong there, but it can be a surprise to discover that bacon, olives, avocados, and many kinds of nuts are also on the list. These foods are listed together because the amount of fat they contain makes them essentially equivalent to pure fat. An eighth of an avocado, a slice of bacon, or a little handful of peanuts can contain as much fat as a pat of butter, and like butter, offers negligible protein and carbohydrate. Hence, when you eat them, you are not eating protein-rich foods; you are eating fat-rich foods.

Some foods not on the exchange lists are also significant contributors of fat to the diet. It can be surprising to see how much of the energy in foods comes from fat—even when you can't see it—that is, from *invisible* fat. For example, 82 percent of an avocado's kcalories is from fat. Anything fried contains abundant fat: potato chips, french fries, fried wonton, fried fish, and many other of people's favorite foods. Many baked goods, too, are high in fat: pie crusts, pastries, biscuits, cornbread, doughnuts, Danish sweet rolls, cookies, and cakes. Chocolate bars contain even more fat kcalories than sugar kcalories. Even cream of mushroom soup when prepared with water, has 66 percent of its kcalories from fat. Surprisingly, abundant fat lurks even on salad bars; you can construct a plate bearing 50 percent of its kcalories from fat without even trying. Not only the salad dressings, but also the mixed salads, are largely fat or oil—the potato salad, the macaroni salad, the coleslaw, and the marinated beans. This is not to condemn the salad bar, but to remind the consumer to choose its items with an awareness of their fat contents. Go ahead and choose the ones you like, but count them as fat.

Fatty Acids and Cholesterol in Foods

In studying the fatty acid contents of foods, a person needs to look mostly at the foods that present the most fat altogether. These foods will have the greatest impact on the fatty acid balance of the diet. The fatty acid contents of typical high-fat foods are shown in Table 4–2. The table is arranged so that you can easily pick out the foods that are highest in polyunsaturates. It shows that the same foods are highest in the essential fatty acid, linoleic acid, and from what is known about food composition, it is likely that these foods will be highest in linolenic acid, too. The fat and fatty acid contents of many other foods are shown in Appendix H.

The length of the carbon chain and the degree of saturation of a fat determine how hard it is at a given temperature. A clue to whether a fat is more or less saturated than another is its hardness at room temperature. Chicken fat, for example, is softer than pork fat, which is softer than beef tallow. Of the three, beef tallow is the most saturated and chicken fat, the least saturated. Polyunsaturated fats melt more readily. Generally speaking, vegetable and fish oils are rich in polyunsaturates, whereas the harder fats—animal fats—are more saturated. Coconut and palm oils are liquids, but it's their short carbon chains, not unsaturation, that makes them liquid. These fats are saturated even though they are of vegetable origin.

Lean meat: chicken without skin, canned tuna.
Medium-fat meat: ground beef, pork loin, liver, eggs.
High-fat meat: commercial hamburger (25–30% fat by weight), country-style ham, cheddar cheese.
See exchange lists, Appendix G.

1 g protein = 4 kcal.
1 g fat = 9 kcal.
1 oz = about 30 g.

Remember that an ounce of meat is not an ounce of protein. An ounce (30 g) of lean meat contains 7 g protein and 3 g fat. The other 20 g are largely water with associated vitamins and minerals.

Nuts are so high in fat that they are listed with butter and bacon in the exchange lists.

The fat on your plate includes *visible fats* and oils, such as butter, the oil in salad dressing, and the fat you trim from meat. It also includes *invisible fat*—it is present, but not very apparent to people, such as the fat that "marbles" a steak, or that is hidden in foods like nuts, cheese, biscuits, avocadoes, olives, fried foods, and chocolate.

Saturated fats have a high melting point and are solid at room or body temperature.

Polyunsaturated fats have a low melting point and are liquid at room or body temperature.

The most polyunsaturated fat melts soonest.

TABLE 4–2

Fatty Acid Contents of Common Fat-containing Foods. Within each group, foods highest in polyunsaturated fats are listed first. As you can see, the linoleic acid content closely parallels the polyunsaturated fat content. Fish oils are not shown because insufficient data were available for this comparison.

Food	Total Fat[a]	Fatty Acids			
		Saturated	Monounsaturated	Polyunsaturated	Linoleic
Animal fats:					
Chicken	100	32	45	18	17
Pork (lard)	100	40	44	12	10
Beef (tallow)	100	48	42	4	4
Avocado	15	2	9	2	2
Butter	81	50	23	3	2
Egg yolk	33	10	13	4	4
Margarine, first ingredient:					
Safflower (liquid)—tub	80	13	16	48	48
Corn oil (liquid)—tub	80	14	30	32	37
Corn oil (liquid)—stick	80	15	36	24	23
Soybean oil (hydrogenated)—stick	81	15	46	14	10
Nuts:					
Walnuts, English	63	7	10	42	35
Walnuts, black	60	5	11	41	37
Brazil nuts	68	17	22	25	25
Pecans	71	6	43	18	17
Peanut butter	52	10	24	15	15
Peanuts	48	9	24	13	13
Salad and cooking oils:					
Safflower	100	9	12	74	73
Sunflower	100	10	21	64	64
Wheat germ	100	17	16	61	61
Corn	100	13	25	58	57
Soybean, unhydrogenated	100	14	24	57	50
Cottonseed	100	26	19	51	50
Sesame	100	15	40	40	40
Soybean, hydrogenated[b]	100	15	43	37	22
Peanut	100	17	47	31	30
Palm	100	48	38	9	9
Olive	100	14	72	9	8
Coconut	100	86	6	2	2
Shortening made from vegetable fat	100	25	44	26	23

[a]The saturated, monounsaturated, and polyunsaturated fatty acids don't add up to 100% of the fat, because there are other, minor fat compounds present.

[b]Common salad and cooking oil for commercial and household use.

Source: Adapted from U.S. Department of Agriculture, Agricultural Research Service, *Fat in Food and Diet,* Agriculture Information Bulletin no. 361 (Washington, D.C.: Government Printing Office, 1977); and H. B. Brown, *Current Focus on Fat in the Diet,* a White Paper (Chicago: American Dietetic Association, 1977).

Cholesterol is found only in animal foods, and these generally are also our major sources of saturated fats. Some animal foods without much total fat can also contain appreciable cholesterol. Thus eggs, milk, and some fish as well as meats appear in Table 4–3, which lists the cholesterol content of selected foods. Many more foods, with their cholesterol contents, appear in Appendix H.

If you wish to make choices consistent with the *Dietary Goals* or *Dietary Guidelines*, you should learn how to read food labels. But don't let words like *vegetable fat* and *unsaturated fat* mislead you. Not all vegetable oils are polyunsaturated. Coconut "oil" and palm "oil," for example, are often used in nondairy creamers, crackers, and frozen desserts, and these oils are really predominantly saturated fats. Other vegetable oils, if they are hydrogenated, have lost their polyunsaturated character. Thus to call a lipid product "vegetable" or "oil" is not the same as to say that it is polyunsaturated.

Since 1978, the FDA has required that the actual sources of fat in foods be listed on labels. There's a loophole, though: the manufacturer may list them as "may be this or this or this," so sometimes you still can't tell what fat is in the food.

Here's the truth. Notice, too, that sugar (disguised as corn syrup solids) is the first and most abundant ingredient.

The fat in milk is mostly saturated fat; the cholesterol content is 33 milligrams per cup of whole milk or 4 milligrams per cup of nonfat milk. Milk is not a high-cholesterol food, certainly, but choosing nonfat in place of whole milk reduces your intakes of both saturated fat and cholesterol.

The fats in meats and eggs are mostly saturated; those in poultry and fish have a better balance between saturated and polyunsaturated fats. As for cholesterol, the foods that contain the highest amounts are organ meats such as liver and kidneys, and eggs. Lower but still detectable levels of cholesterol are contained in beef, ham, lamb, veal, and pork, followed by poultry and fish. Shellfish have been thought to contain high concentrations of cholesterol, but the findings on which this idea was based have been called into question. They contain sterols, but possibly not the kind that have metabolically negative effects, and they may contain much less cholesterol than has been thought in the past.

As a general rule, a meat eater wishing to reduce both saturated fat and cholesterol intake could accomplish these objectives by eating less meat and eggs and more poultry, fish, legumes, and nuts. A vegetarian who uses milk, eggs, and cheese could shift to nonfat milk and low-fat cheese, and could limit butter and egg intake. Pure vegetarians eat a diet very low in fat and consume no cholesterol, because plant foods do not contain it.

Eggs contain about 270 milligrams of cholesterol each, all of it in the yolk. For a person trying to adhere strictly to a low-cholesterol diet, the use of eggs, or at least egg yolks, has to be curtailed. For most people trying to lower blood cholesterol, however, it is not as effective to limit cholesterol intake as to limit saturated fat intake; eggs may still be a valuable part of the diet, because they are inexpensive, useful in cooking, and a source of high-quality protein. An American Heart Association guideline limits eggs to four a week—allowing little room for baked and mixed foods made with eggs, unless eggs as such are omitted altogether.

Each culture has its own favorite food sources of fats and oils. In Canada, rapeseed oil is widely used. Peoples of the Mediterranean (Greeks, Italians, and Spaniards) rely heavily on olive oil, and Asians use the polyunsaturated oil of soybeans. Jewish cookery traditionally employs chicken fat, whereas U.S. south-

Fats in common use. The vegetable oil is polyunsaturated, the olive oil is monounsaturated, the butter is largely saturated, and the margarine, no doubt, is partially hydrogenated.

TABLE 4–3

Cholesterol Content of Common Foods

	Cholesterol (mg)
Fruits/vegetables	0
Grains	0
Milks (1-c serving)	
Whole milk	33
Yogurt (whole milk)	29
Low-fat milk	18
Low-fat yogurt	14
Buttermilk	9
Nonfat milk	4
Cheeses (1-oz serving)	
Cheddar	30
Processed American	27
Swiss	26
Ice creams and puddings (½-c serving)	
Ice cream	30
Pudding	15
Butter (1 tsp)	12
Margarine, all vegetable (1 tsp)	0
Creams (1 tbsp)	
Whipped	20
Sour	8
Half and half	6
Meats (3-oz serving)	
Veal	86
Lamb	83
Beef	80
Pork	76
Chicken	39 to 63
Organ meats (3-oz serving)	
Brains	2,268
Kidneys	425
Liver	372
Eggs (1 large egg)	
Yolk	274
White	0
Fish (3-oz serving)	
Shrimp	128
Lobster	72
Clams	50
Oysters	38
Fish fillet	34 to 75

Source: Adapted from *Cholesterol Information Sheet* (Rosemont, Ill.: National Dairy Council, 1984), and from the previous edition of this textbook.

erners rely heavily on pork fat (lard and bacon).* Elsewhere in the United States, butter and margarine are widely used, and with the recent popularity of fast foods, hydrogenated vegetable oil use has also been increasing.

Artificial Fat: Sucrose Polyester

An artificial fat is beginning to attract public attention even though it is not yet on the market. Invented in the late 1960s, sucrose polyester (SPE) is a synthetic combination of sucrose and fatty acids that looks, feels, and tastes like food fat. Unlike either sucrose or fatty acids alone, however, SPE is indigestible; the body has no way to take it apart. It can therefore be substituted for fats in meals without adding kcalories or promoting a rise in consumers' blood fat levels.

Tests with animals and human beings so far indicate that SPE is safe. Most human subjects are unable to tell the difference between SPE margarine and regular margarine, or between SPE oil and regular oil. Obese subjects find it as satisfying as regular fat in meals and appear not to increase their food energy intakes to compensate for the kcalories they lose by not having regular fat.[3]

Undesirable side effects of SPE use have yet to be discovered. It might, for example, carry fat-soluble vitamins out of the body with it, causing deficiencies. Further tests will tell. But given that high blood cholesterol and obesity are two of our major health problems, SPE is being viewed with hope as a possible help in the treatment of both.

Study Questions

1. What services do the fats in the body provide? What features do they bring to food?
2. Describe the structure of a triglyceride. What are the differences between saturated, unsaturated, monounsaturated, and polyunsaturated fats?
3. What are the special problems of fat digestion and how are they solved?
4. How do phospholipids differ from triglycerides in structure? What roles do phospholipids play in the body and in food?
5. What are the possible roles and destinations of cholesterol in the body?
6. What is the basic structure and purpose of a lipoprotein? What are the differences between the chylomicrons, VLDL, LDL, and HDL?
7. What are the dietary goals regarding fat and cholesterol intake? Which food lists of the exchange system supply fat in abundance? in moderation? not at all?

Notes

1. J. L. Wood and R. G. Allison, Effects of consumption of choline and lecithin on neurological and cardiovascular systems, *Federation Proceedings* 41 (1982): 3015–3021.
2. M. S. Brown and J. S. Goldstein, Lowering plasma cholesterol by raising LDL receptors (editorial), *New England Journal of Medicine* 305 (1981): 515–517.
3. R. Carol, Sucrose polyester: A synthetic fat substitute? *ACSH News and Views*, March-April 1983, p. 10.

*The saturated fat consumption of blacks is cause for concern among health authorities, who note a high incidence of heart disease—both atherosclerosis and high blood pressure—among these people. This high rate of heart disease may be diet related, genetically caused, or both. High blood pressure is related to salt (sodium) intake in some people; thus the *Dietary Goals* and the *Dietary Guidelines* recommend limiting salt intake, a matter taken up in Chapter 11.

These exercises make use of the information you recorded on Forms 1 to 3.

1. How many grams of fat do you consume in a day?

2. How many kcalories does this represent? (Remember, 1 gram of fat contributes 9 kcalories.)

3. What percentage of your total energy is contributed by fat? (To figure this, divide fat kcalories by total kcalories, then multiply by 100.)

4. A dietary guideline says fat should contribute not more than 30 percent of total kcalories. How does your fat intake compare with this

Examine Your Fat Intake

recommendation? If it is higher, look over your food records: what specific foods could you cut down on or eliminate and what foods could you add to your diet to bring your total fat intake into line?

5. How much linoleic acid do you consume? Remembering that linoleic acid is a lipid (energy value, 9 kcalories per gram), calculate the number of kcalories it gives you. What percentage of your total kcalories comes from linoleic acid? The guideline recommends 1 to 3 percent.

6. How much cholesterol do you consume daily? How does your cholesterol intake compare with the suggested limit of 300 milligrams a day? If your intake is high, you might want to read Highlight 4B before arriving at any conclusions regarding the importance of this limit.

HIGHLIGHT FOUR A

Nutrition and Cancer

One out of every four people now alive will eventually contract cancer. Dietary fat is thought to be important in relation to cancer, and this highlight explains why. But diet relates to cancer in several ways, and it is important to get them all in perspective.[1] Current research has been revealing that the ways people eat may make them more or less susceptible to certain kinds of cancer. Constituents in foods may be cancer causing, cancer promoting, or protective against cancer. Also, for the person who has cancer, diet can make a crucial difference to recovery.

Diet and nutrition are not the only factors important in cancer causation, prevention, or recovery. Some cancers are programmed to appear by genes. Other environmental factors are also involved—smoking, for example, and water and air pollution.[2] But many connections exist between nutrition and cancer: what are they, how do we know about them, and how can we apply knowledge of them in our lives?

The steps in cancer development are thought to be:
1. Exposure to a carcinogen.
2. Entry of the carcinogen into a cell.
3. Initiation, probably by the carcinogen's altering the cellular deoxyribonucleic acid (DNA) somehow.
4. Promotion and tumor formation, probably involving several more steps before the cell begins to multiply out of control.

Most people think that the first three steps are the ones that have the nutrition implications. That is, they think that they must learn to avoid eating foods that contain carcinogens.

In particular, many people have learned to fear food additives, believing that they are responsible for diet-related cancer.

Interestingly, however, food additives probably have little to do with the causation of cancer. The law is uncompromising in forbidding the addition to food of any substances that have ever been shown to cause cancer in any animal (see Highlight 13's discussion of the Delaney Clause). Contaminants of food—things that get into foods by accident—may be powerful carcinogens, but the additives permitted in foods are not.

However, foods themselves do contain substances that may have a major influence on whether or not people get cancer. These fall into two categories: promoters, and nutrients that help defeat cancers after initiation.

Several kinds of research have led to what we now know about diet and cancer. The study of whole populations in different areas of the world—epidemiology—provides one source of information on diet and cancer. Another approach is to conduct case-control studies—studies of people who have cancer and of other people as closely matched as possible in age, occupation, and other key variables—to see what differences in their lifestyles may account for the differing cancer incidences. Still another approach is to test possible causes of cancer on animals under controlled laboratory conditions in which all other variables can be ruled out. Each type of study has its limitations and must be interpreted with an awareness of those limitations.

"Now let's see; what's different about the environment in these two places?"

"Now let's see; what was different in these people's lifestyles?"

"Now let's see which of these groups gets cancer."

Epidemiological Studies

A thought-provoking finding from studies of populations comes from the comparison of high-risk and low-risk areas. If only 10 people out of 1,000 get a certain kind of cancer in location X, while 100 out of 1,000 get that same kind of cancer in location Y, researchers are inclined to conclude that 90 percent of the cancers in location Y are caused by some environmental factor and are therefore, in theory, preventable. Comparison of high-risk and low-risk areas suggests that 80 to 90 percent of human cancers may indeed be preventable.[3] We have little or no control over some aspects of our environment, but we can certainly control our food choices, and they may contribute to some part of preventable cancers. Hence the great challenge to nutrition researchers is to discover what dietary differences may exist between people who do and don't get cancer.

Early epidemiological studies showed that the incidence of certain cancers varied both by geographic area and by racial group. Japanese immigration to the United States after World War I provided an especially interesting opportunity for such study. The Japanese living in Japan develop more stomach cancers and fewer colon cancers than people in the United States and other Western countries. However, when Japanese people come to the United States, their children develop both stomach and colon cancers at a rate like that of U.S. citizens. What changes the susceptibility of Japanese immigrants? It probably isn't pollution, because Japan and the United States are both industrial countries. However, something in the environment has changed, and an obvious candidate is diet.

Some other interesting questions arise from this comparison. Curiously, even though the incidence of colon cancer rises in the immigrants, Japanese women of the second generation retain the same rate of breast cancer as women in Japan; a change in breast cancer rates doesn't show up until the third generation.[4] This is in contrast to the fact that, worldwide, breast and colon cancer correlate, rising and falling together in the same population. Does the rate of breast cancer in adulthood reflect the food intakes of childhood, so that it takes more than one generation to bring about a change? Answering one question raises more questions.

Other epidemiological studies provide additional clues for the cancer detectives. For example, Seventh-Day Adventists have a cancer rate remarkably lower than that of the general population. The difference can't be attributed entirely to their nutrition, because members of this religious sect obey rules against smoking and using alcohol, too. But when cancers linked to smoking and alcohol are discounted, Seventh-Day Adventists still have a mortality rate from cancer about one-half to two-thirds that of the rest of the population.

Seventh-Day Adventists' foodways center on a lacto-ovo-vegetarian diet, avoiding hot condiments and spices and expressly forbidding pork, which the Bible speaks of as "unclean meat." Those who don't obey the rules to the letter still eat meat very sparingly. Could their low cancer mortality be due to their low meat intakes, or to their high intakes of vegetables and cereal grains? Could some other dietary factor be responsible? Or could factors other than diet, still unidentified, be the keys to their good health? Seventh-Day Adventists are of a higher-than-average socioeconomic level, and most are college educated. What influence might these factors have on their cancer rates?[5]

In order to track down the factors associated with cancers in some populations, one pair of investigators studied the diets of people in 37 countries. They documented the food available per person per day, as well as other indicators of lifestyle, such as possession of radio receivers and motor vehicles. They found many correlations, but one of the most interesting showed both breast and colon cancer to be strongly associated "with indicators of affluence, such as a high-fat diet rich in animal protein."[6] Other investigators have reported similar findings.

Any attempt to link dietary components with disease should be approached with caution. An increase in one component of the diet causes increases or decreases in others.[7] If a close correlation is shown between a disease and, say, the consumption of animal protein, how can you be sure that the critical factor is the animal protein? It may be increased fat consumption; fat goes with animal protein in foods. Or the disease may occur because of what is crowded out: the vitamins, minerals, or fiber contained in the missing fruits, vegetables, and cereals.

Another problem inherent in population studies is that they depend on dietary recall. People tend to have trouble remembering how much of each food they have eaten.[8] And in the case of cancer studies, the need is not so much to know what the diet is like now, as to know what it was like at an earlier time—say, 30 years ago—when the initiating event may have taken place.[9] In this connection, study of the Seventh-Day Adventists offers hope of clarifying the relationship between animal protein and cancer. Most Seventh-Day Adventists can tell you exactly when they quit eating meat—they quit when they joined the church.

In general, studies of populations have suggested that low cancer rates correlate with low meat and high vegetable and grain intakes. Case-control studies, in which researchers can control some of the variables, have added to what we know about the possible relationships.

Findings from Case-Control Studies

Case-control studies have generally pointed the same way as population studies, and they, too, implicate diet in cancer causation. When 179 Hawaiian Japanese people with colon cancer were carefully matched with 357 Hawaiian Japanese people without cancer, those with cancer were seen to have a strikingly higher consumption of meat, especially beef. An Israeli study showed fiber consumption to be lower in victims of colon cancer than in comparable people who did not have cancer. A study of U.S. blacks with colon cancer showed them to be eating less fiber and more saturated fat than others without cancer. These studies have led reviewers to the view that a diet "high in total fat, low in fiber, and high in beef [is] associated with an increased incidence of large-bowel cancer in man."[10]

Findings from Studies on Animals: Fat and Cancer

After population and case-control studies have tentatively identified a dietary factor, researchers often turn to experiments with laboratory animals. By using animals, researchers can control many variables while manipulating only the diet.

Laboratory studies using animals confirm suspicions that fat, of all dietary components, is uniquely correlated with cancer. For example, K. K. Carroll found that he could increase the number of mammary tumors in rats if he raised their dietary fat.[11] The fat was not initiating the cancers, however; to get the tumors started, Carroll had to expose the animals to a known carcinogen. After that exposure, the high-fat diet made more cancers develop and made them develop earlier than did low-fat diets. Thus fat appeared to be a cancer promoter, rather than an initiator.

People are often surprised to learn that fat may be far more significant in cancer causation than food additives, which have long been suspected and feared. Fat is thought to somehow enhance the process by which cancer gets established in a cell or tissue once the first events have taken place. A high-fat diet may promote cancer in any of a number of ways:

- By causing the body to secrete more of certain hormones (for example, estrogen), thus creating a climate favorable to the development of certain cancers (for example, breast cancer).
- By promoting the secretion of bile into the intestine; bile may then be converted by organisms in the colon into compounds that cause cancer.
- By being incorporated into cell membranes and changing them so that they offer less defense against cancer-causing invaders.

It may not be fat in general, but certain forms of fat, that have these effects. Importantly, it seems that polyunsaturated fat is as responsible as, or even more responsible than, saturated fat for promoting cancer, so the person wishing to apply this information should reduce consumption of all forms of fat. There would appear to be no harm in reducing fat intake to the point where it contributes a maximum of 30 percent of total kcalories, and some cancer researchers suggest an even stricter limit: 20 percent of total kcalories. For the "average American" to accomplish this degree of fat restriction in practice means drastically reducing the amount of fat used in food preparation.

Fiber, Vegetables, and Cancer

In general, wherever the diet is high in fat-rich foods, it is simultaneously low in vegetable fiber. There is a possibility that the absence of fiber promotes cancer independently of the presence of fat. Although these two possibilities are difficult to separate in studies of humans, the association of fat with cancer is stronger than that of fiber-lack with cancer. Still, fiber might help protect against some cancer—for example, by promoting the excretion of bile from the body, or by speeding up the transit time of all materials through the colon so that the colon walls are not exposed for long to cancer-causing substances. That fiber does have an independent protective effect of some kind is supported by evidence from Finland. The Finns eat a high-fat diet, but unlike other such diets, theirs is very high in fiber as well. Their colon cancer rate is low, suggesting that fiber has a protective effect even in the presence of a high-fat diet.[12]

If fat and/or a meat-rich diet are implicated in causation of certain cancers, and if fiber and/or a vegetable-rich diet are associated with prevention, then vegetarians should have a lower incidence of those cancers. They do. The Seventh-Day Adventists have already been mentioned; other vegetarian women also have less breast cancer than do meat eaters. A possible explanation ascribes the difference to lower hormone levels in vegetarians. Vegetarian women excrete more estrogens in their feces, so they probably have lower total body estrogen contents than meat eaters do.[13]

A number of studies have suggested other relationships between cancer and the intake of vegetables, especially certain kinds of vegetables. A study of people in Minnesota and in Norway found less frequent use of vegetables in people with colon cancer; a New York study found, specifically, less use of cabbage, broccoli, and brussels sprouts in colon cancer victims. Similarly, careful comparisons of stomach cancer victims' diets with those of case controls show less use of vegetables in the cancer group—in one case, vegetables in general; in another, fresh vegetables; in others, lettuce and other fresh greens, or vegetables containing vitamin C.[14] One of the suspects for the causation of stomach cancer is nitrosamines, produced in the stomach from nitrites. The vegetables may help keep nitrosamines from forming by contributing vitamin C, which inhibits the conversion of nitrites to nitrosamines.

The possible role of vitamin C in preventing nitrosamine formation might lead consumers to think that they could achieve the same protection by taking the vitamin in pill form. If they did this, though, they would miss out on a dozen other nutrients that probably also have a protective effect. Vitamin C's relation to cancer is further discussed in Highlight 9B.

When environmental causes of another kind of cancer—that of the head and neck—have been sought, the major factor has appeared to be not diet, but rather the combination of alcohol and tobacco consumption. Again, however, some dietary factors have turned up here and there, pointing to a low intake of fruits and raw vegetables in cancer cases, but this time a low intake specifically of the fruits and vegetables that contribute carotene (the vitamin A precursor) and riboflavin. Carotene and its relatives the retinoids are also important in preventing cancers of epithelial origin, including skin cancer.[16]

Among the known actions of vitamin A are the important roles it plays in maintaining the immune function. A strong immune system may be able to prevent cancers from gaining control, even after they have gotten started in the body. Immunity can work even after a tumor has begun to form. Some studies suggest that this may be where vitamin A makes its contribution. In Norway, a five-year prospective study showed the lung cancer incidence to be 60 to 80 percent lower in men with a high vitamin A intake than in those with a low intake. In Japan, a study of 280,000 people showed lung cancer rates to be 20 to 30 percent lower in smokers who ate yellow or green vegetables daily than in those who did not. In ex-smokers who ingested yellow or green vegetables daily, the reduction was much greater, as if the *repair* of damage done by smoking after the initiation of cancer was enhanced by something in the vegetables.[17] A reviewer, impressed by abundant evidence along these lines, says, "No human population at risk for the development of cancer should be allowed to remain in a vitamin A deficient state."[18]

For anyone who might be tempted to think that pills containing vitamin A or carotene might provide the same benefit as green vegetables, it should be pointed out immediately that green vegetables have also been seen to have a protective effect beyond those already discussed for vitamin A, vitamin C, and fiber. The effects of the members of the cabbage family, for example, may be due to their containing substances known as indoles, which may act by

Nitrites and the related compounds, nitrates, are salts that contain nitrite ions. Although some nitrites are used as additives and as fertilizers, they also occur naturally in the environment. They are present in the water supply and are present in high concentrations in many vegetables. They are also made in the human body in quantities much larger than those found in food.

Bacon is permitted to have 120 parts per million of nitrite as sold in the store. Other meats can have 200 parts per million, but most have less than 50 parts per million. Smoked fish can have 500 parts per million nitrate and 200 parts per million nitrite. In contrast, some vegetables contain up to 3,000 parts per million nitrate, and even drinking water sometimes has several hundred parts per million.

It is estimated that people in the United States consume about 200 micrograms of nitrite each day from vegetables, about 2,000 from cured meat, and about 8,500 from their own saliva.[15] We can't avoid them, but we can help to prevent their conversion to nitrosamines (which cause cancer) by eating vitamin C–containing vegetables and fruits along with them. Drink orange juice with your breakfast bacon; eat broccoli with your ham; enjoy fresh fruits and vegetables with every meal. Then don't worry about the amounts of nitrites you eat. Concentrate instead on reducing your intake of food sources of fat, and increasing your intake of fiber. These constituents of food are far more significant in terms of cancer.

By combining vegetables, you can achieve all the vitamins you would receive in a supplement, in addition to other needed nutrients.

What other substances might vegetables contribute to help protect the body against cancer? Among other nutrients known to be important in the functioning of the immune system are vitamin A, vitamin B_6, folacin, pantothenic acid, vitamin B_{12}, vitamin E, iron, zinc, and others.

In the repair of damage to DNA, the B vitamin folacin is necessary, and folacin is found in greater abundance in green vegetables than in any other food, as its root word (*foliage*) attests. Fresh vegetables are preferable to vegetables in any other form, partly because vitamins are lost in processing, and partly because they are a better buy for the nutrients purchased.

A notorious contrast to fresh vegetables are the green pills some companies have been producing that contain dehydrated, crushed vegetable matter. Although advertising for the pills often is accompanied by cancer information, it is revealing to note that no claims of prevention or cure are printed on the labels of the bottles. (By law, labels cannot state claims that are not true, but there are no laws against advertising pills on the same page with cancer information.)

Even if eating the pills were a surefire method for cancer prevention, one of the pills contains nutrients equal to those in only one small forkful of vegetables—minus the losses incurred by processing. Sixty pills, costing $15, deliver vegetable matter worth about $1.50.

---

inducing an enzyme in the host that destroys carcinogens.[19] Green vegetables also contain significant amounts of riboflavin and calcium, and both of these nutrients have been linked to cancer prevention, too.[20]

Cancer Prevention

In 1980, the Food and Nutrition Board of the National Academy of Sciences stated that not enough evidence was available, yet, to justify making any recommendations for the dietary prevention of cancer. Two years later, however, under heavy pressure from the public, the same Academy did publish some provisional recommendations. It was as if they were saying, "This is what we are tempted to recommend, but we don't think we can, yet." The provisional recommendations were entitled "Interim Dietary Guidelines—Diet, Nutrition, and Cancer":

1. Reduce the consumption of both saturated and unsaturated fats.
2. Include fruits (especially citrus fruits), vegetables (particularly carotene-rich and cruciferous vegetables), and whole-grain products in the daily diet.
3. Minimize consumption of foods preserved by salt curing, salt packing, or smoking.
4. Minimize contamination of foods with carcinogens from any source, and continue to evaluate food additives for carcinogenic activity.
5. Reduce the concentration of mutagens in foods when feasible to do so.
6. Consume only moderate amounts of alcohol, if any.

A summary of the evidence that backed these guidelines included these points:

- Attention should also be paid to nitrates and their relatives in foods.
- Toxic substances in drinking water are also of concern.

The concerns about diet that the guidelines addressed included the following:

- *Total energy intake*. Studies on animals show that reduced food intakes reduce cancer incidence at any age, but the evidence is less clear for human beings.
- *Lipids*. Both animal studies and epidemiological studies support the view that high fat intakes increase the incidence of cancers of the breast and colon. Evidence on cholesterol is unclear.
- *Protein*. High protein intakes may be associated with increased risks of certain kinds of cancer, but the evidence is not firm enough, yet, to permit a definitive statement.
- *Carbohydrate*. High carbohydrate intakes may contribute to kcaloric excess (with possible risks already discussed); certain fibers may protect against colorectal cancer.
- *Vitamin A*. Inadequate intakes of vitamin A and/or its relatives (carotenoids) seem to correlate with high incidence of cancers of the lung, bladder, and larynx; by inference, adequate intakes must help protect against these cancers.
- *Vitamin C*. Vitamin C may help prevent formation of carcinogens and thereby protect against cancers of the esophagus and stomach.
- *Other vitamins and minerals*. There are suggestive bits of evidence linking other nutrients to cancer, but no firm conclusions can yet be made.
- *Carotene-rich and cruciferous vegetables*. Consumption of carotene-rich and cruciferous vegetables is associated with a reduced incidence of cancer at several sites.

Other links may exist: between alcohol excess and liver cancer; between alcohol plus cigarette smoking and cancer of the esophagus; between excessive beer drinking and rectal cancer; between certain food contaminants and cancer; and between natural substances in foods and cancer. Additives legally permitted in foods are not implicated in cancer causation.[21]

Obviously, much remains to be learned about the connections between nutrition and cancer. Still, many people working in cancer research believe that

A healthy lifestyle is a balancing act.

we already know enough to take the tentative preventive steps recommended in the "Interim Dietary Guidelines." One pair of reviewers says, "The public is looking for answers regarding this diet-cancer link and will look to anyone willing to provide answers, regardless of his/her qualifications. . . . The recommendations offered here constitute no risk and may help lower the incidence of . . . cancers." To the recommendations made in these guidelines, we would add only one other: Vary your choices. Don't let your diet become monotonous.

This last suggestion is based on an important concept that is specific to the prevention of cancer initiation— dilution. Whenever you switch from food to food, you are diluting whatever is in one food with what is in the others. It is safe to eat *some* processed meats, but don't eat them all the time. Eat many green, yellow, and orange vegetables; they are all needed in the diet for many good reasons. If you include high-fiber foods and reduce your fat intake as well, you have every reason to feel confident that you are providing your body with the best nutrition at the lowest possible risk.

NOTES
1. Parts of this Highlight are adapted from S. R. Rolfes and F. S. Sizer, *Nutrition and Cancer* (a monograph available from Stickley Publishing Co., 210 Washington Square, Philadelphia, PA 19106).
2. A comprehensive, excellent work that offers perspective on the whole subject of cancer causation is A. E. Reif, The causes of cancer, *American Scientist* 69 (1981): 437–447.
3. B. S. Reddy and coauthors, Nutrition and its relationship to cancer, *Advances in Cancer Research* 32 (1980): 238–345.
4. Reddy and coauthors, 1980.
5. R. L. Phillips, Role of life-style and dietary habits in risk of cancer among Seventh Day Adventists, *Cancer Research* 35 (1975): 3513–3522.
6. B. S. Drasar and D. Irving, Environmental factors and cancer of the colon and breast, *British Journal of Cancer* 27 (1973): 167–172.

7. K. K. Carroll, Experimental evidence of dietary factors and hormone-dependent cancers, *Cancer Research* 35, no. 2 (1975): 3374–3383; B. Modan, Role of diet in cancer etiology, *Cancer* 40 (1977): 1887–1891.
8. Modan, 1977.
9. A. B. Miller, Role of nutrition in the etiology of breast cancer, *Cancer* 39 (1977): 2704–2708; B. Armstrong and R. Doll, Environmental factors and cancer incidence and mortality in different countries, with special reference to dietary practices, *International Journal of Cancer* 15 (1975): 617–631.
10. Reddy and coauthors, 1980.
11. Carroll, 1975.
12. E. L. Wynder, Dietary habits and cancer epidemiology, *Cancer* 43 (1979): 1955–1961, as cited by S. H. Brammer and R. L. DeFelice, Dietary advice in regard to risk for colon and breast cancer, *Preventive Medicine* 9 (1980): 544–549.
13. Goldin and coauthors, Effect of diet on excretion of estrogens in pre- and postmenopausal women, *Cancer Research* 41 (1981): 3771–3773.
14. Reddy and coauthors, 1980.
15. R. J. Hickey and R. G. Clelland, Hazardous food additives: Nitrite and saliva? (correspondence), *New England Journal of Medicine* 298 (1978): 1036.
16. J. L. Werther, Food and cancer, *New York State Journal of Medicine*, August 1980, pp. 1401–1408.
17. Werther, 1980.
18. M. B. Sporn, Retinoids and carcinogenesis, *Nutrition Reviews* 35 (1977): 65–69.
19. L. W. Wattenberg, W. D. Loub, L. K. Lam, and J. L. Speier, Dietary constituents altering the responses to chemical carcinogens, *Federation Proceedings* 35 (1976): 1327–1331; L. W. Wattenberg and W. D. Loub, Inhibition of polycyclic aromatic hydrocarbon-induced neoplasia by naturally occurring indoles, *Cancer Research* 38 (1978): 1410–1413.
20. Riboflavin and cancer, in An overview of riboflavin, *Dairy Council Digest* 56, November–December 1985, p. 35; M. Lipkin and H. Newmark, Effect of added dietary calcium on colonic epithelial-cell proliferation in subjects at high risk for familial colonic cancer, *New England Journal of Medicine* 313(1985): 1381–1384.
21. Committee on Diet, Nutrition, and Cancer, National Research Council, *Executive Summary: Diet, Nutrition, and Cancer* (Washington, D.C.: National Academy Press, 1982).

Miniglossary

carcinogen (car-SIN-oh-jen): a cancer-causing substance. A carcinogen is one kind of initiator; another is radiation.
carcin = cancer
gen = gives rise to
cruciferous vegetables: a group of vegetables named for their cross-shaped blossoms. They have been shown to protect against cancer in laboratory animals. Examples are cauliflower, cabbage, brussels sprouts, broccoli, turnips, and rutabagas.
initiating event: an event caused by radiation or chemical reaction that can give rise to cancer.
promoter: a substance that does not initiate cancer, but that favors its development once the initiating event has taken place.

HIGHLIGHT FOUR B

Nutrition and Atherosclerosis

More than half the adults who die in the United States each year die of heart and blood vessel disease (cardiovascular disease, or CVD). The underlying condition that contributes to most of these deaths is artery disease, which is so widespread it has been called an epidemic. What are its causes? How can it be prevented? Can it be reversed?

Artery disease often begins with a condition called "hardening of the arteries," or atherosclerosis. In atherosclerosis, soft mounds of lipid accumulate along the inner walls of the arteries. These plaques gradually enlarge, making the artery walls lose their elasticity and narrowing the passage through them.

Normally, blood surges through the arteries with each beat of the heart, and the arteries expand with each pulse to accommodate the flow. Arteries hardened and narrowed by plaques cannot expand, and so the blood pressure rises. The increased pressure puts a strain on the heart and damages the artery walls further.

As pressure builds up in an artery, the arterial wall may become weakened and balloon out, forming an aneurysm. An aneurysm can burst, and when this happens in a major artery such as the aorta, it leads to massive bleeding and death.

In addition to being elastic, the inner walls of the arteries must be glass smooth so that the blood can move over the surface with as little friction as possible. Clotting of blood is an intricate series of events triggered when the blood moves past a rough surface, such as the edge of a cut. As long as the inner wall of an artery remains smooth, clots will not form in it, but if the plaques encroach on the inside of the artery, their roughness can cause the clotting reactions to begin (see Figures H4B–1 and H4B–2).

A clot thus formed may linger, attached to a plaque, and gradually grow until it shuts off the blood supply to that portion of the tissue supplied by the artery. That tissue may die slowly and be replaced by scar tissue. Or the clot may break loose and travel along the system until it reaches an artery too small to allow its passage. Then the tissues fed by this artery will be robbed of oxygen and nutrients and will die suddenly. When such a clot lodges in an artery of the heart, causing sudden death of part of the heart muscle, we say that the person had a heart attack. When the clot lodges in an artery of the brain, killing a portion of brain tissue, we call the event a stroke.

Atherosclerosis begins early. Fatty streaks have been observed in the aortas of infants less than a year old, and plaques are well developed in most individuals by the time they are 30. No one is free of the condition.[1] The question is not whether you have it, but how far advanced it is and what you can do to retard or reverse it.

Atherosclerosis takes a heavy toll among people in the productive periods of their lives, long before retirement. Many health agencies have devoted millions of hours to the battle against atherosclerosis, but so far all that can be said for sure about its causes is that it is multifactorial in origin. There are many risk factors—perhaps 30 or so in all. The relationships among these many factors are not at all clear. They are only correlations; we do not know what causes what. Furthermore, it is not clear to what extent reducing any of the risk factors will reduce the risk of dying of the disease.

FIGURE H4B–1

Development of atherosclerosis. For photographs of arteries with and without plaques, see Figure H4B–2.

Plaque

Inner Layer (Artery Lining)

Outer Layer (Supportive Tissues)

Middle Layer (Smooth Muscle)

An artery (section) with plaque just beginning to form. Plaques can easily appear in a person as young as 15.

The same artery, years later, half blocked by plaque.

B. Plaques along an artery narrow its diameter and obstruct blood flow. Clots can form, aggravating the problem.

A. A healthy artery provides an open passage for the flow of blood.

FIGURE H4B–2

Plaques in arteries.

C. Atherosclerotic inner surface of a human artery that has been slit open (magnified 2.5 times). The lumps are the plaques.

An analogy may help to make clear the point being made here about correlations and causes. Suppose that there is an outbreak of crime in a certain city—arson, for example. Someone is setting fires, and the police are after him. It is observed that a certain person, Mr. A, is always seen in the neighborhoods when the fires start, and he is deemed guilty of the crimes. However, it may be that a very sneaky individual, Ms. B, is the real culprit and that Mr. A is only following her around. Mr. A is associated with, but is not a causal agent in, the setting of the fires. The evidence against him is only circumstantial (correlational). If the police can show that whenever he is locked up there are no fires, and that whenever he is let out the fires start again, the evidence against him will be stronger. Better yet, they will know for sure if they catch him pouring the gasoline and lighting the match. You may recall that this point has been made before; correlation is not cause. Be careful when you interpret data that imply a causal relationship between foods linked only by association.

The heart gets its nutrients and oxygen not from inside its chambers, but from arteries that lie on its surface. These are the **coronary arteries**.

Risk Factor Studies

Among the many factors linked to atherosclerosis are smoking, gender (being male), heredity (including diabetes), high blood pressure, lack of exercise, obesity, stress, high blood cholesterol, many nutrient excesses and deficiencies, personality characteristics, and more. Some of the risk factors are powerful predictors of heart disease. If you have none of them, the statistical likelihood of your developing CVD in the next 10 or 20 years may be only 1 in 100. If you have three major ones, the chance may rise to over 1 in 20. Table H4B–1 shows one way of calculating your risk score.

Three factors have emerged as the major predictors of atherosclerosis risk:

- Smoking.
- High serum cholesterol (see p. 107).
- High blood pressure (see Chapter 11).

From statistics pooled from many studies on these risk factors, the American Heart Association has published the *Coronary Risk Handbook*. The small portion dealing with six–year predictions for a 45-year-old man is shown in Table H4B–2. The table illustrates dramatically that the chances of having a healthy heart and arteries are much greater if you don't smoke and your blood cholesterol and blood pressure are low.[2]

Another complicating factor in determining risk of atherosclerosis has already been mentioned: the problem of interpreting epidemiological studies. It can be demonstrated that in many countries where the diets are low in fat, the incidence of heart and artery disease is much lower than it is in the United States and Canada. But to attribute the difference in disease rates to the differing diets would be naive. Many other factors also present in developed countries may play a role: urban life; lack of exercise; indeed, lifestyles that differ in many, many respects.

It can be argued that the risk factors all reflect an underlying prior condition. Psychologists point to personality type, and especially the way the person responds to stress, as a potent predictor of risk. People of the personality type called Type A are notorious for being heart attack prone. A Type A person is competitive, strives for achievement, has a sense of time urgency, is inclined to be hostile, suppresses the feeling of fatigue—in short, is uptight, as compared with the more easygoing Type B person. In one type of research, people are scored A or B first and then followed up. The Type A people are found to have more than twice the rate of heart disease than the Type B people have.[3] This is prospective research, and the A-versus-B difference shows up even when the three major risk factors

The Type A person has a sense of time urgency.

TABLE H4B–1

Your Risk of Heart Disease

| | H | E | A | R | T |

Everyone plays the game of health whether he wants to or not. What is your score? Add up the numbers in each category that most nearly describe you.

Heredity	1 No known history of heart disease	2 One relative with heart disease over 60 years	3 Two relatives with heart disease over 60 years	4 One relative with heart disease under 60 years	6 Two relatives with heart disease under 60 years
Exercise	1 Intensive exercise, work, and recreation	2 Moderate exercise, work, and recreation	3 Sedentary work and intensive recreational exercise	5 Sedentary work and moderate recreational exercise	6 Sedentary work and light recreational exercise
Age	1 10–20	2 21–30	3 31–40	4 41–50	6 51–65
Lbs.	0 More than 5 lb below standard weight	1 ±5 lb standard weight	2 6–20 lb overweight	4 21–35 lb overweight	6 36–50 lb overweight
Tobacco	0 Nonuser	1 Cigar or pipe	2 10 cigarettes or fewer per day	4 20 cigarettes or more per day	6 30 cigarettes or more per day
Habits of eating fat	1 0%: No animal or solid fats	2 10%: Very little animal or solid fats	3 20%: Little animal or solid fats	4 30%: Much animal or solid fats	6 40%: Very much animal or solid fats

Your risk of heart attack:

4–9 Very remote.	16–20 Average.	26–30 Dangerous.
10–15 Below average.	21–25 Moderate.	31–35 Urgent danger—reduce score!

Other conditions—such as stress, high blood pressure, and increased blood cholesterol—detract from heart health and should be evaluated by your physician.

Source: Courtesy of Loma Linda University.

TABLE H4B–2

Risk of Developing CVD within Six Years The effect of the three major risk factors are shown alone and in combination for a 45-year-old man.

Smoker	Cholesterol (mg/100 ml[a])	Blood Pressure (mm mercury[b])	Risk (per 100)
No	185	105	1.5
No	185	195	4.4
No	335	195	16.7
Yes	335	195	23.9

[a]Milligrams of cholesterol per 100 ml blood.
[b]The first of the two numbers recorded (for example, *120* in 120/70). The silver column that rises on a blood-pressure instrument is a column of mercury; the height to which it is pushed is marked off in millimeters.
Source: U.S. Senate, Select Committee on Nutrition and Human Needs, *Diet Related to Killer Diseases II, Part 1, Cardiovascular Disease* (hearings), (Washington, D.C.: Government Printing Office), 1977.

already mentioned are taken into account.

Type A people's heart disease seems to arise in the classic way: by blockage of the arteries. The way they react physically to stress may account for the damage. The stress hormones affect blood pressure and blood lipid levels, so the key to prevention may lie in study of the hormones or of the stress response.

Intervention Studies

While research goes on, people want to know what to do *now* to prevent CVD, the devastating disease that kills one out of every two people in the United States. To find out what to do, researchers design intervention studies. Studies of this kind involve tinkering with a cluster of factors (like the obesity–inactivity–smoking–high blood pressure–cholesterol cluster) by altering the items one by one and seeing if any of these alterations leads to reduction in deaths from CVD. A successful intervention study is a major step forward in research; it helps to demonstrate that a risk factor not only accompanies, but causes, a disease.

In some massive intervention studies conducted during the 1970s, thousands of men were persuaded to give up

smoking, take medication to reduce their blood pressure (if it was high), and alter their diets to reduce their cholesterol levels. These studies were complicated by a curious problem, however: everyone else was doing those same things. Word had gotten around to the whole U.S. population that these measures were beneficial. The intervention studies failed to show significant improvement of the experimental groups over controls, perhaps because there *were* no good controls. A retrospective analysis of the impressive downturn in the rate of deaths from CVD between the late 1960s and the late 1970s suggests that a massive, unintentional intervention study may have been spontaneously conducted by the whole U.S. population.

In any case, something certainly seems to have happened in that ten-year period that saved 200,000 lives. At a major conference held in 1979, the experts who had been following the lifestyle changes and trends among people in the United States reported that as a people:
1. We are smoking less.
2. We are controlling our blood pressure better.
3. Our blood cholesterol levels have fallen slightly.

4. We are exercising more.
In other words, independently of the research studies, people have been taking measures that are paying off in lower mortality.[4]

The evidence from review of this happening suggests that reduction of risk factors is advisable for all members of the population, not just for the most heart attack prone. If you divide the population into five groups, from the lowest to the highest risk, more than half the preventable heart disease deaths appear to be in the *middle* three groups.

Which of the risk factors is most important? The balance sheet may look like this:
- A fourth of the reduced risk comes from a moderate reduction in blood cholesterol.
- A fourth comes from better control of high blood pressure—primarily by drugs, but also by diet.
- Half comes from a decrease in the prevalence of cigarette smoking.*[5]

The rest of this highlight focuses on reducing blood cholesterol (see Chapter 11 for more on blood pressure).

How to Lower Blood Cholesterol

Let us first clarify one point: we are talking about blood cholesterol, not the cholesterol in foods.** The most important food factor affecting blood cholesterol is saturated fat, not the cholesterol in foods. The most effective dietary measures to lower blood cholesterol are these:
- Lower your saturated fat intake to 10 percent of total kcalories or less.

*This refers to the reduced risk from CVD only. If risk of death from all causes is measured, serum cholesterol becomes relatively less important (4 percent) and cigarette smoking, considerably more important (65 percent). And exercise is not included, because it isn't one of the "big three" in the heart disease picture.

**Blood, plasma, and *serum* cholesterol all refer to about the same thing. Plasma is simply blood with the cells removed; serum has the clotting factors also removed.

Millions of dollars and decades of effort by hundreds of researchers have yielded many positive findings from risk factor research. Still, as mentioned, the ultimate causes of CVD are unknown. The kind of problem that repeatedly hinders research is illustrated by the story of an investigation conducted in Great Britain.

The researchers, who wanted to relate physical activity to heart attack risk, chose to study bus drivers and bus conductors. They did find, as expected, that the more active people (the conductors) had fewer heart attacks than did the sedentary ones (the drivers). They might have been tempted to conclude that they had found the relationship they were looking for: less activity leads to more heart attacks. But they looked further and found that the drivers were also fatter than the conductors. Perhaps the relationship was that less activity leads to more obesity leads to more heart attacks. They checked further still, however, and found that the drivers had been fatter than the conductors when they started work years before. The conclusion had to be rephrased: fatter people choose less active work. But what, then, caused the heart disease? Conceivably, the drivers might have been headed for CVD as children, even before they became obese. What comes first? Inactivity? No—in this study, it was obesity. What comes before obesity?[6]

The problem illustrated by this study is one that plagues the researcher who is trying to untangle a chain of events and find its beginning. You can see that conclusions drawn from research like this are somewhat shaky. They can always be criticized on the basis that they are retrospective (looking back), so that the researcher cannot tell whether the people who developed the condition might have been self-selected—might have gotten onto the track headed toward heart disease long before the differences (in occupation, for example) were observed. To be free of this criticism, such a study should be prospective. A matched group of people should be selected for study and then followed through time to see what differences develop. Understanding this sampling problem in research will help you evaluate the results of other studies like this one.

concern to researchers in heart disease, because it happens that the oxidation products are highly toxic to arteries. In fact, concentrated oxidized cholesterol can induce lesions in the arteries of experimental animals within 24 hours after it is administered.[7] Many of the earlier experiments that reported cholesterol to be causing heart disease may actually have been flawed by accidental contamination with oxidized cholesterol; if they were, then much of that research is invalid.

Researchers are concerned, too, because oxidation of cholesterol may occur not only in bottles in the laboratory, but also in meats, eggs, and milk products that are exposed to air— especially those that are heavily processed (dehydrated or powdered, for example).[8] Research in progress in the mid-1980s is focused on determining just what oxidation products are formed in foods and what their health effects may be.[9]

The question of whether or not we should attempt to reduce our intakes of dietary cholesterol is thus still open. But while we await answers to that question, what else can we do to reduce our blood cholesterol levels? A host of studies have produced a host of possible answers to this question. Practically every food and nutrient has been studied to see if it raises or lowers blood cholesterol levels, and some of the findings are surprising and interesting. They are summed up in Tables H4B–3 and H4B–4, which are derived from over 50 research studies reported since 1980. It looks as if the person who wishes to use every possible dietary means to lower blood cholesterol would do all of the following:

- Eat fish, especially fatty fish such as mackerel and salmon, often.
- Use milk, and especially fermented milk products such as yogurt, freely.
- Consume abundant legumes of many varieties, including soybeans and chick-peas.

- Partially substitute polyunsaturated for saturated fats. (These two measures should increase your **P:S** ratio to 1 to 1 or greater.)
- Reduce your cholesterol intake to 300 mg a day or less.

There is less agreement about the third of these than about the other two.

A factor that complicates the question of whether we should reduce our intakes of cholesterol from food is an accident that has occurred repeatedly in research on this question. When

purified cholesterol sits in a jar on a laboratory shelf, it changes chemically to a variety of oxidation products. Then, when the scientist takes it off the shelf and mixes it into diets to feed to his experimental animals, it isn't actually cholesterol he is feeding. He may never know this, and if the diets cause plaque formation and heart disease in his animals, he may report that cholesterol is responsible, when in fact it is not.

The fact that cholesterol oxidizes readily on exposure to air is of great

TABLE H4B–3

Nutrients That Raise or Lower Blood Cholesterol[a]

Nutrients and Nutrient Variables That Raise Blood Cholesterol	Nutrients That Have No Effect	Nutrients That Lower Blood Cholesterol
	Carbohydrates	
Sucrose	Starch	Lactose
Fructose	Glucose	
	Fibers	
	Bran (wheat bran)	Citrus pectin
	Cellulose	Oat bran
	Soybean fiber	Guar gum
		Xanthan gum
		Other water-soluble fibers and gums from fruits, legumes, and vegetables
		Hemicellulose
	Lipids	
Saturated fat		Polyunsaturated fat
Trans-fatty acids[b]		Monounsaturated fat
		Artificial fat (sucrose polyester)[c]
	Protein	
Animal protein, especially milk protein	Soybean protein (in some experiments)	Soybean protein (in some experiments)
	Vitamins	
Vitamin C deficiency	Vitamin C; vitamin C megadoses	Vitamin C administered to correct deficiency
	Vitamin E	
	Vitamin B_6[d]	
	Minerals	
Fluoride deficiency		
Other mineral and trace mineral deficiencies or imbalances[e]		
	Water	
Soft water[f]		Hard water[f]
	Other Constituents of Foods	
		Plant sterols
		Flavones (from chick-peas)
		Saponins (from alfalfa)

[a]References available on request; write the authors in care of the publisher.
[b]*Trans*-fatty acids raise blood cholesterol but do not cause atherosclerosis. D. Kritchevsky, Trans fatty acid effects in experimental atherosclerosis, *Federation Proceedings* 41 (1982): 2813–2817.
[c]Sucrose polyester doesn't actively lower blood cholesterol, but works by substituting for saturated fat; which would otherwise raise it. See Chapter 4.
[d]Vitamin B_6 has no effect on blood cholesterol but does inhibit blood clotting. Inhibition of platelet aggregation and clotting by pyridoxal-5´-phosphate, *Nutrition Reviews* 40 (1982): 55–57.
[e]Optimal intakes of all following are necessary to keep cholesterol normal and prevent atherosclerosis: sodium, magnesium, calcium, chromium, copper, zinc, iodine, iron, and selenium. W. Mertz, Trace minerals and atherosclerosis, *Federation Proceedings* 41 (1982): 2807–2812. Magnesium deficiency also causes spasms of coronary arteries. P. D. M. V. Turlapaty and B. M. Alturn, Magnesium deficiency produces spasms of coronary arteries: Relationship to etiology of sudden death ischemic heart disease, *Science* 208 (1980): 198–200.
[f]Perhaps because soft water contains sodium; and hard water, magnesium. R. Masironi and A. G. Shaper, Epidemiological studies of health effects of water from different sources, *Annual Reviews of Nutrition* 1 (1981): 375–400.

TABLE H4B–4

Foods That Raise or Lower Blood Cholesterol[a]

Foods That Raise Blood Cholesterol	Foods That Have No Effect	Foods and Diet Variables That Lower Blood Cholesterol
	Meat, Fish, Poultry	
	Fatty fish (in some experiments)	Fatty fish (in some experiments: salmon sardines, mackerel, kippers, herring, pilchard, trout)
	Dairy Products	
Eggs (in some experiments)	Eggs (in some experiments)	Milk, nonfat milk, fermented milk and milk products
	Vegetables, Fruits	
		Fruits and vegetables Vegetarian diet Garlic[b]
	Legumes	
		Legumes[c] Soy milk [d] Textured soy protein
	Grains	
		Rolled oats and other grains[e]
	Fats, Oils	
Butter Beef fat Other animal fats Hydrogenated fat products		Corn oil Soy oil Cod-liver oil Other fish oils Garlic oil Olive oil
	Other	
Refined sugar Coffee[g]	Hot peppers[f]	Ginseng Weight reduction in obese subjects

[a]References available on request; write the authors in care of the publisher.
[b]Garlic has now been demonstrated to reduce blood cholesterol, slow the development of plaques, inhibit blood clotting, lower LDL, and raise HDL. D. F. Sly, Garlic: A clove a day keeps the doctor away? *Professional Nutritionist*, Fall 1982, pp. 7–10.
[c]Table H4B–3 shows some of the constituents of legumes that may be responsible for their cholesterol-lowering effect.
[d]Soy milk lowered cholesterol "substantially" in subjects above the 50th percentile for North American cholesterol levels, but not in those with lower initial levels. W. A. Check, Switch to soy protein for boring but healthful diet (medical news), *Journal of the American Medical Association* 247 (1982): 3045–3046.
[e]Table H4B–3 identifies some of the components of grains that lower blood cholesterol.
[f]Hot peppers (capsicum) don't lower blood cholesterol but do have an anticlotting effect. S. Visudhiphan and coauthors, The relationship between high fibrinolytic activity and daily capsicum ingestion in Thais, *American Journal of Clinical Nutrition* 35 (1982): 1452–1458.
[g]Although caffeine in animals lowers blood cholesterol, coffee has been shown in one large study to raise it in men. D. S. Thelle, E. Arnesen, and O. H. Forde, The Tromso Heart Study: Does coffee raise serum cholesterol? *New England Journal of Medicine* 308 (1983): 1454–1457. There are many arguments about the meaning of this study. Coffee and cholesterol (correspondence), *New England Journal of Medicine* 309 (1983): 1248–1250.

- Eat generous quantities of fiber-rich fruits and vegetables, including many raw ones.
- Use whole grains (especially oats, and not especially wheat) and sprouts (especially alfalfa sprouts) often.
- Flavor foods liberally with garlic and hot peppers.

Of particular interest are the new findings on fish and fiber. As mentioned in Chapter 4, fish oils contain EPA and other omega-3 fatty acids, which lower blood cholesterol and triglycerides and reduce the tendency of blood to clot.[10] One or two fish dishes a week are all it takes to exert a significant effect,[11] and the fattiest cold-water fish are the most effective: mackerel, herring, sardines, bluefish, salmon, tuna, Pacific oysters, European anchovies, squid, and others.

Dietary fiber may also confer benefits. Persons on high-fiber diets have been shown to excrete more bile acids, sterols, and fat than those on low-fiber diets. One reason for the lowered blood cholesterol levels following a high-fiber regimen is a faster transit time for materials through the gastrointestinal tract, which allows less time for cholesterol absorption. Also, if the body is losing bile acids bound to fiber components, it must simultaneously synthesize new bile acids from its stores of cholesterol; some of these will then be excreted, reducing body cholesterol further. Diets high in fiber are typically low in fat and cholesterol anyway— another advantage to emphasizing fiber.

The various dietary fibers have varying effects on blood cholesterol. The soluble fibers pectin and guar gum have greater cholesterol-lowering effects than the insoluble fibers cellulose and lignin. Indeed, rolled oats and oat bran (rich in soluble fiber) have favorable effects on blood cholesterol, whereas wheat bran (high in cellulose) is far less effective. Apples, pears, peaches, oranges, and grapes are good sources of pectin.

In addition to taking all these positive measures, the person would concentrate on obtaining adequate nutrients from food, and would go easy on eggs, protein-rich foods, and shellfish. These food choices resemble those advocated by the *Dietary Guidelines* (Chapter 2), which thus seem to have mounting evidence in their favor.

How to Raise HDL

While most of the blood cholesterol is carried in the LDL and correlates *directly* with CVD risk, some is carried in the HDL and correlates *inversely* with CVD risk. In fact, for men over 50, the most potent single predictor of heart attack risk may be the HDL level—the higher the level, the lower the risk.[12] While we must exercise the same caution here as formerly (since we don't know for sure if our actions will have any beneficial effect), we can examine the question of how to raise HDL levels.

One way (although we can't do much about this) is to be female. Women have higher HDL levels than men. Another, interestingly, seems to be to stop smoking. Nonsmokers have uniformly higher HDL levels than smokers. Still another is to be in the process of losing weight.

A few investigators have reported that the consumption of moderate amounts of alcohol appeared to raise HDL levels; however, it is becoming apparent that there is more than one kind of HDL, and that the kind of HDL affected by alcohol may not be the "good" kind. But by far the most powerful influence on HDL levels is not a nutrition-related factor at all, but exercise—prolonged, intense, and frequent.

The discovery that exercise raises HDL levels has given great impetus to the physical fitness movement of the 1970s and 1980s, and especially to the popularity of running as a national pastime. The earliest reports were of raised HDL levels in long-distance runners. At first it was thought that only long-distance, endurance-type running had any significant effect, but subsequent reports have suggested that even

Miniglossary

aneurysm (AN-you-rism): the ballooning out of an artery wall at a point where it has been weakened by deterioration.

angina (an JYE nah; some people say ANN-juh-nuh): pain in the heart region caused by lack of oxygen.

aorta (ay-OR-tah): the large, primary artery that conducts blood from the heart to the body's smaller arteries.

atherosclerosis (ath-er-oh-scler-OH-sis): a type of artery disease characterized by patchy nodular thickenings of the inner walls of the arteries, especially at branch points. Atherosclerosis is the major type of **arteriosclerosis** (hardening of the arteries), and the one most influenced by lifestyle factors.
athero = porridge (soft)
scleros = hard
osis = too much

CAD (coronary artery disease): another term for CHD.

CHD (coronary heart disease): atherosclerosis in the arteries feeding the heart muscle.

CVA (cerebrovascular accident): a stroke or aneurysm in the brain.

CVD (cardiovascular disease): a general term for all diseases of the heart and blood vessels. Atherosclerosis is the main form of CVD.

embolus (EM-boh-luss): a thrombus that breaks loose. When it causes sudden closure of a blood vessel, it is an **embolism**.
embol = to insert

IHD (ischemic heart disease): another term for atherosclerosis and its relatives.

ischemia (iss-KEY-me-uh): the deterioration and death of tissue (for example, of heart muscle), often caused by atherosclerosis.

multifactorial: having many causes.

myocardial infarct (MI) (my-oh-CARD-ee-al in-FARKT): the sudden shutting off of the blood flow to the heart muscle by a thrombus or embolism; the same as a heart attack.
myo = muscle
cardium = heart
infarct = blocking off

occlusion (ock-CLOO-zhun): shutting off of the blood flow in an artery.

plaques (placks): mounds of lipid material, mixed with smooth muscle cells and calcium, which are lodged in the artery walls. The same word is also used to describe an entirely different kind of accumulation of material on teeth, which promotes dental caries.

prospective study: researchers take measurements on a number of people now, and then wait for some years to see what differences arise among them.

retrospective study: researchers study a number of people now, and look back at their history to see what may account for the differences among them.

risk factors: factors known to be related to (or correlated with) a disease but not proven to be causal.

thrombus: a stationary clot. When it has grown enough to close off a blood vessel, it is a **thrombosis**. A **coronary thrombosis** is a closing off of a vessel that feeds the heart muscle. A **cerebral thrombosis** is a closing off of a vessel that feeds the brain.
coronary = crowning (the heart)
thrombo = clot
cerebrum = part of the brain

moderate exercise may both lower LDL levels and raise HDL levels if consistently pursued. Evidently, then, it is beneficial even for very sedentary people to become only moderately active.[13]

It seems that the factors affecting the health of the heart and arteries are all tangled together. The exact relationships among them have not yet been worked out; but although we don't know which causes what, all evidence points in the same general direction. For good health, and to avoid CVD, stop smoking; reduce blood pressure and weight, if necessary; eat a balanced, adequate, and varied diet; reduce fat intake, especially saturated fat; increase activity; and—now that you have it all under control—enjoy life.

Although diet and nutrition have been the focus of attention here, it seems important to conclude by taking a broader view of the problem of CVD. Nutrition is obviously not the only factor involved. And CVD deaths are falling while others are on the rise: deaths from accidents, homicides, suicides, lung cancer, and liver disease. The lifestyle of our whole society is implicated in these deaths—it is an urbanized, competitive, industrial society with built-in stresses that have a major impact on health. While we continue focusing on this book's central concern, nutrition, we must acknowledge that society itself may need to change in fundamental ways before we can arrive at ultimate solutions to some of these problems.

Running offers numerous benefits.

The single most important approach to alleviating almost any disease is the reduction of stress. . . . Better still is the elimination of constant worry about your heart, plus the restoration of relaxation and pleasure to your mealtimes. Enjoy food rather than fear it.

Edward R. Pinckney and Cathey Pinckney

NOTES

1. R. L. Holman, H. C. McGill, J. P. Strong, and J. C. Greer, The natural history of atherosclerosis: The early aortic lesions as seen in New Orleans in the middle of the 20th century, *American Journal of Pathology* 34 (1958): 209–234.

2. M. F. Oliver, Diet and coronary heart disease, *British Medical Bulletin* 37 (1981): 49–58. Oliver sets the upper limit of normal for blood cholesterol at 220 milligrams per 100 milliliters.

3. R. H. Rosenman, R. H. Rahe, N. O. Borhanie, and M. Feinleib, Heritability of personality and behavior pattern, *Proceedings of the First International Congress on Twins,* Rome, 1975, as cited by D. C. Glass, Stress, behavior patterns, and coronary disease, *American Scientist* 65 (1977): 177–188.

4. R. J. Havlik and M. Feinleib, eds., *Proceedings of the Conference on the Decline in Coronary Heart Disease Mortality*, NIH publication no. 79–1610 (Washington, D.C.: Government Printing Office, May 1979).

5. J. Stamler, reporting for R. Byington and colleagues, Recent trends of major coronary risk factors and CHD mortality in the United States and other industrialized countries, in Havlik and Feinleib, 1979, pp. 340–380.

6. J. Gorman, A running argument: Does physical activity help prevent heart attacks? *The Sciences*, January-February 1977, pp. 10–15.

7. H. Imai and coauthors, Angiotoxicity and arteriosclerosis due to contaminants of USP-grade cholesterol, *Archives of Pathology and Laboratory Medicine* 100 (1976): 565–572.

8. F. A. Kummerow, Nutrition imbalance and angiotoxins as dietary risk factors in coronary heart disease, *American Journal of Clinical Nutrition* 32 (1979): 58–83.

9. A. M. Pearson and coauthors, Safety implications of oxidized lipids in muscle foods, *Food Technology*, July 1983, pp. 121–128.

10. Fish oils lower plasma triglycerides, according to A. M. Fehily and coauthors, The effect of fatty fish on plasma lipid and lipoprotein concentrations, *American Journal of Clinical Nutrition* 38 (1983): 349–351. They lower cholesterol and slow clotting, according to W. S. Harris and coauthors, in *Nutrition and Heart Disease* (London: Churchill Livingston, 1983), as cited by Fish oils, serum lipids and platelet aggregation, *Nutrition and the MD*, January 1985.

11. D. Kromhout, E. B. Bosschieter, and C. D. Coulander, The inverse relation between fish consumption and 20–year mortality from coronary heart disease, *New England Journal of Medicine* 312 (1985): 1205–1209.

12. Dozens of research articles now support this finding. A typical one is J. G. Brook and coauthors, High-density lipoprotein subfractions in normolipemic patients with coronary atherosclerosis, *Circulation* 66 (1982): 923–926.

13. D. Streja and D. Mymin, Moderate exercise and high-density lipoprotein-cholesterol, *Journal of the American Medical Association* 242 (1979): 2190–2192; W. P. Castelli, Exercise and high-density lipoproteins (editorial), *Journal of the American Medical Association* 242 (1979): 2217.

Protein: Amino Acids

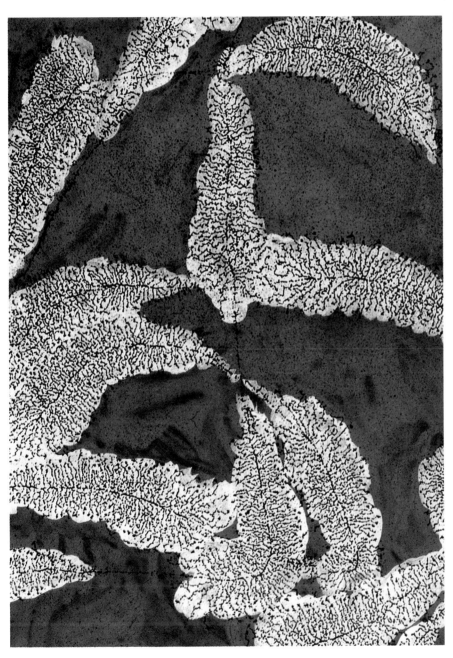

Contents

Enzymes work rapidly and systematically. Part of a cell is shown here, in which about 12 genes (segments of DNA) are being copied into RNA. About 50 enzymes are at work in each gene, creating a Christmas-tree-like formation. Each enzyme is moving along the DNA, making an RNA copy. Those that have moved the farthest have made the longest RNA branches.

One thing protein does *not* do for you is make you thin! See Chapters 7 and 8.

*E*verybody knows that protein is the material of muscles, and that it is important in the diet. It is associated with strength and power, and every cereal box boasts of its presence. In fact, as you will see, protein has been so overemphasized that many people eat more than enough, sometimes at the expense of other nutrients that are equally important. An understanding of the quantity and quality of protein people really need will help put it in its proper place as only one—although a very important one—of the nutrients needed in correct proportions to achieve a balanced diet.

This chapter departs from the organization used for the preceding chapters, jumping right into a description of the chemical structure of protein. The reason is that proteins are far more versatile than carbohydrates or fats in the roles they play in the body, and they derive their versatility from their extraordinary structure. Those who have worked on elucidating the chemical structure of protein have been rewarded with a profound insight into the elegance of nature's designs.

The Chemist's View of Protein

protein: a compound composed of C, H, O, and N atoms, arranged into amino acids linked in a chain. Some amino acids also contain S (sulfur) atoms.

amino (a-MEEN-oh) **acid:** a building block of protein; a compound containing an amino group and an acid group attached to a central carbon atom, which also carries a distinctive side chain.
amino = containing nitrogen

A protein is a chemical compound that contains the same atoms as carbohydrate and lipid—carbon, hydrogen, and oxygen—but protein also contains nitrogen atoms. These C, H, O, and N atoms are arranged into amino acids, which are linked into chains to form proteins. It is easy to construct a protein once we know what an amino acid looks like.

Amino Acid Structure

Like carbohydrates and fats, amino acids contain two or more carbon atoms linked together, but amino acids are different in that they contain nitrogen atoms. Recall that carbons must form four bonds with other atoms; oxygens, two; and hydrogens, one. Nitrogens must form three bonds with other atoms. The structures of all amino acids have three things in common: connected to a central carbon is an amino group (NH_2), an acid group (COOH), and a hydrogen (H). These three parts of the molecule are identical in all amino acids. The central carbon atom also has another atom or group of atoms attached to it, which varies from one amino acid to another.

The side chains on amino acids are what make proteins so varied in comparison with either carbohydrates or lipids. A polysaccharide (starch, for example) is composed of glucose units one after the other. It may be several thousand units long, but every unit in the chain is a glucose molecule just like all the others. In a protein, on the other hand, 22 different amino acids may appear, each differing from the others in the nature of its side chain.* The

Backbone of an amino acid. The asterisk denotes the central carbon.

-N-H
 |
 H

Amino Group

O
||
—C—O-H

Acid Group

---

*It is often said that there are 20 amino acids, but if cystine and ornithine are counted, there are 22. Amino acids sometimes occur in related forms (for example, proline can add an OH group to become hydroxyproline). Chemists can make still other amino acids. We have elected to present (in Appendix C) the structures of the 22 common amino acids as in Nomenclature policy: Abbreviated designations of amino acids, *Journal of Nutrition* 112 (1982): 15.

FIGURE 5–1

Examples of amino acids. Note that the side chains are different in each. The asterisk denotes the central carbon.

Alanine

Aspartic acid

Phenylalanine

simplest amino acid, glycine, has a hydrogen atom in that position. A slightly more complex amino acid, alanine, has an extra carbon with three attached hydrogen atoms. Other amino acids have still more complex side chains. For example, one amino acid may have an acid group, whereas another may have a basic amino group. Still others may have neutral side chains, including some complicated ring structures. These acidic, basic, and neutral groups confer different characteristics on the amino acids. Thus, although the amino acids all share a common starting structure, their properties differ (see Figure 5–1).

Glycine: the side chain is circled. The asterisk denotes the central carbon.

Amino Acid Sequence

Amino acids may be linked together in a great variety of ways to form proteins. They connect by means of a condensation reaction (see p. 58). An OH is removed from the acid end of one amino acid, and an H is removed from the amino group of another. A bond forms between the two amino acids, and the H and OH join to form a molecule of water. The resulting structure is a dipeptide (see Figure 5–2). By the same reaction, the OH can be removed from the acid end of the second amino acid and an H from the amino group of a third to form a tripeptide. As additional amino acids are added to the chain, a polypeptide is formed. Most proteins are polypeptides, 100 to 300 amino acids long.

It would be misleading, however, to end the description here, because in showing the structures on paper, we have drawn a straight, flat chain. Actually, polypeptide chains fold and tangle so that they look not like rods, but like crazy jungle gyms. The sequence of amino acids in a protein determines which specific way the chain will fold.

dipeptide: two amino acids bonded together. The bond between two amino acids is a **peptide bond**.
di = two
peptide = amino acid

tripeptide: three amino acids bonded together by peptide bonds.
tri = three

polypeptide: many (ten or more) amino acids bonded together by peptide bonds. An intermediate string of between four and ten amino acids is an **oligopeptide**.
poly = many
oligo = few

FIGURE 5–2

Formation of a dipeptide. A dipeptide forms as two amino acids are condensed, with the removal of a molecule of water. Condensation reactions have already been shown twice before (pp. 59, 94).

Folding of the Chain

You can best visualize the structure of a protein by keeping in mind that each amino acid side chain has special characteristics that attract it to other side chains. Some side chains are polar (charged), and are attracted to the charges around water molecules (hydrophilic). Other side chains are neutral, and are repelled by water. As amino acids are added to a growing polypeptide, the charged side chains, being hydrophilic, are attracted to positions on the outer surface of the completed protein. The neutral groups, being hydrophobic, tend to tuck themselves inside, away from water. The shape the polypeptide finally assumes is either roughly spherical or fibrous—whichever gives it the maximum stability in water. Finally, two or more of these giant molecules may associate to form a still larger working aggregate. Thus the completed protein is a tangled, complicated chain of amino acids, bristling on the surface with positive and negative charges. Sometimes two, three, or four such chains tangle together to make a giant protein molecule. Hemoglobin, shown in Figure 5–3, is one of the big proteins.

Large protein molecules are fragile; their conformation depends on constant conditions in their surroundings. When they are subjected to heat, acid, or other conditions that disturb their stability, they uncoil or change their shapes, losing their functions. You have seen many examples of this—in the hardening of an egg when it is cooked, in the curdling of milk when it is heated or made acid, and in the stiffening of egg whites when they are whipped.

The change in a protein's shape brought about by heat, acid, or other conditions is known as **denaturation**. Past a certain point, denaturation is irreversible.

There is present in plants and in animals a substance which . . . is without doubt the most important of all the known substances in living matter, and, without it, life would be impossible on our planet. This material has been named Protein.

Gerard Johannes Mulder (1838)

FIGURE 5–3.

The intricate structure of a protein molecule. This molecule represents one molecule of hemoglobin, magnified 27 million times.

The Completed Protein

If you could step onto a carbohydrate molecule like starch and walk along it, the first stepping stone would be a glucose. The next stepping stone would be glucose again, and then glucose, and then glucose, and then glucose. But if you were to walk along a polypeptide chain, your first stepping stone might be a methionine. Your second might be an alanine. The third might be a glycine, and the fourth a tryptophan, then another alanine, and so on. In other words, the units in a protein are varied in both their nature and the sequence in which they appear.

Another analogy compares the amino acids to letters in an alphabet. If you were to try to make a sentence using only the letter *G*, you could only speak gibberish: G-G-G-G-G-G. But with 20–odd different letters available, you can say, "To be, or not to be: that is the question"—or, on a different plane, "The way to a man's heart is through his stomach." The Greek alphabet contains only 24 letters, and all of Homer's work was written with it.

The variety of sequences in which the 22 amino acids can be linked together is even greater than that possible for letters in a sentence, because proteins do not have to be pronounced, as words do. This gives them a tremendous range of possible surface structures, which in turn enables them to perform distinct, individual, and specialized functions. The human body contains an estimated 10,000 to 50,000 different kinds of proteins. Of these thousands, only about 1,000 have been identified,[1] and only about 10 are described in this chapter.

Enzymes: A Function of Protein

When we first mentioned enzymes, we promised that we would look at these magnificent molecules more closely when protein structure had been explained. Let's start by looking at the enzyme maltase.

A typical protein, maltase is a tangled, ball-shaped polypeptide chain, 100 or so amino acids long. The little molecule maltose, on the other hand, is a disaccharide perhaps 100 times smaller. From the point of view of a maltose molecule, then, the enzyme maltase is very large. The small maltose molecule, encountering such an enzyme, would find itself snapping into position on the enzyme surface, a surface custom-designed to fit maltose's contours. On this surface, maltose would soon encounter a molecule of water; as its two glucose parts split apart, the water would also be split apart, its H being added to one glucose and its OH, to the other. Releasing the free glucose, the enzyme would attract other maltoses into that same position and hydrolyze them the same way.

Enzymes and what they do are so fundamental to all life processes that it seems worthwhile to introduce an analogy to clarify two important characteristics they all share. Enzymes are comparable to the clergy and judges who make and dissolve human matrimonial bonds. When two individuals come to a minister to be married, the couple leaves with a new bond between them. They are joined together—but the minister is only momentarily involved in the process

methionine (meth-EYE-oh-neen), **alanine** (AL-uh-neen), **tryptophan** (TRIP-toe-fane or TRIP-toe-fan): amino acids. A complete list of the amino acids, with their structures, appears in Appendix C.

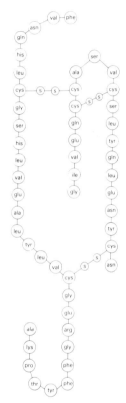

The complete amino acid sequence of insulin, a small protein. S-S represents the cross-links between cysteine molecules, known as disulfide bridges. (For structures and abbreviations of individual amino acids, see Appendix C.)

maltase: the enzyme that hydrolyzes maltose to two glucose units.

maltose: the disaccharide composed of two glucose units (see p. 63).

-ase: a word ending denoting an enzyme. The first part of the word usually identifies the compound the enzyme works on. Thus maltase is the enzyme that works on maltose.

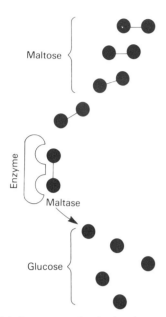

Model of enzyme action (maltase).

synthetase (SIN-the-tase): an enzyme that synthesizes compounds.

protease (PRO-tee-ase): an enzyme that hydrolyzes proteins.

lipase (LYE-pase): an enzyme that hydrolyzes lipids.

The definitions of **carbohydrase, disaccharidase, sucrase, lactase**, and **phospholipase** are self-evident.

catalyst (CAT-uh-list): a compound that facilitates chemical reactions without itself being changed in the process.

enzyme: a protein catalyst.

and remains unchanged. One minister can therefore perform thousands of marriage ceremonies. Similarly, a judge who facilitates the separation of married couples may decree many divorces before retiring or dying.

The minister represents enzymes that synthesize larger compounds from smaller ones—the synthetases, which build body structures. The judge represents enzymes that hydrolyze larger compounds to smaller ones—the proteases, lipases, carbohydrases, disaccharidases, and others. Maltase is a disaccharidase.

The first point to learn is that some enzymes put compounds together, and others take them apart. Since a person is a put-together organism, superbly organized out of billions of molecules designed to make muscle, bone, skin, eyes, and blood cells, you can imagine how numerous and active in the body are the enzymes that put things together. (It is incorrect to think of enzymes as being solely digestive enzymes—those that take things apart.)

The second point is that enzymes are not themselves affected in the process of facilitating chemical reactions. They are catalysts. Biologists and chemists define an enzyme as *a protein catalyst*.

What makes you different from any other human being is minute differences in your body proteins (enzymes, antibodies, and others). These differences are determined by the amino acid sequences of your proteins, which are written into the genetic code of the DNA you inherited from your parents and ancestors. Each person receives at conception a unique combination of genes (DNA codes for protein sequences). The genes direct the making of all the body's proteins, as shown in Figure 5–4. (To see how the protein synthesis machinery fits into the anatomy of a cell, turn to Appendix A.)

Perhaps you have realized by now that the protein story moves in a circle. All enzymes are proteins. All proteins are made of amino acids. Amino acids have to be put together to make proteins. Enzymes put together the amino acids. Only living systems work with such self-renewal. A broken toaster cannot be fixed by another toaster; a car cannot make another car. Only living creatures and the parts they are composed of—the cells—can duplicate themselves.

To follow the circle in nutrition, start with a person eating food proteins. The proteins are broken down in the stomach and intestines by proteins (digestive enzymes) into amino acids. The amino acids enter the cells of the body, where proteins (synthesizing enzymes) put them together in long chains with sequences specified by DNA. The chains fold and become enzymes themselves. These enzymes go to work breaking apart other compounds or putting other compounds together. Day by day, a billion reactions by a billion reactions, these processes repeat themselves, and life goes on.

A Closer Look at Enzyme Action

The following description is an example of the details of enzyme action. We present it to show you how these molecules really work and to give you an insight into the reasons why people need certain nutrients supplied in their foods.

In a biochemical pathway, each compound encounters an enzyme, is converted to another compound that encounters another enzyme, and so forth; the final product may be entirely different from the starting material. In the breakdown of glucose, a six-carbon compound, for example, enzymes add two phosphate groups, alter the arrangement of the atoms, and then split the molecule

FIGURE 5–4

Protein synthesis. The instructions for making every protein in a person's body are transmitted in the genetic information received at conception. This body of knowledge is filed away in the nucleus of every cell. The master file is the DNA (deoxyribonucleic acid), which never leaves the nucleus. The DNA is identical in every cell and is specific for each individual. Each specialized cell has access to the total inherited information but calls on only the instructions needed for its own functions.

To inform the cell of the proper sequence of amino acids for a needed protein, a "photocopy" of the appropriate portion of DNA is made. This copy is messenger RNA (ribonucleic acid), which is able to escape through the nuclear membrane. In the cell fluid it seeks out and attaches itself to one of the ribosomes (a protein-making machine, itself composed of RNA and protein). Thus situated, the messenger RNA presents the sequence in which the amino acids should be linked into a protein strand.

Meanwhile, another form of RNA, called transfer RNA, collects amino acids from the cell fluid and brings them to the messenger. For each of the 22 amino acids, there is a specific kind of transfer RNA. Thousands of these transfer RNAs, with their loads of amino acids, cluster around the ribosomes, like vegetable-laden trucks around a farmers' market awaiting their turn to unload. When an amino acid is called for by the messenger, the transfer RNA carrying it snaps into position. Then the next and the next and the next loaded transfer RNAs move into place. Thus the amino acids are lined up in the right sequence. Then an enzyme bonds them together.

Finally, the completed protein strand is released, the messenger is degraded, and the transfer RNAs are freed to return for another load. It takes many words to describe the events, but in the cell, 40 to 100 amino acids can be added to a growing protein strand in only a second.

A. DNA is in the nucleus of each cell.

B. DNA makes a copy of the portion of itself that has the instructions for the protein the cell needs.

C. RNA leaves the nucleus.

Protein-making Machinery (Ribosome)

D. RNA attaches itself to the protein-making machinery of the cell.

Messenger RNA
Transfer RNA
Amino Acid 1
Amino Acid 2
Amino Acid 3

E. Transfer RNAs carry their amino acids to the messenger RNA, where they are snapped into place.

Protein Strand

F. The completed protein strand is released.

Intermediates in Carbohydrate Metabolism:

Compound A

Compound B

Compound C

in half so that two three-carbon compounds result. One of these is compound A (shown in the margin). The other is converted to compound A, so that the two halves derived from glucose go through an identical process from that point on. Let us look closely at the pathway for four steps thereafter, starting with compound A.

Compound A floats around until it encounters an enzyme that recognizes it. This enzyme has the specialized function of removing hydrogen atoms from molecules of compound A. The encounter results in the altered compound, compound B.

Compound B is released from the enzyme and encounters another enzyme, whose sole mission in life is to remove oxygens from compound B and to substitute amino groups in their place. What results is compound C. The next enzyme removes the phosphate group from the end carbon and replaces it with a hydrogen, leaving compound D.

```
           H
           |
           N - H
      H    |     O
           |     ||
 H-O — C — C — C — O-H
      |    |
      H    H
    Compound D
```

```
      H
      |
    H-N    O
      |    ||
 H-C — C — O-H
      |
      H
    Compound E
```

If you look closely at the picture of compound D, you may recognize its characteristics and not be surprised by the statements that follow. But let us take the process one more step. Another enzyme, whose function is to remove CH_2OH groups from these molecules, forms compound E. Look at this product closely; you have seen it before. It has an amino group at one end, an acid group at the other, and a central carbon carrying two hydrogen atoms. It is the amino acid glycine (p. 135).*

Amazing! The cellular machinery started with a molecule of glucose (a derivative of dietary carbohydrate), made one minute change after another, and transformed it into an amino acid (a member of the protein family).

The lesson to learn from this sequence of events is that the body can make, from glucose and nitrogen-containing compounds, many of the amino acids needed to build body proteins. The amino acid glycine is just one example. Compound D, which precedes glycine on the pathway, is another example: it is the amino acid serine. Thus, among the thousands of tasks that enzymes perform, they even manufacture many of the amino acids they themselves are made of.

Other Roles of Protein

Although the following discussion focuses on protein's roles in the body, other nutrients (vitamins and minerals) cooperate in its tasks. Margin references in this section introduce you to these other nutrients, and later chapters then provide full details on their roles.

Fluid and Acid-Base Balances

Proteins help maintain the body's fluid balance. Fluid is present in several body compartments, chief among them are the space inside the blood vessels; the spaces within the cells; and the spaces between the cells, outside the blood vessels. Fluids flow back and forth between these compartments, and proteins in the fluids, together with minerals, help to maintain the needed distribution of these fluids.

The reasons why proteins in fluids can help determine their distribution in living systems are that proteins are large and attractive to water (hydrophilic). Being large, they cannot pass freely across the membranes that separate the compartments; they are trapped where they are. Being hydrophilic, they keep water molecules near them, which in effect makes them even larger. A cell that "wants" to keep a certain amount of water in its interior space can't move the water around, directly, but it can manufacture proteins to keep inside itself, and those proteins will hold water. Thus the cell uses protein to regulate the distribution of water indirectly. Similarly, the body makes proteins to keep in the

The balance referred to—fluid and electrolyte balance—is fully discussed in Chapter 11.

Minerals are helper nutrients. The attractiveness of protein and mineral particles to water is osmotic pressure; see Chapter 11.

---

*The enzyme that produced compound B was a dehydrogenase; the next enzyme, a transaminase; and the next, a phosphatase.

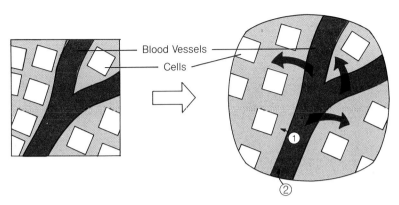

Normal tissue.

Swollen tissue.

Blood Vessels
Cells

FIGURE 5–5

Edema.

1. Fluid leaks into the spaces between the cells.

2. Vascular fluid is replenished (for example, by drinking more) so total vascular fluid remains the same. Total body fluid is now greater but the kidneys don't detect this and don't excrete the excess. The result: swollen tissue. Edema has many causes.

Normal foot and ankle.

Swollen tissue of edema. A thumbprint pressed into the flesh stays there; the fluid flows sluggishly because it is caught between the cells.

bloodstream and in the intercellular spaces, and these proteins help maintain the fluid volume in those spaces.

It once was thought that protein deficiency causes edema, the accumulation of fluid in the spaces between the cells (Figure 5–5 diagrams edema). Now it is known that either can occur without the other.[2] Clearly, other nutrients besides protein, as well as hormones that are affected by malnutrition, are involved in the causation of edema.

Another balance that proteins help maintain is that between acids and bases within the body's fluids. An acid solution is one in which hydrogen ions abound. The more hydrogen ions, the more concentrated the acid. Proteins (and minerals), which have negative charges on their surfaces, attract hydrogen ions, and hydrogen ions in turn attract proteins. As long as the concentration of hydrogen ions—that is, the strength of the acid—stays within certain limits, the proteins maintain their integrity. If the acid becomes too strong, however, the extra positive charges neutralize some of the negative charges on the proteins, changing their internal interactive forces and, so to speak, pulling them out of shape. When this happens, the proteins can no longer function.

Of all the consequences that stem from exceeding the normal limits of the acid-base balance, the most direct and serious is a disturbance of the shapes of the proteins that carry out so many vital body functions. Acidosis and alkalosis can both be lethal if unchecked. The proteins in the plasma, such as albumin, help to prevent these conditions from arising. In a sense, the proteins protect one another by binding or sequestering extra hydrogen ions when there are too many in the surrounding medium and by releasing them when there are too few. This ability to regulate the acidity of the medium is known as the buffering action of proteins.

edema (eh-DEEM-uh): accumulation of fluid in the spaces between the cells. Edema in the abdomen is **ascites** (a-SITE-eez).

acid-base balance: the balance maintained in the body between too much and too little acid. See Chapter 11.

acidosis: too much acid in the blood and body fluids.

alkalosis: too much base in the blood and body fluids.

lethal: causing death.

sequester (see-KWESS-ter): to hide away or take out of circulation.

buffer: a compound that can help keep a solution's acidity or alkalinity constant. See Chapter 11.

diuretic (dye-yoo-RET-ic): a drug that stimulates increased renal water excretion. *renal* = kidney

Development of immunity.

A. The body is challenged with foreign invaders.

B. The body makes the code for manufacturing the antibody.

C. The code makes the antibody.

D. The antibody inactivates the foreign invader.

E. The code remains to make antibodies faster the next time this foreign invader attacks.

The uninformed person may believe that the way to prevent the swelling of edema is to drink less water or to increase excretion by taking a diuretic. If edema has become extreme, these measures, as well as salt restriction, may indeed be a necessary part of treatment. Yet you normally will not cause edema by drinking too much water. The more you drink, the more the kidneys excrete.

This fact illustrates a principle that pervades physiology. The body maintains its own health. Provided that you are healthy to begin with, no drug can render your body more so. Diuretics are not useful as preventive medicine.

The taking of a diuretic does increase water excretion, though, so it causes a sudden weight loss. A person who fails to distinguish between loss of body fat and loss of water may see this as a desirable effect and start using diuretics for this purpose. But because the only loss induced is water loss, the only achievement gained is temporary dehydration.

In edema, water has leaked out of the blood into the tissues and caused swelling. This water is not available to the kidneys to excrete; they can only excrete what is in the bloodstream, which travels through them. Hence the remedy is not to drink less water, but to obtain an accurate diagnosis of the cause of the edema so as to deal with it at its source.

Antibodies and Hormones

Other major proteins found in the blood—the antibodies—act against disease agents. When a body is invaded by a virus—whether it is one that causes flu, smallpox, measles, or the common cold—the virus enters the cells and multiplies there. One virus may produce 100 replicas of itself within an hour or so. These burst out and invade 100 different cells, soon yielding 10,000 virus particles, which invade 10,000 cells. After several hours there may be a million viruses, then 100 million, and so on. If they were left free to do their worst, they would soon overwhelm the body with the disease they cause.

The antibodies, giant protein molecules circulating in the blood, present a defense against viruses, bacteria, and other "foreign agents." Each type of antibody molecule is different and specific, able to combine with and inactivate a specific foreign protein, such as that in a virus coat or bacterial cell membrane. The antibodies work so efficiently that in a normal, healthy individual, the many disease agents that attempt to attack never have a chance to get started. If a million bacterial cells are injected into the skin of a healthy person, fewer than ten are likely to survive for five hours.[3]

Once the body has manufactured antibodies against a particular disease agent (such as the measles virus), the cells never forget how to produce them. The next time that virus invades the body, the antibodies will respond even more quickly. Thus the body acquires immunity against the diseases it is exposed to, by virtue of the molecular memory of the antibody-producing cells.

Hormones are also carried by the blood, and some are made of amino acids. Among them are the thyroid hormone and insulin. The thyroid hormone regulates the body's metabolic rate—the rate of the chemical reactions that yield energy. Insulin regulates the concentration of the blood glucose and its transportation into cells, upon which the functioning of the brain and the nervous system depend. Hormones have many other profound effects, which will become evident as you read further.

Transport Proteins

A special group of the body's proteins specializes in moving nutrients and other molecules into and out of cells. These proteins reside in the membranes of every cell of the body, and each is specific for a certain compound or group of related compounds. Most of these proteins are confined to the cell membranes but can rotate or shuttle from one side to the other. Thus they act as "pumps," picking up compounds on one side of the membrane, depositing them on the other, and thereby permitting the cells to "decide" what substances to take up and what to release.

Examples of well-known transport proteins are the glucose, potassium, and sodium pumps. The first two transport glucose and potassium into cells faster than they can leak out; the sodium pump transports sodium out of cells faster than it can leak in. Thanks to these pumps, higher concentrations of glucose and potassium and a lower concentration of sodium are maintained inside the cells than in the surrounding medium. Laboratory scientists know they are observing pumps at work whenever they find a cell maintaining a concentration gradient of a substance across its membrane. These gradients are of great importance to cells. For example, the sodium-potassium distribution across the membranes of nerve cells makes it possible for nerve impulses to travel—and so for you to think and act.

The mineral calcium enters the body with the help of a protein, too—the calcium-binding protein in the intestinal tract. In fact, almost every water-soluble nutrient seems to have its own transport system in cell membranes. (By contrast, lipids can cross membranes without the help of pumps. A cell can regulate a lipid's distribution by trapping it once it gets where it belongs. The cell attaches the lipid to a protein or other molecule so that it *cannot* move freely across membranes any more.)

The cell membranes' protein machinery can be switched on or off in response to the body's needs. Often hormones do the switching, with a marvelous precision. A familiar example is provided by insulin and glucose. When there is too much glucose in the blood, the pancreas steps up its output of the hormone insulin; the insulin stimulates the cells to take up glucose (and is destroyed in the process); the cells pick up the excess glucose; then, when the blood glucose concentration is normal, the pancreas reduces its insulin output. The blood concentration of calcium is regulated in a similar manner by the hormones calcitonin and parathormone. Hundreds of other body proteins maintain the distribution of hundreds of other substances in the various body spaces.

Other transport proteins, not attached to membranes, move about in the body fluids carrying nutrients and other molecules from one organ to another. You have already read about the lipoproteins, which transport the cumbersome lipid molecules from place to place; the fat-soluble vitamins are also carried by special proteins, and many carriers for the water-soluble vitamins are also becoming known.

antibody: a large protein of the blood and body fluids, produced in response to the invasion of the body by unfamiliar molecules (mostly proteins); it inactivates the invaders and so protects the body.

The thyroid hormone contains iodine, and insulin associates with zinc; these minerals are helper nutrients (see Chapter 12). For a description of many hormones important in nutrition, see Appendix A.

These membrane-associated proteins are variously called **permeases**, **vectorial enzymes**, and **transferases**.

concentration gradient: a difference in concentration of a **solute** (SOLL-yoot), a dissolved substance, on two sides of a selectively permeable membrane.

Calcium concentration is tightly controlled by hormones, as described in Chapter 11.

Lipoproteins: see Chapter 4.

The mineral iron is a nutrient whose handling in the body illustrates especially well how precisely proteins operate. Upon moving into a cell of the intestinal wall, iron is captured by a protein residing in the cell, which will not let go of it unless the iron is needed in the body. Iron leaving the cell to enter the bloodstream is attached to a carrier protein. The carrier, in turn, can pass iron on to a storage protein in the bone marrow or other tissues, which will hold it until it is called for. Then, when it is needed, iron is incorporated into the structure of still another protein in the red blood cells, where it assists in oxygen transport, or into a muscle protein, which helps muscle cells oxidize their energy fuels. At least one protein is similarly involved in the body's handling of calcium. One of this protein's many roles is to relay to cells a sort of message conveyed from other parts of the body by calcium ions.

The protein residing in the intestinal wall cells is **ferritin**; the carrier protein, **transferrin**; the storage protein, **ferritin** again; the red blood cell protein, **hemoglobin**, and the muscle cell protein, **myoglobin**.

The protein that relays calcium's messages is **calmodulin**. See Chapter 11.

Blood Clotting

Blood is unique and wonderful in its ability to remain a liquid tissue even though it carries so many large molecules and cells through the circulatory system. But blood can also turn solid within seconds when the integrity of that system is disturbed. (If it did not clot, a single pinprick could drain your entire body of all its blood, just as a tiny hole in a bucket makes the bucket forever useless for holding water.) When you cut yourself, a rapid chain of events leads to the production of fibrin, a stringy, insoluble mass of protein fibers that plugs the cut and stops the leak. Later, more slowly, a scar forms to replace the clot and permanently heal the cut.

The chain of events is as follows:
1. A phospholipid (**thromboplastin**) is released from blood platelets (small, cell-fragment-like structures in the blood).
2. Thromboplastin catalyzes the conversion of **prothrombin** (a precursor protein made in the liver that circulates in the blood) to **thrombin**.
3. Thrombin then catalyzes the conversion of **fibrinogen** (another circulating precursor protein) to **fibrin**.
   thrombo = clot
   fibr = fibers
   ogen = gives rise to

Vitamin K (involved in the production of prothrombin) and calcium (needed for the blood to clot) are helper nutrients.

Connective Tissue

Proteins help make scar tissue, bones, and teeth. When the construction of a bone or a tooth begins, bone-building cells first lay down a scaffolding made of the protein collagen. Later, they lay down crystals of calcium, phosphorus, fluoride, and other minerals on this matrix to form the hardened bone. When a bone breaks, the bone-building cells begin mending the break by molding a collagen matrix, then laying down the bony material. Collagen is also the mending material in torn tissue, forming scars to hold the separated parts together. It is the material of ligaments and tendons and is a strengthening glue between the cells of the artery walls that helps enable them to withstand the pressure of surging heartbeats.

collagen: the protein material of which scars, tendons, ligaments, and the foundations of bones and teeth are made.
kolla = glue

Vitamin C (needed to form collagen) and minerals (to calcify bones and teeth) are helper nutrients.

Visual Pigments

The light-sensitive pigments in the cells of the retina are molecules of the protein opsin. Opsin responds to light by changing its shape, thus initiating the nerve impulses that convey the sense of sight to the higher centers of the brain.

The list of protein functions here is by no means exhaustive, but it does give some sense of the immense variety and importance of proteins in the body. With this information as background, you are in a position to appreciate the significance of the world's most serious malnutrition problem: protein-kcalorie malnutrition, described later in this chapter.

opsin: the protein of the visual pigments. Vitamin A is a helper nutrient, attached to opsin to form the pigment rhodopsin.

Protein Quality

The role of protein in food is not to provide body proteins directly, but to supply the amino acids from which the body can make its own proteins. Since the body can make glycine and serine for itself, the proteins in the diet need not contain these two amino acids. But there are some amino acids the body can't make at all, and some it can't make fast enough to meet its need. (This is because the body does not possess the genes for the enzymes that could synthesize these amino acids, or because the enzymes it does make work too slowly.) These are the nine essential amino acids. The amino acid arginine is not essential, nor will it serve as a "growth hormone releaser" to make you dream away inches while you sleep.[4]

To make body protein, a cell must have all the needed amino acids available simultaneously. The first important characteristic of a diet with respect to protein is, therefore, that it should supply at least the nine essential amino acids and enough nitrogen for the synthesis of the others.

People usually eat many foods containing protein; each food has its own characteristic amino acid balance; and together, they almost invariably supply more than enough protein and plenty of each individual amino acid. This is true, at least, for those of us privileged to live in the developed countries today, where the food supply is reliable, abundant, and varied. It has not always been true in the past, and even today in most of the world, the protein supply is a crucial factor determining the quality of people's diets and their nutritional health. Where protein-rich foods are scarce and only one is eaten regularly, the quality of that particular food protein is critical to life and health. Therefore, food proteins are tested individually to determine their adequacy for nourishing people who may have to rely on limited amounts of single foods to meet their amino acid needs.

A complete protein is defined as a protein that contains all of the essential amino acids in amounts adequate for human use; it may or may not contain all the others. A high-quality protein is not merely complete; it contains the essential amino acids in amounts proportional to the body's need for them; and it is digestible, so that sufficient numbers of these amino acids reach the body's cells to permit them to make the proteins they need.

Ideally, a diet will supply each amino acid in at least the amount needed for protein synthesis in the body. If one amino acid is supplied in an amount smaller than is needed, the total amount of protein that can be synthesized from the others will be limited. Partial proteins are not made, only complete ones; there is an all-or-none law of protein synthesis. By analogy, suppose that a sign maker plans to make 100 identical signs, each saying LEFT TURN ONLY. He needs 200 *L*s, 200 *N*s, 200 *T*s, and 100 of each of the other letters. If he has only 20 *L*s, he can make only 10 signs, even if all the other letters are available in unlimited quantities. The *L*s limit the number of signs that can be made. Furthermore, the sign maker has no place to keep leftover letters (the body has no storage place for extra amino acids), so if he doesn't get more *L*s right away, he will have to throw away all his other letters.

People eat many different foods containing protein.

complete protein: a protein containing all the amino acids essential in human nutrition in amounts adequate for human use.

high-quality protein: an easily digestible, complete protein whose amino acids fit the pattern needed by human beings.

The sign maker has run out of *L*s, so he can't complete his sign (LEFT TURN ONLY). Similarly, if one essential amino acid is missing, the body can't complete its proteins.

limiting amino acid: the essential amino acid found in the shortest supply relative to the amounts needed for protein synthesis in the body.

A diet that contains an imbalance of amino acids so severe as to limit body protein synthesis is said to be a diet containing protein of poor quality. When the body attempts to use the amino acid supply from such a diet, it wastes many amino acids, because, in the absence of one, it can't use the others—and it has no place to store them. Enzymes strip off the nitrogen-containing amino groups and fix them into the compound urea, which is excreted in the urine. Only the carbon chains remain, and these are used to make glucose or fat, or are oxidized for energy. Urea excreted comes partly from amino acids not retained from food proteins (not built into body proteins) and partly from the breakdown of body protein tissues.

How urea is made: see Chapter 7.

The quality of dietary protein depends not only on whether the protein supplies a balance of the essential amino acids, but also, as mentioned, on the protein's digestibility. An excellent protein by these standards is egg protein, whose nitrogen tends to be retained in the body. Egg protein has been designated the reference protein and has been assigned a biological value of 100 by the Food and Agriculture Organization (FAO) of the United Nations, which sets world standards. In our society, most people consume plenty of protein—in fact, perhaps too much, and eggs don't offer any particular value to our diet. In less-developed nations, though, eggs are valuable. They offer high-quality protein, so that a little goes a long way in a diet that may be marginal or low in protein otherwise. They are relatively inexpensive, and they store well.

digestibility: a measure of the amount of amino acids absorbed from a given protein intake. To learn why "predigested" protein is less digestible than whole protein, even though it is delivered to the body in small fragments, turn to p. 180.

reference protein: egg protein; used by FAO/WHO as a standard against which to measure the quality of other proteins.

Nitrogen Balance Studies

Proteins are needed for the growth and maintenance of all body tissues. Whenever you take a bath, you wash off whole cells from the surface layers of your skin, losing protein. The cells that manufacture hair and fingernails have to synthesize new protein constantly to go into these structures; these processes also result in a net loss of body protein. Protein losses also occur inside your body. When you swallow food, it passes down your intestinal tract. Ultimately, the undigested materials—fiber, water, and waste—leave your body, carrying with them cells that have been shed from the intestinal lining. Both inside and outside you must constantly build new cells to replace those lost from the exposed surfaces. In fact, it is said that a person's skin is replaced totally every seven years.

In addition, proteins are continuously being dismantled in every organ and tissue inside the body. When they break down, they free amino acids to join the general circulation. Some of these may be promptly recycled into body organs; some are deaminated and their amino groups excreted. The constant flux of amino acids from one organ to another by way of the body fluids is known as protein turnover; the protein that participates in this flux is endogenous protein.

protein turnover: the exchange of amino acids among organs within the body.

endogenous protein: the protein in the body.
endo = within
gen = arising

Given either fat or carbohydrate as an energy source, the body can construct many of the materials needed to replace lost cells. But to rebuild protein, the body must eat protein for two reasons: first, because food protein is the only source of the essential amino acids; and secondly, because it is the only practical source of amino nitrogen with which to build the nonessential amino acids.

If the body is growing, it must manufacture more cells than are lost. Children end each day with more blood cells, more muscle cells, and more skin cells than they had at the beginning of the day. So protein is needed both for routine maintenance (replacement) and growth (addition) of body tissue.

The quantity of protein you need depends on the amount of lean tissue in your body. Fat tissue requires relatively little protein to maintain itself, but the muscles, blood, and other metabolically active tissues must be maintained by a continuous supply of essential amino acids. To determine how much protein people need, laboratory scientists have performed nitrogen balance studies.

Protein is the only one of the three energy-yielding nutrients that contains nitrogen. Nitrogen is easy to measure, so it serves as a convenient indicator of the location and amount of protein in food, in the body, and in excreted waste. Nitrogen balance, therefore, indirectly reflects the amount of protein retained and used for protein synthesis.

Normally, healthy adults are in nitrogen equilibrium—they have at all times the same amount of total protein in their bodies. When nitrogen-in exceeds nitrogen-out, they are said to be in positive nitrogen balance; when nitrogen-in is less than nitrogen-out, they are in negative balance. These balances reflect a wide variety of physiological states of the body, both in health and in disease.

Growing children and pregnant women are in positive nitrogen balance; every day they are adding to their bodies new blood, bone, and muscle cells that contain protein. (When a woman gives birth, she suddenly loses most of the protein she has helped her baby to accumulate.) When a woman is lactating, she is in nitrogen equilibrium, but it is a sort of enhanced equilibrium: she is both eating more protein, and excreting more protein in her milk, than before she was pregnant. In contrast, people who are sick are often in negative nitrogen balance; when they have to rest in bed for a long time, their muscles atrophy, and the protein-nitrogen that escapes is excreted in the urine. A circumstance in which positive nitrogen balance might also reflect illness is in kidney disease: an accumulation of urea nitrogen in the blood then reflects a failure of excretion. Negative nitrogen balance in such a case would reflect recovery.

Nitrogen balance studies enable researchers to test the quality of various food proteins. Protein from a single food source is fed (together with adequate kcalories from other foods) in a quantity that would be adequate to meet the body's needs if the protein's amino acid supply were similar to that of egg protein. If, under these conditions, the body starts losing nitrogen, then something is wrong with the protein. Either it isn't being well digested—so that its nitrogen is being excreted in the feces—or it has one or more limiting essential amino acids. If the problem is a limiting essential amino acid, then additional nitrogen will be lost. Lacking enough of some one amino acid to make the proteins they need, the body cells break down the other amino acids they can't use. They derive energy from the carbon skeletons, much as they do from carbohydrate or fat, but they release the amino nitrogens into the bloodstream as the compound ammonia. The liver picks up the ammonia, converts it into urea, a less toxic compound, and returns that to the blood. Finally, the kidneys filter the urea out of the bloodstream; thus, the amino nitrogen ends up in the urine as urea.

Measures of Protein Quality:
1. Chemical Scoring

The simplest way to evaluate a food protein's quality is to study the amino acid composition of the protein itself, in the laboratory. The amino acid composition of a test protein can be compared with the composition of egg protein, and a chemical score can be derived to express the theoretical value of the test protein.

nitrogen balance: the amount of nitrogen consumed (N in) as compared with the amount of nitrogen excreted (N out) in a given period of time. The average amino acid weighs about 6.25 times as much as the nitrogen it contains, so the laboratory scientist can estimate the amount of protein in a sample of food, body tissue, or excreta by multiplying the weight of the nitrogen in it by 6.25.

Nitrogen equilibrium (zero nitrogen balance): N in = N out.
Positive nitrogen balance: N in > N out.
Negative nitrogen balance: N in < N out.

Three terms are used to describe nitrogen excreted from the body: **endogenous** (en-DODGE-en-us) **nitrogen**, meaning "from inside the body," **metabolic nitrogen**, meaning from the intestinal cells, and **exogenous** (ex-ODGE-en-us) **nitrogen**, meaning "from outside the body"—that is, from food. The nitrogen in urine is of two kinds—some from broken-down body proteins (endogenous) and some from food amino acids that got as far as the cells but then didn't get used (exogenous). The nitrogen in feces is also of two kinds—some from intestinal cells and some from food.

chemical score: a rating of the quality of a test protein arrived at by comparing its amino acid pattern with that of a reference protein.

A test protein with a limiting amino acid that is present in only 70 percent of the amount found in egg protein, for example, would receive a chemical score of 70. If you fed the test protein to human beings under carefully controlled conditions in which the total protein fed was just enough to meet the requirements, you would expect that nitrogen would be excreted in the urine equal in quantity to 30 percent of the nitrogen fed. Table 5–1 shows how to use a reference pattern for the nine essential amino acids.

In a world where food is scarce and where many people's diets contain marginal or inadequate amounts of protein, it is important to know which foods contain the highest-quality protein. It is possible to determine the amino acid composition of any protein relatively inexpensively, but unfortunately, chemical scoring does not always reflect accurately the way the body will use a protein. The advantages of chemical scoring are that it is simple and inexpensive, it identifies in one step the limiting amino acid, and it can be used to score mixtures of different proportions of two or more proteins mathematically without having to make them up and test them. Its chief weaknesses are that it fails to predict the digestibility of a protein, which may strongly affect its quality; it relies on a chemical procedure in which certain amino acids may be destroyed, so that the pattern that is analyzed may lack accuracy; and it is blind to other features

TABLE 5–1

A Reference Pattern for Chemical Scoring of Proteins

Essential Amino Acids	Whole Egg Mg Amino Acid per g Nitrogen
Histidine	145
Isoleucine	340
Leucine	540
Lysine	440
Methionine + cystine[a]	355
Phenylalanine + tyrosine[b]	580
Threonine	294
Tryptophan	106
Valine	410
Total	3,210

[a]Methionine is essential and is also used to make cystine. Thus the methionine requirement is lower if cystine is supplied.

[b]Phenylalanine is essential and is also used to make tyrosine if there is not enough of the latter. Thus the phenylalanine requirement is lower if tyrosine is also supplied.

Note: To interpret the table, read, "For every 3,210 units of essential amino acids, 145 must be histidine, 340 must be isoleucine, 540 must be leucine, and so on." To compare a test protein with the reference protein, the experimenter would first obtain a chemical analysis of the test protein's amino acids. Then, taking 3,210 units of the amino acids, she would compare the amount of each to the amount found in 3,210 units of essential amino acids in egg protein. For example, suppose the test protein contained (per 3,210 units) 360 units of isoleucine; 500 units of leucine; 350 of lysine; and for each of the other amino acids, more units than egg protein contains. The two amino acids that are low are leucine (500 as compared with 540 in egg) and lysine (350 versus 440 in egg). The ratio, amino acid in test protein divided by amino acid in egg, is 500/540 (or about 0.93) for leucine and 350/440 (or about 0.80) for lysine. Lysine is the limiting amino acid (lowest ratio compared with egg), so the test protein receives a chemical score of 80.

of the test protein, such as the presence of toxic materials, that would only be revealed by a test in living animals.

2. Biological Value

To determine the actual value of a protein as it is used by the body, it is necessary to measure not only urinary, but also fecal, losses of nitrogen when that protein is actually fed to human beings under test conditions. (Even then, small additional losses from sweat, shed skin, hair, and fingernails will be missed.) This kind of experiment determines the biological value (BV) of proteins, a measure used internationally. The biological values of the proteins in some sample foods are shown in the margin. Generally, a biological value of 70 or above indicates acceptable quality.

In a test of biological value, two nitrogen balance studies are done. In the first, no protein is fed, and nitrogen (N) excretions in the urine and feces are measured. It is assumed that, under these conditions, N lost in the urine is the amount the body always necessarily loses by filtration into the urine each day, regardless of what protein is fed (endogenous N). The N lost in the feces (called metabolic N in the equation) is the amount the body invariably loses into the intestine each day, whether or not food protein is fed. (To help you remember terms: endogenous N is "urinary N on a 0–protein diet"; metabolic N is "fecal N on a 0–protein diet.")

In the second study, an amount of protein slightly below the requirement is fed. Intake and losses are measured. The BV is then derived using this formula:

$$BV = \frac{\{Food\ N - (fecal\ N - metabolic\ N) - (urinary\ N - endogenous\ N)\}}{Food\ N - (fecal\ N - metabolic\ N)} \times 100.$$

The denominator of this equation expresses the amount of nitrogen *absorbed*: food N minus fecal N (excluding the N the body would lose in the feces anyway, even without food). The numerator expresses the amount of N *retained* from the N absorbed: absorbed N (as in the denominator) minus the N excreted in the urine (excluding the N the body would lose in the urine anyway, even without food). Thus it can be more simply expressed:

$$BV = \frac{N\ retained}{N\ absorbed} \times 100.$$

This method has the advantage of being based on experiments with human beings (it can be done with animals, too, of course) and of measuring actual nitrogen retention. But it is also cumbersome, expensive, and often impractical and is based on many assumptions that may not be valid. For example, the subjects used for testing may not be similar physiologically or in terms of their normal environment or typical food intake to those for whom the test protein may ultimately be used. For another example, the fact that protein is retained in the body does not necessarily mean that it is being well utilized. There is considerable exchange of protein among tissues (protein turnover) which is hidden from view when only N intake and output are measured. One tissue could be shorted, and the test of biological value wouldn't detect this.

biological value (BV): the amount of protein nitrogen that is retained from a given amount of protein nitrogen that has been digested and absorbed; a measure of protein quality.

Biological Values of Proteins
Egg	100
Rice	86
Fish	75 to 90
Corn	40

3. Net Protein Utilization

net protein utilization (NPU): the amount of protein nitrogen that is retained from a given amount of protein nitrogen eaten; a measure of protein quality.

Like measurements of BV, determinations of net protein utilization (NPU) involve two balance studies, one on zero and the other on submaximal nitrogen intake. The formula for NPU is:

$$NPU = \frac{\text{Food N} - (\text{fecal N} - \text{metabolic N}) - (\text{urinary N} - \text{endogenous N})}{\text{Food N}} \times 100.$$

The numerator is the same as it is for BV, but the denominator represents food N intake only—not absorbed N. More simply expressed,

$$NPU = \frac{\text{N retained}}{\text{N intake}}.$$

This method has advantages similar to those of BV determinations and is more frequently used, employing animals as the test subjects. A drawback is that if a low NPU is obtained, the test results offer no help in distinguishing between two possible causes: a poor amino acid composition of the test protein or poor digestibility. There is also a limit to the extent to which animal test results can be assumed to be applicable to human beings.

4. Protein Efficiency Ratio

protein efficiency ratio (PER): the grams of weight gained by growing animals per gram of protein fed; a measure of protein quality.

The protein efficiency ratio (PER) is the best-known procedure for evaluating protein quality and is used in the United States as the basis for regulations regarding food labeling and for the protein RDA. Young rats are fed a measured amount of protein and weighed periodically as they grow. The PER is expressed as:

$$PER = \frac{\text{Weight gain (g)}}{\text{Protein intake (g)}}.$$

This method has the virtues of economy and simplicity, but it also has many drawbacks. The experiments are time-consuming; the amino acid needs of rats are not the same as for human beings; and the amino acid needs for growth are not the same as for the maintenance of adult animals (growing animals need more lysine, for example).

The PER is used to qualify statements about daily protein requirements in the United States. You are assumed to eat protein with a PER equal to or better than that of the milk protein casein; if the protein's PER is lower, you need more of the protein. Food labels have to take protein quality into consideration, using the PER of casein as a reference point. If the protein in the package has a PER as great as or greater than that of casein, then 45 grams of that protein is considered to be 100 percent of the U.S. RDA. If its PER is less than that of casein, then there have to be 65 grams of it to meet 100 percent of the U.S. RDA.

For those who choose not to tangle with the formulas for BV and PER, a convenient way to distinguish among proteins is to think of animal proteins as being generally of higher quality than plant proteins. However, the educated

Like all generalizations, the statement that "animal proteins are generally of higher quality" does not quite stand up to close inspection. At least one animal protein is truly incomplete: gelatin. It is low in tryptophan to begin with, and because tryptophan is heat sensitive, it loses what little it does have during processing. Ironically, this is the protein often recommended for correcting cracked nails and dull or brittle hair. The logic is that because these tissues are made of protein, a drink of protein will improve their texture. Even if this were the case, however—and a symptom, you remember, is not a deficiency disease— gelatin supplements would help only if protein containing tryptophan had already been supplied. And if that protein were complete, then the gelatin would not be needed!

vegetarian can design a perfectly acceptable diet around plant foods alone (see this chapter's highlight).

There is one circumstance in which dietary protein—no matter how high the quality—will not be used efficiently by the body and will not support growth: when energy from other energy nutrients is lacking. The body assigns top priority to meeting its energy need, and when no kcalories from other sources are available, it will break down body protein to meet this need. After stripping off the amino nitrogen, it will use the carbon skeletons of amino acids in much the same way it uses those from glucose or from fat. The major reason why it is necessary to have ample carbohydrate and fat in the diet is to prevent this wasting of protein.

Other conditions also affect the body's use of protein. In brief, to be used with maximum efficiency, a protein must contain a suitable amino acid pattern, must be digestible, must be consumed with sufficient kcalories from other sources so that it will not be sacrificed for energy, must be accompanied by the needed vitamins and minerals to facilitate its use, and must be received by a body that is healthy and equipped to use it.

Carbohydrate and fat allow amino acids to be used to build body proteins. This is known as the **protein-sparing action** of carbohydrate and fat.

Energy value of protein: 1 g provides 4 kcal.

Cooking with moist heat leaves proteins digestible, whereas charring reduces digestibility.

protein-kcalorie malnutrition: a deficiency of protein, kcalories, or both, often referred to as **PCM**; also **PEM**, for **protein-energy malnutrition**.

kwashiorkor (kwash-ee-OR-core, kwash-ee-or-CORE): malnutrition caused by protein deficiency in the presence of adequate kcalories.

marasmus (ma-RAZZ-mus): malnutrition caused by inadequate kcalories.

Protein-kCalorie Malnutrition

Protein and kcalories (energy) are involved in every body function. When children are deprived of food and suffer a kcalorie deficit, they degrade their own body protein for energy and thus indirectly suffer a protein deficiency as well as an energy deficiency. Protein and kcalorie malnutrition thus go hand in hand— so often that public health officials have adopted an abbreviation for the overlapping pair: PCM. Cases are observed at both ends of the spectrum, however. The classic protein deficiency disease is kwashiorkor, and the kcalorie deficiency disease is marasmus.

Kwashiorkor: the sickness that invades the first child when the second child is born.

gruel: a thin porridge made by boiling a meal of grains or legumes in water.

Kwashiorkor

The word *kwashiorkor* originally meant "the evil spirit that infects the first child when the second child is born." It is easy to see how this superstitious belief arose among the Ghanaians who named the disease. When a mother who has been breastfeeding her first child bears a second child, she weans the first and puts the second on the breast. The first child soon begins to sicken and die, just as if an evil spirit had accompanied the new baby into the world and set out to destroy the older child. What actually happens, of course, is that protein deficiency follows soon after weaning. Breast milk provides a child with sufficient protein, but the child is generally weaned to a starchy, protein-poor gruel. The gruel does not supply enough amino acids even to maintain a child's body, much less enough to enable it to grow.

Kwashiorkor occurs not only in Africa, but also in Central America, South America, the Near East, and the Far East—and in wealthy, as well as poor, countries. It is probably a mixture of deficiency symptoms from a lack of both protein and zinc, and possibly other nutrients as well. Wherever mother's milk is the only reliable and readily available source of protein and zinc for infants, kwashiorkor threatens them at weaning time. It typically sets in at about the age of two; the child's growth slows down, so that by the time the child is four, he is no taller than he was at two. His hair loses its color, and his skin is patchy and scaly, sometimes with ulcers and sores that fail to heal. His limbs and face become swollen with edema; his belly bulges with fatty liver; he sickens easily and is weak, fretful, and apathetic. Figure 5–6 shows a picture of such a child.

The body follows a priority system when there is not enough protein to meet all its needs. It abandons its less vital systems first. When it cannot obtain

FIGURE 5–6

Kwashiorkor and marasmus.

A. Kwashiorkor. The child at left has the characteristic "moon face" (edema), swollen belly, and patchy dermatitis (from zinc deficiency) often seen with kwashiorkor. At right, the same child after nutritional therapy.

B. Marasmus. The child at left is suffering from the extreme emaciation of marasmus. At right is the same child after nutritional therapy.

enough amino acids from dietary sources, the body switches to a "metabolism of wasting"; it begins to digest its own protein tissues. This way, it can supply the amino acids needed to continue maintaining the vital internal organs and thus keep itself alive. Hair and skin pigments (which are made of amino acids) are dispensable and are no longer manufactured. The skin needs less integrity in a life-or-death situation than the heart does, so skin maintenance stops, and skin sores fail to heal. Many of the antibodies are also degraded so that their amino acids may be used as building blocks for heart, lung, and brain tissue. A child with a depleted supply of antibodies cannot resist infection and readily contracts dysentery, a disease of the digestive tract. Dysentery causes diarrhea, leading to the rapid loss of any nutrients—including amino acids—that the child may be receiving in food. Thus dysentery worsens the protein deficiency, and the protein deficiency in turn increases the likelihood of a second or third or tenth attack of dysentery.

The water loss in diarrhea increases losses of minerals and of the water-soluble B vitamins and vitamin C. Lack of protein carriers for the fat-soluble vitamins creates a deficiency of vitamins A and D as well. The child's inability to manufacture protein carriers for fat often leaves him with fat accumulated in the liver tissue, from which it would normally be carried away. As the liver clogs with fat, its cells lose their ability to carry out their other normal functions, and gradually they atrophy and die.

A malnourished child who contracts measles cannot fight it off. In our country, where protein deficiency is almost never a problem, the child with measles may expect to recover within five to seven days; the kwashiorkor child often dies within the first two days. Other diseases take a similarly heavy toll.

Marasmus

Textbooks usually describe marasmus and kwashiorkor as the two endpoints on a spectrum—lack of kcalories at one end and lack of protein at the other—with PCM occupying the central region. In practice, these distinctions are not so easily made. At all points between marasmus and kwashiorkor, protein deficiency produces symptoms, whether the underlying cause is lack of dietary protein or lack of kcalories to conserve protein. Furthermore, a diet deficient in protein and kcalories is invariably deficient in other nutrients as well.

A marasmic child looks like a wizened little old person—just skin and bones (see Figure 5–6). She is often sick, because her resistance to disease is low. All her muscles are wasted, including the heart muscle, and the heart is weak. Reduced synthesis of key hormones leads to a metabolism so slow that her body temperature is subnormal. Unlike the kwashiorkor child, she has no fat accumulated in her liver, and little or no fat under her skin to insulate against cold. The experience of hospital workers with victims of marasmus is that their primary need is to be wrapped up and kept warm. They also need love, because they have often been severely deprived of maternal attention as well as food.

Unlike the kwashiorkor child, who has been fed milk until weaning, the marasmic child may have been neglected from early infancy. The disease occurs most commonly in children from 6 to 18 months of age in all the overpopulated city slums of the world, and in rural children who have been fed inadequate formulas for too long. Since the brain normally grows to almost its full adult

dysentery (DIS-en-terry): an infection of the gastrointestinal tract caused by an amoeba or bacterium and giving rise to severe diarrhea.

When two variables interact so that each increases the other, they are said to be acting synergistically. Malnutrition and infection are a deadly combination because they work this way.

synergism (SIN-er-jism): the effect of two factors operating together in such a way that their combined actions are greater than the sum of the actions of the two considered separately.

The extent, severity, and causes of world hunger are reviewed in Highlight 13B, together with some approaches to a solution in which individuals can become involved.

FIGURE 5–7

Malnutrition reduces brain cell number. The graph shows the total DNA in cerebellums of children who died at ages up to two and a half years. Those that had suffered malnutrition in infancy had less DNA (a reflection of brain cell number).

Source: M. Winick, P. Rosso, and J. Waterlow, Cellular growth of cerebrum, cerebellum, and brain stem in normal and marasmic children, *Experimental Neurology* 26 (1970): 393–400.

size within the first two years of life, marasmus impairs brain development and so may have a permanent effect on learning ability.

In order to study the effects of PCM on brain growth, one group of researchers analyzed the brain tissue of young children who had died of severe marasmus, as well as brain tissue from otherwise healthy accident victims (children of comparable ages). They found that the number of brain cells of the marasmic children was significantly lower than the number in the well-fed children (see Figure 5–7).[5] Since the number of brain cells does not increase significantly after about the first year of life, children with marasmus may never attain their full intellectual potential, even if they are well fed later.[6]

Protein-kcalorie malnutrition particularly affects vulnerable groups in the community, such as pregnant and lactating women, nursing infants, just-weaned children, and children in periods of rapid growth. These groups have a great need for protein because of the new tissues being formed in their bodies. They need ample kcalories to protect that protein from degradation, yet in many cultures they are the very ones who are denied nourishing food.

Adult PCM

Kwashiorkor is only one of several diseases associated with protein deficiency. Another that is closer to home for most of us is the nutritional liver disease associated with alcoholism. The alcohol abuser, like the kwashiorkor child, consumes abundant kcalories, but up to three-fourths of the kcalories may come from alcohol, a nonprotein substance. Like the kwashiorkor child, the malnourished alcoholic may have a belly swollen with fatty liver; puffy hands, feet, and face; skin sores; and a reduced ability to withstand infection. If the fatty liver goes unremedied for too long, the liver cells ultimately die and are replaced by inert scar tissue. This is the progression to cirrhosis, which is so often caused by alcoholism.

The "beer belly" of the alcoholic is usually rightly attributed to fat, due to an excess intake of kcalories, but it sometimes reflects ascites (edema in the abdomen) or fatty liver.

cirrhosis (seer-OH-sis): irreversible liver damage involving death of liver cells and their replacement by scar tissue.

For more about the effects of alcohol on the liver, see Highlight 7B.

Adult kwashiorkor and marasmus also occur in hospital patients whose diets have been inadequate. A person undergoing surgery or fighting an infection has a greatly increased need of protein and kcalories. At the same time, he may feel too sick to eat or may be fed only liquids or intravenous fluids, which are not nearly nutritious enough even to maintain a healthy body. Hospital malnutrition occurs in up to 50 percent of the patients in some hospitals and increases the risks associated with surgery and infection. Physicians, whose medical school training has until recently almost totally neglected nutrition, are now becoming increasingly aware of its importance in the treatment of the sick. Some hospitals now maintain special staffs to assess the nutrition status of their patients and to provide nutrition support.[7]

Recommended Protein Intakes

Recommended protein intakes can be stated in three ways—as a percentage of total kcalories, as an absolute number (grams per day), or as grams per kilogram body weight. The Senate committee that published the *Dietary Goals for the United States* stated it as a percentage, and recommended that it remain constant at about 12 percent of total kcalories consumed. (They allocated about 58 percent of kcalories or more to carbohydrate, and 30 percent or less to fat.) They reasoned that the intake need not be higher than it already is, and that a reduction, which might require drastic alterations in lifestyle, would not pay off in any predictable benefits.

The Committee on RDA of the Food and Nutrition Board of the National Academy of Sciences states the RDA in grams per day. They consider that a generous protein allowance for a healthy adult would be 0.8 grams per kilogram of appropriate body weight per day. Protein RDA for people of average heights at all ages are presented in the RDA table (inside front cover). If your height is not average, you can compute your own individualized RDA for protein. Suppose your appropriate weight is 50 kilograms, for example; your protein RDA would then be 0.8 times 50, or 40 grams of protein each day. The Canadian recommendation (RNI) for protein is similar to the RDA: 0.82 grams per kilogram for an adult male (see examples in Appendix I). It is 1.3 times the average requirement, to encompass individuals whose needs are above the average.

The committee uses an appropriate reference weight, not the actual weight, for a given height, because it is proportional to the *lean* body mass of the average person. Lean body mass determines protein need. If you gain fat, you gain weight of course, but, as mentioned, fat tissue does not require much protein for maintenance.

In setting the RDA, the committee assumes that the protein eaten will be of high quality (a PER equal to or above that of casein), that it will be consumed with adequate kcalories from carbohydrate and fat, and that other nutrients in the diet will be adequate. The committee also assumes that you are a healthy individual, with no unusual metabolic need for protein.

To calculate the percentage of kcalories you derive from protein:
1. Use your total kcalories as the denominator (example: 1,900 kcal).
2. Multiply your protein *grams* by 4 kcal/g to obtain kcalories from protein as the numerator (example: 70 g protein × 4 kcal/g = 280 kcal).
3. Divide to obtain a decimal, multiply by 100, and round off (example: 280/1,900 × 100 = 15% kcal from protein).

To figure your protein RDA:
1. Look up the appropriate weight for a person of your height (inside back cover). Use this weight as your reference weight.
2. Change pounds to kilograms.
3. Multiply kilograms by 0.8 g/kg.
Example (for a 5'8" medium-frame male):
1. Reference weight: about 150 lb.
2. 150 lb × 1 kg/2.2 lb = 68 kg (rounded off).
3. 68 kg × 0.8 g/kg = 54 g protein (rounded off).

For information on how the RDA was set, see Chapter 2.

The World Health Organization has a task somewhat different from that of the U.S. and Canadian agencies, and this accounts for its lower recommendation: 0.75 grams per kilogram of body weight. WHO must find acceptable levels of nutrient intakes for a world in which poverty makes generous intakes a luxury. WHO carefully defines its protein recommendation in terms of egg or milk protein and also publishes a set of graded recommendations for proteins of lower quality. The difference between the WHO and the Canadian and U.S. recommendations reflects the different realities in the societies for which they were designed.

It is possible to consume too much protein. Animals fed high-protein diets experience a protein overload effect, seen in the hypertrophy of their livers and kidneys. Infants are placed at risk in many ways if fed excess protein.[8] People who wish to lose weight may be handicapped in their efforts if they consume too much protein.[9] The higher a person's intake of such protein-rich foods as meat and milk, the more likely it is that fruits, vegetables, and grains will be crowded out of the diet, making it inadequate in other nutrients. Diets high in protein necessitate higher intakes of calcium as well, because such diets promote calcium excretion.[10] Protein from animal, as opposed to vegetable, food sources may raise serum cholesterol and thus the risk of heart disease; at least as much vegetable as animal protein should be eaten (a 1 to 1 ratio).[11] There are evidently no benefits to be gained by consuming a diet that derives more than 15 percent of its kcalories from protein, and there are possible risks as intakes rise to 20 or more percent of kcalories when kcalories are adequate.[12]

hypertrophy (high-PURR-tro-fee): growing too large.
hyper = too much
trophy = growth
Highlight 7A shows why excess protein doesn't help the body builder to add muscle.

Note the qualification, "when kcalories are adequate," in the statement we just made. Protein intakes can be stated as numbers that vary or as fixed numbers—for example, as a percentage of kcalories, or as an absolute number (grams per day). An absolute number, such as 50 grams a day for a 62–kilogram, moderately active person, offers a reasonable percentage of daily kcalories—but only if the person eats a reasonable *number* of kcalories (say, 2,000 a day). In that case, 50 grams of protein, equal to 200 kcalories, provides 10 percent of the total. But if the person cuts kcalorie intake drastically—to, say, 800 a day—then 200 kcalories from protein is suddenly 25 percent of the total, yet it's still the same absolute number of grams. It's still a reasonable intake, too; it's the kcalorie intake that's not reasonable. Similarly, if the person eats far too many kcalories—say, 4,000—the protein intake represents only 5 percent of the total, yet it's *still* a reasonable intake. Again, it's the kcalorie intake that's unreasonable.

Be careful when judging protein intakes as a percentage of kcalories. Always ask what the absolute number of grams is, too, and compare it with the RDA or some such standard given in grams. Recommendations stated as a percentage of kcalories are only useful when kcalorie intakes are within reason.

Protein in Foods

The foods that supply protein in abundance are those on the milk and meat lists of the exchange system. A cup of milk provides 8 grams of protein; an ounce of the average meat, 7 grams, as shown in Table 2–6 (p. 39). A one-cup portion of legumes, when used as a meat alternate, is treated as having 13 grams of protein in the exchange system (counted as 2 starch and 1 lean meat). As the table also shows, the foods in the vegetable and bread lists contribute small amounts of protein to the diet, but they become significant when several servings are consumed.

The exchange system provides an easy way to estimate the amount of protein a person consumes. Figure 5–8 shows the protein contents of foods, and Figure 5–9 demonstrates the calculation of how much protein is in a day's meals.

The protein RDA represents a generous intake; it is set high enough to cover the estimated needs of most people, even those with unusually high requirements. Still, most people in developed countries such as the United States ingest much more protein than the RDA. This is not surprising when you consider that a single ounce of meat delivers 7 or 8 grams of protein, and that the RDA for an average-sized person is only about 50 grams a day.

To illustrate this point, suppose that *your* recommended protein intake is 50 grams per day. This would divide easily into three meals: 10 grams at breakfast, 20 grams at lunch, and 20 grams at dinner. An egg and a glass of milk at breakfast would exceed the amount allotted for breakfast by half. A chef's salad

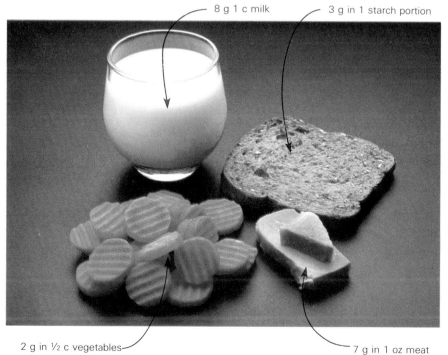

8 g 1 c milk   3 g in 1 starch portion

2 g in ½ c vegetables   7 g in 1 oz meat

FIGURE 5–8

Foods containing protein.
Milk List:
1 c milk contains 8 g protein.
Meat List:
1 oz meat contains 7 g protein.
Vegetable List:
1/2 c vegetables contains 2 g protein.
Starch/Bread List:
1 slice bread, 1 portion cereal, or 1 starchy vegetable contains 3 g protein

FIGURE 5–9

How to estimate protein intake. The values presented in Figure 5–8 provide a way to estimate the amount of protein eaten at a meal or in a day. Using those values, let's estimate the amounts of protein in the meals shown here. (These are the same meals used as examples in Chapters 2, 3, and 4). The fruits and fats (butter) can be assumed to contain no protein; so the only foods to inspect are the meats, milks, grains/starchy vegetables, and vegetables. The exchange system slightly overestimates the protein in these meals. Peas and beans (members of the legume family) contain more protein than other vegetables do. Still the estimate is higher than the actual amount of protein by only 8 percent.

		Protein Grams	
		Estimated	Actual
Breakfast			
1 c oatmeal = 2 starch portions	=	6	6
¼ c raisins = 2 fruit portions	=	0	1
½ c nonfat milk = ½ milk portion	=	4	4
½ grapefruit = 1 fruit portion	=	0	0
		10	11
Lunch			
1 c cooked rice = 3 starch portions	=	9	5
2 c mixed vegetables = 2 starchy vegetables + 2 vegetables	=	10	10
2 oz cheddar cheese = 2 meat portions	=	14	14
⅔ c fresh strawberries = about 1 fruit portion	=	0	0
1 c nonfat milk = 1 milk portion	=	8	8
2 pats butter = 2 fat portions	=	0	0
2 packets sugar	=	0	0
		41	37
Dinner			
3 oz broiled fish = 3 meat portions	=	21	20
½ c green beans = 1 vegetable portion	=	2	1
½ c cooked carrots = 1 vegetable portion	=	2	0
½ c cooked peas = 1 starchy vegetable	=	3	4
2 pats butter = 2 fat portions	=	0	0
1 c nonfat milk = 1 milk portion	=	8	8
		36	33
Snack			
¼ cantaloupe = 1 fruit portion	=	0	1
1 brownie = 1 starch portion	=	3	1
		3	2
Day's total =		90	83

with only **3** ounces of cut-up meat or cheese would more than cover the amount allotted for lunch. A small piece of chicken would suffice for dinner. By the time you added a few vegetables, the recommended second cup of milk, and the four bread and/or cereal items suggested by the Four Food Group Plan, you would have exceeded your protein needs for the day by far. Finally, if you also consumed a cup of legumes besides, you would add over **10** grams more protein to your intake. No wonder most people get more than twice as much protein as they need. This is not harmful—provided that the energy budget is balanced, that fat and cholesterol intakes are not excessive, and that the foods are affordable—but it is not necessary.

Chapter 2 introduced the principles of wise diet planning: adequacy, balance, kcalorie control, nutrient density, and variety. To these should now be added another watchword: moderation.

Study Questions

1. How do proteins differ from carbohydrates and fats in their chemical structure? Describe amino acids in terms of their structure, sequence, and shaping of a protein.
2. What are enzymes? What is their role in chemical reactions?
3. Describe the roles proteins serve in the human body.
4. What determines the quality of dietary protein? How is this measured?
5. Account for the effects of protein-kcalorie malnutrition. Explain why deficiencies of kcalories and protein give rise to many of the same symptoms.
6. What factors are considered in establishing recommended protein intakes?
7. Which food lists of the exchange system supply protein in abundance? in moderation? not at all?

Notes

1. A. Rosenfeld, The great protein hunt, *Science 81*, January–February 1981, pp. 64–67.
2. M. H. N. Golden, Protein deficiency, energy deficiency, and the oedema of malnutrition, *Lancet I* (1982): 1261–1265.
3. R. Y. Stanier, M. Doudoroff, and E. A. Adelberg, *The Microbial World*, 3rd ed. (Englewood Cliffs, N.J.: Prentice-Hall, 1970), p. 784.
4. Fad of the month: Arginine for obesity, *Nutrition and the MD*, May 1985.
5. M. Winick, P. Rosso, and J. Waterlow, Cellular growth of cerebrum, cerebellum, and brain stem in normal and marasmic children, *Experimental Neurology* 26 (1970): 393–400.
6. It is difficult, however, to sort out the effects of nutritional from emotional and intellectual deprivation. J. Cravioto, Nutrition, stimulation, mental development and learning, *Nutrition Today*, September–October 1981, pp. 4–8, 10–15.
7. G. L. Blackburn, B. S. Hopkins, and B. R. Bistrian, The nutrition support service in hospital practice, in *Nutritional Support of Medical Practice*, 2nd ed., eds. H. A. Schneider, C. E. Anderson, and D. B. Coursin (Hagerstown, Md.: Lippincott, 1983), pp. 111–127.
8. Infections and undernutrition, *Nutrition Reviews* 40 (1982): 119–128.
9. Dietary protein and body fat distribution, *Nutrition Reviews* 40 (1982): 89–90.
10. Urinary calcium increases with high protein intakes, perhaps because the protein makes the urine more acidic than usual. A. A. Licata, Acute effects of increased meat protein on urinary electrolytes and cyclic adenosine monophosphate and serum parathyroid hormone, *American Journal of Clinical Nutrition* 34 (1981): 1979–1784.
11. K. K. Carroll, Dietary protein and heart disease, *Nutrition and the MD*, June 1985.
12. High protein diets and bone homeostasis, *Nutrition Reviews* 39 (1981): 11–13.

These exercises make use of the information you recorded on Forms 1 to 3.

1. How many grams of protein do you consume in a day?

2. How many kcalories does this represent? (Remember, 1 gram of protein contributes 4 kcalories.)

3. What percentage of your total kcalories is contributed by protein?

4. The *Dietary Goals* suggest that protein should contribute about 10 to 15 percent of total kcalories. How does your protein intake compare with this recommendation? (Note: if you are on a kcalorie-restricted diet, then a higher percentage of your kcalories should come from protein. See the Self-Study for Chapter 8.) If your protein intake is out of line, what foods could you consume more of—or less of—to bring it into line?

5. Calculate your protein RDA (see p. 155). Is it similar to the RDA for an

SELF-STUDY

Evaluate Your Protein Intake

"average" person your age and sex as shown in the RDA Tables (inside front cover)?

6. Compare your average daily protein intake with your RDA. On the average, about what percentage of your RDA for protein are you consuming each day? If you are "average" and healthy, the RDA is probably a generous recommendation for you, and yet you may be eating more than the recommendation. This means that you may be spending protein prices for an energy nutrient. What substitutions could you make in your day's food choices so that you would derive from carbohydrate, rather

than from protein, the kcalories you need for energy?

7. How many of your protein grams are from animal, and how many from plant, foods? Assuming that the animal protein is all of high quality, no more than 20 percent of your total protein need come from this source. Should you alter the ratio of plant to animal protein in your diet? If you did, what effect would this have on the total *fat* content of your diet?

8. How is your protein intake distributed through the day? (At what times do you eat—how many grams of protein each time?) Do you have amino acids at breakfast time to help maintain your blood glucose supply from carbohydrate? At lunchtime, to replenish dwindling pools? At dinnertime, to sustain you through the evening?

Vegetarianism

The vegetarian has the same nutrition tasks as any other person—planning a diet that will deliver all the needed nutrients within a kcalorie allowance that won't promote weight gain, and choosing a variety of foods that fit the plan. One of the nutrients that meats are famous for is protein—the subject of Chapter 5—and it deserves the vegetarian's attention; so this highlight starts with protein. While on the subject of vegetarianism, though, it covers other nutrients of concern as well.

Protein for Vegetarians

Do vegetarians get enough protein automatically, or must they make special efforts to do so? The answer is yes to both questions—depending on the vegetarian. Some vegetarians (lacto-ovo-vegetarians) omit meat, fish, and poultry from their diets, but use animal products such as eggs, cheese, yogurt, and milk. Others (lactovegetarians) exclude eggs, and the only foods of animal origin they use are milk products. Still others (strict vegetarians, or vegans) allow themselves no foods that come from animals in any form, and restrict themselves to an all-plant diet. Among strict vegetarians are fruitarians, who center their diets on fruits.

Those who eat animal products such as milk and eggs are availing themselves of the highest-quality protein available and need fear no protein deficiencies. Those who eat an all-plant diet may need to give thought to their protein intakes, because plant proteins—at least individually—are of lower quality, and because plants offer less protein per unit (either weight or measure) of food than animal proteins.

Vegans have long been told that they should know how to combine plant proteins that are missing, or are low in, one or more essential amino acids in order to improve the quality of the plant proteins they eat. This strategy is called *mutual supplementation*, and the two protein foods chosen are *complementary proteins*. Mixtures that provide higher-quality protein than the individual protein foods they are made from are shown in Table H5–1. The *amounts* of protein such mixtures provide are ample, too, as shown in Table H5–2.

Studies indicating that mutual supplementation was a necessity for the vegan were first conducted on rats. The protein requirements of human beings are different from those of rats, but the idea that plant proteins are inadequate sources of essential amino acids carried over for years. Now it appears that adequate consumption of the essential amino acids is possible without practicing protein complementation.[1] Plant foods can provide more than enough of all the essential amino acids, and can sustain people in good health, as long as not too many empty kcalories are eaten.

Assuming that the vegan consumes enough kcalories, the possibility of a protein deficiency is remote. Only if she relied heavily on fruits or certain poorly chosen vegetables as the core of the diet might protein deficiency result. Fruits provide adequate kcalories, but they are low in protein. Anyone who can afford fruits, however, can afford other foods

Vegetarians can be as creative with the names of their restaurants as with the dishes they concoct.

TABLE H5–1

Nonmeat Mixtures That Provide High-Quality Protein

Combine		Examples

For the Strict Vegetarian

Cereal grains	+	Legumes	
Barley		Dried beans	Bean taco
Bulgur		Dried lentils	Chili and corn bread
Oats		Dried peas	Lentils and rice
Rice		Peanuts	Peanut butter sandwich
Whole-grain breads		Soy products	Tofu with rice
Pasta			
Cornmeal			

Legumes	+	Seeds and Nuts	
Dried beans		Sesame seeds	Hummus (chick-pea and
Dried lentils		Sunflower seeds	sesame paste)
Dried peas		Walnuts	Split pea soup and
Peanuts		Cashews	sesame crackers
Soy products		Nut butters	

For the Lacto-Ovo-Vegetarian

Eggs or Milk Products	+	Vegetable-Protein Foods	
Eggs		Legumes	Macaroni and cheese
Milk		Nuts	Vegetable omelet
Yogurt		Seeds	Eggplant Parmesan
Cheese		Whole grains	Broccoli with cheese sauce
Cottage cheese		Vegetables	French toast
			Cereal with milk

TABLE H5–2

Protein Sources

Food	Amount	Protein (g)	Energy (kcal)
These are the usual foods people think of when they think of protein:			
Cheese:			
Cheddar	1 oz	7	115
Cottage	½ c	12 to 15	85 to 130
Egg	1 large	7	80
Fish, light and dark, cooked	3 oz	20 to 25	125 to 175
Meat, cooked:			
Ground beef	3 oz	20 to 23	185 to 235
Heart, kidney, liver	3 oz	23 to 28	160 to 215
Pork	3 oz	23 to 28	310
Milk:			
Whole	1 c	9	160
Nonfat	1 c	9	90
Poultry (without skin), light and dark, cooked	3 oz	25	145 to 175

Legumes, high in iron, calcium, and fiber, are an excellent meat alternate.

to supply protein, such as legumes and vegetables. Even advocates of a fruitarian diet use nuts and seeds regularly. The root vegetable cassava, when used as the diet's major staple food, provides another instance of adequate kcalories but inadequate protein; cassava is only about 2 percent protein.

Vegans can improve the quality of protein consumed by practicing mutual supplementation, but they should probably not be overly concerned about it. A wiser use of time and energy is to obtain, prepare, and eat a wide variety of foods from the vegetarian four food groups to obtain adequate kcalories, protein, and other nutrients (see p. 33).

To make obtaining variety easier, convenience foods and other new food products are available for vegetarians. Among them are meat replacements—textured vegetable protein products formulated to look and taste like meat, fish, or poultry. Many of these are designed to match the known nutrient contents of animal-protein foods, but sometimes they fall short. We advise against relying on these products completely, but instead suggest learning to use combinations of whole, natural foods suggested here as well.

An advantage of vegetarian protein foods is that they are often higher than meats in fiber and richer in certain

TABLE H5–2

(continued)

Food	Amount	Protein (g)	Energy (kcal)
These are other good sources of protein that you could use instead:			
Vegetables, cooked:			
Broccoli	1 medium stalk	6	45
Brussels sprouts	1 c	7	55
Cauliflower	1 c	3	30
Greens	1 c	3 to 7	30 to 65
Legumes:			
Dried, cooked	½ c	7 to 8	90 to 115
Mung sprouts, raw	½ c	2	20
Tofu (soybean curd)	4 oz	9	85
Wheat germ	2 tbsp	4	45
You can also get significant quantities of protein from these foods (if you can afford the kcalories):			
Cereal grain products:			
Barley, whole grain, cooked	½ c	4	135
Bran cereal (100% bran), uncooked	½ c	5	90
Breads	1 slice	2 to 3	60 to 80
Cornmeal, unrefined ground, uncooked	½ c	5	215
Pasta, enriched, cooked	1 c	5 to 7	155 to 200
Millet, whole grain, cooked	½ c	3	95
Oatmeal, cooked	1 c	5	130
Rice, cooked	1 c	4 to 5	225 to 230
Unprocessed bran	½ c	4	55
Wheat berries, cooked	½ c	5	110
Wheat, bulgur, cooked	½ c	7	225
Wheat, cracked, cooked	½ c	4	110
Starchy vegetables:			
Corn	1 medium ear or ½ c	3	70
Peas, fresh	1 c	9	115
Potato, baked	1 large	4	145
Winter squash, baked	1 c	4	130
Nuts*	2 tbsp	2 to 5	80 to 115
Nut Butters*	1 tbsp	4	95
Seeds*	2 tbsp	3 to 5	95 to 100
Yeast, brewer's	2 tbsp	6	40 to 45

*These items are high in fat and should be used in moderation.
Source: Adapted from Society for Nutrition Education materials.

Vegetarian meals are colorful, revealing their high vitamin A, vitamin C, and folacin contents.

vitamins and minerals; they are lower in fat as well. Vegetarians can therefore enjoy a nutritious diet that is very low in fat, provided that other high-fat foods like butter, cream cheese, or sour cream are limited, too.

Other Nutrients

Vegetarians naturally consume a greater abundance of some nutrients than other people do—those present in plant foods. It is hard to imagine how a vegetarian could fail to consume enough vitamin A, vitamin C, or folacin, for example, because these are the very vitamins that fruits and vegetables are famous for. However, some vitamins and minerals are of particular concern.

One such vitamin is vitamin B_{12}, which is found only in animal foods and in special nutritional supplements such as yeast grown on vitamin B_{12}-enriched food. The lacto-ovo-vegetarian has no problem getting enough vitamin B_{12}, but the vegan needs a reliable source, such as vitamin B_{12}-fortified soy "milk" or meat replacements. Some vegetarians use seaweeds, fermented soy, and other products in the belief that they provide vitamin B_{12} in adequate amounts, but unless laboratory analyses confirm their hopes, these products are not recommended as reliable sources.[2]

Vitamin B_{12} deficiency takes a long time to develop after a person gives up animal foods, because up to four years' worth can be stored in the body. When it does occur, however, it can irreversibly damage the brain and nerves. A pregnant or lactating vegan should be aware that her infant can develop a vitamin B_{12} deficiency, even if she remains healthy. A deficiency of this vitamin is extraordinarily damaging to developing infants; all vegan mothers must choose their diets carefully to include vitamin B_{12}-fortified products, or take the appropriate supplements.

Another vitamin of concern is vitamin D. Again, the milk drinker is protected (provided the milk is vitamin D fortified, of course), but there is no practical source of vitamin D in plant foods. Regular (not extreme) exposure to the sun will prevent a deficiency, but the homebound or vegans living in a northern climate or smoggy city probably should take vitamin D supplements. Excesses of vitamin D are toxic; the recommended daily amount of 5 micrograms should not be exceeded.

Another nutrient that meats are famous for is iron, and vegetarians don't eat meats. Iron deficiency is widespread among all kinds of people—rich and poor, old and young—and vegetarians are not immune to it, so they should be sure to plan their meals accordingly. Several strategies are useful. Eggs, hummus (chick-pea and sesame seed paste), pumpkin seeds, spinach, legumes, and meat analogs are rich in iron, so some of these foods should be included in every day's diet. Most food group plans for vegetarians recommend two or more servings a day.

Legumes, whole grains, and dark green, leafy vegetables appear to be high in iron when listed on food composition tables, but the iron of these foods is not as absorbable as that of meat. In fact, people absorb three times as much iron from a meal that includes meat as from one that does not, thanks to the MFP factor in meat (see Chapter 12). Vegetarians can compensate completely for the lack of this factor, though, because the vitamin C in fruits and vegetables can also triple iron absorption from other foods eaten at the same meal. Thus another strategy is to include, with the iron sources, foods that are rich in vitamin C.

Oddly enough, the vegetarians who most risk deficiency of iron are those who use milk and milk products in their diets, because those particular foods are poor in iron. They have to be especially careful to use iron-rich legumes and vegetables, and to round out their meals with vitamin C-rich fruits and vegetables, too.

Vegetarians who don't use milk have two other nutrients to attend to that are automatically supplied in the diet of milk users: calcium and riboflavin. It may be impossible for the vegan to entirely meet his calcium needs, unless he uses a food like soy "milk" that has been fortified with calcium. Some people live in areas where these calcium-fortified products are hard to find, but many have solved the problem by using soy-based formula intended for infants. The infant formula is calcium fortified, and can be used in cooking as well as for drinking. Plain, unfortified soy "milk" is a calcium-poor food, but it is rich in iron, protein, and fat. (The unfortified liquid is most closely related to foods high in protein. The calcium-fortified type and infant formula more closely resemble milk.) Other foods that are rich in calcium are tortillas; stone-ground meal; self-rising flour and meal; some nuts, such as almonds; and certain seeds, such as sesame seeds.

As for riboflavin, if dark greens are frequently used in ample servings, the vegan's needs will be met. Nutritional yeast is another rich source of riboflavin for the vegetarian.

Zinc, too, may be a problem nutrient for vegetarians. It is widespread in plant foods, but its availability may be hindered by the fibers and phytates found in fruits and vegetables. The zinc needs of vegetarians and the effects of high-fiber, high-phytate diets on them are subjects of intensive study at the present time, and no clear-cut answers have been arrived at. While research continues, vegetarians are advised to eat varied diets that include whole-grain breads well leavened with yeast, which reduces their phytate content.

Children of Vegetarians

Plant-based diets for children can be nutritionally adequate if sufficient care is taken in planning them, and pediatricians are concerned that vegetarians provide such a diet to promote optimal growth and development in their children. Because of their special needs for growth, infants and children risk nutritional deficiency regardless of the dietary pattern followed. Infants and children on restrictive vegetarian diets are particularly susceptible to nutrient deficiencies and slowed rates of growth and development. Dietary deficiencies most often seen are those related to energy, protein, vitamins D, B_{12}, and riboflavin, and the minerals calcium, iron, zinc, magnesium, and iodine. Symptoms of vitamin and mineral deficiencies and the best food sources of each are given in Chapters 9 through 12.

The fewer foods a vegetarian diet allows, the less likely it can meet nutrient needs. The greatest risk results from undue reliance on a single plant food source. The Zen macrobiotic diet is perhaps the most dangerous of the current diets for growing children.[3] In a series of steps, this diet eliminates animal products and fruits and vegetables, until only brown rice and water are consumed.

Vegetarian diets may be so high in bulk that they may not meet energy needs. The volume of vegetarian foods necessary to meet the energy requirements of infants may exceed the capacity of the infant's stomach. Because of diminished energy intake, protein is then used as an energy source; thus, a protein content equal to the child's RDA becomes marginal.

Assuming energy intakes are adequate, combinations solely of plant foods can be satisfactory for the growth of infants and children. An adequate intake of most vitamins, minerals, and other nutrients can be obtained with legumes (including calcium and B_{12}-fortified soybean formulas), whole-grain products, nuts, seeds, and dark-green leafy vegetables. Legumes provide B vitamins and iron in addition to relatively concentrated protein. Whole grains are a source of thiamin, iron, zinc and other trace minerals, as well as carbohydrate and protein. Nuts and seeds contain B vitamins and iron, and they provide a source of fat. Dark-green leafy vegetables help to supply adequate calcium and riboflavin, which are lacking when dairy products are excluded. Vitamin B_{12} deficiency can be avoided if vitamin B_{12} supplementation in tablet form or in fortified plant foods such as vitamin B_{12}-fortified soy or nut milks are used.

In summary, vegetarian diets that include an adequate number of kcalories in a reasonable volume of food, high quality protein or complementary proteins, plus *available* sources of calcium, iron, and zinc, vitamins D and B_{12}, and recommended levels of other nutrients are believed to be adequate for normal growth and development in infants and children. Still, the repeated occurrences in the literature today of deficiencies of essential nutrients in vegetarian children spotlight the need for careful planning when designing a vegetarian pattern for infants and children.

Benefits of Vegetarianism

Abundant evidence supports the idea that informed vegetarians are more likely than comparable other people to be at the desired weights for their heights, and to have lower blood cholesterol levels, lower rates of certain kinds of cancer, better digestive function, and better health in other ways as well. In a seven-year study of nearly 11,000 British "health-food" consumers, it was concluded that even among people who are "health conscious," vegetarians experience fewer deaths from cardiovascular disease than other such people.[4] Often, vegetarianism goes with a clean-living lifestyle (no smoking, abstinence from alcohol, and an emphasis on supportive family life), so it is impossible to tell whether the dietary practices alone account for all the aspects of improved health. Clearly, however, they contribute to it.

It is apparent that vegetarianism also benefits the earth. A major way to reduce the demands we make on the earth's resources is to depend less on animal-based proteins and to use more plant-based proteins. Today, much rich cropland is used to grow animal feed instead of foods for humans. The animals are then fed these grain and protein feeds in feedlots, where they are fattened much faster than if they had grazed on pastureland. Figure H5–1 shows the different rates at which animals convert feed to edible animal protein. As shown, chickens require about 3 pounds of grain to produce one pound of meat, whereas cattle require 16 pounds of grain to do the same. An argument for vegetarianism, therefore, is that by simply cutting back on our beef consumption and substituting less land-costly plant protein sources, we could make large amounts of land available for human food production. We would also realize other ecological benefits, including decreased water and fertilizer requirements. Irrigation for beef alone requires 4 to 45 times more water than for other field crops.

FIGURE H5–1

A protein factory in reverse.

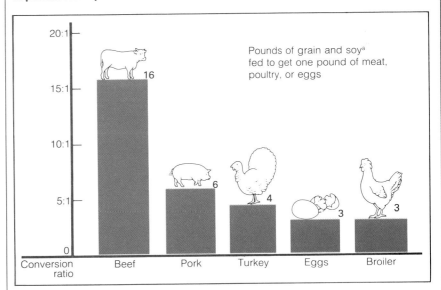

Pounds of grain and soy[a] fed to get one pound of meat, poultry, or eggs

[a]Soy constitutes only 12% of steer feed and 20–25% of poultry feed.

Source: F. M. Lappe, *Diet for a Small Planet* (New York: Ballantine Books, 1975), p. 11. Institute for Food and Development Policy, 1885 Mission Street, San Francisco, CA 94103.

NOTES
1. K. Akers, *A Vegetarian Sourcebook* (New York: Putnam, 1983).
2. Position paper on the vegetarian approach to eating, *Journal of the American Dietetic Association* 77(1980):61–67.
3. R. M. Hanning and S. H. Zlotkin, Unconventional Eating Practices and their Implications, *Pediatric Clinics of North America* 32(1985):429–434.
4. M. L. Burr and P. M. Sweetnam, Vegetarianism, dietary fiber, and mortality, *American Journal of Clinical Nutrition* 36(1982):873.

Miniglossary of Vegetarian Terms

complementary proteins: two or more proteins whose amino acid assortments complement each other in such a way that the essential amino acids missing from each are supplied by the other.

fruitarian: strict vegetarian who centers his or her diet on fruits.

lacto-ovo-vegetarian: vegetarian who omits meat, fish, and poultry from the diet, but uses eggs, cheese, milk, and milk products.

macrobiotic diet: a diet that consists predominately of whole grains and vegetables and claimed by its practitioners to increase spiritual enlightenment.

meat replacement: textured vegetable protein product formulated to look and taste like meat, fish, or poultry. Many of these are designed to match the known nutrient contents of animal-protein foods, but sometimes they fall short.

mutual supplementation: the strategy of combining two protein foods in a meal so that each food provides the essential amino acid(s) lacking in the other.

nutritional yeast: a fortified food supplement containing B vitamins, iron, and protein that can be used to improve the quality of a vegetarian diet.

vegan: vegetarian who omits all animal products (including eggs, cheese, and milk) from the diet; also called strict vegetarian.

Digestion, Absorption, and Transport

6

Contents

The cells of the gastrointestinal tract lining display an intricate architecture that supports their function. Part of one cell is shown here with microvilli at top. The round, dark bodies are lipid droplets (chylomicrons) forming within the cell from recently absorbed lipid fragments. These will be coated with protein and released into the body for transport elsewhere. The slim, striped bodies inside the cell are mitochondria, busily producing energy to fuel the cell's work.

O ne of the beauties of the digestive tract is that it is selective. Materials that are nutritive for the body are broken down into particles that can be assimilated into the bloodstream. Most of those that are not are left undigested and pass out the other end of the digestive tract. In a sense, the human body is doughnut shaped, and the digestive tract is the hole through the doughnut. Only things that penetrate the tract's wall ever enter the doughnut body proper; many things pass through unabsorbed.

The problem of food contaminants, which may be absorbed defenselessly by the body, is the subject of Chapter 13.

Digestion

The digestive system solves many problems for you without your having to make any conscious effort. In fact, the digestive tract is the body's ingenious way of getting the nutrients ready for absorption. Let's consider the problems that are involved:

Diaphragm: see p. 194

1. Human beings breathe as well as eat and drink through their mouths. Air taken in through the mouth must go to the lungs; food and liquid must go to the stomach. The throat must be arranged so that food and liquid do not travel to the lungs.
2. Below the lungs lies the diaphragm, a dome of muscle that separates the upper half of the major body cavity from the lower half. Food must be conducted through this wall to reach the abdomen.
3. To pass smoothly through the system, food must be ground to a paste and must be lubricated with water. Too much water would cause the paste to flow too rapidly; too little would compact it too much, which could cause it to stop moving. The amount of water should be regulated to keep the intestinal contents at the right consistency.
4. For digestive enzymes to break down food, they need it in finely divided form, suspended in a watery solution so that every particle will be accessible. Once digestion is complete and the needed nutrients have been absorbed out of the tract into the body, only a residue remains, which is excreted. It would be both wasteful and messy to excrete large quantities of water with this residue, so some water should be withdrawn, leaving a paste just solid enough to be smooth and easy to pass.
5. The materials within the tract should be kept moving, slowly but steadily, at a pace that permits all reactions to reach completion. The materials should not be allowed to back up, except when a poison or like substance has been swallowed. At such a time, the flow should reverse, to get rid of the poison by the shortest possible route (upward). If infection sets in farther down the tract, the flow should be accelerated, to speed its passage out of the body (downward).
6. The enzymes of the digestive tract are designed to digest carbohydrate, fat, and protein. The walls of the tract, composed of living cells, are also made of carbohydrate, fat, and protein. These cells need protection against the action of the powerful juices that they secrete.

7. Once waste matter has reached the end of the tract, it must be excreted, but it would be inconvenient and embarrassing if this function occurred continuously. Provision must be made for periodic, voluntary evacuation when convenient.

The following sections show how the body elegantly and efficiently solves these problems.

Anatomy of the Digestive Tract

The gastrointestinal (GI) tract is a flexible muscular tube measuring about 26 feet in length from the mouth to the anus. Figure 6–1 traces the path followed by food from one end to the other.

When you swallow a mouthful of food, it first slides across your epiglottis, bypassing the entrance to your lungs. This is the body's solution to problem 1: the epiglottis closes off your air passages so that you don't choke when you swallow.

GI tract: the gastrointestinal tract, or alimentary canal; the principal organs are the stomach and intestines.
gastro = stomach
aliment = food

Miniglossary of Gastrointestinal Terms

epiglottis (epp-ee-GLOTT-iss): cartilage in the throat that guards the entrance to the trachea and prevents fluid or food from entering it when a person swallows (see p. 193).
epi = upon (over)
glottis = back of tongue
trachea (TRAKE-ee-uh): windpipe.
esophagus (e-SOFF-uh-gus): food pipe.
cardiac sphincter (CARD-ee-ack SFINK-ter): sphincter muscle at the junction between the esophagus and the stomach.
cardiac = the heart
sphincter: circular muscle surrounding and able to close a body opening.
sphincter = band (binder)
pylorus (pie-LORE- us): sphincter muscle separating the stomach from the small intestine.
pylorus—gatekeeper
gallbladder and pancreas: see pp. 170–171.
duodenum (doo-oh-DEEN-um, doo-ODD-num): the top portion of the small intestine (about "12 fingers' breadth" long, in ancient terminology).
duodecim = twelve
jejunum (je-JOON-um): the first two-fifths of the small intestine beyond the duodenum.
ileum (ILL-ee-um): the last segment of the small intestine.
ileocecal (ill-ee-oh-SEEK-ul) **valve:** sphincter muscle separating the small and large intestines.
colon (COAL-un): the large intestine. Its segments are the ascending colon, the transverse colon, the descending colon, and the sigmoid colon.
sigmoid = shaped like the letter *S* (*sigma* in Greek)
appendix: a narrow blind sac extending from the beginning of the colon; a vestigial organ with no known function.
rectum: the muscular terminal part of the intestine, from the sigmoid colon to the anus.
anus (AY-nus): terminal sphincter muscle of the GI tract.

FIGURE 6–1

The gastrointestinal tract.

Fiber	Carbohydrate

Mouth

The mechanical action of the mouth crushes and tears fiber in food and mixes it with saliva to moisten it for swallowing.

The salivary glands secrete a watery fluid into the mouth to moisten the food. The salivary enzyme amylase begins digestion:

$$Starch \xrightarrow{amylase} \text{Small polysaccharides, maltose}$$

Esophagus

Fiber is unchanged.

Digestion of starch continues as swallowed food moves down esophagus.

Stomach

Fiber is unchanged.

Stomach acid and enzymes start to digest salivary enzymes, halting starch digestion. To a small extent, stomach acid hydrolyzes maltose and sucrose:

$$Maltose \xrightarrow{HCl} Glucose$$
$$Sucrose \xrightarrow{HCl} \text{Glucose and fructose}$$

Small intestine

Fiber is unchanged.

The pancreas produces carbohydrases and releases them through the pancreatic duct into the small intestine:

$$Polysaccharides \xrightarrow[amylase]{pancreatic} Maltose$$

Then enzymes on the surfaces of the small intestinal cells break these into monosaccharides and the cells absorb them:

$$Maltose \xrightarrow{maltase}$$
$$Sucrose \xrightarrow{sucrase} \left\} \begin{array}{l} \text{Glucose,} \\ \text{fructose,} \\ \text{galactose} \end{array} \right.$$
$$Lactose \xrightarrow{lactase} \text{(absorbed)}$$

Large intestine

Most fiber passes intact through the digestive tract to the large intestine. Here, bacterial enzymes digest some fiber:

$$Some\ fiber \xrightarrow[enzymes]{bacterial} \text{Glucose (absorbed)}$$

Fiber holds water, regulates bowel activity, binds cholesterol and some minerals, carrying them out of the body.

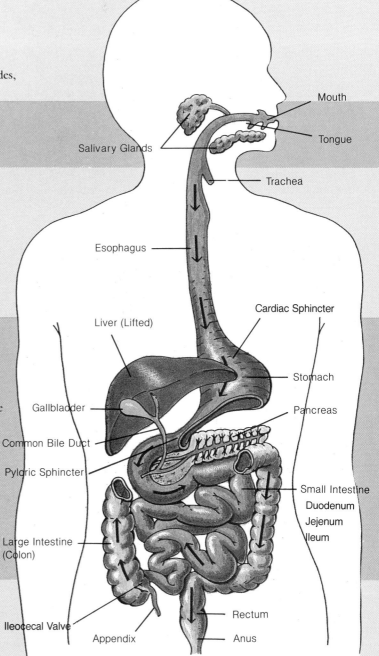

Salivary Glands

Mouth

Tongue

Trachea

Esophagus

Cardiac Sphincter

Liver (Lifted)

Stomach

Gallbladder

Pancreas

Common Bile Duct

Pyloric Sphincter

Small Intestine
Duodenum
Jejenum
Ileum

Large Intestine (Colon)

Ileocecal Valve

Rectum

Appendix

Anus

Fat	Protein	Vitamins	Minerals and Water
Mouth			
Glands in the base of the tongue secrete a lipase known as lingual lipase. Some hard fats begin to melt as they reach body temperature.	Chewing and crushing moistens protein-rich foods and mixes them with saliva to be swallowed.	No action on vitamins takes place in the mouth or esophagus.	The salivary glands add water to disperse and ca... food.
Esophagus			
Fat is unchanged.	No action.	No action.	No action.
Stomach			
The lingual lipase hydrolyzes one bond of triglycerides to produce diglycerides and fatty acids. The degree of hydrolysis of fats by lingual lipase is slight for most fats but may be appreciable for milk fats.	Stomach acid uncoils protein strands and activates stomach enzymes: $$\text{Protein} \xrightarrow[\text{HCl}]{\text{pepsin}} \text{Smaller polypeptides}$$	Intrinsic factor (see Chapter 9) attaches to vitamin B_{12}.	Stomach acid (HCl) acts on iron to reduce it, making it more absorbable (see Chapter 11). The stomach secretes enough watery fluid to turn moist, chewed mass of solid food into liquid chyme.
Small intestine			
The stomach's churning action mixes fat with water and acid. A gastric lipase accesses and hydrolyzes a very little fat. Bile flows in from the liver (via the common bile duct): $$\text{Fat} \xrightarrow{\text{bile}} \text{Emulsified fat}$$ Pancreatic lipase flows in from the pancreas: $$\text{Emulsified fat} \xrightarrow[\text{lipase}]{\text{pancreatic}}$$ Monoglycerides, glycerol, fatty acids (absorbed)	Pancreatic and small intestinal enzymes split polypeptides further: $$\text{Polypeptides} \xrightarrow[\substack{\text{and intestinal}\\\text{proteases}}]{\text{pancreatic}}$$ Dipeptides, tripeptides, and amino acids Then enzymes on the surface of the small intestinal cells hydrolyze these peptides and the cells absorb them: $$\text{Peptides} \xrightarrow[\substack{\text{di- and tri-}\\\text{peptidases}}]{\text{intestinal}} \substack{\text{Amino}\\\text{acids}\\\text{(absorbed)}}$$	Bile emulsifies fat-soluble vitamins and aids in their absorption with other fats. Water-soluble vitamins are absorbed.	The small intestine, pancreas, and liver add enough fluid so that the total secreted into the intestine in a day approximates 2 gallons. Many minerals are absorbed. Vitamin D aids in the absorption of calcium.
Large intestine			
Some fat and cholesterol, trapped in fiber, exits in feces.		Bacteria produce vitamin K, which is absorbed.	More minerals and most of the water are absorbed.

Next, the food slides down the esophagus, which conducts it through the diaphragm (problem 2) to the stomach. There it is retained for a while. The cardiac sphincter at the entrance to the stomach closes behind it so that it can't slip back (problem 5). Then, bit by bit, it pops through the pylorus into the small intestine, and the pylorus, too, closes behind it. At the top of the small intestine it bypasses an opening (entrance only—no exit) from a duct (the bile duct), which is dripping fluids (problem 3) into the small intestine from two organs outside the GI tract—the gallbladder and the pancreas. It travels on down the small intestine through its three segments— the duodenum, the jejunum, and the ileum—a total of 20 feet of tubing coiled within the abdomen. The food is now a liquid substance called chyme.

Having traveled through these segments of the small intestine, the chyme arrives at another sphincter (problem 5 again): the ileocecal valve, at the beginning of the large intestine (colon) in the lower right-hand side of the abdomen. As it enters the colon, it passes another opening. Had it slipped into this opening, it would have ended up in the appendix, a blind sac about the size of your little finger. The chyme bypasses this opening, however, and travels along the large intestine up the right-hand side of the abdomen, across the front to the left-hand side, down to the lower left-hand side, and finally below the other folds of the intestines to the back side of the body, above the rectum.

During chyme's passage through the colon, water is withdrawn, leaving semisolid waste (problem 4). This waste is held back by the strong muscles of the rectum. When it is time to defecate, the muscles relax (problem 7), and the last sphincter in the system, the anus, opens to allow its passage.

To sum up, the path followed is as shown in the margin. This is not a very complex route, considering all that happens on the way.

The Involuntary Muscles and the Glands

You are usually unaware of all the activity that goes on between the time you swallow and the time you defecate. As is the case with so much else that goes on in the body, the muscles and glands of the digestive tract meet internal needs without your having to exert any conscious effort to get the work done.

Chewing and swallowing are under conscious control, but even in the mouth there are some automatic processes you have no control over. The salivary glands squirt just enough saliva to moisten each mouthful of food so that it can pass easily down your esophagus (problem 3). After a mouthful of food has been swallowed, it is called a bolus.

At the top of the esophagus, peristalsis begins. The entire GI tract is ringed with muscles that can squeeze it tightly. Within these rings of muscle lie longitudinal muscles. When the rings tighten and the long muscles relax, the tube is constricted. When the rings relax and the long muscles tighten, the tube bulges. These actions follow each other so that the intestinal contents are continuously pushed along (problem 5). (If you have ever watched a lump of food pass along the body of a snake, you have a good picture of how these muscles work.) The waves of contraction ripple through the GI tract all the time, at the rate of about three a minute, whether or not you have just eaten a meal. Peristalsis, along with the sphincter muscles that surround the tract at key places, prevents anything from backing up (Figure 6–2).

Route followed by nutrients: MOUTH past epiglottis to ESOPHAGUS through cardiac sphincter to STOMACH through pylorus to SMALL INTESTINE (duodenum, with entrance from gallbladder and pancreas; then jejunum; then ileum) through ileocecal valve to LARGE INTESTINE past appendix to RECTUM ending at ANUS.

gland: a cell or group of cells that secretes materials for special uses in the body. Glands may be **exocrine glands**, secreting their materials "out" (into the digestive tract or onto the surface of the skin), or **endocrine glands**, secreting their materials "in" (into the blood).
exo = outside
endo = inside
krine = to separate

The salivary glands are exocrine glands.

bolus (BOH-lus): the portion of food swallowed at one time.

peristalsis (peri-STALL-sis): successive waves of involuntary muscular contraction passing along the walls of the intestine.
peri = around
stellein = wrap

FIGURE 6–2

Peristalsis.

L   C

Cross section of the small intestine. Circular muscles are outside; longitudinal muscles are inside.

Here, the circular muscles are contracting, tightening the tube. The bolus moves ahead of the constriction.

Here, the longitudinal muscles are contracting, and the circular muscles have relaxed, so the tube is loose.

The particle of liquefied food entering the small intestine is called a *bolus*. Peristalsis, which began in the esophagus and stomach, proceeds:

Bolus

Each wave of contraction moves along the GI tract as successive muscle sets contract and relax.

The intestines not only push, but also periodically squeeze their contents at intervals—as if you had put a string around them and pulled it tight. This motion, called segmentation, forces their contents backward a few inches, mixing them and allowing the digestive juices and the absorbing cells of the walls to make better contact with them.

segmentation: a periodic squeezing or partitioning of the intestine by its circular muscles.

Four major sphincter muscles divide the GI tract into its principal divisions. The cardiac sphincter prevents reflux of the stomach contents into the esophagus. The pyloric sphincter, which stays closed most of the time, prevents backup of the intestinal contents into the stomach and also holds the bolus in the stomach long enough so that it can be thoroughly mixed with gastric juice and liquefied. At the end of the small intestine, the ileocecal valve performs a similar function. Finally, the tightness of the rectal muscle is a kind of safety device; together with the anus, it prevents elimination until you choose to perform it voluntarily (problem 7).

The salivary glands.

gastric glands: exocrine glands in the stomach wall that secrete gastric juice into the stomach.
gastro = stomach

chyme (KIME): the semiliquid mass of partly digested food expelled by the stomach into the duodenum.
chymos = juice

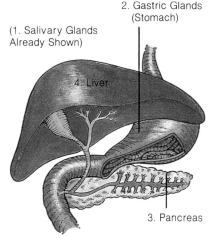

(1. Salivary Glands Already Shown)

2. Gastric Glands (Stomach)

4. Liver

3. Pancreas

Organs that secrete digestive juices.

saliva: the secretion of the salivary glands; the principal enzyme is salivary amylase.

amylase (AM-uh-lace): an enzyme that hydrolyzes amylose (a form of starch). An older name for salivary amylase is ptyalin (TY-uh-lin).

hydrolyze (HIGH-dro-lize): to split by hydrolysis (see p. 59).

Besides forcing the bolus along, the muscles of the GI tract help to liquefy it so that the digestive enzymes will have access to all the nutrients in the bolus. The first step in this process takes place in the mouth, where chewing, the addition of saliva, and the action of the tongue reduce the food to a coarse mash suitable for swallowing. A further mixing and kneading action then takes place in the stomach.

Of all parts of the GI tract, the stomach has the thickest walls and strongest muscles; in addition to the circular and longitudinal muscles, it has a third layer of diagonal muscles that also alternately contract and relax. While these three sets of muscles are all at work forcing the bolus downward, the pyloric sphincter usually remains tightly closed, preventing the bolus from passing into the duodenum. Meanwhile, the gastric glands release juices—a mixture of hydrochloric acid and enzymes—that mix with the bolus. As a result, the bolus is churned and forced down, hits the pylorus, and bounces back. When the bolus is thoroughly liquefied, the pylorus opens briefly, about three times a minute, to allow small portions through. From this point on, the intestinal contents are called chyme. They no longer resemble food.

Diagonal

Longitudinal

Circular

The stomach has three layers of muscles.

The Process of Digestion

One person eats nothing but vegetables, fruits, and nuts; another, nothing but meat, milk, and potatoes. How is it that they wind up with essentially the same body composition? It all comes down to the fact, of course, that the body renders food—whatever it is to start with—into the basic units of carbohydrate, fat, and protein. The body absorbs these units and builds its tissues from them.

To digest the food, four different body organs secrete digestive juices: the salivary glands, the stomach, the liver, and the pancreas. Each of the juices has a turn to promote the breakdown of food to small units that can be absorbed into the body.

Saliva contains not only water and salts, but also amylase, an enzyme that breaks bonds in the straight chains of starch. The digestion of starch thus begins in your mouth. In fact, you can taste the change if you choose. Starch has very little taste, but some maltose is released, conveying a subtly sweet flavor that you may associate with malted milk. If you hold a piece of starchy food like white bread in your mouth without swallowing it, you can taste it getting sweeter as the enzyme acts on it. Saliva also protects the tooth surfaces and linings of the mouth, esophagus, and stomach from attack by molecules that might harm them.[1]

Gastric juice is composed of water, enzymes, and hydrochloric acid. The acid is so strong (pH 2 or below) that if it chances to reflux into the mouth, it burns the throat. The strong acidity of the stomach prevents bacterial growth and kills most bacteria that enter the body with food. It would kill the cells of the stomach as well, but for their natural defenses. To protect themselves from gastric juice, the cells of the stomach wall secrete mucus, a thick, slimy, white polysaccharide that coats the cells, protecting them from the acid and enzymes that would otherwise digest them (problem 6).

All proteins are responsive to acidity; the stomach enzymes work most efficiently in a fluid of pH 2 or lower. However, salivary amylase, which is swallowed with the food, does not work in acid this strong, so the digestion of starch ceases as the acid penetrates the bolus. In fact, salivary amylase becomes just another protein to be digested; its amino acids end up being absorbed and recycled into other body proteins.

The major digestive event in the stomach is the hydrolysis of proteins. Both the enzyme pepsin and the stomach acid itself act as catalysts for this reaction. A gastric lipase accesses and hydrolyzes a very little fat in the stomach; the acid hydrolyzes sucrose to a very small extent; and the attachment of a protein carrier to vitamin B_{12} takes place in the stomach.

gastric juice: the secretion of the gastric glands. The principal enzymes are rennin (curdles milk protein, casein, and prepares it for pepsin action), pepsin (acts on proteins), and lipase (acts on emulsified fats).

A pH of 2 is 1,000 times stronger than a pH of 5. See Chapter 11.

mucus (MYOO-cuss): a mucopolysaccharide (relative of carbohydrate) secreted by cells of the stomach wall. The cellular lining of the stomach with its coat of mucus is known as the mucous membrane. (The noun is *mucus*; the adjective is *mucous*.)

pepsin: a gastric protease. It circulates as a precursor, pepsinogen, and is converted to pepsin by the action of stomach acid.

Vitamin B_{12} and the intrinsic factor: see Chapter 9.

It should be noted here that the strong acidity of the stomach is a desirable condition—television commercials for antacids notwithstanding. A person who overeats or who bolts her food is likely to suffer from indigestion. The muscular reaction of the stomach to unchewed lumps or to being overfilled may be so violent that it causes regurgitation (reverse peristalsis, another solution to problem 5). When this happens, the overeater may taste the stomach acid in her mouth and think she is suffering from "acid indigestion." Responding to television commercials, she may take antacids to neutralize the stomach acid.

Antacids are not, in fact, designed to counteract the stomach's discomfort from overeating or underchewing foods. When our consumer takes an antacid, she simply places a demand on the stomach to secrete more acid to counteract the neutralizer and enable the digestive enzymes to do their work. So the consumer ends up with the same amount of acid in her stomach but has had to work against the antacid to produce it.

Antacids are designed to help relieve symptoms from abnormal conditions, such as the pain felt by an ulcer patient whose stomach or duodenal lining has been attacked by acid. Antacid misuse is similar to the misuse of diuretics already described. The person who overeats or swallows unchewed food had better just keep still until the unhappy stomach has had a chance to cope with the problem it faces. Then the person should repent: learn to chew food more thoroughly, eat it more slowly, and eat less at a sitting.

pancreatic (pank-ree-AT-ic) **juice:** the exocrine secretion of the pancreas, containing enzymes for the digestion of carbohydrate, fat, and protein. (The pancreas also has an endocrine function, the secretion of insulin and other hormones.) Juice flows from the pancreas into the small intestine through the pancreatic duct.

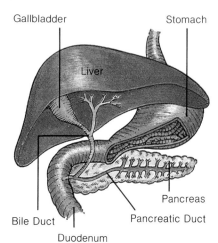

The pancreatic and bile ducts conduct pancreas and liver secretions into the duodenum.

bicarbonate: an alkaline secretion of the pancreas, part of the pancreatic juice. (Bicarbonate also occurs widely in all cell fluids.)

bile: an exocrine secretion of the liver (the liver also performs a multitude of metabolic functions). Bile flows from the liver into the gallbladder, where it is stored until needed.

gallbladder: the organ that stores and concentrates bile. When it receives the signal that fat is present in the duodenum, the gallbladder contracts and squirts bile down the bile duct.

The bacterial inhabitants of the GI tract are known as the **intestinal flora**.
flora = plant growth

By the time food has left the stomach, digestion of all three energy nutrients has begun. But the action really gets going in the small intestine, where the pancreas and liver contribute additional digestive juices by way of ducts leading into the duodenum. The pancreatic juice contains enzymes of all three kinds (protease, lipase, and amylase), plus others, and the cells of the intestinal wall also possess digestive enzymes on their surfaces.

In addition to enzymes, the pancreatic juice contains sodium bicarbonate. The pancreatic juice joins the intestinal contents just after they leave the stomach, and the bicarbonate neutralizes the acidic chyme as it enters the small intestine. From this point on, the contents of the digestive tract are at a neutral or slightly alkaline pH. The enzymes of both the intestine and the pancreas work best at this pH.

Bile, a secretion from the liver, also flows into the duodenum. The liver secretes this material continuously, but it is needed only when fat is present in the intestine. The bile is concentrated and stored in the gallbladder, which squirts it into the duodenum on request. Bile is not an enzyme, but an emulsifier (see Chapter 4); it brings fats into suspension in water so that enzymes can break them down into their component parts. Thanks to all these secretions, the three energy nutrients are digested in the small intestine.

The intestine, being neutral, permits the growth of bacteria. In fact, a healthy intestinal tract supports a thriving bacterial population that normally does the body no harm, and may actually do some good. Bacteria in the GI tract produce a variety of vitamins; three of them (vitamin B_{12}, biotin, and vitamin K) may, on occasion, be of significance to the person surrounding the GI tract. (For example, we sometimes rely on some of the vitamin K our bacteria have produced for us.) Provided that the normal intestinal flora are thriving, infectious bacteria have a hard time getting established and launching an attack on the system.

The small intestine—and, in fact, the entire GI tract—also manufactures and maintains a strong arsenal of defenses against foreign invaders. Several different kinds of defending cells are present there and confer specific immunity against intestinal diseases.

The story of how food is broken down into nutrients that can be absorbed is now nearly complete. All that remains is to recall what is left in the GI tract. The three energy nutrients—carbohydrate, fat, and protein—are the only ones that must be disassembled to basic building blocks before they are absorbed.

Most proteins are broken down to dipeptides, tripeptides, and amino acids before they are absorbed. With this in mind, you will be in a position to refute certain untrue claims made about foods—for instance, "Don't eat food A. It contains an enzyme B that will harm you." Any enzyme you eat becomes but one among thousands of different proteins in your digestive tract. Except for the digestive enzymes, whose design prevents them from being digested while they work, enzymes you eat are simply proteins that are broken down to amino acids identical to those from the other proteins you eat. Your body cannot tell the source of a particular amino acid. Don't be fooled by claims that imply that enzymes you eat will get into your blood and body organs.

The other nutrients—vitamins, minerals, and water—are mostly absorbable as is. The function of undigested residues, such as some fibers, is not to be absorbed, but rather to remain in the digestive tract, mainly to provide a semisolid mass that can stimulate the muscles of the tract so that they will remain strong and perform peristalsis efficiently. Fiber also retains water, keeping the stools soft, and carries bile acids, sterols, and fat with it out of the body, as explained in Chapter 3.

The process of absorbing the nutrients into the body presents its own problems, to be discussed in the next section. For the moment, let's assume that the digested nutrients simply disappear from the GI tract as soon as they are ready. Virtually all are gone by the time the contents of the GI tract reach the end of the small intestine. Little remains but water, a few dissolved salts and body secretions, and undigested materials such as fiber. These enter the large intestine (colon).

In the colon, intestinal bacteria degrade some of the fiber to simpler compounds (Chapter 3). The colon itself actively retrieves from its contents the materials that the conservative body is designed to recycle—much of the water and the dissolved salts (problem 4).

Some vitamins and minerals are slightly altered during digestion. See "Vitamin B_{12}" in Chapter 9 and "Iron" in Chapter 12.

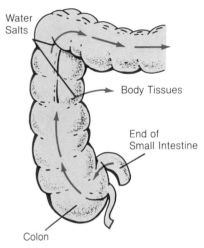

The colon reabsorbs water and salts.

Absorption

Problem: Given an elaborate production in which 1,000 actors are on stage at once, provide a means by which all can exit simultaneously. This is the problem of absorption. Within three or four hours after you have eaten a dinner of beans and rice (or spinach lasagna, or steak and potatoes) with vegetable, salad, beverage, and dessert, your body must find a way to absorb some two hundred thousand million, million, million amino acid molecules one by one, and an equivalent number of monosaccharide, monoglyceride, glycerol, fatty acid, vitamin, and mineral molecules as well.

For the stage production, the manager might design multiple wings that all the actors could crowd into, a dozen at a time. A mechanical genius might somehow design moving wings that would actively engulf the actors as they approached. The absorptive system is no such fantasy; in 20 feet of small intestine, it provides a surface whose extent compares with a quarter of a football field in area, where the nutrient molecules can make contact and be absorbed. To remove them rapidly and provide room for more to be absorbed, a rapid flow of circulating blood continuously bathes the underside of this surface, washing away the absorbed nutrients and carrying them to the liver and other parts of the body.

Anatomy of the Absorptive System

The small intestine is a tube about 20 feet long and an inch or so across. Its inner surface looks smooth and slippery, but viewed through a microscope, it turns out to be wrinkled into hundreds of folds. Each fold is covered with

FIGURE 6–3

Surface features of the small intestinal wall. A. Five folds in the wall of the small intestine. Each is covered with villi. B. Two villi (detail of A). Each villus is composed of several hundred cells. C. Three cells of a single villus (detail of B). Each cell is coated with microvilli. A photograph of part of two cells like these, on neighboring villi is shown in Figure 6-4.

Villi

Microvilli

Capillaries

Lymph Vessel

Vein

Artery

Lymph Duct

A.

B.

C.

villi (VILL-ee, VILL-eye), singular **villus:** fingerlike projections from the folds of the small intestine.

microvilli (MY-cro-VILL-ee, MY-cro-VILL-eye), singular **microvillus:** projections from the membranes of the cells of the villi.

lymph (limf): the body fluid that occupies the spaces between the cells and outside the vascular system. Lymph consists of all the constituents of blood that can escape from the vascular system; it circulates in a loosely organized system of vessels and ducts known as the **lymphatic system**.

thousands of nipplelike projections, as numerous as the hairs on velvet fabric. Each of these small intestinal projections is a villus. A single villus, magnified still more, turns out to be composed of hundreds of cells, each covered with its own microscopic hairs, the microvilli (see Figures 6–3 and 6–4).

The villi are in constant motion. Each villus is lined by a thin sheet of muscle, so that it can wave, squirm, and wriggle like the tentacles of a sea anemone. Any nutrient molecule small enough to be absorbed is trapped in the microvilli and drawn into the cells beneath them. Some partially digested nutrients are caught in the microvilli, digested further by enzymes there, and then absorbed into the cells.

Once a molecule has entered a cell in a villus, the next problem is to transport it to its destination elsewhere in the body. Everyone knows that the bloodstream performs this function, but you may be surprised to learn that there is a second transport system—the lymphatic system. Both of these systems supply vessels to each villus, as shown in Figure 6–3B. When a nutrient molecule has crossed the cell of a villus, it may enter either the lymph or the blood. In either case, the nutrients end up in the blood, at least for a while.

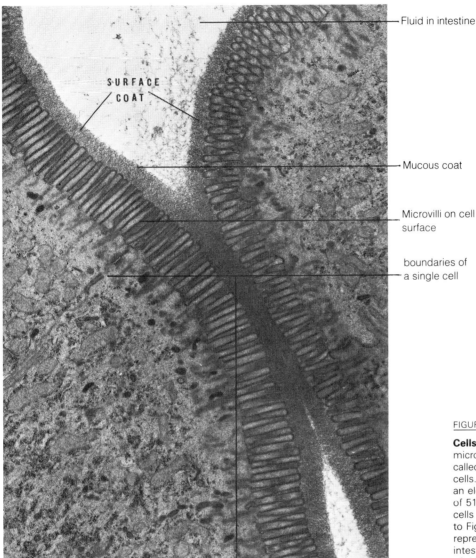

Fluid in intestine

SURFACE COAT

Mucous coat

Microvilli on cell surface

boundaries of a single cell

FIGURE 6–4

Cells of two adjacent intestinal villi. The microvilli and mucous coat are sometimes called the brush border of the intestinal cells. This photograph was taken through an electron microscope at a magnification of 51,000 times. Think how many of these cells there are in the small intestine (refer to Figure 6–3 and notice that even [A] represents but a tiny section of the intestinal wall). The photograph at the start of this chapter represents an even closer view of one of these cells.

A Closer Look at the Intestinal Cells

The cells of the villi are among the most amazing in the body, for they recognize, select, and regulate the absorption of the nutrients the body needs. A close look at these cells is worthwhile, because it will help to explode a number of common misconceptions about nutrition.

Each cell of a villus is coated with thousands of microvilli, which project from the cell's membrane (Figure 6–3C). In these microvilli and in the membrane lie hundreds of different kinds of enzymes and "pumps," which recognize and act on different nutrients. For example, the enzyme lactase, which breaks apart the disaccharide lactose (milk sugar), lies within the cells' microvilli. The presence of lactase at the cell surface ensures the efficient absorption of this sugar; as soon as it is broken into its component parts (glucose and galactose), those parts are easily contacted by the nearby pumps, which move them into the interior of the cell. This arrangement makes it easy for a newborn infant to absorb and use milk sugar, even though his GI tract may in some ways still be immature.

Enzymes for cleaving dipeptides and tripeptides also lie in the surface structures of the intestinal cells. Whole proteins—long polypeptides—are digested to chains a few amino acids in length, out in the fluid of the intestine; once they have been rendered into dipeptides and tripeptides, these fragments are contacted and trapped by the microvilli, which digest them further if necessary. The cells' enzymes then can deliver the final products—amino acids—directly to the pumps, which carry them into the interior of the cells.

There is nothing random about this process. The anatomical arrangement guarantees not only digestion, but also delivery of its products into the body. Digestion and absorption are coordinated.

Some people believe that eating predigested protein (amino acid preparations such as the "liquid protein" products sold to dieters) saves the body the work of having to digest protein, so that the digestive system won't "wear out" so easily. Nothing could be further from the truth. As a matter of fact, the amino acids from whole proteins are better absorbed and utilized than are hydrolyzed amino acid mixtures, because they are released at the rate and in the order that the body can best use.

The absorption of lipids differs from that of amino acids in that pumps are not involved. Cell membranes dissolve lipids easily, because they are made largely of lipid themselves. After the triglycerides have been digested to monoglycerides or to glycerol and fatty acids, for example, they merge into micelles and move into the cells. The cell retains them by reassembling them into triglycerides again.

Another common misconception about digestion is that people shouldn't eat certain food combinations (for example, fruit and meat) at the same meal, because the digestive system can't handle more than one task at a time. The art of "food combining" is based on this idea, and it represents a gross underestimation of the body's capabilities. There is seldom interference between the absorption and utilization of one kind of nutrient and that of another. In fact, they often seem to enhance each other. For example, sugars taken at the same time as protein (within four hours) seem to promote better utilization of the protein. The sugars may slow the digestive process so that it is more complete, or they may provide precursors for some nonessential amino acids so that whole proteins can be produced more readily and retained in the body.

The interaction between the carbohydrate in one food and the protein in another is not unique; there are other interactions that have to do with the vitamins and minerals. For example, the vitamin C in one food enhances the absorption of iron from another. Many other instances of mutually beneficial interactions are presented in later chapters.

As you can see, the cells of the intestinal tract wall are beautifully designed to perform their functions. A further refinement of the system is that the cells of successive portions of the tract are specialized for different absorptive functions. The nutrients that are ready for absorption early are absorbed near the top of the tract; those that take longer to be digested are absorbed farther down. Thus the top portion of the duodenum is specialized for the absorption of calcium and several B vitamins, such as thiamin and riboflavin; the jejunum accomplishes most of the absorption of triglycerides; and vitamin B_{12} is absorbed at the end of the ileum. Medical and health professionals who deal with digestion learn the specialized absorptive functions of different parts of the GI tract so that, when one part becomes dysfunctional, the diet can be adjusted accordingly.

The rate at which the nutrients travel through the GI tract is finely adjusted to maximize their availability to the appropriate absorptive segment of the tract when they are ready. The lowly "gut" turns out to be one of the most elegantly designed organ systems in your body.

Release of Absorbed Nutrients

Once inside the intestinal cells, the products of digestion must be released for transport to the rest of the body. The water-soluble nutrients (including the smaller products of lipid digestion) are released directly into the bloodstream. For the larger lipids and the fat-soluble vitamins, however, access directly into the capillaries is impossible, because they are insoluble in water. The cells assemble the monoglycerides and long-chain fatty acids into larger molecules,

Transport of Nutrients into Blood	
Water-soluble nutrients	
Carbohydrates	
Monosaccharides	Directly into blood
Lipids	
Glycerol	Directly into blood
Short-chain fatty acids	Directly into blood
Medium-chain fatty acids	Directly into blood
Proteins	
Amino acids	Directly into blood
Vitamins	
Vitamins B and C	Directly into blood
Minerals	Directly into blood
Fat-soluble nutrients	
Lipids	
Long-chain fatty acids	Made into triglycerides
Monoglycerides	Made into triglycerides
Triglycerides	To lymph, then blood
Cholesterol	To lymph, then blood
Phospholipids	To lymph, then blood
Vitamins	
Vitamins A, D, E, K	To lymph, then blood

triglycerides. These triglycerides and the other large lipids (cholesterol and the phospholipids) cluster together, forming chylomicrons, and special proteins insert themselves into their surfaces (see p. 105). Finally, the cells release the chylomicrons into the lymphatic system. They can then glide through the lymph spaces until they move to a point of entry into the bloodstream near the heart.

Chylomicrons are one kind of lipoprotein. The lipoproteins were described in Chapter 4.

The Circulatory Systems

Once a nutrient has entered the bloodstream or the lymphatic system, it may be transported to any part of the body and thus become available to any of the cells, from the tips of the toes to the roots of the hair. The circulatory systems are arranged to deliver nutrients anywhere they are needed. Figure 6–5 shows the various ways in which the nutrients get into cells.

The Vascular System

The vascular, or blood circulatory, system is a closed system of vessels through which blood flows continuously in a figure eight, with the heart serving as a pump at the crossover point. The vascular system is diagrammed in Figure 6–6. As the blood circulates through this system, it picks up and delivers materials as needed.

All the body tissues derive oxygen and nutrients from the blood and deposit carbon dioxide and other wastes into it. The lungs are the place for exchange of carbon dioxide (which leaves the blood to be breathed out) and oxygen (which enters the blood to be delivered to all cells). The digestive system is the place for nutrients to be picked up. The kidneys are the place where wastes other than carbon dioxide are filtered out of the blood to be excreted in the urine (see Figure 6–7).

Blood leaving the right side of the heart circulates by way of arteries into the lung capillaries and then back through veins to the left side of the heart. The left side of the heart then pumps the blood out through arteries to all systems of the body. The blood circulates in the capillaries, where it exchanges material with the cells, and then collects into veins, which return it again to the right side of the heart. In short, blood travels this simple route:

■ Heart to arteries to capillaries to veins to heart.

The routing of the blood past the digestive system is unique. The blood is carried to the digestive system (as to all organs) by way of an artery, which (as in all organs) branches into capillaries to reach every cell. However, blood leaving the digestive system goes by way of a vein, not back to the heart, but to another organ: the liver. This vein *again* branches into capillaries, so that every cell of the liver also has access to the blood carried by the vein. (Blood leaving the liver then returns to the heart by way of a vein.) The route is:

■ Heart to arteries to capillaries (in intestines) to vein to capillaries (in liver) to vein to heart.

artery: a vessel that carries blood away from the heart.

capillary (CAP-ill-ary): a small vessel that branches from an artery. Capillaries connect arteries to veins. Exchange of oxygen and nutrients and waste materials takes place across capillary walls.

vein: a vessel that carries blood back to the heart.

The blood arriving at the intestines flows through the **mesentery** (MEZ-en-terry), a strong, flexible membrane that surrounds and supports the abdominal organs.

The vein that collects blood from the mesentery and conducts it to capillaries in the liver is the **portal vein**.
portal = gateway

The vein that collects blood from the liver capillaries and returns it to the heart is the **hepatic vein**.
hepat = liver

FIGURE 6–5

How things get into cells.

Diffusion. Some substances cross membranes freely; water is an example. The concentration of water tends to equalize on the two sides of a membrane; as long as it is higher outside the cell, it flows in; if it is higher inside the cell, it flows out. The cell cannot regulate the entrance and exit of water directly, but can control it indirectly by concentrating some other substance to which water is attracted, such as protein or sodium. Thus the cell can pump in sodium, and water will follow passively. This is the way the cells of the wall of the large intestine act to retrieve water for the body. Since nearly all the sodium is taken into these cells before waste is excreted, nearly all the water is absorbed, too. Small lipids also cross cell membranes by diffusion.

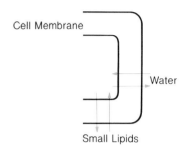

Facilitated diffusion. Other compounds cannot cross the membranes of the intestinal wall cells unless there is a specific carrier or facilitator in the membrane. The carrier may shuttle back and forth from one side of the membrane to the other, carrying its passengers either way, or it may affect the permeability of the membrane in such a way that the compound is admitted. The end result is the same as for diffusion; equal concentrations are reached on both sides. By providing carriers only for the desired compounds, the cell effectively bars all others (except those to which it is freely permeable). Facilitated diffusion is also termed carrier-mediated diffusion or passive transport.
1. Carrier loads particle on outside of cell.
2. Carrier releases particle on inside of cell.
3. Or the reverse.

Active transport. For compounds that must be absorbed actively, the two types of diffusion systems mentioned above will not suffice. The best a cell can do using only diffusion is to move a compound across its membrane until the concentration inside the cell is equal to that outside. An effective means of concentrating a substance inside or outside the cell is to pump it across the membrane, consuming energy in the process. Glucose, amino acids, and other nutrients are absorbed by intestinal wall cells in this manner.
Energy for active transport may be supplied by ATP (see p. 205) or by **cotransport**—a process in which the movement of one substance into the cell somehow facilitates the simultaneous uptake of another. Sodium is known to facilitate glucose uptake this way.
1. Carrier loads particle on outside of cell.
2. Carrier releases particle on inside of cell.
3. Carrier returns to outside to pick up another particle. (Cells can concentrate substances inside or outside their membranes this way.)

Pinocytosis. Pinocytosis involves a large area of the cell membrane, which actively engulfs liquids and "swallows" them into the cell. An occasional whole protein can get into the body this way. This can confer benefits (for example, an infant may receive antibodies from his mother this way) or hazards (allergens can enter this way, on occasion).
1. Liquid contacts cell membrane.
2. Membrane wraps around droplet.
3. Portion of membrane surrounding droplet separates into cell.

FIGURE 6–6

The vascular system. Blood leaves the right side of the heart, picks up oxygen in the lungs, and returns to the left side of the heart. Blood leaves the left side of the heart; goes to the head, or to the digestive tract and then the liver, or to the lower body; then returns to the right side of the heart.

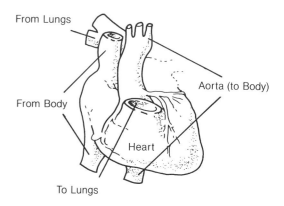

Heart (Anatomically Correct)

From Lungs

Aorta (to Body)

From Body

Heart

To Lungs

*The aorta is the main artery that launches blood on its course through the body. The picture is not anatomically correct but is drawn this way for clarity. The aorta arises behind the left side of the heart and arcs upward, then divides.

Blood Vessel Carrying Blood into Glomerulus

Glomerulus

Capillaries of Glomerulus

Blood Vessel Carrying Blood Away from Glomerulus

Tubules

Blood Vessel Carrying Blood Back to Body

Blood Vessel Carrying Blood Alongside Tubule

To the Bladder

FIGURE 6–7

One of the kidney's many functioning units (nephrons). Blood flows into the entranceway (glomerulus), and some of its fluid, with dissolved substances, is filtered into the tubules (1). Then the blood passes alongside the tubules, which return fluid and substances needed by the body (2). The tubule passes waste materials (urine) on to the bladder (3).

The cleansing of blood in the nephron is roughly analogous to the way you might have your car cleaned up at the service station. First you remove all your possessions and trash so that the car can be vacuumed (1). Then you put back in the car what you want to keep (2) and throw away the trash (3).

An anatomist studying this system knows there must be a reason for this special arrangement. The liver is placed in the circulation at this point so that it will have the first chance at the materials absorbed from the GI tract. (See Figure 6–8.) In fact, the liver has many jobs to do preparing the absorbed nutrients for use by the body. It is the body's major metabolic organ.

You might guess that in addition, the liver may stand as gatekeeper to waylay intruders that might otherwise harm the heart or brain. Perhaps this is why, when people ingest poisons that succeed in passing the first barrier (the intestinal cells) and entering the blood, it is the liver that suffers the damage—from hepatitis virus, from drugs such as barbiturates, from alcohol, from poisons, and from contaminants such as mercury. Perhaps, in fact, you have been undervaluing your liver, not knowing what heroic tasks it quietly performs for you.

Here are *some* of the things the liver does with the nutrients that arrive there:

■ *Carbohydrates.* The liver converts fructose and galactose to glucose, removes excess glucose in response to insulin, makes and stores glycogen, and releases glucose in response to glucagon.

■ *Lipids.* The liver builds and breaks down triglycerides, phospholipids, and cholesterol as needed; packages extra lipids in lipoproteins for export to

FIGURE 6–8

The liver. The routing of the blood ensures that the liver has first crack at all the nutrients absorbed into the bloodstream from the digestive tract:

1. Vessels gather up nutrients and reabsorbed water and salts from all over the digestive tract.
2. These vessels merge into the portal vein, which conducts all absorbed materials to the liver.
3. The hepatic artery brings a supply of freshly oxygenated blood (not loaded with nutrients) from the lungs, to offer oxygen to the liver's own cells.
4. Capillaries branch out all over the liver, making nutrients and oxygen available to all its cells, and giving the cells access to blood from the digestive system.
5. Hepatic veins gather up blood leaving the liver to return it to the heart.

In contrast, lipids absorbed into lymph do *not* go to the liver first. They go to the heart, which pumps them to all the body's cells. The cells can remove the lipids they want, and the liver then has to deal only with the remnants.

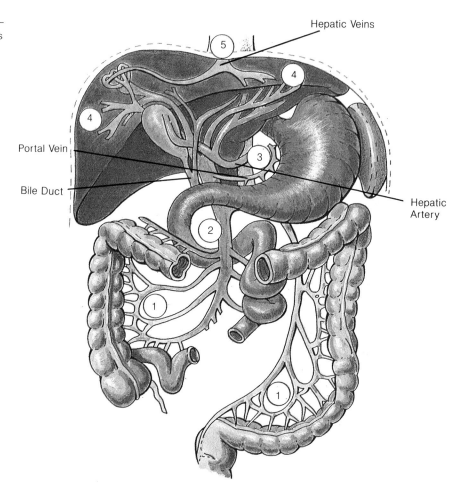

other body organs; manufactures bile to send to the gallbladder for use in digestion; and makes ketone bodies (see Chapter 7) when called for.

- *Protein.* The liver manufactures (nonessential) amino acids that are in short supply; removes from circulation and deaminates those amino acids that are present in excess of need; removes ammonia from the blood and converts it to urea to be sent to the kidneys for excretion; makes other nitrogen-containing compounds the body needs (such as bases used in DNA and RNA); and makes plasma proteins such as albumin, antibodies, clotting factors, and anticlotting factors
- *Other.* The liver detoxifies alcohol, drugs, wastes, and poisons; destroys old red blood cells and makes new ones; stores vitamins, iron, and copper; produces heat; and forms lymph.

The Lymphatic System

The lymphatic system is an open system that can be pictured simply as being similar to the water-filled spaces in a sponge. If you squeeze one end of a sponge, you can force the water to the other end. Between the cells of the body are spaces similar to those in the sponge, and the fluid circulating in them is the lymph. This fluid is almost identical to that of the blood, except that it contains no red blood cells, because they cannot escape through the blood vessel walls. The spaces between the cells are somewhat imprecisely called lymphatic "vessels."

The lymphatic system has no pump; like the water in a sponge, lymph "squishes" from one portion of the body to another as muscles contract and create pressure here and there. Ultimately, much of the lymph collects in a large duct behind the heart. This duct terminates in a vein that conducts the lymph into the heart. Thus materials from the GI tract that enter lymphatic vessels in the villi ultimately enter the blood circulatory system and then circulate through arteries, capillaries, and veins like the other nutrients. In short, nutrients that are first absorbed into lymph soon get into the blood.

The duct that conveys lymph toward the heart is the **thoracic** (thor-ASS-ic) **duct**. The **subclavian vein** connects this duct with the right upper chamber of the heart, providing a passageway by which lymph can be returned to the vascular system.

Once inside the body, the nutrients can travel freely to any destination and can be taken into cells and used as needed. What becomes of them is the subject of the next chapter.

Regulation of Digestion and Absorption

Two marvelous systems coordinate all the digestive and absorptive processes: the hormonal (or endocrine) system and the nervous system. The examples that follow illustrate the principles of the body's regulation of its internal environment.

The stomach normally remains at pH 1.5 or 1.7. How does it stay that way? One of the regulators of the stomach pH is the hormone gastrin, secreted by cells in the stomach wall. The entrance of food into the stomach stimulates these cells to release the hormone. The hormone, in turn, stimulates other stomach glands to secrete the components of hydrochloric acid. When pH 1.5 is reached, the gastrin-producing cells cannot release the hormone, so they stop. The acid itself turns them off. The acid-producing glands, lacking the hormonal stimulus, then stop secreting hydrochloric acid. Thus the system adjusts itself automatically.

Another regulator consists of nerve receptors in the stomach wall. These receptors respond to the presence of food and stimulate activity by both the gastric glands and muscles. As the stomach empties, the receptors are no longer stimulated, the flow of juices slows, and the stomach quiets down.

gastrin: a hormone secreted by cells in the stomach wall. Target organ: the stomach. Response: secretion of gastric juice.

The pylorus opens to let out a little chyme. How does it know when to close? When the pylorus relaxes, acidic chyme slips through. The acid itself touching that muscle on the far side causes the pylorus to close tightly. Only after the chyme has been neutralized by pancreatic bicarbonate and the medium surrounding the pylorus has become alkaline can the muscle relax again. This process ensures that the chyme will be released slowly enough to be neutralized as it flows through the small intestine. This is important, because the small intestine has less of a mucous coating than the stomach does and therefore is not so well protected from acid.

As the chyme enters the intestine, the pancreas adds bicarbonate to it, so that the intestinal contents always remain at a slightly alkaline pH. How does the pancreas

secretin (see-CREET-in): a hormone produced by cells in the duodenum wall. Target organ: the pancreas. Response: secretion of pancreatic juice.

cholecystokinin (coal-ee-sis-toe-KINE-in): a hormone produced by cells of the intestinal wall. Target organ: the gallbladder. Response: release of bile.

enterogastrone (enter-oh-GAS-trone): a hormone believed to be produced by the intestine in response to the presence of fat. Target organ: the stomach. Response: slowing of peristalsis.

The kinds of regulation described are all examples of **feedback** mechanisms: a certain condition demands a response to change that condition. The change produced becomes itself the signal to cut off the response; thus the system is self-corrective.

stress: any threat to a person's well-being. The threat may be physical or psychological, desired or feared, but the reaction is always the same. See *stress response*.

know how much to add? The duodenal contents stimulate cells of the duodenum wall to release the hormone secretin into the blood. As this hormone circulates through the pancreas, it stimulates the pancreas to release its juices. Thus whenever there is an acid in the duodenum, the pancreas responds by sending bicarbonate to neutralize it. When the need has been met, the secretin cells of the duodenal wall are no longer stimulated to release the hormone, the hormone no longer flows through the blood, the pancreas no longer receives the message, and it stops sending pancreatic juice. Nerves also regulate pancreatic secretions.

When fat is present in the intestine, the gallbladder contracts to squirt bile into the intestine, to emulsify the fat. How does the gallbladder get the message that fat is present? Fat in the intestine stimulates cells of the intestinal wall to release the hormone cholecystokinin. This hormone, reaching the gallbladder by way of the blood, stimulates it to contract, releasing bile into the small intestine. Once the fat in the intestine is emulsified and enzymes have begun to work on it, it no longer provokes release of the hormone, and the message to contract is canceled.

The digestion of fat takes longer than that of carbohydrate. When fat is present, intestinal motility slows to allow time for its digestion. How does the intestine know when to slow down? Fat stimulates the release of the hormone enterogastrone, which suppresses the nerves that stimulate GI tract motility, thus keeping food in the stomach longer. You may recall that a mixed breakfast of carbohydrate, fat, and protein is recommended, partly because fat slows the digestion of carbohydrate, helping to keep the blood glucose level steady. Hormonal and nervous mechanisms like these account for much of the body's ability to adapt to changing conditions.

Once you have begun asking questions like these, you may not want to stop until you have become a full-fledged physiologist. For now, however, these few will be enough to make the point. Throughout the digestive system and all other body systems, all processes are precisely and automatically regulated, without your conscious efforts. This leaves you free to compose a symphony or to gaze at the stars instead of tying up your energy in worrying about how much acid to secrete or when to close your pylorus. This remarkable arrangement once prompted the physiologist Claude Bernard to remark, "Stability of the internal environment is the condition of free life." Walter Cannon, another physiologist, wrote a whole book about these processes, aptly entitled *The Wisdom of the Body*.

Stress and Digestion/Absorption

In sudden danger, the body treats digesting food as a low-priority activity; it has more important things to do, such as defending itself, fighting, or running away. Together, the hormonal and nervous systems suppress the digestive activity that they normally coordinate, and instead direct the body's resources to the meeting of danger. This reaction to the necessity presented by environmental change is the famous "fight-or-flight reaction"—the stress response.

Stress can be loosely described as anything that you experience as a threat to your stability or equilibrium. Even eating sugar or walking in the cold is stress, because it demands action to restore the status quo—normal blood glucose level or normal body temperature. Both physical and psychological stresses elicit the body's stress response. Major physical stresses include pain, illness of any kind, surgery, wounds, burns, infections, a very hot or humid climate, toxic compounds, radiation, and pollution. Major psychological stresses are listed in Table 6–1. To be busy is not to be under stress, as long as the busyness does not threaten your equilibrium. Change and threats are what constitute psychological stress.

The stress response begins when a threat to your equilibrium is perceived by the brain. The sight of a car hurtling toward you; the terror that an enemy is concealed around a nearby corner; the excitement of planning for a party, a move, or a wedding; the feeling of pain; or any other such disturbance perceived by the brain serves as an alarm signal. There follows the chain of events depicted in Figure 6–9, which acts through both nerves and hormones to bring about a state of readiness in every body part. The effects all favor physical action (fight or flight). Notice the tremendous array of target organs in Figure 6–9 and in the paragraph that follows.

The pupils of the *eyes* widen so that you can see better; the *muscles* tense up so that you can jump, run, or struggle with maximum strength; breathing quickens to bring more oxygen into the *lungs*, and the *heart* races to rush this oxygen to the muscles, so that they can burn the fuel they need for energy. The *liver* pours forth the needed fuels—glucose and ketone bodies—from its stored supply, and the *fat cells* release fatty acids as alternative fuels. Body *protein tissues* break down to supply amino acids to back up the glucose supply and to be ready to heal wounds if necessary. The *blood vessels* of the muscles expand to feed them better, while those of the *GI tract* constrict; and GI tract glands shut down (digestion is a low-priority process in time of danger). Less blood flows to the *kidney*, so that fluid is conserved; and less flows to the *skin*, so that blood loss will be minimized at any wound site. More *platelets* form, to allow the blood to clot faster if need be. *Hearing* sharpens, and the *brain* produces local opiumlike substances, dulling its sensation of pain, which during an emergency might distract you from taking the needed action. And your *hair* may even stand on end—a reminder that there was a time when our ancestors had enough hair to bristle, look bigger, and frighten off their enemies.

This tightly synchronized, adaptive reaction to threat provides superb support for emergency physical action. You probably remember having had to take such action; you may have performed an amazing feat of strength or speed for a few minutes, and only after it was over noticed that your heart was hammering, your breathing was fast, your fingers were cold, your skin was tingling, your mouth was dry, and the sensation of pain or exhaustion was just beginning to come through as the adrenaline drained away.

Anyone can respond in this magnificent fashion to sudden physical stress for a short time. But if the stress is prolonged, and especially if physical action is not a permitted response to the stress, then it can drain the body of its reserves and leave it weakened, aged, and susceptible to illness. Much of the disability imposed by prolonged stress is nutritional: you can't eat, can't digest your food or absorb nutrients, and so can't store them in reserve for periods of need.

All three energy fuels—carbohydrate, fat, and protein—are drawn upon in increased quantities during stress. If the stress requires vigorous physical action, and if there is injury, all three are used. While the body is busy responding and not eating, the fuels must be drawn from internal sources.

The conservation of *water* at such a time is of utmost importance, as you can deduce from a look at Figure 6–9. The body takes several measures to

stress response: the body's response to stress, mediated by both nerves and hormones initially; begins with an *alarm reaction*, proceeds through a stage of *resistance*, and then leads to *recovery* or, if prolonged, to *exhaustion*. This three-stage response has also been termed the **general adaptation syndrome**.

TABLE 6–1

Events People Perceive as Stressful

People ranked these events, according to how stressful they perceived them to be, on a scale from 1 to 100. Note that some "happy" events are included here. Individual people may score these events higher or lower than the averages shown here.

Life Event	"Stress Points"
Death of spouse	100
Divorce	73
Marital separation	65
Jail term	63
Death of close family member	63
Personal injury or illness	53
Marriage	50
Being fired at work	47
Marital reconciliation	45
Retirement	45
Change in health of a family member	44
Pregnancy	40
Sex difficulties	39
Gain of new family member	39
Business readjustment	39
Change in financial state	38
Death of close friend	37
Change to different line of work	36
Change in number of arguments with spouse	35
Large mortgage or loan	31
Foreclosure of mortgage or loan	30
Change in responsibilities at work	29
Son or daughter leaving home	29
Trouble with in-laws	29
Outstanding personal achievement	28
Wife beginning or stopping work	26
School beginning or ending	26
Change in living conditions	25
Revision of personal habits	24
Trouble with boss	23
Change in work hours or conditions	20
Change in residence	20
Change in schools	20
Change in recreation	19
Change in church activities	19
Change in social activities	18
Small mortgage or loan	17
Change in sleeping habits	16
Change in number of family get-togethers	15
Change in eating habits	15
Vacation	13
Christmas	12
Minor violations of the law	11

Note: Total stress points below 100 for the past six months indicate no cause for concern; totals above 200 suggest an urgent need for stress reduction. Between 100 and 200, intelligent stress management is called for.

Source: Adapted from T.H. Holmes and R.H. Rahe, The social readjustment rating scale, *Journal of Psychosomatic Research* 11 (1967): 213–218, and updated as published in Lifescore, *Family Health,* January 1979, p. 32.

FIGURE 6–9

The stress reaction.

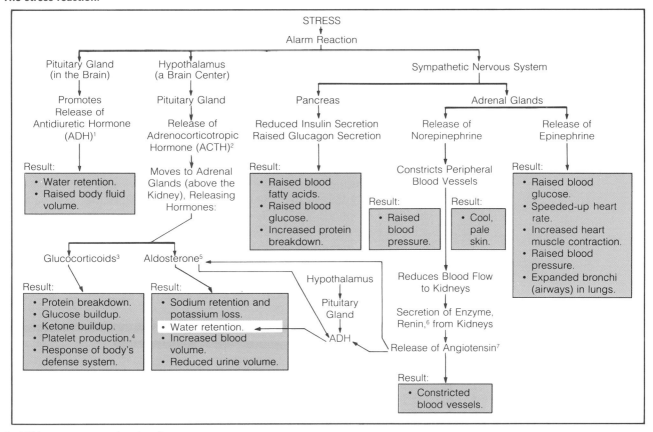

1. ADH prevents water loss in urine.
2. ACTH stimulates the adrenal glands.
3. Glucocorticoids are hormones from the adrenal glands, affecting the body's management of glucose.
4. The platelets are small, cell-fragment-like bodies in the blood that help with blood clotting if injury occurs.
5. The hormone aldosterone, from the adrenal glands, is involved in blood pressure regulation.
6. Renin functions to raise blood pressure by activating angiotensin. (Chapter 11 explains in full.)
7. The hormone angiotensin is involved in blood pressure regulation.

conserve water. One is to retain sodium—but to retain sodium the kidney exchanges, and loses, *potassium*. Thus you need ample stores of potassium to be able to afford this loss.

As for the energy nutrients, *glucose* is taken from stored glycogen in the liver for as long as the supply lasts, but the supply is exhausted within a day. Thereafter, body *protein* provides the only significant continuing glucose supply, and this is drawn primarily from muscle. Amino acids from muscle also have to be used to make scar tissue to heal wounds. Tissues that can do so use *fat* for energy, and in a normally nourished person, fat stores are adequate to meet the need for many days. Chapter 7 displays these processes as they occur during the stress of fasting; for now, what is important to notice is that the body uses not only *dispensable* supplies (those that are there to be used up, so to speak, like stored fat), but also functional tissue that we don't want to lose, like muscle tissue. Two thoughts come to mind. First, in preparation for prolonged periods of stress, we should have as much protein in the muscle as possible. Second, we should take measures to minimize the wasting of muscle during stress.

Another nutrient lost from the body during stress is *calcium* from the bones. The evidence is not completely clear on this, but it has been observed that people lose widely varying amounts of this important bone mineral, depending partly on their hormonal state.[2] Adult bone loss is a common occurrence anyway, so the same considerations apply here as for protein: we want to know, first, how to prepare for these losses, and second, how to minimize them.

The best nutritional preparation for stress is a balanced and varied diet as part of a lifestyle in which exercise plays a constant part. Notice that nothing is said here about supplements or gimmicks. Just eat well to obtain the nutrients and work out regularly to promote their storage, and your body will be as well prepared as it can be to withstand the impact of periods of unavoidable stress.

During severe stress, the appetite is suppressed. We've already said why. It's an adaptive reaction to a *physical* threat, the kind of threat that our ancestors experienced during their evolution. Energy at such a time is needed for fight or flight; it would be wasteful and risky to spend it looking for or eating food. The blood supply has been diverted to the muscles to maximize strength and speed, so even if you swallow food, you may not be able to digest or absorb it efficiently. (In a severe upset, the stomach and intestines will even reject solid food; vomiting and/or diarrhea are their way of disposing of a burden they can't handle.) All of this means that it is poor advice to someone under severe stress to tell them to eat. They can't; and if they force themselves to eat, they can't assimilate what they've eaten.

On the other hand, fasting is itself a stress on the body, and the longer you go without eating, the harder it can be to get started again. So it can be a no-win situation. It is frightening to see the downward spiral people can get into once they have let stress affect them to the point where they can't eat, and not eating makes it harder for them to handle the stress.

It is therefore desirable not to let stress become so overwhelming that eating becomes impossible. Managing stress so that it does not overwhelm is a psychological task, and may require the help of a counselor.

If you can eat, do so, of course. Take only a little if that's all you can handle, and eat more often to keep meeting your energy and nutrient needs. Choose a variety of foods. Drink fluids, too. Although the body conserves fluids during stress, it will excrete what it does not need, and by taking in water you enable your kidneys to excrete the sodium they might otherwise have to retain.

Whenever someone can't eat, there will inevitably be depletion of nutrients. Aside from the protein, calcium, and potassium already mentioned, the nutrients most susceptible to this depletion are the vitamins and minerals that are not stored in substantial quantities. People are aware that some water-soluble vitamins (B vitamins and vitamin C) fall into this category; they are less likely to know that some two dozen minerals do, too. When the question arises whether one should take vitamin supplements during periods of stress, the answer should probably be: Yes, if you can't eat—but not just vitamin supplements. Take a vitamin-mineral preparation that supplies a balanced assortment of all the nutrients that might be needed, not in megadoses, but in amounts comparable to the RDA. And don't forget: the energy nutrients you need don't come in pill form, nor can you obtain the calcium you need from such a pill.

The vitamins and minerals occupy four chapters later in the book, but it seems important to say this much about them here. Generally, people consuming less than about 1,500 kcalories of food per day need such supplements. The

RDA table on the inside front cover shows the amounts to look for, and Appendix J compares national brands.

When the stressful time is over and the body can recover, the opportunity comes to replenish depleted stores. If you have lost weight, you need to gain it back—not just by eating and putting on fat, but by eating and exercising to restore both lean and fat tissue. If you have gained weight, it is time to get back in trim with a combination of diet and exercise. But just as important as nutrition techniques is the learning of attitudes to prevent the next stressful event from being so overwhelming and debilitating.

Common Digestive Problems

The facts of anatomy and physiology presented in this chapter permit easy understanding of some common situations, so a few practical applications will be presented here. Everyone, at one time or another, has to deal with choking on food, vomiting, diarrhea, and constipation; and everyone is familiar with ulcers.

When someone chokes on food, it is because the food has slipped into the air passage and cut off breathing. Food can lodge so securely in the trachea that it cuts off all air. No sound can be made, because the larynx is in the trachea and makes sounds only when air is pushed across it. This has happened often enough so that the event has been given a name: café coronary. The scenario reads like this. A person is dining in a restaurant with friends. A chunk of food, usually meat, becomes lodged in his trachea so firmly that he cannot make a sound. Often he chooses to suffer alone rather than "make a scene in public." If he tries to communicate distress to friends, he must depend on pantomime. The friends are bewildered by his antics and become terribly worried when the victim "faints" after a few minutes without air. They call a doctor or an ambulance. However, by the time the victim arrives at the hospital, he is usually dead—from suffocation. In the past, many of these cases were diagnosed as "death by coronary thrombosis"—thus the name café coronary.

larynx: the voice box (see Figure 6–10).

FIGURE 6–10

Normal swallowing and choking.

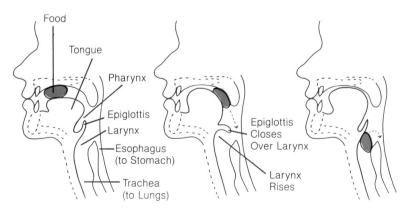

Food in Mouth.

Swallowing.
Food cannot
enter trachea.

Choking.
Food is lodged
in trachea.

To help a person who is choking, first ask this critical question: "Can you make any sound at all?" If the victim makes a sound, relax. You have time to continue with your questioning to see what you can do to help; you are not going to have to make a quick decision. But whatever you do, don't hit him on the back. If you do, the particle may become lodged more firmly in his air passage.

If the choking person who can still make a sound is a child, pick her up by the ankles if you can do so without hurting her, so that gravity can aid the coughing reflex to expel the particle. If the choking person is an adult, lay him on his stomach across a table or bed, with his head and neck off the support and almost vertical to the floor. Again, gravity will help. Now—and not before—you can thump him sharply between the shoulder blades to help dislodge the particle.

If the victim is unable to make a sound, you must act fast. The strategy most likely to succeed is the Heimlich maneuver. Get behind the victim, and put your arms around the lower part of her rib cage. Make a fist with one hand, and place the fist over the spot shown in Figure 6–11. Grasp the wrist of your balled-up hand with your other hand, and give a sudden strong hug. What you are hoping to accomplish with this quick bear hug is to push the diaphragm upward, because this will expel air from the lungs. The hope is that the air will be effective in dislodging the stuck food particle in the same way that built-up gas pressure in a bottle of wine can push the cork out of the bottle. One word of caution: be certain that your fist is in the correct position and is snugly against the person's body, and that you proceed with the hug from that position. Do not slam your fist against the rib cage; this might cause the food to become more securely lodged in the trachea. It would be well to practice this technique at home, for there is no time to hesitate once you are called on to perform this death-defying act.

If all else fails and time is running out, reach into the person's throat to try to pull out the lodged particle. You may scratch the tissues of the throat, but in a life-or-death situation this should not deter you. The scratches will heal if you can only save the person's life.

FIGURE 6–11

The Heimlich maneuver. Press fist on spot marked X, grasp wrist with other hand, and hug. Diaphragm should arch upward, forcing air out of the lungs through the trachea and dislodging the food.

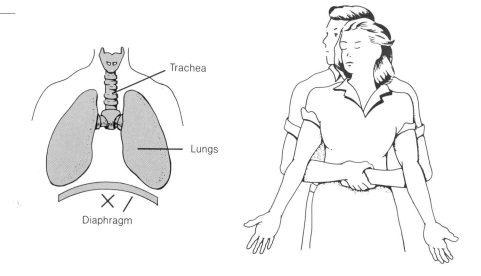

Trachea

Lungs

Diaphragm

Another common digestive mishap is vomiting. Vomiting can be a symptom of many different diseases or may come from any situation that upsets the body's equilibrium, such as air or sea travel. For whatever reason, the waves of peristalsis reverse direction, and the contents of the stomach arc propelled up through the esophagus to the mouth and expelled. If vomiting continues long enough or is severe enough, the reverse peristalsis will carry the contents of the duodenum, with its green bile salts, into the stomach and then up the esophagus. Simple vomiting is certainly unpleasant and wearying for the nauseated person, but it is no cause for alarm. Vomiting is one of the body's adaptive mechanisms to rid itself of something irritating.

Vomiting can be serious, however, and a doctor's care may be needed in some cases. When large quantities of fluid are lost from the GI tract, all the body fluids redistribute themselves so that, eventually, fluid is taken from every cell of the body. Leaving the cells with the fluid are electrolytes that are absolutely essential to the life of the cells, and they must be replaced, which is difficult while the vomiting continues. Intravenous feedings of saline and glucose with electrolytes added are frequently necessary while the doctor is diagnosing the cause of the vomiting and instituting corrective therapy.

In an infant, vomiting is especially serious; a doctor should be contacted soon after onset. Babies have more fluid between their body cells than adults do, so it is much easier to deplete their body water and upset their electrolyte balance than it is with adults.

Projectile vomiting is another kind of vomiting that is not the simple type associated with nausea. In this type, the contents of the stomach are expelled with such force that they leave the mouth in a wide arc, arching far out from the body like a bullet leaving a gun. There are a number of causes for this type of vomiting, and all of them require immediate medical care.

Diarrhea, like vomiting, can incur considerable fluid and electrolyte losses. Diarrhea is the name given to the condition characterized by frequent, loose, watery stools. This sort of stool indicates that the intestinal contents have moved too quickly through the intestines for fluid absorption to have taken place, or that water has been drawn from the cells lining the intestinal tract and added to the food residue. Diarrhea can become serious if it continues. In an infant, it may quickly lead to dehydration so severe as to require emergency medical treatment.

Unlike diarrhea, constipation may not be such a cause for concern. Each person's GI tract responds to food in its own way, with its own rhythm, the fecal matter arriving at the rectal area in a fairly constant number of hours. Each GI tract thus has its own cycle, which depends on its owner's physical makeup and such environmental considerations as the type of food eaten, when it was eaten, and when the person's schedule allows time to defecate. If several days pass between movements, but these movements take place without discomfort, then the person is not constipated, nor did she absorb any "toxins" that would cause irritable behavior. Nor does anyone need to worry about an inability to have daily movements—television commercials notwithstanding.

What, then, is constipation? When a person receives the signal that says to defecate and ignores it, the signal may not return for quite a few hours. In the meantime, water will continue to be withdrawn from the fecal matter, so that when the person does decide to defecate, the bowel movement will be drier and harder. If the movement is hard and is passed with difficulty, discomfort, or

Electrolyte: see Chapter 11.

intravenous (in-tra-VEEN-us): into a vein.

saline (SAY-leen): a salt solution.

constipation: the condition of having painful or difficult bowel movements (elapsed time between movements is not relevant).

defecate (DEF-uh-cate): to move the bowels and eliminate waste.
defaecare = to remove dregs

pain, then it can be said that the person is constipated. (Note that in this definition of constipation, no mention has been made of the amount of time that has elapsed since the previous bowel movement; that is irrelevant.)

Careful review of daily habits may reveal the causes of the constipation. Being too busy to respond to the defecation signal is a common complaint. A person's daily regimen may need to be reexamined with the idea of instituting regular eating and sleeping times that will allow time in the day's schedule, at the dictate of the person's body, to have a bowel movement. This may mean going to bed earlier in order to rise earlier, so that ample time is allowed for a leisurely breakfast and a movement. If discomfort is associated with passing fecal matter, a doctor's help should be sought in order to rule out the presence of organic disease. Once this has been done, dietary or other measures for correction can be considered.

There is a scarcity of laboratory research into the laxative quality of foods. It has been determined, however, that prunes contain a substance shown to be laxative.* If a morning defecation is desired, prune juice should be drunk at bedtime; if the evening is preferred, prune juice could be taken at breakfast.

Another cause of constipation that requires some rearrangement of lifestyle is the lack of physical activity. In modern society many people drive cars or ride buses to work, stand at assembly lines or sit behind desks, then sit in front of a television set in the evening. People who do not have the time or money to work out in a spa are finding that they can park their cars a distance from the office and walk the extra blocks, or they can walk up several flights of stairs rather than take an elevator. With such planning, much exercise can be incorporated into the day. The muscles that are responsible for peristalsis are improved by any activity that increases the muscle tone of the entire body. Another helpful measure may be to increase the fiber content of the diet, as explained in Chapter 3.

Some constipation may be relieved by the addition of fat to the diet. It was previously thought that the success of this regimen was due to its lubricating effect, but it now appears to be due instead to its stimulation of cholecystokinin, which causes bile to be secreted into the duodenum. The bile acts in the same way that a saline laxative does; that is, its high salt content draws from the intestinal wall an abundance of water, which stimulates peristalsis and softens the fecal matter.

Another recommendation for helping to overcome constipation is to increase fluid intake. Since the fluid is reabsorbed in the lower colon, it has been difficult to understand how a greater intake of fluid would soften the fecal matter. However, it has now been suggested that the beneficial effect comes from the physical stimulation of the increased bulk on the upper GI tract, which promotes peristalsis throughout.

These suggested changes in diet or lifestyle should correct chronic constipation without the use of laxatives. One of the fallacies often perpetrated by television commercials is that one person's successful use of a laxative product is a good recommendation for another person to use that product. As a matter of fact, even diet changes that are successful in relieving constipation for one person may increase the constipation of another. For instance, if a person has a spastic type of constipation, in which peristalsis promotes strong contractions

---

*This substance is dihydroxyphenyl isatin.

that close off a segment of the colon and prevent passage, then increasing the fiber in the diet would be exactly the wrong thing to do. A good rule is that if laxatives seem to be indicated, a doctor's advice should be sought.

Another common digestive problem is ulcers of the stomach (gastric ulcers) or duodenum (duodenal ulcers). The term *peptic ulcer* includes both of these. An ulcer is an erosion of the top layer of cells from an area, such as the wall of the stomach or duodenum, leaving the second and succeeding underlying layers of cells exposed, without protection. These exposed cells exude fluid, and anything that touches the eroded area causes pain. The erosion may proceed until the capillaries that feed the area are exposed and bleeding, or until there is a perforation (a hole) in the wall.

Some people naively believe that an ulcer is caused by the secretion of stomach acid, but this is not the case—at least not at first. The stomach lining of a healthy person is well protected by its mucous coat, as you learned earlier in this chapter. Why, then, do ulcers sometimes form? Two factors are required: first, a weakness in the stomach or duodenal wall; then, the secretion of gastric acid to erode the weak spot. We are in the dark with respect to the cause of the initial weakness; it may be poor nutrition, lack of rest, or any other condition (including a genetic flaw) that hinders the maintenance of healthy tissue. But once an ulcer has started to form, the secretion of stomach acid can rapidly make it worse.

What is of interest about ulcers—and the reason why they are included here—is that their origin and development seem to be related more closely to stress than to diet. You may remember that the secretion of digestive juices is regulated by the master coordinators, the hormones and the nerves. Both hormonal secretions and nerve activity are profoundly influenced by a person's mental state. The brain, after all, is composed of nerves, including many that impinge on the endocrine glands. Excessive anxiety and worry may be the cause of the initial lesion of an ulcer; they are clearly related to the excessive acid secretion that makes an ulcer worse.

Sue Rodwell Williams, the author of a widely used textbook on diet therapy, puts it this way: "The individual's particular emotional make-up and his manner of dealing with life's day-to-day problems and challenges, will often be reflected in the functions of his digestive tract. . . . It is not what he eats, it's what is eating him that is important." Williams also reminds her readers to remember that "surrounding every stomach there is a person."[3]

peptic ulcer: an eroded mucosal lesion in the stomach or duodenum.

mucosal (myoo-COH-sul): of the mucous membrane.

lesion: an abnormal change in structure.

The System at Its Best

We have described the anatomy of the digestive tract on several levels: the sequence of digestive organs, the structures of the villi and of the cells that compose them, and the selective machinery of the cell membranes. The intricate architecture of the GI tract makes it sensitive and responsive to conditions in its environment. Knowing what the optimal conditions are will help you to promote the best functioning of the system.

One indispensable condition is good health of the digestive tract itself. This health is affected by such factors of lifestyle as sleep, exercise, and state of mind. Adequate sleep allows for repair, maintenance of tissue, and removal of wastes that might impair efficient functioning. Exercise promotes healthy muscle tone. Mental state profoundly affects digestion and absorption; you should be relaxed and tranquil at mealtimes.

Another factor is the kind of meals you eat. Among the characteristics of meals that promote optimal absorption of nutrients are balance, variety, adequacy, and moderation. Balance means having neither too much nor too little of anything. For example, some fat is needed; fat slows down intestinal motility, permitting time for absorption of some of the nutrients that are slow to be absorbed. A well-planned meal presents you with about 30 percent—but not more—of its energy as fat energy.

Another example of balance is already familiar. Fiber stimulates intestinal motility. With too little fiber, the intestines are likely to be sluggish; they may then fail to mix their contents or fail to bring materials into contact with the sites on the intestinal walls where they can be absorbed. Too much fiber, however, can cause the contents of the intestines to move so fast through the tract that they are not in contact with the walls long enough to be absorbed. A well-planned meal delivers a moderate amount of fiber along with a generous assortment of nutrients.

Variety is important for many reasons, but partly because some food constituents interfere with the absorption of others. Phytic acid was mentioned in Chapter 3 as a compound that often accompanies fiber in foods, and that interferes with the absorption of minerals. Phytic acid is found in whole-grain cereals and legumes, so the minerals in those foods may be to some extent "unavailable." This does not mean that whole-grain cereals are undesirable; they are rightly praised for their nutrient contributions. It does mean, though, that a person who relies too heavily on cereals and legumes may be deriving less of certain minerals from his diet than he would if he were to vary his choices.

As for adequacy—in a sense, this entire book is about dietary adequacy. But here, at the end of this chapter, is a good place to underline the interdependence of the nutrients. It could almost be said that every nutrient depends on every other. All the nutrients work together and are all present in the cells of a healthy digestive tract. To maintain health and promote the functions of the GI tract, you should make balance, variety, adequacy, and moderation features of every day's menus.

Study Questions

1. Describe the problems involved with digesting food and the solutions offered by the human body.
2. Describe the anatomy of the gastrointestinal tract and explain how it facilitates absorption of nutrients.
3. What is the route of blood through the digestive system? Which nutrients enter the bloodstream directly? Which are first absorbed into the lymph?
4. What connections can be made between stress and nutrition?
5. What can you do to maintain a healthy digestive tract?

Notes

1. R. J. Gibbons and I. Dankers, Inhibition of lectin-binding to saliva-treated hydroxyapatite, to buccal epithelial cells, and to erythrocytes by salivary components, *American Journal of Clinical Nutrition* 36 (1982): 276–283.
2. W. H. Griffith, Food as a regulator of metabolism, *American Journal of Clinical Nutrition* 17 (1965): 391–398.
3. S. R. Williams, *Nutrition and Diet Therapy,* 3rd ed. (St. Louis: Mosby, 1977), p. 530.

Nutrition and the Brain

Chapter 6 was devoted to the digestion, absorption, and transport of nutrients. It focused on events in the digestive tract and on the ways that nutrients cross its walls and travel in the bloodstream. A fascinating related area is the study of how nutrients move into the brain and how they affect its functions. Not long ago, most serious-minded scientists would have pooh-poohed the idea that food could affect mood, behavior, or wakefulness. But research not only has shown that food does have such effects, but is beginning to show how the effects are brought about at the molecular level.[1]

How Nutrients Reach the Brain

As the body's master controller, the brain is more completely protected from harmful influences than any other organ. Three barriers separate the brain from direct exposure to what you eat. First, the GI tract cells themselves are selective and are able to protect the body from some harmful substances. Second, all the materials absorbed into the blood circulate through the liver, which selectively removes toxins, drugs, and excess quantities of nutrients before allowing the blood to reach other parts of the body. Thus the blood contents arriving at the brain have already been twice adjusted and cleansed; but the brain presents a third barrier: it has its own molecular sieve to safeguard it further. Called the blood-brain barrier, this protective device normally lets in only those substances the brain cells particularly need: glucose (or ketones), oxygen, amino acids, and other nutrients. The brain cells are capable of making complex molecules for themselves out of the simple building blocks they accept from the passing blood supply. If there is a *deficiency* of an essential nutrient, the brain's supply falls short, of course; the chapters on vitamins and minerals provide examples. But if there is an excess, or if substances are circulating in the body that the brain doesn't need, the contents of brain cells do not usually reflect these fluctuations.

The neurotransmitters, the substances that transmit impulses from one nerve cell to the next, are an exception to the rule that substances in the brain don't reflect blood concentrations. At least some of the neurotransmitters are unusual in being subject to precursor control; that is, the nerve cells respond to a larger or smaller supply of building blocks by making larger or smaller amounts of neurotransmitters. Furthermore, the building blocks (precursors) are able to penetrate the blood-brain barrier, and these building blocks are nutrients derived from food. Thus the food you eat can influence your brain chemistry, to the extent that it produces high concentrations of the precursor nutrients in an available form. These facts link nutrition to brain activity in some intriguing ways. Figure H6–1 depicts a neurotransmitter with

FIGURE H6–1

Tryptophan is converted to the neurotransmitter serotonin in two steps. Serotonin is converted to the inactive product 5–HIAA, and 5–HIAA leaves the brain to be excreted. The chemical drawings shown here are simplified by omission of the Cs and Hs in the ring structures.

its precursor, an amino acid available from the diet.

How Neurotransmitters Work

Nerve cells are elongated structures, analogous to the wires or cables in electrical communications equipment. Each nerve cell has a receiving end, where a stimulus may initiate an electrical impulse, and a transmitting end, where the impulse may be passed on to another nerve cell or to a muscle cell (see Figure H6–2). The electrical impulse can in some cases jump unaided from one cell to the next, but in most cases the gap between cells prevents electrical transmission. This gap is the synapse.

Communication across synapses usually involves neurotransmitters. The first nerve cell (the one sending the impulse) releases a quantity of these molecules, and they diffuse across the synapse to reach the second (receiving) nerve cell. On arrival, they may make the receiving nerve cell either *more* or *less* likely to fire. Thus a neurotransmitter can either *stimulate* or *inhibit* the postsynaptic nerve. If it stimulates it, and the nerve fires, then an electrical impulse starts up and travels along the nerve to the other end, the next synapse. Thus messages are carried along nerves by electrical impulses and from one nerve to the next by chemical compounds, until they result in action (storage or integration of information, or contraction of a muscle) or die away.

A nerve cell "decides" to fire based on inputs from all the other cells in contact with it. If the amount of stimulation relative to the amount of inhibition is great enough to initiate an impulse, then the nerve cell will fire. Figure H6–2 shows a nerve cell causing another to fire by dispatching a neurotransmitter to stimulate it.

Nerve cells manufacture and release amounts of neurotransmitters that, at least in some cases, vary in response to

FIGURE H6–2

How nerve cells transmit messages.

A. The impluse arrives at the end of the first nerve cell. Clustered just inside the nerve cell ending are a multitude of little sacs (vesicles) filled with the neurotransmitter.
B. The vesicles fuse with the nerve cell membrane, releasing the neurotransmitter into the gap between cells (synapse).
C. The neurotransmitter arrives at the receiver cell and (in this instance) stimulates it to generate an impulse that will travel along its length. Simultaneously, the receiver cell destroys the molecules of nuerotransmitter at its membrane, or the transmitter cell takes them up again to reuse them. Total elapsed time: a fraction of a second.

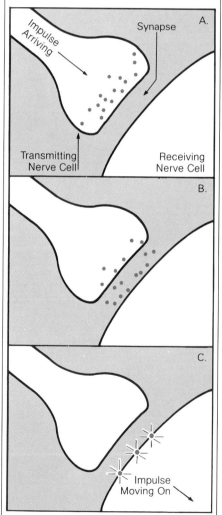

diet. Thus dietary factors affect the overall chemical climate of the brain. If a neurotransmitter's action within a cluster of cells is primarily inhibitory, then an increase in the action of that neurotransmitter will inhibit the cells further. If the same neurotransmitter has an excitatory effect on another group of cells, then an increase will excite them. A change in the supply of a single neurotransmitter apparently increases some kinds of activity and reduces others, thus altering the balance of activities in the brain. Among the diet-responsive neurotransmitters are serotonin, norepinephrine, and acetylcholine. We'll use serotonin as an example of how they all work.

Serotonin

The neurotransmitter serotonin is made in the brain from the essential amino acid tryptophan (Figure H6–1). The amount of serotonin made normally varies with the amount of tryptophan available. Tryptophan availability, in turn, depends on what is eaten (remember, an essential amino acid can't be made in the body). And a lack of tryptophan flowing into the brain can manifest itself in wakefulness and enhanced sensitivity to pain. Animals that have been made tryptophan deficient have a lowered threshold for pain; when they are given a single injection of tryptophan, they manifest a simultaneous restoration of brain serotonin levels and a normalized pain threshold.[2]

The question has been asked—and answered—of exactly how the diet can be adjusted to alter the amount of tryptophan flowing into the brain. It isn't as simple as you might think at first, but experiments with animals have shown what the key factors are.

If tryptophan is fed or injected by itself, as a single amino acid, its concentration in the blood rises, it flows into the brain, and brain serotonin increases proportionately. If protein containing tryptophan is fed, blood tryptophan also rises, but it does *not* flow into the brain. It turns out that some of the other large amino acids in the protein compete with tryptophan for entry into the brain; they use the same carrier.* (Recall that Chapter 5 mentioned specific carriers for specific amino acids—one for the acidic ones, one for the basic ones, and one for the neutral ones.) So protein, even though it contains the amino acid tryptophan, does not effectively enhance brain serotonin synthesis.

On the other hand, if insulin is injected, or if a diet high in carbohydrate (which raises blood insulin) is fed, blood tryptophan rises and enters the brain. It seems that insulin drives the other amino acids, but not tryptophan, into cells, leaving the tryptophan free to enter the brain without competition. Thus, paradoxically, a meal high in carbohydrate, but not one high in protein, causes a rise in tryptophan in both the blood and the brain, and so promotes serotonin synthesis. It's not the total amount of tryptophan, then, but the amount relative to the competing amino acids that affects the brain's serotonin level.[3]

With this knowledge, researchers have some fascinating avenues open to them. Experimentation is active, and its objective is to learn how diet modification can benefit people with sleep disturbances, pain, and depression. Research presently underway is investigating the possibility that the serotonin-using nerves may even provide feedback control of their own tryptophan supply. When the nerve cells have enough serotonin neurotransmission going on, they suppress carbohydrate consumption.[4] When they lack serotonin, perhaps they signal a need for carbohydrate.

*The amino acids that share this carrier are tyrosine, phenylalanine, leucine, isoleucine, and valine.

Stress Eating

The possibilities just mentioned may account for the fact that some people eat more than usual during stress: it may tranquilize or relieve pain in the brain. There are other possibilities, though, and they are entitled to examination. One possible explanation is that, during stress, under the influence of epinephrine, glucose is drawn from stores, the body fails to oxidize it for energy by way of physical exertion, and instead stores it as fat. Glycogen stores are then depleted, even though the glucose hasn't been used for energy. The blood glucose level now falls an hour or two sooner than it otherwise would have, and the person gets hungry and eats sooner. This theory assumes that blood glucose or liver glycogen regulates hunger, and it may not (see Chapter 8).

Another possibility is that the *behavior* of eating helps to relieve stress by occupying the nervous system with a familiar activity that discharges its nerves without doing harm, as fighting might do. The substitution of a familiar and comforting behavior such as eating for a frightening behavior such as fighting is a phenomenon biologists call *displacement activity*, and it is observed in all kinds of animals.

It may also be that eating, or the food eaten, leads to release of substances in the brain that are experienced as soothing. When carbohydrate-containing foods are eaten, it is not only neurotransmitter levels that change. Something else happens, too, that is worth a paragraph of explanation.

It seems that certain stresses lead to the production of substances in the brain that act in the same way as opiates do. (An example of an opiate is the well-known pain-killer, morphine.) Experiments using animals have demonstrated that these opiates promote both eating and reduction of activity. The same opiates are thought to cause a similar reaction in human beings.[5] Some proteins, upon digestion, also apparently release peptides that

Miniglossary of Brain/Nutrition Terms

acetylcholine (ASS-uh-teel COAL-een): a compound related in structure to (and made from) choline (Chapters 4, 9); it serves as one of the brain's principal neurotransmitters.

blood-brain barrier: a barrier composed of the cells lining the blood vessels in the brain, which are so tightly glued to each other that substances can only get through the lining by crossing the cell bodies themselves. Thus the cells can use all their sophisticated equipment and be highly selective in permitting entry.

neurotransmitter: a substance that is released at the end of one nerve cell when a nerve impulse arrives there, diffuses across the gap to the next nerve cell, and alters the membrane of that cell in such a way that it becomes either less or more likely to fire (or does fire).

norepinephrine: a compound related in structure to (and made from) the amino acid tyrosine. When secreted by the adrenal gland, it acts as a hormone; when secreted at the ends of nerve cells, it acts as a neurotransmitter.

precursor control: control of a compound's synthesis by the availability of that compound's precursor. (The more precursor there is, the more of the compound is made.)

serotonin: A compound related in structure to (and made from) the amino acid tryptophan; it serves as one of the brain's principal neurotransmitters.

synapse (SIN-aps): The gap between one nerve cell and the next nerve cell with which it communicates, or between a nerve cell and the muscle cell it stimulates.

have hormonal or opiatelike activity.[6] Much remains to be learned about these substances (known as endogenous and exogenous opiates), but it already seems likely that they may help to explain stress-induced eating. The person who is subject to this behavior and who is threatened with obesity on account of it would be well advised to find an alternative behavior with which to respond to stress—exercise, meditation, listening to music, or the like.

Exercise during stress has at least two other beneficial effects. It builds muscle and bone, promoting the retention of needed nutrients. And it may release the same pain-killing chemicals (endorphins) that stress does, helping to heighten mood.[7]

Research into the roles of nutrients in the brain is relatively new, but has branched out into many lines of investigation. Investigators are studying relationships of several other substances besides tryptophan to neuro-transmission: the mineral iron, the compound choline, and the amino acid tyrosine. The more they learn, the more they want to find out, because so much territory remains to be explored. It is hoped that research into these areas will continue to be supported, not only because they are of interest, but also because they have great potential for enhancing human life.

NOTES

1. R. J. Wurtman and J. J. Wurtman, eds., *Nutrition and the Brain* (New York: Raven, 1977–present).

2. J. D. Fernstrom, Effects of the diet on brain neurotransmitters, *Metabolism* 26 (1977): 207–223; S. H. Zeisel and J. H. Growdon, Diet and brain neurotransmitters, *Nutrition and the MD,* April 1980.

3. Fernstrom, 1977. The reader acquainted with this research may recall that it was at one time thought that *free* tryptophan (tryptophan not bound to albumin) was the key variable, and that therefore other substances that bind albumin, such as fatty acids, might affect tryptophan availability to the brain. The paper cited here presents evidence that the binding of tryptophan to albumin is loose and has little or no effect on its availability to the brain.

4. Zeisel and Growdon, 1980.

5. A. S. Levine and J. E. Morley, Stress-induced eating, in *Food in Contemporary Society*, symposium sponsored by Stokely–Van Camp at the University of Tennessee, Knoxville, May 27–29, 1981, pp. 126–135; J. Slochower and S. P. Kaplan, Anxiety, perceived control, and eating in obese and normal weight persons, *Appetite* 1 (1980): 75–83; J. E. Morley and A. S. Levine, The endorphins and enkephalins as regulators of appetite, in *Food and Contemporary Society,* pp. 136–148; J. E. Morley and A. S. Levine, Stress-induced eating is mediated through endogenous opiates, *Science* 209 (1980): 1259–1261; A. Mandenoff, F. Fumeron, and M. Apfelbaum, Endogenous opiates and energy balance, *Science* 215 (1982): 1536–1538.

6. J. E. Morley, Food peptides: A new class of hormones? (commentary), *Journal of the American Medical Association* 247 (1982): 2379–2380.

7. Run-away pain (Breakthrough), *Health,* April 1982, p. 22.

Metabolism: Nutrient Transformations and Interactions

7

Contents

Muscle cells can work without oxygen, using glycogen for fuel. This strand of muscle is peppered with glycogen (dark spots). Nearby are two mitochondria to oxidize both glycogen and fat breakdown products when oxygen is available.

metabolism: the sum total of all the chemical reactions that go on in living cells. **Energy metabolism** includes all the reactions by which the body obtains and uses the energy from food.
meta = among
bole = change

The mission of this chapter is to shed some light on how the body manages its energy supply. Along the way, it answers some of the questions people often ask about diets. What makes a person gain weight? Are carbohydrate-rich foods more fattening than other foods? What's the best fuel for an athlete? What's the best way to lose weight? Is fasting safe? The answers to these questions lie in an understanding of metabolism.

Metabolism is defined as the sum total of all the chemical reactions that go on in living cells. Energy metabolism includes all the ways the body obtains and uses energy from food. To lay the groundwork for its study, a brief review of the energy nutrients themselves may be helpful. (Protein's amino acids are not, strictly speaking, primarily energy nutrients, but they can flow into energy pathways if needed, so they are included.)

Starting Points

Earlier chapters have introduced carbohydrate, fat, and protein as they are found in foods, and Chapter 6 followed them through digestion to basic units and showed these units moving into the blood. Four of these basic units are seen throughout the metabolic transformations that follow, and they appear again and again in this chapter (see Figure 7–1):

- From carbohydrate—glucose.
- From lipids—glycerol and fatty acids.
- From protein—amino acids.

FIGURE 7–1

Basic units from carbohydrate, lipids, and protein after digestion. Each square represents a carbon atom; the triangles represent nitrogen-containing amino groups.
A. Carbohydrate. During digestion, all available carbohydrates are broken down to monosaccharides and absorbed into the blood. Fructose and galactose are then converted by the liver to glucose (or molecules that are metabolized similarly to glucose). To follow carbohydrate through metabolism, we will simply follow glucose.

B. Lipids. Most of the dietary lipids are triglycerides, composed of two basic units—glycerol and fatty acids. To follow lipids through metabolism, we will follow glycerol and fatty acids.

C. Protein. Protein is ultimately digested to amino acids; these are the units we will follow through metabolism. Amino acids contain different numbers of carbon atoms; we will follow the first two examples given here.

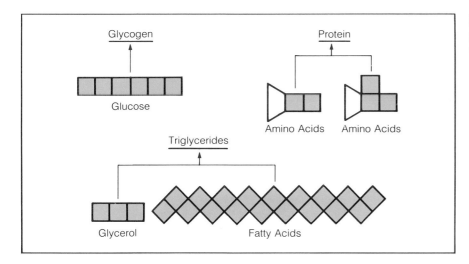

FIGURE 7–2

Basic units used to build body compounds.

Building Body Compounds

You already know what becomes of these basic units when their energy is not needed by the cells; they are used to build body compounds. Glucose units may be joined together to make glycogen chains. Glycerol and fatty acids may be assembled into triglycerides. Amino acids may be used to make proteins. These building reactions, in which simple compounds are put together to form larger, more complex structures, involve doing work and so require energy. They are called anabolic reactions, and are always represented by "up" arrows in diagrams such as those in Figure 7–2.

anabolism (an-ABB-o-lism): reactions in which small molecules are put together to build larger ones. Anabolic reactions consume energy and often involve reduction (Appendix B).
ana = up

Breaking Down Nutrients for Energy

If the body needs energy, it may break apart any or all of these four units into smaller fragments. The breakdown reactions are called catabolic reactions. They release energy and are represented by "down" arrows in diagrams. Much of the body's catabolic work is done with the help of enzymes in the liver cells, and all of the reactions described in this chapter can take place there. Brain, muscle, glandular, and other tissues are also metabolically active.

A special compound is almost always involved when energy transfers are taking place. This compound, available in all cells, is ATP (adenosine triphosphate), the body's quick energy molecule. Figure 7–3 explains how the body

catabolism (ca-TAB-o-lism): reactions in which large molecules are broken down to smaller ones. Catabolic reactions release energy and often involve oxidation (Appendix B).
kata = down

FIGURE 7–3

ATP (adenosine triphosphate), the body's quick-energy molecule. As glucose and fat break down, some of their energy is used to build ATP molecules by attaching phosphate groups to molecules of adenosine diphosphate (ADP). ATP then releases energy when it is hydrolyzed to ADP plus phosphate. ADP has lower energy than ATP; AMP (adenosine monophosphate) has even less.

Note: Glycogen and fat are the body's long-term energy-storage compounds (sort of like bank accounts). ATP is the body's instant energy source, always available in every cell (like pocket money). Cell structures that ATP energy might be used to build include glycogen, fat, proteins, hormones, and others.

Half or more of the total original energy is lost as heat in all such reactions, accounting for the temperature-raising effect of metabolism. ATP can also break apart without doing work, and release all of its energy as heat, if needed.

A. Before ATP is used.

A molecule of ATP with energy contained in the chemical bonds that hold its three phosphate groups in place.

An enzyme complex that can use ATP's energy to do work.

A molecule with a piece to be added to it.

B. During ATP use.

Bond breaks and releases energy.

Energy

Bond forms

A phosphate group breaks off. The energy is used to attach the free piece to the growing molecule.

C. After ATP use.

A molecule of ADP and a free phosphate group are produced as byproducts.

The enzyme complex is now ready to work again.

The growing molecule is now one piece longer.

Glucose has 6 C.
Glycerol has 3 C.
Fatty acids have multiples of 2 C.
Amino acids have 2 or 3 or more C with N attached.
3 C can make glucose; 2 C cannot.

pyruvate (PIE-roo-vate): pyruvic acid, a 3–carbon compound derived from glucose and certain amino acids in metabolism. The term *pyruvate* means a salt of pyruvic acid. (Throughout this book the ending *-ate* is used interchangeably with *-ic acid*; for our purposes they mean the same thing.)

uses ATP as its energy currency, and builds body structures, does other work, or generates heat from it, as needed.

At this point, it must be recalled that although glucose, glycerol, fatty acids, and amino acids are the basic units we get from food, they are composed of still smaller units, the atoms. During metabolism, the body actually separates these atoms from one another. To follow how this takes place, it will help to recall the structures of these compounds, introduced in earlier chapters. There is no need to remember exactly how they are put together; it is enough to remember how many carbons are in their "backbones." Figure 7–1 reviews this information.

A major point to notice in the following discussion is that compounds that have a 3–carbon skeleton can be used to make the vital nutrient glucose. Those that have 2–carbon skeletons cannot.

What happens to these compounds inside of cells can be best understood by starting with glucose. Two new names appear—pyruvate (3 C) and acetyl CoA (2 C)—and the rest of the story falls into place around them.

Glucose

The pathway by which glucose breaks down to smaller compounds is shown in Figure 7–4. Glucose is split in half, releasing energy and forming two 3–

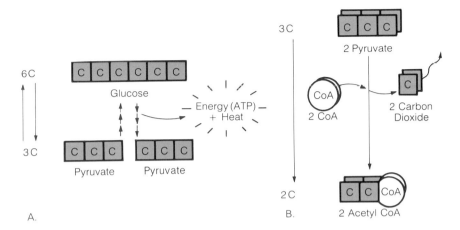

6C

3C

Glucose

— Energy (ATP) —
+ Heat

Pyruvate   Pyruvate

A.

3C

2 Pyruvate

CoA
2 CoA

2 Carbon
Dioxide

2C

2 Acetyl CoA

B.

FIGURE 7–4

The breakdown of glucose to acetyl CoA (major steps).
A. Glucose first splits to two 3–carbon compounds (pyruvate). The pathway is shown as reversible, because 3–carbon compounds such as these can be used to remake glucose. The pathway is known as glycolysis (glucose-splitting).

B. Each pyruvate loses a carbon as carbon dioxide and picks up a molecule of CoA, becoming acetyl CoA. The arrow is shown as one-way (down) because the step is not reversible. Result (from 1 glucose): 2 carbon dioxide and 2 acetyl CoA.

carbon compounds. One is pyruvate, and the other is a 3–carbon compound that is converted to pyruvate, so that two identical halves result from this pathway. While Figure 7–4 shows this as one step, it is actually a pathway called glycolysis (glucose-splitting), which involves several steps and several enzymes.

Should a cell "change its mind" after splitting glucose to pyruvate, it could reverse this pathway (glycolysis); it could put the two halves back together to make glucose again.* For this reason, arrows are shown pointing both up and down between glucose and pyruvate.

If the cell still needs energy, it breaks the pyruvate molecules apart further, cleaving a carbon from each. The lone carbon is combined with oxygen obtained from water molecules to make carbon dioxide, which is released into the blood, circulated to the lungs, and breathed out. The 2–carbon compound that remains is acetate (acetyl CoA).

The carbon removed from pyruvate ends up being combined with oxygen to make carbon dioxide. As carbon dioxide is breathed out, oxygen has to be breathed in to replace it. The person has to breathe oxygen into the lungs, has to attach it to a carrier (hemoglobin) in the red blood cells, and has to bring it to the metabolizing cells to make it available for this purpose. You know you need to breathe harder when you are using energy faster (exercising), but you may not have realized what is happening. Energy nutrients are being broken down to provide that energy, and oxygen is always ultimately involved in the oxidation process.

Should the cell "change its mind" after splitting pyruvate and want to retrieve the shed carbons and remake glucose, it could not do so. The step from pyruvate to acetyl CoA is metabolically irreversible. It is a one-way step, and it is shown with only a "down" arrow in the diagram. Acetyl CoA can be used to make fatty acids or cholesterol, but cannot be used to make glucose.

Finally, acetyl CoA may be split, yielding two more carbon dioxide molecules. This process appears to be a single step in Figure 7–5, but it actually takes

The metabolic breakdown of glucose to pyruvate is **glycolysis** (gligh-COLL-ih-sis).
glyco = glucose
lysis = breakdown

CoA (coh-AY): nickname for a compound described further in Chapter 9. As pyruvate loses a carbon and becomes a 2–carbon compound (**acetate**, or **acetic acid**), a molecule of CoA is attached to it, making **acetyl CoA** (ASS-eh-teel, or ah-SEET-il, coh-AY). For our purposes, acetyl CoA is just "a 2–carbon compound"; the CoA will not be discussed further here.

Carbohydrate can be used:
• For energy.
• For glycogen storage.
• For amino acid synthesis (provided nitrogen is available).
• For fat storage.

---

*The step from glucose to pyruvate is not *literally* reversible. That is, the enzyme that splits glucose can't also put it back together again. But other enzymes can make glucose from 3–carbon compounds, so in this sense it is reversible: the glucose is retrievable.

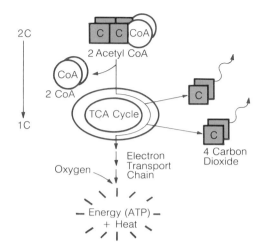

FIGURE 7–5

The breakdown of acetyl CoA. In the TCA cycle (see text and Appendix C), the remaining carbons are converted to carbon dioxide. Each CoA returns to pick up another acetate (coming from glucose, lipids, or protein). Net (from 2 acetate): 4 carbon dioxide.

The reactions by which the complete oxidation of acetyl CoA is accomplished are those of the **TCA** (tricarboxylic acid) or **Krebs cycle** (named for the biochemist who elucidated them) and **oxidative phosphorylation** (also known as the **electron transport chain**). The net result is that acetyl CoA splits, the carbons combine with oxygen, and the energy originally in the acetyl CoA is trapped in ATP and similar compounds, thus becoming available for the body's use.

FIGURE 7–6

Glucose breakdown. These are the processes by which energy from glucose is made available to do the cells' work. Many chemical reactions are involved. Ultimately, glucose is completely disassembled to single-carbon fragments, and the fragments are combined with oxygen to form carbon dioxide. Much of the energy released is trapped and stored in ATP (see Figure 7–3). Details of the TCA cycle and the electron transport chain are shown in Appendix C.

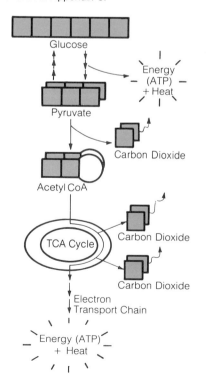

place in a long sequence of reactions, known as the TCA cycle, the details of which are given in Appendix C. The energy released from acetyl CoA during the TCA cycle powers most of the cell's activities.

The whole sequence of steps in glucose breakdown is shown in Figure 7–6. In summary, the main steps in the metabolism of glucose are glucose to pyruvate to acetyl CoA to carbon dioxide. Notice (again) that glucose can only be retrieved from the 3–carbon compounds in this sequence. Later steps are irreversible.

How Fat Enters into Metabolism

Figure 7–7 shows how glycerol and fatty acids enter the pathways of metabolism. The glycerol (3 C) is easily converted to pyruvate (also 3 C, but with a different arrangement of H and OH on the C), and then may go either "up"

Most people spend their entire lives without ever making the acquaintance of pyruvate and acetyl CoA, yet chemists and nutritionists can become quite excited talking about them. The behavior of these two compounds explains the most interesting and important aspects of nutrition and makes it possible to answer questions that interest everyone. For example, in some athletic events the muscles use fat and glucose, while in others they require glucose only. The person who wants to use up body fat during exercise needs to know which is which. For another example, during weight loss, the body derives energy sometimes from body fat and at other times from muscle protein. To avoid using muscle-protein kcalories during a weight-loss program, you have to know how to go about losing weight. It all hinges on which fuels can be converted to glucose and which cannot. The parts of protein and fat that can be converted to pyruvate (3 C) *can* provide glucose for the body; those that are converted to acetyl CoA *cannot* provide glucose. And glucose is all important.

FIGURE 7–7

How lipids enter the metabolic path. Glycerol is converted to pyruvate; fatty acids, to acetyl CoA. Net from an 18–carbon fatty acid: 9 acetyl CoA, which are converted to 18 carbon dioxide molecules.

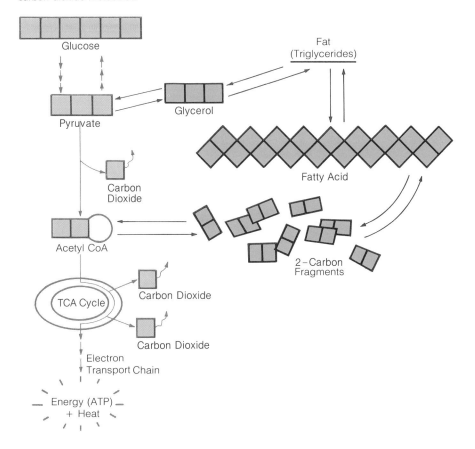

to form glucose or "down" to form acetyl CoA and, finally, carbon dioxide. The fatty acids, however, cannot be broken down to 3–carbon compounds. They are taken apart, *two* carbons at a time, to make acetyl CoA. The arrow from pyruvate to acetyl CoA goes one way (down) only, showing that the fatty acids cannot be used to make glucose.

The significance of this is that fat, for the most part, cannot normally provide energy for the organs (brain and nervous system) that require glucose as fuel. Remember that almost all dietary lipid is triglyceride, and that the typical triglyceride consists of a molecule of glycerol (3 C) and three fatty acids (each about 18 C on the average, or about 54 C in all). True, the glycerol can yield glucose, but that represents only 3 out of 57 parts of the fat molecule—about 5 percent of its weight. Thus, fat is an inefficient source of glucose by itself. About 95 percent of it cannot be converted to glucose at all.

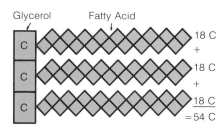

Only 3 of this triglyceride's 57 carbon atoms are in glycerol and can go to glucose.

How Protein Enters the Metabolic Pathway

Amino acids will not enter the energy-yielding pathway being described here if they are used to replace needed body proteins. But if they are needed for

Fat can be used:
- For energy.
- For fat storage.

FIGURE 7–8

How amino acids enter the metabolic pathway. About half are converted to pyruvate (and therefore can be used to synthesize glucose); about half are converted directly to acetyl CoA or bypass CoA completely and go directly into the TCA cycle (and therefore cannot yield glucose). Net from one amino acid: the products depend on the amino acid. See Appendix C.

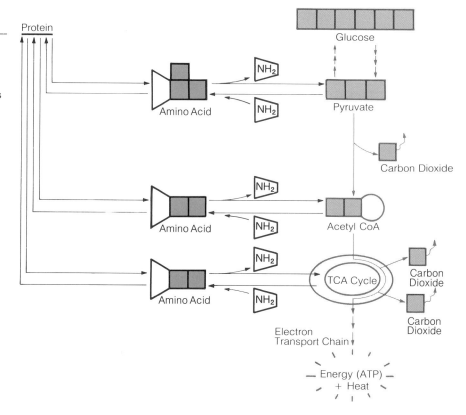

Amino acids can be used in three ways:
- To build body protein.
- For energy—if energy is needed.
- To build body fat—if protein is eaten in excess of need.

The making of glucose from protein or the glycerol portions of triglycerides is **gluconeogenesis** (gloo-co-nee-o-GEN-uh-sis). About 5 percent of fat (the glycerol portion of triglycerides) and about 50 percent of protein (the glucogenic amino acids) can be converted to glucose.
gluco = glucose
neo = new
genesis = making

deamination: removal of the amino (NH₂) group from a compound such as an amino acid.

energy, or if they are consumed in excess of the need for protein, they enter the metabolic pathway as shown in Figure 7–8. They are stripped of their nitrogen (see the next section) and then catabolized in a variety of ways.* The end result is that about half of the amino acids can be converted to pyruvate; the other half go either to acetyl CoA or directly into the TCA cycle. Those that can be used to make pyruvate can provide glucose for the body. Thus protein, unlike fat, is a fairly good source of glucose when carbohydrate is not available; about 50 percent of it can be used this way.

Disposal of Excess Nitrogen

When amino acids are degraded for energy or to make fat, the first step is removal of their nitrogen-containing amino groups, a reaction called deamination. The product is ammonia, chemically identical to the ammonia in the bottled cleaning solutions used in hospitals and industry. It is a strong-smelling and extremely potent poison.

A small amount of ammonia is always being produced by liver deamination reactions. Some of this ammonia is used by liver enzymes in the synthesis of

---

*Some are rearranged to form pyruvate. Others are 4–carbon compounds that are split into two acetyl CoA molecules. One, which contains only 2 carbons after the nitrogen is removed, is rearranged directly to become acetyl CoA. Still others enter the TCA cycle as compounds other than acetyl CoA.

Surplus amino acids cannot be stored in the body as such; they have to be converted to other compounds. Amino acids eaten in excess of need lose their nitrogen-containing amino groups, and most are converted to acetyl CoA (either directly or indirectly, through pyruvate). This acetyl CoA is not broken down further, because energy is not needed. Instead, it is used to make fatty acids and stored in body fat. Thus even the so-called lean nutrient, protein, can add to fat stores if you eat too much of it.

The high-protein dieter objects to the previous statement, saying, "Protein makes you thin!" In fact, many weight-loss diets are based on high protein intakes, making the claim that "Protein will give you energy but will not make you fat. Eat all you want—just stay away from fattening carbohydrates."

One secret of these diets, when they do seem to promote weight loss, is that meals without carbohydrate are in truth so unappetizing that people who ingest them eat much less total food than they normally do. Try eating your breakfast of bacon, eggs, toast, and juice without the toast and juice. Have a ham and cheese sandwich without the bread; try a steak, potatoes, and peas dinner without the potatoes and peas. You'll be surprised how quickly you lose your enthusiasm for the permitted foods. (Some people report, after eating nothing but bacon, eggs, ham, cheese, and steak for a few days, that they start *dreaming* of toast and juice!)

This method of weight loss may sound inviting to the person who wants to lose pounds fast, but the next few sections of this chapter should convince the reader that it's not a safe choice. Meanwhile, it should now be clear that protein, in and of itself, is not nonfattening. People who eat huge portions of meat, even lean meat, and other protein-rich foods may wonder why they have a weight problem. It may be those very foods that are causing the trouble.

There is a message for the athlete, too, in these metabolic facts about protein. *Excess* protein is not a muscle-building food; it's a fat-building food. To the extent that protein is used for energy, carbohydrate would do the job more efficiently. In other words, there is no point in loading up on protein for any reason. Highlight 7A elaborates on nutrition for the athlete.

When amino nitrogen is stripped from amino acids, ammonia is produced. The liver detoxifies ammonia by combining it with another waste product, CO_2, to produce urea before releasing it into the bloodstream. The diagram greatly oversimplifies the reactions; details are shown in Appendix C.

urea (you-REE-uh): the principal nitrogen-excretion product of metabolism. Two ammonia fragments are combined with a carbon-oxygen fragment to form urea.

nonessential amino acids, but what cannot be used is quickly combined with carbon-oxygen fragments to make urea, an inert and less toxic compound.

Urea is released from the liver cells into the blood, where it circulates until it passes through the kidneys. One of the functions of the kidneys is to remove urea from the blood for excretion in the urine. Urea is the body's principal vehicle for excreting unused nitrogen; water is required to keep it in solution. This explains why people who consume a high-protein diet must drink more water than usual, and why the hazard of dehydration is another drawback to the high-protein, low-carbohydrate diet. In fact, the weight loss from water loss

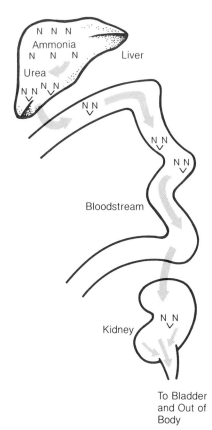

The liver and kidney each play a role in enabling the body to dispose of excess nitrogen. Can you see why the person with liver disease has high blood ammonia, while the person with kidney disease has high blood urea?

is another reason why the diet appears to work, but water loss, of course, is of no value to the person who wants to lose body fat.

Putting It All Together

All the details this chapter has presented so far are combined in Figure 7–9. After a normal mixed meal, if you do not overeat, the body handles the nutrients as shown. The carbohydrate yields glucose; some is stored as glycogen, and some is taken into brain and other cells and broken down to pyruvate and acetyl CoA to provide energy. The acetyl CoA can then enter the TCA cycle to provide more energy. The protein yields amino acids, some of which are used to build body protein. However, if there is a surplus, or if not enough carbohydrate and fat are present to meet energy needs, some amino acids are broken down through the same pathways as glucose to provide energy. Other amino acids enter directly into the TCA cycle, and these, too, can be broken down to yield energy. The fat yields glycerol and fatty acids; some are put together and stored as fat, and others are broken down to acetyl CoA, enter the TCA cycle, and provide energy. In summary, although carbohydrate, fat, and protein enter the TCA cycle by different routes, the cycle is the energy-generating pathway common to all energy-yielding nutrients.

A few hours after the meal, the stored glycogen and fat begin to be released from storage to provide more glucose, glycerol, and fatty acids to keep the energy flow going. When the energy from these compounds has been stored or used, and the body shifts to a fasting mode and begins drawing energy out of storage, it signals hunger; it is time to eat again.

The average person consumes more than a million kcalories a year and expends more than 99 percent of them, maintaining a stable weight for years on end. This remarkable achievement, which many people manage without even thinking about it, could be called the economy of maintenance. The body's energy budget is balanced. Some people, however, eat too little and get thin; others eat too much and get fat. The possible reasons why they do are explored in Chapter 8; the metabolic consequences are discussed here.

The Economics of Feasting

Figure 7–10 shows how metabolism favors fat formation when you eat too much of any energy nutrient—carbohydrate, fat, or protein. Surplus carbohydrate (glucose) is first stored as glycogen, but there is a limit to the capacity of the glycogen-storing cells. Once glycogen stores are filled, the overflow is routed to fat (part A of the figure). Fat cells enlarge as they fill with fat, and their storage capacity seems to be able to expand indefinitely. Thus excess carbohydrate can contribute to obesity.

In the same way, surplus dietary fat can contribute to the fat stores in the body. It may break down to fragments such as acetyl CoA, but if energy flow is already rapid enough to meet the demand, these fragments will not be broken

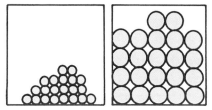

Fat cells enlarge.

FIGURE 7–9

The central pathways of metabolism. Details are in Appendix C.

FIGURE 7–10

How carbohydrate, fat, and protein, eaten in excess, contribute to body fat.
A. Carbohydrate, eaten in excess of need, is broken down to pyruvate and acetyl CoA; these then are built up into fat.
B. Fat, eaten in excess of need, is either stored directly or broken down to pyruvate and acetyl CoA; these then may be built up into different fat molecules.
C. Protein is broken down to amino acids. These, if not used to build body protein, are deaminated, and the nitrogen is excreted as urea; the remaining carbon skeletons are converted to pyruvate and acetyl CoA and then to fat.

down further. Instead, they will be routed to the assembly of triglycerides and stored in the fat cells (part B of the figure).

Finally, surplus protein may encounter the same fate (part C of the figure). If not needed to build body protein or to meet present energy needs, amino acids will be deaminated and their carbon skeletons converted through the intermediates, pyruvate and acetyl CoA, to triglycerides. These, too, swell the fat cells and increase body weight.

Of course, any of these three nutrients is considered as a surplus, only if the total energy intake is also excessive. In other words, it is not carbohydrate or fat or protein alone that contributes to fat formation; it is any or all of these when taken in excess of total energy need.

The Economics of Fasting

Brain, in its rigid vault, cannot store more than a few minutes' worth of glycogen at the most. . . . Hence, the compliant liver expands and contracts. . . .

G. F. Cahill, T. T. Aoki, and A. A. Rossini

Even when you are asleep and totally relaxed, the cells of many organs are hard at work spending energy. In fact, the work that you are aware of—that you do with your muscles during waking hours—represents only about a third of the total energy you spend in a day. The rest is the metabolic work of the cells, for which they constantly require fuel.

The body's top priority is to meet these energy needs, and its normal way of doing so is by periodic refueling—that is, by eating. When food is withdrawn, the body must find other fuel sources in its own tissues. If people choose not to eat, we say they are fasting; if they have no choice (as in a famine), we say they are starving; but there is no metabolic difference between the two. In either case, the body is forced to switch to a wasting metabolism, drawing on its reserves of carbohydrate and fat and, within a day or so, on its vital protein tissues as well. Figure 7–11, parts A and B, show the metabolic pathways operating in the body at the start of a fast.

FIGURE 7–11

Fasting
A. Fasting (early). Liver glycogen has been used up, so body protein (muscle and lean tissue) is breaking down to amino acids that can be converted to glucose for brain and nervous system energy. Those amino acids that generate fat are degraded for energy by the other body cells.
B. Fasting (later). Muscle and lean tissue are still giving up amino acids for conversion to glucose. In addition, the liver is converting fat to ketone bodies. The brain now has two energy sources, and atrophy of lean tissues slows down somewhat.

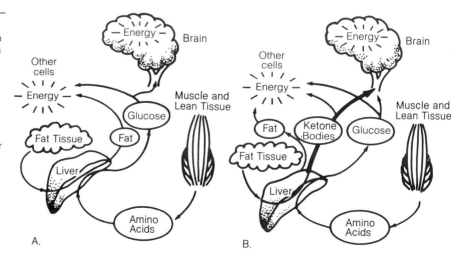

Fuel must be delivered to every cell. As the fast begins, glucose from the liver's stored glycogen and fatty acids from the body's stored fat are both flowing into cells, breaking down to yield acetyl CoA, and delivering energy to power the cells' work. Several hours later, however, most of the glucose is used up, and the liver glycogen is being exhausted.

At this point, most of the cells are depending on fatty acids to continue providing their fuel. But the brain cells cannot; they still need glucose. (It is their major energy fuel, and even if other energy fuel is available, glucose has to be present to permit the energy-metabolizing machinery of the brain cells to work.) Normally, the nervous tissues (brain and nerves) consume about two-thirds of the total glucose used each day—about 400 to 600 kcalories' worth.[1] About one-fifth of the energy the body uses when it is at rest is used for the brain.

The brain's special requirement for glucose poses a problem for the fasting body. The body can use its stores of fat, which may be quite generous, to furnish most of its cells with energy, but for the brain and nerves, it must supply energy in the form of glucose. This is why body protein tissues, such as muscle and liver, always break down to some extent during fasting. Only those amino acids that yield 3–carbon pyruvate can be used to make glucose; and to obtain them, whole proteins must be broken down. The other amino acids, which can't be used to make glucose, are used in place of some fat as an energy source. This is an expensive way to gain glucose, but to extract a molecule of glycerol from a triglyceride obligates the body to dispose of some 50 or 60 carbons' worth of fatty acids, which is even more expensive. In the first few days of a fast, body protein provides about 90 percent of the needed glucose, and glycerol, about 10 percent. If body protein loss were to continue at this rate, death would ensue within three weeks.

As the fast continues, the body adapts by producing an alternate energy source, ketone bodies, by condensing together acetyl CoA fragments derived from fatty acids. Normally produced and used in only small quantities, ketone bodies can serve as a fuel for some brain cells. Ketone body production rises until, at the end of several weeks, it is meeting about half or more of the nervous system's energy needs. Still, many areas of the brain rely exclusively on glucose, and body protein continues to be sacrificed to produce it.[2]

During fasting, appetite may be suppressed. It has been thought that ketosis caused loss of appetite. The theory was that it would be an advantage to a person in a famine to have no appetite, because the search for food would be a waste of energy. When the person finds food and eats carbohydrate again, the body shifts out of ketosis, the hunger center gets the message that food is again available, and appetite returns. This hypothetical chain of events has served as justification for weight-loss routines, such as fasting and fad diets, that cause ketosis. However, it may be that any kind of food restriction, with or without ketosis, leads a person to adapt by losing appetite. An ordinary low-kcalorie diet can induce the same effect.[3]

Formation of ketone bodies:

2 acetyl CoA

$(+H\text{-}O\text{-}H)$ $(-2\ CoA)$

A ketone (keto-acid) $(+2\ H\text{-}CoA)$

This ketone may lose a molecule of carbon dioxide to become another ketone:

Acetone

Or, the keto-acid may add 2 hydrogens, becoming a related compound (a ketone body). See Appendix C for more details.

Acetone (ASS-uh-tone) is familiar to some as the solvent used in nail-polish remover. "Acetone breath" indicates that a person is in ketosis.

ketone (KEE-tone) **body:** a compound formed during the incomplete oxidation of fatty acids. Ketones contain a C=O group between other carbons; when they also contain a COOH (acid) group, they are called keto-acids. These and compounds related to them as in the figure are ketone bodies. Small amounts of ketone bodies are a normal part of the blood chemistry, but when their concentration rises, they spill into the urine. The combination of high blood ketone bodies (ketonemia) and ketone bodies in the urine (ketonuria) is termed **ketosis.**

Figure 7–11, part B, shows the metabolism of late fasting. While the body is shifting to the use of ketone bodies, it simultaneously reduces its energy output and conserves both its fat and lean tissue. As the lean (protein-containing) organ tissue shrinks in mass, it performs less metabolic work, reducing energy expenditures. As the muscles waste, they do less work, reducing energy expenditures further. Because of the slowed metabolism, the loss of fat falls to a bare minimum—less, in fact, than the fat that would be lost on a low-kcalorie diet.[4] Thus, although weight loss during fasting may be quite dramatic, fat loss may be less than when at least some food is supplied.

The adaptations just described—slowing of energy output and reduction in fat loss—occur in the starving child, the fasting religious person, and the malnourished hospital patient, and help to prolong their lives. The physical symptoms of marasmus include wasting, slowed metabolism, lowered body temperature, and reduced resistance to disease (see Chapter 5).

The body's adaptations to fasting are sufficient to maintain life for a long period. Mental alertness need not be diminished, and even physical energy may remain unimpaired for a surprisingly long time. Still, fasting is not without its hazards, as physician-supervised fasting has revealed. Among the multitude of changes that take place in the body are:

- Sodium and potassium depletion.
- An increase in body uric acid.
- A rise in blood cholesterol.
- A decrease in thyroid hormone.

The same alterations are seen in low-carbohydrate dieting (next section). Renewed food intake, especially of carbohydrate, results in dramatic changes in the body's salt and water balance, accounting for most of the wide swings in body weight seen in people on fasts or low-carbohydrate diets.[5]

The Low-carbohydrate Diet

An economy similar to that of fasting prevails in the person who consumes a low-carbohydrate diet. Advocates of the low-carbohydrate diet would have you believe there is something magical about ketosis, something that promotes faster weight loss than a regular low-kcalorie diet. In fact, the low-carbohydrate diet presents the same problem as a fast. Once the body's available glycogen reserves are spent, the only significant remaining source of energy in the form of glucose is protein. The low-carbohydrate diet usually provides some protein from food, but some is still taken from body tissue. The onset of ketosis is the signal that this wasting process has begun.

The Protein-sparing Fast

A variant on fasting is the technique of ingesting only protein. The hope is that the protein will spare lean tissue and that the person will break down body fat at a maximal rate to meet other energy needs. The protein does spare the lean tissues to some extent from being used to provide glucose, but also is largely used for glucose itself, just as dietary carbohydrate would be. The idea sounded good when it was first suggested for use with very obese people, but it has met with mixed results. It seems effective only after considerable lean tissue has

Fasting = living on body fat and body protein.

Low-carbohydrate dieting = living on dietary and body fat and dietary and body protein almost exclusively.

Protein-sparing fasting = living on dietary and body protein, and body fat.

People are attracted to the low-carbohydrate diet because of the dramatic weight loss it brings about within the first few days. They would be disillusioned if they realized that much of this weight loss is a loss of glycogen and protein together with quantities of water and important minerals. A dieter who boasts of losing 7 pounds in two days on a low-carbohydrate diet must be unaware that at best, a pound or two is fat, and 5 or 6 pounds are lean tissue, water, and minerals. Once off the diet, the dieter's body will avidly devour and retain these needed materials, and the weight will zoom back to within a few pounds of the starting point.

A warning is suggested by these facts. Beware of those who promote quick-weight-loss schemes. Learn to distinguish between loss of *fat* and loss of *weight*.

already been lost, at which time the body may be conserving itself quite efficiently anyway, and the fast has not been shown more effective than a mixture of protein and carbohydrate.[6] Furthermore, it has a low long-term success rate; most people regain the lost weight.[7] Thus the protein-sparing fast has to be judged at best a moderate success and at worst a failure, for the ultimate criterion of success in any weight-loss program is maintenance of the new low weight.

The idea of a protein-sparing fast originated with some responsible physicians who experimented carefully with it, using whole foods naturally rich in protein, such as fish and lean beef. Unfortunately, the idea was then seized upon and misused with the publication of a popular book, *The Last Chance Diet*, in 1977.[8] Fad dieters, usually without any medical supervision, drank liquid protein potions prepared from low-quality sources, or consumed very low kcalorie, high-protein diets and lost dramatic amounts of weight—including, of course, lean tissue, water, and vital minerals. Within the year, 11 deaths had been ascribed to the fad, and since then, many more have died. High-biological-value protein supplements were used by some of the victims—so the quality of the protein was not alone responsible for the deaths.[9] Mineral deficiencies were suspected as contributing factors.

The term *protein-sparing* has been used in another connection. Malnourished hospital patients also lose body protein, and this is especially likely, and especially dangerous, if they are simultaneously fighting infection, which prevents the body from going into ketosis. Physicians make every effort to prevent the loss of vital lean tissue by supplying amino acids as well as glucose in some form—through a vein if the patient can't eat. The effort to provide protein-sparing *therapy* in these circumstances should not be confused with the profiteering of faddists who promote the protein-sparing *fast*.

Moderate Weight Loss

Your body's cells and the enzymes within them have the task of converting the energy nutrients you eat into those you need. They are extraordinarily versatile. They relieve you of having to compute exactly how much carbohydrate, fat, and protein to eat at each meal. As you have seen, the body's remarkable machinery

Low-kcalorie dieting = living on food and body fat.

1 lb = 3,500 kcal. A pound of body fat (adipose tissue) is actually composed of a mixture of fat, protein, and water and yields 3,500 kcal on oxidation. A pound of pure fat (454 g) would yield 4,086 kcal at 9 kcal/g.

can convert either carbohydrate (glucose) or protein to fat. To some extent, it can convert protein to glucose. To a very limited extent, it can even convert fat (the glycerol portion) to glucose. But a grossly unbalanced diet or one that is severely limited in kcalories imposes hardships on the body. If energy intake is too low or if carbohydrate and protein energy is undersupplied, the body is forced to degrade its own lean tissue to meet its glucose need.

Someone who wants to lose body fat must be reconciled to the hard fact that there is a limit to the rate at which fat tissue will break down, just as there is a limit to the rate at which fat tissue can be deposited. The maximum rate, except for a very large, very active person, is 1 to 2 pounds a week. To design a moderate diet requires adjusting energy balance so that energy intake is reduced, energy output is increased, or both. To achieve weight loss that actually reflects body-fat loss, the most effective means is to adopt a balanced, low-kcalorie diet supplying all three energy nutrients in reasonable amounts while increasing energy expenditure by getting more exercise. In effect, this means adjusting the energy budget so that intake is 500 to 1,000 kcalories per day less than output. A person who wants to gain weight needs to make the opposite adjustment.

It might seem that the effort to lose or gain weight would involve tedious counting of kcalories, but this is not the case. The next two sections show how energy input and energy output can be estimated and balanced to achieve either weight loss, gain, or maintenance.

Metabolism During Exercise

Up to now, the metabolic activities described have been those that take place all the time, even in the body at rest. Metabolism during exercise involves an interplay among three factors: the supply of oxygen to the muscles, and the supply of the two muscle fuels, glucose and fatty acids.[10] The lungs pass oxygen to the blood, which carries it to the muscles. The glucose used as muscle fuel is derived chiefly from glycogen stored within the muscle itself, while the fatty acids come partly from fat inside the muscles and partly through the bloodstream from fat in other storage depots. The nervous and hormonal systems orchestrate the interplay, conducting subtle changes to support the exercising person's exertion according to how strenuous and how extended it is.

Of the three factors mentioned above, oxygen is usually the limiting factor. For the muscles to use the body's virtually unlimited supply of body fat to fuel their work, they must have ample oxygen, because the breakdown of fatty acids is a strictly aerobic process.

The heart and lungs can provide only so much oxygen and only so fast. When the muscles' exertion is great enough that their energy demand outstrips their oxygen supply, they can no longer rely solely on the aerobic process of fat breakdown to provide that energy. They must draw more heavily on their limited supply of glucose, a more versatile energy fuel that can be metabolized without oxygen to produce the ATP required for muscle movement. When the muscles

aerobic (air-ROE-bic): requiring oxygen.

FIGURE 7–12

Anaerobic glucose metabolism and the production of lactic acid.

A. In anaerobic metabolism, the first few steps of glucose breakdown in the muscles take place without oxygen, until pyruvate (pyruvic acid) has been produced.

B. Because the circulation can't bring them oxygen fast enough, the muscle cells convert the pyruvic acid to the temporary waste product lactic acid. Lactic acid is released into the blood.

C. The liver can reconvert lactic acid to glucose and release it, so that the muscles can use it again. The cycle by which energy stored in liver is made available for muscle use is called the Cori cycle.

D. The heart and lungs, having access to oxygen, can reconvert lactic acid to pyruvate and oxidize it aerobically for energy.

need an anaerobic energy source, glucose is released from muscle glycogen at lightning speed to meet the demand. Glucose can make some of its energy available to the body without involving oxygen; it can break down as far as pyruvate without oxygen's being involved.

You may have heard the name of one of the waste products generated when glucose is oxidized in the absence of oxygen: lactic acid. Figure 7–12 shows that lactic acid is produced from pyruvic acid when not enough oxygen is available to oxidize pyruvic acid all the way to carbon dioxide and water. Both acids accumulate in the muscles, causing fatigue and pain; both can be disposed of only when oxygen is once again available to permit their complete oxidation.*

Some muscle cells specialize in anaerobic, others in aerobic work. An example of the first type of muscle cells is the type involved in intense, prolonged exertion such as that of the weight-lifter, whose muscles must tighten and stay tight for many seconds at a time. The muscle cells specialized for such an effort are called fast-twitch muscle fibers; they are so packed with glycogen between times that they appear white under the microscope. Slow-twitch muscle fibers are the kind that contract and relax many times in a few seconds, such as those a basketball player or sprinter uses. These burn predominantly fat as fuel and appear red when magnified.

Although glucose differs from fat in that it can supply some energy without the use of oxygen, glucose still requires oxygen to be metabolized completely and to deliver its full energy potential. The first split, to pyruvate, yields very

anaerobic (AN-air-ROE-bic): requiring no oxygen.

lactic acid or **lactate**: a temporary product of anaerobic glucose metabolism.

pyruvic (pie- ROO-vic) **acid**: another name for pyruvate, a breakdown product of glucose that can be produced anaerobically.

Two types of muscle fibers:
fast-twitch muscle fibers: packed with glycogen, white in appearance, adapted for predominantly anaerobic work—that is, intense uninterrupted contractions.
slow-twitch muscle fibers: containing less glycogen, interlarded with fat, red in appearance, adapted better for aerobic work—that is, alternating contraction and relaxation.

*The lactic acid transported out of the muscle during work is sent to the liver where a molecule of glucose is synthesized from each two molecules of lactic acid. The glucose can be released by the liver and transported to the muscle to be used as an anaerobic energy source. This pathway is known as the Cori cycle and is a method for disposing of toxic lactic acid by using it as raw material for new synthesis of glucose (or, as the physiologists say, as substrate for gluconeogenesis).

oxygen debt: the oxygen needed to completely metabolize a substance produced when the body performs exercise so demanding that the circulation can't bring oxygen to the muscles fast enough. It is repaid by rapid breathing after the activity stops.

little energy; most is still tied up in the pyruvate molecules. During anaerobic metabolism, the breakdown of glucose goes only as far as pyruvate without oxygen—and that is as far as it can go. At the point when the heart and lungs can't keep up with the need, the body begins to incur an oxygen debt. Oxygen is needed to complete the metabolism of pyruvate.

You can sense when this is happening as you exert yourself. During moderate exercise, your circulatory system has no trouble keeping up with the need for oxygen. You breathe deeply and easily. But sometimes the exercise is so demanding that your muscles burn, you can't seem to breathe fast enough, and your heart is racing. This is when your body is building up the oxygen debt.

Later, the debt comes due. If exercise continues and wastes build up further, you start feeling short of breath, you pant, and finally you must stop or at least slow down "to catch your breath" and replenish your oxygen supply. If you do not, your muscles will cramp, signifying "no more lactic acid can be accommodated here." When you have caught your breath, you can fully break down lactic acid by reconverting it to pyruvate and running it through the TCA cycle; you are thus producing energy aerobically once again.

A strategy for dealing with lactic acid buildup is to relax the muscles at every opportunity, so that the circulating blood can carry it away (see Figure 7–12). A muscle will last much longer if it can contract and relax at intervals—for example, between tennis strokes or between hiking steps. Football players last longer if their coach calls time outs for huddles at intervals, too.

Breathing is thus important to performance. The more oxygen you can bring to the muscle, the longer it can work aerobically, getting all the available energy from its stored glucose. This is why athletes, to get in the best possible shape, have to condition their cardiovascular and respiratory systems—that is, do aerobic exercise that requires prolonged, speeded-up breathing and a rapid heartbeat, and not just short-term exercises such as weight-lifting that essentially increase only muscle strength.

At the end of an event, the athlete continues to breathe fast; the heart continues pounding for some time because oxygen is still being circulated to the tissues to help break down the accumulated lactic acid. The carbon dioxide that results stimulates the brain to keep the heart and lungs speeded up until the lactic acid has been disposed of.

Study Questions

1. Define metabolism, anabolism, and catabolism; give an example of each.
2. Name the four basic units used by the body after digestion in metabolic transformations.
3. What is the body's quick energy molecule and how is it used?
4. Summarize the main steps in the metabolism of glucose, fatty acids, glycerol, and amino acids.
5. Describe how a surplus of the three energy nutrients contributes to body fat stores.
6. Define ketosis. What adaptations does the body make during a fast?
7. Distinguish between a loss of *fat* and a loss of *weight* on a low-carbohydrate diet.
8. Define aerobic and anaerobic metabolism. Explain why oxygen rather than the two muscle fuels is the usual limiting factor for metabolism during exercise.

Notes

1. G. F. Cahill, T. T. Aoki, and A. A. Rossini, Metabolism in obesity and anorexia nervosa, in *Nutrition and the Brain*, vol. 3, eds. R. J. Wurtman and J. J. Wurtman (New York: Raven Press, 1979), pp. 1-70.

2. R. A. Hawkins and J. F. Biebuyck, Ketone bodies are selectively used by individual brain regions, *Science* 205 (1979): 325-327.

3. J. C. Rosen and coauthors, Comparison of carbohydrate-containing and carbohydrate-restricted hypocaloric diets in the treatment of obesity: Effects on appetite and mood, *American Journal of Clinical Nutrition* 36 (1982): 463-469.

4. M. F. Ball, J. J. Canary, and L. H. Kyle, Comparative effects of calorie restriction and total starvation on body composition in obesity, *Annals of Internal Medicine* 67 (1967): 60-67.

5. Cahill, Aoki, and Rossini, 1979.

6. T. B. Van Itallie and M.-U. Yang, Current concepts in nutrition: Diet and weight loss, *New England Journal of Medicine* 297 (1977): 1158-1161.

7. Morbid obesity: Long-term results of therapeutic fasting, *Nutrition Reviews* 36 (1978): 6-7.

8. R. Linn and S. L. Stuart, *The Last Chance Diet* (New York: Bantam Books, 1977).

9. T. B. Van Itallie and M.-U. Yang, Cardiac dysfunction in obese dieters. A potentially lethal complication of rapid, massive weight loss, *American Journal of Clinical Nutrition* 39 (1984): 695-702.

10. The section on metabolism during exercise is adapted from F. S. Sizer and E. N. Whitney, *Life Choices: Health Concepts and Strategies* (St. Paul, Minn.: West, in press).

HIGHLIGHT SEVEN A

Nutrition and Fitness

People engage in exercise and sports at all levels—from occasional weekend walks to daily five-mile runs and more. This highlight is written to show the effects of nutrition on fitness—and the reverse, for there is a two-way relationship. Optimal nutrition contributes to athletic performance and conversely, regular exercise contributes to a person's ability to use and store nutrients optimally. The two together are indispensable to a high quality of life.

It should be noted, though, that nutrition and exercise training are not the only factors that contribute to athletic success. For keen competition, some people's genetic heritage equips them better from the outset. The quality of training is of major importance; so, too, is motivation. But in the context of these factors, anyone who is keenly interested in fitness is bound to be interested in nutrition as well.[1] This highlight begins with a consideration of fuels and how they are best used, building on the information about metabolism presented in the last chapter. Then it delves into the problems of muscle building and weight control; goes on to discuss the importance of vitamin-mineral nutrition; and concludes with a discussion of the most important nutrient of all: water.

Fuels for Athletic Activity

Chapter 7 described two stored fuels muscles draw on when they are working: the glycogen and fat (triglycerides) they have stored within their cells. They also use circulating glucose and fat (fatty acids) during exercise; and on rare occasions, protein. They go through the entire repertoire in the course of a long, demanding event such as a marathon; in shorter events, they don't switch fuels as often. During low or moderate intensity activity, muscle cells use predominantly fat as fuel; during intense activity, they use glycogen; and after glycogen is used up, fat and small amounts of protein. The details are best illustrated by following a marathon racer through the course of the race.[2]

If the racer starts off without a warm-up, the muscles will begin by using glycogen intensively. This is because the heart and lungs haven't started working hard enough to supply sufficient oxygen to support aerobic activity. Pyruvic, lactic, and other acids begin to accumulate, and within five minutes, 20 percent of the muscles' glycogen will have been burned up. However, the cardiovascular system will now have begun to work efficiently, and aerobic activity takes over. The racer experiences this shift as a relief from initial discomfort: the "second wind." The acids are oxidized, together with fat, both from inside the muscle cells and from fatty acids released from adipose cells elsewhere in the body. Henceforth, for as long as possible, the body burns a mixture of all four fuels— fat from the two sources just mentioned, and glucose from both

---

The body wants to be fit. Given the chance, it will respond with the strength and vigor that comes from proper exercise, nutrition, and rest.

Ellington Darden

---

within and outside the muscle. Throughout the race the muscles continue to require some glucose to support their activity.

The racer in prime condition can use fat the longest and at the exercise level of the highest intensity. As the intensity increases, though, fat supplies less and less, and glycogen more and more, of the energy need. After 40 to 60 minutes of racing, the free fatty acids in the blood are at six times the levels at which they started, and if the runner stops at any point after this, ketosis ensues.

A marathon race goes on for miles farther—so far, in fact, that finally, after about 20 miles, the runner "hits the wall"— experiences sudden, disabling fatigue. The only recourse is to slow down, for from this point on, the intensity of the exercise can only be as great as what aerobic fuel, fat, can support. Glucose released from the liver may still supply some energy for muscle work; and at this point protein tissue breakdown may also help maintain blood glucose, but it can't keep up with the needs of a racer at full tilt.

Marathon racers have learned that the ultimate limit to their endurance is the amount of glycogen they can pack away in their muscles before the race. This knowledge has led to the technique of glycogen loading—a strategy that uses a specific pattern of exercise and diet to trick the muscles into storing more glycogen than they normally do. Extra glycogen stored in muscle prolongs the time during which the marathoner can run the fastest and postpones exhaustion.

Most sports-minded people don't run marathons, so for them, the total

A Note on Glycogen Loading

When the technique of glycogen loading was first introduced, athletes were taught to reduce their carbohydrate intake for several days by eating meals high in protein and fat, and simultaneously to exercise heavily to deplete the muscle glycogen stores. The exercise had to involve the same muscles as those that would be working in the event. The second step was to reduce exercise intensity and switch abruptly to a diet high in carbohydrate for three days. Muscle glycogen stores rebounded to about two to four times the normal level and thus provided fuel that would last longer in an endurance event. In a hot climate, glycogen loading may confer an additional advantage, because glycogen holds a lot of water. As it breaks down, it releases this water, helping to meet the athlete's fluid needs.[3]

Until the mid-1970s, the hazards of this practice were unknown. Now, unfortunately, it is clear that there are hazards. The heart is a muscle, and it becomes packed with glycogen just as the skeletal muscles do; cardiac pain results, as well as generalized muscle pain and weight gain. It is strongly suggested that marathoners not load more than about three times a year, due to the effects on heart function. Most exercise physiologists recommend a different routine. Don't restrict carbohydrate and then rebound, they say; just eat a diet generally high in carbohydrate, and exercise intensively until two or three days before competition. Then ease off on the exercise and eat, for a day or so, meals especially high in carbohydrate. This method also keeps muscle glycogen high, but not so high as to cause any apparent ill effects.

---

amount of glycogen they store is not important. Still, they may deplete their glycogen stores during training for an endurance activity such as long-distance running, cycling, or swimming. If they do, they may experience increasing fatigue as the days of training go on. One reason for this is that it takes 48 hours or more to restore muscle carbohydrate to its pre-exercise level after it has been completely exhausted. Exercise is good training and normally promotes muscle building, but in the days immediately before an important competitive event, it is desirable to take a periodic day's rest, if possible. Ease off on training in the days immediately before competition.

To this point, the contributions of diet to athletic performance have been emphasized. Fitness also contributes to nutrition status, by altering the way dietary materials are used. In particular, muscle conditioning increases the muscles' ability to burn fat as fuel; the muscles build up more fat-metabolizing machinery in response to demand. A microscopic look at muscles shows that they respond to training by becoming crowded with mitochondria—intricately organized bodies inside the cells that contain the enzymes for aerobic metabolism (the TCA cycle). Muscle cells packed with mitochondria burn fat at a higher-intensity exercise level than poorly conditioned muscles, and will go much longer before starting to use glycogen. The point at which the body starts using glycogen is the beginning of the end, because glycogen stores are limited, whereas fat stores are (in effect) unlimited.

Conditioned muscles also burn fat more rapidly all day long, even between periods of exertion. People whose muscles are in good shape thus find it easier to keep off excess fat; that is, conditioning helps with weight control.

Fat, in contrast to glycogen, is an aerobic fuel, as we've said before. Fat deposits therefore supply energy for moderate, but not for intense, muscular work. Long, slow, moderately intense activities such as long walks are most effective as an adjunct to a weight-loss effort, because fat is continuously oxidized for the duration of these activities.

Protein Needs of the Conditioned Body

A fuel *not* useful for athletic competition is protein. Muscles are made largely of protein, but they can't use it efficiently as fuel; besides, it's a structural material and has more important uses. Many experiments have shown that extra protein in the diet confers no advantage on the athlete in terms of strength, endurance, or speed.

To become and stay fit, do you need to eat more protein than others? Yes and no. Athletes do, in fact, use a little more protein in their activities than nonathletes, but only a little more—perhaps 10 percent. The margin of safety built into the protein recommendation for all people is high enough to cover the athlete's need, so the recommended protein intake is not higher for the athlete than for anyone else—and most people eat so much protein, anyway, that the chances of even marginal deficiency are virtually nonexistent. To protect muscle protein (to avoid losing more than you can easily replace), you need to be sure to eat enough protein-sparing kcalories to meet your energy needs. If your energy needs are very high, then, what you need is extra kcalories, not extra protein.

To *build* muscle requires positive nitrogen balance (this was explained in Chapter 5), but even that doesn't mean eating more protein. There is no way to make muscles grow just by eating more protein. Excess protein can cause dehydration, because the discarded amino groups, combined into urea, require water to be excreted with them. Cells won't respond to excess protein by helplessly accepting it; they respond to the hormones that regulate them and to the demands put upon them, and then they select the nutrients they need from what is offered. So the way to make muscle cells grow is to put a demand on them—that is, to make them work. They will respond by taking up nutrients, amino acids included, so that they can grow. In summary, don't *push* protein at them, but exercise them in order to demand that they *pull* protein in for themselves. Then just eat an ordinary, adequate diet.

Energy Needs and Weight Control

Depending on the sport, an athlete in active training and competition may have extraordinarily high energy needs. Football players, for example, seem to average close to 6,000 kcalories a day during the football season, with some days' intakes topping 10,000 kcalories.[4] With the increased energy expenditure goes increased need for the B vitamins used to generate energy in metabolism. The increased intake, therefore, shouldn't be just any high-kcalorie food, but should be food rich in B vitamins as well—breads, cereals, fruits, vegetables, and other protective foods. It is a rare individual who can eat over 5,000 kcalories of nutrient-dense food in only three meals a day; five to six meals make the task easier.[5] Food, sufficient to provide this much energy, will also supply the vitamins and minerals needed to go with it— provided the selection is balanced and varied.

Chapter 8 is devoted to weight control for everyone, but a few words especially for the athlete are appropriate here. First of all, the recommended weight for an athlete is whatever weight and body composition achieves the optimum ratio of muscle strength to body mass. When the muscles are in top condition for performance of the chosen sport, the amount of body fat and total body weight should be whatever the muscles can carry most easily. Too little fat can make the body susceptible to too-rapid heat loss; too much creates a drag on motion. The ideal body composition is considered to

Muscles grow in response to work, not to protein feeding alone.

be about 15 percent fat for men in most sports, and 20 percent or more for women; less fat is considered ideal for runners, more for swimmers.

Sometimes seasonal sports or competitions require that an athlete gain or lose weight rapidly to fit into a weight category. An athlete who wants to gain weight in a hurry and doesn't care whether it is muscle or fat can add kcalories of any kind to the diet to achieve the desired gain. Because fat in foods is more energy-dense than protein or carbohydrate, athletes can most easily gain weight by eating a high-fat diet. This technique is an abuse of the body, though. The weight gained is mostly fat, and it increases the risk of heart disease, to which athletes are not immune. The healthy way to gain weight is to build oneself up by patient and consistent training, and at the same time to eat nutritious foods containing enough extra kcalories to support the weight gain.

A pound of muscle mass contains about 2,500 to 3,000 kcalories' worth of material. To gain a pound of muscle requires about a week of hard workouts, and an energy intake 3,000 kcalories above the amount sufficient to support that work. If you eat a big snack of foundation foods between meals, you can eat 700 to 800 extra kcalories a day this way, thus achieving a weight gain of 1 to 1½ pounds, mostly muscle, in a week.

Remember to cut *down* on kcalories between and after training periods. Muscles respond to reduced demand by losing mass. It would be magical thinking to believe that the mass simply disappears. In fact, the cells slowly atrophy, and the materials they are made of (mostly carbohydrate, fat, and protein) become available as potential fuel for other body cells. Of course, this fuel will be stored as fat unless it is expended in activity. It should be no surprise, then, that a heavily muscled individual of 20 who stops working out but keeps on eating like a football player in training can become an oversized, flabby, and obese person at 30. It is not literally true that the person's "muscle has turned to fat," but it is true that muscle has been lost and fat has been gained.

Losing weight, like gaining it, can be done wisely or unwisely. To achieve ideal body composition—the optimum ratio of muscle strength to body mass— you must reduce only body fat, and you can't do this for more than a very few weeks at a rate faster than about 2 pounds a week. Hurry-up techniques, such as sauna bathing, exercising in a plastic suit (to sweat the fat off), using diuretics or cathartics, or inducing vomiting, achieve faster weight loss only by causing dehydration, and dehydration seriously impairs performance. The hazards of fasts and fad diets have already been described, but a reminder should be repeated here. What is achieved by quick-weight-loss dieting is loss of lean tissue, glycogen, bone minerals, and fluids—all materials vital to healthy body functioning. Abnormal heart rhythms have been seen in healthy adults after only ten days of fasting. (Sometimes, however, an athlete obviously has heart disease, either hereditary or acquired. Diet can't always be blamed for sudden deaths in athletes.)

Athletes, like all people in our society, are susceptible to the eating disorders anorexia nervosa and bulimia.

These conditions, which arise in people overly responsive to the cultural ideal of thinness, are fully described in Highlight 8.

Even if it is achieved by healthy methods, extreme weight loss can be hazardous to the athlete, as to any person. Occasionally one hears that an "elite runner"—in superb physical condition and at the peak of his career—has died suddenly at the end of an intensive exercise session. In each case, the person had been severely restricting kcalories and had reached a new, all-time-low weight, while at the same time breaking his own previous records for distance or time. Heart failure caused the deaths.[6] Severe kcalorie restriction, weight loss, mineral losses, and hard training seem to have been contributing factors, possibly in combination with a primary heart abnormality to start with.[7]

Female athletes sometimes experience menstrual irregularity or even complete stoppage of the menstrual cycle. Athletic amenorrhea resembles the amenorrhea seen in women with anorexia nervosa or in the world's undernourished women and has been thought to be due to loss of body fat. The theory is that a certain minimum amount of body fat is necessary to support the making and using of the female hormones, which are fat-like compounds themselves. However, low body fat may not be the only cause; a stress-induced change in the brain's regulation of sex hormone output may be responsible for athletic amenorrhea.

A severe loss of bone calcium may accompany athletic amenorrhea, endangering the integrity of the skeleton in women who have allowed themselves to become too thin. Athletic osteoporosis also suggests hormonal involvement. In any case, the possible relationship of amenorrhea to body weight serves as a reminder that all athletes should keep in mind the definition of ideal weight already mentioned: the optimum ratio of muscle strength to body mass. Optimum means neither too much *nor too little* body mass.

Vitamins and Minerals for Athletic Activity

To maximize endurance, a competitor must pay attention not only to fuel reserves in the muscle, but also to the muscle's ability to use that fuel. That means maximizing all of the following:

- Aerobic capacity (by heart and lung conditioning)—for oxygen delivery.
- Hemoglobin levels (by optimal iron and protein nutrition)—because the protein hemoglobin, with iron in its structure, is the blood's oxygen carrier.
- Metabolic regulators (by optimal vitamin and mineral nutrition).
- Muscular fat-using ability (by muscular conditioning).
- Fluids and electrolytes—to provide the optimal environment for the muscles to work in.

Every vitamin and mineral is important in these connections.

The B vitamins are the metabolic regulators referred to above. Some of them directly coordinate energy metabolism and the need for them is proportional to energy expenditure. A person who expends 4,000 kcalories a day needs twice as much of these vitamins as someone who spends 2,000 kcalores. The B vitamins are named and described in detail in Chapter 9 where their food sources are also listed. Choices of complex carbohydrate foods in a diet relatively low in fat and empty kcalories assure B-vitamin intakes proportional to energy intakes.

Several B vitamins, as well as vitamins A, C, E, and many minerals are involved in making the oxygen-carrying red blood cells and the hemoglobin molecules with which they are filled. The mineral iron is a part of hemoglobin. Inadequacies of these can cause different kinds of anemia (described in Chapter 9), reducing the blood's ability to carry oxygen to exercising muscles.

The most common anemia in women is iron-deficiency anemia, caused by an iron intake inadequate to compensate for the monthly losses incurred by menstruation. Women have to make special efforts to obtain adequate iron, and many have depleted stores. If they restrict kcalories, they are almost certain to lose more iron than they replace. Even those who eat large amounts of food have to choose their foods with attention to iron contents. Ideal meals for this purpose include iron sources such as meats, legumes, and dark green vegetables combined with iron absorption-enhancing factors such as (again) meats and foods rich in vitamin C. Chapter 12 contains abundant suggestions for obtaining sufficient iron from foods; for people diagnosed iron-deficient, supplements should be prescribed.

An apparent anemia can also occur in athletes that reflects no reduction in hemoglobin supply, but rather an increase in the plasma volume.[8] The causes of athletes' anemia have not yet been determined, nor is it agreed whether it is a desirable effect of normal physiology or a pathological change. But it is known that plasma volume can increase during periods of heavy training because the kidney conserves sodium and water at these times.

Adequate electrolytes are essential for fluid balance, a crucial factor in athletic performance. When sodium is retained, potassium is lost. There has been some concern that potassium depletion might occur in people who engage in vigorous activity day after day, particularly if the activity involves sweating. The ordinary diet can easily supply enough potassium to cover the athlete's needs if designed according to guidelines similar to those just described for iron. (Chapter 11 offers more; see "Potassium.")

This brief treatment of vitamins and minerals for the athlete is intended to demonstrate the importance of nutrition for athletes as for all people who care about their health, and not to imply that special supplements are needed except for diagnosed medical conditions. A diet composed of a variety of nutritious foods offers the best support for athletic performance.

The Pregame Meal

The meal before a competitive event is an issue of heated debate. Many coaches and athletes believe intensely in special food rituals. For example, a football team can't play without breakfasting first on T-bones. A swim team is forbidden milk at the meet because it "causes cotton mouth." A bicyclist takes two tablespoons of honey before the race and savors the sweet on her tongue as she pedals away. Do these rituals work?

Scientifically, no particular food confers a special benefit before an athletic contest. A meal of steak may boost morale, but it is high in fat and may take so long to digest that it hinders performance. The idea that milk causes cotton mouth is pure superstition. Honey demands water from the blood to dilute it, a handicap during exertion. Although it is tempting to hope that a rise in blood glucose from a sugary snack will lend an athlete greater energy, actual study of runners shows that a sugar drink taken directly before exercise can *reduce* athletic endurance by 25 percent.[9]

In summary, some rituals have little effect, and some can impair performance. However, if a harmless but scientifically unproven practice gives a competitor a morale boost or extra confidence, it can make the difference between winning and losing a game, and so should be respected. People may have special, personal meanings associated with certain foods, but none has any unusual power to promote speed, endurance, or any other performance factor.

"*None* has any special power? Not even bee pollen? Surely this book must be out of date. Bee pollen has been proven to boost athletic performance."

This book, like any book, can contain erroneous information. When it does, it will be apologetically corrected. But so far, bee pollen is looking like any other health fad. One Finnish runner claimed it gave him the edge, long ago, in the 1972 Olympics in which he won a gold medal. It has sold with inflated claims ever since, but no one has gained any benefits from using it. In fact, bee pollen causes an allergic reaction in susceptible people, varies widely in composition from area to area and from one harvest to the next, is composed of at least 50 percent sugar, and sells for up to $24 per pound.

A claim may have been made many times, but that doesn't make it true. Some scientific "facts" have been "validated" only by conversation, not by experimentation.

Does it matter at all, then, what the meal before an event consists of? Olympic training tables are laden with foods such as breads, pasta, rice, potatoes, and fruit juice. These are good choices, because they are high in carbohydrate and low in fat, protein, and fiber. (Fiber is normally highly desirable, but not right before physical exertion, because, like the others listed here, it stays in the digestive tract too long and attracts water out of the blood.) Competitors eat as much of these foods as they can, because they supply energy without burdening the body. And they know it's especially important to include plenty of fluid. Foods like gelatin, juices, and Popsicles all deliver fluid with carbohydrate (Table H7-1 gives some examples of snacks to support top performance).

Any meal should be finished a good three or four hours before the event, because digestion requires routing the blood supply to the digestive tract to pick up nutrients. By the time the contest begins, the circulating blood should be freed from that task, and should be available instead to carry oxygen and fuel to the muscles. A person who eats a snack closer to competition time is especially advised to make it mostly carbohydrate with very

little protein and fat, because these are too slowly digested. Better yet, just fill up your fluid banks with beverages lacking sugar, such as water, diet sodas, or tea or coffee that is unsweetened or sweetened with artificial sweetener. To repeat, sweets immediately before the game can impair performance; fluids will enhance it.

Alcohol and Caffeine

Alcohol or other drugs and sports are always a dangerous combination. Judgment is crucial to the safety of the swimmer, skier, horseback rider, jogger, biker, or any other sports participant. Many recreation fatalities, like drownings, are caused by misjudgments, and alcohol and drugs are often responsible. They also cause the body to react much more slowly when action is needed. The connection is clear: decreased judgment and slowed reactions can be fatal in sports.

Alcohol has exactly the wrong effect on fluid balance, too—it is a diuretic that causes the excretion, rather than the retention, of water. It also induces losses of many minerals. Highlight 7B is devoted entirely to alcohol and nutrition, and makes these and many other details clear.

TABLE H7A–1

Sample Pregame Snacks

These foods, to be eaten three to four hours before competition, do *not* have many vitamins or minerals and are not suggested for inclusion in the daily diet. The hours before competition are too late for vitamins and minerals, but the special needs for energy and fluid can be met by eating the following snacks.

Sample Snack #1

Food	Serving Size	Energy (kcal)	Approximate % of Energy Donated by Carbohydrate
White bread	2 slices	140	74
Jam or jelly	2 tbsp	130	100
Gelatin dessert	1 c	70	97
Grape juice	1 c	165	100
Total		505	94
Sample Snack #2			
Spaghetti and tomato sauce (canned, plain)	1 c	190	80
Roll (white flour)	1	85	71
Popsicle (3 oz)	2	140	100
Limeade	1 c	100	100
Total		515	90
Sample Snack #3			
Banana	1	100	100
Sweetened dry cereal	¾ c	115	90
Skim milk	½ c	45	53
Cranberry juice cocktail	⅔ c	109	100
Gumdrops	1 oz	100	100
Total		469	95

Note: Substitutions can be made for cereal (1 c), spaghetti (1 c), or bread (2 slices):

    1 c white or flavored rice.
    1 3-inch-diameter muffin (plain).
    1 piece angel food cake.
    3 small pancakes and syrup.

To substitute liquids (gelatin, juices, limeade), use 1 c for each: 1 c any sugar-sweetened beverage.

Caffeine is also a diuretic. Many people like to meet their fluid needs with fluids containing caffeine because caffeine gets fat mobilization started before the event, helping to spare glycogen a little longer than otherwise. Others avoid it because the diuretic effect not only promotes the loss of water, vitamins, and minerals from the body but also necessitates urinating sooner than otherwise. To get around this problem still others prefer tablets (without water) containing caffeine. Caffeine used this way is classified as drug use and is forbidden in Olympic competition. There seems to be no harm, though, in the ordinary person's drinking a cup of coffee before going for an informal walk, run, or swim. This initiates use of the most efficient fuel mixture right from the start, rather than making the transition after the activity has begun.

The Athlete's Liquid Needs

Muscles heat up during heavy exertion. With inadequate circulation, the exercising muscle cramps. An adequate fluid intake is most important to prevent heat disorders from disabling the athlete. Fluid is needed to maintain the plasma volume so that blood can penetrate the muscles and carry the heat away, and also to permit sweating. The evaporation of sweat is the body's primary means of releasing heat during exercise in a hot environment.

Dehydration can disable the athlete more seriously than any other nutrition factor. Maintaining fluid balance is crucial to successful performance, because the first symptom of dehydration is fatigue. A rapid water loss equal to 5 percent of the body weight can reduce muscular work capacity by 20 to 30 percent. It is recommended that the competitor replenish fluid during an event by drinking 1/5 strength orange juice or a balanced fluid and electrolyte mixture at intervals.

Salts are lost when fluid is lost through sweating, but replacement need not be immediate and shouldn't be by way of salt tablets. A person can sweat away as much as 9 pounds of fluid and still perform well, provided he drinks enough water, even without salt. A rule of thumb is to drink close to a pound of fluid (14 to 16 ounces) for each pound of body weight lost during an activity.[10]

After intensive competition, your thirst is not an adequate guide to the amount of fluid you need, because your stomach will get full and signal "stop drinking" before your body is fully rehydrated. People sometimes stay dehydrated for several days beyond sports competitions. It is therefore recommended that you weigh yourself before the event, and when it is over, weigh yourself again on the same scale. Then measure out the amount of fluid you'll need to restore your body weight (remember, "a pint's a pound, the world around"), and be sure to drink it all the same day.

As for salt loss, when the event is over, eating regular food can make it up. At that point, replacement of magnesium and potassium may be more important than replacement of sodium; this means consuming nutrient-dense, not empty-kcalorie, beverages and foods. Fruits, fruit juices, *fresh* vegetables, and unprocessed foods of all kinds are especially good sources of these minerals, as later chapters make clear. Salt tablets are still unnecessary, even if they've been given the scientific-sounding name "electrolyte pills."

You may be wondering how this statement can be made when the makers of Gatorade and other "sweat replacers" claim that their mixtures of water and glucose, sodium, chloride, potassium, magnesium, and calcium enter the system "faster than water" and help football players win games. Actually, although such mixtures do resemble sweat in composition (except for the glucose) and do satisfy thirst, they are probably absorbed less rapidly, not more rapidly, than water, because the glucose in them delays absorption.

Also, some people think the sugar would elicit the secretion of insulin, which opposes release of both glycogen and fat for use as fuel. However, once an athlete is warmed up and working out, dilute glucose solutions ingested at intervals apparently do not increase insulin secretion.[11] Moreover, except for the case of the marathon runner, the body of a trained athlete stores extra amounts of the minerals in question and can ordinarily replenish them with food and fluids after the competition is over.[12] Furthermore, a person who sweats heavily (say, two liters) during competition *cannot* replace the lost fluid even by drinking that much, because the body can't absorb more than 4/5 liter in an hour. The best fluid to take during a marathon event is *diluted* juice (for example, one part orange juice plus four parts water) or plain, cool water in small quantities. However, there is probably no great harm in the moderate use of sweat replacers. The sugar in them tastes good, and they may bolster morale.

Pills, Powders, and Potions

People can disagree endlessly about nutrition and performance, but to those who have researched it, the subject doesn't generate much disagreement.

Still, claims are everywhere that promote the taking of a multitude of powders, syrups, granules, and pills to increase strength, endurance, speed, and skill. To distinguish fact from fiction, when you hear such claims being made, ask the person speaking where the facts came from. Generally, you'll get the most valid information from an informant who has taken college or even graduate school courses in the science of nutrition.

Here are a few questions to ask yourself about any health gimmick, product, or device that you see advertised, or that someone tries to sell you:

- Is the promised action of the product based on magical thinking? ("Eat all you want and lose weight." "Develop a trim body with no exercise.")
- Does the promotion claim that "doctors agree" or "research has determined" without clarification? Which doctors? What research?
- Does the promotion state that hormones, drugs, or nutrient doses useful in correcting an abnormal condition are needed to make the normal, healthy person more fit?
- Does the promoter use scare tactics to pressure you into buying the product? ("It's the only one available without poisons.")

Miniglossary

athletes' amenorrhea (ay-men-or-REE-uh): the failure in female athletes to menstruate.
a = without
menor = menstrual cycle
athletes' anemia: anemia seen in athletes; cause unknown.
athletic osteoporosis: bone loss seen in women athletes, especially runners with anorexia.
glycogen loading: a technique of inducing muscles to store more glycogen than they normally do, by manipulating the diet's carbohydrate levels.
mitochondria (mye-toe-KON-dree-uh): intracellular bodies with a highly organized structure containing many internal membranes; on the membranes are mounted the enzymes that conduct aerobic metabolism (the TCA cycle and the electron transport chain). Mitochondria are abundant in all cells, but especially in the cells of conditioned muscles.

- Does the promoter promise quick and easy physical changes?
- Is the product being sold or promoted by a self-styled health adviser who has no acceptable credentials, a crusading organization, or a faith-healing group?
- Is the product advertised as having a multitude of different beneficial effects? ("Makes bigger muscles; gives that 'pumped-up feeling'; improves digestion, coordination, and breathing.")
- Does the sponsor claim persecution by the medical community and the government because they do not accept this wonderful discovery?
- Is the product available only from the sponsor by mail order and with payment in advance?
- Does the promoter use many case histories or testimonials from grateful users?
- Is the product a special or "secret" formula not available from any other source?

If you answer yes to one or more of these questions, it's your warning signal that you may be dealing with quackery.

The recommendations made in this highlight are simple, commonsense suggestions. To sum up, a normal varied diet is best for the athlete, as for anyone else. Athletes eat more food to get the extra kcalories they need, and if they choose their foods with reasonably good judgment, they can easily get the protein, vitamins, and minerals they need as well. An adequate fluid intake is indispensable to successful performance.

Notes

1. We are indebted to Professor Stanley Winter, of Golden West College, Huntington Beach, California, for his thoughtful and informative critique of this highlight. Parts of the highlight were adapted from F. S. Sizer and E. N. Whitney, *Life Choices: Health Concepts and Strategies* (St. Paul, Minn.: West, in press), Chapter 7.

2. Details of the description that follows are from R. Locksley, Fuel utilization in marathons: Implications for performance—Medical Staff Conference, University of California, San Francisco, *Western Journal of Medicine* 133 (1980): 493–502.

3. G. R. Hagerman, Nutrition in part-time athletes, *Nutrition and the MD*, August 1981.

4. S. Short and W. R. Short, Four-year study of university athletes' dietary intake, *Journal of the American Dietetic Association* 82 (1983): 632–645.

5. Energy intake and exercise, *Nutrition and the MD*, August 1981.

6. T. J. Bassler, Body build and mortality (letter to the editor), *Journal of the American Medical Association* 244 (1980): 1437.

7. Nutrition and the QT interval, *Lancet*, 22 June 1985, p. 1431.

8. "Anaemia" in athletes, *Lancet*, 29 June 1985, pp. 1491–1492.

9. K. Keller and R. Schwarzkopf, Preexercise snacks may decrease exercise performance, *The Physician and Sportsmedicine*, April 1984, pp. 89–91.

10. Hagerman, 1981.

11. S. Wintsch, Beading the heat, *Science 81*, February 1981, pp. 80–82.

12. Wintsch, 1981.

HIGHLIGHT SEVEN B

Alcohol and Nutrition

One of the many drugs—and often the most important one—that enters people's lives as they arrive at their teen and adult years is alcohol. With the understanding of metabolism gained from Chapter 7, the student is in a position to understand at a deep level just how alcohol affects nutrition status.

If liver cells could talk, they would describe the alcohol of intoxicating beverages as demanding, egocentric, and disruptive of the liver's normally efficient way of running its business. For example, liver cells prefer fatty acids as their fuel, and they like to package excess fatty acids into triglycerides and ship them out to other tissues, but when alcohol is present, they are forced to use it and let the fatty acids accumulate, sometimes in huge stockpiles.

Alcohol affects every organ of the body, but the most dramatic evidence of its disruptive behavior appears in the liver. This is the only organ whose cells can oxidize alcohol for fuel to any great extent. All other cells are affected by the presence of alcohol but can do practically nothing about getting rid of it. Liver cells make nearly all of the body's alcohol-processing machinery—

namely, the enzyme alcohol dehydrogenase and the MEOS, described on page 235. Alcohol dehydrogenase can convert alcohol to acetaldehyde, which can in turn be converted to acetyl CoA, the compound that all energy nutrients become on their way to being used as fuel. But we are getting ahead of our story. Let's start at the beginning, when alcohol first enters the body in a beverage, and follow it until it leaves or is made into useful acetyl CoA.

Alcohol in Beverages

To the chemist, *alcohol* refers to a class of compounds containing reactive hydroxyl (OH) groups. The glycerol to which fatty acids are attached in triglycerides is an example of an alcohol to a chemist. But to the average person, *alcohol* refers to the intoxicating ingredient in beer, wine, and hard liquor (distilled spirits). The chemist's name for this particular alcohol is *ethyl alcohol*, or *ethanol*. Glycerol has three carbons with three hydroxyl groups attached; ethanol has only two carbons and one hydroxyl group. For the remainder of this highlight, we will be discussing alcohol, but you will know that we are really talking about a particular alcohol—ethanol.

Ethanol arises naturally from carbohydrates when certain microorganisms metabolize them in the absence of oxygen—a process called fermentation. Since all plants contain carbohydrate, all can serve as the starting material for fermentation. Many different plants are used by different societies to produce alcoholic beverages; the most familiar are grapes and other berries (used to make wine), apples (fermented or hard cider), and grains (beer and various distilled liquors). Wines, ciders, and beers are used as is, after fermentation, whereas the so-called hard liquors are made by further distilling the products of fermentation, so as to concentrate the alcohol. Thus grain mashes can be distilled further to yield the whiskeys— bourbon (at least half from corn), rye (from rye), scotch (from barley), vodka (from wheat, rye, corn, or potatoes), rum (from cane products such as molasses), and brandy (from wine). Hard liquors may then be served with mixers such as carbonated beverages or fruit juices (cocktails), or they may be sweetened with herbs and spices (liqueurs, or after-dinner drinks). Wine and beer have a relatively low percentage of alcohol, whereas whiskey, vodka, rum, and brandy may be as much as 50 percent alcohol.

The alcohols affect living things profoundly, partly because they act as lipid solvents. They can dissolve the lipids right out of cell membranes, destroying the cell structure and thereby killing the cells. For this reason, most alcohols are toxic, or poisonous; by the same token, because they kill microbial cells, they are useful as disinfectants.

```
      H
      |
   H-C-OH
      |
   H-C-OH
      |
   H-C-OH
      |
      H
```
Glycerol is an alcohol.

```
   H            H
   |            |
 H-C-H       H-C-H
   |            |
 H-C-H         OH
```
Ethanol is the alcohol in beer, wine, and distilled spirits.

Ethanol, like the other alcohols, is toxic—but less so than some. Sufficiently diluted and taken in small enough doses, it produces euphoria—an effect that people seek—not with zero risk, but with a low enough risk (if the doses are low enough) to be tolerable. Used to achieve these effects, alcohol is a drug—that is, a substance that can modify one or more of the body's functions. Like all drugs, alcohol offers some benefits; it also has tremendous abuse potential.

Benefits of Alcohol Use

The beneficial effects of alcohol have long been appreciated and praised. Wine, beer, and other fermented beverages have given pleasure and relaxation to people for more than 5,000 years. Only recently have we begun to learn exactly how the little molecule ethanol acts in our bodies, but people have always known that it affects their mood, sensations, and behavior. Because it alters mood, alcohol has many uses. Taken in moderation, alcohol relaxes people, reduces their inhibitions, and encourages desirable social interactions.

The term *moderation* is important in the statement just made. Just what is moderation in the use of alcohol? We can't name an exact amount of alcohol per day that would be appropriate for everyone, because people differ in their tolerance levels, but authorities have attempted to set a limit that is appropriate for most healthy people: not more than three drinks a day for the average-sized, healthy man, or two drinks a day for the average-sized, healthy woman. This amount is supposed to be enough to produce euphoria without incurring any long-term harm to health. Doubtless some people could consume slightly more; others could definitely not handle nearly so much without significant risk.

Alcohol in any beverage has the same sought-after effects. In addition, wine in particular is credited with some special effects. Grape juice has a proven antiviral effect that carries over when the grape juice is made into wine.[1] The high potassium content of grape juice is beneficial to people with high blood pressure; when the grape juice is made into wine, the potassium remains in the wine, so this effect also carries over. Dealcoholized wine also increases the absorption of potassium, calcium, phosphorus, magnesium, and zinc; so does wine, but the alcohol in it promotes the *excretion* of these minerals, so the dealcoholized version is preferred.[2] If people who are accustomed to drinking wine give it up, they can still enjoy these benefits by learning to drink moderate amounts of fruit juices or dealcoholized wine in its place.

Alcoholic beverages also affect the appetite. Usually, they reduce it, making people unaware that they are hungry, but in people who are tense and unable to eat, small doses of wine taken 20 minutes before meals improve the appetite. Certain acid compounds in the wine, known as congeners, are credited with this effect. For undernourished people and for people with severely depressed appetites, wine may facilitate eating even when psychotherapy fails to do so. At the same time, because it relaxes people, wine may help obese people lose weight. Its success in that connection is thought to stem from its ability to relieve emotional stress, which is a common reason for overeating. Again, certain congeners in wine may contribute to the tranquilizing effect; some are said to be nearly 100 times more effective than alcohol.[3] French wine also contains a compound which is known to lower liver lipids and cholesterol.[4]

Several research studies have also shown that wine and beer contribute an important trace mineral—silicon—to people's diets. In wine-drinking countries, this is thought to be a factor that contributes to favorable cardiovascular mortality. This doesn't mean that people have to drink wine to obtain the silicon they need, of course, but where their diets lack silicon and their wine happens to supply it, the wine gets the credit.[5] Most wines are also low in sodium and high in potassium, and some are low enough in sugar to be useful in the diets of persons with diabetes. Wine adds kcalories, of course, but there is something to be said for its kcalories as opposed to those of, say, sour cream. (Sour cream is almost pure fat and is virtually empty of nutrients.) People who want to enhance their meals with a luxury item they enjoy could easily do worse than to add a glass of wine.*

An example of the beneficial use of alcohol is provided by the experience of the staff at a hospital for the aging,** where three-fourths of the male clients were incontinent (unable to control their bladders) and needed safety restraints to hold them in their wheelchairs. Needless to say, these clients became depressed. The staff decided to serve beer, cheese, and crackers six times a week in the late afternoon in hopes that this would improve morale and perhaps encourage the men to enjoy themselves and socialize more. Within two months, only one fourth were incontinent, only 12 percent needed safety restraints, and most had become able to walk around unaided. Group activity more than tripled. The staff attributed the change to the "socializing" effect of the cocktail hour.[6]

---

*Wine has 200 other substances in it, some of which may be beneficial. It is low in sodium and in some cases may be high in calcium, iron, or other valuable nutrients. The virtues of wine are well described (possibly even without bias) by the Wine Institute in its publication *Wine and Medical Practice, A Summary* (for distribution only to the medical profession), San Francisco, Calif.: Wine Institute, 1979.

**The hospital described here is the Cushing Hospital, near Boston.

This example shows that alcoholic beverages can be beneficial when used to improve people's morale. Another example: after President Eisenhower had his first heart attack, his physician recommended that he have a drink or two of cognac every evening. The purpose was to relax him and enable him to achieve a daily escape from the pressures of the presidency. Such uses of alcohol can prolong life and good health, although a person might be even better off learning how to relax without chemical help in the face of such pressures.

You may have heard that drinking, at least moderately, improves the heart's health by raising the blood concentration of HDL (high-density lipoproteins), the indicator of a low risk of heart attack (see Chapter 4). It turns out, though, that two classes of HDL exist—one class associated with lowered heart disease risk, and another associated with moderate drinking. Alcohol raises one type of HDL, but it's not the type that reduces heart disease risk.[7] This, then, cannot be counted among the benefits of alcohol use, but the others seem real.

Alcohol in the Body

From the moment alcohol enters the body in a beverage, it is treated as if it has special privileges. Foods sit around in the stomach for a while, but not alcohol. The tiny alcohol molecules need no digestion; they can diffuse as soon as they arrive, right through the walls of the stomach, and they reach the brain within a minute. You can feel euphoric right away when you drink, especially if your stomach is empty. When your stomach is full of food, the molecules of alcohol have less chance of touching the walls and diffusing through, so you don't feel the effects of alcohol so quickly. If you don't want to become intoxicated at parties, then, eat the snacks provided by the host. Carbohydrate snacks are best suited for

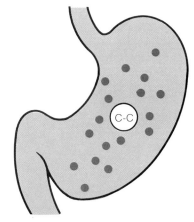

The alcohol (C-C) in a stomach filled with food has a low probability of touching the walls and diffusing through.

slowing alcohol absorption. High-fat snacks help, too, because they slow peristalsis.[8] But when the stomach contents are emptied into the duodenum, it doesn't matter that plenty of food is mixed with the alcohol. The alcohol is absorbed rapidly anyway, "as if it were a V.I.P. (Very Important Person)."[9]

Alcohol Arrives in the Liver

The capillaries that surround the digestive tract merge into the veins that carry the alcohol-laden blood to the liver. Here the veins branch and rebranch into capillaries that touch every liver cell. As already mentioned, liver cells are the only cells in the body that can make enough alcohol dehydrogenase to oxidize alcohol at an appreciable rate. However, there is a limit to the amount of alcohol anyone can process in a given time. This limit is set by the number of molecules of the enzyme alcohol dehydrogenase that reside in the liver. If more molecules of alcohol arrive at the liver cells than the enzymes can handle, the extra alcohol must wait. It enters the general circulation and moves on past the liver. From the liver, it is carried to all parts of the body, circulating again and again

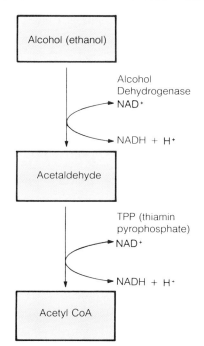

The conversion of alcohol to acetyl CoA.

through the liver until enzymes are available to convert it to acetaldehyde.

The rate at which alcohol dehydrogenase can work limits the rate of the body's handling of alcohol. The type of enzyme produced varies with individuals, depending on the genes they have inherited. Some racial groups—for example, Asians—have genetic information that causes them to produce atypical forms of alcohol dehydrogenase and its partner enzyme acetaldehyde dehydrogenase. This difference explains why some persons are made too uncomfortable by alcohol to become addicted.* High levels of

---

*Alcohol dehydrogenase, although atypical, works as fast as normal in Asians, but their acetaldehyde dehydrogenase works more *slowly*, so that they suffer from a kind of acetaldehyde poisoning. D. P. Agarwal, S. Harada, and H. W. Goedde, Racial differences in biological sensitivity to ethanol: The role of alcohol dehydrogenase and acetaldehyde dehydrogenase enzymes, *Alcoholism: Clinical and Experimental Research* 5 (1981): 12–16.

FIGURE H7B-1

A simplified version of the glucose-to- energy pathway, showing the entry of ethanol into the pathway.
The coenzyme NAD which is the active form of niacin, is the only one included.

If more molecules of alcohol arrive at the liver cells than the enzymes can handle, the extra molecules must wait.

acetaldehyde in the brain and other tissues are responsible for many of the punishing effects of alcohol abuse.

The amount of alcohol dehydrogenase present is also affected by whether you eat or not. Fasting for as little as a day causes degradation of the enzyme (protein) within the cells, and can reduce the rate of alcohol metabolism by half. Drinking on an empty stomach thus not only lets the drinker feel the effects more promptly, but also brings about higher blood alcohol levels for longer periods of time and increases the effect of alcohol in anesthetizing the brain.

Alcohol dehydrogenase oxidizes alcohol to acetaldehyde. Simultaneously, it reduces a molecule of NAD, converting it to NADH.* (The N in NAD is a form of niacin, one of the B vitamins.) The related enzyme acetaldehyde dehydrogenase reduces another NAD to NADH while it

oxidizes acetaldehyde to acetyl CoA, the compound that enters the TCA cycle to generate energy.* Thus whenever alcohol is being metabolized in the body, NAD is consumed, and NADH accumulates. Chemists describe the consequence by saying that the body's "redox state" is altered, because NAD can oxidize, and NADH can reduce, many other body compounds. During

alcohol metabolism, NAD becomes unavailable for the multitude of reactions for which it is required.

Figure H7B-1 is a drawing of the pathway from glucose to energy, showing the many places along the way that require NAD. It shows that for glucose to get completely metabolized, the TCA cycle must be operating, and NAD must be present. If these conditions are not met (and when alcohol is present, they may not be), the pathway will be blocked, and traffic will back up—or an alternate route will

*More awkwardly (but more accurately) stated, NAD^+ is converted to $NADH + H^+$. For simplicity's sake, the description here is stated as if one hydrogen is added to NAD, but really, two are added to NAD^+.

*All cells possess acetaldehyde dehydrogenase, so this step can take place elsewhere besides the liver.

Acetyl CoAs are blocked from getting into the TCA cycle by the high level of NADH. Instead of being used for energy, they become building blocks for fatty acids.

be taken. There are physical consequences to such changes in the normal flow of traffic from glucose to available energy. Think about some of these as you follow the pathway.

In each step of alcohol metabolism in which NAD is converted to NADH, hydrogen ions accumulate, resulting in a dangerous shift of the acid-base balance toward acid. The accumulation of NADH depresses the TCA cycle, so that pyruvate and acetyl CoA build up. The excess acetyl CoA then takes the route to the synthesis of fatty acids, and fat clogs the liver so it cannot function.[10]

The body's altered redox state interferes with the process by which the liver generates glucose from protein. The unavailability of glucose from this source, together with the overabundance of acetyl CoA molecules blocked from getting into the TCA cycle, sets the stage for a shift into ketosis. The making of ketone bodies consumes acetyl CoA, but some ketone bodies are acids, so they push the acid-base balance further toward acid.

The surplus of NADH also favors the conversion of pyruvate to lactic acid, which serves as a temporary storage place for hydrogens from NADH. The conversion of pyruvate to lactic acid restores some NAD, but a lactic acid

buildup has serious consequences of its own. It adds still further to the body's acid burden and interferes with the excretion of uric acid, causing goutlike symptoms.

The presence of alcohol alters amino acid metabolism in the liver cells. Synthesis of some proteins important in the immune system slows down,

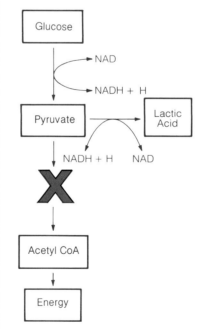

Pyruvate is converted to lactic acid if the pathway to acetyl CoA is blocked.

weakening the body's defenses against infection. Synthesis of lipoproteins speeds up, increasing blood triglyceride levels.

Protein deficiency can develop, both from the depression of protein synthesis in the cells, and from poor diet. Normally the cells would at least use the amino acids that one happened to eat, but the drinker's liver deaminates the amino acids and channels their carbon backbones into fat or ketones. Eating well does not protect the drinker from protein depletion. One has to stop drinking alcohol for complete protection.

The synthesis of fatty acids also accelerates as a result of the liver's exposure to alcohol. Fat accumulation can be seen in the liver after a single night of heavy drinking. Fatty liver, the first stage of liver deterioration seen in heavy drinkers, interferes with the distribution of nutrients and oxygen to the liver cells. If the condition lasts long enough, the liver cells will die, and the area will be invaded by fibrous scar tissue—the second stage of liver deterioration, called fibrosis. Fibrosis is reversible with good nutrition and abstinence from alcohol, but the next (last) stage—cirrhosis—is not.

Alcohol affects every tissue's metabolism of nutrients in other ways as well. Stomach cells oversecrete the immune system's inflammation-producing agent histamine, and acid, becoming vulnerable to ulcer formation. Intestinal cells fail to absorb thiamin, folacin, and vitamin B_{12}. Liver cells lose efficiency in activating vitamin D, and alter their production and excretion of bile. Rod cells in the retina, which normally process vitamin A alcohol to its aldehyde form needed in vision, find themselves processing ethanol to acetaldehyde instead. The kidney excretes increased quantities of magnesium, calcium, potassium, and zinc.

Acetaldehyde interferes with metabolism, too. It dislodges vitamin

B$_6$ from its protective binding protein, so that it is destroyed, causing a vitamin B$_6$ deficiency and, thereby, lowered production of red blood cells.

The liver's V.I.P. treatment of alcohol is reflected in its handling of drugs, as well as nutrients. In addition to the enzyme alcohol dehydrogenase, the liver possesses an enzyme system that metabolizes *both* alcohol and drugs— any compounds that have certain chemical features in common. Called the MEOS, this system handles only about one fifth of the total alcohol a person consumes, but the MEOS enlarges if repeatedly exposed to alcohol. This may not make the drinker able to handle much more alcohol at a time than before, because the total alcohol-metabolizing ability of the MEOS is small, but the effect on the ability to metabolize drugs is considerable.

When the MEOS enlarges, it makes the body able to metabolize drugs much faster than before. This can make it confusing and tricky to work out the correct doses of medications. The doctor who prescribes sedatives every four hours, for example, assumes that the MEOS will dispose of the drug at a certain predicted rate. Well and good; but in a client who is a heavy drinker, the MEOS is adapted to metabolizing large quantities of alcohol. It therefore metabolizes the drug extra fast. The drug's effects wear off unexpectedly fast, leaving the client undersedated. Imagine the doctor's alarm if the client wakes up on the table during an operation! A skilled anesthesiologist always asks clients about their drinking patterns before putting them to sleep.

An enlarged MEOS will oxidize drugs *faster* than expected, but only as long as there is no alcohol in the system. If the person drinks and uses the drug at the same time, the drug will be metabolized more *slowly* and so will be much more potent. The MEOS is busy disposing of alcohol, so the drug can't be handled till later; and the dose may build up to where it greatly oversedates, even kills, the user.

Ethanol Arrives in the Brain

Alcohol is a narcotic. It was used for centuries as an anesthetic because of its ability to deaden pain. But it wasn't a very good anesthetic, because one could never be sure how much a person would need and how much would be a lethal dose. As new, more predicable anesthetics were discovered, they quickly replaced alcohol. However, alcohol continues to be used today as a kind of anesthetic on social occasions, to help people relax or to relieve anxiety. People think that alcohol is a stimulant, because it seems to make them lively and uninhibited at first. Actually, though, the way it does this is by sedating *inhibitory* nerves, which are more numerous than excitatory nerves. Ultimately, it acts as a depressant, and sedates all the nerve cells.

When alcohol flows to the brain, it sedates the frontal lobe first, the reasoning part. As the alcohol molecules diffuse into the cells of this lobe, they interfere with reasoning and judgment. If the drinker drinks faster than the rate at which the liver can oxidize the alcohol, then the speech and vision centers of the brain become narcotized, and the area that governs reasoning becomes more incapacitated. Later, the cells of the brain responsible for large-muscle control are affected; at this point, people "under the influence"

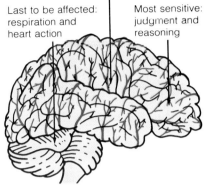

Alcohol's effects on the brain. Alcohol is rightly termed an anesthetic, because it puts brain centers to sleep in order: first the cortex; then the emotion-governing centers; then the centers that govern muscular control; and, finally, deep centers that control respiration and heartbeat.

(labels on figure:) Next most sensitive: muscular control. Last to be affected: respiration and heart action. Most sensitive: judgment and reasoning.

stagger or weave when they try to walk. Finally, the conscious brain is completely subdued, and the person "passes out." Now, luckily, the person can drink no more; this is lucky because a higher dose's anesthetic effect could reach the deepest brain centers that control breathing and heartbeat, and the person could die. Table H7B-1 shows the blood alcohol levels that correspond with progressively greater intoxication.

We've called it lucky that the brain centers respond to alcohol in the order just described, because one passes out before one can drink a lethal dose. It is possible, though, to drink fast enough

TABLE H7B–1

Alcohol Doses and Brain Responses

Number of Drinks	Blood Alcohol (%)	Effect on Brain
2	0.05	Judgment impaired
4	0.10	Control impaired
6	0.15	Muscle coordination and reflexes impaired
8	0.20	Vision impaired
12	0.30	Drunk, out of control
14 or more	0.50 to 0.60	Amnesia, finally death

that the effects of alcohol continue to accelerate after one has gone to sleep. The occasional death that takes place during a drinking contest is attributed to this effect. The drinker drinks fast enough, before passing out, to receive a lethal dose.

Liver cells are not the only cells that die with excessive exposure to alcohol; brain cells are particularly sensitive. When liver cells have died, others may later multiply to replace them, but there is no regeneration of brain cells. This is one reason for the permanent brain damage observed in some heavy drinkers.

Alcohol depresses production of antidiuretic hormone (ADH) by the pituitary gland in the brain. All people who drink have observed the increase in urination that accompanies drinking, but they may not realize that they can easily get into a vicious cycle as a result. Loss of body water leads to thirst. Thirst leads to more drinking—but drinking of what? The only fluid that will relieve dehydration is water, but the thirsty person welcomes any cold fluid, even concentrated alcohol, because it relieves the dry mouth associated with thirst. If a person tries to use concentrated alcoholic beverages to quench thirst, however, it only becomes worse. The smart drinker, then, either drinks beer (which contains plenty of water), or drinks wine or hard liquor with mixers or chasers. Better still, the drinker limits the total amount consumed.

The water loss caused by depression of antidiuretic hormone involves loss of more than just water and some alcohol. With water loss there is a loss of such important minerals as magnesium, potassium, calcium, and zinc (see Chapters 11 and 12). These minerals are vital to the maintenance of fluid balance and to many chemical reactions in the cells, including muscle contraction. For the person made sick by excessive alcohol intake and requiring detoxification, repletion therapy has to be instituted early to bring magnesium and potassium levels back to normal as quickly as possible.

With these changes in mind, it is time to take a look at alcohol consumption from the social view and at the malnutrition that results from excessive drinking.

Drinking and Drunkenness

If you want to drink socially, you should drink slowly, with food, and should sip, not gulp, your drinks. If the alcohol molecules dribble slowly enough into the liver cells, the enzymes will be able to handle the load. Spacing of drinks is important, too. It takes about an hour and a half to metabolize one drink, depending on your body size, on previous drinking experience, on how recently you have eaten, and on how you are feeling at the time.

If you want to help a friend sober up, there is no reason to wear yourself out walking your friend around the block. The muscles have to work harder, but since they can't metabolize alcohol, they can't help clear it from the blood. Time is the only thing that will do the job; each person has a particular level of the enzyme alcohol dehydrogenase, and it clears the blood at a steady rate. This is not true for most nutrients. If you bring in more of a nutrient, generally the body can promptly step up the rate at which it metabolizes that nutrient. But not with alcohol.

Nor will it help your friend to drink a cup of coffee. Caffeine is a stimulant, but it won't speed up the metabolism of alcohol. The police say ruefully, "If you give a cup of coffee to a drunk, you'll just have a wide-awake drunk on your hands."

So far we have mentioned only one way that the blood is cleared of alcohol—metabolism by the liver. However, about 10 percent of the alcohol is excreted through the breath and in the urine. This fact is the basis for the breathalyzer test for drunkenness administered by the police. The amount of alcohol in the breath is in proportion to that still in the bloodstream. In most states, legal drunkenness is set at 0.15 percent, although many states are lowering the criterion to 0.10 percent—especially as statistics accumulate that show a relationship between alcohol use and industrial and traffic accidents.

The lack of glucose for the brain's function and the length of time needed to clear the blood of alcohol account for some diverse consequences of drinking. Responsible aircraft pilots know that they must allow 24 hours for their bodies to clear alcohol completely, and refuse to fly any sooner. Major airlines enforce this rule. Women who may become pregnant are warned to abstain from the use of alcohol, because it severely threatens the development of the fetus's central nervous system. The fetal brain grows at the rate of 100,000 new brain cells a minute, so deprivation of even a few minutes' oxygen supply can have an adverse impact. One of the effects of an acute dose in experimental animals is to collapse the umbilical cord temporarily, depriving the developing fetus of oxygen.[11] This can occur even before a woman is aware that she is pregnant.

You may have heard the story of the country woman who kept saying "Amen!" as the preacher ranted about one sin after another; but when he got to her favorite sin, she whispered to her husband that the preacher had "quit preachin' and gone to meddlin'." We've tried to stick to scientific facts, so the only "meddlin'" that we'll do is to urge you to look again at the accompanying drawing of the brain and note that judgment is affected first when someone drinks. A person's judgment may tell him that he should limit himself to two drinks at a party, but the first drink may take his judgment away, so that he has many more. The failure to stop drinking as planned, on repeated occasions, is a danger sign that indicates that the person should not drink at all.

Drinking and Malnutrition

It has been estimated that more than 9 million people in the United States abuse alcohol to the point that their personal relationships, their jobs, or their health is impaired. One of the health hazards is malnutrition. Alcohol depresses appetite by the euphoria it produces, as well as by its attack on the mucosa of the stomach, so that heavy drinkers usually eat poorly, if at all. With a large portion of their energy fuel coming from the empty kcalories of alcohol, they find it difficult to obtain the essential nutrients. Thus some of their malnutrition is due to lack of food—but even if they eat well, the direct effects of alcohol will take their toll. Alcohol hinders the absorption, alters the metabolism, and increases the excretion of many nutrients, so that malnutrition can occur even in the well-fed drinker.

Ethanol interferes with a multitude of chemical and hormonal reactions in the body—many more than have been enumerated here. The point of this highlight, however, was not to summarize every effect of alcohol; the point was to offer a reward to the reader for learning the basics of metabolism explained in Chapter 7. The understandings gained permit a profound appreciation of processes like those described here.

Miniglossary

alcohol dehydrogenase: a liver enzyme that converts ethanol to **acetaldehyde** (ass-et-AL-duh-hide). The MEOS also oxidizes alcohol.

antidiuretic hormone (ADH): a hormone produced by the pituitary gland in response to dehydration (or a high sodium concentration in the blood); stimulates the kidneys to reabsorb more water and so excrete less. This ADH should not be confused with the enzyme alcohol dehydrogenase, which is sometimes also abbreviated ADH.

cirrhosis (seer-OH-sis): advanced liver disease, in which liver cells have died, hardened, and turned orange; often associated with alcoholism.
cirrhos = an orange

congeners (CON-jen-ers): compounds in alcoholic beverages that confer their chemical individuality on them—responsible in part for their flavor, aroma, hangover-producing, and tranquilizing effects, among others.

drink: a dose of any alcoholic beverage that delivers ½ oz of pure ethanol: 3 to 4 oz of wine; 8 to 12 oz of beer; 1 oz hard liquor (whiskey, scotch, rum, or vodka).

drug: a substance that can modify one or more of the body's functions.

euphoria (you-FORE-ee-uh): a feeling of great well-being, which people often seek through the use of drugs such as alcohol.
eu = good
phoria = bearing

fatty liver: an early stage of liver deterioration seen in several diseases, including kwashiorkor and alcoholic liver disease. Fatty liver is characterized by accumulation of fat in the liver cells.

fermentation: the oxidation of carbohydrate in the absence of atmospheric oxygen, a process that yields alcohol as the end product.

fibrosis: an intermediate stage of liver deterioration seen in several diseases, including viral hepatitis and alcoholic liver disease. In fibrosis, the liver cells lose their function and assume the characteristics of connective tissue cells (fibers).

gout (GOWT): accumulation of uric acid crystals in the joints.

MEOS (microsomal ethanol oxidizing system): a system of enzymes in the liver that oxidize not only alcohol, but also several classes of drugs. (The **microsomes** are tiny particles of membranes with associated enzymes that can be collected from broken-up cells.)
micro = tiny
soma = body

narcotic (nar-KOT-ic): any drug that dulls the senses, induces sleep, and becomes addictive with prolonged use.

proof: a way of stating the percentage of alcohol in distilled liquor. Liquor that is 100 proof is 50% alcohol; 90 proof is 45%, and so forth.

Notes

1. J. Konowalchuk and J. I. Speirs, Virus inactivation by grapes and wines, *Applied and Environmental Microbiology*, December 1976, pp. 757–63; A vintage medicine, *New York Times*, 12 June 1977, p. E7.

2. J. B. McDonald, Not by alcohol alone, *Nutrition Today*, January/February 1979, pp. 14–19.

3. D. J. Forkner, Should wine be on your menu? *Professional Nutritionist*, Spring 1982, pp. 1–3.

4. P. N. Chaudhari and V. G. Hatwalne, Effect of epicatechin on liver lipids of rats fed with choline deficient diet, *The Indian Journal of Nutrition and Dietetics* 14 (1977): 136–39.

5. R. M. Parr, Silicon, wine, and the heart, *Lancet* 17 May 1980, p. 1087.

6. W. J. Darby, The benefits of drink, *Human Nature*, November 1978, pp. 31–37.

7. Alcohol and plasma lipids, *Nutrition and the MD*, August 1984.

8. A. B. Eisenstein, Nutritional and metabolic effects of alcohol, *Journal of the American Dietetic Association* 81 (1982): 247–251.

9. F. Iber, In alcoholism, the liver sets the pace, *Nutrition Today*, January-February 1971, pp. 2–9.

10. C. S. Lieber, Liver adaptation and injury in alcoholism, *New England Journal of Medicine* 288 (1973): 356–361.

11. A. B. Mukherjee and G. D. Hodgen, Maternal ethanol exposure induces transient impairment of umbilical circulation and fetal hypoxia in monkeys, *Science* 218 (1982): 700–702.

Energy Balance and Weight Control

8

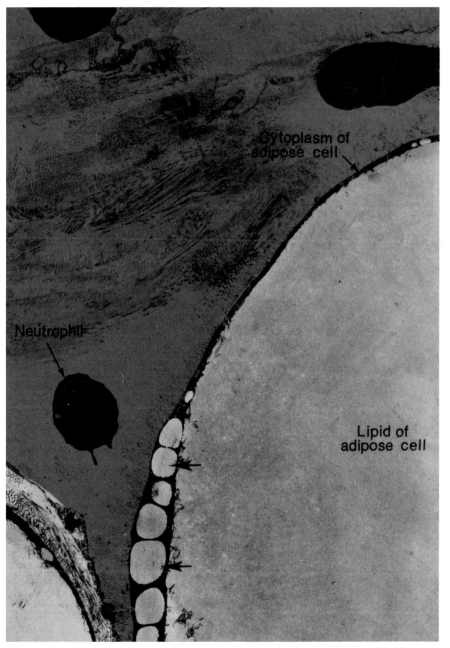

Cytoplasm of adipose cell

Neutrophil

Lipid of adipose cell

Fat cells can expand immensely as their fat stores increase. Here is a portion of a fat cell, embedded in connective tissue. The cell material (cytoplasm) is pushed to the very edge of the cell; the center is a giant fat reservoir. New fat being synthesized first forms small droplets near the edge of the cell (arrows); then the droplets merge into the central reservoir.

O besity is a major malnutrition problem, and something of a mystery. It seems simple enough: some people eat too much and get fat. But why and how obesity occurs and what can be done about it are matters for much speculation, debate, and frustration. For the obese person who has earnestly tried every known means of losing weight only to fail, frustration can turn to despair. Equally mysterious is the problem faced by the underweight person, who finds it as hard to gain weight as a fat person does to lose it.

This chapter emphasizes the problems of overweight and obesity, partly because they have been more intensively studied and partly because they are a more widespread health problem in the developed countries. This does not imply that the underweight person faces a less difficult problem, but underweight receives far less research emphasis except when caused by sickness. Whenever information is available on underweight, it is presented here. The highlight that follows this chapter delves into the eating disorders anorexia nervosa and bulimia.

Overweight and underweight both result from unbalanced energy budgets. The overweight person has consumed food energy in excess over expenditures and has banked the surplus in body fat. The underweight person has not consumed enough, and so has depleted fat stores. Energy itself doesn't weigh anything and can't be seen, but when it exists in the form of chemical bonds in nutrients or body fat, the material that it holds together is both heavy and visible.

The amount of fat you might deposit or withdraw from "savings" on any given day depends on your energy balance for that day—the amount you consume (energy in) versus the amount you expend (energy out). You can reduce your fat deposits by withdrawing more energy from them than you put in. A pound of body fat stores 3,500 kcalories. To lose it, you must experience a deficit; you must take in 3,500 kcalories less than you expend. To lose that pound in a week, you need to achieve an average deficit of 500 kcalories a day.

Bomb calorimeter.

calorimetry (cal-o-RIM-uh-tree): the measurement of energy as heat.
calor = heat
metron = measure
When an organic substance such as food is burned, the energy in the chemical bonds that held its carbons and hydrogens together is released in the form of heat. The amount of heat released can be measured; this direct measure of the amount of energy that was stored in the food's chemical bonds is termed **direct calorimetry**.

As the chemical bonds in food are broken, the carbons (C) and hydrogens (H) combine with oxygen (O) to form carbon dioxide (CO_2) and water (H_2O). Measuring the amount of oxygen consumed in the process gives an indirect measure of the amount of energy released, termed **indirect calorimetry**.

Energy In: The kCalories in Food

To find out how many kcalories are in a food, a laboratory scientist can burn the food in a bomb calorimeter. This device can reveal kcalorie values in two ways. Either it directly measures the heat given off (and kcalories are units of energy defined in terms of heat), or it measures the amount of oxygen consumed in the burning, an indirect measure of the energy released.

The number of kcalories in a food as determined by direct calorimetry is higher than the number of kcalories that same food would give to the human body. The body does not metabolize all the food all the way to carbon dioxide and water, as the calorimeter does. Calorimeter-derived values are corrected for this discrepancy, so that they state accurately the number of kcalories a food provides to the body, thus permitting researchers to make useful tables presenting the energy values of foods.

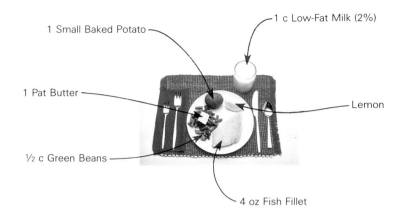

1 Small Baked Potato

1 c Low-Fat Milk (2%)

1 Pat Butter

Lemon

½ c Green Beans

4 oz Fish Fillet

FIGURE 8–1.

kCalorie quiz. In case you'd like to try guessing how many kcalories are in the meal depicted here, the answer is provided in Figure 8–2.

Another way to arrive at food energy values is to compute them from the amounts of protein, fat, and carbohydrate (and alcohol, if present) found in them. Some of the kcalorie values in the table of food composition in Appendix H were derived by bomb calorimetry, and many were derived by calculation from their energy-nutrient contents.

If you want to be able to estimate the kcalorie values of foods roughly, an exchange system such as the one described in Chapter 2 provides a simple method. The foods depicted in Figure 8–1, for example, could be found one by one in Appendix H, but it is quicker to translate them into exchanges and add up the kcalorie values to get a rough idea of the number. (See Figure 8–2.) With some practice, you can look at any plate of food and "see" the number of kcalories on it. Only seven values need be learned as a start toward gaining this skill.

Remember:
1 g carbohydrate = 4 kcal.
1 g fat = 9 kcal.
1 g protein = 4 kcal.
1 g alcohol = 7 kcal.

Food kCalorie Values	
1 c nonfat milk	90 kcal
(1 c low-fat milk)	(120 kcal)
(1 c whole milk)	(150 kcal)
1/2 c vegetable[a]	25 kcal
1 portion[a] fruit (unsweetened)	60 kcal
1 portion grain or starchy vegetable	80 kcal
1 oz lean meat (1 exchange)	55 kcal/oz[b]
(1 oz medium-fat meat)	(75 kcal/oz)
(1 oz high-fat meat)	(100 kcal/oz)
1 fat (1 tsp fat or oil)	45 kcal
1 tsp sugar	20 kcal

[a]For the distinction between vegetables and starchy vegetables, the sizes of fruit portions, and other details, see the exchange lists in Appendix G. An introduction to the exchange system was given in Chapter 2.

[b]An ounce is not a typical serving of meat. Typical servings are 3, 4, or more ounces. A 4-oz portion of lean meat would be 220 kcal; of medium-fat meat, 300 kcal, of high-fat meat, 400 kcal.

FIGURE 8–2.

Quiz answers. We figure about 490 kcalories for the meal.

80 kcal — 120 kcal
45 kcal — 0 kcal
25 kcal — 220 kcal

Note: Appendix H values yield a total of about 432 kcal, lower because these foods are low-kcalorie choices within the exchange groups. Any answer within about 50 to 100 kcal of this is a good estimate.

1 c lowfat milk	120 kcal
½ c green beans	25
1 small potato (1 starchy vegetable)	80
1 pat butter (1 fat)	45
4 oz fish (4 lean meat, assuming no fat is added), at 55 kcal/oz	220
Lemon wedge	0
	490 kcal

For the U.S. and Canadian energy allowances, see Appendix I.

Energy Out: The kCalories the Body Spends

Counting the kcalories in the food you eat tells you your energy income, but to balance your budget, you also need to know your expenditure. How can you count the kcalories you expend in a day? One way is to assume you are a "typical citizen" of the United States or Canada, and to use the numbers their governments use as standards for population studies.

Government Recommendations

The U.S. Committee on RDA and the Canadian Ministry of Health and Welfare have published recommended energy intakes for various age-sex groups in their populations. These are useful for population studies, but the range of energy needs for any one group is so broad that it is impossible even to guess an individual's needs from them without knowing something about the person's lifestyle. The U.S. recommendation for a woman, for example, assumes she is 20 years old, stands 5 feet 4 inches tall, weighs about 120 pounds, and typically engages in light activity. Women who fit this description need between 1,700 and 2,500 kcalories a day to maintain their weight. The man used as a reference figure is 20 years old, stands 5 feet 10 inches tall, weighs 154 pounds, engages in light activity, and needs 2,500 to 3,300 kcalories a day. Taller people need proportionately more, and shorter people proportionately fewer, kcalories to balance their energy budgets. Older people generally need fewer kcalories, with the number diminishing by about 5 percent per decade beyond age 30. Light activity, for both women and men, means sleeping or lying down for eight hours a day, sitting for seven hours, standing for five, walking for two, and spending two hours a day in light physical activity.

Although very few people fit these descriptions exactly, most fall close to the mean. For adults it is believed that an 800–kcalorie range covers most individuals, but the total span of needs is broad, and some have energy needs outside this range. In fact, in any group of 20 similar people with similar activity levels, one will expend twice as much energy per day as another.[1] Clearly, it is impossible to pinpoint any person's energy need within such a wide range without knowing more.

Diet Record Method

To obtain an individualized estimate of your energy needs, the best means is to monitor your food intake and body weight over a period of time in which your activities are typical of your lifestyle. If you keep a strictly accurate record of all the food and beverages you consume for a week or two, and if your weight does not change during that time, you can assume that your energy budget is balanced. Records have to be kept for at least a week, however, because intakes fluctuate from day to day. (On about half the days you eat less, on the other half more, kcalories than the average.)

Laboratory Methods

Modern physiologists describe human energy expenditure as thermogenesis—the generation of heat. The body converts the energy of food to the energy of the temporary storage molecules, ATP (see p. 206), with about 50 percent efficiency. Then, when ATP energy is used to do work (chemical, electrical, osmotic, or mechanical), about 50 percent of its energy is lost as heat. Thus the overall efficiency of the human body in converting food energy to work is 25 percent; the other 75 percent of food energy appears as heat.[2] The work itself, once done, generates heat as well, so a body's total heat production provides an index of the amount of energy it is spending.

Because heat is always a by-product of energy expenditure, a device that measures escaping heat gives a direct measure of the energy being spent. Early efforts to make this kind of measurement involved putting a person inside an insulated, tightly sealed room with water circulating in pipes in the ceiling. The rise in the water's temperature indicated the amount of energy being generated by the person's body. Inside the room, the person could be at rest or engaged in an activity such as studying or bicycle riding.

This clumsy and expensive method can be replaced by a portable, practical backpack oxygen tank using the principle that the amount of oxygen consumed and carbon dioxide expelled is in direct proportion to the heat released. The subject breathes in and out through a tube while resting or moving about doing various activities. This advance makes it possible to measure the energy expended during a wider range of physical activities. Laboratory studies of energy output by human beings have been so extensive that tables are now available giving averages for people engaged in different activities (see Table 8–1 for an example). People vary, though, and energy expenditures derived from these tables do not always apply to particular individuals.

Estimation from Metabolism and Activities

The two major contributors to human energy output under normal conditions are metabolic processes and voluntary activities. A way of estimating the total energy you spend is to estimate each of these components individually, then add them together.

The first component, metabolic energy, is by far the largest item in most people's energy budgets. It consists of the energy spent to keep the heart beating, the lungs inhaling and exhaling air, the cells conducting their metabolic activities, the nerves generating their continuous streams of electrical impulses—in short, to keep all the processes going on that support life.

The basal metabolic rate (BMR) is the rate at which energy is spent for these maintenance activities, usually expressed as kcalories per hour. This rate varies from one person to the next, and may vary for one individual with a change in circumstance or physical condition. The rate is lowest when a person is sleeping undisturbed, but since periodic tossing and turning increase it, it is usually measured with the subject lying down in a room with a comfortable temperature and not digesting any food. (The difference from sleep can be discounted in all but the most precise laboratory measurements.)

The metabolic contribution to energy expenditure normally amounts to at least two-thirds of the energy spent in a day. People often do not realize that

thermogenesis: the generation of heat; used in physiology and nutrition studies as an index of how much energy the body is spending. Four categories of thermogenesis account for the total energy a body spends:
- Basal thermogenesis (similar to basal metabolic rate, described below).
- Exercise-induced thermogenesis (generation of heat by physical activity).
- Diet-induced thermogenesis—energy used while metabolizing food.
- Adaptive thermogenesis (adjustments in energy expenditure related to environment and physiological events such as cold, overfeeding, trauma, and changes in hormone status).

Energy spent during an activity appears as heat.

basal metabolism: the total energy output of a body at rest after a 12–hour fast. Also called **basal metabolic rate (BMR). The resting metabolic rate (RMR)** is similar, but may be measured after less than 12 hours of fasting.

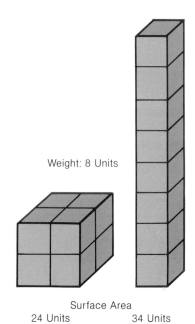

Weight: 8 Units

Surface Area
24 Units　　　34 Units

Both weigh the same, but the tall, thin structure will lose more heat to its surroundings.

thyroxin (thigh-ROX- in): a hormone secreted by the thyroid gland; it regulates the BMR.

Normally, unless muscular activity is very strenuous and prolonged, it demands less energy than metabolism.

so much of their energy is going to support the basic work of their bodies' cells, because they are unaware of all the work these cells do to maintain life.

The metabolic rate is highest in the young, and decreases by about 2 percent per decade after growth has stopped. (A decrease in voluntary activity as well brings the total reduction in energy expenditure to 5 percent per decade.) It is also higher in people with larger surface areas; of two people who weigh the same, the taller, thinner person will have the faster metabolic rate, reflecting a greater skin surface through which heat is lost by radiation.

The metabolic rate is lower in general in older people and in females, but it is untrue to say that "age always slows metabolism," or that "males always have a faster metabolic rate." The key to the difference is the amount of lean body tissue, or fat-free mass, because lean tissue is more active metabolically than fat tissue, even during rest. A young woman, an older woman, and an older man can have as rapid a metabolic rate as a young man if they have the same amount of lean tissue. Your energy requirement, therefore, need not decline much during aging. You need not stop exercising as you grow older, and if your BMR falls by 2 percent per decade, that's only 10 percent in 50 years—perhaps 120 kcalories per day overall.*

Fever increases the energy needs of cells, raising the metabolic rate by 7 percent for each degree Fahrenheit. By the same token, fasting and constant malnutrition lower metabolic output; prolonged starvation reduces the total amount of metabolically active lean tissue in the body.

The hormones epinephrine and thyroxin also affect the BMR. During stress, the cells' responses to epinephrine increase their energy needs and thus raise the metabolic rate. As for thyroxin, it is the chief hormone that governs the BMR. The more thyroxin secreted, the greater the energy used to support the cells' basal activities.

To sum up, BMR is higher in people with greater lean body mass, in people who are tall for their weight, in people with fever or under stress, and in people with high thyroid gland activity. It is lowered by loss of lean tissue due to inactivity, fasting, or malnutrition. The box on the next page shows how basal metabolic energy can be estimated from a person's weight and sex.

The second component of energy output is physical activity voluntarily undertaken and achieved by use of the skeletal muscles. The amount of energy needed for an activity like playing tennis or studying for an exam depends on how many muscles are involved, and on how intensely and how long they have to work. Table 8–1 shows the amounts of energy spent on various activities by the average individual.

As disheartening as it may be to discover, intense mental activity requires only slightly more energy than resting, even though it may make you very tired. Contraction of muscles, on the other hand, uses up a great many kcalories. In addition to the muscles involved in moving the body, the heart must beat faster to send nutrients and oxygen to the muscles, and the lungs must move faster to get rid of the carbon dioxide and bring in additional oxygen.

A heavier person usually uses more energy to perform a task than does a lighter person, because it takes extra effort for the heavier person to move the additional body weight. However, other factors may alter the amount of energy

---

*Assume a 2,000 kcal/day requirement. Of that, two-thirds is for BMR—say, 1,200 kcal. A loss of 10% of that over five decades is 120 kcal.

Estimation of Energy Output

Basal Metabolism. Use the factor 1.0 kcalories per kilogram of body weight per hour for men, or 0.9 for women (men usually have more muscles than women, by virtue of the way their hormones govern their physical development). Example (for a 150–pound man):

1. Change pounds to kilograms:

   150 lb ÷ 2.2 lb/kg = 68 kg.

2. Multiply weight in kilograms by the BMR factor:

   68 kg × 1 kcal/kg/hr = 68 kcal/hr.

3. Multiply the kcalories used in one hour by the hours in a day:

   68 kcal/hr × 24 hr/day = 1,632 kcal/day.

Energy for BMR equals 1,632 kcalories per day.

Voluntary Muscular Activity. The following figures are crude approximations based on the amount of muscular work a person typically performs in a day. To select the one appropriate for you, remember to think in terms of the amount of *muscular* work performed; don't confuse being *busy* with being *active.*

- For sedentary (mostly sitting) activity (a typist), add 40 to 50 percent of the BMR.
- For light activity (a teacher), add 55 to 65 percent.
- For moderate activity (a nurse), add 65 to 70 percent.
- For heavy work (a roofer), add 75 to 100 percent or more.

If the man we used for an example were a clerk, we could estimate the energy he needs for physical activities by multiplying his BMR kcalories per day by 50 percent:

   1,632 kcal/day × 50% = 816 kcal/day.

Energy for activities equals 816 kcalories per day.
Total. The man in our example spends, in a day:

   1,632 kcal/day + 816 kcal/day = 2,448 kcal/day.

Because the exact figure is based on several estimates, i   bly best to express the man's needs as falling within a 100-kcalc

Total energy equals about 2,400 to 2,500 kcalories p

spent, such as the person's skill or efficiency at perfo   't the
task itself, but the moving of muscles, that demand   You
can estimate the energy needed for activities by us   ered
in the box.

The total energy a person spends in a da   wo
components together. The box shows that the   )ut
2,400 to 2,500 kcalories per day on his BMR

TABLE 8-1

Energy Spent on Various Activities

	Energy Spent, Including Metabolic Energy (kcal/kg/hr)	Energy Spent, Exclusive of Metabolic Energy (kcal/kg/hr)
Sleeping	0.9	0
Awake, lying still	1.1	0.1
Sitting quietly	1.3	0.3
Eating	1.5	0.5
Writing	1.5	0.5
Standing, relaxed	1.8	0.8
Dressing	2.0	1.0
Driving car	2.2	1.2
Washing dishes	2.2	1.2
Ironing	2.2	1.2
Typing rapidly	2.2	1.2
Doing laundry by machine	2.4	1.4
Walking (3 mph)	3.3	2.3
Vacuuming floor	4.2	3.2

Note: To obtain the total energy you spend in a day, keep a diary of all activities expressed as hours or parts of hours, until you have recorded exactly 24 hours of activity. Figure the total kcalories per kilogram spent on each activity for the time involved. Multiply each by your body weight in kilograms, and add all together.

Diet-induced thermogenesis is also sometimes called the specific dynamic effect (SDE) or specific dynamic activity (SDA) of food.

Some energy expenditure, not taken into account in this estimate, is that required for the body to manage food. When food is taken into the body, many cells that have been dormant begin to be active. The muscles that move the food through the intestinal tract speed up their rhythmic contractions; the cells that manufacture and secrete digestive juices begin their tasks. All these cells and others need extra energy as they come alive to participate in the digestion, absorption, and metabolism of food. This stimulation of cellular activity is diet-induced thermogenesis, and is generally thought to represent about 6 to 10 percent of the total food energy taken in. For purposes of rough estimates, diet-induced thermogenesis can be ignored; the 10 percent it might contribute to total energy output is smaller than the probable errors involved in estimating energy input from food or output for activities.

Finally, another category of energy expenditure is the energy required for adaptation to changed circumstances (adaptive thermogenesis, mentioned earlier). When the body has to adapt to physical conditioning, cold, overfeeding, trauma, or other types of stress, it has extra work to do, building the necessary tissues and secreting the necessary enzymes and hormones. Normally, this energy need not be taken into account in estimating a person's needs, but there are circumstances in which it makes a considerable difference. For example, a thin person who undertakes to try to gain weight may have to eat considerably more than 3,500 kcalories above normal energy expenditures to gain a pound. Another example: the person who undertakes a physical conditioning program may unexpectedly lose weight at first, even while increasing food intakes to cover apparent added energy expenditure.

Energy Balance: Weight Loss and Gain

In the average person, a deficit of 500 kcalories a day brings about loss of body fat at the rate of a pound a week; of 1,000 kcalories, 2 pounds a week. Extraordinarily active people, by virtue of their high energy expenditures, or extremely obese people, by virtue of the metabolic demands made by the sheer bulk of their body cells and the energy cost of moving their bodies, can lose weight faster. For those who are only slightly overfat, the maximum possible rate of fat loss is 1 to 2 pounds a week, which for most people means an intake of about 1,000 to 1,500 kcalories a day. Below 1,200 kcalories, the dieter will be losing lean tissue, and at such a restricted kcalorie level, the diet planner is hard put to achieve adequacy for all the vitamins and minerals. (The person of below-average height will need to adjust these numbers in proportion to his height.)

These principles are simple, but putting them into practice is more difficult than you might imagine. Obesity and underweight are complex problems with social and psychological ramifications, as well as the metabolic ones just described. The next sections deal with the factors that contribute to the problems of overweight and underweight and then provide some practical pointers for the person who wants to lose or gain weight.

Definition of Obesity

Once upon a time, the definition of obesity was simple. A person's weight could be compared with that in the ideal weight tables. If the actual weight were 20 percent or more above the ideal weight, then the person was obese. Now (to tell a long story in a few words), the term *ideal weight* is no longer in use, and the definition of obesity is no longer simple.

Among the problems were these. Weight depends on a person's frame size— but how do you measure frame size? Weight doesn't matter as much as body composition, and especially body fat content, but how do you measure body fat content? How much body fat there is doesn't matter as much as where it is located on the body, but how do you tie this to ideal weight and the definition of obesity? Anyway, the 1959 ideal weight tables listed the wrong weights; a reevaluation of the statistics on which they were based showed that the weights should have been higher, and higher weights were published in 1983. Then the basis on which the 1983 weights had been arrived at was challenged.

After much discussion and review of the evidence at a Consensus Development Conference on Obesity in 1985, the experts have settled on some temporary working procedures and have agreed that more research is needed:

body mass index (BMI): an index of a person's weight in relation to height, determined by dividing the weight in kilograms by the square of the height in meters:

$$BMI = \frac{weight\ (kg)}{height^2\ (m)}.$$

- They will continue defining obesity as 20 percent above the insurance company table weights, using either the 1959 tables or the 1983 tables.
- If a person is deemed obese by this rough indicator, the physician should apply a more sensitive indicator, the body mass index (BMI). A body mass index of greater than 27.2 in men or 26.9 in women indicates the need for weight loss. See Figure 8–3.
- Diabetes (non-insulin-dependent type), hypertension, and high blood cholesterol also indicate the need for weight loss.
- The severity of the obesity also depends on factors associated with it, such as the distribution of the body fat; social, economic, and ethnic status; and age.[3]

The problem of using weight as an indicator of health or risk status is greatest for weights near the average (presumably desirable) weights. The problem is that body weight says so little about body composition. A person who doesn't seem to weigh too much may be too fat; a person who does seem to weigh too much may not be. A dancer or an athlete, whose muscles are well developed and whose bones have become well mineralized by responding to constant stress,

FIGURE 8–3.

Nomogram for body mass index. Weights and heights are without clothing. With clothes, add 5 pounds for men or 3 pounds for women, and 1 inch in height for shoes. Draw a straight line from your height (left) to your weight (right). At the point where it crosses the BMI line, read your body mass index. A body mass index greater than 27.2 for men or 26.9 for women indicates obesity.

Source: B. T. Burton and W. R. Foster, Health implications of obesity, an NIH Consensus Development Conference, *Journal of the American Dietetic Association* 85 (1985): 1117–21.

may weigh the same as a sedentary person with a similar figure, yet the dancer or athlete may be at the right weight, and the sedentary person may be too fat. There is no easy way to look inside a person and see the bones and muscles.

There are other problems with the ideal weight concept. Even supposing everyone had the same percentage of body fat, the use of the word *ideal* demands an answer to the question "ideal for what?" The weights in the tables were never shown to be ideal *for* anything; they were considered desirable on the basis of a correlation. They were, simply, the weight ranges that correlated with the greatest longevity in the population studied. The population studied was a population of insured people, and people who buy life insurance may be unlike others in terms of their health. Their weights had only been taken once, if ever; some had only reported their weights verbally and not been weighed. The weights were taken at the time they submitted their applications for life insurance, not years later when, by dying, they provided the statistics the life insurance companies used to generate the weight tables. All of this makes it clear that when a person's weight is compared with the table weight, it is not being measured against a standard, but simply compared with the average weight found years ago in a population of people who lived quite long after that until they died.

The determination of frame size represents an attempt to deal with the problem of people's differing bone and muscle structures. Now: how to measure frame size? Researchers have attempted to answer several questions, in order to ensure that they are doing it right. First, does bone mass correlate with muscle mass (that is, do people with bigger bones also have greater muscle mass)? Reassuringly, the answer to that question seems to be yes.[4] That means it should be possible to measure a bone to obtain an estimate of the body's fat-free mass.

Next, what bone to measure? It has to be one that correlates with fat-free mass, but not with body fat. Six frame measures have been suggested, including the breadth of the elbow bone, the distance between the hip bones, the breadth of the wrist bone or that of the ankle bone, and measures at the shoulder and knee. The wrist and ankle breadths seem to be associated *least* with total body fat, but the insurance height-weight tables use the breadth of the elbow bone as an index of frame size (see Table 8–2). They chose this particular measurement because a recent survey had provided extensive reference values for elbow breadth in U.S. adults.[5] Unfortunately, though, elbow breadths tend to be greater in fatter people—or, to put it the other way around, people with larger elbow bones tend to be fatter. This may mean that a large frame, determined this way, is itself a risk factor.[6]

The struggle continues. Research is directed toward making the height-weight tables useful in assessing obesity and its risks. Meanwhile, they have limited usefulness, but every bathroom and every doctor's office seems to have a scale, and the tables will doubtless continue to be used. If you choose to use them, be sure to add an inch to your barefoot height (you are assumed to be wearing shoes with 1-inch heels), and adjust for clothing (the tables assume 3 to 5 pounds for clothes).

If the weight tables cause frustration in would-be users, perhaps that reaction brings with it a benefit—it leads them to ask deeper questions about the state of the body most compatible with good health and long life. Simple answers don't await the asker, but when answers do come, they will doubtless have to do with body composition.

Two people of the same sex, height, and age may weigh the same, yet one may be too fat and the other may not be.

frame size: the size of a person's bones and musculature. A person with a large frame can weigh more than one the same height with a small frame before risk begins to increase.

TABLE 8–2

How to Determine Your Body Frame by Elbow Breadth

To make a simple approximation of your frame size, do the following. Extend your arm, and bend the forearm upward at a 90-degree angle. Keep the fingers straight, and turn the inside of your wrist away from the body. Place the thumb and index finger of your other hand on the two prominent bones on *either side* of your elbow. Measure the space between your fingers against a ruler or a tape measure.[a] Compare the measurements with the following standards.

These standards represent the elbow measurements for medium-framed men and women of various heights. Measurements smaller than those listed indicate you have a small frame, and larger measurements indicate a large frame.

Men

Height in 1-Inch Heels	Elbow Breadth
5 ft 2 inches to 5 ft 3 inches	2½ to 2⅞ inches
5 ft 4 inches to 5 ft 7 inches	2⅝ to 2⅞ inches
5 ft 8 inches to 5 ft 11 inches	2¾ to 3 inches
6 ft 0 inches to 6 ft 3 inches	2¾ to 3⅛ inches
6 ft 4 inches and over	2⅞ to 3¼ inches

Women

Height in 1-Inch Heels	Elbow Breadth
4 ft 10 inches to 4 ft 11 inches	2¼ to 2½ inches
5 ft 0 inches to 5 ft 3 inches	2¼ to 2½ inches
5 ft 4 inches to 5 ft 7 inches	2⅜ to 2⅝ inches
5 ft 8 inches to 5 ft 11 inches	2⅜ to 2⅝ inches
6 ft 0 inches and over	2½ to 2¾ inches

[a]For the most accurate measurement, have your physician measure your elbow breadth with a caliper.

Source: Metropolitan Life Insurance Company. An alternative means of measuring frame size appears in Appendix E.

Body Composition

Several laboratory techniques for estimating body fatness have been developed. One way is to determine the body's density (weight compared with volume). Lean tissue is denser than fat tissue, so the more dense a person's body is, the more lean tissue it must contain. Weight is measured with a scale; volume measurement involves submerging the whole body in a large tank of water and measuring the amount of water displaced. From the density, an estimate of the percentage of body fat can be derived. This technique is not available in the typical home or doctor's office, for obvious reasons, but is in wide use on university campuses that pursue exercise physiology research.

Another way to estimate body fat is to inject a water-soluble substance that is easy to detect and measure, and allow it to penetrate into the lean tissues (it will not mix into the fat tissues). A blood sample taken soon after will show the extent to which the substance has been diluted, providing an estimate of the amount of lean tissue.

A simpler way to obtain an estimate of the amount of body fat is by taking a fatfold measure. The assessor lifts a fold of skin from the back of the arm, from the back, or from other body surfaces and measures its thickness with a caliper that applies a fixed amount of pressure. The fat under the skin in these regions represents about half of the body's total fat tissue, and on most people

The fatfold test is a practical procedure for determining total body fat.

it is roughly proportional to total body fat. If the person gains body fat, the fatfold increases proportionately; if the person loses fat, it decreases. The fatfold test is a practical diagnostic procedure in the hands of trained people and is in increasingly wide use. Table 8–3 presents percentiles for fatfold measures for males and females. Generally speaking, people whose fatfold measurement exceeds the 95th percentile are considered obese.

The major limitation of the fatfold test is that fat may be thicker under the skin in one area than another. A pinch at the side of the waistline may not yield the same measurement as a pinch on the back of the arm. This limitation can be overcome by taking the average of a number of different fatfolds.

There is another complication, too: fat around the abdomen may represent a greater risk to health than fat elsewhere on the body. Abdominal fat is closest to the portal circulation; when it is mobilized, it goes directly to the liver, where it is made into cholesterol-carrying LDL; and it has been shown to correlate, more closely than fat located elsewhere on the body, with an increased incidence of diabetes and coronary heart disease.[7] Fatfold measurements do not take this fat distribution difference into account. A simple comparison of the waist to the hip measurement may become a standard part of the assessment of body fatness in years to come.[8]

fatfold test: a clinical test of body fatness in which the thickness of a fold of skin on the back of the arm (on the triceps), below the shoulder blade (subscapular), or in other places is measured with a caliper. The older, less preferred, term for this is **skinfold test**.

TABLE 8–3

Triceps Fatfold Percentiles (millimeters) for Males and Females.

Age	Male					Female				
	5th	25th	50th	75th	95th	5th	25th	50th	75th	95th
1– 1.9	6	8	10	12	16	6	8	10	12	16
2– 2.9	6	8	10	12	15	6	9	10	12	16
3– 3.9	6	8	10	11	15	7	9	11	12	15
4– 4.9	6	8	9	11	14	7	8	10	12	16
5– 5.9	6	8	9	11	15	6	8	10	12	18
6– 6.9	5	7	8	10	16	6	8	10	12	16
7– 7.9	5	7	9	12	17	6	9	11	13	18
8– 8.9	5	7	8	10	16	6	9	12	15	24
9– 9.9	6	7	10	13	18	8	10	13	16	22
10–10.9	6	8	10	14	21	7	10	12	17	27
11–11.9	6	8	11	16	24	7	10	13	18	28
12–12.9	6	8	11	14	28	8	11	14	18	27
13–13.9	5	7	10	14	26	8	12	15	21	30
14–14.9	4	7	9	14	24	9	13	16	21	28
15–15.9	4	6	8	11	24	8	12	17	21	32
16–16.9	4	6	8	12	22	10	15	18	22	31
17–17.9	5	6	8	12	19	10	13	19	24	37
18–18.9	4	6	9	13	24	10	15	18	22	30
19–24.9	4	7	10	15	22	10	14	18	24	34
25–34.9	5	8	12	16	24	10	16	21	27	37
35–44.9	5	8	12	16	23	12	18	23	29	38
45–54.9	6	8	12	15	25	12	20	25	30	40
55–64.9	5	8	11	14	22	12	20	25	31	38
65–74.9	4	8	11	15	22	12	18	24	29	36

Adapted from A. R. Frisancho, New norms of upper limb fat and muscle areas for assessment of nutritional status, *American Journal of Clinical Nutrition* 34 (1981):2540–2545.

Even after you have a body fatness estimate, problems arise. For example, how do you interpret it? What is the "ideal" amount of fat for a body to have? The question—ideal for what?—has to be answered first.

For competitive athletes, especially endurance athletes, the ideal is relatively easy to define. The amount of fat in the body should be above the minimum needed for essential functions such as providing fuel, insulation, and normal fat-soluble hormone activity. Otherwise it should be as low as possible, so as not to contribute excess weight for the muscles to carry. A man of normal weight may have, on the average, 15 percent, and a woman, 20 percent, of the body weight as fat. Endurance athletes consider it ideal to have lower fat percentages than these.

For an Alaskan fisherman, the ideal percentage of body fat is probably higher. Fat provides an insulating blanket, and in some settings, heat loss from the body handicaps performance. In those settings, such a blanket confers an advantage. For a woman starting a pregnancy, the ideal percentage of body fat may be different again; it is known that the outcome of pregnancy is compromised if the woman begins it with too little body fat. Below a certain threshold body fat content, some individuals become infertile, develop depression or abnormal hunger regulation, or become unable to keep warm. These thresholds are not the same for each function or in all individuals, and much remains to be learned about them.

Just as there is a minimum percentage of body fat that is ideal for a given individual, there is also a maximum, and this too may differ from person to person. One major factor that determines where to draw the line is the blood pressure. Extra fat tissue means that the heart must work harder to pump blood through miles of extra capillaries that feed that fat tissue. Some people can tell you exactly at what weight their blood pressure begins to rise; when they lose weight to below that threshold, their blood pressure becomes normal again. Other risk indicators also rise and fall with body fatness—blood glucose and blood cholesterol, for example. For those in whom these signs appear with added fat, weight reduction is most critical.

The uncertainties surrounding the definition of ideal body composition reflect the newness of the branch of nutrition science that studies body weight and its regulation. The best definition of obesity would be body fatness significantly in excess of that consistent with optimal health, determined by a reliable measure, but the techniques to pinpoint it accurately are still to be worked out. With this understanding, you should be able to apply the appropriate number of grains of salt to rules of thumb such as these:

- A fatfold over 1 inch thick reflects obesity.
- A person whose weight is 10 to 20 percent above the weight on the life insurance tables is overweight; more than 20 percent above is obese.
- Each inch by which your waist measurement exceeds your chest (not bust) measurement will take two years off your life.

Besides having all the health implications that it does, body weight is also a social and personal matter. In some societies fatness is desired; it is equated with prosperity, comfort, and security. In others it is despised; it is considered undisciplined to be fat. The person seeking a single, authoritative answer to the question "How much should I weigh?" is therefore bound to be disappointed. None can tell you *exactly* how much you should weigh—but with health as

of nutrition science concerned
t control is **bariatrics**
icks).
weight

excessive body fatness, presently
ned by comparing body weight
e life insurance tables. The person
weight is 20% above the table
t is considered obese and should be
ated further. Treatment is indicated if
ody mass index exceeds 27.2 (men)
6.9 (women) or if there is high blood
essure, high blood cholesterol, or
iabetes. Ten percent above the table
weight is **overweight**; 10% below the
table weight is **underweight**.

a value, at least you have a starting framework. Your weight should fall within a range. Below the bottom end or above the top end of the range, your athletic performance, fertility (in women), health, or longevity would be adversely affected. Within the range, the weight to pick is up to you. Your own standards are important.

The Problem of Obesity

However you define it, obesity does occur to an alarming extent and is increasing in the developed countries. For example, in the United States some 10 to 25 percent of all teenagers and some 25 to 50 percent of all adults are obese.

Obesity brings many health hazards with it. Insurance companies report that fat people die younger from a host of causes, including heart attacks, strokes, and complications of (type II) diabetes.* In fact, among adults, gaining weight often appears to precipitate diabetes. Fat people more often have high blood cholesterol (a risk factor for coronary heart disease), hypertension, complications after surgery, gynecological irregularities, and the toxemia of pregnancy. For men, the risk of cancers of the colon, rectum, and prostate gland rises with obesity; for women, the risk of cancers of the breast, uterus, ovaries, gallbladder, and bile ducts is greater. The burden of extra fat strains the skeletal system, aggravating arthritis— especially in the knees, hips, and lower spine. The muscles that support the belly may give way, resulting in abdominal hernias. When the leg muscles are abnormally fatty, they fail to contract efficiently to help blood return from the leg veins to the heart; blood collects in the leg veins, which swell, harden, and become varicose. Extra fat in and around the chest interferes with breathing, sometimes causing severe respiratory problems. Gout is more common, and even the accident rate is greater for the severely obese.

Beyond all these hazards is the risk incurred by millions of obese people throughout much of their lives—the risk of ill-advised, misguided dieting. Some fad diets are more hazardous to health than obesity itself. One survey of 29,000 claims, treatments, and theories for losing weight found fewer than 6 percent of them effective—and 13 percent dangerous![9]

Social and economic disadvantages also plague the fat person. Obese people are less often sought after for marriage, pay higher insurance premiums, meet discrimination when applying for college admissions and jobs, can't find attractive clothes so easily, and are limited in their choice of sports. For many, guilt, depression, withdrawal, and self-blame are inevitable psychological accompaniments to obesity.

Although obesity is a severe physical handicap, it is unlike other handicaps in two important ways. First, mortality risk is not linearly related to excess weight. Instead, there is a threshold at which risk dramatically increases. Being

---

*The greater the degree of overweight, the higher the excess death rate, especially in the young. Consensus Panel addresses obesity question, *Journal of the American Medical Association* 254 (1985): 1878.

FIGURE 8–4.

Threshold weight. The relationship of risk to weight is not linear (A), but curvilinear (B). Underweight and overweight are both associated with greater health risks than normal weight (middle of the curve). At the threshold weight, risk rises abruptly.

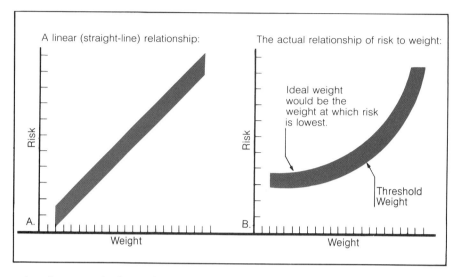

only a few pounds above this threshold weight may cause blood pressure, blood glucose, and blood lipids to zoom upward. The concept of a danger zone of weight is illustrated in Figure 8–4. Second, obesity is highly reversible, and if it is corrected in time, some of its risks are, too. Mortality rates (from insurance data) are no higher for the formerly obese than for the never obese. Prevention is desirable, but where it has failed, treatment is needed.

Causes of Obesity

Energy is not stored in fat until the body's energy needs have been met. Excess body fat can accumulate only when kcalories are eaten beyond those needed for the day's metabolic, muscular, and digestive activities. To put it bluntly, obesity results from overeating.

Why, though, do people overeat? Is it a hunger problem? An appetite problem? A satiety problem? Is it genetic? Metabolic? Environmental? Is it a matter of habits learned in early childhood? Is it psychological? Might all these factors play a role? To tell the truth, we do not know the cause.

In general, two schools of thought address this problem. One attributes obesity to inside-the-body causes; the other, to environmental factors. One currently popular inside-the-body theory is the so-called set-point theory. Noting that many people who lose weight on reducing diets subsequently return to their original weight, some researchers have suggested that the body "wants" to maintain a certain amount of fat and regulates eating behaviors and hormonal actions to defend its "set point." This theory is compelling in its simplicity, but the question whether scientific evidence supports its reality in human beings is still open.

The other point of view is that obesity is environmentally determined. Proponents of this view hold that we overeat because we are pushed to do so by factors in our surroundings—foremost among them, the availability of a multitude of delectable foods. The two views are not mutually exclusive, and research with animals suggests that both are possible. Some obesity may arise from one cause and some from the other, and there is no reason why they should not both be operating, even in the same person.

The next sections summarize current obesity research without coming to a final conclusion as to cause. Several lines of investigation seem promising, and the findings that are emerging suggest that no single answer will ever be found; obesity is multifactorial.

Development of Obesity

One way to approach the question of what causes obesity is to ask whether it is hereditary. In some animals, at least one kind of obesity is hereditary: strains of rats exist that are genetically fat, and they tend to be fat in any environment—that is, no matter what kind or variety of food is offered. In human beings, family histories show no such clear relationships; experimental manipulations are not practicable, but twin studies offer insights. For example, identical twins can be located who have been raised in different families, one family fat and the other thin. If genes determine fatness, then both twins will become equally fat or thin. But if the environment is responsible, then each twin will resemble the family he grows up in. Another approach is to study adopted children, to see whether they resemble their natural or adoptive parents. Studies of both kinds suggest that the tendency to obesity is inherited, but that the environment is influential in the sense that it can prevent or permit the development of obesity when the potential is there.

Another approach is to ask whether obesity is initiated in childhood and then—whether hereditary or environmental or both—persists into adulthood. In other words, do fat babies become fat adults? Obesity does run in families; and clearly, eating habits learned in childhood tend to persist throughout life. Food-centered families encourage such behaviors as overeating at mealtimes, rapid eating, excessive snacking, and eating to meet needs other than hunger. Children readily imitate overeating parents, and their behavior at the table tends to persist outside the home. Obese children have been observed to take more bites of food per interval of time and to chew them less thoroughly than their nonobese schoolmates. But several longitudinal studies have shown that fat babies don't always become fat adults; sometimes they grow out of their obesity.

Research on fat cells suggests a possible reason why early-onset obesity is especially resistant to treatment. Simply stated, early overfeeding is thought by some researchers to stimulate fat cells so that they increase abnormally in *number*. The number of fat cells is thought to become fixed by adulthood; if it is, then a gain in weight thereafter can take place only through an increase in the *size* of the fat cells. A person with an abnormally large number of fat cells is thought likely to be abnormally hungry and to overeat for that reason. On the other hand, a person who gains weight in adulthood supposedly has a normal number

Children readily imitate overeating parents.

A longitudinal study is one in which the subjects are studied over time—for example, in 1960 and again in 1970 and in 1980.

fat cell theory: the theory that during the growing years, fat cells respond to overfeeding by increasing in number; that the number of fat cells becomes fixed before adulthood, and that the number regulates hunger, so that an individual overfed during infancy or childhood will always overeat.

Obesity due to increased number of fat cells is **hyperplastic obesity**. Obesity due to increased size of fat cells is **hypertrophic obesity**.

of fat cells and therefore normal hunger regulation. Such a person needs only to reduce the size of the cells to return to normal weight.

The fat cell theory has been heavily criticized on several grounds. Fat cells are hard to count, and researchers disagree as to whether new cells are being formed at certain periods or whether small, empty fat cells are being recruited as new storage cells. Even the critics agree, however, that there are certain periods in life when body fat increases more rapidly than lean tissue: early infancy (up to about two years), again during preadolescence (and throughout adolescence in girls), and possibly again during the third trimester of pregnancy. The multiplication of fat cells that takes place at these times may be irreversible, so preventive efforts are most important during these times. Fat is hard enough to lose, no matter when it is gained.

Once a person becomes obese, the situation does tend to perpetuate itself, but this is true even if the excess fat is gained during adulthood. When fat cells enlarge, they become sluggish in responding to insulin, the hormone that promotes the making and storage of fat. The excess glucose remains in the bloodstream longer than normal and stimulates the insulin-producing cells of the pancreas to secrete more insulin. When the fat cells finally respond, they store more fat than normal in response to the raised insulin level. As if this were not enough, the enlarged fat cells are also less sensitive to other hormones that promote fat breakdown. Weight loss restores insulin levels to normal, but it first has to be achieved against these odds.

Hunger and Appetite Regulation

Whether or not the fat-cell theory is supported by research findings to come, it deals with an important question: what regulates hunger? Whatever sets the stage for excess fat accumulation, the fat is gained because we put food into our mouths. A vast amount of research has been devoted to finding out what stimulates and governs eating behavior. Why do we start to eat? Why do we eat as much as we do? Why do we stop?

An important distinction exists between hunger, appetite, and satiety. Hunger is said to be physiological (an inborn instinct) whereas appetite is psychological (a learned response to food). The two are not the same. We have all experienced appetite without hunger: "I'm not hungry, but I'd love to have a piece." The too-thin person may often experience the reverse, hunger without appetite: "I know I'm hungry, but I don't feel like eating." Hunger is a negative experience (and we may eat in order to avoid it); appetite is positive. As for satiety, which signals that it is time to stop eating, it vies with hunger and appetite for the distinction of being recognized as the primary regulator of eating behavior. One view holds that eating behavior is turned on all the time, except when the satiety signal turns it off. But the exact nature of the satiety signal is not known.

The stomach participates in signaling satiety. Nerves responsive to the stretching of the stomach wall fire when the stomach is full, transmitting a message to the brain. Even animals without stomachs get hungry, though, so clearly an empty stomach is not the only cue to hunger.

Whether hunger, appetite, or satiety regulates eating behavior (and there are other possibilities discussed below), two questions arise. First, what molecular or other messengers make us feel these sensations? Second, where in the body

hunger: the physiologic need to eat; a negative, unpleasant sensation.

appetite: the desire to eat, which normally accompanies hunger; by itself, a pleasant sensation.

satiety (sat-EYE-uh-tee): the feeling of fullness or satisfaction at the end of a meal, which prompts a person to stop eating.

are they received? Many theories have been put forth to answer the first question. The glucostatic theory of hunger regulation proposes that the blood glucose level determines whether we are hungry or sated; the lipostatic theory states that the size of our fat stores dictates how much we eat; and the purinergic theory proposes that the circulating levels of purines, molecules found in DNA and RNA, govern hunger.[10] Careful measurement of blood levels of glucose show that they do not account for the starting and stopping of eating, however, and glucose researchers are now pursuing the possibility that exhaustion of liver glycogen may somehow convey the signal "Eat." If fat cells regulate hunger in some way, the level may be set by the number of fat-storing enzymes (lipoprotein lipase, described in Chapter 5) on the fat cells' surfaces, but the messenger the cells might send to the brain has yet to be identified. As for the purinergic theory, it is relatively new and untested.

Other ideas as to what molecules might be the regulators of eating behavior include the endogenous opiates (more about them later) and a variety of hormones. It has long been known that the GI tract produces several hormones that serve to notify the pancreas, the gallbladder, and the intestine that food is present and must be dealt with. A flurry of findings during the early 1980s brought forth many reports that these same hormones, now numbering some 20 or 30, are also produced in the brain after meals. Perhaps, in the brain, they signal satiety.

That brings us to the question of where in the brain these messages are received. One brain area stands out as a regulator for food behavior—the hypothalamus—but it is not the only one involved. At one time, it was thought that the front-central hypothalamus was the "satiety center," and that the sides were the "hunger centers," but that is an oversimplification. The hypothalamus integrates many kinds of signals received from the rest of the body, including information about the blood's temperature, sodium content, and glucose content. It is certainly important in regulating eating, because damage to the hypothalamus produces derangements in eating behavior and body weight—in some cases causing severe weight loss, in others vast overeating. In the person with a normal hypothalamus, however, eating behavior seems to be a response not to a single signal arriving at some one location in the hypothalamus, but to a whole host of signals. Somehow these many inputs become integrated into a "final common path"—the act of eating.

These findings leave open the question whether overeating is determined by an inherited, internal regulatory defect, or is a learned behavior. Chances are that the answer will be different for different individuals. Research efforts presently in progress in the study of hunger and appetite are illustrated in Figure 8–5.

Considerable evidence supports the view that at least in some cases of obesity, internal regulatory mechanisms are abnormal. Considerable evidence also supports the view that in many cases, overeating can be explained psychologically. The next two sections oversimplify the picture by presenting, separately, the inside-the-body view and then some outside-the-body possibilities.

Set-Point Theory

Many experiences with both animals and human beings suggest that somehow, the body chooses a weight that it wants to be and defends that weight. When

glucostatic theory of hunger regulation: the theory that blood levels of glucose determine when people eat.
gluco = glucose
stasis = staying the same

lipostatic theory of hunger regulation: the theory that when the body's total fat stores are depleted, they store more fat, and eating behavior is turned on.
lipo = fat

purinergic theory of hunger regulation: the theory that circulating purines regulate eating behavior.
erg = driving force

Among the hormones produced in the brain as well as the GI tract after meals are cholecystokinin (COAL-ee-sis-to-KINE-in), the messenger that communicates the arrival of fat to the gallbladder and pancreas; and calcitonin, a hormone that responds to blood calcium level (see Chapter 11).

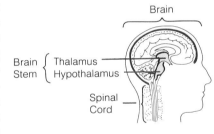

hypothalamus (high-po-THALL-uh-mus): a brain center that integrates signals about the blood's temperature, glucose content, and other conditions.

set point: the point at which controls are set (for example, on a thermostat). In the case of body weight, the set point is that point above which the body tends to lose weight and below which it tends to gain weight.

FIGURE 8–5.

Hunger and appetite. This is a partial list of the factors thought to be operating to control food intake.

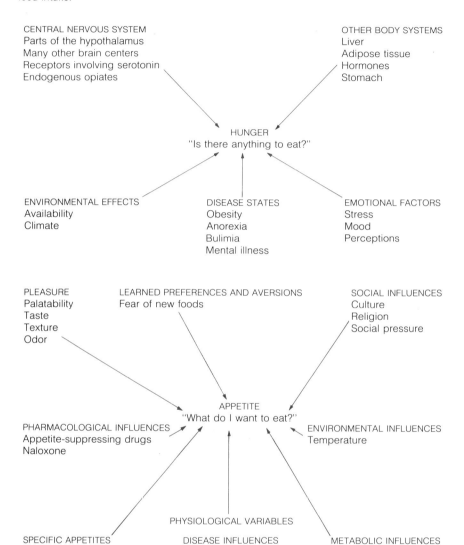

Source: Adapted from T. W. Castonguay and coauthors, Hunger and appetite: Old concepts/new distinctions, *Nutrition Reviews* 41, April 1983, pp. 101–110.

subjects in an experiment are made to overeat so that they gain weight, they spontaneously lose weight back to whatever is normal for them as soon as the experiment is over. And when animals undergo surgical removal of fat tissue, they compensate afterward by depositing more fat until they are back where they started from.[11] Children recovering from malnutrition gain weight faster than their age mates for a spell of "catch-up growth"; then as soon as they are at the right weight, they gain at the normal rate. People who give up smoking often gain a fixed amount of weight—say, 20 pounds—and then stop gaining and maintain their weight at the newly set level. All these examples illustrate the body's tendency to settle at a weight plateau for long periods of time. The plateau may change from time to time with changed circumstances, but the new level then tends to stay as fixed as the old one did.

The possibility hasn't been ruled out that people's eating and exercise habits account for the phenomenon of set point, with no other factors entering in. But another possibility also exists: that their metabolism compensates for changes in eating or exercise in a way that at first looks mysterious, but that can be explained.

To understand how a metabolic shuttle might waste energy, remember that chemical reactions take place in the body with an efficiency less than 100 percent. That is, the starting energy is never entirely retained in the products of reactions; some is always converted to heat, so that the products contain less energy than the reactants. In a metabolic pathway in which substance A is converted to B, to C, to D, the most energy-efficient way to perform the reaction is just that way: A–B–C–D. Should some vacillation take place between A and D (for example, A–B–C–B–C–B–C–D), then more energy would be lost than one might predict. Suppose, now, that A is the energy in food, and that D is the amount of that energy ultimately stored in body fat. You can see that the amount stored could depend on the number of heat-losing steps that take place between A and D. Should one person efficiently store food energy in body fat with no extra moves, and another person shuttle it back and forth and radiate off a lot of it as heat, the two might eat the same amount, and exercise the same amount, but still not end up weighing the same. Within the same person, furthermore, the amount of shuttling might be different at different times (say, depending on how much the person ate and exercised), so that body weight might be kept pretty much the same, regardless of food energy intake and activity level.

Another way that energy conservation versus wastage can be controlled is by way of so-called futile cycles. Suppose that in a series of metabolic reactions, some energy is transferred into a compound such as ATP (see Chapter 7) and some is lost as heat. ATP then contributes its energy to the building of body fat. Now suppose that the enzyme that is supposed to capture the energy in that reaction fails to do so, but lets it escape as heat. Considerably less fat storage might take place in response to the eating of a given number of kcalories of food energy.

Many of the body's metabolic reactions are coupled reactions—that is, reactions in which the breakdown of a compound is coupled with the making of another. The coupling of energy nutrient breakdown with ATP generation at several points along the metabolic pathway is an example. The coupling of ATP breakdown with fat synthesis is another example. Uncoupling of certain reactions is known to take place under certain circumstances; perhaps the body uses it to maintain its set-point weight in the face of varying food energy intakes and exercise levels. Figure 8–6 shows diagrammatically how uncoupling might work.

Thyroid hormone helps to regulate the body's metabolic rate by bringing about changes from conservative to "wasteful" metabolism. In the cold, for example, the body produces more heat. People say their metabolism speeds up.

shuttling: going back and forth. In a metabolic pathway in which (for example) substance A is converted to B, then C, then D, shuttling might occur as follows: A to B to C to B to C to B to C to D. Extra moves on a metabolic path cause extra loss of energy as heat, leaving less to be stored.

futile cycles: metabolic pathways in which energy is spent without accomplishing work.

coupled reaction: a pair of chemical reactions that occur simultaneously, with the energy released by one reaction consumed by the other.

uncoupling: the separation of a coupled reaction so that all the energy released is lost without doing work.

FIGURE 8–6.

Coupled and uncoupled reactions. The same amount of energy is spent in A as in B, but in A it accomplishes work, while in B, it is "wasted." Energy "wasted" is not stored in body fat and, therefore, does not contribute to obesity.

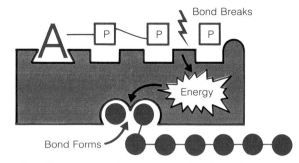

A. A coupled reaction. The energy in ATP is harnessed to do work—forming a chemical bond in another compound.

B. Uncoupling. ATP is split as in A, but its energy is lost as heat, rather than doing work.

brown fat: tissue cells whose enzymes can oxidize energy compounds without using the energy released to do work (see *uncoupling*); the energy is released as heat. In human beings, the predominant type of fat is **white fat**, of which the main function is to store energy for the body's work.

Actually, the thyroid hormone signals the metabolic pathways to uncouple at key places to generate heat energy rather than to store that energy as fat.

Coupled and uncoupled reactions take place when fat breaks down, too. In fact, there are two kinds of fat—the ordinary kind, called white fat, used to store energy for use in doing the body's work, and another kind, brown fat, that serves as a reserve for generating heat when needed. Hibernating animals store much of their energy in brown fat and metabolize it during the winter months to keep their bodies warm. Human babies are born with some brown fat around their shoulders and upper backs, and it has been thought that some adults might have more brown fat than others, accounting for their differing rates of energy conservation and heat loss.[12]

These and other metabolic theories have been advanced to explain how the body might be able to "choose" whether to store or spend energy, and may provide clues to the way it maintains its weight. A person who eats more than usual on a given day may metabolize the food faster (more wastefully) than usual, and gain less weight than expected. A person who eats less than usual might conserve more, that day, and so lose less weight than expected. Such mechanisms might help to explain why gaining and losing weight are equally hard to do for a person at the set-point weight, and may also help to account for the mysterious plateaus at which both weight gainers and weight losers tend to get stuck.

Environment and Behavior

Earlier, we mentioned that some rats were genetically obese, no matter what they were fed; and the previous section presented the possibility that some human beings might also be stuck with obesity for internal, metabolic reasons. As you might expect, some direct evidence suggesting alternative possibilities is available, on both animals and human beings. The environmental obesity model is supported by experiments with "cafeteria rats." Ordinary rats, fed regular rat feed, are of normal weight (for rats), but if those very same rats are offered free access to a wide variety of tempting, rich, highly palatable foods, they greatly overeat and become obese. Evidently, the behavior of eating, which occurs appropriately in response to internal hunger signals, can be triggered by external stimuli at times when it is not appropriate.

Some obese people are prone to eating in response to external stimuli. Rather than responding only to internal, visceral hunger cues, they seem to respond helplessly to such external factors as the time of day ("It's time to eat") or the availability, sight, and taste of food. This is the basis of the external cue theory.

Experiments under controlled conditions bear this out. If lean and fat people are offered their meals in monotonous liquid form from a feeding machine, they respond differently. The lean people eat enough to maintain their weight, but the fat people drastically reduce their food intake and lose weight. When kcalories are added to the formula, the lean people adjust their intake to continue maintaining weight as if they had an internal kcalorie counter, but the obese people continue drinking the same volume of formula as before, and stop losing weight.[13]

The implications for treatment of obesity are obvious. Such people need to learn several strategies—to avoid places where the "eat me" signals that food sends out are too overwhelming; to create environments for themselves where food stimuli are at a minimum, and to learn to say no in circumstances where tempting but unneeded foods are offered. Today's environment is not conducive to weight control. The very same TV station that displays the slim athletic bodies of male and female models offers mountains of delectable, technicolor food in its commercials. Fast food places, complete with tempting aromas, line our main streets; and kitchen appliances such as the hamburger cooker and the doughnut maker make it all too easy to prepare and impulsively eat high-kcalorie foods.

If the behavior of eating is appropriate as a response only to internal hunger sensations, and is inappropriate when triggered by chance offerings of food, it is even more inappropriate when triggered by psychological stimuli. Yet the behavior easily becomes conditioned to occur automatically in response to a wide variety of inappropriate stimuli, because food itself rewards the eater with its good taste and calming effects. The program is built in, in the brain's response to stressors such as pain, anxiety, arousal, excitement, even the presence of food. On experiencing these stimuli, the brain responds by producing endogenous opiates. They soothe pain and lessen arousal, and they have two effects on energy balance. They enhance appetite for palatable foods, and they reduce activity.[14] Combine these effects with a tendency to be supersensitive to particular stressors anyway, and one is all the more likely to gain weight in response to stress.

Some obese people respond to anxiety, or in fact to any kind of arousal, by eating. Significantly, however, if they are able to give a name to their aroused condition, thereby gaining a feeling that they have some control over it, they

Cafeteria rats.

external cue theory: the theory that some people eat in response to such external factors as the presence of food or the time of day rather than to such internal factors as hunger.

endogenous opiates: morphinelike compounds produced in the brain in response to pain, stress, certain drugs, and other circumstances. They act as internal tranquilizers, reducing arousal level.

The term **arousal** has been used several times. The general meaning is self-evident, but in the sense in which it is used here, it refers to heightened activity of certain brain centers associated with excitement and anxiety.

are not as likely to overeat.[15] Highlight 6 described another link between food molecules and brain sensations—the neurotransmitter serotonin, produced in response to the eating of carbohydrate—and no doubt there are others.

Hunger and appetite are also intimately connected to deep emotional needs such as the primitive fear of starvation and the infant's association of food with mother love. Yearnings, cravings, and addictions with profound psychological significance can express themselves in people's food behavior. An emotionally insecure person might eat rather than call a friend and risk rejection. Another might use eating to relieve boredom or to ward off depression.

Stress eating may appear in different patterns; some people eat excessively at night, while others characteristically go on an eating binge during an emotional crisis. The overly thin often react oppositely. Stress hormones cause them to reject food and thus become thinner. Clearly, investigations of the chemical, hormonal, and neural mechanisms involved in the body's responses to different stimuli hold much promise for a future understanding of eating behavior.

Inactivity

The many possible causes of obesity mentioned so far all relate to the input side of the energy equation. What about output? People may be obese because they eat too much, but another possibility is that they spend too little energy. In fact, underactivity is probably the most important single contributor to the obesity problem in our country. The control of hunger/appetite actually works quite well in active people and only fails when activity falls below a certain minimum level. Obese people under close observation are often seen to eat less than lean people, but they are sometimes so extraordinarily inactive or efficient in their way of moving that they still manage to have an energy surplus.

No two people are alike either physically or psychologically, and the causes of obesity may be as varied as the people who are obese. Many causes may contribute to the problem of obesity in a single person. Given this complexity, it is obvious that there is no panacea. The top priority should be prevention, but where prevention has failed, the treatment of obesity must involve a simultaneous attack on many fronts.

The Treatment of Obesity

The only realistic and sensible way for the obese person to achieve and maintain ideal weight is to cut kcalories, to increase activity, and to maintain this changed lifestyle for life. This is a tall order. Fewer than a third of those who lose weight manage to keep it off in the long run. To succeed means modifying all the attitudes and behaviors that have contributed to the problem in the first place, sometimes against internal and external pressures that can't be changed. Still, it can be and has been done successfully. A three-pronged approach works best: diet, exercise, and behavior modification.

The way a person loses weight is a highly individual matter. Two weight-loss plans may both be successful and yet have little or nothing in common. To heighten the sense of individuality, the following sections are written in terms of advice to "you." This is not intended to put "you" under pressure to take it personally, but to give you the illusion of listening in on a conversation in which an obese person (with, say, 50 pounds to lose) is being competently counseled by someone familiar with the techniques known to be effective. Bullets at intervals highlight the principles involved.

Diet

No particular diet is magical, and no particular food must either be included or avoided. You are the one who will have to live with the diet, so you had better be involved in its planning. Don't think of it as a diet you are going "on"—because then you may be tempted to go "off." The diet can be called successful only if the pounds do not return. Think of it as an eating plan that you will adopt for life. It must consist of foods that you like, that are available to you, and that are within your means.

- Keep in mind that you will want to maintain your lost weight. Practice the needed behaviors as you go.

Dr. Bruce Bistrian, who has worked extensively with weight loss, reports that to be successful, people have to learn not one, but two sets of behaviors: first, weight loss; then, maintenance of the lost weight. They are separate problems, and of the two, maintenance is the more difficult to manage.[16] If you adopt an "eating plan" rather than "a diet," you can be practicing maintenance behaviors all the time you are losing weight. You will be ready to succeed for the rest of your life, once you arrive at your goal weight.

- Be involved in planning your own program.

The balance of a weight-loss diet is different from that of a maintenance diet. When you are maintaining weight, the ideal balance is thought to be 15 percent of kcalories from protein, 30 percent or less from fat, and 55 percent or more from carbohydrate. These amounts are supposed to deliver enough protein to more than meet your RDA and a small enough amount of fat not to compromise your health.

When you cut kcalories in order to lose weight, you have to be careful not to cut your protein amount below the RDA, and you should leave enough fat in your diet to provide satiety. As a result, *percentages* of protein and fat kcalories in the diet are higher than in a maintenance diet, although the total *amounts* are about the same (and the carbohydrate amount is lower). Table 8–4 shows a sample weight-loss diet.

- Adopt a realistic plan.

Choose a kcalorie level you can live with. If you maintain your weight on 2,000 kcalories a day, then you can certainly lose a pound a week on a 1,200 kcalorie diet. A deficit of 500 kcalories a day for seven days is a 3,500–kcalorie deficit—enough to lose a pound of body fat. Make a slightly larger deficit, if the expected weight-loss rate means a lot to you. There is not much point in hurrying, though, because you will never go "off" this eating plan (you will

TABLE 8–4

A Sample Balanced Weight-Loss Diet[a]

Exchange Item	Number of Exchanges	Carbohydrate (g)	Protein (g)	Fat (g)
Starch/Bread	4	60	12	trace
Meat (lean)	5	0	35	15
Vegetables	4	20	8	0
Fruit	4	60	0	0
Milk (nonfat)	2	24	16	trace
Fat	3	0	0	15
Total		164 g	71 g	30 g

[a]This 1,250-kcal diet typifies the balance recommended for a weight-loss diet: approximately 50% carbohydrate, 25% protein, and 25% fat. (Carbohydrate supplies 656 kcal; protein, 284 kcal; and fat, 270 kcal.) When the dieter returns to a maintenance plan by adding mostly carbohydrate foods, the ratio will resemble the 15% protein, 30% fat, and 55% carbohydrate recommended for a maintenance diet.

only modify it)—and nutritional adequacy can't be achieved for the average person on fewer than 1,200 kcalories—1,000 at the very least.

This recommendation is made for the reference woman, 5 feet 4 inches tall, goal weight about 120 pounds. A smaller woman (5 feet tall) with a goal weight of 100 pounds could perhaps go proportionately lower (100 is 5/6 of 120, so she could take 5/6 of the kcalories—900 to 1,000 kcalories). A larger man (5 feet 10 inches, goal weight 160 pounds) should perhaps not go as low (160/120 of 1,200, or 1,600 kcalories, might be a better kcalorie level for him). No nutrient intake recommendations have been made for non-standard-sized people; the appropriate assumption might be that smaller people need smaller amounts of nutrients and so can get by on fewer kcalories.

Put diet adequacy high on your list of priorities. This is a way of putting yourself first. "I like me, and I'm going to take good care of me" is the attitude to adopt. This means including low-kcalorie foods that are rich in valuable nutrients: tasty vegetables and fruits; whole-grain breads and cereals; a limited amount of lean protein-rich foods like poultry, fish, and eggs; nutritious meat substitutes like dried beans and peas; and low-fat dairy products such as cottage cheese and nonfat milk. Within these categories, learn what foods you like and use them often. If you plan resolutely to include a certain number of servings of food from each of these categories each day, you may be so busy making sure you get what you need that you will have little time or appetite left for high-kcalorie or empty-kcalorie foods.

Tasty vegetables and fruits are an important part of a weight control plan.

- Make the diet adequate.
- Emphasize high nutrient density.
- Individualize. Use foods you like.
- Stress dos, not don'ts.

The carbohydrate-containing foods you eat should be largely unrefined, complex-carbohydrate foods of low energy density. People who eat these foods in abundance have been observed to spontaneously eat for longer times and to eat 33 percent fewer kcalories than when eating foods of high energy density.[17] The satiety signal indicating that you are full is sent after a 20-minute lag, so you can eat a great deal more than you need before the signal reaches your brain. Conversely, underweight people need to learn to eat more food within the first 20 minutes of a meal.

Confirming these statements, one research study reported that the eating of soup at either lunch or dinner reduces people's rate of eating. People who eat fewer than 20 kcalories per minute tend to lose more weight. The single suggestion that they include soup in their meals helped the subjects to lose a pound a week.[18]

■ Select carbohydrate-rich foods high in bulk. Use soups often.

At least a fourth of the kcalories in your diet should come from fat, to make your meals more satisfying. At least a third of the fat should be polyunsaturated—soft margarine, salad dressing, mayonnaise, or the like. Read the label to be sure of the kind of fat. And measure your fat with extra caution. A slip of the butter knife adds even more kcalories than a slip of the sugar spoon. And speaking of empty kcalories, omit sugar, pure fat and oil, and alcohol altogether—if you are willing. Let your carbohydrate come from starchy foods and your fat from protein-rich foods. Table 8–4 shows how you can plan a diet using the exchange system.

Take well-spaced weighings so you can see your progress. If you see a weight gain and you know you have strictly followed your diet, this probably represents a shift in water weight. Many dieters experience a temporary plateau after about three weeks—not because they are slipping, but because they have gained water weight temporarily while they are still losing body fat. The fat you are hoping to lose must be combined with oxygen (oxidized) to make carbon dioxide and water if it is to leave the body. The oxygen you breathe in combines with the carbons of the fat to make carbon dioxide, and with the hydrogens to make water. The carbon dioxide will be breathed out quickly, but the water stays in the body for a longer time. The water takes a while to leave the cell, then works its way into the lymph system, and finally enters the bloodstream. Finally, after the water arrives in the blood, the kidneys "see" it and send it to the bladder for excretion; meanwhile, you have a weight gain, because the water weighs more than the fat that was oxidized.* If you faithfully follow your diet plan, one day the plateau will break. You can tell from your frequent urination.

■ Anticipate a plateau (have realistic expectations from the start).

A dieter who undertakes an exercise program may arrive at a plateau for another reason: gain in muscle mass at the expense of body fat. The next section discusses the role of exercise in a weight control program.

Exercise

Some people who want to lose weight hate the very idea of exercise. Obese people often—understandably—do not enjoy moving their bodies. They feel heavy, clumsy, even ridiculous. A word to reassure them: weight loss, at least to a point, is possible without exercise. But even if you choose not to alter your habits at first, let your mind be open to the possibility that you will want to

No matter how much you huff and puff, you can't just shake it off, rock it off, roll it off, knock it off or bake it off. . . . The only way is to eat less and exercise more.

American Medical Association

*Water weight accumulates during fat oxidation because 1 fatty acid weighing 284 units leaves behind water weighing 324 units—14% more.

Benefits of Exercise:
• Increased expenditure of energy.
• Long-term increase in resting metabolic rate.
• Appetite control.
• Stress reduction.
• Control of stress-induced eating.
• Increased self esteem.
• Psychological and physical well-being.

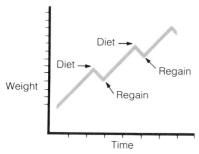

Weight / Time

The ratchet effect. Each round of dieting, without exercise, is followed by a rebound of weight to a higher level than before.

ratchet effect: a popular term for the effect that repeated cycles of weight loss and gain, without exercise, have on body composition, in which the body fat content increases and kcaloric needs fall after each round, making the next round of weight loss harder.

Two more benefits of regular exercise:
• Conditioned body burns more body fat during exercise than unconditioned one.
• Short-term increase in metabolism.

take up some activity later on. As the pounds come off, moving your body becomes a pleasure, as does letting others see you move.

■ Pave the way for later changes.

The contributions exercise makes to a weight-control program are several. Exercise alters body composition in a desirable direction, and thereby alters metabolism, making daily energy needs higher even during rest. It spends energy directly, too, and it helps control appetite that might otherwise be unruly. Exercise also offers the psychological benefits of looking and feeling healthy, and reduces stress and stress-induced eating. Increased self-esteem accompanies these benefits, and this tends to support a person's resolve to persist in a weight-control effort—rounding out a beneficial cycle.

Weight loss without exercise can have a negative effect on body composition. No doubt you've heard someone say as a joke, "I've lost 200 pounds, but I was never more than 20 pounds overweight." What this person means is that frequent, intermittent dieting, alternating with weight gain, is an expected pattern of life. Such a person may not realize that with each bout of dieting she trades in small amounts of healthy lean body tissue for a slightly higher body fat content.

A person who diets without exercising loses both lean and fat tissue, as described earlier. A person who gains weight without exercising gains mostly fat; the lean is gone forever. Thus, after a round of weight loss and regain, the body may weigh the same as before, but it contains more fat tissue and less lean. More likely, if the person's eating habits haven't changed, the body will wind up weighing *more* each time than the last, the so-called ratchet or "yoyo" effect of dieting.

As we've said, compared with lean tissue, fat tissue is relatively inactive metabolically. Metabolic activity uses up food energy. Thus the more lean tissue you develop, the faster your metabolism becomes, the more energy you spend, and the more you can afford to eat. This brings you both pleasure and nutrients. The ratchet effect reverses the situation. If you initially weighed 160 pounds, lost down to 130 pounds, and then returned to your initial weight, all without exercising, you would now have less lean tissue than you did when you weighed 160 the first time. Less lean tissue means that your metabolism is slower. So, if you eat as you did at 160 pounds before, you will now gain fat rather than maintain your weight.

Even when a person follows a medically sound low-kcalorie diet, dieting without exercise causes losses of lean body mass. The only way to avoid lean body losses while losing fat is to include *both* vigorous exercise and sensible dieting in your plan. As it happens, this is also the way to lose fat the fastest.

It must be clear by now that exercise, by shifting body composition toward more lean tissue, speeds up the metabolism *permanently*—that is, for as long as you keep your body conditioned. Exercise has two other beneficial effects we haven't mentioned.

First, the conditioned body is "trained" to use fatty acids, rather than glucose, as fuel; therefore, after you've become conditioned, you'll tend to burn more body fat during exercise than you did when you were out of condition. The best kind of exercise for building up your fat-burning equipment is not severely strenuous, but easy-paced to moderate exercise of long duration (30 minutes or more). Furthermore, the more muscle and lean tissue you have, the more fat you will burn—all day long, even when you are resting.

Second, on any given day, an intensive bout of exercise will speed up the metabolism *temporarily*—for a day or so. The metabolism is stimulated by about 25 percent for as long as three hours after an intensive bout of exercise, and may still be running 10 percent faster two days later.

Table 8–5 shows the energy in foods and shows how far you must run or how long you must walk to "work them off." People can take such charts out of context and say, "An apple and a glass of milk will cost me an hour of running . . . hmm, I think I'll skip lunch." Don't let the table fool you into thinking only in terms of kcalories. First, such charts refer only to kcalories eaten in *excess* of your daily maintenance level or the lower kcaloric level chosen for a weight-loss diet. Second, your body needs nutritious foods during weight loss as much as ever. So eat the apple, drink the milk, go do your workout, and know that you've found the best of both worlds.

Keep in mind that if exercise is to help with weight loss, it must be active exercise—voluntary moving of muscles. Being moved passively, as by a machine at a health spa or by a massage, does not increase kcalorie expenditure. The more muscles you move, the more kcalories you spend.

People sometimes ask about "spot reducing." Can you lose fat in particular locations? Unfortunately, muscles don't "own" the fat that surrounds them. All body fat is shared by all the muscles and organs, so "spot-reducing" exercises that work only the flabby parts won't help reduce the fat located there. There is some good news, though: tightening muscles in trouble spots by way of a balanced, all-over exercise program will help the appearance of the fatty areas.

Another thing to keep in mind is that the number of kcalories spent in an activity depends more upon your weight than on how fast you can do the exercise. For example, a person who weighs 120 pounds and runs a 6-minute mile burns off 83 kcalories. That same person, ambling along for a mile in 10 minutes, burns almost the same amount—76 kcalories. Similarly, a 220-pound person spends 148 kcalories on the 6-minute mile, and only a little less—136 kcalories—on the 10-minute amble. The rule seems to be that you don't have

TABLE 8–5

Activity Cost of Eating Foods beyond kCalorie Need[a]

To work off the kcalories from this food eaten beyond your energy need	You have to walk:	or jog:	or wait:
Cookie, chocolate chip (50 kcal)	10 min	3 min	39 min
Ice cream, ⅔ cup (200 kcal)	38 min	11 min	2½ hr
T-bone steak, 8 oz (800 kcal)	2½ hr	41 min	10¼ hr
Pizza, gooey, 1 slice (300 kcal)	1 hr	15 min	3¾ hr
Beer or cola beverage, 12 oz (150 kcal)	29 min	8 min	2 hr
Caramel candy, 1 oz, or potato chips, 10 chips (115 kcal)	22 min	6 min	1½ hr
Chocolate-coated peanuts, 8 (160 kcal)	31 min	8 min	2 hr

[a]For a 150-lb person, the energy cost of walking at 3.5 mph is 5.2 kcal/min; of running, is 19.4 kcal/min; and of reclining, is 1.3 kcal/min.

to work fast to use up energy effectively. If you choose to walk the distance instead of run, you'll use up about the same energy; it'll just take you longer.

You may have heard the suggestion that you incorporate more exercise into your daily schedule in many simple, small-scale ways. Park the car at the far end of the parking lot; use the stairs instead of the elevator; do a deep knee bend each time you get up from your chair. These strategies don't add up to many kcalories each, but over a year's time they become significant. If you also incorporate regular aerobic exercise into your schedule (see Highlight 7A), your heart and lungs, as well as your muscles, will be fit.

Behavior Modification

Some psychologists view human behavior as regulated by environmental factors. In simple terms, they see each behavior as sandwiched between two environmental conditions, those that precede it and those that follow it—the antecedents and the consequences:

$$A \text{ (antecedents)} \rightarrow B \text{ (behavior)} \leftrightarrow C \text{ (consequences)}$$

A behavior occurs in response to antecedents (cues or stimuli); the more intense they are, the more likely the behavior is to occur. The behavior leads to consequences, and the more intense these are, the more or less likely the behavior is to occur again. Behavior modification involves manipulating these environmental conditions so as to favor the repeated occurrence of a desired behavior and extingush the occurrence of unwanted behaviors.

Behavior modification can be used to change the behaviors of overeating and underexercising that lead to and perpetuate obesity. Figure 8–7 illustrates

FIGURE 8–7.

Behavior modification model. See text for explanation.

Source: Adapted from R. B. Stuart and B. Davis, *Slim Chance in a Fat World, Behavioral Control of Obesity* (Champaign, Ill.: Research Press, 1972), Figure 2, p. 76.

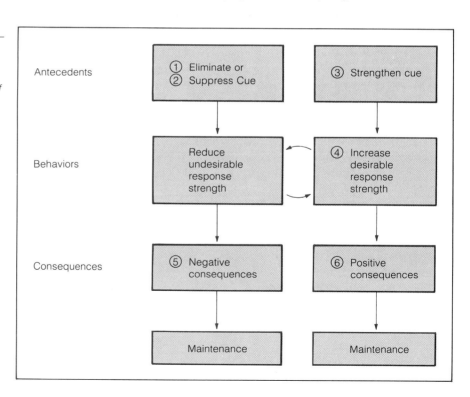

strategies to modify antecedents, behaviors, and consequences to reduce the frequency of overeating behaviors and increase the frequency of desirable eating behaviors. The discussion that follows attends to each of the figure's parts, following the example of a classic book in the field, *Slim Chance in a Fat World*.[19]

First, behavior modification experts say, you should establish a baseline. Keep a diary, like that shown in Figure 8–8. This will provide you with clues from which you can tell what your particular eating stimuli, or cues, are.

Now, set about eliminating the cues that prompt you to eat inappropriately. They may be manifold: watching TV, talking on the telephone, passing a convenience store or a vending machine, being offered food, and many more. Resolve to respond no longer to these cues by eating, but to respond only to one set of cues designed by you: one particular place in one particular room. No other place should stimulate you to eat. This strategy heads the list of elimination steps recommended:

- Eat only in one place, in one room.
- Don't buy problem foods (shop when you aren't hungry).
- Don't serve rich sauces and toppings at the table.
- Let spouses and children buy, store, and serve their own sweets.
- Clear plates directly into the garbage.
- Create obstacles to the eating of problem foods (for example, make it necessary to unwrap, cook, and serve each one separately, allowing time for resistance to develop).

Second, set about suppressing those cues to inappropriate eating behavior that you can't eliminate. For example, if one or more family members tend to push you to eat the wrong things, solicit behavioral cooperation from them. Don't ask that they point out what you do wrong; that doesn't work.

- Ask others to provide you with positive cues to desired behavior.
- Ask others to provide you with positive reinforcement when you eat acceptably.
- Have others nearby when you eat.
- Minimize contact with excessive food (serve individual plates; don't put serving dishes on the table; leave the table when finished).
- Make small portions of food look large (spread food out; serve on small plates).
- Control states of deprivation (plan and eat regular meals; don't skip meals; avoid getting tired; avoid boredom by keeping cues to interesting activities in plain sight).

Third, strengthen the cues to appropriate eating:

- Keep a variety of appropriate foods available.
- Provide feedback about how much to eat (learn appropriate portion sizes when substituting).
- Save allowable foods from meals for snacks (and these should be your only snacks).
- Prepare allowable foods attractively.

Fourth, alter the response itself. Overeaters eat faster than others, so:

- Slow down (pause for two to three minutes; put down utensils; swallow before reloading the fork; always use utensils).

FIGURE 8–8.

Food diary. The record reveals problem areas, the first step towards solving problems.

Fifth, arrange as far as possible to have negative consequences follow inappropriate eating behavior. Scolding is *not* a negative consequence (it is a form of attention giving, which is positive), so don't ask to be scolded:

- Ask that others respond neutrally to your deviations (make no comment). This is a negative consequence, because it withholds attention.
- Bring into focus the aversive consequences of overeating.

Sixth and finally, make sure that positive consequences, including material rewards, follow upon your exhibition of the desired behaviors:

- Update records of food intake, exercise, and weight change regularly.
- Arrange for material reinforcement (rewards for each unit of behavior change or weight loss).
- Provide social reinforcement (ask to be encouraged).

You may find it helpful to join a group such as Take Off Pounds Sensibly (TOPS), Weight Watchers (WW), or Overeaters Anonymous (OA). A modest expenditure for your own health and well-being is well worth while (but avoid expensive, quick-weight-loss, "magical" rip-offs, of course). Many dieters find it helpful to form their own self-help groups, and it often helps to enlist a family member's participation and cooperation.

If you are especially sensitive to social situations where you feel you have to eat, it will also help to have some assertiveness training. Learning to say "No, thank you" might be one of your first objectives. Learning not to "clean your plate" might be another.

- Learn and practice assertiveness.

From all the behavior changes available to you, you can choose the ones to begin with. Don't try to master them all at once. No one who attempts too many changes at one time is successful. Set your own priorities. Pick one trouble area that you think you can handle, start with that, and practice your strategy until it is habitual and automatic. A new habit as simple as switching from whole to nonfat milk may take a week of effort and practice before you get used to it. Then you can select another trouble area to work on.

- Use small-step modification.

Enjoy your new, emerging self. Inside every fat person, a thin person is waiting to be freed. Get in touch with—reach out your hand to—your thin self, and help that self to feel welcome in the light of day.

Finally, be aware that it can be harder to maintain weight loss than to lose weight. People who lose weight often regain all that they have lost—and more. Paradoxically, those who lose the most (more than 40 pounds) have the greatest tendency to zoom up to levels higher above their starting points than people who have lost less weight. On arriving at the goal weight after months of self-discipline and new habit formation, the victorious weight loser must at all cost avoid "celebrating" by resuming old eating habits. They are gone forever—remember? Membership in an ongoing weight-control organization such as Overeaters Anonymous or Weight Watchers, as well as continued participation in regular sports or other physical activity, can provide indispensable support for the formerly fat person who wants to remain trim.

Inside of every fat person, a thin person is waiting to be freed.

The three-part approach to weight loss, just described, is effective. Diet and exercise shift energy balance so that more kcalories are being spent than taken in; the exercise maintains or even builds the lean body so that fat is preferentially lost and metabolic energy needs remain high; and the behavior modification retrains habits so that once the weight is lost, it will not return. Magical alternatives to this systematic, hard-work approach have been offered time and again over the centuries—ways to "shrink the stomach," to eat "negative kcalories," to "eat all you want and lose weight"—but they are born of wishful thinking. They are effective only when they directly affect the kcalorie balance. If they can be said to be successful in any sense, it is only because they are popular, not because they work. The next section of this chapter addresses alternative strategies for losing weight; as you will see, some have limited usefulness, and some are not useful at all.

Treatments of Obesity: Poor Choices

One choice people sometimes make is to take "water pills." The idea that excess weight is due to water accumulation is appealingly simple, and indeed, temporary water retention, seen in many women around the time of the menstrual period, may make a difference of several pounds on the scale.* If water retention is a problem, a physician can prescribe a diuretic and possibly a mild degree of salt restriction. But the obese—that is, overfat—subject has a *smaller* percentage of body water than the person of normal weight. If such a person takes a self-prescribed diuretic, the scale may show a few pounds of loss for half a day, but the loss will be water, not fat, and the price may be dehydration.

diuretic (dye-you-RET-ic): a drug that promotes water excretion; popularly, a "water pill."
dia = through
ure = urine

Then there are other drugs—both prescription and over-the-counter varieties. Some doctors prescribe amphetamines ("speed") to help with weight loss, such as Dexedrine and Benzedrine. These reduce appetite—but only temporarily. Typically, the appetite returns to normal after a week or two, the lost weight (and often more) is regained, and the user then has the problem of trying to get off the drug without gaining more weight. It is generally agreed that these drugs cause a dangerous dependency and are of little or no usefulness in treating obesity.[20]

People also buy over-the-counter medications to help with weight loss. The FDA has given approval to the over-the-counter weight control aid: phenyl-propanolamine hydrochloride (as in Dexatrim and Appedrine), but may soon withdraw it, because this drug is an amphetamine. The only other drug it approves is benzocaine with caffeine. It considers bulk producers or fillers safe, but questions their effectiveness. It has withheld approval for grapefruit diet pills, and states, as this book does, that the only demonstrated way to lose weight is to eat fewer kcalories than your body uses.[21]

Some strategies for losing weight have limited usefulness.

---

*Oral contraceptives may have the same effect. They may also promote actual fat gain in some women. A woman who has this problem should consult her physician about switching brands.

A multitude of other drugs are presently under investigation: hormones and hormonelike compounds, inhibitors of nutrient absorption, inhibitors of fat synthesis, promoters of fat breakdown, other modifiers of metabolism—in short, every kind of agent that researchers can imagine might be effective in any way against obesity. Tests in humans of any of these would be premature at present, and results in animals are not encouraging. Side effects, in many cases, are severe. In short, at present, no known drug is both safe and effective, and many are hazardous. Even diet pills, long thought safe and widely used, have been shown not to be safe for all users; serious illness has been ascribed to the taking of diet pills containing phenylpropanolamine hydrochloride. The only effective appetite-reducing agent to which tolerance does not develop in time is cigarette smoking—and that, of course, entails severe hazards of its own too numerous to mention.

Nor do starch blockers allow you to eat your favorite carbohydrate foods and derive no kcalories from them. Uncooked wheat and kidney beans contain inhibitors of the starch-digesting enzyme amylase, and when these inhibitors are purified and fed to rats, they excrete some starch and gain less weight than controls. But tests on human beings show no inhibition of starch digestion whatsoever;[22] the pills may cause nausea, vomiting, diarrhea, and stomach pains, but don't block starch digestion.

People have also been trying glucomannan, a preparation derived from a vegetable (konjak tuber) used in Japanese cuisine. The Japanese are said to have used konjak for weight control for 1,500 years—but in a controlled experiment reported in 1982, glucomannon was ineffective.[23]

Someday a pill may be developed that is effective against overeating and obesity. None of those described here is a likely candidate. One that may be promising is the opiate antagonist naloxone hydrochloride, which blocks stress-induced eating in animals, and possibly also in humans.[24] Extensive testing will be required to determine whether naloxone hydrochloride can be safely used for this purpose.

Perhaps the most promising antiobesity agent presently being tested is the artificial fat (sucrose polyester) described in Chapter 4. It remains to be seen, however, whether long-term use will facilitate permanent weight loss or whether, like artificial sweeteners, sucrose polyester will become a mere addition to the diet.

Other gimmicks that don't help with weight loss are found in salons and spas. Hot baths do not speed up the basal metabolic rate so that pounds can be lost in hours. Steam and sauna baths do not melt the fat off the body, although they may dehydrate a person so that his weight on the scales changes dramatically. Machines intended to jiggle parts of the body while the person leans passively on them provide pleasant stimulation, but no exercise, and so no expenditure of energy. Brushes, sponges, and massages intended to break down "cellulite" do nothing of the kind, because there is no such thing as cellulite.[25]

What about hormones? Hormones are powerful body chemicals and many affect fat metabolism, so it has long been hoped that a hormone might be found that would promote weight loss. Several have been tried, but with testing, all have proven ineffective and often hazardous as well. Thyroid hormone, in particular, causes loss of lean body mass and heart problems except when medically prescribed for the correction of a thyroid deficiency— and thyroid deficiency is very seldom the cause of obesity.

Among the hormones advertised as promoting weight loss is HCG (human chorionic gonadotropin), a hormone extracted from the urine of pregnant women.

Being passively moved provides no expenditure of energy.

cellulite (SELL-you-leet): supposedly a lumpy form of fat; actually a fraud. The skin sometimes appears lumpy in fatty areas of the body because strands of connective tissue attach the skin to underlying structures. These points of attachment may pull tight where the fat is thick, making lumps appear between them. The fat itself is not different from fat anywhere else in the body. So, if you lose the fat there, you lose the lumpy appearance.

HCG has legitimate uses; for example, it can stimulate ovulation in a woman who has had difficulty becoming pregnant. But it has no effect on weight loss and does not reduce hunger. A rash of "clinics" run by "doctors" that sprang up on the West Coast during the 1970s advertised tremendous success using HCG in the treatment of obesity. These outfits seem to have had one element in common. They prescribed an extremely rigid low-kcalorie diet, which accounted for their apparent effectiveness. The American Medical Association and the California Medical Association have concluded that the claims made for HCG are groundless and that the side effects are unknown and probably dangerous.

Still another approach to weight control is surgery, which some obese people request out of sheer desperation. One operation, bypass surgery, involves shortening the small intestine to reduce absorption. Another operation involves stapling the stomach to make it smaller.

Gastric stapling is in increasing use in preference to bypass surgery, because it forces the person to eat less rather than causing malabsorption. Still, although the theory is pleasingly simple, stapling involves hazards in practice; stomach tissue is damaged, scars are formed, staples pull loose. The person contemplating surgery should think long and hard before submitting to it.

Desperation of the same kind leads some clients to request that their jaws be wired shut so that they will be forced to consume a liquid diet. This does bring about weight loss, but when the wires are removed, there is "relentless weight gain . . . until the prewiring weight has been reached."[26] Other medical treatments for obesity include: supervised fasting as mentioned in Chapter 7; insertion of a stomach balloon; and surgical removal of fat pads for figure remodeling.

Last, but not least, among poor choices in obesity treatment are the fad diets. Most of them are low-carbohydrate diets, of which the hazards have already been described in Chapter 7. Table 8–6 rates presently popular diets according to sound nutrition principles.

human chorionic gonadotropin (core-ee-ON-ic go-nad-o-TROPE- in), or **HCG**: a hormone extracted from the urine of pregnant women; believed (incorrectly) to promote fat breakdown.

The Problem of Underweight

Much of what has been said about obesity applies to underweight as well. No serious hazards accompany mild degrees of underweight. In fact, the only causes of death seen more often in thin people than in normal-weight people are wasting diseases such as tuberculosis and cancer. (Suicide is more common among underweight people, but the underweight is not thought to be a cause. The severe depression probably came first and caused anorexia, or lack of appetite.)

The causes of underweight may be as diverse as those of overeating. Hunger, appetite, and satiety irregularities may exist; there may be contributory psychological factors in some cases and metabolic ones in others. Clearly there is a genetic component. Habits learned early in childhood, especially food aversions, may perpetuate themselves. The demand for kcalories to support physical activity and growth often contributes to underweight; an extremely active boy during his adolescent growth spurt may need more than 4,000 kcalories a day to maintain his weight. Such a boy may be too busy to take time to eat. The underweight person states with justification that it is as hard to gain a pound

anorexia (an-o-REX-ee-uh): lack of appetite.
an = not
orexis = appetite

TABLE 8–6

Weight-Loss Diets Compared

With a balanced perspective on foods and a sense of what's important in diet planning and what's not, you can evaluate the many different diets people consume. Here's a summary of the questions you might ask. Start with 100 points, and subtract if any of these criteria are not met:

1. Does the diet provide a reasonable number of kcalories (enough to maintain weight; not too many; and if a reduction diet, not fewer than 1,200 kcal for the average-sized person)? If not, give it a **minus 10.**
2. Does it provide enough, but not too much, protein (at least the recommended intake or RDA, but not more than twice that much)? If not, **minus 10.**
3. Does it provide enough fat for satiety, but not so much fat as to go against current recommendations (say, between 20 and 35% of the kcalories from fat)? If not, **minus 10.**
4. Does it provide enough carbohydrate to spare protein and prevent ketosis (100 g of carbohydrate for the average-sized person)? Is it mostly complex carbohydrate (not more than 20% of the kcalories as concentrated sugar)? If no to either, **minus 5**; if no to both, **minus 10.**

Diet Name and Description	Question 1: kCalories	Question 2: Protein
Dr. Atkins' Diet Revolution. A low-carbohydrate/high-protein diet that allows unlimited protein and fat, but severely limits carbohydrate. See p. 216 for hazards of a very low carbohydrate intake. In addition to these hazards, the diet is high in total fat, saturated fat, and cholesterol. The omission of breads and cereals and the large reduction of fruits, vegetables, and milk characterize the diet. Similar to this diet are *Dr. Atkins' Superenergy Weight Reduction Diet* and others.	Yes	No, excessive protein MINUS 10
Banana-Milk Diet (also called the *Johns Hopkins Diet*). A daily diet of six bananas and three glasses of milk plus vitamin and mineral supplements.	No, provides less than 1,000 kcal MINUS 10	No, low protein MINUS 10
Beverly Hills Diet. A diet that allows, for the first ten days, no food other than specific fruits. Timing and combining of foods are claimed to cause weight loss, with no scientific basis for the claims. Sometimes causes diarrhea and excess gas in the digestive tract because of laxative nature of fruit. Physicians warn that shock, low blood pressure, and perhaps death may result.	No, low kcalories MINUS 10	No, low protein MINUS 10
Complete Scarsdale Medical Diet plus *Dr. Tarnower's Lifetime Keep-Slim Program.* Touted as a no-hunger, no-pills way to lose 20 lb in two weeks. The plan is a two-weeks-on, two-weeks-off low-carbohydrate, ample-protein diet of about 1,100 kcal/day.	Yes	No, provides approximately 216% of the protein needs MINUS 10
Cambridge Diet. A powdered formula sold directly to the public through "counselors" (nonmedical people who have used the diet) for use three times daily. One day's worth of the formula provides 33 g protein, 40 g carbohydrate, and 3 g fat. Any diet of such low kcaloric value carries serious health hazards (p. 217), in addition to the low-carbohydrate diet effects. The powder is fortified with vitamins and minerals.	No MINUS 10	No, low protein MINUS 10
Fasting (ZIP Diet). A fast in which water is allowed. See pp. 214–216 for a complete discussion of effects.	No MINUS 10	No MINUS 10
High Roughage Reducing diet (Dr. David Rubin). Inclues the addition of 2 tsp of bran to be taken with water at each mealtime. The foods provided by the menus are low-fat, low-kcalorie items, with few milk products. Closely related is *Dr. Siegal's Natural Fiber Permanent Weight-Loss Diet,* but he requires nine "heaping" tablespoons of bran daily. The diarrhea that may result from high bran levels can cause serious medical problems if it continues for several days.	Yes	Yes
I Love New York Diet (Myerson and Adler).[a] A diet based on a New York City Health Department plan. A strict diet built around the Four Food Group Plan. Alternates periods of 700 kcal/day and 1,500 kcal/day.	Although the average intake is 1,100 kcal/day, periods of severe restriction are included MINUS 5	Yes

5. Does it offer a balanced assortment of vitamins and minerals from whole food sources in all four food groups (see Chapter 1)? If a food group is omitted (for example, meats), is a suitable substitute provided? The four food groups are milk/milk products; meat/fish/poultry/eggs/legumes; fruits/vegetables; and grains. For *each* food group omitted and not adequately substituted for, **minus 10.**
6. Does it offer variety, in the sense that different foods can be selected each day? If you'd class it as "monotonous," give it a **minus 10.**
7. Does it consist of ordinary foods that are available locally (for example, in the main grocery stores) at the prices people normally pay? Or does the dieter have to buy special, expensive, or unusual foods to adhere to the diet? If you'd class it as "bizarre" or "requiring unusual foods," **minus 10.**

Question 3: Fat	Question 4: Carbohydrate	Question 5: Food Groups	Question 6: Variety	Question 7: Ordinary Foods	Total Score
No, excessive fat MINUS 10	No, inadequate carbohydrate MINUS 10	No, three food groups omitted MINUS 30	No, monotonous MINUS 10	Yes	30 points
No, low fat MINUS 10	Yes	No, two food groups omitted MINUS 20	No, monotonous MINUS 10	Yes	40 points
No, low fat MINUS 10	No, no starch MINUS 10	No, three food groups omitted MINUS 30	No, monotonous; omits most food groups other than fruits MINUS 10	No, requires tropical fruits in large quantites and later suggests lobster and steak MINUS 10	10 points
No, meat has a high fat percentage MINUS 10	No, carbohydrate level is 30% of need MINUS 5	No, milk group omitted MINUS 10	Yes	Yes	65 points
No, low fat MINUS 10	No, low carbohydrate MINUS 10	No food allowed on a regular basis MINUS 40	No variety MINUS 10	No ordinary food; expensive formula required MINUS 10	0 points
No MINUS 10	No MINUS 10	No MINUS 40	No MINUS 10	No MINUS 10	0 points
Yes	Yes	Half the milk allowance MINUS 5	Yes	Requires bran MINUS 5	90 points
Yes	Yes	Yes	Yes	Yes	95 points

TABLE 8–6

(continued)

Diet Name and Description	Question 1: kCalories	Question 2: Protein
Kempner's Rice Diet A diet originally developed to treat hypertension; involves eating rice and fruit. Blood pressure can be reduced by the diet, which may be dangerous for normal individuals. Vitamin and mineral supplements are recommended.	Yes	No, low protein MINUS 10
Magic Mayo Diet (Grapefruit Diet). A very low carbohydrate, high-fat, high-meat, very low kcalorie diet with no milk—doubtless a diet less than magic. One-half grapefruit is required before each meal, and false claims are made about this food's ability to "burn" kcalories in other foods. The diet is in no way associated with the Mayo Clinc.	No MINUS 10	No, too high MINUS 10
Nathan Pritikin's Maximum Weight Loss Diet. Originally aimed at curing ills. This diet severely restricts fat, limits protein to below the recommended levels, and limits dairy products severely. Several levels of kcalories are available from 700 to 1,200 per day.	Choosing any plan except 1,200 kcal will not provide the recommended level MINUS 5	No, too low MINUS 10
New Canadian High-Energy Diet.[b] Written by a professional dietitian, a diet that uses the exchange system to ensure adequate nutrient intake, while emphasizing complex carbohydrate foods. High energy comes from nutritional adequacy and from the carbohydrate.	Yes	Yes
Rotation Diet. A diet developed by a clinical psychologist who is not a nutrition professional. The diet alternates 600, 900, and 1,200 kcalorie-per-day intakes (higher for men) in the first three weeks, then allows moderate intakes for a week, and starts over. It also includes unlimited quantities of selected fruits and vegetables.	Two weeks of severe kcalorie restriction is ill advised MINUS 5	Not likely to have sufficient protein, especially in view of carbohydrate restriction MINUS 5
Dr. Stillman's Quick Inches Off Diet. A high-carbohydrate, low-protein diet that is claimed by the author to allow dieters to reduce fat in desired body areas. No meats or milk products are allowed.	?	No, too low MINUS 10
UCLA Diet (California Slim).[c] Developed at the UCLA Center for Health Enhancement, Education, and Research. The diet is basically a low-fat, controlled-portion diet of 1,200 kcal/day that allows unlimited salads and emphasizes fresh vegetables and fruits.	Yes	Yes
Weight Watchers. Emphasizes behavior change and support groups, along with a balanced diet based on the four food groups and exchange system. Processed, prepared dishes such as frozen entrées and other products can be used instead of home-prepared foods.	Yes	Yes

Other (name): _____

[a]P. H. Harper, The I love New York diet (book review), *Journal of Nutrition Education* 14, (1982): 127.
[b]S. Cohen-Rose and C. P. Rose, *The New Canadian High-Energy Diet* (Montreal: Corona Publishers, 1983).
[c]UCLA Center for Health Enhancement, Education, and Research, Los Angeles, as cited in *Health,* May 1982, p. 43.

Question 3: Fat	Question 4: Carbohydrate	Question 5: Food Groups	Question 6: Variety	Question 7: Ordinary foods	Total Score
No, low fat MINUS 10	Yes	No meat or milk allowed MINUS 20	No, monotonous MINUS 10	Yes	50 points
Yes, but so low in kcalories that total fat is low MINUS 10	No, too low MINUS 10	No milk or grains allowed MINUS 20	No, monotonous MINUS 10	Yes	30 points
No, too low MINUS 10	Yes	No, meat and milk groups restricted MINUS 5 MINUS 5	YES	No, dieters are urged to use "Pritikin breads" and other products MINUS 10	55 points
Yes	Yes	Yes	Yes	Yes	100 points
No, too little fat, half the time MINUS 5	No, too little carbohydrate, half the time MINUS 5	No, insufficient milk likely, half the time MINUS 5	Yes	Yes	75 points
No MINUS 10	Yes	No, meat and milk omitted MINUS 20	No, monotonous MINUS 10	Yes	50 points
Yes	Yes	Yes	Yes	Yes	100 points
Yes	Yes	Yes	Yes	Yes; although Weight Watchers produces a line of prepared foods, they are not aggressively marketed, and the program is designed to be followed without them.	100 points

as for an obese person to lose one. So much energy may be spent adapting to a higher food intake that as many as 750 to 800 extra kcalories a day may be needed to gain a pound a week.[27]

Strategies recommended for weight gain center mostly on increasing food intake and using foods that provide as many kcalories in as small a volume as possible so as not to get uncomfortably full. Recommended are nutritious, high-kcalorie milk shakes; liberal servings of meat, bread, and starchy vegetables; and desserts. Whereas the weight loser is urged to select the lowest-kcalorie items from each category, the gainer is encouraged to pick the highest-kcalorie items. Moreover, while the weight loser is taught to eat slowly and fill up on bulky foods at the beginning of a meal, the person who wants to gain weight must do the opposite: eat faster, and eat the higher-kcalorie items first.

An effective strategy for gaining weight is to snack systematically between meals. A 400-kcalorie milk shake at midmorning and a 700-kcalorie sandwich plus shake between lunch and dinner can help to promote a weight gain rate of 1 1/2 to 2 pounds a week. No known pill, shot, hormone, or surgical procedure will increase weight safely, and a reduction in activity is not recommended unless the condition is so severe as to threaten overall health.

As with weight loss, the person attempting a weight gain must anticipate a plateau. At that time a further increase in food intake will be necessary to continue to gain.

An extreme underweight condition known as anorexia nervosa is sometimes seen in young people, usually young women, who exercise heroic self-denial in order to control their weight. They actually go to such an extreme that they become severely undernourished, finally achieving a body weight of 70 pounds or even less. The distinguishing feature of the anorexic, as opposed to other very thin people, is that the starvation is intentional.

Anorexia nervosa is one of two eating disorders that are becoming widespread in our society today. The other is bulimia—compulsive overeating. These two disorders are the subject of the highlight that follows this chapter.

Study Questions

1. Discuss the limitations for the definition of ideal or desirable weight.

2. How do you calculate the total energy that a person spends in a day?

3. List the factors that tend to increase the risk of obesity. What are the dangers of excess weight?

4. What considerations are essential to any successful weight loss program?

5. Discuss strategies suitable for achieving weight gain.

6. Describe the behavior modification techniques recommended for changing an individual's dietary habits.

7. What are the benefits of increased physical activity in a weight loss program?

Notes

1. Refractory obesity and energy homeostasis, *Nutrition Reviews*, November 1983, pp. 349–351.

2. Refractory obesity, 1983.

3. Consensus panel addresses obesity question, *Journal of the American Medical Association* 254 (1985): 1878; A. R. Frisancho and P. N. Flegel, Relative merits of old and new indices of body mass with reference to skinfold thickness, *American Journal of Clinical Nutrition* 36 (1982): 697–699.

4. T. B. Van Itallie, When the frame is part of the picture (editorial), *American Journal of Public Health* 75 (1985): 1054–1055.

5. First National Health and Nutrition Examination Survey (HANES I), as cited by Van Itallie, 1985.

6. J. H. Himes and C. Bouchard, Do the new Metropolitan Life Insurance weight-height tables correctly assess body frame

iets can be planned using the exchange system to gain weight, lose weight, or stay the same. For practice in the use of this convenient system, try planning two diets, one for weight maintenance or gain, the other for weight loss.

Diet for Weight Maintenance or Gain

1. Set your daily energy level. If you choose to maintain weight, it should be equal to your daily energy expenditure (see p. 245). If you wish to gain weight, it should be at least 500 kcalories above that.

Practice Diet Planning

2. Decide on the proportions in which protein, fat, and carbohydrate kcalories will be represented in the diet. A suggested ratio is about 10 to 15 percent of the energy from protein, not more than 30 percent from fat, and the rest from carbohydrate. Given the daily kcalorie level you chose, how many kcalories will you allot to each nutrient?
3. Translate these kcalorie amounts into grams. (Remember, 1 gram of protein

or carbohydrate = 4 kcalories; 1 gram of fat = 9 kcalories.) Enter these gram amounts and your intended kcalorie total at the top of Form 6. (Appendix K)
4. Now decide how many exchanges of milk, vegetables, and fruit you'd like to have each day; enter these numbers in the form; and compute the number of grams of carbohydrate, protein, and fat they will deliver (don't compute kcalories yet). See p. 39 or Appendix G for the exchange system values. (Caution: Use pencil. You'll want to change these numbers several times before you finalize your plan.)

Only one more set of foods—the

and body fat relationships? *American Journal of Public Health* 75 (1985): 1076–1079.

7. Consensus panel, 1985.

8. M. Ashwell, T. J. Cole, and A. K. Dixon, Obesity: New insight into the anthropometric classification of fat distribution shown by computed tomography, *British Medical Journal* 290 (1985): 1692–1694.

9. M. Simonton, An overview: Advances in research and treatment of obesity, *Food and Nutrition News,* March–April 1982.

10. A. S. Levine and J. E. Morley, Purinergic regulation of food intake, *Science* 217 (1982): 77–79.

11. G. A. Bray and L. A. Campfield, Metabolic factors in the control of energy stores, *Metabolism* 24 (1975): 99–117.

12. N. J. Rothwell and M. J. Stock, Regulation of energy balance, in *Annual Review of Nutrition,* vol. 1, eds. W. J. Darby, H. P. Broquist, and R. E. Olson (Palo Alto, Calif.: Annual Reviews, 1981), pp. 235–256.

13. T. B. Van Itallie and R. G. Campbell, Multidisciplinary approach to the problem of obesity, *Journal of the American Dietetic Association* 61 (1972): 385–390.

14. A. Mandenoff, F. Fumeron, and M. Apfelbaum, Endogenous opiates and energy balance, *Science* 215 (1982): 1536–1538.

15. J. Slochower and S. P. Kaplan, Anxiety, perceived control, and eating in obese and normal weight persons, *Appetite* 1 (1980): 75–83.

16. B. R. Bistrian, The medical treatment of obesity (editorial), *Archives of Internal Medicine* 141 (1981): 429–430.

17. K. H. Duncan, J. A. Bacon, and R. L. Weinsier, The effects of high and low energy density diets on satiety, energy

intake, and eating time of obese and nonobese subjects, *American Journal of Clinical Nutrition* 37 (1983): 763–767.

18. H. A. Jordan, L. S. Levitz, K. L. Utgoff, and H. L. Lee, Role of food characteristics in behavioral change and weight loss, *Journal of the American Dietetic Association* 79 (1981): 24–29.

19. R. B. Stuart and B. Davis, *Slim Chance in a Fat World: Behavioral Control of Obesity* (Champaign, Ill.: Research Press, 1972).

20. A. C. Sullivan, C. Nauss-Karol, and L. Cheng, Pharmacological treatment, in *Obesity,* ed. M. R. C. Greenwood (New York: Churchill Livingston, 1983), pp. 123–158.

21. Diet plans, *Consumer News,* February 1976.

22. G. W. Bo-Linn and coauthors, Starch blockers: Their effect on kcalorie absorption from a high-starch meal, *New England Journal of Medicine* 307 (1982): 1413–1416.

23. L. Sanders, But do they work? *Health,* September 1982, pp. 29, 52, 62.

24. A. S. Levine and J. E. Morley, The shortening pathways to appetite control, *Nutrition Today,* January–February 1983, pp. 6–14.

25. D. C. Fletcher, What is cellulite? (letter to the editor), *Journal of the American Medical Association* 235 (1976): 2773. The FDA concurs, in its leaflet: L. Fenner, Cellulite: Hard to budge pudge, HHS publication no. FDA 80–1078 (Washington, D.C.: Government Printing Office), reprint from *FDA Consumer,* May 1980.

26. A. E. Kark, Jaw wiring, *American Journal of Clinical Nutrition* 33, supplement no. 2 (February 1980): 420–424.

27. Questions doctors ask, *Nutrition and the MD,* June 1978.

bread exchanges—contribute any carbohydrate to the diet. Select the number of bread exchanges that will bring your total carbohydrate intake close to the amount you want. Adjust the numbers of these four exchanges until they seem reasonable to you.

Suggestions: Diets for adults should include two to three milk exchanges daily, two or more vegetable exchanges, and at least two and preferably more fruit exchanges. The number of bread exchanges is variable, but the bread list includes many nutritious foods containing complex carbohydrates. It is not unusual for women's diets to include four to six bread exchanges and for men's to include twice as many or even more. High-kcalorie diets can have many more of all of these carbohydrate-containing exchanges.

If you have a special fondness for sugar or sugar-containing foods, add a line to Form 6 under Bread, and allow yourself some "sugar exchanges" (see p. 76). At the end of this step, you should have a carbohydrate gram total within about 10 percent of the number you planned in step 3.

5. Subtotal the protein grams delivered by these four types of foods. Only one more list of foods—the meat exchanges—will contribute any protein to the diet. Select the number of meat exchanges you need to bring your total protein intake close to what you planned in step 3.

Note: The recommended intake of carbohydrate is high compared with what many people are used to. Planners often find that once they have completed step 4 of this procedure they have almost used up their protein allowance and must therefore drastically limit their consumption of meat exchanges. If it works out this way for you, you have two choices. You can accept the dictates of this pattern and resolve to limit your intake of meats and meat alternates accordingly. Or you can increase the number of protein

grams you will allow yourself (step 3) and reduce carbohydrate and/or fat to keep the kcalorie level within bounds.

At the end of this step, you should have a protein gram total that agrees (within 10 percent) with your plan of step 3.

6. Subtotal the fat grams delivered by these five categories of foods. Now use the fat exchanges to bring your total fat intake up to the level planned in step 3.

7. Fill in the kcalorie amounts contributed by the exchanges you have selected, and check to see that the total agrees (within 10 percent) with the kcalorie level you set in step 1. The completed form now indicates the total exchanges of each type that you will consume on each day of your diet.

8. Distribute the exchanges you have selected into a meal pattern like that on Form 7. You may want to plan four to six meals a day or to have only one snack; if so, or if you have other preferences, make your own form.

9. Finally, to see how your diet plan might work out on an actual day, make a sample menu. Look over the exchange lists and choose foods you would like to eat that fit the pattern you worked out in step 8. For example:

My meal pattern for breakfast specifies:

    1 fruit exchange.
    2 starch/bread exchanges.
    1 milk exchange.
    1 sugar exchange.
    1 fat exchange.

So I might choose:

    1/2 cup orange juice.
    3/4 ounce dry cereal and
    1 slice bread, toasted.
    1/2 cup milk on the cereal and
    1/2 cup milk in a glass.
    1 teaspoon sugar on the cereal.
    1 pat margarine on the toast.

Diet for Weight Loss

1. Set your daily kcalorie level. If you wish to lose a pound a week, set it 500

kcalories per day below your energy need (p. 245). You could set it higher or lower than this, but on no account should you set it below 1,000 kcalories per day unless your height is below average (see p. 264.).

2. Decide on the proportions in which protein, fat, and carbohydrate kcalories will be represented in the diet. A suggested ratio is that offered in Table 8–4: about 50 percent of the kcalories from carbohydrate, and 25 percent each from protein and fat.

3. Translate these kcalorie amounts into grams, as in the previous diet plan, and enter them and your kcalorie level into Form 6.

4. Now, using pencil on Form 6, decide on the number of carbohydrate-containing exchanges you'll have, as in step 4 of the first plan. Try to include two milk, two vegetable, and at least two fruit exchanges, and make up the rest of your carbohydrate intake with bread exchanges. Allow no sugar unless you really can't do without it. At the end of this step you should have a carbohydrate gram total within about 10 percent of the number you planned in step 3.

5. Now subtotal the protein grams you have so far, and bring your total protein intake up to the level of your plan by adding meat exchanges. At the end of this step, you should have a protein gram total that agrees (within 10 percent) with your plan of step 3.

6. Now subtotal the fat grams you have so far, and add fat exchanges to bring your total fat intake up to the level planned in step 3.

7. Fill in the kcalorie amounts contributed by the exchanges you have selected, and check to see that the total agrees (within 10 percent) with the kcalorie level you set in step 1.

8. Distribute the exchanges into a meal pattern, using Form 7 or your own form based on your own preferences.

9. Make a day's sample menus, as in step 9 of the first plan.

Eating Disorders and Society

Julie is 18 years old. She has always been a beautiful girl and a superachiever in school. She prides herself on her fine figure and watches her diet with great care. She exercises daily, maintaining a heroic schedule of self-discipline. She is thin, but she is not satisfied with her weight and is determined to lose more. She is 5 feet 6 inches tall and weighs 85 pounds. She has anorexia nervosa.

Julie is unaware that she is undernourished, and she sees no need to obtain treatment. But her friends and family have become concerned about her. She stopped menstruating (developed amenorrhea) several months ago and has become very moody. She insists that she is too fat, although her eyes lie in deep hollows in her face. She denies that she is ever tired, although she is obviously close to physical exhaustion. Her family is reluctant to push her, but has insisted that she see a psychiatrist. The psychiatrist has evaluated her case and has decided to hospitalize her. This step may save her life.

Anorexia Nervosa

The incidence of anorexia nervosa in our country and in other industrially advanced countries is steadily increasing. The disease now occurs in almost 1 of every 100 women.[1] Those who have studied it are convinced that the predisposition to it is inherited, and that our particular culture favors its development.[2] It is four to five times more common in identical than in nonidentical twins. People with anorexia nervosa often have a history of complications surrounding the time of their birth; they also have a higher birthweight and greater prevalence of obesity before they become anorexic than do people who never develop the disease. Nineteen out of 20 people with anorexia are young women, and the incidence is increasing.

A characteristic cluster of family and social circumstances often, though not always, surrounds the person with anorexia. Such a family is described as being dominated by the mother and values achievement and outward appearances more than an inner sense of self-worth and self-actualization. The young person values her parents' opinion highly and tries hard to please them, works hard, and shows a high degree of perfectionism. The parents cherish and indulge the child, so the intermeshing of needs is tight.

An absentee or distant father is often seen in the anorexic girl's family. Young women look to their male parents for important feedback on their self-worth, and when they don't receive it, tend to be oversensitive to negative cultural influences such as the drive for thinness and the view of emaciation as beautiful.[3] Julie's father has alcoholism, and her mother left him a year ago. Julie loves both parents and wants very much to please them. She identifies so strongly with their ideals and goals for her that she sometimes feels she has no identity of her own. She can't get in touch with her own feelings, and she sometimes feels like a robot. She earnestly desires to control her own destiny, but she feels controlled by others.

Anorexia resembles an addiction. The characteristic behavior is obsessive and compulsive, and often there are other addictions in the family, as exemplified by Julie's father's alcoholism. When Julie eats, she does so for external reasons. As a child, when she cried with hunger, her parents didn't respond by feeding her. Rather, they fed her on a rigid schedule. They forced food on her at times when she didn't want it, insisting that she eat it; and they withheld it when she was hungry, thus overriding her internal hunger signals. Julie lost the ability to detect her own hunger signals, and as she grew up, she became a person who felt she had to control her eating from outside as her parents had done.

As almost always happens, Julie began to develop anorexia within half a year after her menstrual periods started. Julie was distressed by the signs that she was turning into a woman and afraid of the changes that were taking place in her body. If she remained thin, she felt, she might escape being enveloped in a woman's body with hips, belly, and breasts—which frightened and revolted her. Julie's anorexia has tightened the bonds between herself and her mother, stabilizing her in a juvenile state and making it unnecessary for either of them to deal with the other problems that they face in their lives.

You may wonder how a person as thin as Julie could possibly continue to diet. Julie controls her food intake with tremendous discipline. She avoids carbohydrates and fats as if they were poison and eats strictly limited amounts of lean meat and low-kcalorie vegetables. She knows the number of kcalories per serving of dozens of different foods, and thinks and talks about food constantly. She cooks elaborate meals for her mother and her mother's friends, but she never partakes of them herself. If she feels that she has gained an ounce of weight, she runs or jumps rope until she is sure she has exercised it off. Her favorite sports are solitary sports; she doesn't participate in team sports. Once in a while she slips and eats more than she intends to, and when she has done that, she takes laxatives to hasten the exit of the food from her system. She is unaware that this doesn't work, because her other ways of staying thin are so effective. Her preoccupation with foods reveals that she is starving and is desperately hungry; the reason she doesn't eat is because of her fierce determination to achieve self-control, not because she isn't hungry.

When Julie looks at herself in the mirror, she sees herself as fat. The psychiatrist who tested her gave her a visual self-image test, and she drew a picture of herself that was grossly distorted. The psychiatrist took this as an index of the severity of her illness, knowing that the more she overestimated her body size, the more resistant she would be to treatment, and the more unwilling to examine her faulty values and misconceptions.[4] When asked to draw her best friend, Julie rendered an accurate image.

Physical abnormalities in anorexia nervosa include many hormonal aberrations. People with the disorder always have amenorrhea, and in 25 percent of cases, that symptom precedes the weight loss.[5] Young men with the disorder lose their sex drive and become impotent. To resume normal cycling, a female must gain body fat to at least 17 percent of her body weight. Sometimes it requires 22 percent fat content before periods may resume, and some never restart even after they have gained the weight. It isn't clear whether the hormonal change is first or whether stress precedes the hormonal change. Up to three out of every four women

in concentration camps and all women on death row have amenorrhea. The early teen years are a stressful time, and many teen girls may be uncertain about their own ability to fill the all-encompassing female role in modern society—as homemaker, wife, mother, lover, professional, natural beauty, etc. Roles are changing much more rapidly for females than males today and traditional guidelines no longer exist. The likely sequence in the development of anorexia nervosa is stress; then hormonal abnormalities; then food restriction, amenorrhea, and weight loss.[6]

Once the victim has undertaken her rigorous dieting routine, physical effects of starvation begin to set in. Thyroid hormone secretion becomes abnormal. Adrenal secretions, growth hormone, and blood pressure-regulating hormones also are abnormal. Heart function changes drastically. The heart pumps less efficiently, the muscle becomes weak and thin, the chambers diminish in size, and the blood pressure falls. Heart rhythms may change, with a characteristic abnormality appearing on the heart monitor. Sudden stopping of the heart, perhaps due to lean tissue loss and mineral deficiencies, accounts for many cases of sudden death among severely emaciated subjects.

The person with anorexia nervosa also has many abnormalities of immune function, but does not have more numerous infections than contemporaries. There may be anemia. As the person becomes thinner and thinner, abnormalities of the GI system also occur. Peristalsis becomes sluggish, and if the person eats too fast, the stomach becomes overfull, because it empties abnormally slowly. The lining of the digestive tract atrophies, and on eating food again the person may have diarrhea, because the system can't absorb nutrients well. The pancreas becomes unable to secrete many enzymes, as does the lining of the intestinal tract.

Other starvation effects include altered serum lipid levels, high concentrations of vitamin A and carotene in the blood, reduced blood proteins, an increased amount of fine body hair, skin dryness, and decreased skin and core temperatures. The electrical activity of the brain becomes abnormal, sleep is disturbed, and bad dreams are common. The person with anorexia nervosa may complain of never feeling rested.

Anorexia nervosa is hard to diagnose, because nearly everyone in our society is engaged in the "pursuit of thinness." Some women *without* weight loss meet all the criteria for the diagnosis of anorexia nervosa based on their eating attitudes and behaviors, as if they had a subclinical or premorbid disorder. Anorexia-like thought patterns are common among fashion models, long-distance runners, and dancers. Because our society favors thinness, it may even help a person who exhibits this behavior to obtain personal or vocational goals. Many young women, on learning of the disorder, state that they wish they had "a touch" of it, in order to get thin.

It takes a skilled clinician to make a diagnosis. Denial runs high among people with anorexia, and they deceive their families effectively. Usually, the clinician has to employ diagnostic tests to make a differential diagnosis using a scheme of comparisons between this disease and other similar ones. Table H8–1 shows the diagnostic criteria for anorexia nervosa.

Therapies for anorexia nervosa include insight-oriented therapy, cognitive behavior therapy, behavior modification, and family therapy. When they are compared, it is found that the therapy itself is not the key factor, but the spirit in which it is given: "The effectiveness of the [therapist]-patient interaction determines the outcome."[7]

Treatment is aimed at restoring adequate nutrition, avoiding medical complications, and altering the

TABLE H8–1

Diagnostic Criteria for Anorexia Nervosa

Intense fear of becoming obese, which does not diminish as weight loss progresses.
Disturbance of body image (example: claiming to "feel fat," even if emaciated).
Weight loss of at least 25% of original body weight. (If under 18 years of age, weight loss of at least 25% of original body weight plus projected weight gain expected from growth charts.)
Refusal to maintain body weight over a minimal normal weight for age and height.
No known physical illness that would account for the weight loss.

Source: American Psychiatric Association, *Diagnostic and Statistical Manual of Mental Disorders,* 3rd ed. (Washington, D.C.: American Psychiatric Association, 1980), p. 69.

psychological and environmental patterns that have supported or permitted the emergence of anorexia. Treatment programs of recent date have been more successful than in the past, and residential treatment centers specializing in eating disorders are often especially successful. Medical, psychiatric-psychological, and nutrition personnel are all needed and should work together as a team. The person who works most closely with the client should aim at four goals:

- To support her own feeling of autonomy—her feeling that she can control her own life, feel her own feelings, and choose her own behaviors.
- To earn her trust by being honest, acknowledging that the treatment for anorexia may be uncomfortable at first, and that for a while things may seem worse before they begin to get better; to acknowledge the client's feelings about this, too.
- To involve the family, so that they will not continue to reinforce maladaptive behavior, but will help the client gain weight by providing positive reinforcement.
- To make connections with other health-care agencies, depending on individual needs.

Some people have to go to the hospital. The malnutrition of anorexia nervosa can be so severe as to throw a person into severe electrolyte imbalance, create tremendous metabolic stress by way of infection, cause depression to the point of suicide, and even stop the heart. Programs that force-feed by tube have not been successful and in fact may traumatize and cause further harm. Even if they bring about weight gain, it is only temporary. Psychiatric hospitalization may be considered, but will benefit the person only if it is part of a more general treatment program.

Appropriate nutritional treatment is crucial. It need not be as aggressive as the remediation of malnutrition caused by other medical conditions, but it must be tailored to the client's needs. People with anorexia nervosa are usually younger than people with other medical conditions and are usually not ill with other diseases, so they are under less physical stress. Seldom are they willing to feed themselves, but if they are, chances are they can recover without other interventions. It is suggested that subjects be classed as being at low, intermediate, or high risk, depending on how they score on several indicators of protein-kcalorie malnutrition.* Low-risk people need nutritional counseling by a dietitian and psychological counseling

*Indicators of protein-kcalorie malnutrition: the percentage of body fat, serum albumin, serum transferrin, and immune reactions.

simultaneously. Intermediate-risk people may need nutritional supplements such as high-kcalorie, high-protein formulas besides ordinary meals but may not have to be hospitalized. The initial goal is to provide 250 to 500 kcalories above the daily energy requirement—about the maximum that most people are willing and able to accept. Drugs may be used to improve gastric motility and help people become able to tolerate larger meals. If the risk is high, then hospitalization is indicated, daily kcalorie supplementation may be greater, and tube feeding may have to be instituted. The hope is that the person will gain about 1 to 2 kilograms (2 to 4 pounds) a month. For a person who refuses to eat, forcible methods may be necessary to forestall death. These are in the hands of the physician and will not be described here. Drug therapies may be used as accompaniment.

Treatment outcomes are better than they used to be. Three-quarters of those in treatment may regain weight up to within 25 percent of the desired weight. Half to three-quarters may resume normal menstrual cycles. About two-thirds fail to eat normally on follow-up, but they may eat better than they did before. About 6 percent die, 1 percent by suicide.*

Social and family relationships may remain impaired. It seems that anorexia nervosa can adversely affect a person's social, psychological, and family functioning for life. Table H8–2 shows the factors that predict the degree of recovery from anorexia nervosa.

*This is from a review of 19 studies on about 1,000 clients over a five-year period. Other deaths are from infection; heart disease; lung disease; and iatrogenic causes including aspiration, electrolyte imbalance from intravenous therapy, and vitamin D poisoning. M. A. Balaa and D. A. Drossman, Anorexia Nervosa and Bulimia: The Eating Disorders, *Disease-a-Month* (Chicago: Year Book Medical Publishers, 1985), p. 34.

TABLE H8–2

Long-Term Prognostic Factors in Anorexia Nervosa

Good prognosis
  High educational achievement
  Early age at onset
  Good educational adjustment
  Improvement in body image after weight gain

Poor prognosis
  Late age at onset
  Continued overestimation of body size
  Premorbid obesity
  Self-induced vomiting or bulimia
  Laxative abuse
  Low social class
  Long duration of illness
  Disturbed parental relationship
  Male sex
  Marriage
  Marked depression, obsessional behavior, or somatic complaints

No effect on prognosis
  Premorbid personality type or psychological disturbance
  Hyperactivity
  Degree of weight loss
  Pharmacotherapy

Source: D. A. Drossman, D. A. Ontjes, and W. D. Heizer, Anorexia nervosa, *Gastroenterology* 77 (1979): 1115.

Bulimia

Bulimia is more common than anorexia nervosa, and more common in males. The possibility exists that only the reporting of bulimia is increasing, but the incidence seems to be rising. In any case, a survey of 300 middle- to upper-class suburban women shoppers in Boston taken in 1984 showed that over 10 percent reported a history of bulimia, and almost 5 percent were currently practicing it.[8] Among college women, the incidence may range anywhere from 5 to 20 percent.

Bulimia occurs in women of all ages, but is more common in those under 30 years old. Fewer than one-third discuss their eating difficulties with their doctors, and only 2.5 percent receive medical treatment. Only 5 percent of people with bulimia meet the criteria for anorexia nervosa, and fewer than 1 percent are actively anorexic. The case of Sophie will illustrate the plight of the person with bulimia.

Sophie is a charming, intelligent woman of normal weight who thinks constantly about food. She alternately starves herself and binges, and when she has eaten too much she vomits. Probably few people would fail to recognize these characteristics as the description of bulimia, for although the disease was recognized and named only in 1980, it has received much media attention. Until 1979 it was thought to be a variant of anorexia nervosa. Now

it is generally recognized as a separate entity. Diagnosis is not difficult, because no other diseases present similar symptoms (see Table H8–3).

Like the "typical" person with bulimia, Sophie is single, Caucasian, and in her early 20s. She is well educated and close to her ideal body weight. She binges periodically, and when she does so, it is in secret, usually at night, and lasts an hour or more. Sophie seldom lets binging interfere with her work or social activities, although a third of all bingers do; she is like most people with bulimia (60 percent), in that she starts the binge after having gone through a period of rigid dieting, so that her eating is accelerated by her hunger. Each time, she eats anywhere from one to many thousands of kcalories of food containing little fiber or water, smooth in texture, and high in sugar and fat, so that it is easy to consume vast amounts rapidly, with little chewing. Typically, she chooses cookies, cake, ice cream, or bread, although sometimes she binges on atypical foods—for example, vegetables—when she is dieting. After the binge, she pays the price of having swollen hands and feet, bloating, fatigue, headache, nausea, and pain.

The binge itself is not like normal eating. It is not primarily a response to hunger, apparently, and the food is not consumed for its nutritional value. It is a compulsion and usually occurs in several stages: "anticipation and planning, anxiety, urgency to begin, rapid and uncontrollable consumption of food, relief and relaxation, disappointment, and finally shame or disgust."[9]

As Sophie repeats and repeats this behavior, she faces more and more serious consequences, including medical ones. Fluid and electrolyte imbalance caused by vomiting can lead to abnormal heart rhythms and injury to the kidneys, which have to cope with the altered balance. Infections of the bladder and kidneys can lead to kidney

> If Lenny and my parents wouldn't give me any attention, I would turn to someone who could love me back. Food loved me back.
>
> Richard Simmons

TABLE H8–3

Diagnosis of Bulimia

Recurrent episodes of binge eating.
At least three of the following:
1. Consumption of high-kcaloric, easily ingested food during a binge.
2. Inconspicuous eating during a binge.
3. Termination of eating episodes by abdominal pain, sleep, social interruption, or self-induced vomiting.
4. Repeated attempts to lose weight by severely restrictive diets, self-induced vomiting, or use of cathartics or diuretics.
5. Frequent weight fluctuations greater than 10 pounds due to alternating binges and fasts.
Awareness that the eating pattern is abnormal and fear of not being able to stop eating voluntarily.
Depressed mood and self-deprecating thought following eating binges.
Bulimic episodes not due to anorexia nervosa or any known physical disorder.

Source: American Psychiatric Association, *Diagnostic and Statistical Manual of Mental Disorders*, 3rd ed. (Washington, D.C.: American Psychiatric Association, 1980), pp. 70–71.

failure. Vomiting causes irritation and infection of the pharynx, esophagus, and salivary glands; erosion of the teeth; and dental caries. The esophagus may rupture or tear, as may the stomach. Sometimes the eyes become red from pressure on vomiting. The hands may be bruised and lacerated from scraping on the teeth while inducing vomiting.

Some people use cathartics—violent laxatives that can injure the lower intestinal tract. Others use emetics to induce vomiting; it was these that caused the death of popular singer Karen Carpenter in 1983.

What makes a person become bulimic? Again Sophie is typical. From early in her childhood, she has been a high achiever, with a strong feeling of dependence on her parents. Her mother is a bright, well-educated woman who abandoned a promising career in order to stay home and raise the family; she has taught her children a high degree of respect for their father, who is a powerful but distant figure. Sophie experiences considerable social anxiety, and has difficulty in establishing personal relationships. She is sometimes depressed, and often exhibits impulsive behavior. Some people with bulimia

exhibit antisocial behavior, including drug abuse, kleptomania, and sexual promiscuity.

Unlike Julie, Sophie is aware of the consequences of her behavior, feels that it is abnormal, and is deeply ashamed of it. She feels inadequate, unable even to control her eating, and so she tends to be passive and to look to men for confirmation of her sense of worth. When rejected, either in reality or in her imagination, her bulimia becomes worse; in fact, many women point to real or imagined male rejection as the event that triggered the first big diet and subsequently the first binge.[10] If Sophie gets carried away by bulimia, she may not only experience a deepening of her depression, but may move on to drug or alcohol abuse.

A food-centered society that favors thinness in women puts a woman in a bind. Bulimia has been described as socially sanctioned and almost required among upper-class women who must attend many dinners and cocktail parties. Typically, they have been raised in families that encouraged hearty eating, and there is much socializing around the dinner table. Food is always involved in celebrations and also is used to console the family during periods of

mourning. When a child raised in such a setting is also made socially conscious and is told she must become thin, she may perceive that she has little alternative but to celebrate or mourn with the family; indulge in vast quantities of food; and then vomit, crash diet, or fast to "undo" her possible weight gain.

Bulimia is in many respects easier to treat than anorexia nervosa, because it seems to be more of a chosen behavior. People with bulimia know that their behavior is abnormal, and many are willing to try to cooperate. A number of approaches have been described, but little study has shown, yet, which might be most effective. It is suggested that the most important goal is to help the person gain control over binge-eating—a task more easily assigned than carried out, since the trigger that starts the binge has not been identified. Warning signs are times of family stress, and especially times of real or perceived rejection. One strategy is obvious: since most binges begin after a round of strict dieting, the person needs to learn to eat a quantity of nutritious food sufficient to nourish her body and leave her satisfied without bringing on the anathema of weight gain. Such an approach has been used successfully in the treatment of many people with severe bulimia; it requires that they eat no less than 1,500 kcalories a day.[11]

Drug therapy may accompany psychotherapy for bulimia. Almost 90 percent of people with bulimia are clinically depressed, and about half have a biochemical abnormality not otherwise seen except in severe undernutrition, although their body weights are near normal.* Antidepressant medication doesn't help them all, but is indicated and useful for some.

*The abnormality referred to is an abnormal dexamethasone suppression test. Balaa and Drossman, 1985.

Long-term follow-up studies remain to be undertaken. It isn't clear what becomes of people with bulimia in later life. Possibly, there are roughly three categories: college students who engage in the disorder briefly and then recover; binge/vomiters who also begin during college and who require more intensive therapy and hospitalization; and older people who have chronic and stable bulimia and whose binge-eating and vomiting patterns are regular and established. These people might be said to be socially adjusted, in a way, because their behavior fits in with their other activities.

Eating Disorders and Society

Both anorexia nervosa and bulimia are relatively new diseases. Anorexia nervosa was first described 100 years ago; bulimia was first defined as a medical disorder only in 1980. Both are known only in developed nations and become more prevalent as wealth increases. Some people point to the vomitoriums of ancient peoples and claim that bulimia is nothing new, but the two are actually quite distinct. The ancient people were eating for pleasure, without guilt, and in the company of others; they vomited so that they could rejoin the feast. Bulimia is a disease of isolation and is always accompanied by self-hate and low self-esteem. The causes of both bulimia and anorexia nervosa are unknown, but one school of thought labels them social problems. The common negative experiences that lead privileged young women to self-destructive eating patterns include the internalization of a message of their own low worth, and the idealizing of some unachievable, "perfect" image.

If asked today, Julie might describe herself as proud of her achievements in dieting, eager to achieve more, and resentful of her confinement in the hospital. She has, after all, made significant progress toward achieving society's goal for her—to be thin.

Sophie, on the other hand, would describe herself as unhappy, because she has failed to control her eating. She is longing for the time when she'll be happy—that is, when she's thin. It's not uncommon in our society for some women to develop a kind of Cinderella complex—to hide behind obstacles, real or imaginary, waiting and hoping for some event or some person to "bring them happiness." The reasoning goes like this: "I'll be happy when someone marries me (or when I have more money, a house, a child). I can't find someone to marry me until I meet him/her. I can't meet new people because I'm shy. People reject me because I'm too fat (not beautiful, too thin, too poor, too short, too tall). Someday my problems will go away, someone will marry me, and *then* I'll be happy." Caught in a trap of her own making, waiting for a preconceived stamp of approval from outside herself, such a person can't grow, and through stagnation and a negative attitude, she may repel the very people with whom she could otherwise share life's enjoyments.

At so tender an age as 12 years, beautifully growing, normal-weight female youngsters are already worried that they are too fat. Most are "on diets." Magazines, newspapers, and television all present two-dimensional, contrived, camera-ready women, flaws concealed, unreasonably thin, worthy only so long as they are lovely to look at; these are perceived as ideal. The message is clear—only with *this* kind of body are you acceptable. The way you are isn't good enough. You should become like the cover girl who doesn't sweat; doesn't grow hair on her slender legs; has firm, small breasts, a flat stomach, a perfect face, small feet; and is always perfectly happy. If *you*, young woman, are not perfectly happy, it is because your body is not beautiful enough. Anorexia nervosa and bulimia are not a form of rebellion against such unreasonable expectations, but rather the exaggerated acceptance of them.

Slowly, society is changing. Recognition of the success and desirability of a growing number of outstanding women in such traditionally male-dominated fields as athletics, science, law, and politics has raised women's collective self-esteem. Perhaps anorexia nervosa and bulimia are diseases of society in transition, and they may once again become unknown to medical literature as feminine roles and ideals change. Prevention may be most effective if begun very early in children's lives. Warnings to children that the Madison Avenue female figure is simply an advertising gimmick designed to sell products, and not an

Miniglossary

anorexia nervosa: a disorder seen (usually) in teenage girls, involving self-starvation to the extreme.
an = without
orex = mouth
nervos = of nervous origin
bulimia (alternative spelling **bulemia**) (byoo-LEEM-ee-uh): recurring binge eating. Some people call this **bulimarexia** (byoo-lee-ma-REX-ee-uh); others reserve the latter term for bulimia with emaciation probably caused by purging after binging.
buli = ox
orex = mouth
cathartic: a strong laxative.
emetic (em-ETT-ic): a agent that causes vomiting.
purgative: see *cathartic*.

ideal with which to compare one's own living body, may be of some help. The simple concept—to respect and value your own uniqueness—may be lifesaving for a future generation.

Deep inside there had always been a small child begging for my attention. . . . All I gave her was food. Now I give her love.

Eda LeShan

NOTES:
1. M. A. Balaa and D. A. Drossman, Anorexia Nervosa and Bulimia: The Eating Disorders, *Disease a Month*, (Chicago: Year Book Medical Publishers June 1985), pp. 1–52.
2. Balaa and Drossman, 1985, p. 12.
3. K. McCleary, Eating disorders: Daddy Dearest, *American Health*, January–February 1986, p. 86.
4. H. Bruch, Anorexia nervosa, *Nutrition Today*, September–October 1978, pp. 14–18.
5. Balaa and Drossman, 1985, p. 10.
6. Balaa and Drossman, 1985, p. 20.
7. Balaa and Drossman, 1985, p. 33.
8. H. G. Pope, Jr., J. I. Hudson, and D. Yurgelun-Todd, Anorexia nervosa and bulimia among 300 suburban women shoppers, *American Journal of Psychiatry* 141 (1984): 2, as cited by Balaa and Drossman, 1985.
9. Balaa and Drossman, 1985, p. 38.
10. M. Baskind-Lodahl and J. Sirlin, The gorging-purging syndrome: Bulimarexia, *Psychology Today,* March 1977, pp. 50–52, 82, 85.
11. S. Dalvit-McPhillips, A dietary approach to bulimia treatment, *Physiology and Behavior* 33 (1984): 769–775.

The Water-Soluble Vitamins: B Vitamins and Vitamin C

9

Contents

Collagen—made with the help of vitamin C—is the body's major connective material. Here, strands of collagen lie tangled near a muscle fiber membrane disrupted by freezing and chemical etching.

The B vitamins and vitamin C are entitled to individual attention, but the whole array of them is presented here first to show you the "forest" in which they are the trees. They come together in foods, they work together in the body, and there is much to be learned from viewing them as a group.

First of all, together with vitamin C, the B vitamins form a natural group of nutrients known as the water-soluble vitamins. They got their names from the labels *B* and *C* on the test tubes into which they were first collected. Later, test tube B turned out to have more than one vitamin in it; the fractions were given subscripts (B_1, B_2, and so on); and later still, most of them received names.

The water-soluble vitamins are present in the watery compartment of foods, and they are distributed into the water-filled compartments of the body. Most of them, except for vitamin B_{12}, can easily be excreted in the urine if their blood concentration rises too high—in contrast to the fat-soluble vitamins, which tend to be tucked away in storage places. As a consequence, the water-soluble vitamins become deficient more readily, but are also less likely to reach toxic levels than the fat-soluble vitamins. People have been known to overdose on all of them, and to suffer toxicity symptoms, but it's not so easy to do.

The B vitamin riboflavin is a yellow compound so bright that it is easy to see in a water solution. Since excesses of the B vitamins are excreted, bright yellow urine may signify the presence of this vitamin. If you are in the habit of taking a multivitamin supplement "to avoid deficiencies" and your diet is otherwise adequate in riboflavin, you may notice this effect. In fact, the extra dose will do nothing for you but increase the loss of dollars in your urine.

In summary, the water-soluble vitamins are, for the most part, carried in the bloodstream, excreted in urine, needed in frequent small doses, and unlikely to be toxic, except when taken in very large quantities. Exceptions occur, but these generalizations are worth remembering.

Vitamin ads would have you believe that vitamins also give you energy. They don't—and they are the first of the nutrients discussed in this book that don't. The energy nutrients, which we have dealt with up to now, can be used as fuel, but the vitamins only help to burn that fuel; they do not serve as fuel themselves. If you tried to live only on water and vitamins, you would quickly become a wreck.

It is true, though, that without B vitamins you would lack energy. Some of the B vitamins serve as helpers to the enzymes that release energy from carbohydrate, fat, and protein; they stand alongside the metabolic pathways, so to speak, and help to keep the disassembly lines moving. In an industrial plant they would be called expediters. Other B vitamins help cells to multiply, and this is especially important in populations of cells with short life spans that must replace themselves rapidly. Such are the red blood cells, and the cells lining the GI tract—both key members of the team of cells that deliver energy to all the body's tissues.

The B Vitamins: Coenzymes

Each B vitamin plays several roles in metabolism; the roles they play as coenzymes are the best understood. Coenzymes are small nonprotein molecules that associate closely with enzymes. Some coenzymes form part of the enzyme structure, in which case they are known as prosthetic groups; others are associated more loosely with the enzyme. Some participate in the reaction being performed and are chemically altered in the process, but they are always regenerated sooner or later. Others are unaltered but form part of the active site of the enzyme. There are differences in details, but one thing is true of all. Without the coenzymes, the enzymes cannot function.

The consequences of a failure of metabolic enzymes can be catastrophic, as you will realize if you study the pathways of metabolism depicted in Figure 9–1. The abbreviations for some of the coenzymes that keep the processes going

coenzyme (co-EN-zime): a small molecule that works with an enzyme to promote the enzyme's activity. Many coenzymes have B vitamins as part of their structure.
co — with

prosthetic (pros-THET-ic) **group**: a coenzyme that is physically part of (attached to) its enzyme.
prosth = in addition to

An enzyme before attachment of its coenzyme or prosthetic group, is a nonfunctional **apoenzyme** (APE-oh-enzyme). With the coenzyme or prosthetic group attached, it becomes the active holoenzyme (HOLE-oh-enzyme).
apo = detached
holo = whole

active site: that part of the enzyme surface on which the reaction takes place.

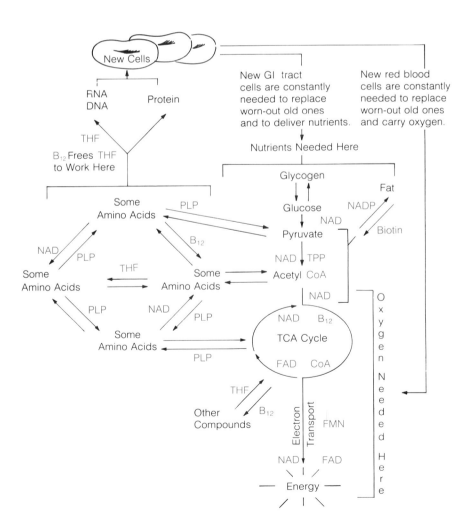

FIGURE 9–1.

Some metabolic pathways and the coenzymes that facilitate the reactions (schematic). For further details, see Appendix C.

TABLE 9–1

Names and Roles of the B Vitamins

Vitamin Name	Coenzyme Form	Enzymes Assisted	Other Roles
Thiamin (vitamin B_1)	Thiamin pyrophosphate (TPP).	Pyruvate decarboxylase; alpha-keto acid decarboxylases; transketolases; aldehyde transferases.	As thymidine triphosphate (TTP) or TPP, occupies a site on the nerve cell membrane that either is or is adjacent to a sodium channel.
Riboflavin (vitamin B_2)	Flavin mononucleotide (FMN) and flavin adenine dinucleotide (FAD); also a prosthetic group on some enzymes.	Enzymes involved in TCA cycle and electron transport: dehydrogenases, oxidases, and reductases.	
Vitamin B_6 (pyridoxal, pyridoxine, pyridoxamine)	The phosphate forms of these: pyridoxal phosphate (PLP) and pyridoxamine phosphate (PMP).	60 enzymes, including transaminases, racemases, decarboxylases, cleavage enzymes, synthetases, dehydrases, and desulfhydrases.	
Niacin (nicotinic acid, nicotinamide, niacinamide, vitamin B_3)	Nicotinamide adenine dinucleotide (NAD) and the phosphate form (NADP).	Dehydrogenases in metabolism of fat, carbohydrate, and amino acids; other dehydrogenases; enzymes involved in synthesis of fats and steroids.	A bond in NAD breaks to provide energy for DNA repair. Nicotinic acid may be a component of the glucose tolerance factor (Chapter 12).
Folacin (folic acid or folate, also known as pteroylglutamic acid)	Dihydro and tetrahydro forms of folate (DHF and THF) and polyglutamate forms of the folates (that is, folates with numbers of glutamates attached); THF is the carrier of one-carbon units.	Enzymes that move one-carbon units at different levels of oxidation from place to place. These one-carbon units arise primarily from metabolism of amino acids and are used to interconvert amino acids and to synthesize purines and pyrimidines needed to make new RNA and DNA preparatory to cell division.	

TABLE 9–1

(continued)

Vitamin Name	Coenzyme Form	Enzymes Assisted	Other Roles
Vitamin B$_{12}$ (cobalamin and related forms)	Methylcobalamin and coenzyme B$_{12}$ (deoxyadenosyl-cobalamin).	The enzyme that removes a methyl group from methyl folate, regenerating THF; the enzyme that converts a precursor (homocysteine) to the amino acid methionine; an enzyme in the TCA cycle.	
Biotin	Becomes attached to enzyme. First, converted to biotinyl adenylate; this condenses with apoenzyme to form holoenzyme. The reaction is mediated by another enzyme, holoenzyme synthetase.	Carboxylases (including one that converts acetyl CoA to a precursor of cholesterol); transcarboxylases; decarboxylases.	
Pantothenic acid	Coenzyme A and others.	Condensing enzymes, addition enzymes, transferases, and others. Example: the enzyme that converts pyruvate to acetyl CoA.	

are shown in the figure; the vitamins and their coenzyme names are given in Table 9–1.

Look at the first step in the now-familiar pathway of glucose breakdown. Some of the enzymes involved in the breakdown of glucose to pyruvate require the coenzyme NAD. Part of this molecule is a structure the body cannot make. Hence it must be obtained from the diet; it is an essential nutrient (Chapter 1). This essential part is the B vitamin niacin. The way NAD works is shown in Figure 9–2.

In other words, to take glucose apart the cells must have certain enzymes. For the enzymes to work, they must have the coenzyme NAD. To make NAD, the cells must be supplied with niacin (or a closely related compound they can alter to make niacin). The rest of the coenzyme they can make without outside help.

The next step in glucose catabolism is the breakdown of pyruvate to acetyl CoA. The enzymes involved in this step require NAD plus another coenzyme, TPP. The cells can manufacture the TPP they need from thiamin, but thiamin

niacin (NIGH-a-sin): a B vitamin. Niacin can be eaten preformed or can be made in the body from its precursor, tryptophan, one of the amino acids (see pp. 145). The active coenzyme forms are NAD and NADP (see Table 9–1).

thiamin (THIGH-uh-min): a B vitamin. The coenzyme form is TPP (see Table 9–1).

FIGURE 9–2.

Coenzyme action. Each coenzyme is specialized for certain kinds of chemical reactions. NAD⁺ (containing niacin), for example, can accept hydrogen atoms removed from other compounds and can lose them to compounds that ultimately pass them to oxygen. In many steps during the catabolism of glucose, hydrogens are removed and NAD⁺ participates this way. A model of the way NAD⁺ works with an enzyme to remove hydrogens is shown here.

A. An enzyme with coenzyme NAD⁺ encounters a molecule containing two hydrogens.

B. A complex is formed.

C. The hydrogens are removed from the molecule and attached to NAD⁺, forming NADH + H⁺. The enzyme releases NADH + H⁺ and the molecule.

D. Later the NADH + H⁺ donates the hydrogens to another compound and returns to its enzyme again as NAD⁺.

pantothenic (PAN-to-THEN-ic) **acid**: a B vitamin. The principal active form is coenzyme A, called "CoA" throughout Chapter 7. See Table 9–1.

biotin (BY-oh-tin): a B vitamin, which forms a prosthetic group on the enzymes it works with.

riboflavin (RIBE-o-flay-vin): a B vitamin. The coenzyme forms are FMN and FAD (see Table 9–1).

vitamin B₆: a family of compounds— pyridoxine, pyridoxal, and pyridoxamine. The active forms are PLP and PMP (see Table 9–1).

folacin: (FOLL-a-sin): a B vitamin. The chief coenzyme form is THF.

is a compound they cannot synthesize, so it must be supplied in the diet. Thiamin is the vitamin part of the coenzyme TPP.

Another coenzyme needed for this step is coenzyme A, or CoA for short. As you have probably guessed, the cells can make CoA except for an essential part of it that must be obtained in the diet. This essential part—the vitamin part—is pantothenic acid. Still another coenzyme, biotin, forms part of the enzyme complex involved in converting pyruvate to acetyl CoA; that is, it is a prosthetic group on the enzyme.

These and other coenzymes are involved throughout all the metabolic pathways. FAD, needed in the TCA cycle, is synthesized in the body, but part of its structure, the vitamin riboflavin, must be obtained in the diet. PLP is required for a multitude of interconversions of amino acids, a crucial step in the making of the iron-containing portion of hemoglobin for red blood cells, and many other reactions; it is made from vitamin B₆. THF, made from the vitamin folacin, is required for the synthesis of new genetic material and therefore new cells.

$$
\begin{array}{ccc}
\text{H} & & \\
| & & \\
\text{H-C-O-H} & \text{H-C=O} & \text{H-C=O} \\
| & | & | \\
\text{H} & \text{H} & \text{O-H} \\
\text{Methanol} & \text{Formaldehyde} & \text{Formic acid}
\end{array}
$$

These are three one-carbon compounds, each more oxidized (having fewer hydrogens or more oxygens) than the one before. The folate coenzymes can carry all of them. The folate coenzymes are versatile enough to do this because they can exist at three different levels of oxidation. Their three forms are folate, dihydrofolate (which has two more hydrogens than folate), and tetrahydrofolate (which has four more hydrogens than folate). See Appendix C.

The vitamin B_{12} coenzyme, in turn, has to free THF from a chemical form in which it tends to get stuck, so vitamin B_{12} is also necessary for the formation of new cells. Thus every coenzyme is involved, directly or indirectly, in energy metabolism. Some are facilitators of the energy-releasing reactions themselves; others help build new cells to deliver oxygen and nutrients, which permit the energy pathways to run.

Now suppose the body's cells lack one of these B vitamins—niacin, for example. Without niacin, the cells cannot make NAD. Without NAD, the enzymes involved in every step of the glucose-to-energy pathway will fail to function. Since it is from these steps that energy is made available for all the body's activities, everything will begin to grind to a halt. This is no exaggeration. The deadly disease pellagra, caused by niacin deficiency, produces the devastating "four Ds": dermatitis, which reflects a failure of the skin to maintain itself; dementia (insanity), a failure of the nervous system; diarrhea, a failure of digestion and absorption; and death. These are only the most obvious, observable consequences of deficiency; it affects every organ in the body, because all are dependent on the energy pathways. As you can see, niacin is like the horseshoe nail for want of which a war was lost. All the vitamins are like such horseshoe nails.

In summary, these eight B vitamins play many specific roles in helping the enzymes to perform thousands of different molecular conversions in the body. They are active in carbohydrate, fat, and protein metabolism and in the making of DNA and thus new cells. They are found in every cell and must be present continuously for the cells to function as they should.

Metabolism, Assessment, and Interdependence

In 1937, the coenzyme form of thiamin was first discovered and isolated. Since then, the world of vitamins and enzyme action has opened up, revealing its intricacies, and permitting medicine and science to put vitamins and enzymes to use in a multitude of ways. The examples that follow are selected to illustrate three principles. First, once the precise action of a nutrient is known, it becomes possible to test for its presence by measuring that action. Second, the nutrients are interdependent; they affect each other's absorption, metabolism, and excretion, so that an apparent deficiency of one may reflect a deficiency or abnormality in the action of another. Third, the nutrients are small molecules, and drugs are, too; drugs often get into the same spots where the nutrients are acting and interfere with those actions, changing nutrient requirements.

To provide all the details now known about the absorption, metabolism, and interrelationships of the B vitamins would require more pages than remain in this book and would burden the reader with specialized knowledge beyond the level appropriate for the beginning study of nutrition. But to omit them all would be to deprive the reader, leaving the curtains closed on a colorful and dramatic theater of action that fascinates its audience. A compromise is attempted here: a few illustrative examples, a sneak peek at the scene in which nutritional biochemists spend their days.

Thiamin's coenzyme, TPP, helps break down pyruvate to acetyl CoA, as already mentioned. The step involves transferring a keto group to oxygen. TPP can also help enzymes transfer keto groups to other compounds; such enzymes

vitamin B_{12}: a B vitamin. Its active form is coenzyme B_{12}.

For want of a nail, a horseshoe was lost.
For want of a horseshoe, a horse was lost.
For want of a horse, a soldier was lost.
For want of a soldier, a battle was lost.
For want of a battle, the war was lost,
And all for the want of a horseshoe nail!
Mother Goose

The dermatitis of pellagra. The skin darkens and flakes away as if it were sunburned. In kwashiorkor there is also a "flaky paint" dermatitis, but the two are easily distinguishable. The dermatitis of pellagra is bilateral and symmetrical, and occurs only on those parts of the body exposed to the sun.

When a drug displaces a vitamin from its site of action, it renders the vitamin ineffective. The drug is then said to be acting as a vitamin **antagonist.**

are known as transketolases. One such enzyme is active in the red blood cells: erythrocyte transketolase.*

Blood is easy to sample and to work with in the laboratory, so it is logical to use a test of erythrocyte transketolase to see if thiamin's coenzyme is present and doing its job. The cells in a test tube are given the starting material, an alpha-keto acid, and the rate of its disappearance or the rate of appearance of the product is measured. (A control, in which the enzyme is working as expected, is run simultaneously to provide a standard for comparison.) If the enzyme is fully equipped with all the TPP it needs, it will work at the maximal rate. If it works slowly, then a thiamin deficiency is suspected. The clincher is to add TPP to the test tube: if the reaction rate speeds up, then this is good evidence that a deficiency did, indeed, exist. Erythrocyte transketolase activity has proven to be a practical test for the diagnosis of thiamin deficiency.

If a deficiency is found, the clinician still has to determine whether it is primary (inadequate intake) or secondary (impaired absorption or metabolism, or excessive excretion). The intestine absorbs thiamin passively unless the concentration is low; then it calls into play an active transport process that requires sodium and ATP. Several enzymes are involved: one splits the ATP to obtain its energy to transport the thiamin across the intestinal wall; another adds phosphate after the thiamin has arrived, making it into TPP. Lack of sodium, any antacid, any disease that disturbs the structures in the intestinal wall, or any drug that interferes with the actions of the needed enzymes can impair thiamin absorption. The effect of antacids points to the need for moderation in their use (and suggests one reason why they should not be used as calcium supplements, a subject discussed further in Chapter 11). Folacin is known to be involved in thiamin absorption, although the exact site of action is not known.[1] A folacin deficiency therefore causes a thiamin deficiency, and even thiamin supplements don't correct it until after the folacin deficiency has been corrected.

Riboflavin's coenzyme roles are listed in Table 9–1; an enzyme in the red blood cells can be used to assess its activity. Like thiamin at low concentrations, riboflavin is absorbed by active transport, and once it is inside the cells of the small intestine, it receives a phosphate group to keep it there. It travels in the blood bound to a protein of its own, and its metabolism is affected by many hormones and drugs. The enzymes it assists are needed for the metabolism of many other nutrients. Its role in the TCA cycle has already been mentioned; it is also required for the metabolism of vitamin B_6, folacin, niacin, and vitamin K.[2] Thus deficiency of riboflavin is invariably tangled up with deficiencies of other nutrients.

Vitamin B_6 and its coenzyme forms all occur in foods. They interconvert freely in the intestine and in the cells, and any of them can be absorbed, transported, and conveyed into cells without a special carrier. Once they are inside, the cells can hold them there by adding phosphate groups to them. In the cells, large amounts bind to various proteins, but attempts to use these proteins as a

Assessment test for thiamin status: erythrocyte transketolase activity.

Assessment test for riboflavin status: erythrocyte glutathione reductase activity.

---

*The step from pyruvate to acetyl CoA involves removal of a carbon with its associated oxygen (a keto group) and adding them to another oxygen to form carbon dioxide; it is known as *oxidative decarboxylation*. TPP can help catalyze this reaction with any organic acid that has a keto group in the position right next to its terminal carbon (the alpha position); thus chemists name TPP's exact specialty the oxidative decarboxylation of *alpha-keto acids*. Enzymes that transfer keto groups are known as *decarboxylases* or *transketolases*.

There are two things the reader of details like this can do with them. One is to simply learn the details. The other is to obtain meaning or significance from them. The purpose of presenting these details is to lay the groundwork for several statements of their significance to consumers. Assessment of vitamin status is possible, using specific and accurate techniques. It is also difficult and complicated. It seems worthwhile to provide enough detail to make this apparent, because much misunderstanding and misinformation surrounds the evaluation of people's vitamin status. This is particularly important with vitamin B$_6$, as this chapter's first Highlight makes clear. To self-diagnose, or to be misdiagnosed, with a vitamin B$_6$ deficiency can prove hazardous to health. A person who wants a nutrition assessment should take care to have it performed correctly.

means of assessing vitamin B$_6$ status have met with frustration. Test results are confounded by the subjects' hormonal state, the tests are difficult and expensive to perform, and the results don't seem to reflect reliably body stores of the vitamin.

Among the many drugs that interact with vitamin B$_6$, alcohol stands out. When the body breaks down alcohol, it first produces acetaldehyde, a toxic compound that must quickly be broken down further. Acetaldehyde knocks PLP loose from its enzymes; once loose, PLP breaks down to an excretion product; then the kidneys dispose of it. Thus alcohol actively promotes the destruction of vitamin B$_6$ and its loss from the body.

Another drug that acts as a vitamin B$_6$ antagonist is INH, a potent inhibitor of the growth of the tuberculosis bacterium.* INH has saved countless lives, but as a vitamin B$_6$ antagonist, it binds and inactivates the vitamin, inducing a deficiency. Whenever INH is used to treat tuberculosis, supplements of vitamin B$_6$ must be given to protect the client from deficiency.

Niacin and its amide are freely absorbed from food, converted easily in all tissues to their coenzyme forms, used in multitudinous reactions, and converted to other compounds for excretion in urine. Assessment of niacin status is usually based on measurement of these breakdown products after the administration of a test dose of niacinamide; the less niacin that is excreted, the more the body must have needed, and the greater the deficiency must have been.

Large doses of nicotinic acid and nicotinamide act like drugs in the nervous system, and on blood lipids and blood glucose. A careful review of the evidence shows that, despite hope to the contrary, the vitamin does not help cure schizophrenia or learning disorders in children.[3]

Nicotinic acid in large doses has been found to raise HDL in some people, and this has given hope that it might be useful to help prevent atherosclerosis. Unfortunately, the HDL increase arises not from an increase in the making of HDL, but from a reduction in their breakdown, and it doesn't seem to reduce mortality from heart disease. Meanwhile, high doses of nicotinic acid may injure

Tests for vitamin B$_6$ nutriture: The tryptophan load test involves feeding an overload of the amino acid tryptophan, which requires vitamin B$_6$ for disposal, and then measuring the rate of disappearance of tryptophan from the blood or its excretion in the urine. The measurement of PLP in serum involves creating a test solution using a PLP-dependent apoenzyme and adding a sample of the subject's blood. The more PLP there is in the blood, the faster the enzyme will work.

Assessment test for niacin status: urinary metabolites NMN (N-methyl nicotinamide) or 2-pyridone, or preferably both.

When a normal dose of a nutrient clears up a deficiency condition and gives rise to a normal blood concentration, the nutrient is having a **physiological effect.** When a megadose (100 times larger than normal) overwhelms some system and acts like a drug, the nutrient is having a **pharmacological effect.**

*INH stands for isonicotinic acid hydrazide.

the liver, cause peptic ulcer, and produce lab evidence of diabetes, so self-dosing would seem ill-advised.[4]

Folacin occurs in foods mostly with many glutamates attached (the polyglutamate form described in Table 9–1). The intestine prefers to absorb the folacin with only one glutamate attached (the monoglutamate form), sometimes with a methyl group attached. Enzymes on the surfaces of the intestinal cells hydrolyze the polyglutamate and then may attach the methyl group; special transport systems take up either form (the monoglutamate with and without a methyl group); and then both forms travel freely in the blood. The liver absorbs most of them, and treats the two forms in different ways. To the plain monoglutamate, it adds additional glutamates, thus converting it into the polyglutamate form for storage. As for the methyl form, the liver secretes most of it into bile, and ships it to the gallbladder, whence it returns to the intestine again—an enterohepatic circulation route like that of bile itself. Should the methyl folate be needed within the body, the methyl group would have to be removed—and the enzyme that removes it requires another B vitamin as a coenzyme: vitamin B_{12}, to be discussed next.

The cells of organs other than the liver also absorb the monoglutamate form of folate and add glutamates to it to keep it from escaping. They hydrolyze it back to the monoglutamate to release it again.

This complicated transportation and conversion system for the folates is vulnerable to interference from a number of sources. For one thing, since one form of folacin is actively secreted back into the intestinal tract with bile, it has to be reabsorbed repeatedly. If it is not—if something interferes with absorption, such as injury to the GI tract cells—then folacin will be rapidly lost from the body. Such is the case in the person whose GI tract is injured by alcohol abuse; folacin deficiency rapidly develops and, ironically, impairs the GI tract further. The folacin coenzymes, remember, are active in cell multiplication—and the cells lining the GI tract are among the most rapidly multiplying cells in the body. Without the ability to make new cells, the tract rapidly deteriorates, and not only loses folacin more rapidly, but also fails to absorb other nutrients. The replacement of blood cells also falters in a folacin deficiency, because it, too, requires rapid cell multiplication; hence the resulting anemia.

Knowledge of these details permits assessment of folate status. To obtain accurate information, three lab tests are necessary. One measures free folate in the blood; the second measures folacin in the red blood cells (which reflects the amount stored in the liver); and the third checks on vitamin B_{12} status—because without enough vitamin B_{12}, folacin can be trapped inside of tissue cells.[5]

Vitamin B_{12} requires an "intrinsic factor"—a compound made inside the body—for absorption from the intestinal tract into the bloodstream. The design for this factor is carried in the genes. The intrinsic factor is synthesized in the stomach, where it attaches to the vitamin; the complex then passes to the small intestine and is gradually absorbed.

Certain people have in their genetic makeup a gene for the intrinsic factor that becomes defective, usually in midlife. Without the intrinsic factor, they can't absorb the vitamin even though they are taking enough in their diets, and so they develop deficiency symptoms. In such a case, or when the stomach has been injured and cannot produce enough of the intrinsic factor, vitamin B_{12} must be supplied to the body by injection to bypass the block in the intestinal

Assessment tests for folate status: free folate, erythrocyte folate, and vitamin B_{12} status.

intrinsic: inside the system. The intrinsic factor is a glycoprotein made in the stomach that aids in the absorption of vitamin B_{12}.

glycoprotein: a protein with sugar (glucose) molecules attached.

tract. The vitamin B_{12} deficiency caused by lack of intrinsic factor is known as pernicious anemia.

One of the most obvious vitamin B_{12}–deficiency symptoms is the anemia of folacin deficiency, characterized by large, immature red blood cells. (Vitamin B_{12}, remember, is needed to free folacin; without it, folacin can't help manufacture red blood cells.) Either vitamin B_{12} or folacin will clear up this condition. However, vitamin B_{12} also functions in maintaining the sheath that surrounds and protects nerve fibers and in promoting their normal growth, as well as in producing mature red blood cells. Thus a deficiency of vitamin B_{12} causes not only anemia, but also a creeping paralysis of the nerves and muscles, which begins at the extremities and works inward and up the spine. This symptom is not detectable from a blood test, and the paralysis cannot be remedied by administering folacin. Early detection and correction are necessary to prevent permanent nerve damage and paralysis.

Assessing vitamin B_{12} status is not simple. A preferred test is to measure the amount of DNA made by blood cells from raw material presented to them in a test tube in the presence and absence of vitamin B_{12} added from outside. The greater the difference the added vitamin makes, the more deficient the cells must have been to begin with.[6]

These examples, using the six best-known B vitamins, illustrate the depth of knowledge that has been gained about the B vitamins in the last half century. Additional details about them, and also about biotin and pantothenic acid, appear in Table 9–1.

pernicious anemia: vitamin B_{12} deficiency caused by lack of intrinsic factor.
pernicious = evil

Assessment test for vitamin B_{12}: The DNA synthesis test is known as the deoxyuridine suppression test (DUMP test—from the abbreviation for the chemical name of DNA's raw material, deoxyuridine monophosphate).

B Vitamin Deficiencies and Toxicities

Oddly enough, although we know a great deal about their individual molecular functions, we are unable to say precisely why a deficiency of one B vitamin produces one disease whereas the deficiency of another produces another. With the deficiency of any B vitamin, many body systems become deranged, and similar symptoms may appear. Removing a number of "horseshoe nails" can have such disastrous and far-reaching effects that it is difficult to imagine or predict the results.

Deficiencies of single B vitamins seldom show up in isolation. After all, people do not eat nutrients singly; they eat foods, which contain mixtures of nutrients. If a major class of foods is missing from the diet, the nutrients contributed by that class of foods will all be lacking to varying extents. In only two cases have dietary deficiencies associated with single B vitamins been observed on a large scale in human populations and been given disease names. One of these diseases, beriberi, was first observed in the Far East when the custom of polishing rice became widespread. Rice contributed 80 percent of the kcalories consumed by the people of those areas, and rice hulls were their principal source of thiamin. When the hulls were removed in the effort to make the rice whiter and more pleasing to the people, beriberi spread like wildfire. It was believed

Tests were initiated by the results of my studies on a chicken disease similar to beriberi. I was able to establish that that disease is caused by feeding certain grains, especially rice. Only polished rice (raw or boiled) proved to be harmful; unpolished rice was tolerated quite well by the chickens. . . . From these experiments I drew the conclusion that the cuticles probably contain a substance or substances which neutralize the harmful influence of the starchy nutriment.

C. Eijkman, 1897

beriberi: the thiamin-deficiency disease; it pointed the way to discovery of the first vitamin, thiamin.

The edema of beriberi. Thiamin deficiency also sometimes produces a "dry" beriberi, without edema, for reasons not well understood. Another marked symptom is inability to walk, manifested by collapse of the lower limbs when the person tries to stand.

pellagra (pell-AY-gra): the niacin-deficiency disease.
pellis = skin
agra = seizure

to be caused by an infectious agent, and medical researchers wasted much time and energy seeking a microbial cause before they realized that the problem was not what was present in the food, but what was absent from it. It is curious that words such as *refined* and *polished* should refer both to upper-class people and to inferior foods. Chapter 2 told a similar story about bread in North America: refined bread lacks many vitamins and minerals, and "enriched" bread does not fully compensate for the losses.

The other disease, pellagra, became widespread in the U.S. South in the early part of this century, in people who subsisted on a low-protein diet whose staple grain was corn. This diet was unusual in that it supplied neither enough niacin nor enough of its amino acid precursor tryptophan to make up the deficiency. An excess of the amino acid leucine probably also contributes to deficiency; leucine inhibits a key enzyme that converts tryptophan to NAD and speeds up the activity of another enzyme that breaks tryptophan down.[7]

Even in these cases, the deficiencies were not pure. When foods were provided containing the one vitamin known to be needed, the other vitamins that may have been in short supply came as part of the package.

Once vitamin research was well under way and other B vitamins had been discovered, the clarification of their functions was often greatly helped by laboratory experiments in which animals or human volunteers were fed diets devoid of one vitamin. The effect of the deficiency of that vitamin could then be studied to determine what functions it normally performed. Other deficiency diseases were discovered in this way and have since been observed to occur outside the laboratory.

Table 9–2 sums up a few of the better-established facts about B vitamin deficiencies. A look at the table will make another generalization possible. Different body systems depend to different extents on these vitamins. Processes in nerves and in their responding tissues, the muscles, depend heavily on glucose metabolism and hence on thiamin; thus paralysis sets in when this nutrient is

Significantly, beriberi and pellagra were eliminated by supplying foods—not pills. Although both diseases were attributed to single vitamins, both were likely to have been deficiencies of several vitamins in which one vitamin happened to stand above the rest. Giving one B vitamin to people with a multiple deficiency may make latent deficiencies of other B vitamins become overt.

Pushers of vitamin pills make much of the fact that vitamins are vital and indispensable to life. But human beings obtained their nourishment from foods for centuries before there were vitamin pills. If your diet lacks a vitamin, the natural solution is to adjust it so that food supplies that vitamin.

Pushers of so-called natural vitamins would have you believe that their pills are the best of all because they are purified from real foods rather than synthesized in a laboratory. But if you think back on the course of human evolution, you may conclude that it really is not natural to take any kind of pills at all. In reality, the finest, most complete vitamin "supplements" available are meat, fish, poultry, eggs, legumes, nuts, milk and milk products, vegetables, fruits, and grain products. Any time you hear the suggestion made that you should meet your vitamin needs by taking pills, look out. Someone may be trying to sell you something you don't need.

It really isn't natural to take any kind of pills.

lacking. The replacement of red blood cells and GI tract cells occurs at a rapid pace and involves much making of DNA; this depends on folacin and vitamin B_{12}, so two of the first symptoms of a deficiency of either of these nutrients are a type of anemia and GI tract deterioration. But again, each nutrient is important in all systems, and these lists of symptoms are far from complete.

The skin and the tongue appear to be especially sensitive to vitamin B deficiencies, but you should note that the listing of these items in Table 9–2 gives them undue emphasis. Remember that in a medical examination these are two body parts that are visible. If the skin is degenerating, other tissues beneath it may be, too. Similarly, the mouth and tongue are the visible part of the digestive system; if they are abnormal, there may well be an abnormality throughout the GI tract. What is really happening in a vitamin deficiency happens inside the cells of the body; what the doctor sees and reports are its outward manifestations.

Major, epidemic-like deficiency diseases such as pellagra and beriberi are no longer seen in the United States and Canada, but lesser deficiencies of nutrients, including the B vitamins, sometimes are observed. When they occur, it is usually in people whose food choices are poor because of poverty, ignorance, illness, or poor health habits like alcohol abuse.

The case of folacin deficiency illustrates some additional points about nutrient deficiencies in general. They arise not only because of deficient intakes, but also for other reasons. Folacin deficiency may result not only from an inadequate intake, but also from impaired absorption or unusual metabolic need for the vitamin. Deficiencies from all three causes are common.

Tongue symptoms of B vitamin deficiency. The tongue is smooth due to atrophy of the tissues (glossitis). This person has a folacin deficiency.

TABLE 9–2

B Vitamins—Deficiency Symptoms

Vitamin	Disease	Deficiency Syndrome		Technical Terms for Symptoms
		Area Affected	Main Effects	
Thiamin	Beriberi	Nervous system	Mental confusion Peripheral paralysis Loss of ankle and knee jerk reflexes	
		Muscles	Weakness Wasting Painful calf muscles	
		Cardiovascular system	Edema Enlarged heart Death from cardiac failure	
Riboflavin	Ariboflavinosis	Facial skin	Dermatitis around nose and lips Cracking of corners of mouth	Cheilosis (kee-LOH-sis)
		Eyes	Hypersensitivity to light Reddening of cornea	Photophobia
		GI tract	Magenta tongue	
Niacin	Pellagra	Skin	Bilateral symmetrical dermatitis, especially on body parts exposed to sun	
		Tongue	Loss of surface features, swelling, edema	Glossitis (gloss-EYE-tis)
		GI tract	Diarrhea	
		Nervous system	Irritability Mental confusion, progressing to psychosis or delirium	
Vitamin B$_6$	(No name)	Skin	Dermatitis Cracking of corners of mouth Irritation of sweat glands	Cheilosis
		Tongue	Smoothness (atrophy of surface structures)	Glossitis
		Nervous system	Abnormal brainwave pattern Convulsions	
Folacin	(No name)	Tongue	Smoothness, swelling, cracks	Glossitis
		GI tract	Diarrhea (loss of villi and their enzymes)	
		Nervous system	Fatigue, depression, confusion	
		Blood	Anemia (characterized by large cells)	Macrocytic anemia
		Immune system	Suppression; infections likely	
Vitamin B$_{12}$	(No name[a])	Tongue	Smoothness, swelling, cracks	Glossitis
		Blood	Anemia (characterized by large cells)	Macrocytic anemia
		Skin	Hypersensitivity	
		Nervous system	Degeneration of peripheral nerves	
Pantothenic acid	(No name)	GI tract	Vomiting, GI distress	
		Nervous system	Insomnia, fatigue	
Biotin	(No name)	Skin	Scaly dermatitis, drying, loss of hair	
		Nervous system	Depression, lassitude, muscle pains	
		GI tract	Anorexia, nausea	
		Cardiovascular system	Abnormal heart action	

[a]The name *pernicious anemia* refers to the vitamin B$_{12}$ deficiency caused by lack of intrinsic factor, but not to that caused by inadequate dietary intake.

It is more and more apparent that you cannot observe a symptom and automatically jump to a conclusion regarding its cause. The warning was given earlier (in Chapter 4) that skin rashes are a symptom, not a disease. As you have seen, deficiencies of linoleic acid, riboflavin, niacin, and vitamin B_6 can all cause rashes. A deficiency of vitamin A can, too. Because skin is on the outside, where you and your doctor can easily look at it, it is a useful indicator of things-going-wrong-in-cells. But by itself, a skin symptom tells you nothing about its possible cause.

The same is true of anemia. We often think of anemia as being caused by an iron deficiency, and often it is. But anemia can also be caused by a folacin or vitamin B_{12} deficiency; by digestive tract failure to absorb any of these nutrients; or by such nonnutritional causes as infections, parasites, cancer, or loss of blood. So be careful. You can often recognize a false claim by the implication that a specific nutrient will always cure a given symptom.

A person who feels chronically tired may be tempted to self-diagnose iron-deficiency anemia, and self-prescribe an iron supplement. But the iron supplement will relieve tiredness only if the symptom is caused by iron-deficiency anemia. If the problem is a folacin deficiency, taking iron will only prolong the period in which the tiredness persists. A person who is better informed may decide to take a vitamin supplement with iron, covering the possibility of a vitamin deficiency. But there may be a nonnutritional cause of the symptom. If the cause of the tiredness is actually hidden blood loss due to cancer, the postponement of a diagnosis may be equivalent to suicide.

anemia: literally, "too little blood." Anemia is any condition in which there are too few red blood cells, or the red blood cells are immature or too small, or they contain too little hemoglobin to carry the normal amount of oxygen to the tissues. It is not a disease itself, but can be a symptom of many different disease conditions, including many nutrient deficiencies, bleeding, excessive red blood cell destruction, defective formation, and other causes.
an = without
emia = blood

An inadequate intake is seen in babies fed goat's milk, which is notoriously low in folacin. Overconsumers of alcohol or other empty-kcalorie items are vulnerable, and deficiency can also be precipitated by any condition that requires cell multiplication to speed up: multiple pregnancies (twins and triplets), cancer, skin-destroying diseases such as chicken pox and measles, burns, blood loss, GI tract damage, and more. A too-low intake is also theoretically possible in anyone whose diet does not include generous amounts of folacin-rich foods.

Toxicities of the B vitamins are also observed. High doses of thiamin, taken by injection, cause a nervous system hypersensitivity reaction. Niacin in large doses (75 milligrams or more) dilates the capillaries and causes a tingling effect which, if intense, can be painful; the effect is known as the "niacin flush." The alternative form of niacin, niacinamide, doesn't have this effect.

High doses of folacin have been reported to have adverse effects, but research reports are inconsistent. The other B vitamins seem relatively innocuous with one notable exception, vitamin B_6, which has been reported to cause severe impairment of the sensory nerves in doses of 500 milligrams a day or more. Highlight 9A is devoted to the controversy surrounding vitamin B_6 supplements and their toxicity.[8]

Niacin toxicity symptoms:
- niacin flush
- heartburn, nausea
- vomiting, diarrhea
- ulcer activation
- liver malfunction
- low blood pressure
- fainting

Requirements and Food Sources

The preceding sections have shown both the great importance of the B vitamins in promoting normal, healthy functioning of all body systems and the severe consequences of deficiency. Now you may want to know how to be sure you are getting enough of these vital nutrients. This section offers some practical pointers regarding requirements and food sources. A section at the end of the chapter provides pointers on shopping, storing, and cooking foods to maximize their vitamin value.

The RDA for thiamin is 1.5 milligrams for men 19 to 22 years old, and 1.4 milligrams for older men. For women 19 to 22, it is 1.1 milligrams, and for older women 1.0 milligram. The RDA for special groups are shown in the RDA table (inside front cover).

Because thiamin is used for energy production, more is needed when energy expenditure is high. In fact, the thiamin requirement can be stated in terms of milligrams per 1,000 kcalories. Provided that you are consuming enough kcalories to meet your energy needs—and obtaining those kcalories from thiamin-containing foods—your thiamin intake will adjust automatically to your need. However, people who derive a large proportion of their kcalories from empty-kcalorie items like sugar or alcohol may suffer thiamin deficiency. A person who is fasting or who has adopted a very low kcalorie diet needs the same amount of thiamin as on a regular diet; stores last about two months, and needs change very little during fasting, because they are proportional to energy expenditure, not to energy intake.[9] Table 9–3 shows the thiamin amounts in different types of foods.

Thiamin RDA: 0.5 mg/1,000 kcal (women). 0.6 mg/1,000 kcal (men). Canadian recommendation: 0.4 mg/1,000 kcal (both sexes); perhaps more for older adults.

A Note on Looking to Foods for Single Nutrients

Table 9–3 is the first of a long series of tables that will present the nutrients in foods, one by one, through the next four chapters. If you looked at only one or a few of these tables, you might get the wrong impression: that you should think in terms of single nutrients and learn which foods supply each one. Realistically, though, people cannot eat for single nutrients, and the tables are not intended to show you how to do so. Withhold judgment for a while, until you see the effect of all the tables taken together. A conclusion can be shown about how to eat, after surveying the whole array of nutrients in foods, and this will be done in Chapter 13.

Here's a sneak preview of the conclusion: vegetables and other plant foods deserve more emphasis in the diet than they have traditionally been given in our society. They are capable of supplying more than adequate amounts of most nutrients for many fewer kcalories than are meats and animal products. A discussion of how this works for the single nutrient thiamin follows, but it works similarly for all nutrients.

TABLE 9–3

Thiamin In Foods

Foods Ranked by Thiamin Per Serving	Thiamin Per Serving (mg)	Energy Per Serving (kCal)	Foods Ranked by Thiamin Per 100 kCalories	Thiamin Per Serving (mg)	Thiamin Per 100 kCal (mg)
Brewers yeast (1 tbsp)	1.25	25	Brewers yeast (1 tbsp)	1.25	5.00
Pork chop, broiled (3.1 oz)	0.87	275	Romaine lettuce, chopped (1 c)	0.06	0.67
Ham, canned roasted (3 oz)	0.82	140	Ham, canned roasted (3 oz)	0.82	0.59
Sunflower seeds, dry (¼ c)	0.82	205	Wheat germ, raw (¼ c)	0.38	0.56
Green peas, cooked (1 c)	0.46	146	Mushrooms, raw sliced (1 c)	0.08	0.44
Black beans, cooked (1 c)	0.43	225	Cooked Canadian bacon (2 pc)	0.38	0.44
Blackeyed peas, cooked (1 c)	0.40	190	Asparagus, cooked (1 c)	0.18	0.41
Watermelon (1 sl)	0.39	152	Sunflower seeds, dry (¼ c)	0.82	0.40
Cooked Canadian bacon (2 pc)	0.38	86	Green peas, cooked (1 c)	0.46	0.37
Hamburger patty, bun (4 oz)	0.38	445	Pork chop, broiled (3.1 oz)	0.87	0.32
Wheat germ, raw (¼ c)	0.38	68	Alfalfa seeds, sprouted (1 c)	0.03	0.30
Oysters, raw (1 c)	0.29	160	Looseleaf lettuce (1 c)	0.03	0.30
Sirloin steak, lean (8 oz)	0.29	480	Mustard greens, cooked (1 c)	0.06	0.29
Peas, dry split, cooked (1 c)	0.28	230	Tomato, whole raw (1)	0.07	0.29
Oatmeal, cooked (1 c)	0.26	145	Acorn squash, boiled (1 c)	0.24	0.29
Acorn squash, boiled (1 c)	0.24	83	Bean sprouts, fresh (1 c)	0.09	0.28
Baked potato, whole (1)	0.22	220	Broccoli, cooked (1 c)	0.13	0.28
Winter squash, baked (1 c)	0.21	96	Cauliflower, cooked (1 c)	0.08	0.27
Peanuts, dried unsalted (1 oz)	0.19	161	Watermelon (1 sl)	0.39	0.26
Asparagus, cooked (1 c)	0.18	44	Cabbage, raw shredded (1 c)	0.04	0.25
Tofu soybean curd (1 block)	0.18	86	Bok choy cabbage, cooked (1 c)	0.05	0.25
Broccoli, cooked (1 c)	0.13	46	Zucchini squash, cooked (1 c)	0.07	0.24
Kidney beans, canned (1 c)	0.13	230	Turnip greens, cooked (1 c)	0.07	0.24
Orange, fresh medium (1)	0.11	60	Winter squash, baked (1 c)	0.21	0.22
Cantaloupe melon (½)	0.10	94	Summer squash, cooked (1 c)	0.08	0.22
Honeydew melon (1/10)	0.10	45	Honeydew melon (1/10)	0.10	0.22
Whole wheat bread (1 sl)	0.10	70	Tofu soybean curd (1 block)	0.18	0.21
Millet, cooked (½ c)	0.10	54	Blackeyed peas, cooked (1 c)	0.40	0.21
Whole milk (1 c)	0.09	150	Parsley, chopped fresh (1 c)	0.04	0.20
Nonfat milk or yogurt (1 c)	0.09	86	Green beans, cooked (1 c)	0.09	0.20
Green beans, cooked (1 c)	0.09	44	Millet, cooked (½ c)	0.10	0.19
Bean sprouts, fresh (1 c)	0.09	32	Black beans, cooked (1 c)	0.43	0.19
Cauliflower, cooked (1 c)	0.08	30	Orange, fresh medium (1)	0.11	0.18
Mushrooms, raw sliced (1 c)	0.08	18	Oatmeal, cooked (1 c)	0.26	0.18
Summer squash, cooked (1 c)	0.08	36	Oysters, raw (1 c)	0.29	0.18
Zucchini squash, cooked (1 c)	0.07	29	Celery, outer stalk (1)	0.01	0.17
Tomato, whole raw (1)	0.07	24	Whole wheat bread (1 sl)	0.10	0.14
Turnip greens, cooked (1 c)	0.07	29	Peanuts, dried unsalted (1 oz)	0.19	0.12
Chicken breast, roasted (½)	0.06	142	Peas, dry split, cooked (1 c)	0.28	0.12
Mustard greens, cooked (1 c)	0.06	21	Cantaloupe melon (½)	0.10	0.11
Romaine lettuce, chopped (1 c)	0.06	09	Nonfat milk or yogurt (1 c)	0.09	0.10
Bok choy cabbage, cooked (1 c)	0.05	20	Baked potato, whole (1)	0.22	0.10
Sole/flounder, baked (3 oz)	0.05	120	Hamburger patty, bun (4 oz)	0.38	0.09
Cabbage, raw shredded (1 c)	0.04	16	Whole milk (1 c)	0.09	0.06
Parsley, chopped fresh (1 c)	0.04	20	Sirloin steak, lean (8 oz)	0.29	0.06
Miso (3 tbsp)	0.03	88	Kidney beans, canned (1 c)	0.13	0.06
Looseleaf lettuce (1 c)	0.03	10	Sole/flounder, baked (3 oz)	0.05	0.04
Alfalfa seeds, sprouted (1 c)	0.03	10	Chicken breast, roasted (½)	0.06	0.04
Apple, fresh medium (1)	0.02	80	Miso (3 tbsp)	0.03	0.03
Celery, outer stalk (1)	0.01	06	Apple, fresh medium (1)	0.02	0.03
Cheddar cheese (1 oz)	0	114	Cheddar cheese (1 oz)	0	0

Table 9–3 shows the thiamin amounts in different types of foods as compared with the kcalories they contribute. The left side of the table ranks typical foods by the thiamin in single servings; the right side, by the thiamin per 100 kcalories. The left side shows that, of foods commonly eaten, those richest in thiamin per serving are meats of the pork/ham family, and legumes (peas and beans). Large servings of these contribute large amounts of kcalories, however; thiamin doesn't come at a low kcalorie cost in these foods.

A food is a thiamin "bargain" if it contributes more thiamin relative to your need than kcalories relative to your need of kcalories. The best thiamin bargains, by this definition, are listed first on the right side of the table. Vegetables appear significantly more often in the thiamin-per-100-kcalorie list than in the thiamin-per-serving list of foods, because they have so many fewer kcalories in a serving. If you were to eat large quantities of vegetables, you could obtain significant amounts of thiamin from them, even though they don't make large contributions per serving. Depending on the bulk of the food you can eat, and how many kcalories you can afford to eat, you might want to choose foods from both rank orders.

If you study the table while thinking about your own food habits, you will probably conclude that many of the foods you like and eat daily contribute some thiamin, but none by itself can meet your total need for a day. A useful guideline is to eliminate empty-kcalorie foods from your diet and to include ten or more different servings of nutritious foods each day, assuming that on the average each serving will contribute about 10 percent of your need. Foods chosen from the bread and cereal group should be either whole-grain or enriched.

The recommended daily riboflavin intake for adult men aged 19 to 22 is 1.7 milligrams a day; for older men it is 1.6 milligrams a day. For women 19 to 22, it is 1.3 milligrams a day, and for older women it is 1.2 milligrams a day. The differences depend on how much energy people expend daily. (Like thiamin, riboflavin needs are stated in terms of milligrams per 1,000 kcalories.) Children's needs rise rapidly during their growing years. Teenagers, because they are very active, need more riboflavin than adults.

Unlike thiamin, riboflavin is not evenly distributed among the food groups. The major contributors in most people's diets are milk and meat, because they offer the largest amounts of riboflavin per serving and because people eat several servings a day. The need for riboflavin provides a major reason for including milk in some form in every day's meals; no other food that is commonly eaten can make such a substantial contribution in a single serving.

Table 9–4 shows the riboflavin in foods per serving, and also per 100 kcalories. Clearly, milk, milk products such as cheese, and organ meats dominate the top of the per-serving list, with a few meats and exceptionally nutritious vegetables scattered among them. However, the per-100-kcalorie list includes many dark-green, leafy vegetables near the top of the rank order. For adequate intakes of riboflavin, people can depend on *generous* servings of many different kinds of vegetables. A cup of cooked broccoli, for example, offers only 0.32 milligrams of riboflavin, whereas an 8-ounce sirloin steak offers 0.70 milligrams. Still, for most people, the broccoli would be a better source of riboflavin—two cups would provide nearly as much riboflavin as the steak at a much lower kcalorie cost (92 kcalories for the broccoli, 480 for the steak). Most people derive about half their riboflavin from milk and milk products, about a fourth from meats, and most of the rest from leafy green vegetables and whole-grain

Riboflavin RDA:
0.6 mg/1,000 kcal or a minimum of 1.2 mg/day (U.S.).
0.5 mg/1,000 kcal (Canada).

These are among the many dairy foods supplying riboflavin.

TABLE 9–4

Riboflavin In Foods

Foods Ranked by Riboflavin Per Serving	Riboflavin Per Serving (mg)	Energy Per Serving (kCal)	Foods Ranked by Riboflavin Per 100 kCalories	Riboflavin Per Serving (mg)	Riboflavin Per 100 kCal (mg)
Beef liver, fried (3 oz)	3.52	185	Beef liver, fried (3 oz)	3.52	1.90
Braunschweiger sausage (2 pcs)	0.87	205	Mushrooms, raw sliced (1 c)	0.32	1.78
Sirloin steak, lean (8 oz)	0.70	480	Brewers yeast (1 tbsp)	0.34	1.36
Mushroom pieces, cooked (1 c)	0.46	42	Mushroom pieces, cooked (1 c)	0.46	1.10
Ricotta cheese, part skim (1 c)	0.46	340	Beet greens, cooked (1 c)	0.42	1.05
Nonfat milk + solids (1 c)	0.43	91	Spinach, cooked (1 c)	0.42	1.02
Oysters, raw (1 c)	0.43	160	Broccoli, cooked (1 c)	0.32	0.70
Cottage cheese, lowfat 2% (1 c)	0.42	205	Romaine lettuce, chopped (1 c)	0.06	0.67
Beet greens, cooked (1 c)	0.42	40	Bok choy cabbage, cooked (1 c)	0.11	0.55
Spinach, cooked (1 c)	0.42	41	Dandelion greens, cooked (1 c)	0.18	0.51
1% lowfat milk (1 c)	0.41	102	Asparagus, cooked (1 c)	0.22	0.50
Whole milk (1 c)	0.40	150	Nonfat milk + solids (1 c)	0.43	0.47
Buttermilk (1 c)	0.38	99	Mustard greens, cooked (1 c)	0.09	0.43
Nonfat milk or yogurt (1 c)	0.34	86	Braunschweiger sausage (2 pcs)	0.87	0.42
Goat milk (1 c)	0.34	168	Nonfat milk or yogurt (1 c)	0.34	0.40
Brewers yeast (1 tbsp)	0.34	25	1% lowfat milk (1 c)	0.41	0.40
Mushrooms, raw sliced (1 c)	0.32	18	Looseleaf lettuce (1 c)	0.04	0.40
Broccoli, cooked (1 c)	0.32	46	Alfalfa seeds, sprouted (1 c)	0.04	0.40
Pork roast (3 oz)	0.30	187	Buttermilk (1 c)	0.38	0.38
Peach halves, dried (10)	0.28	311	Bean sprouts, stir fried (1 c)	0.22	0.35
Roast ham (3 oz)	0.22	133	Turnip greens, cooked (1 c)	0.10	0.34
Almonds, whole dried (1 oz)	0.22	167	Parsley, chopped fresh (1 c)	0.06	0.30
Asparagus, cooked (1 c)	0.22	44	Oysters, raw (1 c)	0.43	0.27
Bean sprouts, stir fried (1 c)	0.22	62	Whole milk (1 c)	0.40	0.27
Corned beef, canned (3 oz)	0.20	185	Green beans, cooked (1 c)	0.12	0.27
Ground beef, 10% fat (3 oz)	0.18	230	Tomato, whole raw (1)	0.06	0.25
Dandelion greens, cooked (1 c)	0.18	35	Strawberries, fresh (1 c)	0.10	0.22
Salmon, smoked (3 oz)	0.17	150	Cottage cheese, lowfat 2% (1 c)	0.42	0.20
Turkey (3 oz)	0.15	145	Goat milk (1 c)	0.34	0.20
Green beans, cooked (1 c)	0.12	44	Summer squash, cooked (1 c)	0.07	0.19
Bok choy cabbage, cooked (1 c)	0.11	20	Roast ham (3 oz)	0.22	0.17
Cheddar cheese (1 oz)	0.11	114	Pork roast (3 oz)	0.30	0.16
Strawberries, fresh (1 c)	0.10	45	Sirloin steak, lean (8 oz)	0.70	0.15
Chicken breast, roasted (½)	0.10	142	Ricotta cheese, part skim (1 c)	0.46	0.14
Blackeyed peas, cooked (1 c)	0.10	190	Almonds, whole dried (1 oz)	0.22	0.13
Kidney beans, canned (1 c)	0.10	230	Corned beef, canned (3 oz)	0.20	0.11
Turnip greens, cooked (1 c)	0.10	29	Salmon, smoked (3 oz)	0.17	0.11
Mustard greens, cooked (1 c)	0.09	21	Turkey (3 oz)	0.15	0.10
Sole/flounder, baked (3 oz)	0.08	120	Cheddar cheese (1 oz)	0.11	0.10
Summer squash, cooked (1 c)	0.07	36	Peach halves, dried (10)	0.28	0.09
Whole wheat bread (1 sl)	0.06	70	Whole wheat bread (1 sl)	0.06	0.09
Cantaloupe melon (½)	0.06	94	Ground beef, 10% fat (3 oz)	0.18	0.08
Romaine lettuce, chopped (1 c)	0.06	9	Orange, fresh medium (1)	0.05	0.08
Tomato, whole raw (1)	0.06	24	Chicken breast, roasted (½)	0.10	0.07
Parsley, chopped fresh (1 c)	0.06	20	Sole/flounder, baked (3 oz)	0.08	0.07
Oatmeal, cooked (1 c)	0.05	145	Cantaloupe melon (½)	0.06	0.06
Orange, fresh medium (1)	0.05	60	Blackeyed peas, cooked (1 c)	0.10	0.05
Peanuts, dried unsalted (1 oz)	0.04	161	Kidney beans, canned (1 c)	0.10	0.04
Looseleaf lettuce (1 c)	0.04	10	Oatmeal, cooked (1 c)	0.05	0.03
Alfalfa seeds, sprouted (1 c)	0.04	10	Apple, fresh medium (1)	0.02	0.03
Apple, fresh medium (1)	0.02	80	Peanuts, dried unsalted (1 oz)	0.04	0.02

or enriched bread and cereal products, but people who eat abundant, large servings of vegetables can obtain sufficient riboflavin to meet the RDA for many fewer kcalories.

Table 9–4 illustrates another point of interest. Compare the various milk items listed and note that, on both sides of the table, the lower-fat items have the higher amounts of riboflavin. It stands to reason: riboflavin is a water-soluble vitamin. The less fat there is in a given volume, the more water there will be, and therefore the more water-soluble nutrient.

Riboflavin can be destroyed by light. For this reason, milk is seldom sold (and should not be stored) in transparent glass or translucent plastic containers. Cardboard or opaque plastic containers protect the riboflavin in the milk from light.

Recommended niacin intakes are stated in "equivalents," a term that requires explanation. Niacin is unique among the B vitamins because it can be obtained from another nutrient source—protein. The amino acid tryptophan can be converted to niacin in the body: 60 milligrams of tryptophan (by a rough approximation) yields 1 milligram of niacin. Thus a food containing 1 milligram of niacin and 60 milligrams of tryptophan contains the equivalent of 2 milligrams of niacin, or 2 milligram equivalents.

The RDA for niacin for men aged 19 to 22 is 19 milligram equivalents; for older men it is 18. For women 19 to 22, it is 14 milligram equivalents, and for older women, 13. Infants', children's, and teenagers' needs are proportional not to their size, but to their energy output.

Tables of food composition list only the preformed niacin in foods, although people actually derive the vitamin from both niacin itself and dietary tryptophan. However, tryptophan is first used to build needed body proteins, and only that available thereafter is used to make niacin. Thus calculating the amount of niacin available from the diet is a complicated matter. A means of obtaining a rough approximation is shown in the margin, but the simplest assumption is that if the diet is adequate in complete protein, it will supply enough niacin equivalents to meet the daily need.

Milk, eggs, meat, poultry, and fish contribute about half the niacin equivalents consumed by most people, and about a fourth come from enriched breads and cereals. Table 9–5 shows that even when ranked by niacin content per 100 kcalories, fish and poultry still come out near the top of the list of niacin sources. Mushrooms and greens are among the richest vegetable sources (per kcalorie) for the person who eats abundant amounts of them.

Because the vitamin B_6 coenzymes play many roles in amino acid metabolism, dietary needs are roughly proportional to protein intakes. The RDA for adult men is 2.2 milligrams a day; for women, 2.0 milligrams; this is enough to handle 100 grams of protein. There is some possibility that older people have a greater need for vitamin B_6 than young adults.

Table 9–6 shows the vitamin B_6 contents of foods per serving, and per 100 kcalories. Meats, legumes, vegetables, fruits, and grains all offer vitamin B_6, but the foods that are richest in the vitamin on a per-kcalorie basis are clearly the vegetables (see right side of table). The generalization is gaining strength that vegetables, if eaten in sufficient quantities, can provide significant amounts of many nutrients.

Folacin occurs in foods in both bound and free forms. The bound form is folacin combined with a string of amino acids (glutamic acid), known as the

niacin equivalents: the amount of niacin present in food, including the niacin that can theoretically be made from its precursor, tryptophan, present in the food.

Niacin RDA: 6.6 mg equiv./1,000 kcal or a minimum of 13 mg equiv. (U.S.).
7.2 mg equiv./1,000 kcal (Canada) and not less than 14.4 mg equiv.

To obtain a rough approximation of your niacin intake:

1. Calculate total protein consumed (g).
2. Subtract your recommended protein intake to obtain "leftover" protein usable to make niacin (g).
3. Divide by 100 to obtain the amount of tryptophan in this protein (g).
4. Multiply by 1,000 to express this amount of tryptophan in milligrams.
5. Divide by 60 to get niacin equivalents (mg).
6. Finally, add the amount of niacin obtained preformed in the diet (mg).

Vitamin B_6 RDA: 0.02 mg/g protein (U.S.). 15 μg as pyridoxine per gram of protein (Canada).

TABLE 9–5

Niacin In Foods

Foods Ranked by Niacin Per Serving	Niacin Per Serving (mg)	Energy Per Serving (kCal)	Foods Ranked by Niacin Per 100 kCalories	Niacin Per Serving (mg)	Niacin Per 100 kCal (mg)
Tuna, canned (3 oz)	13.20	135	Mushroom pieces, cooked (1 c)	6.96	16.57
Beef liver, fried (3 oz)	12.30	185	Mushrooms, raw sliced (1 c)	2.88	16.00
Chicken breast, roasted (½)	11.80	142	Wheat bran (¼ c)	2.43	12.79
Sirloin steak, lean (8 oz)	9.92	480	Brewers yeast (1 tbsp)	3.16	12.64
Hamburger patty, bun (4 oz)	7.85	445	Tuna, canned (3 oz)	13.20	9.78
Halibut, broiled (3 oz)	7.70	140	Chicken breast, roasted (½)	11.80	8.31
Mushroom pieces, cooked (1 c)	6.96	42	Beef liver, fried (3 oz)	12.30	6.65
Pink salmon, canned (3 oz)	6.80	120	Pink salmon, canned (3 oz)	6.80	5.67
Oysters, raw (1 c)	6.00	160	Halibut, broiled (3 oz)	7.70	5.50
Peach halves, dried (10)	5.69	311	Asparagus, cooked (1 c)	1.90	4.32
Salmon, broiled/baked (3 oz)	5.50	140	Salmon, broiled/baked (3 oz)	5.50	3.93
Lamb chop, braised (3 oz)	5.29	238	Oysters, raw (1 c)	6.00	3.75
Ground beef, 21% fat (3 oz)	4.90	245	Bok choy cabbage, cooked (1 c)	0.73	3.65
Braunschweiger, sausage (2 pcs)	4.78	205	Shrimp, boiled (3.5 oz)	3.70	3.39
Turkey (3 oz)	4.63	145	Turkey (3 oz)	4.63	3.19
Sardines, canned (3 oz)	4.60	175	Romaine lettuce, chopped (1 c)	0.28	3.11
Pork chop, broiled (3.1 oz)	4.35	275	Tomato, whole raw (1)	0.74	3.08
Peanuts, dried unsalted (1 oz)	4.02	161	Mustard greens, cooked (1 c)	0.61	2.90
Hash brown potatoes (1 c)	3.78	340	Sardines, canned (3 oz)	4.60	2.63
Shrimp, boiled (3.5 oz)	3.70	109	Broccoli, cooked (1 c)	1.18	2.57
Potato, microwaved with skin (1)	3.46	212	Summer squash, cooked (1 c)	0.92	2.56
Baked potato, whole (1)	3.32	220	Peanuts, dried unsalted (1 oz)	4.02	2.50
Brewers yeast (1 tbsp)	3.16	25	Braunschweiger sausage (2 pcs)	4.78	2.33
Mushrooms, raw sliced (1 c)	2.88	18	Peach, fresh medium (1)	0.86	2.32
Crab meat, canned (1 c)	2.60	135	Green peppers, whole (1)	0.41	2.28
Wheat bran (¼ c)	2.43	19	Cauliflower, cooked (1 c)	0.68	2.27
Asparagus, cooked (1 c)	1.90	44	Lamb chop, braised (3 oz)	5.29	2.22
Sole/flounder, baked (3 oz)	1.60	120	Looseleaf lettuce (1 c)	0.22	2.20
Cantaloupe melon (½)	1.53	94	Spinach, cooked (1 c)	0.88	2.15
Kidney beans, canned (1 c)	1.50	230	Parsley, chopped fresh (1 c)	0.42	2.10
Broccoli, cooked (1 c)	1.18	46	Sirloin steak, lean (8 oz)	9.92	2.07
Whole wheat bread (1 sl)	1.07	70	Turnip greens, cooked (1 c)	0.59	2.03
Summer squash, cooked (1 c)	0.92	36	Ground beef, 21% fat (3 oz)	4.90	2.00
Spinach, cooked (1 c)	0.88	41	Crab meat, canned (1 c)	2.60	1.93
Peach, fresh medium (1)	0.86	37	Peach halves, dried (10)	5.69	1.83
Green beans, cooked (1 c)	0.77	44	Hamburger patty, bun (4 oz)	7.85	1.76
Tomato, whole raw (1)	0.74	24	Green beans, cooked (1 c)	0.77	1.75
Bok choy cabbage, cooked (1 c)	0.73	20	Potato, microwaved with skin (1)	3.46	1.63
Cauliflower, cooked (1 c)	0.68	30	Cantaloupe melon (½)	1.53	1.63
Mustard greens, cooked (1 c)	0.61	21	Pork chop, broiled (3.1 oz)	4.35	1.58
Turnip greens, cooked (1 c)	0.59	29	Whole wheat bread (1 sl)	1.07	1.53
Parsley, chopped fresh (1 c)	0.42	20	Baked potato, whole (1)	3.32	1.51
Green peppers, whole (1)	0.41	18	Sole/flounder, baked (3 oz)	1.60	1.33
Orange, fresh medium (1)	0.37	60	Hash brown potatoes (1 c)	3.78	1.11
Oatmeal, cooked (1 c)	0.30	145	Kidney beans, canned (1 c)	1.50	0.65
Romaine lettuce, chopped (1 c)	0.28	9	Orange, fresh medium (1)	0.37	0.62
Nonfat milk or yogurt (1 c)	0.22	86	Nonfat milk or yogurt (1 c)	0.22	0.26
Looseleaf lettuce (1 c)	0.22	10	Oatmeal, cooked (1 c)	0.30	0.21
Whole milk (1 c)	0.20	150	Apple, fresh medium (1)	0.11	0.14
Apple, fresh medium (1)	0.11	80	Whole milk (1 c)	0.20	0.13
Cheddar cheese (1 oz)	0.02	114	Cheddar cheese (1 oz)	0.02	0.02

TABLE 9–6

Vitamin B₆ In Foods

Foods Ranked by Vitamin B₆ Per Serving	Vitamin B₆ Per Serving (mg)	Energy Per Serving (kCal)	Foods Ranked by Vitamin B₆ Per 100 kCalories	Vitamin B₆ Per Serving (mg)	Vitamin B₆ Per 100 kCal (mg)
Sirloin steak, lean (8 oz)	.77	480	Brewers yeast (1 tbsp)	.40	1.60
Navy beans, cooked dry (1 c)	.72	225	Bok choy cabbage, cooked (1 c)	.30	1.50
Baked potato, whole (1)	.70	220	Spinach, cooked (1 c)	.44	1.07
Watermelon (1 sl)	.69	152	Turnip greens, cooked (1 c)	.26	0.89
Potato, microwaved with skin (1)	.69	212	Mustard greens, cooked (1 c)	.18	0.85
Salmon, broiled/baked (3 oz)	.68	140	Cauliflower, cooked (1 c)	.24	0.80
Banana, peeled (1)	.66	105	Broccoli, cooked (1 c)	.31	0.67
Salmon, smoked (3 oz)	.59	150	Green peppers, whole (1)	.12	0.66
Chicken breast, roasted (½)	.52	142	Banana, peeled (1)	.66	0.62
Soy beans, cooked dry (1 c)	.50	235	Asparagus, cooked (1 c)	.26	0.59
Potato, microwaved, no skin (1)	.50	156	Parsley, chopped fresh (1 c)	.10	0.50
Sunflower seeds, dry (¼ c)	.46	205	Salmon, broiled/baked (3 oz)	.68	0.48
Spinach, cooked (1 c)	.44	41	Zucchini squash, cooked (1 c)	.14	0.48
Tuna, canned (3 oz)	.42	135	Watermelon (1 sl)	.69	0.45
Figs, dried (10)	.42	477	Cabbage, raw shredded (1 c)	.07	0.43
Trout, broiled (3 oz)	.41	175	Chicken livers, simmered (1)	.12	0.40
Brewers yeast (1 tbsp)	.40	25	Salmon, smoked (3 oz)	.59	0.39
Turkey (3 oz)	.39	145	Tomato, whole raw (1)	.09	0.37
Ground beef, 10% fat (3 oz)	.39	230	Chicken breast, roasted (½)	.52	0.36
Pork chop, broiled (3.1 oz)	.35	275	Summer squash, cooked (1 c)	.12	0.33
Cantaloupe melon (½)	.31	94	Mushrooms, raw sliced (1 c)	.06	0.33
Broccoli, cooked (1 c)	.31	46	Romaine lettuce, chopped (1 c)	.03	0.33
Beef liver, fried (3 oz)	.31	185	Cantaloupe melon (½)	.31	0.33
Bok choy cabbage, cooked (1 c)	.30	20	Potato, microwaved with skin (1)	.69	0.32
Sole/flounder, baked (3 oz)	.28	120	Potato, microwaved, no skin (1)	.50	0.32
Turnip greens, cooked (1 c)	.26	29	Navy beans, cooked dry (1 c)	.72	0.32
Asparagus, cooked (1 c)	.26	44	Baked potato, whole (1)	.70	0.31
Cauliflower, cooked (1 c)	.24	30	Tuna, canned (3 oz)	.42	0.31
Mustard greens, cooked (1 c)	.18	21	Collards, cooked (1 c)	.06	0.30
Wheat germ, raw (¼ c)	.17	68	Looseleaf lettuce (1 c)	.03	0.30
Zucchini squash, cooked (1 c)	.14	29	Turkey (3 oz)	.39	0.26
Summer squash, cooked (1 c)	.12	36	Wheat germ, raw (¼ c)	.17	0.25
Green peppers, whole (1)	.12	18	Trout, broiled (3 oz)	.41	0.23
Chicken livers, simmered (1)	.12	30	Sole/flounder, baked (3 oz)	.28	0.23
Whole milk (1 c)	.10	150	Sunflower seeds, dry (¼ c)	.46	0.22
Parsley, chopped fresh (1 c)	.10	20	Soy beans, cooked dry (1 c)	.50	0.21
Nonfat milk or yogurt (1 c)	.10	86	Ground beef, 10% fat (3 oz)	.39	0.17
Tomato, whole raw (1)	.09	24	Beef liver, fried (3 oz)	.31	0.16
Peanuts, dried unsalted (1 oz)	.08	161	Sirloin steak, lean (8 oz)	.77	0.16
Orange, fresh medium (1)	.08	60	Green beans, cooked (1 c)	.07	0.15
Green beans, cooked (1 c)	.07	44	Orange, fresh medium (1)	.08	0.13
Cabbage, raw shredded (1 c)	.07	16	Pork chop, broiled (3.1 oz)	.35	0.12
Apple, fresh medium (1)	.07	80	Nonfat milk or yogurt (1 c)	.10	0.11
Mushrooms, raw sliced (1 c)	.06	18	Figs, dried (10)	.42	0.08
Collards, cooked (1 c)	.06	20	Apple, fresh medium (1)	.07	0.08
Whole wheat bread (1 sl)	.05	70	Whole wheat bread (1 sl)	.05	0.07
Oatmeal, cooked (1 c)	.05	145	Whole milk (1 c)	.10	0.06
Kidney beans, canned (1 c)	.05	230	Peanuts, dried unsalted (1 oz)	.08	0.05
Romaine lettuce, chopped (1 c)	.03	9	Oatmeal, cooked (1 c)	.05	0.03
Looseleaf lettuce (1 c)	.03	10	Kidney beans, canned (1 c)	.05	0.02
Cheddar cheese (1 oz)	.02	114	Cheddar cheese (1 oz)	.02	0.01

polyglutamate form. This has to be hydrolyzed to the monoglutamate ("free" folacin) before the intestine can absorb it.

Canada's recommendation for daily intake is stated in terms of "free folate (folacin)." It is 210 micrograms a day for adult men and 165 micrograms for women. The U.S. recommendation for adults is stated in terms of all forms of folacin, of which about half is freed for use in the body. Hence, the recommendation is 400 micrograms a day. The need for folacin rises considerably during pregnancy and whenever cells are multiplying, so the recommendations for pregnant women are higher. The typical diet in the United States probably delivers about 600 micrograms daily.

Although estimates of folacin in foods are thus less reliable than those of some other nutrients, you can still tell from tables of food composition which foods are likely to be the best sources. Table 9–7 shows that folacin is especially abundant in vegetables, legumes, and seeds, and that milk, milk products, and meats are not notable for their folacin contents. On a per-100-kcalorie basis, leafy vegetables are especially notable, clustering at the top of the right side of the table.

Among the poor in the United States and in other parts of the world, folacin deficiency due to inadequate intake is probably the most common of all vitamin deficiencies. Folacin deficiency anemia is especially common among pregnant women. Some authorities recommend that in pregnancy a folacin supplement, as well as an iron supplement, should be given as a preventive measure.

The risks of overdosing with folacin are greater than those for the other B vitamins discussed so far. They arise from the close relationship between folacin and vitamin B_{12}. Without enough vitamin B_{12}, folacin can be trapped inside of cells, therefore the symptoms of folacin deficiency can be caused by vitamin B_{12} deficiency, even in the presence of adequate folacin.

According to the RDA, adults need about 3 micrograms of vitamin B_{12} a day; the Canadian recommendation for adults is 2 micrograms. This is the tiniest amount imaginable—three-millionths of a gram, and a gram would not even fill a quarter teaspoon. The ink in the period at the end of this sentence probably weighs about 3 micrograms. But what seems like such a tiny amount to the human eye contains billions of molecules of vitamin B_{12}, enough to provide coenzymes for all the enzymes that need its help.

Vitamin B_{12} is unique among the nutrients in being found almost exclusively in animal flesh and animal products. Anyone who eats reasonable amounts of meat is guaranteed an adequate intake, and lacto-ovo-vegetarians (if they use enough milk, cheese, and eggs) are also protected from deficiency. "Enough" means a cup of milk or 3 ½ ounces of cheese or one egg in a given day.[10] Microorganisms can make available their own vitamin B_{12}, so yeast grown in a vitamin B_{12}-enriched environment is a good source.

Vegans usually have normal vitamin B_{12} status.[11] Researchers have wondered why, since by definition, they eat no foods from animal sources. Many hypotheses have been advanced to account for this finding. Perhaps vegans' intestinal bacteria produce vitamin B_{12} for them to absorb. Perhaps they continually reabsorb the vitamin B_{12} they have. Perhaps they ingest bacteria containing the vitamin with their foods or drinking water. It appears that some plant foods do provide significant amounts of vitamin B_{12}—among them, soybeans, mung beans and mung bean sprouts, comfrey leaves, peas, whole wheat, ground nuts, lettuce, and alfalfa.[12] Why they contain the vitamin is not known; perhaps in some cases

Note: Recommended folacin intakes are stated in micrograms (µg). A microgram is a thousandth of a milligram or a millionth of a gram.

The U.S. RDA for folacin, 400 µg, can also be stated as 0.4 mg.
Canada: 210 µg (men).
        165 µg (women).

Of these three vegetables, the cauliflower is the richest in folacin.

Note: Recommended vitamin B_{12} intakes are stated in micrograms. 3 µg is 0.003 mg, three-millionths of a gram.
RDA: 3.0 µg.
Canada: 2.0 µg.

Foods Ranked by Folacin Per Serving	Folacin Per Serving (μg)	Energy Per Serving (kCal)	Foods Ranked by Folacin Per 100 kCalories	Folacin Per Serving (μg)	Folacin Per 100 kCal (μg)
Brewers yeast (1 tbsp)	313	25	Brewers yeast (1 tbsp)	313	1,252
Spinach, cooked (1 c)	262	41	Spinach, fresh chopped (1 c)	109	908
Asparagus, cooked (1 c)	176	44	Romaine lettuce, chopped (1 c)	76	844
Turnip greens, cooked (1 c)	171	29	Spinach, cooked (1 c)	262	639
Lima beans, cooked (1 c)	170	260	Turnip greens, cooked (1 c)	171	590
Beef liver, fried (3 oz)	150	185	Parsley, chopped fresh (1 c)	110	550
Blackeyed peas, cooked (1 c)	142	190	Asparagus, cooked (1 c)	176	400
Pinto beans, cooked (1 c)	137	265	Collards, cooked (1 c)	55	275
Parsley, chopped fresh (1 c)	110	20	Cabbage, raw shredded (1 c)	40	250
Spinach, fresh chopped (1 c)	109	12	Dandelion greens, cooked (1 c)	82	234
Navy beans, cooked dry (1 c)	108	225	Broccoli, cooked (1 c)	107	233
Broccoli, cooked (1 c)	107	46	Cauliflower, cooked (1 c)	64	213
Beets, cooked (1 c)	98	52	Bean sprouts, fresh (1 c)	63	197
Sunflower seeds, dry (¼ c)	85	205	Beets, cooked (1 c)	98	188
Kidney beans, canned (1 c)	85	230	Bok choy cabbage, cooked (1 c)	32	160
Dandelion greens, cooked (1 c)	82	35	Alfalfa seeds, sprouted (1 c)	12	120
Cantaloupe melon (½)	80	94	Bean sprouts, stir fried (1 c)	72	116
Romaine lettuce, chopped (1 c)	76	9	Zucchini squash, cooked (1 c)	30	103
Great northern beans (1 c)	74	210	Summer squash, cooked (1 c)	36	100
Bean sprouts, stir fried (1 c)	72	62	Green beans, cooked (1 c)	42	95
Winter squash, baked (1 c)	69	96	Wheat germ, raw (¼ c)	62	91
Cauliflower, cooked (1 c)	64	30	Honeydew melon (1/10)	39	87
Bean sprouts, fresh (1 c)	63	32	Cantaloupe melon (½)	80	85
Wheat germ, raw (¼ c)	62	68	Beef liver, fried (3 oz)	150	81
Tofu soybean curd (1 block)	55	86	Mushrooms, raw sliced (1 c)	14	78
Collards, cooked (1 c)	55	20	Blackeyed peas, cooked (1 c)	142	74
Grapefruit juice, fresh (1 c)	52	96	Winter squash, baked (1 c)	69	72
Green beans, cooked (1 c)	42	44	Orange, fresh medium (1)	40	67
Orange, fresh medium (1)	40	60	Green peppers, whole (1)	12	67
Cabbage, raw shredded (1 c)	40	16	Celery, outer stalk (1)	4	67
Honeydew melon (1/10)	39	45	Lima beans, cooked (1 c)	170	65
Summer squash, cooked (1 c)	36	36	Tofu soybean curd (1 block)	55	64
Bok choy cabbage, cooked (1 c)	32	20	Strawberries, fresh (1 c)	28	62
Zucchini squash, cooked (1 c)	30	29	Grapefruit juice, fresh (1 c)	52	54
Peanuts, dried unsalted (1 oz)	30	161	Pinto beans, cooked (1 c)	137	52
Strawberries, fresh (1 c)	28	45	Tomato, whole raw (1)	12	50
Sirloin steak, lean (8 oz)	19	480	Navy beans, cooked dry (1 c)	108	48
Whole wheat bread (1 sl)	16	70	Sunflower seeds, dry (¼ c)	85	41
Nonfat milk or yogurt (1 c)	14	86	Kidney beans, canned (1 c)	85	37
Mushrooms, raw sliced (1 c)	14	18	Great northern beans (1 c)	74	35
Whole milk (1 c)	12	150	Whole wheat bread (1 sl)	16	23
Tomato, whole raw (1)	12	24	Peanuts, dried unsalted (1 oz)	30	19
Green peppers, whole (1)	12	18	Nonfat milk or yogurt (1 c)	14	16
Alfalfa seeds, sprouted (1 c)	12	10	2% lowfat milk (1 c)	12	10
2% lowfat milk (1 c)	12	121	Sole/flounder, baked (3 oz)	10	8
Sole/flounder, baked (3 oz)	10	120	Whole milk (1 c)	12	8
Oatmeal, cooked (1 c)	10	145	Oatmeal, cooked (1 c)	10	7
Cheddar cheese (1 oz)	5	114	Apple, fresh medium (1)	4	5
Celery, outer stalk (1)	4	6	Cheddar cheese (1 oz)	5	4
Apple, fresh medium (1)	4	80	Sirloin steak, lean (8 oz)	19	4
Chicken breast, roasted (½)	3	142	Chicken breast, roasted (½)	3	2

bacteria in their roots make the vitamin—and the plants then translocate it to their edible parts. In tempeh, a fermented soybean product, vitamin B_{12} is produced whenever a certain bacterial species is present during the fermentation process.[13]

Both pantothenic acid and biotin are widespread in foods, and there seems to be no danger that people who consume a variety of foods will suffer deficiencies. Claims that these vitamins are needed in pill form to prevent or cure disease conditions are at best unfounded and at worst intentionally misleading.

In a very few instances under unusual circumstances, biotin deficiencies have been seen in human adults. Recommendations for daily intakes are therefore made, but they are not as firm as the RDA. They are "estimated safe and adequate daily dietary intakes."

Invariably biotin deficiencies have been associated with artificial feeding— that is, feeding mixtures of purified nutrients, lacking biotin, into a vein in hospital clients who couldn't eat. Even under such circumstances, a client would normally not experience deficiency, because the bacteria in the GI tract can synthesize enough biotin to meet the host's needs. However, in the hospital, antibiotics are often given, and these kill the intestinal bacteria.

Researchers can induce a biotin deficiency in animals or human subjects by feeding them raw egg whites, which contain a protein that binds biotin. However, it takes more than two dozen raw egg whites to produce the effect; and cooking denatures the protein. Occasional drinkers of eggnog have nothing to fear from raw egg whites.

Biotin is important metabolically, and some genetic disorders greatly increase the need for it. Individuals born with an inherited metabolic disorder involving biotin can develop deficiency symptoms and will benefit from therapeutic doses.

Pantothenic acid and biotin: deficiencies are unlikely in humans.

Estimated safe and adequate intake of biotin (U.S.): 100–200 μg
Canada: 1.5 μg/kg body weight.
Estimated safe and adequate intake of pantothenic acid (U.S.): 4–7 mg.
Canada: 5–7 mg.

The protein **avidin** in egg whites binds biotin.
avid = greedy

B Vitamin Relatives

A trio of compounds sometimes called B vitamins are inositol, choline, and lipoic acid. These are not essential nutrients for humans, although deficiencies can be induced in laboratory animals in order to study their functions. Like the B vitamins described above, they serve as coenzymes in metabolism. Even if they were essential for humans, supplements would be unnecessary, because they are abundant in foods.

When used as drugs, choline and its relative lecithin have some important beneficial effects on several disease conditions that affect memory and muscular coordination.* These particular diseases are responsive not because they are caused by deficiencies of choline or lecithin, but because large doses of these nutrients are acting pharmacologically, in a different way altogether from normal doses.

Lecithin, remember, contains choline as part of its structure. See Chapter 4.

---

*The two diseases most intensively investigated have been Alzheimer's disease and tardive dyskinesia. Some five others may be ameliorated by choline or lecithin (phosphatidylcholine). J. L. Wood and R. G. Allison, Effects of consumption of choline and lecithin on neurological and cardiovascular systems, *Federation Proceedings* 41 (1982): 3015–3021.

For a rational way to compare different vitamin-mineral supplements, turn to Appendix J.

Animals are biologically similar to human beings, but not identical.

Health-food purveyors make much of inositol, choline, and lipoic acid, insisting that we must supplement our diets with them. Some vitamin companies include them in their formulations in hopes that you will read the label and conclude that their vitamin pill is more "complete" than someone else's. These incorrect notions arise from an unjustified application of findings from animal studies to human beings. Animals are useful for nutrition research, and their nutrient needs are often the same as ours, but not always. We cannot always arrive at correct conclusions as to what an animal research finding means to us without performing some tests directly on human beings. To weigh the relevance of nutrition information derived from animal studies, ask yourself if the finding has been proven applicable to human beings. (There's more about the applicability of research using animals in later chapters.)

The beneficial effects of choline and lecithin on these diseases have led to many false claims—"Lecithin improves memory" and the like—with a consequent rush to buy and consume bottles of it. As a result, medical practitioners have been able to witness and report on the effects of overdoses of these compounds. They can cause not only short-term discomforts such as GI distress, sweating, salivation, and anorexia, but also long-term health hazards from disturbance of the nervous and cardiovascular systems.[14]

In addition to choline, inositol, and lipoic acid, other substances have been mistaken for essential nutrients for humans because they are needed for growth by bacteria or other forms of life. These substances include:

- PABA (para-aminobenzoic acid).
- Bioflavonoids (vitamin P or hesperidin).
- Ubiquinone.

Other names you may hear are vitamin B_5 (another name for pantothenic acid), vitamin B_{15} (also called "pangamic acid," a hoax), vitamin B_{17} (Laetrile, a fake "cancer cure" and not a vitamin by any stretch of the imagination), "vitamin B_T" (carnitine, an important piece of cell machinery, but not a vitamin), and more. There is another water-soluble vitamin, however, of great interest and importance—vitamin C.

Vitamin C

scurvy: the vitamin C–deficiency disease.

Two hundred fifty years ago, any man who joined the crew of a seagoing ship knew he had only half a chance of returning alive—not because he might be slain by pirates or die in a storm, but because he might contract the dread disease scurvy. As many as two-thirds of a ship's crew might die of scurvy on a long voyage. Only ships that sailed on short voyages, especially around the Medi-

If you read or hear a report of a substance having a beneficial or harmful effect, it is an oversimplification to conclude that the substance is "good" or "bad." You must ask what dose was used. Two corollaries to this statement might be the following:

- A substance that is poisonous at a high concentration may be an essential nutrient at a lower concentration.
- A nutrient needed at a low concentration may be toxic at a high concentration.

The drawings in the margin show three possible relationships between dose levels and effects. In (A), as you progress in the direction of more, the effect gets better and better, with no end in sight. (Real life is seldom, if ever, like this.) In (B), as you progress in the direction of more, the effect reaches a maximum and then a plateau, becoming no better with higher doses. In (C), as you progress in the direction of more, the effect reaches an optimum at some intermediate dose and then declines, showing that too much is as bad as too little. (C) represents the situation with nutrients—and nutrient-like compounds such as choline and lecithin.

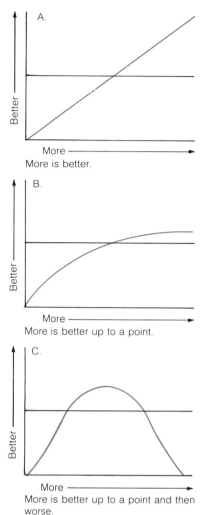

A.
More is better.

B.
More is better up to a point.

C.
More is better up to a point and then worse.

terranean Sea, were safe from this disease. It was not known at the time that the special hazard of long ocean voyages was that the ship's cook used up his provisions of fresh fruits and vegetables early and relied for the duration of the voyage on cereals and meat brought along as provisions.

The first nutrition experiment conducted on human beings was devised in 1747 to find a cure for scurvy. James Lind, a British physician, divided 12 sailors with scurvy into six pairs. Each pair received a different supplemental ration: cider, vinegar, sulfuric acid, sea water, oranges and lemons, or a purgative mixed with spices. The ones receiving the citrus fruits were cured within a short time. Sadly, it was 50 years before the British Navy made use of Lind's experiment by requiring all vessels to carry sufficient limes for every sailor to have lime juice daily. British sailors are still nicknamed "limeys" as a result of this tradition.

The antiscurvy "something" in limes and other foods was dubbed the antiscorbutic factor. Nearly 200 years later, the factor was isolated from lemon juice and found to be a six-carbon compound similar to glucose. It was named ascorbic acid. Shortly thereafter it was synthesized, and today hundreds of millions of vitamin C pills are produced in pharmaceutical laboratories each year and sold for a few dollars a bottle.

antiscorbutic factor: the original name for vitamin C.
anti = against
scorbutic = causing scurvy

ascorbic acid: one of the two active forms of vitamin C (see Figure 9–3). Many people refer to vitamin C by this name.
a = without
scorbic = having scurvy

Metabolic Roles of Vitamin C

Vitamin C, like all the vitamins, is a small organic compound needed by human beings in minute amounts daily. Being organic, it is convertible to several different forms, two of which are active (see Figure 9–3). It is water soluble, and like most of the B vitamins, it is excreted rapidly when excesses are taken. But unlike the B vitamins, its mode of action is different in different situations. In some settings it may act as a coenzyme or cofactor, assisting a specific enzyme

FIGURE 9-3.

Active forms of vitamin C. The reduced form can lose two hydrogens with their electrons, becoming oxidized. The electrons may then reduce some other compound.

Ascorbic Acid (Reduced Form)   Dehydroascorbic Acid (Oxidized Form)

collagen: the characteristic protein of connective tissue.
kolla = glue
gennan = to produce

Collagen is unique among body proteins, because it contains large amounts of the amino acid hydroxyproline, the hydroxy derivative of proline.

Proline

Hydroxyproline

antioxidant: a compound that protects others from oxidation by being oxidized itself.

Chemists describe this action of vitamin C as maintaining the "oxidation-reduction equilibrium" or "redox state" and as participating in "electron transport."

in the performance of its job. In others, it may act in a more general way—for example, as an antioxidant.

Vitamin C helps to form the protein collagen. Brief mention was made of this protein in Chapter 6; it is the single most important protein of connective tissue. Collagen serves as the matrix on which bone is formed. It forms scars; when you have been wounded, collagen glues the separated tissue faces together. The material that holds cells together is largely made of collagen; this function is especially important in the artery walls, which must expand and contract with each beat of the heart, and in the walls of the capillaries, which are thin and fragile and must withstand a pulse of blood every second or so without giving way.

Collagen, like all proteins, is formed by the stringing together of a chain of amino acids. An amino acid used in abundance to make collagen is proline. After proline is added to the chain, an enzyme hydroxylates it (adds an OH group to it), making hydroxyproline. Vitamin C is essential for the hydroxylation step to occur.

Vitamin C acts as an antioxidant, as mentioned. An antioxidant is any substance that can reduce (donate electrons to) another substance; when it reduces the other substance, it simultaneously becomes oxidized itself.

Many substances found in foods and important in the body can be altered or even destroyed by oxidation. (An example in Chapter 4 was oils that turn rancid when exposed to air.) Vitamin C—because it can be destroyed itself—can protect other substances from this destruction. Vitamin C is like a bodyguard for oxidizable substances; it stands ready to sacrifice its own life to save theirs. Unemotionally, the chemists call such a bodyguard an antioxidant.

Because of its antioxidant property, vitamin C is sometimes added to food products, not to improve their nutritional value, but to protect important constituents in the products. In the cells and body fluids, it probably helps to protect other molecules, and in the intestines, it protects ferrous iron by maintaining the neighborhood in the appropriately reduced state. It also promotes the absorption of iron, a function fully discussed in Chapter 12.

Vitamin C is involved in the metabolism of several amino acids. Some of these amino acids may end up being converted to hormones—notably, norepinephrine and thyroxin.

The adrenal glands contain a higher concentration of vitamin C than any other organ in the body, and during emotional or physical stress they release large quantities of the vitamin together with the hormones epinephrine and norepinephrine. What the vitamin has to do with the stress reaction is unclear; it is known that some physical stresses increase vitamin C needs, but psychological stress alone does not appear to increase needs above the RDA.

Vitamin C is also needed for the synthesis of thyroxin, which regulates the rate of metabolism. The metabolic rate speeds up under extreme stress and also when the body needs to produce more heat—for example, in fever or cold weather. Thus infections and exposure to cold increase needs for vitamin C. Perhaps its involvement in the fever response to infection explains the vitamin's possible effects on cold prevention and symptom reduction. (Highlight 9B explores these effects, as well as the relationship between vitamin C and cancer.)

In scurvy, protein metabolism may be altered, resulting in negative nitrogen balance. No one knows why this occurs, but the involvement of vitamin C with amino acids provides a notable example of the way nutrients of different classes cooperate with one another to maintain health.

Vitamin C Deficiency

In both the United States and Canada, vitamin C deficiency is still seen, despite the past century's explosion of nutrition knowledge. In the United States, the Ten-State Survey showed evidence of unacceptable serum levels of vitamin C in about 15 percent of all age groups studied, with symptoms of outright scurvy showing up in 4 percent. The more recent Nationwide Food Consumption Survey showed intakes below two-thirds of the RDA for 20 to 30 percent of all persons surveyed. Especially in infants, teenagers, and people over 60 years of age, intakes of vitamin C were much lower than the RDA (less than 50 percent). In Canada, many Eskimos and Indians and some members of the general population have deficiency symptoms. Evidently we all need to make efforts to obtain enough of this vitamin.

With an adequate intake, the body maintains a fixed pool of vitamin C and rapidly excretes any excess in the urine. With an inadequate intake, the pool becomes depleted at the rate of about 3 percent a day. Obvious deficiency symptoms don't begin to appear until the pool has been reduced to about a fifth of its optimal size, and this may take two months or more to occur. Thus the first sign of a developing vitamin C deficiency is a lowered serum or plasma vitamin C concentration. A low intake as revealed by the diet history is the cue that prompts the diagnostician to request a clinical test to measure the body's vitamin C levels.

As the pool size continues to fall, latent scurvy appears. Two of the earliest signs of a vitamin C deficiency are related to its role in maintaining capillary integrity. The gums around teeth bleed easily, and capillaries under the skin break spontaneously, producing pinpoint hemorrhages. Atherosclerotic plaques grow rapidly in the arteries. If the vitamin levels continue to fall, the symptoms of overt scurvy appear. Failure to promote normal collagen synthesis causes further hemorrhaging. Muscles, including the heart muscle, may degenerate. The skin becomes rough, brown, scaly, and dry. Wounds fail to heal because scar tissue will not form. Bone rebuilding is not maintained; the ends of the long bones become softened, malformed, and painful, and fractures appear. The teeth may become loose in the jawbone, and fillings may loosen and fall out. Anemia is frequently seen, and infections are common. There are also characteristic psychological signs, including hysteria and depression. Sudden death is

Assessment tests for vitamin C: Vitamin C shifts unpredictably between the plasma and the white blood cells known as leukocytes; thus a plasma or serum determination may not accurately reflect the body's pool. The appropriate clinical test may be a measurement of leukocyte vitamin C. A combination of both tests may be more reliable than either one alone.

Scorbutic gums. Unlike other lesions of the mouth, scurvy presents a symmetrical appearance without infection.

Infant scurvy. This is the characteristic "scorbutic pose," with legs bent and thighs rotated open. The infant's joints are painful, and she will cry if made to move.

latent: the period in disease when the conditions are present but before the symptoms have begun to appear.
latens = lying hidden

overt: out in the open, full-blown.
ouvrire = to open

likely, occasioned by severe atherosclerosis or by massive bleeding into the joints and body cavities.

Once diagnosed, scurvy is readily reversed by vitamin C. Moderate doses in the neighborhood of 100 milligrams per day are all that are needed; the scurvy is cured within about five days. Thereafter, as before, only 10 milligrams a day are sufficient to prevent its reappearance.

Recommended Intakes of Vitamin C

How much vitamin C is enough? Allowances recommended by different nations vary from as low as 30 milligrams per day in Britain to 60 milligrams per day in the United States and Canada and 75 in West Germany. The requirement—the amount needed to prevent the appearance of the overt deficiency symptoms of scurvy—is well known to be only 10 milligrams, but 10 milligrams a day apparently does not saturate all the body tissues, because larger intakes have been observed to increase the body's total vitamin C pool. At about 60 milligrams per day, the pool size in the average person stops responding to further increases in intake, and at 100 milligrams per day, 95 percent of the population probably reaches tissue saturation. After the tissues are saturated, all added vitamin C is excreted.[15]

It may seem strange that of West Germany and Britain, two similar industrialized nations, one should recommend two and a half times the vitamin C intake of the other. In view of the wide range of possible intakes, however, the German and British recommendations are not so far apart. Both are generously above the minimum requirement, and both are well below the level at which toxicity symptoms might appear. The range of possible intakes, illustrated in the margin, shows that all the allowances are in the same ballpark. In contrast, the recommendation by Dr. Linus Pauling and others that people should take 2 to 4 grams a day (or even 10 grams) is clearly way up in the clouds.

It is important to remember that recommended allowances for vitamin C, like those for all the nutrients, are amounts intended to maintain health in healthy people, not to restore health in sick people. Unusual circumstances may increase nutrient needs. In the case of vitamin C, a variety of physical stresses deplete the body pool and may make intakes higher than 60 milligrams or so desirable. Among the stresses known to increase vitamin C needs are infections; burns; extremely high or low temperatures; toxic levels of heavy metals such as lead, mercury, and cadmium; and the chronic use of certain medications, including aspirin, barbiturates, and oral contraceptives.[16] After a major operation (such as removal of a breast) or extensive burns, when a tremendous amount of scar tissue must form during healing, the amount needed may be as high as 1,000 milligrams (1 gram) a day or even more.

Vitamin C Toxicity

The easy availability of vitamin C in pill form and the publication of a book recommending intakes of over 2 grams a day (see Highlight 9B) have led

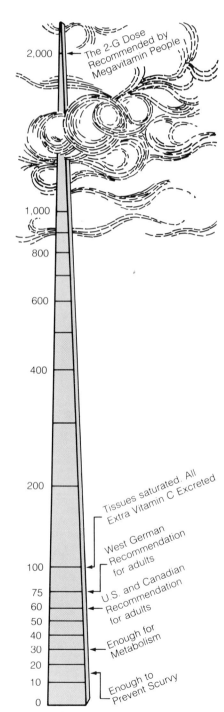

Recommendations for vitamin C intake (mg).

thousands of people to take vitamin C megadoses. Not surprisingly, instances have surfaced of vitamin C's causing harm.

Some of the suspected toxic effects of megadoses have not been confirmed. Among these are formation of stones in the kidneys, upset of the body's acid-base balance, destruction of vitamin B_{12} resulting in a deficiency, and interference with the action of vitamin E. Research and reasoning have demonstrated that these effects are theoretically possible, but no cases of their actual occurrence in human beings have yet been seen with intakes as high as 3 grams a day.

Other toxic effects, however, have been seen often enough to warrant concern. Nausea, abdominal cramps, and diarrhea are often reported. Several instances of interference with medical regimens are known. The large amounts of vitamin C excreted in the urine obscure the results of tests used to detect diabetes, giving a false positive result in some instances and a false negative result in others. People taking medications to prevent their blood from clotting may unwittingly abolish the effect of these medicines if they also take massive doses of vitamin C.

People of certain genetic backgrounds are more likely to be harmed by vitamin C megadoses than others. Some black Americans, Sephardic Jews, Asians, and certain other ethnic groups have an inherited enzyme deficiency that makes them susceptible to any strong reducing agent. Megadoses of vitamin C can make their red blood cells burst, causing hemolytic anemia. Those with sickle-cell anemia may also be vulnerable to megadoses of vitamin C. In sickle-cell anemia, the hemoglobin protein is abnormal; it responds to a reducing agent by assuming a shape that distorts the red blood cells, making them clump and clog capillaries. Those who have a tendency toward gout and those who have a genetic abnormality that alters the way they break down vitamin C to its excretion products are more prone to forming stones if they take megadoses of C.

The body of a person who has taken large doses of vitamin C for a long time may adjust by limiting absorption and destroying and excreting more of the vitamin than usual.[17] If the person then suddenly reduces intake to normal, the accelerated disposal system may not be able to put on its brakes fast enough to avoid destroying too much of the vitamin. It has been suggested that adults who discontinue megadosing may develop scurvy on intakes that would protect a normal adult, but evidence is scanty on this point. If it occurs, it is not unlike the withdrawal reaction seen in drug and alcohol abusers when they discontinue drug use.

After reviewing the published research on large doses of vitamin C, the National Nutrition Consortium reported in 1978 that there are probably very few instances in which taking more than 100 to 300 milligrams a day is beneficial. Adults may not be exposing themselves to very severe risks if they choose to dose themselves with 1 to 2 grams a day, but above 2 grams, "genuine caution should be exercised," and amounts above 8 grams per day may be "distinctly harmful. It is irresponsible and inexcusable to proclaim that ascorbic acid is safe in any amounts that may be ingested."[18]

In conclusion, the range of safe vitamin C intakes seems to be broad, as is typical for water-soluble vitamins. Between the absolute minimum of 10 milligrams a day and a reasonable maximum of perhaps 1,000 milligrams, nearly everyone should be able to find a suitable intake. People who venture outside these limits do so at their own risk.

Vitamin C RDA:
U.S.: 60 mg.
Canada: 60 mg (men).
        40 mg (women).

Remember the distinction between the *requirement* and the recommended *allowance or standard* (see pp. 18–19).

Vitamin C is inactivated and degraded by several routes, and sometimes a product along the way is oxalate, which can form stones in the kidneys. People can also have oxalate crystals in their kidneys that are not due to vitamin C overdoses.

The anticlotting agents with which vitamin C interferes are such anticoagulants as warfarin and dicumarol.

gout: a metabolic disease in which crystals of uric acid precipitate in the joints.

withdrawal reaction: a reaction to withdrawal (usually of a drug) that reveals that the user has become dependent. One infant is reported to have been born of a mother who took massive doses of vitamin C. The infant developed **rebound scurvy** on an intake that would have been adequate for the average infant.

Vitamin C in Fruits and Vegetables

When nutritionists say "vitamin C," people think "oranges" . . .

But these foods are actually richer in vitamin C for their kcalorie cost.

staple: a food kept on hand at all times and used daily or almost daily in meal preparation.

The inclusion of intelligently selected fruits and vegetables in the daily diet guarantees a generous intake of vitamin C. Even those who wish to ingest amounts well above the recommended 30 to 60 milligrams can easily meet their goals this way. If you drink a double portion of orange juice at breakfast, choose a salad for lunch, and include a stalk of broccoli and a potato on your dinner plate, you will exceed 300 milligrams even before counting the contributions made by incidental other sources. Clearly, then, you would have no need for vitamin C pills unless you wanted to join the ranks of the megadosers.

Table 9–8 shows the amounts of vitamin C in various common foods and reveals that the citrus fruits are rightly famous for being rich in vitamin C, but certain vegetables and some other fruits are in the same league: broccoli, brussels sprouts, greens, cabbage, cantaloupe, and strawberries. You have to eat larger servings of the vegetables than of the fruits to get the same amount of the vitamin, but you can do this without consuming excess kcalories. A single serving of any of these provides more than 30 milligrams of the vitamin.

The humble potato is an important source of vitamin C in Western countries, not because a potato by itself meets the daily needs but because potatoes are such a popular staple and are eaten so frequently that overall they make substantial contributions. They provide about 20 percent of all the vitamin C in the U.S. diet. Some young men report french fries as their only regular source of vitamin C, and yet because they eat so many, they receive the recommended amount.

No vitamin C is found in seeds, only in growing plants. Thus grains (breads and cereals) contain negligible amounts of the vitamin. Milk (except breast milk) is also a notoriously poor source.

Animal foods don't normally contribute much vitamin C to the diet. For this reason, if for no other, fruits and vegetables must be included in any diet to make it adequate. Organ meats (liver, kidneys, and others) contain some, but most people don't eat large quantities of these. Raw meats also contain vitamin C, but again, these are rare in the U.S. diet. Raw meats and fish make enough of a contribution of vitamin C to be significant in the diets of the Inuit people of Alaska and Canada, and in Japanese cuisine, but in most of Canada and the United States, fruits and vegetables are necessary to supply vitamin C.

Shopping, Storing, and Cooking to Maximize Vitamin Value

Knowing all that this chapter has presented so far is not enough to guarantee good nutrition with respect to the water-soluble vitamins. A few practical pointers are in order.

TABLE 9–8

Vitamin C In Foods

Foods Ranked by Vitamin C Per Serving	Vitamin C Per Serving (mg)	Energy Per Serving (kCal)	Foods Ranked by Vitamin C Per 100 kCalories	Vitamin C Per Serving (mg)	Vitamin C Per 100 kCal (mg)
Papaya, whole fresh (1)	188	117	Green peppers, whole (1)	95	528
Orange juice, fresh (1 c)	124	111	Parsley, chopped fresh (1 c)	54	270
Cantaloupe melon (½)	113	94	Cauliflower, cooked (1 c)	68	230
Broccoli, cooked (1 c)	98	46	Bok choy cabbage, cooked (1 c)	44	220
Brussels sprouts, cooked (1 c)	97	60	Broccoli, cooked (1 c)	98	213
Green peppers, whole (1)	95	18	Cabbage, raw shredded (1 c)	33	206
Grapefruit juice, fresh (1 c)	94	96	Strawberries, fresh (1 c)	85	189
Strawberries, fresh (1 c)	85	45	Mustard greens, cooked (1 c)	35	167
Oysters, raw (1 c)	72	160	Brussels sprouts, cooked (1 c)	97	162
Orange, fresh medium (1)	70	60	Papaya, whole fresh (1)	188	161
Cauliflower, cooked (1 c)	69	30	Romaine lettuce, chopped (1 c)	13	144
Mango, fresh (1)	57	135	Turnip greens, cooked (1 c)	40	138
Parsley, chopped fresh (1 c)	54	20	Pink/red grapefruit (½)	47	127
Asparagus, cooked (1 c)	50	44	Cantaloupe melon (½)	113	120
Watermelon (1 sl)	47	152	Orange, fresh medium (1)	70	117
Pink/red grapefruit (½)	47	37	Asparagus, cooked (1 c)	50	114
Tomato juice, canned (1 c)	45	42	Orange juice, fresh (1 c)	124	112
Bok choy cabbage, cooked (1 c)	44	20	Tomato juice, canned (1 c)	45	107
Turnip greens, cooked (1 c)	40	29	White grapefruit (½)	39	100
Spinach, cooked (1 c)	40	41	Grapefruit juice, fresh (1 c)	94	98
White grapefruit (½)	39	39	Spinach, cooked (1 c)	40	98
Tomatoes, whole canned (1 c)	36	47	Tomato, whole raw (1)	22	92
Mustard greens, cooked (1 c)	35	21	Sauerkraut, canned (1 c)	35	80
Sauerkraut, canned (1 c)	35	44	Tomatoes, whole canned (1 c)	36	77
Cabbage, raw shredded (1 c)	33	16	Honeydew melon (⅟₁₀)	32	71
Honeydew melon (⅟₁₀)	32	45	Dandelion greens, cooked (1 c)	19	54
Butternut squash, baked (1 c)	31	83	Raspberries, fresh (1 c)	31	52
Raspberries, fresh (1 c)	31	60	Celery, large outer stalk (1)	3	50
Baked potato, whole (1)	26	220	Oysters, raw (1 c)	72	45
Winter squash, baked (1 c)	24	96	Bean sprouts, fresh (1 c)	14	44
Pineapple chunks, fresh (1 c)	24	76	Mango, fresh (1)	57	42
Beef liver, fried (3 oz)	23	185	Butternut squash, baked (1 c)	31	37
Tomato, whole raw (1)	22	24	Pineapple chunks, fresh (1 c)	24	32
Dandelion greens, cooked (1 c)	19	35	Watermelon (1 sl)	47	31
Bean sprouts, fresh (1 c)	14	32	Green beans, cooked (1 c)	12	27
Romaine lettuce, chopped (1 c)	13	9	Winter squash, baked (1 c)	24	25
Green beans, cooked (1 c)	12	44	Summer squash, cooked (1 c)	9	25
Summer squash, cooked (1 c)	9	36	Baked potato, whole (1)	26	12
Apple, fresh medium (1)	8	80	Beef liver, fried (3 oz)	23	12
Celery, large outer stalk (1)	3	6	Apple, fresh medium (1)	8	10
Nonfat milk or yogurt (1 c)	2	86	Nonfat milk or yogurt (1 c)	2	2
Whole milk (1 c)	2	150	Whole milk (1 c)	2	1
Sole/flounder, baked (3 oz)	1	120	Sole/flounder, baked (3 oz)	1	1
Brewer's yeast (1 tbsp)	0	25	Brewer's yeast (1 tbsp)	0	0
Whole wheat bread (1 sl)	0	70	Whole wheat bread (1 sl)	0	0
Kidney beans, canned (1 c)	0	230	Chicken breast, roasted (½)	0	0
Peanuts, dried unsalted (1 oz)	0	161	Cheddar cheese (1 oz)	0	0
Chicken breast, roasted (½)	0	142	Kidney beans, canned (1 c)	0	0
Sirloin steak, lean (8 oz)	0	480	Peanuts, dried unsalted (1 oz)	0	0
Cheddar cheese (1 oz)	0	114	Sirloin steak, lean (8 oz)	0	0

One of the best ways to eat vegetables is raw.

HTST (high temperature–short time): Every 10° C (18° F) rise in processing temperature gives approximately a tenfold increase in microbial destruction while it only doubles nutrient losses.

To see the effect of canning and draining off canning water on thiamin in foods, look at Appendix H, items 563 and 564 (3 oz raw clams versus 3 oz canned clams). Or check the thiamin in items 891 and 890 (½ c green peas, cooked from frozen versus ½ c canned green peas). While you're looking, what other effects of canning on thiamin do you see?

If you buy and prepare your own food, you have choices to make in the grocery store. How can you purchase the most nutritious foods there? Must you buy only fresh foods? Are canned foods OK? How do frozen foods compare?

In general, food processing involves a trade-off: it makes food safer and produces foods with a longer usable lifetime than fresh food, but at the cost of some vitamin and mineral losses. In some instances, however, processed food has the edge over its unprocessed counterpart, even in terms of nutritional quality.

Canning is one of the better methods for preserving food against the microbes (bacteria, fungi, and yeasts) that might otherwise spoil it, but canned foods, unfortunately, do have fewer nutrients. Like other heat treatments, the canning process is based on time and temperature. Each small increase in temperature has a major killing effect on microbes with only a minor effect on nutrients. By contrast, long treatment times are costly in terms of nutrient losses. Therefore, industry chooses high temperature–short time (HTST) treatments for canning.

To answer the question of how much of a food's nutritional value is lost in canning, food scientists have performed many experiments. They have paid particular attention to the three very vulnerable water-soluble vitamins—thiamin, riboflavin, and vitamin C.

Acid stabilizes thiamin, but heat rapidly destroys it; therefore, the foods that lose the most thiamin during canning are the low-acid foods like lima beans, corn, and meat. Up to half, or even more, of the thiamin in these foods can be lost during canning. The majority of canned foods, however, retain up to 80 percent of their thiamin for up to a year of storage. Unlike thiamin, riboflavin is stable to heat, but sensitive to light; so glass-packed, not canned, foods are most likely to lose riboflavin. Vitamin C's special enemy is an enzyme (ascorbic acid oxidase) present in fruits and vegetables, as well as in microorganisms. By destroying this enzyme, HTST processes such as canning actually aid in preserving vitamin C. As for the fat-soluble vitamins, they are relatively stable and are not affected much by canning.

Minerals are unaffected by heat processing, because they can't be destroyed, as vitamins can be. However, both minerals and the vitamins can be lost when

The nutrient contents of canned foods are usually shown as "solids and liquids." It is important to use the canning water to reheat canned foods, because its vitamin contents are already in balance with those in the foods, and it will not, therefore, leach further nutrients from the food during the reheating process. If you throw away the liquid from a canned food, you are throwing away all the nutrients that have leaked into that liquid, often as much as half of some of the nutrients. A bit of southern folk wisdom related to the cooking of "greens" (dark green vegetables) is to pour off the liquid and drink it rather than throwing it away; this is known as drinking the "pot liquor." The user of canned vegetables who can think of a way to use the "liquor"—for example, by saving it to make soups, cook rice, or moisten casseroles—is displaying similar wisdom.

they move into canning or cooking water that is then thrown away. Losses are closely related to the extent to which food tissues have been broken, cut, or chopped; the amount of water present; and the length of time the food is in contact with the water.

The higher prices on nationally advertised canned foods reflect the cost of the advertising, not the nutritional quality of the product. The less expensive, generic products generally provide comparable nutrients. Although taste differences may dictate your preference for one brand over another, the assumption that the less expensive brands are necessarily nutritionally inferior is incorrect. However, if you buy canned foods with nutrition information on their labels, you can choose the ones with the higher nutrient contents. By so doing, you are encouraging the food manufacturer both to put nutrition information on labels, and to take care in the processing of foods so as to minimize nutrient loss during processing.

An alternative to canning, as a means of preserving food, is freezing. The freezing process itself does not destroy nutrients, but losses may occur during the steps taken in preparation for freezing, such as blanching, washing, trimming, or grinding. Vitamin C losses are especially likely, because they occur whenever tissues are broken and exposed to air (oxygen destroys vitamin C). Uncut fruits, especially if they are acidic, don't lose their vitamin C; strawberries, for example, may be kept frozen for over a year without losing much vitamin C.

Overall, freezing is an excellent way to preserve nutrients. If foods are frozen and stored under proper conditions, they will often contain more nutrients when served at the table than fresh fruits and vegetables that have lost nutrients during transportation and storage in the store and at home.

An important point to remember in connection with freezing, however, is that to be really frozen, a food has to be kept at a temperature colder than 32 degrees Fahrenheit or 0 degrees centigrade. Destruction of vitamin C occurs

When you buy a refrigerator or freezer, you have the choice whether to buy the self-defrosting variety or the kind you have to defrost yourself. Few people are aware of the significance of the difference to the nutritional quality of their frozen foods. A self-defrosting freezer periodically cycles to a temperature warm enough to melt the ice that has accumulated on its walls. In the process, it partially thaws some of the frozen foods it contains, destroying the vitamin C. This may not be a problem if you keep frozen foods only a day or so, or if you eat fruits and vegetables in such abundance that your vitamin C intake is well above your minimum requirement. Some consumers feel, however, that the convenience of the self-defrosting feature is not worth the price it incurs in nutrient losses. A good freezer doesn't accumulate much ice, they say, and you have to defrost it every now and then for cleaning, anyway.

Whatever the choice you make, it is a good idea to be aware of the difference. Manufacturers of household appliances, after all, don't make it their concern to protect your nutritional health; that's your responsibility.

"Fresh" means fresh from the field.

rapidly at warmer temperatures. Food may seem frozen at 2 degrees centigrade, but much of it is actually unfrozen, and enzyme-mediated changes can occur. Under these conditions, the vitamin C in a frozen food can be completely lost in as short a time as two months.

In general, for frozen foods, the lower the temperature, the longer the storage life and the greater the nutrient retention. If you want to maximize the nutritive value of the foods you store at home, invest in a freezer thermometer, monitor the temperature of your frozen-food storage place, and keep it below freezing. Zero to five degrees Fahrenheit costs more in electricity, but is preferable nutritionally to the 20 degrees usually recommended.

Canned and frozen foods are the most widely used, but we use other processed foods, too. Dried or dehydrated foods have their own special characteristics. Drying eliminates microbial spoilage (because microbes need water to grow), and it greatly reduces the weight and volume of foods (because foods are mostly water). Furthermore, drying doesn't cause major nutrient losses. Vacuum puff drying and freeze drying, which take place in cold temperatures, conserve nutrients especially well.

During the drying of fruits such as peaches, grapes (raisins), and plums (prunes), sulfur dioxide is added to prevent browning. Sulfur dioxide happens to help preserve vitamin C as well, but it is highly destructive of thiamin. The overall effect of its addition is probably beneficial, because most sulfured, dehydrated products are not major sources of thiamin anyway.

Some food products, particularly snack foods, have undergone a process known as extrusion. In this process, the food is heated, ground, and pushed through various kinds of screens to yield different shapes, usually bite-size or smaller, like pieces of breakfast cereal or the "bits" you sprinkle on salad. Considerable nutrient losses occur during extrusion processes, and nutrients are usually added to compensate. But foods this far removed from the original fresh state may still be lacking significant nutrients, and you should not rely on them as major components of the diet (staples). Enjoy them, but only as occasional snacks and as additions to enhance the appearance, taste, and variety of meals.

These pointers have addressed the questions people most often ask about processed foods. A generalization you may find useful in selecting and preparing foods is as follows. As food quality (appearance, taste, and texture) deteriorates, there is often a corresponding deterioration in nutrient content. For example,

This discussion has covered the subject of shopping for food in the grocery store, but there's another kind of store it hasn't fully dealt with—the convenience store. Many of the foods sold there are snack foods low in nutrient density and high in sugar, salt, and fat. Some people call these foods *junk foods*. One reference to them is in Highlight 14, where an argument is presented suggesting that the consumption of a *junk diet* may be linked, through the effects of nutrient deficiencies, to behavioral abnormalities in children. It's OK to buy low-quality foods now and then, but you need to keep them under control. Do most of your shopping in a place where you can buy *real* foods, *food* foods—the grocery store.

THE WATER-SOLUBLE VITAMINS 325

when a food smells bad, the odor reveals that oxidative or enzymatic changes have occurred—the same kinds of reactions as those that have adverse effects on nutrients. Thus some of the unprocessed foods sold as "natural food" may be a poor choice in spite of the claims made for them. If they have lost their freshness, they may well have lost much of their vitamin content too, because "no processing" means no measures have been taken to prevent oxidative and enzymatic changes. Thus your common sense, which tells you that a food "doesn't look quite right," can usually be trusted to give you valid information concerning a food's nutrient content.

In modern commercial processing, losses of vitamins seldom exceed 25 percent. In contrast, losses in food preparation at home and in restaurants can be 100 percent, and it is not unusual to see losses in the 60 to 75 percent range. You can see that while the kinds of foods you buy certainly make a difference, what happens to them in the kitchen makes a major difference, too.

Once you have brought nutritious foods home from the store, you have the task of storing and preparing them so that they deliver the nutrients to you when you eat them. Because vitamin C is one of the most vulnerable of the vitamins, it can be used to demonstrate the principles involved, but remember, all the water-soluble vitamins deserve the same care as vitamin C.

Vitamin C is an organic compound synthesized and broken down by enzymes found in the fruits and vegetables that contain it. Like all enzymes, these have a temperature optimum. They work best at the temperatures at which the plants grow, normally about 70 degrees Fahrenheit (25 degrees centigrade), which is also the room temperature in most homes. After a fruit has been picked, synthesis of vitamins (which has depended on a continued influx of energy from sunlight) largely stops; degradation continues. Chilling the fruit slows the degradation. To protect the vitamin C content, fruits and vegetables should be vine ripened (if possible), chilled immediately after picking, and kept cold until they are used.

Because it is an acid and an antioxidant, vitamin C is most stable in an acid solution, away from air. Citrus fruits, tomatoes, and many juices are acid enough to favor its stability. As long as the skin is uncut or the can is unopened, the vitamin is protected from air, but if you store a cut vegetable or fruit or an opened container of juice, cover it with an airtight wrapper and store it in the refrigerator.

Being water soluble, vitamin C readily dissolves into the water in which cut vegetables are washed, boiled, or canned. If the water is discarded, as much as half of the vitamin is poured down the drain with it. To minimize this kind of loss, steam vegetables over water rather than in it, or boil them in a volume of water small enough to be reabsorbed into them by the time they are cooked. Of course, if the water is used in the food or soaks back into it, as in soup, preserves, or fruit pies, a larger volume of water can be used. To prevent losses during washing, wash the food before cutting it. To minimize the oxidation of vitamin C, avoid high temperatures and long cooking times.

Steam vegetables over water rather than in it.

All these factors represent legitimate concerns to which industrial food processors rightly pay attention. Awareness of them has brought about changes in many commercial products: fortification of instant mashed potatoes with vitamin C to replace that lost during processing, and flash heating and freezing of vegetables to minimize enzymatic losses. Saving a small percentage of the vitamin C in foods can mean saving several hundred pounds of the vitamin a day; for people whose intakes are otherwise marginal, this can make a crucial difference.

Meanwhile, however, in your own kitchen, a law of diminishing returns operates. Most vitamin C losses under reasonable conditions are not catastrophic. (For example, reconstituted orange juice typically retains 80 percent of its original vitamin C activity after eight days of storage.) You need not fret and worry over small vitamin losses that occur in your kitchen; you may waste time that is valuable to you in other ways. You can be assured that if you start with plenty of foods containing ample amounts of vitamin C, and you are reasonably careful in their preparation, you will receive enough vitamin C, and a bounty of the other nutrients that they contain.

Study Questions

1. For thiamin, riboflavin, niacin, vitamin B_6, folacin, vitamin B_{12}, pantothenic acid, biotin, and vitamin C, state:
   - its chief function in the body
   - the deficiency symptoms characteristic of it
   - significant food sources for it
2. What is the relationship of tryptophan to niacin?
3. Which B vitamins are involved in anemia?
4. What risks are associated with megadoses of vitamin C?
5. Discuss the pros and cons of using fresh versus processed foods with respect to vitamin value. Discuss the loss of vitamins in the handling and cooking of foods.

Notes

1. V. Tanphaichitr and B. Wood, Thiamin, in *Present Knowledge in Nutrition,* 5th ed. (Washington, D.C.: The Nutrition Foundation, 1984), pp. 273–281.

2. R. S. Rivlin, Riboflavin, in *Present Knowledge in Nutrition,* 5th ed. (Washington, D.C.: The Nutrition Foundation, 1984), pp. 285–302.

3. B. S. N. Rao and C. Gopalan, Niacin, in *Present Knowledge in Nutrition,* 5th ed. (Washington, D.C.: The Nutrition Foundation, 1984), pp. 318–331.

4. Rao and Gopalan, 1984.

5. C. Wagner, Folic acid, in *Present Knowledge in Nutrition,* 5th ed. (Washington, D.C.: The Nutrition Foundation, 1984), pp. 332–346.

6. V. Herbert, Vitamin B_{12}, in *Present Knowledge in Nutrition,* 5th ed. (Washington, D.C.: The Nutrition Foundation, 1984), pp. 347–364.

7. Rao and Gopalan, 1984.

8. J. Hathcock, Vitamin safety, a current appraisal, *Vitamin Issues V* (Nutley, N.J.: Hoffman-LaRoche, 1985), p. 2.

9. M. Brin and J. C. Bauernfeind, Vitamin needs of the elderly, *Postgraduate Medicine* 63, no. 3 (1978): 155–163.

10. A. M. Immerman, Vitamin B_{12} status on a vegetarian diet, a critical review, *World Review of Nutrition and Dietetics* 37 (1981): 38–54.

11. Immerman, 1981.

12. Immerman, 1981; K. H. Steinkraus and coeditors, *Handbook of Indigenous Fermented Foods* (New York and Basel: Marcel Dekker, 1983), p. 40.

13. I. T. H. Liem, K. H. Steinkraus, and T. C. Cronk, Production of vitamin B_{12} in tempeh, a fermented soybean food, *Applied and Environmental Microbiology* 34 (1977): 773–776.

14. J. L. Wood and R. G. Allison, Effects of consumption of choline and lecithin on neurological and cardiovascular systems, *Federation Proceedings* 41 (1982): 3015–3021.

15. A. Kallner, D. Hartmann, and D. Hornig, Steady-state turnover and body pool of ascorbic acid in man, *American Journal of Clinical Nutrition* 32 (1979): 530–539.

16. F. Clark, Drugs and vitamin deficiency, *Journal of Human Nutrition* 30 (1976): 333–337; Committee on Safety, Toxicity, and Misuse of Vitamins and Trace Minerals, National Nutrition Consortium, *Vitamin-Mineral Safety, Toxicity, and Misuse* (Chicago: American Dietetic Association, 1978).

17. Toxicity of vitamin C megadoses, *Nutrition and the MD,* October 1980.

18. Committee on Safety, Toxicity, and Misuse of Vitamins and Trace Minerals, 1978, p. 17.

Several of these exercises make use of the information you recorded on Forms 1 to 3.

1. Look up and record your recommended intake of thiamin (from the RDA tables on the inside front cover or from the Canadian recommendations in Appendix I). Also record your actual intake, from the average derived on Form 2. What percentage of your recommended intake did you consume? Was this enough? What foods contribute the greatest amount of thiamin to your diet? If you

Evaluate Your Intakes of B Vitamins and Vitamin C

consumed more than the recommendation, was this too much? Why or why not? In what ways would you change your diet to improve thiamin intake?

2. Repeat exercise 1 using riboflavin as the subject.

3. Estimate your niacin intake using the method outlined on p. 308. Did you consume enough niacin preformed in foods to meet your recommended intake? If not, did you consume enough extra protein to bring your intake up to the recommendation? What do you suppose are the limitations on this means of estimating niacin intake?

4. Repeat exercise 1 using each of the other B vitamins and vitamin C as the subject.

Vitamin B₆: Does it Cure PMS and Other Ills?

To illuminate this highlight's subject, we have created a monster. His name is Dr. Dover. He is a holistic health practitioner with questionable credentials; it isn't clear what kind of a degree he has, but he is not an M.D.; he does not have a Ph.D. in nutrition or biochemistry; and he is not an R.D. (registered dietitian).

Dr. Dover hasn't had much experience, but he is a nice young man, and is accumulating a sizable practice composed of people who are dissatisfied with their "regular doctors," who, they feel, don't know enough about nutrition. Dr. Dover is a great nutrition enthusiast, and these days is especially energetic in promoting vitamin B₆.

Our story is oversimplified. No one, we sincerely hope, is as outrageous a practitioner as Dr. Dover. But there are people out there who are making the kinds of mistakes he makes, and we'd like to alert you to them.

In the course of telling this story, we first present a wide array of symptoms that have been associated with vitamin B₆ deficiency. You have to read to the end to see that *none of these symptoms is sufficient evidence by itself that a vitamin B₆ deficiency exists*. All *may* reflect such a deficiency; but they may have other, possibly life-threatening causes.

Our conclusion is that, in all cases, the connections with vitamin B₆ are interesting and worth pursuing, but that no applications are possible now. Anyone who has a suspected deficiency of vitamin B₆ should have a valid blood or urine test to confirm or deny its reality, and *then* take appropriate action. No one should take vitamin B₆ supplements until such a test has demonstrated low B₆ status. And anyone taking such supplements should be warned that, in amounts above 200 milligrams a day, they can lead to toxic effects within a few weeks.

Finally, it's worth pointing out that *this kind of story could be told as well about any other vitamin or mineral*. All can be and have been misused this way. Vitamin B₆ won the spotlight here because it is of great current interest. Ten years ago, vitamin C or vitamin E would have occupied this place. Ten years from now some other nutrient will have its name in lights.

Symptoms Associated with Vitamin B₆ Deficiency

Juanita gets sick in Chinese restaurants; Joann has pain in her left hand. Harriet is taking oral contraceptives, and James has had a heart attack and fears another. George has sores in his mouth, Angela is becoming senile, and Margie feels miserable before her menstrual period. What do all these people have in common? All have visited Dr. Dover, who has recommended that they take a gram a day of vitamin B₆. Some of them are getting better, and some are beginning to get sicker than they were to begin with, because they are beginning to suffer the toxic effects of an overdose. What are the bases for Dr. Dover's recommendations, and what are the risks associated with them?

Chinese Restaurant Syndrome

Whenever Juanita eats Chinese food, she reacts within an hour. She feels warm, stiff, weak, and tingly in the limbs; gets a headache and feels light-headed; and gets a stomachache or sensations like heartburn. Dr. Dover has told her she is suffering from Chinese restaurant syndrome, a sensitivity to the flavor enhancer monosodium glutamate (MSG) used in Asian cookery, and has suggested she take megadose supplements of vitamin B₆. What are the chances that he's right?

He *could* be right in thinking Juanita may have a vitamin B₆ deficiency. In 1981 a group of researchers, speculating that Chinese restaurant syndrome might be a manifestation of borderline vitamin B₆ deficiency, sought out 27 students who didn't take vitamin supplements and who, by a clinical test, were in poor vitamin B₆ status. They tested the students to see if they were sensitive to MSG; of the 27, 12 were, and 15 were not. They then tested the 12 students further: they gave vitamin B₆ (50-milligram doses each day for three months) to 9 of them and an inert placebo (see p. 340) to the other 3 without telling them which was which. At the end of that time, 8 of the 9 who had received the vitamin were no longer sensitive to MSG, while all 3 of the untreated subjects still reacted adversely to it.[1]

This one report is the basis for Dr. Dover's recommendation to our friend Juanita that she take a gram a day of vitamin B₆. He didn't test her, though, to see if she had a deficiency of this or any other vitamin or mineral, and the dose he is recommending is dangerously high. You can see why he thinks it might work—but remember, the people in the one experiment reported were selected *because* they were deficient in vitamin B₆. The researchers didn't look for other people who had Chinese restaurant syndrome. And don't forget the one subject whose reaction didn't change; she proves that there are nonresponders to B₆. Even after her vitamin B₆ status became entirely normal, she wasn't cured. Also, the dose the researchers used was 50 milligrams a day. Dr. Dover is recommending 1,000 milligrams, 20 times as much. It may be dangerous for Juanita to keep taking these huge doses of vitamin B₆, and they may not even affect her sensitivity to MSG.

Carpal Tunnel Syndrome

Joann's left hand is almost useless to her. When she unthinkingly moves it, it hurts so much she cries out. Her physician has been considering surgery, to relieve the pressure on her wrist nerves that is causing the pain, but now that she has visited Dr. Dover, she has decided to try taking megadose supplements of vitamin B₆ first to see if they help. What are the chances that they will?

A report published in 1978 is probably the basis for Dr. Dover's recommendation to Joann. The report reviewed a case in which a 40-year-old man with carpal tunnel syndrome was brought relief with vitamin B₆ supplements of 100 milligrams per day for 10 to 11 weeks. At the same time, an enzyme in his red blood cells that was dependent on vitamin B₆ as a coenzyme went from abnormal to normal in its action. When he was given a placebo for nine weeks, both his physical state and the enzyme activity deteriorated; when he was given the real vitamin again, both were restored to normal. The man seemed to have been eating a vitamin B₆–deficient diet for ten years or more, and RDA levels of vitamin B₆ (2 milligrams a day) were not enough to correct his deficiency.[2]

The researchers who reported this case also reviewed evidence that other

people with carpal tunnel syndrome may have vitamin B₆ deficiencies. Anyone reading their report, which was published in a reputable journal, would be inclined to test any client with carpal tunnel syndrome for a possible vitamin B₆ deficiency. However, tests on 13 clients by other investigators have seemed to indicate that vitamin B₆ does not relieve carpal tunnel syndrome.[3]

Anyway, the trouble with Dr. Dover's approach in Joann's case is that he performed no such test. Perhaps he couldn't; not being a licensed medical doctor, perhaps he didn't have access to the necessary laboratory facilities. More likely, he may not have known what test to use or how to interpret the results. In any case, he blindly "prescribed" vitamin B₆ for Joann without collecting any evidence to confirm or reject his "diagnosis," and without investigating any other possible causes of her pain. If Joann's symptoms result from another cause, her visits to Dr. Dover will have wasted time and money and will have needlessly prolonged her suffering.

Oral Contraceptives

Dr. Dover has advised Harriet to take vitamin B₆ supplements on the basis that "oral contraceptive users need more than the RDA." The hormones in oral contraceptives affect the way the body handles tryptophan (an amino acid), so that substances appear in the urine that would normally be metabolized in the body. Vitamin B₆ assists in the metabolism of tryptophan, and when women on the Pill take added B₆, the abnormality largely disappears. This suggests, but does not prove, that women on the Pill have a vitamin B₆ requirement greater than the RDA of 2 milligrams a day, although not greater than 5 milligrams.[4] Larger doses might bring about undesirable alterations in amino acid metabolism and might even interfere with the effectiveness of the Pill's hormones, since the vitamin, in megadose amounts, interferes with the action of

this class of hormones generally.[5] Dr. Dover hasn't tested Harriet to see if she has the abnormality that indicates a B₆ need, and he is way out on a limb in recommending 1,000, rather than 5, milligrams a day.

Blood Clotting

James, who has had a heart attack and fears another, is now dosing himself with vitamin B₆ on Dr. Dover's advice. Dr. Dover suspects that James may have a vitamin B₆ deficiency because such deficiencies have been observed to cause injuries in the arteries of monkeys, dogs, rats, and rabbits. High doses of the vitamin (perhaps 40 milligrams a day) may modify a protein that affects platelet aggregation so that blood clots are less likely to form.[6] The tests showing this effect were performed on blood samples in test tubes, however, not in human beings, and experiments will have to address many more research questions before they can assess the safety or effectiveness of vitamin B₆ supplements to prevent clotting, or determine the appropriate dose. It would be unsafe to recommend supplements to anyone based on this little bit of knowledge. A doctor's first duty is to "do no harm"; only after he is certain of that can he propose steps that *may* do good. Vitamin B₆ may do good in some instances like this, but it isn't clear yet that it does no harm.

Still, it would certainly do no harm to try to determine whether James's vitamin B₆ status is normal. If James has a deficiency, it would be a shame to overlook it. But Dr. Dover didn't check James's diet or his blood enzyme levels for evidence of a deficiency. He only connected James's symptoms in his mind with the possibility of a deficiency. On that basis he recommended megadose supplements. Hardly responsible medicine.

Oral Lesions

George has sores in his mouth and is now, on Dr. Dover's advice, taking vitamin B_6 supplements to cure them. Dr. Dover must have reasoned that, because oral lesions are a manifestation of vitamin B_6 deficiency,[7] George must have such a deficiency. This was sloppy thinking. Practically every vitamin and mineral deficiency and many other conditions cause oral lesions of one kind or another; that they are a problem for George only indicates that he needs a diagnosis, not that he needs vitamin B_6.

What would a responsible clinician do, faced with the same physical finding? We could demonstrate the diagnostic procedure for any of the symptoms being discussed here; we'll use mouth sores as an example for all of them. A responsible clinician would follow a procedure that goes something like this:

Finding: *Sore mouth.*

Question: *Where are the sores?*[8]

If they are on one place only, they may indicate a problem as simple as a jagged tooth, or as serious as cancer. If they are all over the tongue, they suggest glossitis, which may reflect any of many different kinds of infection, allergy, or nutrient deficiency.

Question: *Are the sores discolored?*

If they are creamy yellow and easy to scrape off, they may reflect oral thrush, a fungus disease. The doctor's next question will be "Have you been taking antibiotics recently?"—because, if you have, thrush is especially likely to develop. If they don't scrape off, and if they are painful, the next questions are:

Question: *Do you feel ill? Do you have a temperature of 100 degrees or above?*

Illness and fever with these sores may reflect a viral infection. Similar sores without illness and fever may be mouth ulcers or canker sores.

The doctor keeps asking questions until she has sorted all possible causes of mouth sores into two categories: "no" and "possible." Then she systematically pursues the "possibles" one by one using a priority system and her judgment of the client's individual situation to decide which to pursue first. She thinks in terms of these considerations:

- *Urgency.* If this is the diagnosis, is it imperative to find out quickly? (Example: cancer.)
- *Cost.* If not urgent, how expensive is the test? (The less expensive tests can be performed first. Maybe the more expensive ones won't be necessary.)
- *Simplicity.* As with cost, the simpler tests can be performed first.
- *Probability of being correct.* If the doctor is virtually certain that a particular diagnosis is correct, she may perform this test first.

What a far cry this kind of thinking is from that of Dr. Dover! His thinking seems to have been: "Mouth sores, huh? Well, mouth sores can mean vitamin B_6 deficiency. Let's try a B_6 supplement and see if it works." We can hope that Dr. Dover won't be allowed to practice for very much longer. Perhaps an angry client will sue him successfully for malpractice and put him out of business. And we can hope that this client won't have to pay for the privilege with an advanced case of mouth cancer.

Aging of the Brain

Dr. Dover has suggested that Angela, who seems to be becoming senile, should take vitamin B_6 supplements. Vitamin B_6 deficiency has been shown to cause alterations in the brain cells of rats, suggesting premature aging of the brain;[9] and it is known that older people in general have an increased likelihood of vitamin B_6 deficiency.[10] But to demonstrate degenerative brain changes in animals, the researchers virtually had to deprive them totally of the vitamin; total absence of the vitamin is *not* seen in human populations, and is surely not the case for Angela. (On the other hand, people live much longer than rats, so time is available for the effects of slight vitamin deficiency to accumulate.) Angela should certainly be checked for vitamin B_6 deficiency—but then, her entire nutrition profile should be studied, and she should also go through a standard diagnostic workup including questions about chest infections, urinary tract infections, depression, use of drugs, alcohol use, and other possibilities.

Premenstrual Syndrome

Margie, too, is taking vitamin B_6 supplements on Dr. Dover's advice. She suffers from premenstrual syndrome (PMS), and he has given her the hope that vitamin B_6 will cure it.

No one, as of this writing, knows what causes PMS. Vitamin B_6 seems related to it somehow, but many other nutrients are, too. This section discusses not only vitamin B_6, but all known possibilities.

Margie's PMS, which is a typical case, involves sore breasts, a backache, and a headache. She cries easily, is irritated and depressed. She tends to binge on sweets. Predictably, every month, it comes on, stays a week to ten days, and then mysteriously disappears like a cloud lifting a few hours after her menstrual period has begun. One out of every three women recognizes some of these symptoms as hers.

Is poor nutrition the cause of all this? Some people are tempted to think so; others think not. Research into the relationships between PMS and nutrition is new, with few, if any, conclusions reached as yet. But some interesting questions have been raised and partially answered.

Because the hormones that dominate the premenstrual weeks promote sodium and water retention, some doctors prescribe diuretics to get rid of the excess sodium and water. Some researchers have reported that diuretics relieve all PMS symptoms except painful breasts, but others have tried to confirm this finding and failed. Possibly the placebo effect has confounded the work: women in treatment, who expected to feel better, may have felt better whether they were given diuretics or not. The placebo effect is discussed further in Highlight 9B; it can be so strong that it can make a nutrient *seem* to relieve PMS symptoms even for several months in a row, and yet the nutrient may not in reality be a cure for those symptoms.*

Magnesium may have some connection with PMS. When magnesium status was studied in "normal" and PMS subjects, the levels of this mineral in the red blood cells were found to be lower in the PMS group.[11] One might jump to the conclusion that "people with PMS need more magnesium," but this may not be the case at all. The subjects' diets weren't studied, so it's impossible to tell whether they had a dietary deficiency, were absorbing less, or were excreting more magnesium. In fact, it's possible that the women's total body contents of magnesium hadn't changed, but that there had been a shift of magnesium from the red blood cells into some other body compartment. Red blood cells, like all cells, "decide" what their contents should be; that is, they actively take in or reject available substances in response to signals from elsewhere—hormones, for example. The PMS group might have too much or too little of some other substance, and this difference might cause their red blood cells to take up less magnesium. Clearly, on the basis of the one finding, it is impossible to say whether people with PMS need more magnesium, or less, or more or less of something else.

Vitamin B_6 has been a prime candidate for relieving PMS, based on at least two different complex lines of logic. One argument is that women with PMS may have abnormally high levels of the hormone prolactin (this remains to be confirmed), and that high prolactin levels cause PMS (this is not established as fact). Possibly (from another report), high doses of vitamin B_6 depress prolactin. Based on these three ifs, megadoses of vitamin B_6 might relieve PMS.[12]

The other chain of reasoning is that women with PMS have an abnormal ratio of estrogen to progesterone, and that this *might* cause a "relative vitamin B_6 deficiency," because estrogen displaces vitamin B_6 from its preferred sites on enzyme surfaces. Also, estrogen speeds up a process that requires vitamin B_6.

Trials of vitamin B_6 in PMS have had such mixed results as to invoke despair in the hearts of all but the most cheerful investigators. The most positive evidence is from trials with one woman with a vitamin B_6 deficiency who claimed that her PMS symptoms were responsive to vitamin B_6 supplements. Investigators gave her the vitamin (50 milligrams per day) and a placebo in alternate months for six months without telling her and also without knowing, themselves, which was which until the end of the study (a double-blind experiment). She experienced relief from her symptoms consistently with the vitamin and not with the placebo, showing clearly, they said, that in her case PMS was related to vitamin B_6.[13] Thus the vitamin may have real, beneficial effects on PMS when a deficiency of the vitamin exists. The old lesson of basic nutrition is reinforced here: a vitamin will clear up symptoms—but only if they are caused by a deficiency of that vitamin.

Vitamin E deficiency is another candidate for contributor to PMS, and one creditable attempt has demonstrated that vitamin E has some effectiveness in relieving one symptom often experienced in PMS—sore breasts. The research involved 75 women; it was a double-blind, placebo-controlled study; and its results suggested that vitamin E (300 mg) brought relief while the placebo did not.[14] However, some women *without* PMS also have sore breasts that can sometimes be relieved by vitamin E.[15] Possibly the correct logic is that vitamin E deficiency can cause sore breasts, and the menstrual cycle can make them worse; but *not* that vitamin E deficiency causes PMS.

Vitamin A deficiency, too, has been blamed for PMS. Vitamin A helped a woman once in 1947, and occasional reports of its therapeutic effectiveness have appeared since then. Surely, though, the past 40 years would have been enough time to confirm if it were so, that vitamin A deficiency was the cause of PMS, or that vitamin A megadoses would cure it. Attempts to demonstrate these possibilities have failed, and no recommendations regarding vitamin A can be made on the basis of evidence collected to date.[16]

In summary, based on these reports, there is reason to investigate these nutrients further: magnesium, vitamin B_6, and vitamin E. Other, nonnutritional avenues also deserve much more attention. They include hormone imbalances (some that affect the blood glucose level), and brain chemicals (endorphins) that affect perceptions and moods.[17]

Meanwhile, medical and health professionals, under pressure to make recommendations *now* for their clients with PMS, are trying a number of shots in the dark:

Natural progesterone and lithium carbonate . . . methyltestosterone (for headache); minor tranquilizers; "Relaxation for Living" classes; regular breakfasts; aspirin; orgasm; bromocriptine; scientific information and emotional support; potassium; calcium, alone or with magnesium; special diets (low-sodium, high-protein, high-fiber); amphetamine; ibuprofen; and hiding in your room.[18]

---

*"There is a very striking placebo effect in this disorder. Symptoms often disappear during a woman's first month on sugar pills," but gradually return over the next four to five months. R. L. Reid, as quoted by E. R. Gonzalez, Premenstrual syndrome: An ancient woe deserving of modern scrutiny (medical news), *Journal of the American Medical Association* 245 (1981): 1393–1396.

Practitioners other than doctors have still other remedies to offer. Evening primrose oil, for instance. At least two companies selling it—one in Nova Scotia, the other in Massachusetts—are claiming a fantastic success rate in treating PMS with it. It is said to be "the only natural source, besides mother's milk," of gamma-linolenic acid. Women "whose tissues are depleted of it" are urged to take primrose oil capsules twice a day for two or three months, and they will become "symptom free."[19]

Gamma-linolenic acid is not the same as the essential fatty acid linoleic acid (see Chapter 4), but is made from it in the human body. "Tissue depletion" is said to occur when there is inadequate conversion of linoleic to gamma-linolenic acid, a circumstance that arises often in PMS sufferers, according to the promoters of primrose oil.[20] They have only a little research to base their claims on,[21] and many questions remain unanswered. Gamma-linolenic acid doesn't occur naturally in foods, and surely our cave ancestors didn't eat bucketsful of primroses. Why do so many women (and not men) have "tissue depletion"? And—very importantly—when research is performed by independent investigators, who are *not* making their livings from the sales of primrose oil, will it confirm the effectiveness of gamma-linolenic acid in relieving the symptoms of PMS?

Before we can really know what to recommend to women who suffer with PMS, several kinds of studies will have to be done. One type of study will have to answer the question, How do the diets of women with PMS differ from those of women unaffected by PMS? One report suggests that women with PMS eat more refined sugar and salt, and less of several nutrients, than "normal" women—in other words, that they tend to choose foods of lower nutrient density, and have lower intakes of B vitamins, iron, and zinc as a

consequence.[22] However, the study may be biased, because its chief author is employed by a company that sells nutrient supplements. Without several more such studies, carefully performed by a variety of independent investigators, we can't really know what the typical nutrition status of PMS women is. When we do know, we will still have to ask whether nutrition abnormalities cause, or result from, PMS. Nor do we yet have enough information on PMS sufferers' nutrient status derived from lab work. Most important is to answer the basic question, what are the metabolic defects in PMS? Is there one cause or are there several causes that would imply different solutions for different people?

One thing seems clear: the woman with PMS should look to her diet. Like any other person suffering from any other symptoms, she may not have complete control over her condition, but her diet *is* under her control. If she has any nutrient deficiencies, then she isn't doing all she can to help herself be well.

All menstruating women can benefit from some recent findings on nutrition and the menstrual cycle. Many women just plain get hungry during the week or two before their periods. Reliable research shows that two things happen during that time:

- Basal metabolic rate speeds up.[23]
- Appetite and kcalorie intake pick up.[24]

About 20 percent of the women in two studies indicated, when asked, that their appetites increased before their periods,[25] but in fact most or all women may actually eat more during this time without being aware that they do. They report that they crave sweets, and when their food intakes are actually measured, they are seen to be eating an average of 500 kcalories a day more during the ten days prior to their periods than during the ten days after—principally from carbohydrate.[26]

There's at least one application of these findings that seems obvious at

first glance. Many women attempt to restrict their kcalories, sometimes severely, in the effort to control their weight. During the two weeks following their periods, they may find this relatively easy to do, but during the two weeks before their next periods, they may find it very hard, because they are fighting a natural, hormone-governed increase in metabolic rate, appetite, and even craving for carbohydrate. Given the complex, sometimes guilt-ridden feelings about food that many women have, they are at a great disadvantage trying to fight these forces. Women need to know that the increased hunger and carbohydrate craving that precede menstruation are natural, probably universal biological phenomena, and not signs of their own incompetence, inadequacy, or neuroticism. Rather than attempt to restrict kcalorie intakes rigidly to some fixed amount throughout the month, any woman whose appetite is affected by the cyclic rhythm of her hormones would do better to relax and go with it: increase kcalories during the two weeks before her period, and reduce them during the two weeks after.

Finally, the same advice holds for women with PMS as for women or men with any other health problem or need. Be sure to get adequate sleep and adequate exercise. Eat well, and be sensible about your intakes of sugar, caffeine, salt, alcohol, and any other "abuse-able" substances. If you have reason to think your nutrient intakes are inadequate and you *can't* rectify them by eating foods, then fall back on a daily supplement for a while. But avoid megadoses. Stay with the moderate amounts available in an ordinary multivitamin-mineral supplement. And be very, very skeptical when people who can pocket your money in return for their goods tell you their products will relieve your symptoms. Watch out for snake-oil salespeople; there are a lot of them out there.

How Widespread Are Vitamin B_6 Deficiencies?

Vitamin B_6 was discovered only about 50 years ago, and the human need for it has been known for only 30 years. Research into its metabolic roles is currently very active, and much remains to be learned. The RDA has been set, tentatively, at 2.0 milligrams a day for women and 2.2 milligrams for men— enough to cover the high protein intake of our typical diet. These amounts are as likely to be too high as to be too low. Dependency can be induced in adults fed a normal diet supplemented with 200 milligrams a day of vitamin B_6 for a month.[27]

The Nationwide Food Consumption Survey, concluded just prior to 1980, found vitamin B_6 intakes below 70 percent of the RDA in about half of the people surveyed. No one quite knows what to make of this finding. An extreme interpretation is that one out of every two people has a less-than-optimal, or even inadequate, intake of vitamin B_6. At the other extreme is the view that no one is really deficient in vitamin B_6. Food contents of vitamin B_6 are still being worked out. No one knows how well the body absorbs vitamin B_6 from different foods, so even if we know how much you ingest, we can't guess how much you absorb. No one knows how much of an impact food processing and cooking has on the vitamin. The first research findings on these subjects are just now being published.

The Nationwide Food Consumption Survey asked only about intakes; it sought no lab data to show if low intakes were reflected by physical abnormalities. When lab data are sought, they indicate that vitamin B_6 deficiencies are real among these groups:

- Some pregnant women.
- Some oral contraceptive users.
- Older people.
- Alcohol abusers.
- People with kidney disease.
- People with Down's syndrome (a type of mental retardation).
- People taking certain prescription medications.*

Also, a few individuals have rare genetic diseases that greatly increase their needs for vitamin B_6.[28] Among the population at large, findings suggest that at least some of those with low intakes are paying a physical price.**

The conclusion seems reasonable that some of the many symptoms we started with are related, at least in part, to real vitamin B_6 deficiencies. Perhaps, then, Dr. Dover's head is screwed on right when he suggests vitamin B_6 supplements to Margie, Joann, and all his other patients. What harm does it really do to try and see?

Risks of Megadoses

The first major report of toxic effects of vitamin B_6 appeared in 1983; since then, similar reports have followed. The first report told of seven individuals who had been taking more than 2 grams a day of vitamin B_6 for two months or more, most of them attempting to cure the edema of PMS. Some simply self-prescribed it; some were following their gynecologists' advice; one had a prescription from an "orthomolecular psychiatrist," and one was taking it after reading about it in a health magazine. The cases were similar,

---

*Isoniazid (INH), penicillamine, corticosteroids, and anticonvulsants.
**For example, in one study where half of the subjects were receiving less than 70 percent of the RDA, a third of them also had low lab values; A. Kirksey and coauthors, Vitamin B_6 nutritional status of a group of female adolescents, *American Journal of Clinical Nutrition* 31 (1978): 946–954. In another study, only about 20 percent had low intakes (the criterion used was stricter), and again, about a third had low lab values; S. C. Vir and A. H. G. Love, Vitamin B_6 status of the hospitalized aged, *American Journal of Clinical Nutrition* 31 (1978): 1383–1391.

---

with only minor variations. They started with numb feet, then lost sensation in their hands, then became unable to work. Later, in some cases, their mouths became numb. In all but two cases they had started with much lower doses, found they didn't work, and progressed to higher and higher doses seeking an effect. They may have suffered irreversible nerve damage. Their symptoms began clearing up after withdrawal of the supplements, but it was uncertain that they would completely disappear.[29]

Since then, 16 more cases have been reported, in which doses as low as 200 milligrams, taken for a long time, caused "pins and needles," numbness of the hands, difficulty walking, and other symptoms. When they stopped taking the vitamin, patients reported improvement but not complete disappearance of their symptoms.[30] Then followed a report on 58 women who were taking 50 to 300 milligrams a day of vitamin B_6. In these women, other symptoms—in fact, those normally associated with PMS— improved or disappeared on *stopping* taking the vitamin: depression, headaches, tiredness, bloatedness, irritability, and neuropathy.[31] The evidence seems to be mounting that high doses of this vitamin are ill-advised.

Personal Strategy

Vitamin B_6 is the wonder vitamin of the decade. It deserves its place in the sun; it is a versatile performer in the drama of metabolism. But its fans are overly enthusiastic when they want it to be the star of every show. It is only one of many nutrients that work together, and there are some roles it can't play. It can cure its own deficiency symptoms, and possibly, in high doses, it can act as a drug, but it can't work miracles.

Deficiencies of vitamin B_6 do exist in our population. That means that marginal deficiencies also exist, causing symptoms that have not been well characterized yet, and are probably not always recognized, even by reputable, skilled physicians and dietitians. Increased public awareness of the importance of this vitamin is leading in a desirable direction—toward detection and correction of deficiencies and relief from the symptoms they cause.

Dr. Dover is, in one sense, in the forefront of medical and nutrition practice in that he is aware of the possibility of vitamin B_6 deficiencies among the people who consult him. But he is making three dangerous mistakes in "prescribing" vitamin megadoses to Juanita, Joann, and all his other clients. He hasn't tested for chemical signs of vitamin B_6 deficiency. He hasn't checked their diets to see whether primary deficiencies are a real possibility. And he is recommending a frighteningly high dose.

Rather than follow the risky course of consulting a Dr. Dover, if you or anyone you know suspects a vitamin B_6 deficiency, consult an R.D. and an M.D. The R.D., if worthy of the credential, will check your diet history. The M.D., if nutrition-wise, will check for clinical and biochemical signs of vitamin B_6 deficiency. And both should review your medical and drug history for interactions of diseases and medications with the vitamin. If they have reason to believe you have a vitamin B_6 deficiency, *and once they have excluded other diagnoses,* they will recommend a therapeutic dose supplement for a finite period of time— probably 50 to 200 milligrams for not more than six to ten weeks. Meanwhile, they will counsel you on improving your diet so that supplementation will not continue to be necessary, and they will advise you to come back for follow-up and further diagnostic work if B_6 replacement proves ineffective.

Miniglossary

carpal tunnel syndrome: tingling and numbness in part of the hand and wrist and shooting pains up the arm caused by swelling of tissue surrounding a nerve that passes through the wrist bones. Possible causes include fluid accumulation and hormone imbalances, as well as vitamin B_6 deficiency.

Chinese restaurant syndrome: an intolerance reaction that may occur in one out of several hundred people 20 minutes after the ingestion of the additive MSG (monosodium glutamate, or Accent). Symptoms include burning sensations, chest and facial flushing and pain, and throbbing headache.

syndrome: a cluster of symptoms.

NOTES
1. Possible vitamin B_6 deficiency uncovered in persons with the "Chinese restaurant syndrome," *Nutrition Reviews* 40 (1982): 15–16.
2. K. Folkers, Biochemical evidence for a deficiency of vitamin B_6 in the carpal tunnel syndrome based on a crossover clinical study, *Proceedings of the National Academy of Sciences USA* 75 (1978): 3410–3412.
3. R. D. Scheyer and D. C. Haas, Pyridoxine in carpal tunnel syndrome, *Lancet,* July 1985, p. 42.
4. The vitamin B_6 requirement in oral contraceptive users, *Nutrition Reviews* 37 (1979): 344–345.
5. Does pyridoxal phosphate have a non-coenzymatic role in steroid hormone action? *Nutrition Reviews* 38 (1980): 93–95.
6. Inhibition of platelet aggregation and clotting by pyridoxal-5'-phosphate, *Nutrition Reviews* 40 (1982): 55–57.

7. S. Bapurao, L. Raman, and P. G. Tulpule, Biochemical assessment of vitamin B_6 nutritional status in pregnant women with orolingual manifestations, *American Journal of Clinical Nutrition* 36 (1982): 581–586.
8. The fragment of a differential diagnosis that follows is from J. R. M. Kunz, ed., *The American Medical Association Family Medical Guide* (New York: Random House, 1982), p. 140.
9. E. J. Root and J. B. Longenecker, Brain cell alterations suggesting premature aging induced by dietary deficiency of vitamin B_6 and/or copper, *American Journal of Clinical Nutrition* 37 (1983): 540–552.
10. S. C. Vir and A. H. G. Love, Vitamin B_6 status of the hospitalized aged, *American Journal of Clinical Nutrition* 31 (1978): 1383–1391.
11. G. E. Abraham and M. M. Lubran, Serum and red cell magnesium levels in

A Note on Seeking Therapy for PMS

The American Council on Science and Health advises women seeking treatment for PMS to be skeptical of clinics or practitioners who:
- Claim 100 percent success rates.
- Claim to be able to diagnose the condition with tests on blood, urine, or hair.
- Offer a "secret formula".
- Charge inordinately high prices.
- Fail to warn about possible risks or side effects of a particular therapy.
- Fail to inform that treatment with progesterone, other steroid hormones, bromocriptine, spironolactone, pyridoxine (vitamin B_6), vitamin E, evening primrose oil, or magnesium are still experimental and that some of these approaches have not been proven safe.

Source: Adapted from ACSH, as cited by *Nutrition Forum*, November 1985, p. 84.

patients with premenstrual tension, *American Journal of Clinical Nutrition* 34 (1981): 2364–2366.

12. D. Y. Jones and S. K. Kumanyika, Premenstrual syndrome: A review of possible dietary influences, *Journal of the Canadian Dietetic Association* 44 (1983): 194–203.

13. J. A. Mattes and D. Martin, Pyridoxine in premenstrual tension, *Human Nutrition: Applied Nutrition* 36A (1982): 131–133.

14. R. S. London and coauthors, The effect of alpha-tocopherol on premenstrual symptomatology: A double-blind study. *Journal of the American College of Nutrition* 2 (1983): 115–122.

15. E. R. Gonzalez, Vitamin E relieves most cystic breast disease; may alter lipids, hormones (medical news), *Journal of the American Medical Association* 244 (1980): 1077–1078.

16. R. L. Reid and S. S. C. Yen, Premenstrual syndrome, *American Journal of Obstetrics and Gynecology* 139 (1981): 85–104.

17. Reid and Yen, 1981.

18. Gonzalez, 1980.

19. The primrose path, *Health,* February 1983, p. 17. The article referred to "gamma linoleic acid," but gamma-*linolenic* acid is correct.

20. M. G. Brush and coauthors, Abnormal essential fatty acid levels in plasma of women with premenstrual syndrome, *American Journal of Obstetrics and Gynecology,* 150 (1984): 363–366.

21. D. F. Horrobin, The role of essential fatty acids and prostaglandins in the premenstrual syndrome, *Journal of Reproductive Medicine* 28 (1983): 465–468.

22. G. S. Goei, J. L. Ralston, and G. E. Abraham, Dietary patterns of patients with premenstrual tension, *Journal of Applied Nutrition* 34 (1982): 4–11.

23. S. J. Solomon, M. S. Kurzer, and D. H. Calloway, Menstrual cycle and basal metabolic rate in women, *American Journal of Clinical Nutrition* 36 (1982): 611–616.

24. S. P. Dalvit, The effect of the menstrual cycle on patterns of food intake, *American Journal of Clinical Nutrition* 34 (1981): 1811–1815.

25. J. H. Morton and coauthors, A clinical study of premenstrual tension, *American Journal of Obstetrics and Gynecology* 65 (1953): 1182–1191; H. Sutherland and I. Stewart, A critical analysis of the premenstrual syndrome, *Lancet* 1 (1965): 1180–1183, as cited by Jones and Kumanyika, 1983.

26. S. P. Dalvit-McPhillips, The effect of the human menstrual cycle on nutrient intake, *Physiology and Behavior* 31 (1983): 209–212.

27. Food and Nutrition Board, Committee on Recommended Allowances, *Recommended Dietary Allowances,* 9th ed. (Washington, D.C.: National Academy of Sciences, 1980), p. 97.

28. H. E. Sauberlich, Clinical aspects of vitamin B_6 (pyridoxine) metabolism, *Nutrition and the MD,* March 1983.

29. H. Schaumberg and coauthors, Sensory neuropathy from pyridoxine abuse, *New England Journal of Medicine* 309 (1983): 445–448.

30. More B_6 toxicity reported, *Nutrition Forum,* November 1985, p. 84.

31. K. Dalton, Pyridoxine overdose in premenstrual syndrome, *Lancet,* 18 May 1985, pp. 1168–1169.

Vitamin C: Rumors Versus Research

When Dr. Linus Pauling published his book *Vitamin C and the Common Cold* in 1970, he started a storm of controversy that raged for a decade.[1] Newspaper headlines screamed VITAMIN C CURES COLDS; others yelled back VITAMIN C NO EFFECT. One "famous scientist" said this, another that. Meanwhile, behind the scenes, teams of researchers in laboratories and hospitals across the world went to work designing and executing controlled experiments to determine whether, in fact, vitamin C has any therapeutic or preventive effect against the viruses that cause the myriad disorders collectively called the cold.

Since then some hundreds of articles have been published in the research journals, numbering several thousands of pages. Hundreds of people have been tested in a variety of experimental designs, and some conclusions have been reached. Meanwhile, Dr. Pauling has gone on to make additional claims for vitamin C; he urges that any client diagnosed as having cancer should immediately start taking 10 grams a day.[2] More research studies have followed, and the cancer question is generating as much controversy as the common cold.

The purpose of this highlight is primarily to make you aware of the difficulties inherent in attempting to discover whether a nutrient (or any therapeutic approach) remediates symptoms or cures a disease. New findings on the efficacy of various treatments appear every week, but always, the same kinds of questions have to be answered before their usefulness can be evaluated. Research on vitamin C and colds illustrates particularly well what those questions are. Along the way, the relationship of vitamin C to colds will be clarified. As for cancer, more nutrients than just vitamin C are involved, and Highlight 4A attempts to put them all in perspective.

In most studies on the efficacy of vitamin C, two groups of people are selected. Only one group is given vitamin C; both are followed to determine whether the vitamin C group does better in terms of colds or cancer than the control group. A number of pitfalls are inherent in an experiment of this kind; they must be avoided if the results are to be believed.

Controls

First, the two groups must be similar in all respects except for vitamin C dosages. Most important, both must have the same track record with respect to colds, to rule out the possibility that an observed difference might have occurred anyway. (If group A would have caught twice as many colds as

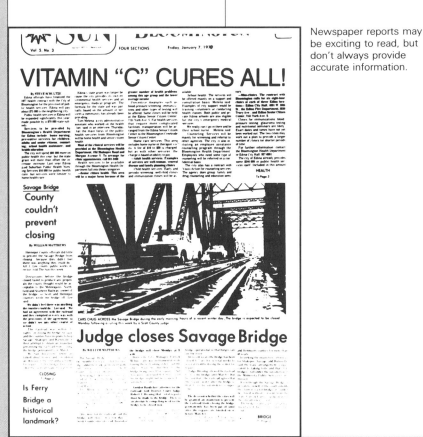

Newspaper reports may be exciting to read, but don't always provide accurate information.

group B anyway, then the fact that group B happened to receive the vitamin proves nothing.) Also, in experiments involving a nutrient, it is imperative that the diets of both groups be similar, especially with respect to that nutrient. (If those in group B were receiving less vitamin C from their diet, this fact might cancel the effects of the supplement.) Similarity of the experimental and control groups is one of the characteristics of a well-controlled experiment and is accomplished by randomization, a process of choosing the members from the same starting population by throws of the dice or some such method involving chance.

Sample Size

To ensure that chance variation between the two groups does not influence the results, the groups must be large. (If one member of a group of five people catches a bad cold by chance, he will pull the whole group's average toward bad colds; but if one member of a group of 500 catches a bad cold, it will not unduly affect the group average.) In reviewing the results of experiments of this kind, always ask whether the number of people tested was large enough to rule out chance variation. Statistical methods are useful for determining the significance of differences between groups of various sizes.

Placebos

If a person takes vitamin C for a cold and believes it will cure him, the chances of recovery are greatly improved. The administration of any pill that the taker believes is medicine hastens recovery in about half of all cases.[3] This phenomenon, the effect of faith on healing, is known as the placebo effect. In experiments designed to determine whether vitamin C actually affects prevention of, or

In discussing these subtleties of experimental design, our intent is not to make a research scientist out of you, but to show you what a far cry real scientific validity is from the experience of your neighbor Mary (sample size, one; no control group), who says she takes vitamin C when she feels a cold coming on and "it works every time." (She knows what she is taking, she has faith in its efficacy, and she tends not to notice when it doesn't work.) Before concluding that an experiment has shown that a nutrient cures a disease or alleviates a symptom, you have to ask yourself these questions:

- Was there a control group similar in all important ways to the experimental group?
- Was the sample size large enough to rule out chance variation?
- Was a placebo effectively administered (blind)?
- Was the experiment double blind?

These are a few, but not all, of the important variables involved in studying the efficacy of a "cure." With them in mind, let's review the literature to see how successfully Dr. Pauling's vitamin C theory has stood the test of experimentation.

recovery from, colds or cancer, this mind-body effect must be rigorously controlled.

To control for the placebo effect, the experimenters must give pills to all participants, some containing vitamin C and others, of similar appearance and taste, containing an inactive ingredient (placebos). All subjects must believe they are receiving the vitamin so that the effects of faith will work equally in both groups. If it is not possible to convince all subjects that they are receiving vitamin C, then the extent of unbelief must be the same in both groups. An experiment conducted under these conditions is called blind.

Double-Blind Experiments

The experimenters, too, must not know which subjects are receiving the placebo and which are receiving the vitamin C. Being fallible human beings and having an emotional investment in a successful outcome, they tend to hear what they want to hear and so to interpret and record results with a bias in the expected direction. This is not

No matter how convincing a personal experience may sound, it doesn't have the validity of scientific research.

dishonest, but is an unconscious shifting of the experimenters' perceptions of reality to agree with their expectations. To prevent it, the pills given to the subjects must be coded by a third party, who does not reveal to the experimenters which subjects received which medication until all results have been recorded quantitatively.

Reviewing the Evidence

In 1975, Dr. Thomas C. Chalmers, a physician, reviewed the data from 14 clinical trials of vitamin C in the treatment and prevention of the common cold.[4] Of the trials, five were poorly controlled, in Chalmers's judgment; nine were reasonably well controlled in that the subjects given vitamin C and those given placebos were randomly chosen. In addition, eight of these nine studies were double blind. When the data from these eight studies were pooled, there was a difference of one-tenth of a cold per year and an average difference in duration of one-tenth of a day per cold in favor of those subjects taking vitamin C. In two studies, the effects of vitamin C seemed to be more striking in girls than in boys.

In one study, a questionnaire given at the conclusion revealed that a number of the subjects had correctly guessed the contents of their capsules. A reanalysis of the results showed that those who received the placebo *who thought they were receiving vitamin C* had fewer colds than the group receiving vitamin C *who thought they were receiving the placebos!*

Other reviewers who have assembled and looked at all the evidence, as Dr. Chalmers did, have reached the same conclusions. At the start of the 1980s, reports of additional experiments were still coming out, and most were consistent with previous findings. The balanced picture emerging from the reviews seems to indicate that the effects of the vitamin, if any, are small.

The statistical effect of vitamin C on colds in the kinds of populations studied has been small. Meanwhile, what has the research on cancer shown so far?

Vitamin C and Cancer

In 1976, Dr. Pauling and his associate Dr. Cameron reported that they had administered vitamin C to 100 cancer clients in the Vale of Leven, Scotland, and had prolonged their survival rate. As compared with 1,000 similar clients who had been in the same hospital in earlier years and who had lived only 50 days, these clients lived 210 days.[6] In response, a group of researchers at the Mayo Clinic in Rochester, Minnesota, conducted a study to test the validity of this finding. The Mayo Clinic researchers criticized the earlier study on several grounds. It was not legitimate to use former clients as controls; most importantly, they said the control subjects should have been chosen randomly from the *same* population as those given vitamin C, to make sure they were similar. They therefore conducted a randomized, controlled, double-blind trial, giving vitamin C to 60 clients and a placebo that tasted and looked similar to 63

The writer of popular science articles rarely reports on such reviews of literature, because they are cold, objective, and give many viewpoints, rarely stressing one. They are not, therefore, sensational enough to sell in the marketplace. Who wants to read a scholarly, conservative, textbooklike report in a newspaper? What usually appears in the newspaper or on TV is the report of one experiment that obtained a significant result. "Professor So-and-So of the Such-and-Such Lab at the Etcetera University," the commentator may say, "has found that vitamin C does make a difference after all, at least for little girls. In a double-blind, co-twin study, in which one of each pair of twins received vitamin C and the other a placebo, the youngest girls, but not the boys, receiving vitamin C had significantly shorter and less severe illnesses than their twins. . . ."

If you chose to look up the source of the report, you would probably find that the study had been conducted as described and that the little girls had indeed had fewer colds than the little boys.[5] But the researchers themselves did not jump to the conclusion that vitamin C makes a difference. In an admirable effort to put their finding in perspective, they pointed out, "One should be aware that, as the number of tests increases, the possibility of obtaining a 'significant' result by chance alone is also increased." In other words, the experiment would have to be repeated and the same result seen several times more before it could be accepted as real. The general public may be made uneasy by scientists who admit that their results are inconclusive, but the scientific community prefers total honesty to dogmatic statements.

The scientist who reports a "significant" finding from a single experiment is not being dishonest. The term *significant* means that statistical analysis suggests that the findings probably didn't arise from a chance event, but from the experimental treatment being tested. The human significance, or meaning, of her findings is apparent only after the piece of research is added into the total picture. Sources you should turn to for a broad and balanced picture of the available information are the journals, the indexes, and the reviews of literature (see Figure H9B–1). If you are relying on a single source for your information, ask yourself, "Is this one viewpoint? Or is it a balanced picture?"

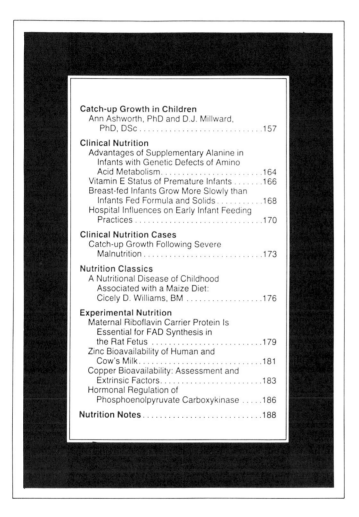

Nutrition Reviews

Volume 44   May 1986   Number 5

Reviews   To find a critique of all the important work on a subject, you can turn to a journal of reviews like the one shown here. One major review appears in *Nutrition Reviews* every month. It is followed by a bibliography that provides references to all of the original work reviewed.

FIGURE H9B–1.

Sources of reliable nutrition information.

Journals   Reports of single experiments are presented in journals like the *Journal of the American Medical Association.*

N VITAMIN A VITAMIN B-6	C DIETARY DEFICIENCY/ NUTRIT 96257
ITAMIN C THE EFFECT OF	C EITHER ALONE OR IN THE PRE 92222
VELOPMENT SYNTHESIS/	C ENHANCEMENT OF BROOD RE 2622
OKINETICS/ CHANGES OF	C EXCRETED INTO URINE AFTER 24681
RVIEW HUMAN VITAMIN A	C FIBER FAT PROTEIN FOOD FRE 61002
ION VITAMIN A VITAMIN E	C FOLIC-ACID MARGINAL DEFICI 88726
SE SYRUPS COPPER IRON	C FOOD QUALITY STORAGE NUT 12341
VITAMIN B-1 VITAMIN B-2	C HEMOGLOBIN IRON TRANSFER 61001
MANCE/ SUPPLEMENTAL	C IN SWINE DIETS FEED INTAKE 270
ABOLIC-DRUG MATERNAL	C INTAKE MILK VOLUME URINE R 24984
OF DIFFERENT LEVELS OF	C INTAKE ON THE VITAMIN C CO 24984
REATMENT/ EFFECTS OF	C INTAKE ON WHOLE BLOOD PLA 88735
RI HUMAN MILK AND THE	C INTAKES OF BREAST-FED INFA 24984
IAMIN RIBOFLAVIN NIACIN	C IRON CALCIUM SODIUM PHOSP 61004
AIN LUMBAR PUNCTURE/	C LEVELS IN CEREBROSPINAL FL 6207
ISONIDAZOLE VITAMIN E	C METABOLIC-DRUG DNA DAMA 5491
/ LONG-TERM STUDY ON	C NO EFFECT ON EXPERIMENTAL 5247
OTEIN CARBOHYDRATES	C OCCUPATION/ EFFECT OF FOO 33782
NGES OF CONSTITUENTS	C OIL CONTENTS FIBER DRY MAT 85643
T OF ALOE WITH RNA AND	C ON ADJUVANT ARTHRITIS HUM 79962
FECTS OF HIGH DOSES OF	C ON THE COURSE AND RESULT 107424
ASTIC-DRUG/ EFFECTS OF	C ON TUMOR INDUCTION ... DIE 88075
IDES SAP ...NS TANNINS	YSACCHARIDES/ ... 42911
FOR SI ... RELEASE	TS VITAMI... 61623

Index   You can look up a large number of experiments on a single topic in an index of abstracts. The part of a page shown here, from *Biological Abstracts,* lists all recently published titles containing the term *vitamin C* and gives each one a reference number. The number refers to a short summary of the reported work, which also tells exactly where it was published. The indexes will lead you to reports of experiments in many different journals. New volumes of *Biological Abstracts* come out semimonthly. *Nutrition Abstracts and Reviews,* a monthly publication, would also contain titles including the word *vitamin C.*

clients. Clients in both groups worsened at the same rate and died at the same times. The authors concluded, "We cannot recommend the use of high-dose vitamin C in patients with advanced cancer who have previously received radiation treatment or chemotherapy."[7]

Dr. Pauling angrily jumped on the authors for their conclusion, pointing out that they had not fairly tested his hypothesis. His clients had relatively strong immune systems, because they had not had the debilitating cancer treatments (radiation or chemotherapy) that the Mayo clients had had. The question whether large doses of vitamin C prolong survival time in cancer clients whose immune systems are not already severely damaged remains to be tested in a randomized, controlled, double-blind trial.[8]

Since the Mayo study, a few other reports have trickled in, relating to the vitamin's effect on cancer. According to the *Medical Tribune* (a newspaper, not a journal), a Japanese researcher administered various doses of vitamin C to 99 terminal cancer clients who were "untreatable by any conventional forms of cancer therapy." Those receiving 5 to 30 grams a day lived an average of 6.1 times longer than those receiving 4 grams a day or less.[9] No mention was made of whether the study was double blind, so its validity is impossible to assess. It is mentioned here in hopes that the reader will be reminded to view it, and all other such studies, with skepticism unless the full details are given and stand up to close inspection. The question remains open whether vitamin C helps with cancer at all, but one result is clear from the Mayo study. It did not help with advanced cancer clients who had received radiation or chemotherapy.

As this is written, a further attempt to define the effect of vitamin C, if any, on cancer is being made by researchers using a randomized, controlled, double-blind design. Because cancer takes so long (20 years) to develop, the researchers are studying a cancer precursor instead: polyps in the colon. Within a few years, enough data should be in to indicate whether the vitamin C approach to cancer treatment is a hopeful one.[10]

The big questions—Does vitamin C prevent or cure colds? Does it cure cancer or prolong the survival of cancer victims?—remain to be answered. Researchers are hard at work in many labs and clinics pursuing greater understanding of what the vitamin does and doesn't do. This highlight cannot give a final answer on such a subject, but it has fulfilled its two promises: to make you aware of the difficulties inherent in this kind of research, and to show you the kinds of research questions that will have to be answered before we know what vitamin C does.

While you await reports of the next controlled, double-blind studies on carefully defined and randomized groups of clients, you may wonder what doses of vitamin C to take, yourself, in light of what is already known. The decision is entirely up to you, but in case you should choose to aim for an intake of several hundred milligrams a day (say, ten times the RDA), this reminder is in order. You can easily obtain this amount of vitamin C by including many vitamin C–rich vegetables and fruits in your daily diet. There is no need to take any kind of pills.

Miniglossary

blind experiment: one in which the subjects do not know whether they are members of the experimental or the control group.
control group: a group of individuals similar in all possible respects to the group being experimented on, except for the experimental treatment. Ideally, the control group receives a sham treatment while the experimental group receives a real one.
double-blind experiment: one in which neither the subjects nor those conducting the experiment know which subjects are members of the experimental group and which are serving as control subjects, until after the experiment is over.
placebo (pla-SEE-bo): an inert, harmless medication given to provide comfort and hope.
placere = to please
placebo effect: the healing effect that faith in medicine, even inert medicine, often has.
polyp (POLL-ip): in this case, a mushroomlike growth that can progress to cancer.
randomization: a process of choosing the members of the experimental and control groups in a random fashion.
replication: repeating an experiment and getting the same results. The skeptical scientist, on hearing of a new, exciting finding, will ask, "Has it been replicated yet?" If it hasn't, he will withhold judgment regarding its validity.

NOTES
1. L. C. Pauling, *Vitamin C and the Common Cold* (San Francisco: W. H. Freeman, 1970).
2. L. Pauling, Vitamin C therapy of advanced cancer (letter to the editor), *New England Journal of Medicine* 302 (1980): 694; N. Horwitz, Now Japanese report 6-fold survival jump in terminal cancer with ascorbate megadoses, *Medical Tribune,* July 22, 1981.
3. This finding is widely agreed on; it is discussed, among other places, in the debate on vitamin C in *Nutrition Today,* March–April 1978.
4. T. C. Chalmers, Effects of ascorbic acid on the common cold, *American Journal of Medicine* 58 (1975): 532–536.
5. J. Z. Miller and coauthors, Therapeutic effect of vitamin C: A co-twin control study, *Journal of the American Medical Association* 237 (1977): 248–251.
6. E. Cameron and L. Pauling, Supplemental ascorbate in the supportive treatment of cancer: Prolongation of survival times in terminal human cancer, *Proceedings of the National Academy of Science USA* 73 (1976): 3685–3689.
7. E. T. Creagan and coauthors, Failure of high-dose vitamin C (ascorbic acid) therapy to benefit patients with advanced cancer, *New England Journal of Medicine* 301 (1979): 687–690.
8. Pauling, 1980.
9. Horwitz, 1981.
10. W. R. Bruce and coauthors, Strategies for dietary intervention studies in colon cancer, *Cancer* 47 (1981): 1121–1125.

The Fat-Soluble Vitamins: A, D, E, and K

10

Contents

The eye's light-sensitive pigments lie in layers in the rods and cones. This is a cone cell between two rod cells. At the tip of the cone (top) is a stack of discs packed with pigment containing vitamin A (retinal). Beneath the tip lies a bundle of spaghetti-like mitochondria prepared, when light hits the cone, to produce the energy needed to stimulate the next cell to initiate a nerve impulse.

. . . how remarkable it is that you can see things.

I remember well the time when the thought of the eye made me cold all over.

Charles Darwin

Has it ever occurred to you how remarkable it is that you can see things? As an infant you were enchanted with the power this gave you. You closed your eyes and the world disappeared. You opened them and made everything come back again. Later you forgot the wonder of this, but the fact remains that your ability to see brings everything into being for you, more so than any of your other senses. Light reaching your eyes puts you in touch with things outside your body, from your friend sitting near you to stars in other galaxies.

Has it ever occurred to you how extraordinary it is that a child grows? From a mere nothing, a speck so tiny that it is invisible to the naked eye, each person develops into a full-size human being with arms and legs, teeth and fingernails, a beating heart and tingling nerves. Years go into the making of an adult human being, with each day bringing changes so gradual they seem undetectable. Only if you are absent during a part of this process do you notice it on your return and remark to a child, "My, how you've grown!"

And when did you last think about your breathing? In, out, in, out, day and night, year after year, you take in the oxygen you need and release it, disposing of the used-up carbons whose energy moves you and keeps you alive. The nutrients discussed in this chapter—vitamins A, D, E, and K—are vital for these and other processes that you may often take for granted.

Vitamin A, D, E, and K are the fat-soluble vitamins, different from the water-soluble vitamins in several ways. They are found in the fat and oily parts of foods. They tend to move into the liver and adipose tissue and remain there, rather than being regularly excreted, as most of the water-soluble vitamins are. Their storage in the body makes it possible to survive for days, weeks, or even months or years without them; an *average* daily intake is all one has to aim for. The risk of toxicity is greater, at least for three of them (A, D, and K), than it is for the water-soluble vitamins.

Vitamin A

retina (RET-in-uh): the layer of light-sensitive cells lining the back of the inside of the eye; consists of rods and cones.

pigment: a molecule capable of absorbing certain wavelengths of light, so that it reflects only those that we perceive as a certain color.

rhodopsin (ro-DOP-sin): the light-sensitive pigment of the rods in the retina.

iodopsin (eye-o-DOP-sin): the light-sensitive pigment of the cones in the retina. Both rhodopsin and iodopsin contain retinal; the protein portions of the pigments differ.

retinal (RET-in-al): the aldehyde form of vitamin A, active in the eye. For the structure of this and other forms, see Appendix C.

Vitamin A has the distinction of being the first fat-soluble vitamin to have been recognized. It may also be one of the most versatile, because of its role in several important body processes.

Foremost, and best known, of vitamin A's roles is its role in vision. At the place where light hits the retina of the eye, profoundly informative communication occurs between the environment and the person. The eye receives the light and transforms it into signals that travel to the interior of the brain. There a mental picture forms of what the light conveys (Figure 10−1). For this to happen, the eye must perform a remarkable transformation of light energy into nerve impulses. The transformers are the molecules of pigment (rhodopsin, iodopsin, and others) in the cells of the retina. A portion of each pigment molecule is retinal, a compound the body can synthesize only if vitamin A or its relatives are supplied by the diet.

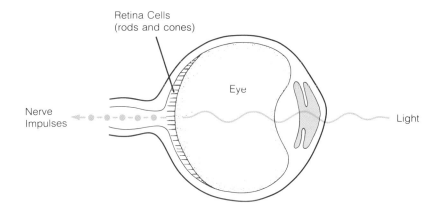

FIGURE 10–1.

The eye. As light enters the eye, pigments within the cells of the retina absorb the light and generate nerve impulses that travel into the brain.

A mechanical genius could not have designed such a system better. Light itself cannot be conducted through the solid material of the brain, so it is changed into signals transmitted by nerves. But light comes in different colors (wavelengths), which convey needed information. To keep the colors sorted out, the eye uses different light-sensitive cells (cones) to receive them. Blue light is absorbed by one set of cells, green by another, and yellow-red by a third. By day, combinations of these give the full range of color vision. By night, the light entering the eye is of low intensity, and the set of cells (rods) that can receive this light are of one kind only; so by night a person can normally discern only the presence of light, not its color.

The pigment molecules inside the cells absorb the light. Each pigment molecule is composed of a protein called opsin bonded to a molecule of retinal. When a particle of light energy (a photon) enters the eye, it is absorbed by the retinal portion of the pigment molecule, which responds by changing shape. It shifts from a *cis* to a *trans* configuration, as fatty acids do during hydrogenation (p. 99). In the process, it changes color, too, becoming bleached. In its altered form, retinal cannot remain bonded to opsin and so is released. This disturbs the shape of the opsin molecule.

This shape change disturbs the membrane of the cell inside of which the pigment is packed, permitting charged ions to enter and leave the cell. The cell hyperpolarizes (that is, the electrical differential across its membrane increases), and an electrical impulse travels along the cell's length. At the other end of the cell, the impulse is transmitted to a nerve cell, which conveys it deeper into the brain. Thus the message is sent.

Meanwhile, back in the retina and once again in the dark, the changed molecule of retinal is converted back to its original form and rejoined to opsin to regenerate the pigment rhodopsin. Many molecules of retinal are involved in this process. There are about 6 to 7 million cone cells and 100 million rod cells in the retina, and each contains about 30 million molecules of visual pigment. Repeated small losses incurred by visual activity necessitate the constant replenishment of retinal from the blood, which brings a new supply from the body stores. Ultimately, vitamin A and its relatives in food are the source of all the retinal in the pigments of the eye.

Bright light seen suddenly, when the eyes are dark-adapted, destroys much more retinal than light seen by day, for three reasons. First, the pupil is wide

cones: the cells of the retina that respond to bright light and are responsible for color vision.

rods: the cells of the retina that respond to dim light and convey black-and-white vision.

opsin (OP-sin): the protein portion of the visual pigment molecule.

photon (FOE-ton): a particle of light energy. Depending on its wavelength, a photon conveys different colors of light.

Light (photon) hits pigment.

Retinal changes shape and is released from opsin. Opsin changes shape.

open at night, to allow as much light as possible to enter the eye. Second, a shadowing pigment that protects the rods by day withdraws at night, leaving them exposed. Third, there are many more rods than cones. Hence, if a bright light suddenly shines at night through the wide-open pupil onto the unprotected rods, much of the pigment in them is bleached and momentarily inactivated. More retinal than usual is freed, and more is lost. A moment passes before the pigments regenerate and sight returns. You no doubt remember being "blinded" on occasion by a flashlight shining directly into your eyes. People who must do a lot of night driving, facing headlights from oncoming cars, thus need an increased amount of vitamin A. The more flashes of light they face, the more vitamin A they lose.

The eye is not designed for night driving or, in general, for accommodating itself to bright light at night. The mechanisms of vision evolved over millions of years, before humankind had harnessed electricity and lit up the night with headlights, beacons, and streetlights. In nature, animals in the wilderness have no need to adapt to sudden flashes of bright light at night, because they occur so seldom.

Vitamin A is undeniably an important nutrient, if for no other reason than that it plays a vital role in vision. But only one-thousandth of the vitamin A in the body is in the retina. Much more is in the body's skin and linings.

It is important that each of these surfaces be smooth: the linings of the mouth, stomach, and intestines; the linings of the lungs and the passages leading to them; the linings of the urinary bladder and urethra; the linings of the uterus and vagina; the linings of the eyelids and sinus passageways. The cells of all these surfaces—epithelial cells—secrete a smooth and slippery substance (mucus) that coats and protects them from invasive microorganisms and other harmful particles. The mucous lining of the stomach also shields its cells from digestion by the gastric juices. In the upper part of the lungs, the epithelial cells possess little whiplike hairs (cilia), which continuously sweep the coating of mucus up and out, so that any foreign particles that chance to get in are carried away by the flow. (When you clear your throat and swallow, you are excreting this waste by way of your digestive tract.) In the vagina, similar cells sweep the mucus down and out. During an infection in any of these locations, these surface cells secrete more mucus and become more active, so that a noticeable discharge occurs; when you cough it up, blow your nose, or wash it away, you help to rid your body of the infective agent.

Vitamin A plays a role in maintaining the integrity of the mucous membranes. When vitamin A is not present, the cells that secrete mucus diminish in number and activity, and the tissue becomes defenseless against infection. On many surfaces (with the important exception of the GI tract lining), the cells

mucosa (myoo-COH-suh): the membranes, composed of cells, that line the surfaces of body tissues.

urethra (you-REE-thruh): the tube through which urine from the bladder passes out of the body.

The cells on the surface are known as **epithelial** (ep-i-THEE-lee-ul) **cells.**

mucus (adjective **mucous**): a class of substances secreted by the epithelial cells of the mucosa; mucopolysaccharide. (A **mucopolysaccharide** is a polysaccharide that contains amine groups and others in its structure; see Appendix C.)

Healthy body lining

Body lining in Vitamin A deficiency

are displaced by cells containing the protein keratin—the hard, inflexible protein of hair and nails. Within the body, the mucous membranes line an area larger than a quarter of a football field; so this function of vitamin A accounts for most of the body's vitamin A need. As you might predict, greater losses of vitamin A occur during infection than under normal conditions.

Vitamin A is also essential for healthy skin, another 1 or 2 square meters of body surface. Thus all surfaces, both inside and out, are maintained with the help of vitamin A. And it has still another role to play during growth.

The organs and body parts all grow at different rates with different timings. The brain, for instance, reaches 90 percent of its adult size by the time a child is two, but the testes are still baby-size when a male enters his teens. Body parts do not just "get bigger"; bones are a case in point.

To enlarge the interior of a brick fireplace, the first thing you have to do is remove some of the old bricks. Similarly, to make a bone larger requires remodeling, as Figure 10–2 shows. To convert a small bone into a large bone, the bone-remodeling cells must "undo" some parts of the small bone as they go.

Vitamin A is required for the undoing. Some of the cells involved in bone formation are packed with sacs of degradative enzymes that can take apart the structures of bone. With the help of vitamin A in a sensitively regulated process, these cells release their enzymes, which eat away at selected sites in the bone, removing the parts that are not needed as the bone grows longer. (A similar process occurs when a tadpole loses its tail and becomes a frog. As you know, the tail doesn't simply fall off; rather it is resorbed, "growing" shorter and shorter until it disappears. As a fetus you also had a tail and lost it, a process that depended on vitamin A.)

Vitamin A's role in promoting good night vision, the health of mucous membranes and skin, and the growth of bone are well known. Other roles include parts it plays in:

- Reproduction.
- Maintaining the stability of cell membranes.
- Helping the adrenal glands to synthesize a hormone (corticosterone).
- Helping to ensure a normal output of the hormone thyroxin from the thyroid gland.
- Helping to maintain nerve cell sheaths.
- Assisting in immune reactions.
- Helping to manufacture red blood cells.

Vitamin A research still in progress is yielding many new details of how this nutrient functions in the body. Three different forms of vitamin A are active in the body: retinol (an alcohol), retinal (an aldehyde), and retinoic acid (see Figure 10–5 later in this chapter). Each has its own special binding proteins in the cells in which it works. There is also a special zinc-containing binding protein to pick up vitamin A from the liver, where it is stored, and to carry it in the blood. Cells that will receive and use vitamin A also have special receptors for it, as if it were fragile and had to be passed carefully from hand to hand without being dropped.

Each form of vitamin A triggers specific reactions in cells that are set up to respond to it. Retinol and retinoic acid, for example, act like hormones; they travel into cells, cross the nuclear membrane, and interact with DNA,

keratin (KERR-uh-tin): a water-insoluble protein; the normal protein of hair and nails. Keratin-producing cells may replace mucus-producing cells in vitamin A deficiency.

These sacs of degradative enzymes are **lysosomes** (LYE-so-zomes).
lyso = to break
soma = body

The cells are **osteoclasts** (see p. 349).

FIGURE 10–2.

Growth of bone. As bone lengthens, vitamin A helps remove old bone.

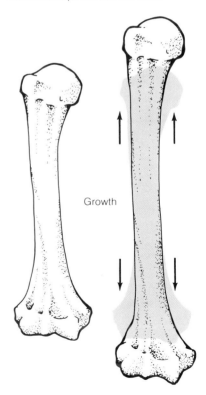

Growth

causing certain genes to express their coded instructions and make specific proteins.

Vitamin A Deficiency

Vitamin A assessment: The vitamin A-carrying protein referred to is **retinol-binding protein (RBP)**, and a measure of its blood level, if not complicated by protein deficiency, is a sensitive indicator of vitamin A nutrition status. Other indicators: serum vitamin A and serum carotene.

Either zinc deficiency or vitamin A deficiency can cause the symptoms of vitamin A deficiency, because zinc is part of the protein that mobilizes vitamin A from the liver. Zinc is also part of the enzyme that converts retinol to retinal in the eye. If zinc status is adequate, vitamin A deficiency depends on the adequacy of vitamin A stores. Up to a year's supply of vitamin A may be stored in the body, 90 percent of it in the liver. If you stop eating good food sources of the vitamin, deficiency symptoms will not begin to appear until after your stores are depleted. Then, however, the consequences are profound and severe. Table 10–1 itemizes some of them. Some have to do with the role of vitamin A in vision, some with its functions in epithelial tissue, and some with its part in growth; others are as yet unexplained.

TABLE 10–1

Vitamin A Deficiency

Area Affected	Main Effects	Technical Name for Symptoms
Eye		
Retina	Night blindness	
Membranes	Failure to secrete mucopolysaccharide causes changes in epithelial tissue	**Hyperkeratinization**
General	Drying (mildest form)	**Xerosis**
	Triangular grey spots on eye	**Bitot's spots**
	Irreversible drying and degeneration of the cornea causes blindness (most severe)	**Keratomalacia**
	The eye's symptoms of vitamin A deficiency are collectively known as:	**Xerophthalmia.**
Skin	Hair follicles plug with keratin, forming white lumps	**Hyperkeratosis**
GI tract	Changes in lining; diarrhea	
Respiratory tract	Changes in lining; infections	
Urogenital tract	Changes in lining favor calcium deposition, resulting in kidney stones, bladder disorders	
	Infections of bladder and kidney	
	Infections of vagina	
Bones	Bone growth ceases; shapes of bones change; joints are painful	
Teeth	Enamel-forming cells malfunction; teeth develop cracks and tend to decay; dentin-forming cells atrophy	
Nervous system	Brain and spinal cord grow too fast for stunted skull and spine; injury to brain and nerves causes paralysis	
Immune system	Depression of immune reactions	
Blood	Anemia, often masked by dehydration	

enamel: the hard mineral coating of the outside of the tooth, composed of calcium compounds embedded in a fine network of keratin fibers.

dentin: the softer material underlying the enamel of the tooth, composed of calcium compounds embedded in a network of collagen fibers.

For a picture of tooth structure, see p. 66.

If the blood bathing the cells of the retina does not supply sufficient retinal to rapidly regenerate visual pigments bleached by light, then a flash of bright light at night will be followed by a prolonged spell of night blindness. This is one of the first detectable signs of vitamin A deficiency. Because night blindness is easy to test, it aids in diagnosis of the condition. (Of course, it is only a symptom, and may indicate some condition other than vitamin A deficiency.) Figure 10–3 shows how night blindness can be tested.

The body's smooth skin and body cavity linings become rough in vitamin A deficiency, as mucus-producing cells are shouldered aside by keratinized cells. In the eye this process leads to drying and hardening of the cornea, which may progress to permanent blindness. In the mouth, drying and hardening of the salivary glands make them susceptible to infection; failure of mucous secretion in the mouth may lead to loss of appetite. Mucous secretion in the stomach and intestines is reduced, hindering normal digestion and absorption of nutrients, causing diarrhea, and so indirectly worsening the deficiency. Infections of the respiratory tract, the urinary tract, and the vagina are also made more likely by vitamin A deficiency. The outer body surface hardens, too: the skin becomes dry, rough, and scaly. Around each hair follicle an accumulation of hard material makes a lump.

Because growth and development of the brain and eyes are most rapid in the fetus and in the very young infant, the effects of vitamin A deficiency are most severe at and around the time of birth. For example, in a child of one or

night blindness: slow recovery of vision after flashes of bright light at night; an early symptom of vitamin A deficiency.

The epithelial surface hardens with keratin in a process known as **keratinization**. (In the GI tract, this doesn't occur, but mucus-producing cells dwindle, and mucus production declines.) The progression of this condition to the extreme is **hyperkeratinization** or **hyperkeratosis**. *hyper* = too much

In the eye, the symptoms of vitamin A deficiency are collectively known as **xerophthalmia** (zer-off-THAL-mee-uh). *xero* = dry *ophthalm* = eye

An early sign is **xerosis** (drying of the cornea); the latest and most severe stage is **keratomalacia** (total blindness). *malacia* = softening, weakening

cornea (KOR-nee-uh): the transparent membrane covering the outside of the front of the eye.

FIGURE 10–3.

Night blindness.

In dim light, you can make out the details in this room. You are using your rods for vision.

A flash of bright light momentarily blinds you as the pigment in the rods is bleached.

You quickly recover, and can see the details again in a few seconds.

With inadequate vitamin A, you do not recover but remain blind for many seconds.

Follicular hyperkeratosis.

The accumulation of this hard material, keratin, around each hair follicle is **follicular hyperkeratosis.**

follicle (FOLL-i-cul): a group of cells in the skin from which a hair grows.

two, stunted growth of the skull may cause crowding of the brain (which is growing rapidly at that age), mimicking the signs of a brain tumor. Tooth growth may also be abnormal. Crooked teeth in a child may reflect a vitamin A deficiency suffered by its mother while its jawbones were forming during her pregnancy.

Damage to the eyes is also most pronounced in the young. Worldwide, half a million children go blind every year from xerophthalmia—a preventable condition. Countless more children suffer from the less obvious signs of vitamin A deficiency such as stunted growth, decreased appetite, and increased infections and illness. It is estimated that 20 to 35 percent of all childhood mortality may be related to vitamin A deficiency.[1]

In the United States, the problem of vitamin A deficiency is all too common. The Ten-State Survey (described in Chapter 1) revealed that a third of the children under six who were examined had less than the recommended vitamin A intakes. Hispanics and blacks exhibited the most pronounced evidence of deficiency. In the more recent Nationwide Food Consumption Survey, similarly, about a third of the population surveyed had intakes below two-thirds of the RDA. Some subgroups of the Canadian population are also deficient, notably Canadian and Eskimo women, especially during their pregnancies.

A major source of vitamin A is vegetables, and a probable reason for widespread deficits of vitamin A in children is their refusal to eat vegetables. A section of Chapter 15 emphasizes the importance of encouraging children to like vegetables and suggests practical ways to ease their acceptance.

Vitamin A Toxicity

Vitamin A toxicity occurs when all the binding proteins for vitamin A are swamped, and free vitamin A attacks the cells. Such effects are not likely if you depend on foods for your nutrients, but if you take pills or supplements containing the vitamin, toxicity is a real possibility. Overdoses have serious effects on the same body systems that exhibit symptoms in vitamin A deficiency (see Table 10–2). Children are most likely to be affected, because they need less,

TABLE 10–2

Vitamin A Toxicity

Disease	Area Affected	Main Effects
Hypervitaminosis A[a]	Bones	Increased activity of osteoclasts causes decalcification, joint pain, fragility, stunted growth, and thickening of long bones; pressure increases inside skull, mimicking brain tumor; headache
	Blood	Red blood cells lose hemoglobin and potassium; menstruation ceases; clotting time slows; bleeding is easily induced
	Immune system	Stimulation of immune reactions
	Nervous system	Loss of appetite; irritability; fatigue; restlessness; headache; blurred vision; nausea; vomiting; muscle weakness; interference with thyroxin
	Muscles	Soreness after exercise
	GI tract	Nausea; vomiting; abdominal pain; diarrhea; weight loss
	Skin	Dryness; itching; peeling; rashes; dry, scaling lips; cracking and bleeding of lips; nosebleeds; loss of hair; brittle nails
	Liver	Jaundice; enlargement; massive accumulation of fat and vitamin A[b]
	Spleen	Enlargement

[a]A related condition, hypercarotenemia, is caused by the accumulation of too much of the vitamin A precursor carotene in the blood, which turns the skin yellow. Hypercarotenemia is not, strickly speaking, a toxicity symptom; it does no harm and is readily visible.

[b]If liver impairment is severe, the "classic" signs seen in skin and hair may be masked. Masked hypervitaminosis A and liver injury, *Nutrition Reviews* 40 (1982): 303–305.

osteoclasts: the cells that destroy bone during its growth. Those that build bone are **osteoblasts**.
osteo = bone
clast = break
blast = build

jaundice (JAWN-diss): yellowing of the skin; a symptom of liver disease, in which bile and related pigments spill into the bloodstream.

they are smaller and more sensitive to overdoses, and it is easy to give them too much in pill form or in other concentrates. The availability of breakfast cereals, instant meals, fortified milk, and chewable candylike vitamins—each containing 100 percent or more of the recommended daily intake of vitamin A—makes it possible for a well-meaning parent to provide several times the daily allowance of the vitamin to a child in a few hours. Serious toxicity is seen in small infants when they are given more than ten times the recommended amount every day for weeks at a time. A child may also overdose, liking vitamin pills and thinking of them as candy.

There is a wide range of vitamin A intakes in which neither deficiency nor toxicity symptoms appear. Recommended intakes in both the United States and Canada are set at about double the minimum necessary to prevent deficiency. Doubtless, many people need not consume amounts this high. The exact upper limit of safety cannot be determined exactly, because people's tolerances to overdoses vary. Probably the amount of added vitamin A that anyone can tolerate depends on the length of time it is taken and on how much of the vitamin has already accumulated before overdosing begins. Alcohol use makes vitamin A toxicity more likely. Larger people can tolerate higher doses as Figure 10–4 implies; the toxicity is stated for doses relative to kilograms of body weight.

FIGURE 10-4.

Vitamin A deficiency and toxicity. As the dose increases from zero, normalcy is reached. A range of intakes is safe. Then toxicity is reached. For reference, 100 μg/kg body weight would equal about 7,000 RE for a 150-pound person.

Source: Adapted from J. Hathcock, Vitamin safety: A current appraisal, *Vitamin Issues* V (Nutley, N.J.: Hoffman-LaRoche, 1985), Figure 1.

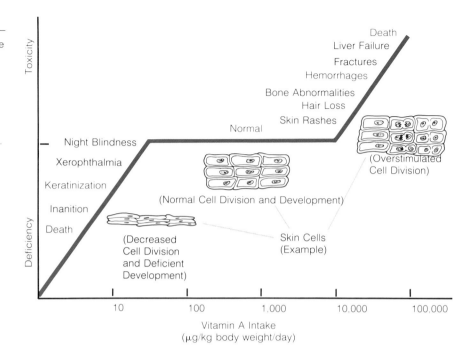

In one case, toxic effects were reported in a person who took daily doses 10 times the recommended intake for only one month;[2] but in others, it may take 40 times the recommended intake for several months to elicit symptoms of toxicity.[3] The National Nutrition Consortium advises that adults should avoid intakes of more than 5 to 10 times the recommended amounts to ensure safety.[4] In general, it makes sense to get half or more of your vitamin A from plant sources.

Adolescents should be warned that massive doses of vitamin A taken internally will have no beneficial effect on acne, but may cause the miseries itemized in Table 10-2. The belief that vitamin A cures acne arises from the knowledge that it is needed for the health of the skin. As with all nutrients, however, the vitamin promotes health when enough is supplied; more than enough has no further beneficial effects.

A new topical acne medicine, Accutane, is made from vitamin A but is chemically different from over-the-counter vitamin A. Accutane is effective against the deep lesions of cystic acne. It is highly toxic, especially during growth, and causes serious birth defects in the infants of women who have taken it during their pregnancies.

Some of vitamin A's relatives may have a preventive role with respect to cancer, as explained in Highlight 4A. Retinol itself is not one of these, but this doesn't stop gullible people from taking massive doses of vitamin A in the hope of preventing cancer. It is expected that more cases of vitamin A toxicity will be reported in the years to come, but it is hoped that no reader of this book will be among them.[5]

It is possible to suffer toxicity symptoms only when excess amounts of the preformed vitamin from animal foods or supplements are taken. The precursor, beta-carotene, which is available from plant foods, is not converted to vitamin A rapidly enough in the body to cause toxicity, but is instead stored in fat depots as carotene. Being yellow in color, it may accumulate under the skin to such an extent that the overdoser actually turns yellow (hypercarotenemia).

Vitamin A in Foods

Vitamin A terminology is in a period of transition. Vitamin A occurs in a number of different forms, and these convert to the active forms in the body with different efficiencies. In animal foods, vitamin A occurs as retinol-like compounds, which convert to retinol and its relatives in the body with high efficiency. In plant foods, no biologically active, preformed vitamin A occurs, but plant pigments known as carotenoids can be converted to vitamin A by the liver with a lower efficiency. The most active of the carotenoids is beta-carotene. When beta-carotene is split, it yields two molecules, one of which is converted to retinol. Figure 10–5 diagrams the common forms of the vitamin A family.

The active form of vitamin A used for reference is retinol, and the recommended amounts of vitamin A are stated in terms of retinol equivalents (RE). As of 1980, both U.S. and Canadian authorities were using this terminology and were recommending 1,000 RE per day for adult men and 800 RE for women.

preformed vitamin A: vitamin A in its active form.

precursor: a compound that can be converted into active vitamin A (see also p. 96). Another name for vitamin precursors is **provitamins**

beta-carotene: a vitamin A precursor found in plants.

retinol: one of the active forms of vitamin A, similar to retinal. Retinol is an alcohol; retinal is an aldehyde.

RE (retinol equivalent): a measure of vitamin A activity; the amount of retinol that a vitamin A compound will yield after conversion in the body.

FIGURE 10–5.

Vitamin A and beta-carotene. In this diagram, corners represent carbon atoms as in all previous diagrams in this book. A further simplification, here, is that methyl groups (CH_3) are understood to be at the ends of the lines extending from corners.

Retinol, the Alcohol Form

Retinal, the Aldehyde Form

Retinoic Acid, the Acid Form

Beta-carotene

tively, a diet including more or larger servings of medium sources would ensure an ample intake. No doubt you can find food sources of the vitamin that appeal to you and can easily calculate the minimum amounts you should eat to meet your needs.

The fruit and vegetable family is, of course, one of the four food groups. Its importance for meeting vitamin A needs is reflected in the recommendation that adults have at least four servings a day, including at least one dark green or deep orange item every other day.

Fast foods are notable for their *lack* of vitamin A. Anyone who dines frequently on hamburgers, french fries, shakes, and the like is advised to emphasize vegetables heavily—and not just salads—at other meals.

One animal food notable for its vitamin A content is liver. A moment's reflection should reveal the reason for this. Vitamin A not needed for immediate use is stored in the liver.* Some nutritionists recommend that people include a serving of liver in their diets every week or two, partly for this reason.

People sometimes wonder if vitamin A toxicity can result from using liver too frequently. This problem has been observed in the Arctic, where explorers who have eaten large quantities of polar bear liver have become ill with symptoms suggesting vitamin A toxicity. Presumably, it could happen closer to home if someone ate liver daily for weeks on end, but that would be too much of a good thing. Liver is an extremely nutritious food, and its periodic use is highly recommended.

Recall that folacin, too, is found most abundantly in dark green vegetables.

Foods rich in vitamin A.

Parathormone and calcitonin: see p. 388. Collagen: see p. 316.

mineralization (calcification): the process in which calcium, phosphorus, and other minerals crystallize on the collagen matrix of a growing bone, hardening the bone.

Vitamin D

Vitamin A helps to remodel bones; vitamin D helps to mineralize them. It is a member of a large and cooperative bone-making and maintenance team made up of nutrients and other compounds, including vitamin C; the hormones parathormone and calcitonin; the protein collagen, which underlies and supports bone; and the minerals calcium, phosphorus, magnesium, and fluoride, which compose the inorganic part of bone.

Blood calcium is very active metabolically. It has been estimated that about a fourth of the calcium in the blood is exchanged with bone calcium every minute. The special function of vitamin D is to help make calcium and phosphorus available in the blood that bathes the bones, to be deposited as the bones harden (mineralize).

Vitamin D raises blood concentrations of these minerals in three ways: by stimulating their absorption from the GI tract; by helping to withdraw calcium from bones into the blood; and by stimulating calcium retention by the kidneys. The star of the show is calcium itself; vitamin D is a director. A description of how calcium moves from food into the blood and into and out of bone is reserved for Chapter 11, where a closer view of the whole system is provided.

---

*Liver is not the only organ that stores vitamin A. The kidneys, adrenals, and other organs do, too, but liver is the only one commonly eaten.

The object here is to make you aware of the importance of vitamin D, the risks of deficiency and toxicity, and the ways in which the vitamin can be obtained.

Vitamin D is different from all the other nutrients in that the body can synthesize it with the help of sunlight. Therefore, in a sense, vitamin D is not an essential nutrient. Given enough sun, you need consume no vitamin D at all in the foods you eat. Rather, it is like a hormone—a compound manufactured by one organ of the body that has effects on another. And like certain hormones, it can actually enter a cell, cross the nuclear membrane, attach to specific receptors on the DNA or its protein wrapping, and promote the synthesis of specific proteins.

The liver manufactures a vitamin D precursor, which is released into the blood and circulates to the skin. When ultraviolet rays from the sun hit this compound, it is converted to previtamin D_3, which works its way back into the interior of the body. Slowly, then, over the next 36 hours, the previtamin is converted with the help of the body's heat to vitamin D_3. Two more steps occur before the vitamin becomes fully active. First, the liver adds an OH group, and then the kidney adds another OH group at specific locations to produce the active vitamin. (This is why diseases affecting either the liver or the kidney exhibit symptoms of bone deterioration.) Active vitamin D then promotes the making of several proteins that help with calcium transport into the intestinal cell, and assists these proteins in their action. It also has specific attachment sites in the brain, parathyroid glands, bone, and kidney, where it is thought to regulate the production of proteins that manage calcium homeostasis. In the pancreas, it affects insulin secretion.

There are two ways to meet your vitamin D needs. You can synthesize it yourself with the help of sunlight, or you can eat foods containing the preformed vitamin—chiefly animal foods. A plant version of vitamin D (ergosterol) may also yield an active compound, vitamin D_2 (ergocalciferol), on irradiation, but animal food containing vitamin D are considered more reliable sources.

The precursor of vitamin D made in the liver is 7–dehydrocholesterol, which is made from cholesterol. This is one of the body's many "good" uses for cholesterol.

The technical name for the final product, active vitamin D, is 1,25–dihydroxycholecalciferol—**cholecalciferol** or **dihydroxy vitamin D** for short.

ergocalciferol: the plant version of cholecalciferol.

Vitamin D Deficiency and Toxicity

Both inadequate and excessive vitamin D intakes take their toll in the United States and Canada, despite the fact that the vitamin has been known for decades to be essential for growth and toxic in excess. The Ten-State Survey conducted in the late 1960s revealed that nearly 4 percent of the children under six who were examined showed evidence of vitamin D deficiency, with several cases of overt rickets. (The more recent Nationwide Food Consumption Survey did not assess vitamin D.) The National Nutrition Survey in Canada revealed low intakes of vitamin D in women and children, but no overt cases of rickets—although they may exist in persons not tested. Worldwide, rickets still afflicts large numbers of children.

The symptoms of an inadequate intake of vitamin D are those of calcium deficiency, shown in Table 10–4. The bones fail to calcify normally and may be so weak that they become bent when they have to support the body's weight. A child with rickets who is old enough to walk characteristically develops bowed legs, often the most obvious sign of the disease.

Adult rickets, or osteomalacia, occurs most often in women who have low calcium intakes and little exposure to sun, and who go through repeated pregnancies and periods of lactation. The bones of the legs may soften to such an

Assessment of vitamin D: No accurate measure is available for individuals. A serum enzyme (alkaline phosphatase) is used in surveys.

rickets: the vitamin D–deficiency disease in children. A rare type of rickets, not caused by vitamin D deficiency, is known as **vitamin D–refractory rickets.**

osteomalacia (os-tee-o-mal-AY-shuh): the vitamin D–deficiency disease in adults. *osteo* = bone
mal = bad (soft)
Osteomalacia may also occur in calcium deficiency; see Chapter 11.

vitamin E deficiency to see if there is a common thread. It is by these means that vitamin E has been shown to be ineffective in the treatment of such diseases as muscular dystrophy, reproductive failure, and heart disease.

In summary, when a symptom has been shown to be caused by a nutrient deficiency in several species of laboratory animals, this fact can be used as a pointer toward the existence of the same relationship in humans. However, until a deficiency symptom can be produced in human subjects by a diet deficient in the nutrient and then cured by the restoration of that nutrient, it cannot be claimed that the symptom is caused by the lack of that nutrient.

Vitamin E Toxicity

All kinds of people take vitamin E supplements for all kinds of reasons. As a result, some signs of toxicity are now known or suspected, but toxicity is not common or marked as it is with vitamins A and D. "Possible GI disturbances" are reported in some people who consume more than 600 milligrams a day. High doses may interfere with drugs used to oppose unwanted blood clotting; people given anticoagulant therapy should report their vitamin E use to their physicians.[16]

Vitamin E Intakes and Food Sources

tocopherol (tuh-KOFF-er-all): a kind of alcohol (see Appendix C). Alpha-tocopherol is one of several forms of tocopherol, and D-alpha-tocopherol is the "right-handed" version.

Vitamin E recommended intakes:
U.S. men's RDA: 10 mg.*
women's RDA: 8 mg.
Canadian RNI for
men aged 19 to 24: 10 mg.
older men: 7 mg.
women aged 19 to 24: 7 mg.
older women: 6 mg.

Vitamin E is a kind of alcohol, namely a tocopherol. Several tocopherols occur in foods; the most active is alpha-tocopherol. Alpha-tocopherol occurs in two mirror-image forms, D and L (remember D- and L-sugars in Chapter 3), of which the D form is more active. Different forms of vitamin E differ in their activity; to reconcile them, the recommended intake is, as of 1980, expressed in terms of "the amount of vitamin E activity equivalent to that of 10 milligrams of D-alpha-tocopherol." Many people were surprised when, in 1980, the RDA for vitamin E appeared to have dropped from the 15 units recommended in 1974 to 10 units. Actually, the units changed, and 15 of the old units give the same activity as 10 of the new ones. The amount of vitamin E recommended is the same.

A person's need for vitamin E is higher if the amount of PUFA consumed is higher. Fortunately, vitamin E and the polyunsaturates tend to occur together in the same foods.

Vitamin E is widespread in foods. About 60 percent of the vitamin E in the diet comes directly or indirectly from vegetable oils in the form of margarine, salad dressings, and shortenings; another 10 percent comes from fruits and vegetables; smaller percentages come from grains and other products. Soybean oil and wheat germ oil have especially high concentrations of vitamin E; cot-

---

*The RDA is expressed in milligrams of D-alpha-tocopherol equivalents. One milligram equivalent has the biological activity of 1 mg D-alpha-tocopherol. The RNI is expressed in the same units, relative to which beta- and gamma-tocopherol and alpha-tocotrienol have activities of one-half, one-tenth, and one-third the activity, respectively.

tonseed, corn, and safflower oils rank second, with a tablespoon of any of these supplying more than 10 milligrams (more than the RDA) of the vitamin. Other oils contain less (for example, peanut oil supplies about half as much per tablespoon). Animal fats such as butter and milk fat have negligible amounts of vitamin E.

Vitamin E is readily destroyed by heat processing and oxidation, so fresh or lightly processed foods are preferable as sources of this vitamin. Processed and convenience foods can contribute to a vitamin E deficiency if their use continues over several years.

Vitamin K

Vitamin K seems to act primarily in the blood clotting system. There, its presence can make the difference between life and death. At least 13 different proteins and the mineral calcium are involved in making a blood clot, and vitamin K is essential for the synthesis of at least four of these proteins, among them prothrombin, made by the liver as a precursor of the protein thrombin.

When any of these factors is lacking, blood cannot clot, and hemorrhagic disease results; if an artery or vein is cut or broken under these circumstances, bleeding goes unchecked. (As usual, this is not to say that the cause of hemorrhaging is always vitamin K deficiency. Another cause is hemophilia, which is not curable by vitamin K.) Deficiency of vitamin K may occur under abnormal circumstances when absorption of fat is impaired (that is, when bile production is faulty, or in diarrhea). The vitamin is sometimes administered before operations to reduce bleeding in surgery but is only of value at this time if a vitamin K deficiency exists. Toxicity is not common but can result when water-soluble substitutes for vitamin K are given, especially to infants or to pregnant women.* Toxicity symptoms include red cell hemolysis, jaundice, and brain damage.

Long known only for its role in blood clotting, vitamin K is now known to have another function. It participates with vitamin D in synthesizing a bone protein that helps to regulate blood calcium levels.[17]

Vitamin K can be made within your GI tract—but not by you. In your intestinal tract there are billions of bacteria, which normally live in perfect harmony with you, doing their thing while you do yours. One of their "things" is synthesizing vitamin K that you can absorb. You are not dependent on bacterial synthesis for your vitamin K, however, since many foods also contain ample amounts of the vitamin, notably liver (of course), green leafy vegetables, members of the cabbage family, and milk.

The body resists vitamin K deficiency, and it is seldom seen except when an unusual combination of circumstances conspire to bring it about. When it does

Assessment of vitamin K: Blood clotting time is measured—the prothrombin time. If vitamin K is deficient, clotting is slow.

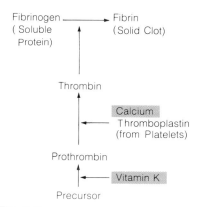

The clotting process.

K stands for the Danish word *koagulation* ("coagulation" or "clotting").

Prothrombin and thrombin: see p. 144.

hemorrhagic (hem-o-RAJ-ik) **disease:** the vitamin K–deficiency disease.

hemophilia: a hereditary disease having no relation to vitamin K, but caused by a genetic defect that renders the blood unable to clot because of lack of ability to synthesize certain clotting factors.

hemolysis: see p. 359.

jaundice (hyperbilirubinemia): yellowing of the skin, due to spillover of bile pigments (**bilirubin**) from the liver into the general circulation. When these pigments invade the brain, the condition is **kernicterus**.

---

*A toxic dose of a vitamin K compound causes the liver to release a bile pigment into the blood (hyperbilirubinemia), and leads to jaundice of certain areas of the brain (kernicterus). Vitamin K, in *Vitamin-Mineral Safety, Toxicity, and Misuse* (Chicago: American Dietetic Association), 1978, pp. 11–12.

The bacterial inhabitants of the digestive tract are known as the **intestinal flora**. *flora* = plant inhabitants

sterile: free of microorganisms, such as bacteria.

The synthetic substitute usually given for vitamin K is **menadione** (men-uh-DYE-own); see Appendix C.

Vitamin K recommended intakes:
U.S. suggestion for adults: 70 to 140 µg.
Canada makes no recommendation.

occur, however, it can be fatal. The scenario goes like this: a client is in the hospital; he has been given antibiotics to prevent or overcome infection; and he is being fed a formula diet that does not include vitamin K. The antibiotics have killed his intestinal bacteria, and his vitamin K stores are depleted. Now he goes into surgery, and when he bleeds, his blood fails to clot normally, so he bleeds to death. The combination of antibiotics, unsupplemented formula diet, and surgery raises a warning flag and requires that clotting time be checked before surgery is performed.[18]

Brand-new babies are commonly susceptible to a vitamin K deficiency, for two reasons. First, a baby is born with a sterile digestive tract; she has her first contact with intestinal bacteria as she passes down her mother's birth canal, and it takes the bacteria a day or so to establish themselves in the baby's intestines. Second, a baby may not be fed at the very outset (and breast milk is a poorer source of vitamin K than cow's milk). A dose of vitamin K (usually in a water-soluble form similar but not identical to the natural vitamin) may therefore be given at birth to prevent hemorrhagic disease of the newborn; it must be administered carefully to avoid toxic overdosing. People taking sulfa drugs, which destroy intestinal bacteria, may also become deficient in vitamin K.

Sometimes people have to take drugs to oppose blood clotting—for example, when the clotting mechanism is overly active and threatens to block arteries. In such cases, anticoagulant medications are prescribed. Cases are on record in which a person's intake of vitamin K from large amounts of green, leafy vegetables was high enough to oppose the action of a prescribed anticoagulant. A person taking anticlotting drugs should not make major changes in the amounts of greens consumed without warning the physician.

Study Questions

1. List the fat-soluble vitamins. What characteristics do they have in common? How do they differ from the water-soluble vitamins?
2. Summarize the symptoms of vitamin A deficiency.
3. What is meant by vitamin precursors? Name the precursors of vitamin A and tell in what classes of foods they are located.
4. What is the chief function of vitamin D? What are the richest sources of this vitamin?
5. What are the chief functions of vitamins E and K in the body? What are the chief symptoms of deficiency of vitamin E? Of vitamin K?

Notes

1. U.S. House of Representatives, Select Committee on Hunger, *Vitamin A: An Urgent Nutritional Need for the World's Children* (Washington, D.C.: Government Printing Office, 1985).

2. S. J. Yaffe and L. J. Filer, Jr. (American Academy of Pediatrics, Joint Committee Statement on Drugs and on Nutrition), The use and abuse of vitamin A, *Pediatrics* 48 (1971): 655–656.

3. D. R. Davis, Using vitamin A safely, *Osteopathic Medicine* 3 (October 1978): 31–43.

4. National Nutrition Consortium, Committee on Safety, Toxicity, and Misuse of Vitamins and Trace Minerals, *Vitamin-Mineral Safety, Toxicity, and Misuse* (Chicago: American Dietetic Association, 1978).

5. Masked hypervitaminosis A and liver injury, *Nutrition Reviews* 40 (1982): 303–305.

6. J. G. Bieri and M. C. McKenna, Expressing dietary values for fat-soluble vitamins: Changes in concepts and terminology, *American Journal of Clinical Nutrition* 34 (1981): 289–295; Food and Nutrition Board, Committee on Recommended Allowances, *Recommended Dietary Allowances*, 9th ed. (Washington, D.C.: National Academy of Sciences, 1980), pp. 56–57.

7. M. F. Holick, J. A. MacLaughlin, and S. H. Doppelt, Regulation of cutaneous previtamin D₃ photosynthesis in man: Skin pigment is not an essential regulator, *Science* 211 (1981): 590–593.

8. C. J. Dillard and coauthors, Effects of exercise, vitamin E, and ozone on pulmonary function and lipid peroxidation, *Journal of Applied Physiology* 45 (1978): 927–932.

T hese exercises make use of the information you recorded in Self-Study 1.

1. Look up and record your recommended intake of vitamin A. Note that this recommendation is stated in RE units.

2. What percentage of your recommended intake of vitamin A did you consume? Was this enough? What foods contribute the greatest amount of vitamin A to your diet? What percentage of your intake comes from plant foods? If you consumed more than the recommendation, was this too much? Why or why not? In what ways would you change your diet to improve

Evaluate Your Intake of Fat-Soluble Vitamins

it in this respect?

3. Appendix H does not show vitamins D, E, and K, but you can guess at the adequacy of your intake. For vitamin D, answer the following questions. Do you drink fortified milk (read the label)? Eat eggs? Fortified breakfast cereal? Liver? Are you in the sun frequently? (Remember, though, that

excessive exposure to sun can cause skin cancer in susceptible individuals.)

4. For vitamin E, consider the foods you ate in 24 hours. Vitamin E often accompanies linoleic acid in foods. Did you consume enough linoleic acid? (The recommendation is 1 to 3 percent of total kcalories from linoleic acid, as specified in Self-Study 4).

5. For vitamin K, does your diet include 2 cups of milk or the equivalent in milk products every day? Does it include leafy vegetables frequently (every other day)? Do you take antibiotics regularly (which inhibit the production of vitamin K by your intestinal bacteria)?

9. F. Umeda and coauthors, Inhibitory effect of vitamin E on lipoperoxide formation in rat adrenal gland, *Tohoku Journal of Experimental Medicine* 137 (1982): 369–377.

10. C. F. Nockels, Protective effects of supplemental vitamin E against infection, *Federation Proceedings* 38 (1979): 2134–2138; B. E. Sheffy and R. D. Schultz, Influence of vitamin E and selenium on immune response mechanisms, *Federation Proceedings* 38 (1979): 2139–2143.

11. Effect of vitamin E on prostanoid biosynthesis, *Nutrition Reviews* 39 (1981): 317–320.

12. Vitamin E in clinical nutrition, *Nutrition and the MD*, October 1982.

13. M. A. Guggenheim, Vitamin E deficiency diseases, *Vitamin Nutrition Information Service*, RCD 3813A/III, Hofmann-La Roche, Inc., Nutley, NJ 07110.

14. D. P. R. Muller, J. K. Lloyd, and O. H. Wolff, Vitamin E and neurological function, *Lancet*, 29 January 1983, pp. 225–228.

15. R. E. Gillilan, B. Mondell, and J. R. Warbasse, Quantitative evaluation of vitamin E in the treatment of angina pectoris, *American Heart Journal* 93 (April 1977): 444–449.

16. J. Hathcock, Vitamin safety: A current appraisal, *Vitamin Issues V* (Nutley, N.J.: Hofmann-LaRoche, 1985), p. 4.

17. The active form of vitamin D stimulates the synthesis of a vitamin K–dependent bone protein, *Nutrition Reviews* 39 (1981): 282–283.

18. Intestinal microflora, injury and vitamin K deficiency, *Nutrition Reviews* 38 (1980): 341–343.

HIGHLIGHT TEN

Vitamin, Mineral, and Other Supplements

Billions of dollars are spent on vitamin pills in the United States each year. Two-thirds of our citizens use them. Some people buy them because their doctors have told them to, but most people decide independently that they need them.[1] One person takes a single pill every morning, expecting it to deliver all the vitamins needed for the day. Another puts together a veritable arsenal of pills and powders in a pattern tailored to a personally selected standard.

Who's right? Or is it necessary to take vitamin pills at all? Many takers of the single daily pill seem to view it as a kind of nutrition insurance. This practice does little harm even to the pocketbook, compared to extreme practices. However, most people can learn to adjust their diets and meet their nutrient needs much better from foods than from pills, and with a much more solid guarantee that they are really getting the balance of nutrients they need.

The person to worry about is the one with the huge stockpile of nutrient preparations. Before breakfast, this person takes, say, 2 grams of vitamin C, 2 grams of vitamin E, several tablespoons of "nutritional yeast," some kelp tablets, a capsule of vitamins A and D, a spirulina tablet, several spoons of lecithin, some green pills, and assorted other pills containing trace minerals, and sprinkles desiccated liver, powdered bone, bone meal, and wheat germ on some granola, followed by powdered nonfat milk. Such practices reveal that the person wants pills and powders to play a role that is better entrusted to food. (Not all the choices just listed are

Who is better nourished?

equally questionable, however. The wheat germ, granola, and milk are nutritious foods.)

Such a person is persuaded that ordinary foods will not supply all the nutrients necessary to optimal health. Even granting that there were no magic in health foods, this person still might depend on the use of pills and powders: "I need them because I may have unusually high needs for vitamins and minerals; and besides, it can't hurt to take a little extra." These beliefs are typical of nutrition faddism, which is born of inadequate knowledge applied with sincere interest. Let's take a close look at the statement, "I may have unusually high needs."

Nutrition Individuality

Biologically speaking, no two people are exactly alike except identical twins, and no two people have exactly the same nutrient needs. You may need a bit more vitamin C than your friend, and your friend a bit more protein than you, to maintain peak health. Not only are people different biologically, but their different lifestyles affect their nutrient needs. Even identical twins, if

they live differently, may not have identical needs. If one of them has a highly stressful job, for example, that one may need a bit more of certain nutrients than the other; but rarely (in only 2 to 3 percent of cases*) is a person's need above the RDA. These differences between individuals—which are nothing more than normal variations—may make our nutrient requirements differ as much as twofold or threefold, one from another; that is, you may need up to twice or three times as much vitamin C as your friend does, if your friend's requirements are near the bottom end of the range and yours are near the top.

One person may even need seven times as much of a nutrient as someone else, but to say this is to display the full range of needs from the very lowest to the very highest. That is, the comparison is between someone with extraordinarily small needs and someone with extraordinarily high ones.[2] Such a comparison cannot be used as the basis for recommending that any normal person take doses of nutrients seven or so times higher than the *average* requirement. Still less does

---

*The theory behind the RDA is that it should be set 2 standard deviations to the right of the mean requirement for each nutrient. This would leave 5 percent of the population outside the range covered by the RDA—2.5 percent on the low side, 2.5 percent on the high side. Thus only 2.5 percent of the population would have needs above the RDA. Actually, for most nutrients, the RDA committee did not have enough data to set the RDA this accurately, but the range they chose may be even broader on this account, and the people left out would be fewer.

this comparison suggest that a person take nutrient doses seven times higher than the RDA.

In some instances, *very* large differences in nutrient needs are seen. Some people are born with rare genetic defects that keep them from using certain nutrients in the normal way. These people may have extraordinarily high or low nutrient requirements, differing tenfold or a hundredfold from the average. But these are rare defects indeed. Only one person in 10,000 may have such a defect, and it demands diagnosis if the person is to live a normal life.

Illness also imposes differences in nutrient requirements. Under the stress of surgery or high fever or after suffering extensive burns, a person's needs for protein are much greater than usual, up to perhaps five times normal, and the needs for vitamins and minerals may be increased even more. Some prescription and over-the-counter medicines also increase specific vitamin and mineral needs.

What we are concerned with here, however, are normal variations, and these do not justify the taking of large quantities of vitamins and minerals in concentrated form by the normal, healthy person. Foods contain enough vitamins and minerals so that a reasonably careful selection of them will supply all that most people need. The food group plan described in Chapter 2 provide a healthful balance of nutrients: enough to meet the needs of people at the top of the range of normal variation.

"But," the supplement taker may say, "that argument is based on too many assumptions for my comfort. You assume that the foods you speak of have the nutrients in them—whereas they may be poor in nutrients. You assume that they haven't lost those nutrients in cooking—when in fact they could be cooked to pieces and have no nutritional value." You might counter that ordinary grocery store foods, if they are whole foods, can be nutritious (see Highlight 2). You might point out that losses in cooking are moderate if you are careful (Chapter 9). You might say that the choice of a variety of foods from day to day minimizes the risk of suffering a lack of nutrients in case one item chosen should happen to be nutrient-poor. But the debate between the self-doser and the ordinary-food user goes on and on.

One other aspect of the self-dosing practice should at least be mentioned here: the risks of toxicity. The self-doser said, "Besides, it can't hurt." But people vary in their tolerances for high doses of nutrients, just as they vary in their thresholds for deficiencies, and toxicity from overdoses of vitamins and minerals may be more common than we realize. One physician, reporting several cases of harm from vitamin overdoses in his local community, warns that the cases we hear about are just the tip of the iceberg.[3] Even an alert physician who is on the lookout for such cases may not spot them all, and is likely to catch only those resulting from short-term megadose effects. Chronic nutrient toxicity, in which the effects develop subtly and slowly, is hard to detect.[4] Most of the nutrients, even including some of the water-soluble B vitamins, are now known to have toxic effects when taken in sufficient excess,[5] and the amounts people take are sometimes preposterously high.

It is important to try to answer this question for those who choose to take supplements: How much of a particular nutrient in a supplement is safe? Or, how high is too high? A possible guideline is to think of the original cave dweller, who had to depend only on foods for life and health. If the foods available to the cave dweller *could* have supplied the amount of a nutrient being advocated, then perhaps it is not unsafe for us, the cave dweller's descendants, to ingest that amount ourselves. By this standard, the doses some people take are clearly excessive. To obtain 840 milligrams of vitamin E from its best food source, wheat germ, for example, you would have to eat 15 pounds of wheat germ—yet some people take supplements containing more than 840 milligrams of vitamin E every day. To obtain 5 grams of vitamin C, you would have to eat 19 pounds of oranges, yet some people consume more than that much vitamin C daily from supplements.

Since our ancestors survived for centuries without nutrient supplements, and arrived successfully at the point of producing us, this argument runs, we clearly need no more vitamins or minerals than what *we* can obtain from food. That much, but not more, would be reasonable to look for in a supplement.

And, come to think of it, if all we need can come from food, why not just get it from food?

How Vitamins Are Promoted

Three-fourths of the public believe that extra vitamins provide more pep and energy. Twenty-six percent use nutrient supplements on their own initiative, without a physician's advice.[6] If it is not necessary to do this, why have so many people been bamboozled into believing that it is? The idea of nutrition individuality described earlier provides fuel for the kinds of claims made by pill pushers. Other fuel comes from the notion that "you should try it [a fad] even though it didn't work for me." Dr. V. Herbert, professor of medicine and pathology at Hahnemann Medical Center in Philadelphia, has noted many other earmarks of faddism. Dr. Herbert says you can tell it may be a quack talking if the person tries to persuade you:

- That you should buy something you would not otherwise buy.
- That your disease condition is due to a faulty diet.
- That you have a "subclinical" deficiency.

- That, in fact, you should take supplements of any kind.
- That you should take "natural" vitamins.[7]

The last of these notions—that "natural" vitamins are of more virtue than synthetic vitamins—is not a valid claim. The body cannot tell whether a vitamin in the bloodstream came from an organically grown cantaloupe or from a chemist's laboratory. Pills made from the melon and from some chemical in the lab may differ from one another in their *other* ingredients, but insofar as they contain a certain vitamin, they are identical. If either kind of pill has an advantage of any kind, it is as often the synthetic as the "natural" pill. In one instance, vitamin C from *synthetic* pills was found to be absorbed better than that from "natural" pills, because something in the "natural" pills was interfering with the absorption of the vitamin.[8] In another case, the "natural" pills were found to be so weak that synthetic vitamin C had to be added to them to bring the concentration up to acceptable levels.[9]

In any case, there is nothing natural about a pill, no matter what its source. If we define *natural* more carefully and insist that the word be used only to refer to foods, not pills, and only to foods in their original, farm-grown state, then we can make a statement that will hold up to critical inspection. The natural food (like a cantaloupe) may be better for you than any pill—not because it has better vitamin C in it, but because it conveys "fringe benefits" along with the vitamin C: carbohydrate; fiber; and fluid with dissolved calcium, potassium, and many other nutrients. "There is no advantage to eating a nutrient from one source as opposed to another, but there may be fringe benefits to eating that nutrient in a natural food as opposed to a purified nutrient preparation."[10]

With all there is to be said against the use of vitamin pills, is there anything to be said *for* them? Yes, when a doctor prescribes them, and yes, in at least two other instances:

- When your energy intake is below about 1,500 kcalories, (for the average-size person), so that you can't eat enough total food to be sure of meeting your vitamin needs.
- When you know that—for whatever reason—you are going to be eating irregularly for a limited time.

On these occasions, a single, balanced vitamin-mineral pill should suffice. It is important to remember that, if vitamins are needed, minerals will be needed, too, and a "vitamin pill" is not enough. A vitamin-mineral supplement is called for. (For a listing and comparison of available vitamin-mineral supplements, turn to Appendix J.)

A problem that remains for the reader who is persuaded of the view presented here is "How do I tell my friends about this?" Trying to persuade a pill-popping friend not to take pills and powders can easily turn into the unfortunate experience of losing the friend. As one nutrition professor has put it, "Isn't it amazing how when you explain to someone that what they have accepted as fact is not so, they become

People don't always appreciate your showing them why they are wrong.

angry with you rather than with the person who gave them the inaccurate information in the first place?"[11] Yes, it is amazing—and painful. But the response is not surprising when you recall that the person who has paid his own money as the price for believing a bogus "fact" has a personal stake in having the fact be true.

To avoid alienating the people we are trying to reach with valid information, we can adopt several strategies. For one thing, we can always acknowledge the validity of the feelings and values that underlie the faddist's practices. Then we can distinguish between practices that are dangerous and those that are merely neutral. We can ignore the neutral ones and confront only the dangerous ones. Finally, we can make ourselves responsible for learning the facts of the matter as thoroughly as we can, getting them all in perspective, and communicating them clearly.

In closing, it may be of interest to demonstrate how nutrition knowhow would rank the items selected by the pill-and-powder breakfaster described at the start. They can be sorted into groups as follows:

- *Most risky*: The A and D capsules and the minerals, because overdoses are a real possibility and have serious ill effects.*
- *Second*: The powdered bone (the calcium from such a source is poorly absorbed, and some bone meal has been found to contain high levels of lead[12]); and the kelp tablets (the urine of people who use kelp tablets has been found to contain raised concentrations of arsenic, a poison

---

*Even potassium chloride, which is sold in health-food stores, has caused death in a baby whose mother had read the book *Let's Have Healthy Children* by Adelle Davis and had given the supplement to the infant, as the book suggested, for colic. M. Stephenson, The confusing world of health foods, *FDA Consumer*, July–August 1978, pp. 18–22.

and a possible cancer-causing agent[13]).

- *Third*: The vitamin C and the vitamin E. The doses are high enough to be toxic in some individuals.
- *Fourth*: The spirulina and the lecithin. Spirulina has some vitamin B_{12}, but some of the vitamin B_{12}–like compounds in it may actually compete with the vitamin B_{12} from other sources, rendering the vitamin less effective. Also, spirulina does not suppress appetite.[14] As for lecithin, doses taken as supplements have caused nausea and GI distress in the takers, as Chapter 4 described.
- *Fifth*: The desiccated liver and the green pills. These are probably neutral items (although some risks could still come to light). It is easy to get the same nutrients delivered in ordinary foods, but there may be no harm in taking them in this form.
- *Sixth*: The nutritional yeast and the granola. Using them is probably a neutral practice. Live baker's yeast cells, used to leaven bread, consume nutrients, but nonliving, brewer's yeast cells do not. Brewer's yeast is grown specially as a nutrient

Keep your own counsel if it isn't sought—unless a nutrition practice is dangerous.

Miniglossary

desiccated liver: dehydrated liver; a powder sold in health-food stores and supposed to contain, in concentrated form, all the nutrients found in liver. Possibly not dangerous, this supplement has no particular nutritional merit, and grocery store liver is considerably less expensive. *Desiccated* means "totally dried."

granola: a cereal made from mixed oats and other grains.

green pills: pills containing dehydrated, crushed vegetable matter. One pill contains nutrients equal to those in one small forkful of fresh vegetables—minus losse incurred by processing. Sixty pills costing $15 deliver vegetable matter worth about $1.50.

kelp: a kind of seaweed used by the Japanese as a foodstuff. Kelp tablets are made from dehydrated kelp.

normal variation: the variation normally expected in a biological system. Nutrient needs, for example, normally vary over a twofold or threefold range from the mean, although individuals are much more likely to have needs falling near the mean than near the extreme. See Chapter 2, Figure 2–2.

nutritional yeast: a preparation of yeast cells, often praised for its high nutrient content. Yeast is a concentrated source of B vitamins, as are many other foods. The type of yeast used is brewer's, not baker's, yeast; see items 993 and 992 in Appendix H, and the end of this highlight.

powdered bone; **bone meal**: two among many nutrient supplements intended to supply calcium and other bone minerals. (Chapter 11 discusses calcium supplements.)

spirulina: a kind of alga ("blue-green manna") said to be highly nutritious and to suppress appetite. It is not more nutritious than other algae, and it does not suppress appetite.

subclinical: a nutrient deficiency that has no visible or otherwise detectable (clinical) symptoms. It is possible for such a deficiency to develop (see the discussion of loss of iron from body stores in Chapter 1), but the term is often used as a scare tactic to persuade consumers to buy nutrient supplements they don't need.

wheat germ: a part of the wheat grain, rich in nutrients.

supplement, particularly for vegetarian diets; it is a good source of protein, B vitamins, and iron. Added to cereal, it improves the cereal's protein quality—important for the vegetarian, whose total protein intake may be nearer the minimum needed than is the meat eater's intake. Granola is a fairly nutritious cereal, although it has drawbacks. It contains coconut oil, a saturated fat; it contains more sugar than most people realize; it is sticky, and so is unpopular with dentists concerned about sugar and tooth decay; and it is high in kcalories.

- *Last*: The wheat germ and the powdered nonfat milk. These are nutritious foods, they can be bought in the grocery store, and the nonfat milk in particular is an economical source of valuable nutrients.

In counseling the user, you might praise the value system that puts such a high premium on health. Then you might reinforce the use of wheat germ and powdered nonfat milk, agreeing that these foods are nutritious, reasonable in cost, and delicious. When you are sure of your listener's openness to whatever else you might have to say, you might offer a caution about the use of the potent supplements listed first, but keep your own counsel about the remaining ones unless you are asked. This way you probably will not lose a friend, and you may provide a substantial boost to exactly what she treasures most—her good health.

NOTES
1. H. G. Schutz and coauthors, Food supplement usage in seven Western states, *American Journal of Clinical Nutrition* 36 (1982): 897–901.
2. R. Dubos, The intellectual basis of nutrition science and practice, paper presented at the NIH conference on the biomedical and behavioral basis of clinical nutrition, Bethesda, Md., 19 June 1978, and reprinted in *Nutrition Today*, July–August 1979, pp. 31–34.
3. Santa Barbara physician warns of vitamin overdosing, *California Council against Health Fraud Newsletter*, March–April 1983, p. 2.

All substances are poison. The right dose differentiates a poison and a remedy.

Paracelsus (16th century)

4. Nutrient toxicity: A special report, *Nutrition Reviews* 39 (1981): 249–256.
5. L. Alhadeff, C. T. Gualtieri, and M. Lipton, Toxic effects of water-soluble vitamins, *Nutrition Reviews* 42 (1984): 33–40.
6. P. L. White, Food faddism, *Contemporary Nutrition* 4 (February 1979).
7. V. Herbert, The health hustlers, in *The Health Robbers*, eds. S. Barrett and G. Knight (Philadelphia: George F. Stickley, 1976).
8. O. Pelletier and M. O. Keith, Bioavailability of synthetic and natural ascorbic acid, in *The Nutrition Crisis: A Reader*, ed. T. P. Labuza (St. Paul, Minn.: West, 1975), pp. 192–200.
9. A. Kamil, How natural are those "natural" vitamins? *Co-op News*, 13 March

1972, p. 3, reprinted in *Nutrition Reviews/Supplement: Nutrition Misinformation and Food Faddism*, July 1974, p. 34.
10. Position paper on food and nutrition misinformation on selected topics, *Journal of the American Dietetic Association* 66 (1975): 277–279.
11. A. E. Harper, Science and the consumer, *Journal of Nutrition Education* 11 (October–December 1979): 171.
12. The FDA has requested that bone meal makers place a warning label on the product to protect infants, young children, and pregnant and lactating women; but as of early 1983, only 1 in 50 had complied. FDA request for lead warning rejected, *Nutrition Week*, 9 June 1983, p. 6.
13. M. Stephenson, The confusing world of health foods, *FDA Consumer*, July–August 1978, pp. 18–22.
14. V. Herbert and G. Drivas, *Spirulina* and vitamin B_{12}, *Journal of the American Medical Association* 248 (1982): 3096–3097; Spirulina discounted (Update), *FDA Consumer*, September 1981, p. 3.

Water and the Major Minerals

11

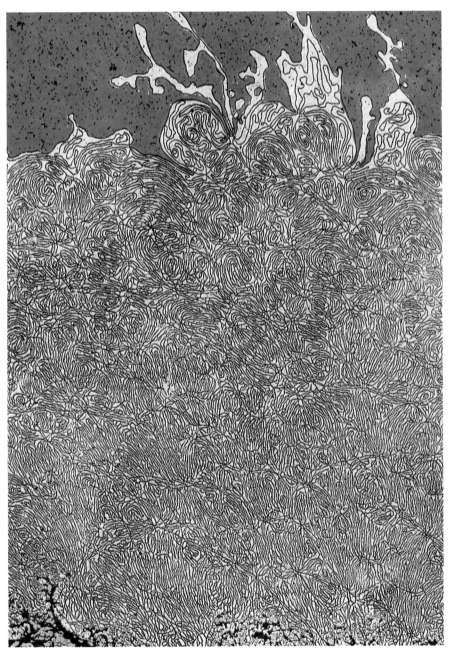

The mineral phosphorus abounds in DNA. The tremendous, orderly tangle shown here is part of a chromosome consisting of long loops of DNA attached to a core of protein (dark area at bottom).

The body's water cannot be considered separately from the minerals dissolved in it. One can drink pure water, but in the body, that water mingles with minerals to become fluids in which all life processes take place. This chapter begins by discussing water and the minerals that give the body fluids their character, then considers some other properties of major mineral nutrients.

The body fluids provide the medium in which all of the cells' chemical reactions take place; they participate in many of these reactions, and supply the means for transporting vital materials to cells and carrying waste products away from them. Every cell is bathed in a fluid of the exact composition that is best for it. Each of these fluids is constantly undergoing loss and replacement of its constituent parts as cells withdraw nutrients and oxygen from them and excrete carbon dioxide and other waste materials into them. Yet the composition of the body fluids in each compartment remains remarkably constant at all times. The fluid between the cells, for example, always has a high concentration of sodium and chloride ions and lower concentrations of about eight other major ions. The intracellular fluid always has high potassium and phosphate concentrations and lower concentrations of other ions. These special fluids regulate the functioning of cells; the cells in turn regulate the composition and amounts of the fluids. The entire system of cells and fluids remains in a delicate but firmly maintained state of dynamic equilibrium.

The maintenance of this balance is so important that it is credited with our ability and that of other animals to live on land. It is thought that we had single-celled ancestors that depended on the seawater they lived in to provide nutrients and oxygen and to carry away their waste. We have managed, over the course of our 2-billion-year evolutionary history, to internalize the ocean—to continue bathing our cells in a warm nutritive fluid that keeps them alive. The amounts of salts in our body fluids, and the fluids' temperature, are believed to be the same as in the ocean—not as it is now, but as it was at the time when our ancestors emerged onto land. The ocean has since become more salty, but we still carry the ancient ocean within us.

Water constitutes about 55 to 60 percent of an adult's body weight and a higher percentage of a child's. As for the major minerals, Figure 11–1 shows the amounts found in the body. The major minerals (those to the left of the line in the figure) are discussed in this chapter; the trace minerals (to the right of the line) are discussed in Chapter 12. All of the major minerals strongly influence the body's fluid balances and blood pressure.

The ocean—a nutritive fluid that keeps cells alive.

Salt does not refer only to sodium chloride, but also to ionic compounds, as defined later.

It was assuredly not chance that led Thales to found philosophy and science with the assertion that water is the origin of all things.

Lawrence J. Henderson

Body Fluids

The body fluids form a river coursing through the arteries, capillaries, and veins, carrying a heavy traffic of nutrients and waste products. Fluids also fill the cells and the spaces between them. Water molecules also nestle inside the body's giant proteins, glycogen, and other macromolecules, helping to form their struc-

FIGURE 11–1

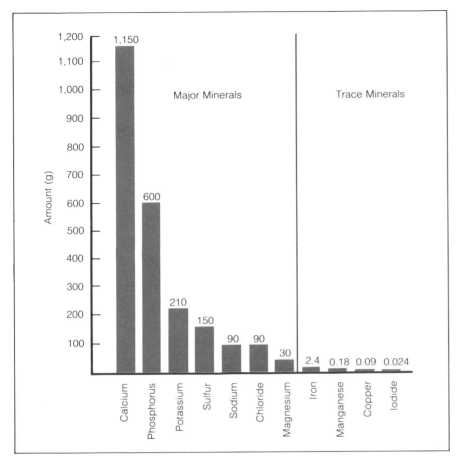

The amounts of minerals in a 60-kilogram human body. A line separates the major minerals from the trace minerals. The major minerals are those present in amounts larger than 5 grams (a teaspoon). A pound is about 454 grams; thus only calcium and phosphorus appear in amounts larger than a pound. There are more than a dozen trace minerals, although only four are shown here.

ture, and it participates actively in many chemical reactions. Fluids also serve many other functions:

- They serve as the solvent for minerals, vitamins, amino acids, glucose, and a multitude of other small molecules.
- They act as lubricants around joints.
- They serve as shock absorbers inside the eyes, spinal cord, and amniotic sac in pregnancy.
- They aid in the body's temperature maintenance.

The total amount of fluid in the body is homeostatically regulated to remain constant, thanks to delicate balancing mechanisms. Imbalances can occur—dehydration and water intoxication—but they are restored to normal as promptly as the body can manage it. Both intake and excretion are subject to regulation.

Thirst and satiety govern water intake, apparently sensed by the mouth, hypothalamus, and stomach. When the blood is too concentrated (having lost water, but not salt and other solutes), its solutes attract water out of the salivary glands. The mouth becomes dry as a result, and you drink to wet your mouth. The hypothalamus also monitors the concentration of the blood, and when it finds it too high, initiates impulses that stimulate drinking behavior. The stomach

dehydration: loss of too much fluid from the body.

water intoxication: the condition in which body water contents are too high.

The term **water balance** refers to the balance between water intake and excretion (conceptually similar to *nitrogen balance*).

Water follows salt and other solutes, moving in the direction of higher osmotic pressure (see p. 376).

TABLE 11–1

Water Balance

Water Intake	ML
Liquids	550 to 1,500
Foods	700 to 1,000
Metabolic water	200 to 300
	1,450 to 2,800

Water Output	ML
Kidneys	500 to 1,400
Lungs	350
Feces	150
Skin	450 to 900
	1,450 to 2,800

may also play a role: thirsty animals drink until nerves in their stomachs, known
as stretch receptors, are stimulated enough to turn off the drinking. More must
be learned about these mechanisms, but it is clear from what we know already
that thirst adjusts to provide a water intake that exactly meets the need.

Thirst lags behind water lack. A water deficiency that develops slowly can
switch on drinking behavior in time to prevent serious dehydration, but one that
develops fast may not. Also, thirst itself does not remedy a water deficiency; you
have to notice that you are thirsty, pay attention, and take the time to get a drink.
Therefore, the thirst mechanism works imperfectly. The athlete, the long-distance
casual runner, the gardener in hot weather, or the elderly person whose attention
wanders can experience serious dehydration; they need to learn to notice con-
sciously their need for water and drink promptly in response to it.

The mechanism of water excretion involves the brain and the kidneys. The
cells of the hypothalamus, which monitor salt concentration in the blood, stimulate the pituitary gland to release a hormone, antidiuretic hormone (ADH),
whenever the body's salt concentration is too high. ADH stimulates the kidneys
to hold back (actually, to reabsorb) water, so that it recirculates rather than
being excreted. Thus the more water you need, the less you excrete. There are
also cells in the kidney itself that are responsive to the salt concentration in the
blood passing through them. When they sense a too-high salt concentration,
they too release a substance. By a roundabout route, this substance also causes
the kidneys to retain more water (see Figure 11–5, later in this chapter). Again,
the effect is that when more water is needed, less is excreted.

These renal excretion mechanisms cannot work by themselves to maintain
water balance unless you drink enough water. This is because the body must
excrete a minimum amount of water each day—the amount necessary to carry
away the waste products generated by a day's metabolic activities. Above this
amount (a minimum of about 500 milliliters a day—that is, about a pint), the
amounts of water you excrete can be adjusted to balance your intake. If you
drink more water, the urine merely becomes more dilute. Hence drinking plenty
of water is never a bad idea.

In addition to the obvious dietary source, water itself, nearly all foods contain
water (see p. 3). In addition, water is generated from the energy nutrients in
foods (recall that the carbons and hydrogens in these nutrients combine with
oxygen during metabolism to yield carbon dioxide, CO_2, and water, H_2O).
Daily water intake from these three sources totals, on the average, about 2 ½
liters (about 2 ½ quarts). Similarly, in addition to the water excreted via the
kidneys, some water is lost from the lungs as vapor, some in feces, and some
from the skin. The losses of all of these also total about 2 ½ liters a day, on the
average. Table 11–1 shows how intake and excretion naturally balance out.

The body uses minerals to help regulate the distribution, composition, and
acidity of its fluids. This regulation is vital to the life of the cells, for all cells
must be continuously bathed in fluid both within and without.

Fluid and Electrolyte Balance

Water molecules move freely across cell membranes. Cells have no way to hold
onto them directly; they slip through all barriers. However, the cells are able
to move salts around, and water follows salt, so the cells move water by this
indirect means.

Salts are referred to as electrolytes when their behavior in water is of interest. When salts dissolve, their positive and negative ions separate (dissociate) and move about independently throughout the water. (Pure water conducts electricity poorly, but ions efficiently carry electrical current, hence the term *electrolyte*.) A solution of common table salt (NaCl) in water is an electrolyte solution.

Many salts, or electrolytes, are important in the body besides sodium chloride. Table 11–2 lists some of the most important electrolytes and reveals that in some, the anions are not single atoms, but molecules that bear an overall negative charge. It also reveals that, of the mineral ions involved in electrolyte balance, some are found chiefly outside cells (notably sodium and chloride), some inside (notably potassium, magnesium, phosphorus, and sulfur), and some are relatively evenly distributed (such as calcium).

In any fluid with dissolved electrolytes, as in any other substance, there will always be the same number of positive and negative charges. If an anion enters a cell, a cation must accompany it or another anion must leave so that electroneutrality will be maintained.

For example, in serum the numbers of cations and anions both equal 155 milliequivalents per liter (mEq/l). Of the cations, sodium ions make up 142 milliequivalents per liter, and potassium, calcium, and magnesium ions make up the remainder. Of the anions, chloride ions number 103 milliequivalents per liter, bicarbonate ions number 27, and the rest are provided by phosphate ions, sulfate ions, organic acids, and protein.

Water molecules are attracted to electrolytes because water molecules are "polar." This means that although each water molecule bears a net charge of zero, the oxygen side of the molecule is slightly negatively charged, and the hydrogens are slightly positively charged. Figure 11–2 shows the result in an electrolyte solution: both positive and negative ions attract clusters of water molecules around them.

salt: a compound composed of charged atoms or molecules (ions). An example is potassium chloride (K^+Cl^-). Exceptions: a compound in which the cations are H^+ is an acid (example H^+Cl^-, hydrochloric acid); a compound in which the anions are OH^- is a base (example K^+OH^-, potassium hydroxide).

cation (CAT-eye-un): a positively charged ion.

anion (AN-eye-un): a negatively charged ion.

For a closer look at ions, see Appendix B.

A salt that dissolves in water and dissociates is an **electrolyte**.

dissociation: physical separation of a compound into ions.

electrolyte solution: a solution that can conduct electricity.

Na = sodium.
Cl = chlorine.

chloride: the ionic form of chlorine, Cl^-. (For metals, the same term applies to the neutral form and to the ion. For example, *sodium* refers to both Na and Na^+.)

TABLE 11–2

Important Body Electrolytes

Electrolyte	Extracellular Concentration (mEq/l)	Intracellular Concentration (mEq/l)
Cations		
Sodium (Na^+)	142	10
Potassium (K^+)	5	150
Calcium (Ca^{++})	5	2
Magnesium (Mg^{++})	3	40
	155	202
Anions		
Chloride (Cl^-)	103	2
Bicarbonate (HCO_3^-)	27	10
Phosphate ($HPO_4^=$)	2	103
Sulfate ($SO_4^=$)	1	20
Organic acids (lactate, pyruvate)	6	10
Proteins	16	57
	155	202

A **milliequivalent (mEq)** is the amount of a substance that contains the same number of charges as 1 mg of hydrogen. The number of milliequivalents is a more useful measure than milligrams or grams when we are considering ions, because we are primarily interested in the number of charges present. If two solutions contain the same number of milliequivalents, they contain the same number of charges.

FIGURE 11-2

Water follows salt.

A. Water is polar, because the negatively charged electrons which bond the hydrogens to the oxygen spend most of their time near the large oxygen atom. This results in the oxygen being slightly negative and the hydrogen positive (see Appendix B).

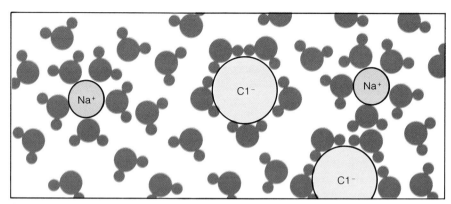

B. In an electrolyte solution, therefore, water molecules are attracted to both anions and cations. Notice that the negative oxygen atoms of the water molecules are drawn to the sodium cation (Na^+) here, while the positive sides of the water molecules are drawn to the chloride ions (Cl^-).

This tendency of water to follow solutes such as ions is known as the **osmotic pressure** of a solution. Water flows *toward* the higher osmotic pressure. The substances dissolved in the water that creates this pressure are the **solutes** (SOLL-yutes).

Other terms used to describe electrolyte solutions:
isotonic (having the same concentration of solute and therefore the same osmotic pressure as human body fluid), **hypertonic** (having a higher osmotic pressure than human body fluid), and **hypotonic** (having a lower osmotic pressure than human body fluid). Saline (salt) solutions used in the hospital are made isotonic to human blood.

The cell membrane is **selectively permeable**; that is, it permits only the solvent (water) to pass freely. Solutes (such as sodium ions) have to be actively transported or else cannot get across the membrane easily. Osmotic pressure moves water across the membrane whenever the concentrations of solutes on the two sides of the membrane are not equal.

For more about the cell-membrane pumps, see Chapter 5.

As mentioned earlier, water follows salt. More precisely, water may move freely from one place to another, but tends to remain wherever solutes such as sodium chloride are concentrated. Water will tend to concentrate on one side of a barrier rather than another, only if solute is concentrated on that side, and if the barrier separating the two fluid solutions is permeable to water but not permeable (or less freely permeable) to the solute. Figure 11-3 shows this principle in operation.

You have seen this force at work if you have ever put salad dressing on lettuce an hour before eating it. When you came back to the salad, the lettuce was wilted, and there was water in the salad bowl. The high concentration of salt (and therefore low concentration of water) in the dressing caused water to move out of the cells. They collapsed (the lettuce wilted), and the water puddled in the salad dish. Sugar would have caused the same reaction. You can prevent this by coating the lettuce lightly with oil before adding the salty dressing. The oil acts as a barrier against the salt, and prevents it from pulling water out of the lettuce.

The divider between the water inside and outside a cell is the cell membrane. The cell cannot pump water directly across its membrane, but it does have proteins in its membrane that can move sodium ions from one side of the membrane to the other. (Negative ions follow.) When these proteins, known as sodium pumps, are active, they pump out sodium faster than it can diffuse into the cell. Water then follows the ions. Cells also have potassium pumps. When they are active, they pump in potassium, and water follows. By maintaining the concentrations of sodium, potassium, and other electrolytes inside and outside its boundaries in this manner, the cell can regulate the amount of water it contains.

The maintenance of fluid and electrolyte balance requires that the amounts of various salts in the body remain nearly constant. If they are lost, they must be replaced from external sources—meaning, of course, foods and beverages.

The salt needed in the largest quantity is sodium chloride; a review of Table 11-2 will reveal the reason. Sodium and chloride are the body's principal extracellular cation and anion; therefore they are first to be lost when fluid is lost by sweating, bleeding, or renal or fecal excretion.

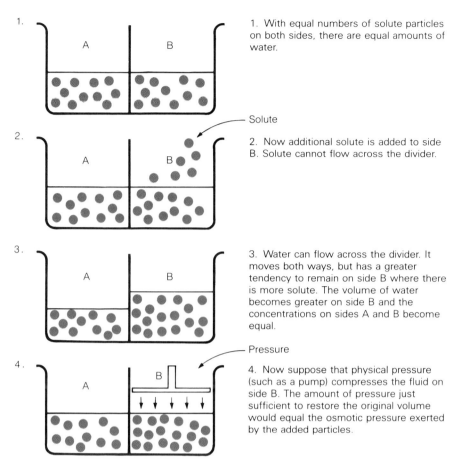

1.

A B

1. With equal numbers of solute particles on both sides, there are equal amounts of water.

2.

A B

Solute

2. Now additional solute is added to side B. Solute cannot flow across the divider.

3.

A B

3. Water can flow across the divider. It moves both ways, but has a greater tendency to remain on side B where there is more solute. The volume of water becomes greater on side B and the concentrations on sides A and B become equal.

4.

A B

Pressure

4. Now suppose that physical pressure (such as a pump) compresses the fluid on side B. The amount of pressure just sufficient to restore the original volume would equal the osmotic pressure exerted by the added particles.

FIGURE 11–3

Osmotic pressure. Water flows in the direction of the higher concentration of solute.

It is not known whether any regulating system other than the kidneys governs the body's salt contents. We have thirst to govern our intake of water, but do we have a salt hunger to govern our intake of sodium? Salt hunger is well known in plant-eating animals like cattle, which will travel long distances to a salt lick when they have been depleted of sodium. The tongue, in both animals and humans, is equipped with taste receptors that respond only to the salty taste. Animals know instinctively when to seek this stimulus, but humans may seek it when they have no need. Future research may determine whether a true salt hunger operates in humans. Discussion of food sources of minerals is reserved for later in this chapter.

There are four kinds of taste receptors on the tongue: those sensitive to salty, sweet, sour, and bitter flavors.

The body neither helplessly absorbs nor helplessly excretes electrolytes. It has highly evolved regulatory mechanisms to help ensure that its content of each mineral stays within bounds. Regulation occurs chiefly at two sites: the GI tract and the kidney.

The GI tract pours minerals continuously into its upper portions (stomach and small intestine) with the digestive juices and bile it secretes. It then reabsorbs them in its lower segment (the colon) as needed. In a day, a total of 8 liters (8 quarts) of fluids are recycled this way, providing ample opportunity for the regulation of electrolyte balance.

The kidney's control of water excretion has already been described. If you drink too little water or eat too much salt, your extracellular fluid (including your blood) becomes hypertonic. The brain receives the signal, secretes ADH, and the kidney responds by retaining water. The urine volume is small, so the urine is a concentrated solution of excretion products. In the reverse situation, the urine becomes more dilute.

To control electrolyte excretion, the kidney depends on the adrenal gland to signal any change needed in the blood level of an electrolyte. The hormone aldosterone carries the message. Aldosterone promotes sodium reabsorption and potassium excretion from the kidney tubule, if the body's sodium level is low.

The ability of the kidneys to regulate the sodium and water content of the body is remarkable. Sodium is absorbed easily from the intestinal tract; it then travels in the blood, where it ultimately passes through the kidneys. The kidneys filter all the sodium out, and then with great precision return to the bloodstream the exact amount of sodium needed. Normally, the amount excreted equals the amount ingested that day. About 30 to 45 percent of the body's sodium is thought to be stored on the surface of the bone crystals, where it is easy to recover if the blood level drops.

The blood level of sodium rises after a person eats heavily salted foods or meals very high in carbohydrate.* The high blood level stimulates thirst receptors in the brain, and the person drinks until the sodium-to-water ratio reaches a target level. Then the extra water is excreted by the kidneys together with the extra sodium.

Thus you are well protected from imbalances of water and electrolytes. However, you may encounter situations in which such large amounts of fluid and electrolytes are rapidly lost that your kidneys, thirst instinct, and cell membranes cannot compensate. Vomiting, diarrhea, heavy sweating, burns, wounds, and the like may result in such great fluid losses that a medical emergency results.

Fluid and Electrolyte Imbalance

The details of electrolyte balance are among the most important ones that medical students must learn. These details are taught in physiology courses and in medical and nursing curricula. Everyone, however, should appreciate the importance of the balance and the principles by which it is maintained, and be aware of the situations that threaten it. When any of these gets out of control, the appropriate action is to seek medical help. We usually take water and salts for granted and ignore them, but the loss of water and salts can more rapidly result in life threatening conditions than any of the other nutrients considered in this book.

A few examples will illustrate (see Table 11–3). Suppose, for example, that the kidneys are poisoned and fail to respond to aldosterone when it calls for sodium retention and potassium excretion. Sodium will be lost (and the extracellular fluid volume will decline), while potassium will be retained (and the intracellular fluid volume will increase). Or suppose that fluid is lost by vomiting or diarrhea—a situation in which sodium is lost wholesale but potassium is not

*Overeating of carbohydrate results in sodium retention, probably mediated by effects of insulin and glucose on the kidney's regulatory mechanisms. Conversely, starvation, carbohydrate-free, and low-carbohydrate diets increase sodium excretion. S. F. Hull, Body fluid and electrolyte balance, *Dietetic Currents, Ross Timesaver* 12 (1985): 3–4.

TABLE 11–3

Different Causes of Fluid and Electrolyte Imbalance (Examples)

Cause	Effect on Fluid and Electrolyte Balance	Effect on Fluid Volumes	
		Extra-cellular	Intra-cellular
Kidney poisoning	Sodium loss, potassium retention	↓	↑
Vomiting, diarrhea	Sodium loss (potassium unchanged), water loss	↓	(little change)
Glycosuria (sugar excretion in urine)	Water loss	↓	↓

returned in exchange for it. The extracellular fluid volume will decline, but the intracellular fluid volume will remain unchanged. Now suppose that water is pulled out of the body by a solute not normally excreted (for example, glucose, in the person with uncontrolled diabetes). A disproportionate amount of water will be lost relative to electrolytes, and the fluid volume will decline both inside and outside the cells. All three situations are types of dehydration, but each requires a different remedy: restore sodium and restrict potassium in the first; restore sodium and water in the second; restore only water in the third.

Acid-Base Balance

The body uses ions not only to help maintain water balance, but also to help regulate the acidity (pH) of its fluids. Some of the electrolyte mixtures in the body fluids, as well as the proteins, protect the body against changes in acidity by acting as buffers—substances that can neutralize newly introduced acids or bases. The pH scale is shown in Figure 11–4.

The body's most important buffering systems are mixtures of electrolytes in solution. For example, the blood contains sodium ions (+) and bicarbonate ions (−). When a strong acid is added to this solution, it forms two products: a salt, which is neutral, and a different acid, carbonic acid. It so happens that carbonic acid breaks down to carbon dioxide and water, so the end products are neither acidic nor basic. The lungs expel the carbon dioxide, and the kidneys excrete the water and salt (see margin next page).

The body's buffer systems serve as a first line of defense against changes in the fluids' acid-base balance. The lungs, skin, GI tract, and kidneys provide other defenses. If acid builds up regardless, the respiration rate speeds up, and more carbon dioxide is exhaled. If base builds up, the respiration rate slows, so that carbon dioxide, which is being formed all the time by cellular respiration, will form additional carbonic acid to balance it.

The skin can excrete acid in sweat, and the specialized tear ducts can alter the composition of tears. The stomach excretes acid as well. These are of minor but not negligible importance, but the chief regulatory organ is the kidneys.

The kidneys help to adjust acid-base balance by selecting which ions to retain and which to excrete. Their work is so complex that whole books have been

pH: The concentration of H^+ ions (see Appendix B). The lower the pH, the stronger the acid. Thus at pH 2, a solution is a strong acid and at pH 6, a solution is a weak acid (pH 7 is neutral). A pH above 7 is alkaline, or basic (a solution in which OH^- ions predominate).

ion: see Appendix B.

buffer: a substance or mixture capable of neutralizing both acids and bases and thereby capable of maintaining the acidity or alkalinity of a solution.

FIGURE 11–4

The pH scale.

Note: Each step is ten times as concentrated in base (1/10 as much acid, or H$^+$) as the one below it.

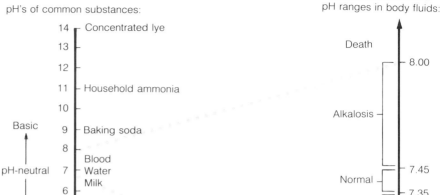

pH's of common substances:

pH	Substance
14	Concentrated lye
13	
12	
11	Household ammonia
10	
9	Baking soda
8	
7	Blood / Water / Milk
6	
5	Coffee
4	Orange juice
3	Vinegar
2	Lemon juice / Gastric juice
1	
0	Battery acid

Basic ↑ pH-neutral ↓ Acid

Normal and abnormal pH ranges in body fluids:

Death — 8.00
Alkalosis
Normal — 7.45 / 7.35
Acidosis
Death — 6.8

The bicarbonate/carbonic acid buffering system starts with sodium bicarbonate dissociated in water:

$$Na^+ \qquad \underset{O}{\overset{O}{\underset{|}{\overset{\parallel}{C}}}} {-}O{-}H$$

When acid is added:

$$H^+ \qquad Cl^-$$

The sodium and chloride electrically balance each other (as salts always do):

$$Na^+ \qquad Cl^-$$

What's left is another acid:

$$H^+ \qquad \underset{O}{\overset{O}{\underset{|}{\overset{\parallel}{C}}}} {-}O{-}H$$

This releases carbon dioxide, which is expelled in the breath:

$$O = C = O$$

What's left is water:

$$H{-}O{-}H$$

A Note on Acid-Formers and Base-Formers

In connection with the acidity of the urine, some foods have been called "acid-forming" and others "base-forming." This concept has won wide acceptance, but its practical implications are unclear. It is true that when foods are burnt to ash and the ashes are put in water, solutions of different pH's may result; but the acidity of the urine when these same foods are eaten cannot be predicted from that. The ashing of foods drives off gases containing nitrogen, sulfur, and other elements which, when metabolized in the body, produce compounds that dissolve in the fluids and affect their pH. To make things more complicated, the metabolic byproducts of the constituents of foods differ depending on how they are metabolized. Also, the body has other ways of excreting acid than in the urine, as just described. The notion that the "acid-forming" and "base-forming" effects of foods on the urine can be predicted from the composition of their ashes oversimplifies the case.

The theory that diets can be designed around such foods to produce a more acidic or basic urine seems not to have been established by actual research. Such diets have been used, however, for two chief purposes. One is to inhibit the growth of bacteria causing a bladder infection; the other is to reduce the likelihood of certain stones forming in the kidney (some stones precipitate from acid, others from basic solutions). These diets are seldom used any more. For bacterial infections, antibacterial drugs are preferred; for stone formation, strategies proven effective are to increase water intake so as to produce a dilute urine in which precipitation of any kind of stone will be less likely, and to limit intake of the constituents of the stone.

written on renal physiology, but their net effect is easy to sum up. The *body's* total acid burden remains nearly constant; and to a great extent, it is the acidity of the *urine* that is affected by what you ingest.

Sodium, Other Minerals, and High Blood Pressure

The body has to maintain a certain blood pressure to sustain the lives of its cells. The pressure of the blood against the walls of the capillaries ensures that fluids carrying nutrients and oxygen move into the tissues to deliver their cargo. Figure 11–5 shows that, when blood reaches the capillaries, whose thin walls permit fluid to cross them, much of its fluid and small dissolved molecules exit, and the concentration of cells and large proteins in the remaining blood becomes maximal. Fluids from the tissues, thanks to the osmotic pressure of the concentrated blood, then seep back into the capillaries, now carrying carbon dioxide and other waste materials. Thus the cells' needs for supply and removal of materials are met. The blood pressure also helps ensure that the fluids of the blood are pushed into the kidney tubules as blood passes through them. Then

Pumping pressure from the heart.

Fluid can't cross thick wall of artery.

Artery

Start of capillary. Fluid can cross thinner wall.

1. Blood pressure forces fluid across wall at start of capillary. Small organic molecules (glucose, amino acids) and salts move out with the water. Proteins and cells remaining are becoming more concentrated in the fluid that remains in the blood. Osmotic "pull" is increasing. Blood pressure is decreasing.

At midpoint of capillary, osmotic "pull" balances blood pressure and there is no net flow of fluid across capillary wall.

Solute now so concentrated that it attracts fluid back into the capillary by osmotic pressure. Small molecules (waste products) accompany the fluid.

2. End of capillary.

Vein

FIGURE 11–5

Two kinds of pressure in the capillaries. One (mechanical pressure from the heart) ensures that fluid leaves the capillary to nourish the surrounding tissues. The other (osmotic pressure) ensures that fluid returns to the vascular system.

the kidney selectively retrieves materials to return to the blood and excretes the waste in the urine (see Figure 6–7 in Chapter 6).

Blood Pressure Regulation

When the blood pressure falls, the lives of all the body's cells are threatened. The kidneys detect the lowered pressure and immediately set in motion a mechanism to raise the blood pressure again. Figure 11–6 shows how this mechanism works.

Normally, this response of the kidneys is highly adaptive. In dehydration, for example, a true "water deficiency" exists. By constricting the blood vessels and conserving water and sodium, the kidney-initiated mechanism ensures that blood pressure is maintained until more water can be drunk.

Sometimes, however, the kidneys are fooled. They experience a "water deficiency" when there is none. Then they retain water, increase the blood volume and raise the blood pressure with harmful effects—a maladaptive response. Most often, the cause is atherosclerosis, which narrows the arteries in the kidney as elsewhere, making it hard for the heart to push blood through them. In effect, this deprives the kidneys of their blood supply just as if the blood pressure were too low. In response to poor circulation of fluid, the kidneys release the enzyme renin, leading to a rise in blood pressure. This improves the blood flow through the kidneys, but now the heart has to pump extra hard to push the extra fluid around against resistant arteries all over the body. Added weight (obesity) raises the pressure further, and extra adipose tissue means miles of extra capillaries through which the blood must be pumped. The combination of high blood pressure, obesity, and hardened arteries is deadly.

High Blood Pressure

In 10 percent of cases, hypertension is caused by recognized kidney disease, and is called secondary hypertension, but in 90 percent, the cause is unknown. The vast majority of cases are called *essential* hypertension, meaning that the disease process must be primary. Among the causes suspected are several genetic mechanisms, tension from anxiety (which affects the nervous and hormonal systems controlling blood pressure), and many nutrition factors.[1]

Hypertension is mysterious in another way, too: you can't tell by feel if you have it. Since even mild hypertension exerts harmful wear and tear on the heart and arteries over the long term, it is important to know that you have it, so as to be able to take preventive measures if necessary. Figure 11–7 shows how to interpret your blood pressure.

The mineral sodium has been implicated so strongly in the causation of high blood pressure that many people have been led to believe it alone is to blame. Findings such as these incriminate sodium (but withhold judgment for a moment):

1. Populations with high intakes of sodium have more high blood pressure (for example, the Japanese).
2. Populations that eat little or no salt have normal blood pressure (even some vegetarian groups in our society).
3. Severely restricting sodium reduces high blood pressure; adding sodium back to the diet restores high blood pressure.[2]

Atherosclerosis is the subject of Highlight 4B.

hypertension: high blood pressure. People sometimes confuse hypertension with stress, but hypertension is an internal, and stress an external, condition. Stress may cause hypertension in sensitive people, however.

Secondary hypertension is high blood pressure caused by (that is, secondary to) kidney disease (10 percent of cases). Primary, or essential, hypertension is of unknown origin (90 percent of cases) and can cause kidney disease.

"High" blood pressure is defined differently for different purposes. Here, if the higher of the two numbers is over 140 or if the lower is over 90, it is considered to be too high.

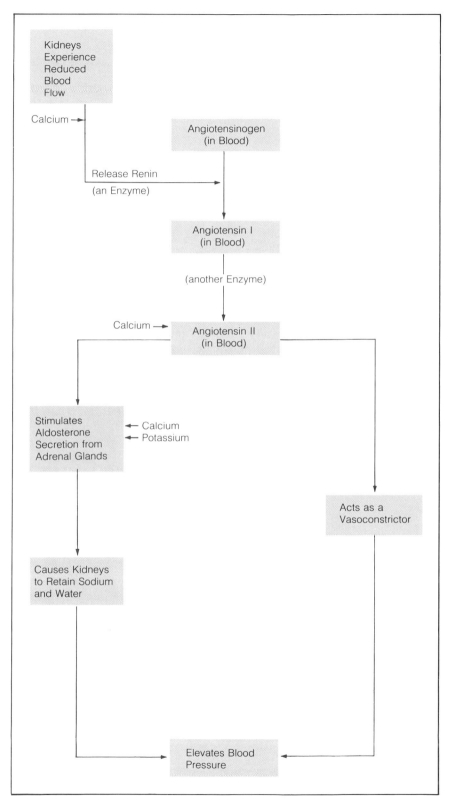

FIGURE 11–6

Blood pressure regulation.
Angiotensinogen is present in the blood at all times. When the kidneys release renin, it is converted to the active form that raises blood pressure as shown. Calcium and potassium are involved at the points indicated.

FIGURE 11–7

How to interpret your blood pressure.
The heart has a two-step beat: the **systole** (SIS-toe-lee) and the **diastole** (dye-ASS-toe-lee). The systole creates a higher pressure in the arteries. Both are recorded, the systole first, diastole second (example: 105/70). "High blood pressure" is defined differently for different purposes, but generally, if the higher number is over 140, or if the lower is over 90, the blood pressure is considered too high.

| 105 | ← | This is the systolic pressure. If this number is above 140, you may have hypertension. |

This is the diastolic pressure, the more sensitive indicator of hypertension. Interpret this number as follows:

| 70 | ← | |

Less than 85	Normal blood pressure
85 to 89	High normal blood pressure
90 to 104	Mild hypertension
105 to 114	Moderate hypertension
115 or more	Severe hypertension

Source: Adapted from R. W. Miller, The fight against heart disease, Part 1: Diet, exercise and other keys to a healthy heart, *FDA Consumer*, February 1986, pp. 8–13.

hard water: water containing high concentrations of calcium and magnesium.

soft water: water containing a high sodium concentration.

When water is softened, its magnesium and calcium ions are exchanged for sodium. Two sodiums (Na$^+$) replace one calcium (Ca^{++}) or magnesium (Mg^{++}), so the number of particles doubles. The harder the water to begin with, the more sodium the softened water will finally have.

It is not a disaster to have high blood pressure, but it is important to know your blood pressure so you can control it.

4. A nationwide program to control blood pressure, including sodium reduction, has seemed to lower blood pressure in many individuals.[3]
5. People in areas with soft water (which contains sodium) have higher (average) blood pressure than people in areas with hard water (which contains calcium and magnesium).
6. Genetically sodium sensitive strains of animals are known; their blood pressure is greatly affected by dietary sodium. Some humans (perhaps 20 percent) are genetically sensitive also.[4]

Blood pressure regulation is not simple, however. Other factors are involved. Items 1 and 2, above, show correlations, not evidence of cause. With respect to item 3, people with *normal* blood pressure usually do not show an increase when fed large amounts of salt, at least over a short course of time. With respect to item 4, drugs were used to lower blood pressure, and the independent effect of sodium restriction, if any, is unknown. As for item 5, who is to say that it is the sodium in soft water that accounts for the difference? Perhaps it is some other mineral, or perhaps the calcium and magnesium in *hard* water protect against high blood pressure.

The only findings that seem to hold up strongly are that some people are sensitive to sodium and tend to have high blood pressure, and that they can lower it by reducing their salt intakes. Since not all these people know who they are (and you can't tell by "feel" when you have high blood pressure), some authorities contend that the whole population should be encouraged to reduce its salt intakes. The government's *Dietary Goals*, the *Dietary Guidelines for Americans*, and the Canadian government's guidelines recommend reducing sodium intakes based on this assumption.

Setting sodium aside for a moment, what are the other diet-related factors that affect blood pressure? Obesity is one, as already mentioned (see Chapter 8, especially). Several other minerals are also involved—notably, potassium, calcium, magnesium, and cadmium.

Dietary Factors Affecting Blood Pressure

When sodium is retained in the body, potassium is traded for it. Even subjects with normal blood pressure, if fed very large quantities of sodium over a long time period, ultimately show a rise in blood pressure—but at the same time, their potassium excretion is increasing. ~~Fed potassium simultaneously with the sodium, they do not have a rise in blood pressure.~~[5]

Population studies show sodium being traded for potassium in a different sense. People who eat many foods high in sodium (processed foods, for example) necessarily eat fewer potassium-containing foods (such as fruits and whole vegetables) at the same time. ~~Potassium is the "intracellular cation,"~~ remember, and this is true in plants as well as in animal bodies. ~~When foods are processed, their cells are disrupted, and they spill their potassium contents. Thus they lose potassium, then they gain sodium when salt is~~ added. The more whole and unprocessed a food is, the more ideal (probably) its potassium-to-sodium ratio is. Conversely, the more processed a food is, the poorer the ratio. Table 11–4 shows how dramatically the potassium-to-sodium ratio is affected by processing in all classes of foods.

Calcium and magnesium are implicated in blood pressure regulation because of the hard water versus soft water observation already mentioned. It has also been reported that both calcium intakes and blood levels are low in people with high blood pressure. ~~In fact, the lower the calcium intake, the higher the blood pressure~~—a stronger argument that calcium is responsible.[6] ~~The contaminant cadmium is leached from pipes into~~ water, especially soft water, and may ~~contribute to high blood pressure.~~[7] Other food- and drink-related factors implicated

TABLE 11–4

Whole Unprocessed Foods versus Processed Foods—Potassium and Sodium Contents

Food	Amount	Potassium (mg)	Sodium (mg)	Potassium-to-Sodium Ratio
Milk Foods				
Milk	1 c	370	122	3:1
Chocolate pudding (cooked from mix)	1 c	354	343	1:1
Chocolate pudding (instant)	1 c	335	820	1:2
Meats				
Beef roast (cooked)	3 oz	279	42	7:1
Corned beef (canned)	3 oz	51	803	1:16
Chipped beef	3 oz	170	3660	1:22
Vegetables				
Corn (cooked)	1 c	304	71	4:1
Creamed corn (canned)	1 c	248	671	1:3
Sugar-coated cornflakes	1 c	27	262	1:10
Fruits				
Peaches (fresh)	1 peach	202	1	202:1
Peaches (canned)	1	333	5	67:1
Peach pie	1 piece	201	201	1:1
Grains				
Whole-wheat flour	1 c	444	4	100:1
Whole-wheat bread	1 slice	68	132	1:2
Doughnut, snack cake	1	23	125	1:5

in the blood pressure connection are chloride, alcohol, protein, and fatty acids.[8] Under experimental conditions, PUFA lower blood pressure slightly, probably by way of their effect on prostaglandins. All of these findings point toward the advisability of using a diet similar to that suggested for the maintenance of overall health and for the prevention of atherosclerosis, diabetes, and cancer—that is, a diet consisting largely of whole foods, minimally processed, and low in fat and salt.

Such a diet, and especially sodium restriction, may be especially important for people who have a genetic sensitivity to sodium that leads to hypertension. How many people this represents is a much-debated question, but one in five seems to be a conservative estimate; by age 65 it may be half of all individuals. Black Americans are significantly more at risk than other groups. This being the case, perhaps we should all curtail our sodium intakes, as the authorities mentioned earlier suggest.

For people with hypertension already present, possible strategies are to use blood-pressure lowering drugs, diet and other changes, or both. It is generally agreed that for moderate and severe hypertension, drugs are advisable, but debate surrounds the question whether drugs are necessary to treat mild hypertension. Clearly many people with mild hypertension can control it by means of lifestyle changes alone, and probably even those who have to use drugs should also adopt these lifestyle changes:

- Weight reduction.
- Sodium restriction.
- Adequate intakes of potassium, calcium, and magnesium.*
- Other dietary changes (low fat, high fiber).
- Exercise.
- Relaxation.
- Moderation in alcohol use.[9]

Sodium and Salt in Foods

No RDA has been set for sodium, because there is no sodium shortage in the diet. Intakes of 1.1 to 3.3 grams per day (1,100 to 3,300 mg) are considered safe and adequate for adults. Intakes vary widely, especially because of cultural differences in diets. Asians, who liberally use soy sauce and monosodium glutamate (MSG, or Accent) for flavoring, consume about 30 to 40 grams of salt per day; most people in the United States average about 6 to 18 grams per day. Vegetarians, depending on their food preferences, can consume much less.

Soft water can add appreciable sodium to people's diets, and it appears to contribute to a higher incidence of high blood pressure and heart disease in areas where it is used. The National Academy of Sciences has suggested a standard for public water allowing no more than 100 milligrams of sodium per liter. This limit would ensure that the water supply would add not more than 10 percent to the average person's total sodium intake. The American Heart Association has recommended a more conservative standard of 20 milligrams per liter, to protect heart and kidney clients whose sodium intakes must be

Recommended intakes of sodium:
U.S. suggested intake: 1,100 to 3,300 mg.
Canada's RNI: 35 mg/kg.

5 g salt is about 2 g sodium.
1 g salt = ⅕ tsp.

---

*The literature review from which we obtained this set of recommendations said "potassium, calcium, and magnesium supplementation." We have taken the liberty of restating it in terms of foods.

restricted. At present, about half the U.S. population drinks water containing more than 20 milligrams per liter.

The *Dietary Guidelines* recommends that we limit our sodium intake to not more than 5 grams of added salt a day (that is, salt added by manufacturers and consumers above and beyond that already in the food as grown). In practice, this would mean avoiding highly salted foods and removing the salt shaker from the table. The notes in the margin provide general suggestions for avoiding sodium in foods for the person who wishes to do so.

Persons who wish to avoid salt need to know that what they pour from the salt shaker may be only a third of the total salt they consume. One-fourth to one-half comes from processed food, to which salt is added as a preservative and flavoring agent. As of July 1, 1986, all foods that bear nutrition labels must state their sodium contents; sodium-conscious consumers can easily learn to read them as shown in Figure 2–3 in Chapter 2. The serious sodium avoider must also stay away from fast-food places and Asian restaurants and stop using many canned, frozen, and instant foods at home. (On the positive side, unprocessed, whole foods are lower in sodium—and higher in potassium—than most people realize.)

Processed foods do not always taste salty. Most people are surprised to learn that a serving of cornflakes contains more sodium than a serving of cocktail peanuts—and that a serving of chocolate pudding contains still more. The reason the peanuts taste saltier is because the salt is all on the surface, where the tongue's sensors immediately pick it up.

Foods seem far less tasty without salt, at first. With practice, however, people can learn to enjoy the flavors of many unsalted foods and, where spices are needed, to make liberal use of sodium-free spices like those listed in Table 11–5. If you persist long enough (say, two months) in eating a low-salt diet, your taste threshold for salt will actually change so that your preferred level is lower.[10]

The person who wishes to use diet to prevent high blood pressure should probably not only reduce sodium intake, but emphasize positive actions as well:

- Eat plenty of fresh fruits and vegetables, because they are rich in potassium (as well as many other vitamins and minerals, of course).
- Eat a variety of foods, including good food sources of calcium and magnesium.
- Maintain ideal weight.
- Use alcohol in moderation.

Calcium

Unlike sodium, calcium is not so abundant in the diet, and deficiencies are widespread in human societies. The price you pay for neglecting to obtain enough calcium throughout early and middle life is extensive degeneration of the skeleton in old age—adult bone loss, which leads to crippling deformities, irreparable fractures, and even death. Nearly all people suffer some bone loss as they grow older, and serious fractures result in about one of every three people

To avoid too much sodium:

- Learn to enjoy the unsalted flavors of foods.
- Cook with only small amounts of added salt.
- Add little or no salt to food at the table.

Cut down on:

- Foods prepared in brine, such as pickles, olives, and sauerkraut.
- Salty or smoked meats, such as bologna, corned or chipped beef, frankfurters, ham, luncheon meats, salt pork, sausage, and smoked tongue.
- Salty or smoked fish, such as anchovies, caviar, salted and dried cod, herring, sardines, and smoked salmon.
- Snack items such as potato chips, pretzels, salted popcorn, and salted nuts and crackers.
- Bouillon cubes; seasoned salts (including sea salt); and soy, Worcestershire, and barbecue sauces.
- Cheeses, especially processed types.
- Canned and instant soups.
- Prepared horseradish, catsup, and mustard.

Read labels. You may be surprised to learn that some processed foods that contain no table salt and don't taste salty have lots of sodium. Look for the word *soda* or *sodium* or the symbol *Na* on labels. Examples are *sodium* bicarbonate (baking *soda*), mono*sodium* glutamate, most baking powders, di*sodium* phosphate, *sodium* alginate, *sodium* benzoate, *sodium* hydroxide, *sodium* propionate, *sodium* sulfite, and *sodium* saccharin.—USDA

TABLE 11–5

Sodium-free Spices and Flavorings

Allspice	Onion powder
Almond extract	Paprika
Bay leaves	Parsley
Caraway seeds	Pepper
Cinnamon	Peppermint extract
Curry powder	Pimiento
Garlic	Rosemary
Garlic powder	Sage
Ginger	Sesame seeds
Lemon extract	Thyme
Mace	Turmeric
Maple extract	Vanilla extract
Marjoram	Vinegar
Mustard powder	Walnut extract
Nutmeg	

The regulators are hormones from the parathyroid and thyroid glands, as well as vitamin D. One, **parathormone,** raises blood calcium. The other, **calcitonin,** lowers it by inhibiting release of calcium from bone. The hormonelike **vitamin D** raises blood calcium by acting at the three sites listed.

calcium rigor: hardness or stiffness of the muscles caused by high blood calcium.

calcium tetany: intermittent spasms of the extremities due to nervous and muscular excitability caused by low blood calcium.

over 65. It is therefore urgent to understand the necessity of obtaining adequate calcium in food from the early years on throughout adulthood. Simply stated: drink plenty of milk daily—and if you can't, find and use ample substitute calcium sources daily.

The urgency of obtaining enough calcium has to be learned through education, because the body sends no signals saying it is deficient. Most nutrient deficiencies make themselves known by way of symptoms that can be felt or seen, such as pain, skin lesions, tiredness, and the like. But a developing calcium deficiency is utterly silent; it becomes apparent only when a hip or pelvic bone suddenly shatters into fragments that cannot be reassembled. No evidence of a developing calcium deficiency can be found in a blood sample, because blood calcium remains normal no matter what the bone content may be. Nor does depletion of bone calcium show up on an x-ray until it is so far advanced as to be virtually irreversible.

Figure 11–8A shows a hipbone sliced lengthwise so that you can see the lacy network of calcium-containing crystals inside the bone. These are the deposits in the body's calcium bank, which are drawn on whenever the supply from the day's diet runs short. Invested in savings during the milk-drinking years of childhood, these calcium deposits provide a nearly inexhaustible fund of calcium; 99 percent of the body's calcium is stored in the bones. Figures 11–8B and C show the effects of bone loss on the spine and on a person's height. The skeleton literally sags and shrinks when bone material is lost.

The other one percent of the body's calcium is in the blood and body fluids, where its concentration is tightly controlled by a system of hormones and vitamin D. Whenever the blood calcium concentration rises too high, these agents promote its deposit into bone. Whenever the blood concentration falls too low, the regulatory system acts in three locations to correct it:

- Intestine: increase calcium absorption.
- Bone: increase calcium release.
- Kidney: reduce calcium excretion.

Thus blood calcium returns to normal.

Food calcium never affects blood calcium, but this is not to say that blood calcium never changes. It does change, but in response to changed regulatory control, not to diet. When blood calcium rises above normal, the result is known as calcium rigor: the muscle fibers contract and cannot relax. Similarly, calcium levels may fall below normal in the blood, causing calcium tetany—also characterized by uncontrolled contraction of muscle tissue due to a change in the stimulation of nerve cells. These conditions do not (we repeat) reflect a dietary lack or excess of calcium; they are caused by a lack of vitamin D or by glandular malfunctions that result in abnormal amounts of the hormones that regulate blood calcium concentration.

On the other hand, a chronic *dietary* deficiency of calcium or a chronic deficiency due to poor absorption over the course of years can diminish the savings account in the bones. Because this is an important concept, we repeat once more: it is the bones, not the blood, that are depleted by calcium deficiency.

Roles of Calcium

The calcium that circulates in the body fluids plays many roles. Some calcium is found in close association with cell membranes, where it helps to regulate the

FIGURE 11–8

Normal and osteoporotic bone.

A. Cross section of bone. The lacy structural elements are **trabeculae** (tra-BECK-you-lee), which can be drawn on to replenish blood calcium.

B. A healthy spine and one that has deteriorated from adult bone loss (osteoporosis). Notice how the vertebrae are crumbling.

C. Effects of osteoporosis on a woman's height. On the left is a woman at menopause and on the right, the same woman 30 years later. Notice that collapse of her vertebrae has shortened her back; the length of her legs has not changed.

Source: Adapted from *Why Should Adults Drink Milk?* (Tallahassee, Fla.: Nutrition Company, 1983).

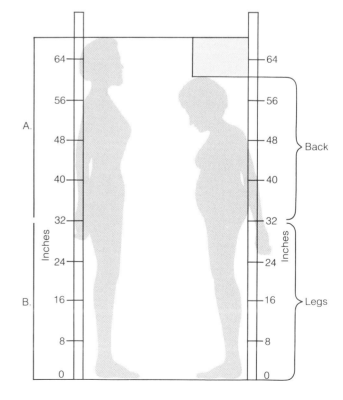

transport of other ions in and out. It is essential for muscle action and so helps maintain the heartbeat. Calcium must be present between nerve and nerve, and between nerve and muscle, for the reception and interpretation of nerve impulses; and when it enters cells, it delivers important messages to intracellular receptors (see Figure 11–9).

Among the messages calcium delivers are several that have to do with blood pressure. It regulates the tone of muscles in the blood vessel walls. It also helps govern the secretion of the blood pressure regulators aldosterone, angiotensin II, and renin.[11]

Calcium must also be present if blood clotting is to occur, because it is one of the 14 factors directly involved in this process. (The other 13 are proteins; vitamin K is needed, too, for the synthesis of some of these proteins.) Calcium also acts as a cofactor for several enzymes.

As for the calcium in bone, it plays two important roles. One, as already mentioned, is to serve as a bank to prevent alteration of the all-important blood calcium concentration. And the bones, of course, hold the body upright and serve as attachment points for muscles, making motion possible.

cofactor: a mineral element that, like a coenzyme, works with an enzyme to facilitate a chemical reaction. The cofactor occurs at the active site, maintains the structural integrity of the protein, and may also facilitate the enzyme's catalytic activity.

Coenzyme: see p. 291.

FIGURE 11–9

How calcium delivers messages. Calcium is concentrated outside cells, and an inactive protein, **calmodulin** (cal-MOD-you-lin), is concentrated inside them. Calmodulin will become active only when calcium is attached to it; then it becomes a messenger that tells other proteins what to do. The system serves as interpreter for nerve-mediated messages arriving at cells. Here's how it works. The brain initiates a message by sending an electrical impulse along a nerve (sodium rushes in and potassium rushes out, changing the electrical potential along the nerve). The electrical impulse arrives at the nerve ending and depolarizes the membrane at the receiving cell. Until then, the proteins (calmodulin and others) have been inactive (1).

Calcium enters the receiving cell and attaches to calmodulin, making it active (2). Calmodulin now tells other cellular proteins what to do (3). On receiving the message, a cell that is programmed to start dividing in response to nerve messages will do so. A cell that is programmed to manufacture and release secretory products will do that. A muscle fiber will contract. Thus, while sodium and potassium carry the messages along nerves, calcium permits them to be received and translated into action.

Afterwards, calcium is rapidly expelled from the cell by membrane pumps, and the proteins become inactive again (4).

Calcium is abundant; so is calmodulin. The reaction is one of the fastest in the body. Even hormones cannot work so fast.

Source: Adapted from W. Y. Cheung, Calmodulin, *Scientific American* 246 (1982): 62–70.

Calcium Deficiency

The disease rickets has been mentioned in connection with vitamin D deficiency. Often in rickets, the amount of calcium in the diet is adequate, but it passes through the intestinal tract without being absorbed into the body, leaving the bones undersupplied. Vitamin D deficiency, by depressing the production of the calcium-binding protein, is the most common cause of rickets. (The symptoms were listed in Table 10–4.) In children, the failure to deposit sufficient calcium in bone causes growth retardation, bowed legs, and other skeletal abnormalities. In adults, the disease may set in after a normal childhood during which calcium intake and absorption were adequate, and after the skeleton has become fully calcified. Prolonged inadequate calcium uptake during adulthood, whether due to vitamin D deficiency or to calcium deficiency, may cause the gradual and insidious removal of calcium from the bones. The result is altered composition or reduced density of the bones in old age, which makes them fragile.

Many older people are severely afflicted with osteoporosis. The causes seem to be multiple, but inadequate storage of calcium during the growing years is a factor always present. This fact underscores the importance of prevention: drink plenty of milk while you are young to have strong bones in later life, and continue drinking milk throughout adulthood to avoid losing calcium. A net calcium loss occurs in many adults, especially women after menopause or hysterectomy, suggesting that hormonal changes are responsible. Many minerals and vitamins are required to form and stabilize the structure of bones, including magnesium, fluoride, vitamin A, and others. Any of these may be essential for preventing osteoporosis. One obvious line of defense, however, is to maintain a lifelong adequate intake of calcium.

Food Sources of Calcium

The recommended intake of calcium, arrived at by way of balance studies, is 700 to 800 milligrams (0.7 to 0.8 grams) per day for adults in both the United States and Canada. Adults can stay in balance on intakes lower than this if they adapt over a long period of time to lower intakes, and the World Health Organization recommends only 400 to 500 milligrams per day for adults. However, high protein intakes increase calcium excretion, and in the United States and Canada, where diets are rich in protein, 700 to 800 milligrams for adults and 1,200 for pregnant and lactating women seems to be a protective recommendation. Authorities advocate even more—1,200 to 1,500 milligrams a day—for women over 50. To obtain 1,500 milligrams of calcium from milk, one of its richest sources, a woman would have to drink more than 5 cups. The minimum number of kcalories one would have to ingest to do this would be 90 per cup, using nonfat milk—or 450 kcalories in all.

Table 11–6 shows that calcium is found almost exclusively in three classes of foods—milk/milk products, green vegetables, and a few fish and shellfish. The green vegetables look best in terms of calcium per 100 kcalories. Nonfat milk offers about 300 milligrams of calcium in an 88-kcalorie cup, for example, while greens (depending on the variety chosen) offer 100 or more milligrams in a 20-kcalorie cup. The greens would therefore seem to be the better choice per kcalorie, but a complication enters in—absorption. It isn't clear to what extent calcium is absorbed from green vegetables, while calcium is known to

rickets: the calcium deficiency (or vitamin D–deficiency) disease in children.

Altered composition of the bones is reflected in **osteomalacia,** the condition in which the bones become soft (see p. 355). Osteomalacia is sometimes called **adult rickets.**

Reduced density of the bones results in **osteoporosis** (oss-tee-oh-pore-OH-sis)— literally, "porous bones."

Chapter 16 shows that exercise, too, is important in the prevention of osteoporosis.

Recommended intakes of calcium:
  U.S. adults' RDA: 800 mg.
  Canadian RNI for women: 700 mg.
                          men: 800 mg.

The Four Food Group Plan recommends daily milk servings:

- Children under 9   2 to 3 c
- Children 9 to 12   3+ c
- Teenagers   4+ c
- Adults   2 c
- Pregnant women   3+ c
- Lactating women   4+ c
- Older women   3+ c

TABLE 11–6

Calcium In Foods

Foods Ranked by Calcium Per Serving	Calcium Per Serving (mg)	Energy Per Serving (kCal)	Foods Ranked by Calcium Per 100 kCalories	Calcium Per Serving (mg)	Calcium Per 100 KCal (mg)
Sardines, canned w/bones (3 oz)	371	175	Bok choy cabbage, cooked (1 c)	158	790
Kefir (1 c)	350	160	Turnip greens, cooked (1 c)	198	683
Goat milk (1 c)	326	168	Spinach, cooked (1 c)	244	595
Shrimp, boiled (3.5 oz)	320	109	Collards, cooked (1 c)	113	565
Nonfat milk + solids (1 c)	316	91	Spinach, canned (1 c)	271	542
1% milk + solids (1 c)	314	105	Mustard greens, cooked (1 c)	104	495
Romano cheese (1 oz)	302	110	Spinach, fresh chopped (1 c)	55	458
Nonfat milk or yogurt (1 c)	302	86	Dandelion greens, cooked (1 c)	147	420
1% lowfat milk (1 c)	300	102	Beet greens, cooked (1 c)	165	413
Whole milk (1 c)	291	150	Seaweed, kelp, raw (1 oz)	48	400
Buttermilk (1 c)	285	99	Parsley, chopped fresh (1 c)	78	390
Chocolate milk, whole (1 c)	280	210	Broccoli, cooked (1 c)	178	387
Swiss cheese (1 oz)	272	107	Looseleaf lettuce (1 c)	38	380
Spinach, canned (1 c)	271	50	Nonfat milk or yogurt (1 c)	302	351
Spinach, cooked (1 c)	244	41	Nonfat milk + solids (1 c)	316	347
Cheddar cheese (1 oz)	204	114	Parmesan cheese (1 tbsp	69	300
Muenster cheese (1 oz)	203	104	1% milk + solids (1 c)	314	299
Oysters, raw (1 c)	202	160	Shrimp, boiled (3.5 oz)	320	294
Turnip greens, cooked (1 c)	198	29	1% lowfat milk (1 c)	300	294
Broccoli, cooked (1 c)	178	46	Buttermilk (1 c)	285	288
Salmon, canned w/bones (3 oz)	167	120	Romano cheese (1 oz)	302	275
Beet greens, cooked (1 c)	165	40	Swiss cheese (1 oz)	272	254
Bok choy cabbage, cooked (1 c)	158	20	Celery, outer stalk (1)	14	233
Cottage cheese, lowfat 2% (1 c)	155	205	Kefir (1 c)	350	219
Dandelion greens, cooked (1 c)	147	35	Sardines, canned w/bones (3 oz)	371	212
Soy beans, cooked dry (1 c)	132	235	Okra pods, fresh-cooked (8)	54	200
Collards, cooked (1 c)	113	20	Cabbage, raw shredded (1 c)	32	200
Tofu soybean curd (1 block)	108	86	Muenster cheese (1 oz)	203	195
Mustard greens, cooked (1 c)	104	21	Whole milk (1 c)	291	194
Parsley, chopped fresh (1 c)	78	20	Goat milk (1 c)	326	194
Almonds, whole dried (1 oz)	75	167	Cheddar cheese (1 oz)	204	179
Kidney beans, canned (1 c)	74	230	Salmon, canned w/bones (3 oz)	167	139
Parmesan cheese (1 tbsp)	69	23	Summer squash, cooked (1 c)	48	133
Green beans, cooked (1 c)	58	44	Chocolate milk, whole (1 c)	280	133
Spinach, fresh chopped (1 c)	55	12	Green beans, cooked (1 c)	58	132
Okra pods, fresh-cooked (8)	54	27	Tofu soybean curd (1 block)	108	126
Orange, fresh medium (1)	52	60	Oysters, raw (1 c)	202	126
Summer squash, cooked (1 c)	48	36	Cauliflower, cooked (1 c)	34	113
Seaweed, kelp, raw (1 oz)	48	12	Orange, fresh medium (1)	52	87
Looseleaf lettuce (1 c)	38	10	Cottage cheese, lowfat 2% (1 c)	155	76
Cauliflower, cooked (1 c)	34	30	Soy beans, cooked dry (1 c)	132	56
Cabbage, raw shredded (1 c)	32	16	Almonds, whole dried (1 oz)	75	45
Cantaloupe melon (½)	29	94	Kidney beans, canned (1 c)	74	32
Sirloin steak, lean (8 oz)	26	480	Cantaloupe melon (½)	29	31
Whole wheat bread (1 sl)	20	70	Whole wheat bread (1 sl)	20	29
Oatmeal, cooked (1 c)	20	145	Oatmeal, cooked (1 c)	20	14
Peanuts, dried unsalted (1 oz)	17	161	Apple, fresh medium (1)	10	13
Celery, outer stalk (1)	14	6	Sole/flounder, baked (3 oz)	13	11
Sole/flounder, baked (3 oz)	13	120	Peanuts, dried unsalted (1 oz)	17	11
Chicken breast, roasted (½)	13	142	Chicken breast, roasted (½)	13	9
Apple, fresh medium (1)	10	80	Sirloin steak, lean (8 oz)	26	5

be very well absorbed from milk. Milk is therefore recommended for daily consumption by all members of the population. To make it easier for people to obtain the calcium they need from milk, the dairies are experimenting with a form of milk fortified so as to deliver twice as much calcium as regular milk; 1 cup would therefore do the job of 2.

Besides milk, another dairy food that contains comparable amounts of calcium is cheese. One slice of cheese (1 ounce) contains about two-thirds as much calcium as a cup of milk—at a kcalorie cost of 80 to 120 kcalories. Cottage cheese offers less calcium for more kcalories, and is a poor source by this standard; for the person who can eat unlimited kcalories, though, it can help meet the calcium need.

Milk and milk products need not be taken as such; there are ways to conceal them in foods. For children and adults who can afford the kcalories, ice cream, ice milk, and whole milk yogurt are acceptable substitutes for regular milk, and puddings, custards, and baked goods can be prepared in such a way that they also contain appreciable amounts of milk. Powdered nonfat milk, which is an excellent and inexpensive source of protein, calcium, and other nutrients, can be added to many foods (such as cookies and meatloaf) in preparation; this is probably the best way for older women to obtain the calcium they need beyond the amount they can practicably get from liquid milk.

The word *daily* should be stressed with respect to food sources of calcium. Because of the body's limited ability to absorb calcium, it cannot handle massive doses periodically, but instead needs frequent opportunities to take in small amounts. The word *milk products* should also be stressed, rather than dairy products. Butter and cream contain negligible calcium, because calcium is not soluble in fat.

Many factors affect calcium absorption. The stomach's acidity favors it by helping to keep calcium soluble. Vitamin D aids in calcium absorption by helping to make the necessary calcium-binding protein. (It is no accident that milk is chosen as the vehicle for fortification with vitamin D.) The lactose in milk also seems to facilitate calcium absorption by a mechanism as yet unknown.[12] Calcium levels are lower in breast milk than in cow's milk, but babies absorb calcium better from breast milk, possibly because of its higher lactose content.

The body is able to regulate its absorption of calcium by altering its production of the calcium-binding protein. More of this protein is made if more calcium is needed. Thus you will absorb more when you need more. This system is most obviously reflected in the increased absorption by a pregnant woman, who absorbs 50 percent of the calcium from the milk she drinks instead of only 30 percent, as she formerly did. Similarly, growing children absorb 50 to 60 percent of ingested calcium; when their growth slows or stops (and their bones no longer demand a net increase in calcium content each day), their absorption falls to the adult level of about 30 percent.

An important relationship exists between calcium and phosphorus. Each is better absorbed if they are ingested together. Authorities differ on the ratio that might best favor health, but it seems probable that most would agree on a 1:1 ratio; perhaps any ratio from 3:1 to 1:3 is all right.

Some foods contain binders that combine chemically with calcium and other minerals such as iron and zinc to prevent their absorption, carrying them out of the body with other wastes. For example, phytic acid renders the calcium (as well as iron and zinc) in certain foods less available than it might be otherwise; oxalic acid also binds calcium and iron. Phytic acid is found in oatmeal and

Milk and milk products are rightly famous for their calcium contents.

binders: chemical compounds occurring in foods, that can combine with nutrients (especially minerals) to form complexes the body cannot absorb. **Phytic** (FIGHT-ic) and **oxalic** (ox-AL-ic) **acids** are examples of such binders. See Chapter 3 for more about phytic acid.

Assessment of calcium: serum calcium does not detect bone mineral loss. Methods of assessing bone minerals are under development.

milk allergy: the most common food allergy; caused by the protein in raw milk. Milk allergy is sometimes overcome by cooking the milk to denature the protein, sometimes "cured" by abstinence from, and gradual reintroduction to, milk. See also the discussion of lactose intolerance, p. 63.

milk intolerance: digestive or other system symptoms, experienced subjectively after consuming milk. It can be due to the lactose content of the milk, but other chemical substances or contaminating toxins can also produce intolerance to milk in individuals capable of efficient digestion of lactose.

other whole-grain cereals, and oxalic acid, in beets, rhubarb, and spinach, among other foods.[13] Fiber in general seems to hinder calcium absorption, so the higher the diet is in fiber, the higher it should be in calcium. This fact doesn't affect the overall value of high-fiber foods; they are nutritious for many reasons, but they are not useful as calcium sources.[14]

Protein also affects calcium status, as already mentioned, but not by affecting absorption. The greater the amount of protein in the diet, the greater the amount of calcium excreted in the urine.[15] This is why recommended intakes of calcium in the United States and Canada (where protein intakes are often double those recommended) are greater than for people in countries whose protein intakes are lower. Another piece of advice, not often given but worth considering, is to eat less protein.

To sum up, positive calcium balance is favored by vitamin D, phosphorus (in up to a 1:1 ratio), and lactose. It is opposed by high-fiber foods and diets high in protein.

Milk Substitutes and Calcium Supplements

Some people are allergic to milk; others are lactose intolerant and can't drink it for that reason. For them, and especially the children among them, calcium-rich substitutes must be found. Whatever substitute is chosen has an important role to play in supplying the nutrients otherwise supplied by milk. Among the possible substitutes are: boiled milk, goat's or other species' milk, enzyme-treated milk, calcium-fortified soy milk, milk products such as plain yogurt and cheese, nondairy foods containing the nutrients of milk, imitation milk, and supplements.

In theory, it should be easy to choose the appropriate milk substitute. If the person is allergic to milk, then, in theory, the milk protein is the offending substance, and a substitute with altered or different proteins must be found. If the person is intolerant to lactose, then a lactose-free substitute is needed. It is often difficult, however, to determine why someone tolerates milk poorly. Milk intolerance can occur for unknown reasons other than allergy or lactose intolerance.[16] Both the kinds and amounts of milk any given person can tolerate can only be determined by experimenting. In practice, therefore, the selection of a substitute may have to proceed by trial and error.

Milk protein is denatured when milk is boiled. Some cases of milk allergy can be solved by this simple means. Plain, boiled milk tastes strange to a person who is accustomed to drinking fresh milk but may be acceptable to an unpre-

A generalization that has been gaining strength throughout this book is supported by the information given here about calcium. A balanced diet that supplies a variety of foods is the best guarantee of adequacy for all essential nutrients. All food groups should be included, and none should be overused. In our culture, calcium is usually lacking wherever milk is underemphasized in the diet—whether through ignorance, simple dislike, fad dieting, lactose intolerance, or allergy. By contrast, iron is usually lacking whenever milk is overemphasized, as Chapter 12 shows.

judiced child. Alternatively, liquid or powdered milk can be cooked into foods such as custards, baked goods, and meat loaf.

Goat's milk proteins differ somewhat from cow's milk proteins and may be tolerated by the person who can't tolerate cow's milk. Nutritionally, the two milks are similar in most respects; both should be fortified with vitamins A and D, however, to be compatible with the standard diet.

The treatment of milk with enzymes to digest its lactose offers a possible solution to the problem of lactose intolerance. The enzyme preparation (LactAid) can be purchased over the counter and mixed with the milk before the milk is served. Another possible alternative is low-lactose milk, if available.

If a deficiency of the digestive enzyme lactase is the problem, the intolerance is usually not absolute. In fact, the majority of individuals with a lactase deficiency experience no discomfort when they drink eight ounces of milk.[17] Those who do, can often handle small amounts of milk periodically throughout the day— up to half a glass each time. Fermented dairy products offer the same nutrients as milk but with a lower lactose content, because in fermenting the milk, bacteria use the lactose as an energy source to do their work. Fermented dairy products' lactose contents compare with the lactose in milk as shown in Table 11–7.

A product people sometimes wonder about is acidophilus milk. To give the end of the story first, it is *not* useful for lactose-intolerant individuals. It was developed on the theory that *L. acidophilus* bacteria could be added to milk to compete against other bacteria that might otherwise grow there or that might grow in the intestines after the milk was ingested. However, if *L. acidophilus* bacteria were allowed to grow in the milk and ferment the lactose, they would produce a sour byproduct, lactic acid. (The human intestinal enzyme that digests lactose, in contrast, produces the monosaccharides it is made of, glucose and galactose.) Therefore, *L. acidophilus* bacteria are grown in another medium and then harvested and added to milk, where they are not allowed to act any further. Acidophilus milk tastes sweet because its sugars are sweet, but its composition is the same as that of milk.

acidophilus (acid-OFF-ih-lus) **milk:** milk to which a culture of *Lactobacillus acidophilus* has been added. The theory is that the presence of these bacteria in the milk, and in the intestines after the milk is drunk, prevents the growth of other bacteria that might be harmful.

TABLE 11–7

Lactose Contents of Dairy Products.

Note that these are all fermented dairy products. A nonfermented milk product like ice cream has about the same amount of lactose per protein as milk (1½ cups have 93% of the lactose in 1 cup of milk).

Dairy Product	Serving Size to Equal 1 c Milk in Protein	Amount of Lactose as Compared to that in 1 c Milk
Yogurt	1 c	75%[a]
Strawberry yogurt	1 c	39%[b]
Pasteurized processed cheese food	3 tbsp	33%[b]
Grated American cheese	¾ oz	25%[b]
Cottage cheese	¼ c	14%[a]
Aged cheddar cheese	2 cu in	6%[a]
Swiss cheese	1 oz	trace[b]
Extra sharp cheddar cheese	2 cu in	trace[b]

[a]Calculated from A. D. Newcomer, Lactase deficiency, *Contemporary Nutrition* (April, 1979).

[b]Calculated from D. E. Lee and C. B. Lillibridge, A method for qualitative identification of sugars and semiquantitative determination of lactose content suitable for a variety of foods, *American Journal of Clinical Nutrition* 29 (1976): 428–440.

Not only dairy products but also certain meats and vegetables can be used to help supply the nutrients of milk. If foods are to be chosen to help replace milk in the diet, their calcium and riboflavin contents should be the basis for making the choice, because milk and milk products normally supply about 75 percent of people's intake of calcium and about 40 percent of their riboflavin. In most foods, the two nutrients occur together, so a selection made on the basis of calcium contents will serve both purposes. Foods to emphasize could be selected from Table 11–6. Many of these foods supply ample amounts of vitamin A as well, but their vitamin D contents are variable. The growing child who is outdoors daily can make his or her own vitamin D, given adequate exposure to sunlight (see page 357). A sick child needs a vitamin D fortified milk substitute or a vitamin supplement.

The alternatives offered for milk, so far, have been superior in the sense that they are whole dairy products or foods that offer many nutrients besides the ones listed in the tables. An inferior alternative is imitation milk. Imitation milk varies, but typically consists of water, sugar, vegetable fat, a source of protein (casein or soy, usually), and flavoring agents and stabilizers. Whatever is listed first on the label is the predominant ingredient. Imitation milk may be lower in protein than milk (for example, 1 percent rather than 3.5 percent) and may not supply the nutrients typical of milk. A milk substitute is satisfactory only if it provides high-quality protein, calcium, phosphorus, riboflavin, and vitamins A and D in quantities comparable to those in fortified fresh milk. Use of imitation milks in the diets of children and infants is generally undesirable. Figure 11–10 presents a decision tree for persons seeking a milk substitute.

Figure 11–10 recommends calcium supplements only as a last resort. The reason is simply that they are not foods. They do not offer the variety of nutrients foods do, and their calcium is not, for the most part, absorbed as well as that from milk. Whenever possible, a person would do better to do the thinking and make the effort necessary to obtain calcium from suitable substitutes in some kind of food form. However, some people cannot be persuaded to do this, and for them, the only question worth addressing is the question of how the various supplements available compare with each other.

Calcium comes in combination with a number of different anions in organic and inorganic salts. The organic salts include the lactate, the gluconate, and the citrate; the inorganic salts include the carbonate, the phosphate, and others. The carbonate is 40 percent calcium and the gluconate, only 9 percent—so you have to swallow fewer pills to get the needed calcium from the carbonate. On the other hand, the organic salts are probably better absorbed, especially by older people. Unfortunately, how much better is not established. Acid aids in calcium absorption, and calcium carbonate is an antacid, requiring the healthy stomach's secretion of sufficient hydrochloric acid to help it get into the system. Older people's stomach acid secretion tends to slow down, so that if they take calcium carbonate pills on an empty stomach, they may absorb only one-tenth as much calcium as they would from the calcium citrate. The effect is abolished by taking calcium carbonate with a full breakfast, so this is probably the strategy to adopt.[18]

Regular vitamin-mineral pills contain only small amounts of calcium, as you can tell by checking the label. Don't be fooled; the label may list some number of milligrams of calcium that sounds like a lot, but the U.S. RDA for calcium is a thousand milligrams (equal to a gram).

Read the label, and don't be fooled by the mention of calcium. Use the RDA as a yardstick.

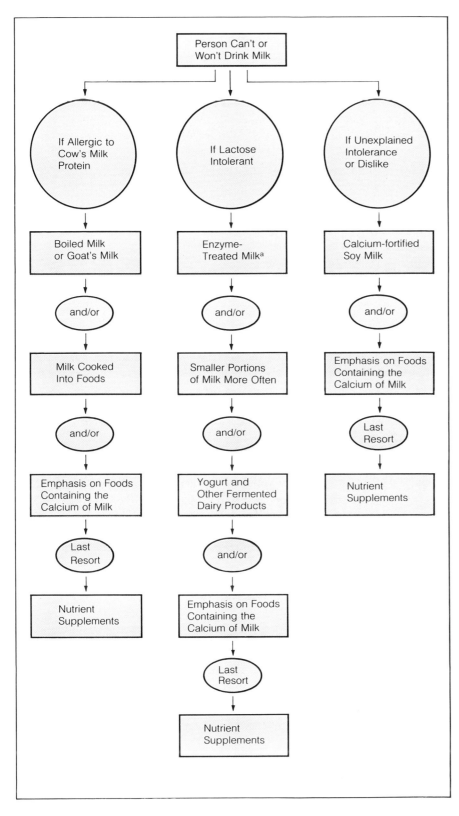

FIGURE 11–10

Choosing a milk substitute.

Source: Adapted from E. N. Whitney and C. B. Cataldo, *Understanding Normal and Clinical Nutrition* (St. Paul, Minn.: West, 1983), pp. 559–568.

[a]You can buy milk already treated or add the enzyme (LactAid) yourself. Enzyme treatment may not reduce lactose content sufficiently to relieve symptoms, and you may have to try the other alternatives.

Calcium pills only contain calcium; they do not offer the other nutrients that accompany calcium as fringe benefits in a food such as milk—thiamin, riboflavin, niacin, potassium, phosphorus, vitamin A, protein, and all the rest. There is another reason why this book urges milk, rather than supplements, as a calcium source. Calcium carbonate, an antacid, counteracts not only the absorption of calcium, but also the absorption of iron, another mineral that is likely to be deficient in people's diets. For these reasons, foods are preferred.

If supplements must be used, then here are some guidelines. Take any calcium salt recommended, being careful to read its calcium contents correctly. A 1-gram pill does not offer 1 gram of calcium; it offers 1 gram of a calcium salt, of which calcium is a part. Do not take dolomite, bone meal, or oyster shells, as their composition varies from one source to another, and some have been found to be contaminated with heavy metal poisons such as arsenic and lead. Take the supplement several times a day in divided doses rather than all at once, to improve absorption. Take it with a meal each time, and work out a system that will prompt you to take it, every time.

Phosphorus

Phosphorus is the mineral in second largest quantity in the body. About 85 percent of it is found combined with calcium in the crystals of the bones and teeth. There it occurs as calcium phosphate, one of the compounds in the crystals that give strength and rigidity to these structures.*

The concentration of phosphorus in blood plasma is less than half that of calcium: 3.5 milligrams per 100 milliliters of plasma. But as part of one of the body's major buffers (phosphoric acid and its salts), it is found in all body cells. It is a part of DNA and RNA, the genetic code material present in every cell. Thus phosphorus is necessary for all growth, because new DNA and RNA have to be made to provide the building instructions whenever new cells are formed.

Phosphorus also plays many key roles in energy transfers occurring during cellular metabolism. Many enzymes and the B vitamins become active only when a phosphate group is attached. (The B vitamins, you will recall, play major roles in energy metabolism.) ATP itself, the energy carrier of the cells, contains three phosphate groups and uses these groups to do its work (see Figure 7–3 in Chapter 7).

Some lipids contain phosphorus as part of their structure. These phospholipids help to transport other lipids in the blood; they also reside in cell membranes, where they affect transport of nutrients into and out of the cells.

Animal protein is the best source of phosphorus, because phosphorus is so abundant in the energetic cells of animals. The recommended intakes for phosphorus are the same as those for calcium: 700 to 800 milligrams per day for adults. Deficiencies are unknown.

Recommended intakes of phosphorus are the same as for calcium:
U.S. adults' RDA: 800 mg.
Canadian RNI for women: 700 mg.
men: 800 mg.

*The suffix -ate in *calcium phosphate* indicates that the phosphorus has undergone a chemical reaction with oxygen and is bonded to it.

Chlorine

The element chlorine occurs as a poisonous gas, but when it combines with sodium in salt, it is not poisonous, but is part of a life-giving compound. It occurs in salt as the negative chloride ion.

The chloride ion is the major negative ion of the fluids outside the cells, where it is found mostly in association with sodium. Chloride can move freely across membranes and so is also found inside the cells in association with potassium. Its role in balancing the pH of the blood has already been described.

In the stomach, the chloride ion is part of hydrochloric acid, which maintains the strong acidity of the stomach. The cells that line the stomach continuously expend energy to push chloride into the stomach fluid. One of the most serious consequences of vomiting is the loss of acid from the stomach, which upsets the acid-base balance.

A chlorine compound is added to public water to reduce its bacterial count before it flows through pipes into people's homes. The compound turns to the deadly poisonous gas chlorine, kills dangerous microorganisms that might otherwise spread disease, and then evaporates, leaving the water safe for human consumption. The addition of chlorine to public water is one of the most important public health measures ever introduced in the developed countries and has eliminated such waterborne diseases as typhoid fever, which once ravaged vast areas, killing thousands of people.

Chlorine is never naturally lacking in the diet. It abounds in foods as part of sodium chloride and other salts. The only way in which people can suffer a chloride deficiency is through human error; a case is on record in which chloride was mistakenly omitted from infant formula and caused widespread illness before it was discovered.

Recommended intakes of chloride:
  U.S. suggestion: 1,700 to 5,100 mg.
  Canadian RNI: 50 mg/kg.

Potassium

Potassium, as mentioned earlier, is the body's principal intracellular electrolyte, important in maintaining the fluid volume inside cells, and the acid-base balance. Cell membranes are relatively permeable to it, 100 times more so than to sodium or chloride, but as it leaks out, a highly active cell membrane pump promptly shuttles it back in, in exchange for sodium. It is important that potassium remain inside cells, for if the cells were to give up to the blood only 6 percent of the potassium they contain, it would stop the heart.[19]

During nerve transmission and muscle contraction, potassium and sodium briefly exchange places across the cell membrane. The cell then quickly pumps them back into place. This makes sodium and potassium critical in the transmission of messages along nerves and from nerves to muscles, as well as in the

The pump referred to actively exchanges sodium for potassium across the cell membrane, maintaining a strong concentration gradient of each. It uses ATP (Chapter 7) as an energy source and is known as the **sodium-potassium ATPase** (A-T-P-ase).
ase = an enzyme that splits compounds (in this case, ATP)

Assessment of potassium: serum potassium.

Recommended intakes of potassium:
   U.S. suggestion: 1,875 to 5,625 mg
   (1.9 to 5.6 g).
   Canadian RNI: 70 mg/kg.

These foods are rich in potassium per kcalorie.

response of muscles, including the heart muscle, to those messages. Potassium is also known to play a catalytic role in carbohydrate and protein metabolism, but the exact nature of this role is not known.

The relationship of potassium and sodium in maintaining the blood pressure is not entirely clear. Abundant evidence supports the simple view that the two minerals have opposite effects, but occasional experiments produce contradictory findings.[20] In any case, it is clear that increasing the potassium in the diet can promote sodium excretion under most circumstances, and thereby lower the blood pressure.[21] A lifelong intake of foods low in sodium and high in potassium protects against essential hypertension and is thought to be a major reason for the low blood pressure seen in vegetarians.[22]

High blood pressure is often treated using diuretics—drugs that act on the kidney to promote fluid excretion. The object is to lower the body's total fluid volume, including the level of fluids (and thereby the pressure) in the vascular system. Different diuretics work differently, and they have different effects on body potassium levels. Some promote water excretion directly by way of an effect on the ADH system. With these, sodium is not excreted, but potassium is, and it must be replaced; these are known as potassium-wasting diuretics. Others promote sodium excretion, and thereby water excretion indirectly, by way of an effect on the aldosterone system. As sodium exits, potassium is returned to the system, so replacement is not needed. All persons whose blood pressure is high enough to warrant diuretic use should reduce their sodium intakes to help lower their blood pressure and should follow a doctor's or dietitian's instructions regarding potassium.[23]

A deficiency of potassium from getting too little in the diet is unlikely, but high-sodium diets low in fresh fruits and vegetables can make it a possibility. Abnormal conditions such as diabetic acidosis or loss of large volumes of water can cause potassium deficiency. One of the earliest symptoms is muscle weakness.

Gradual potassium depletion might occur when a person sweats profusely day after day and fails to replenish his potassium stores. The authors of one study have recommended that a person who sweats heavily and often should eat five to eight servings of potassium-rich foods each day.[24] However, attempts to demonstrate this need have failed: even four days of heavy sweating and a low-potassium diet fail to deplete body potassium stores, as measured in plasma and muscle.[25] Furthermore, anyone who sweats heavily due to hard work or exercise presumably also eats well. Such a person, in a day, could eat 20 or 30 servings of 100 kcalories each (see Table 11–8), and many of them could easily be potassium rich.

When body potassium is depleted, its concentration in the blood and in the muscle cells falls, but its concentration in the central nervous system remains unchanged.[26] The brain and nerves have a way of protecting themselves from changes they cannot tolerate; apparently potassium is too crucial to their function to be allowed to vary. Blood and muscle potassium appear to be used as stores from which potassium can be released gradually to keep the nervous system's supply constant.[27]

Because potassium is found inside of all living cells, both plant and animal, and because cells break open when foods are processed, many of the richest sources of potassium are whole foods of all kinds—fruits, vegetables, grains, meats, fish, and poultry. Potassium is also abundant in fresh milk. Table 11–8 shows the potassium contents of foods.

TABLE 11–8

Potassium In Foods

Foods Ranked by Potassium Per Serving	Potassium Per Serving (mg)	Energy Per Serving (kCal)	Foods Ranked by Potassium Per 100 kCalories	Potassium Per Serving (mg)	Potassium Per 100 kCal (mg)
Peach halves, dried (10)	1,295	311	Bok choy cabbage, cooked (1 c)	630	3,150
Lima beans, cooked (1 c)	1,163	260	Spinach, cooked (1 c)	838	2,044
Winter squash, baked (1 c)	1,071	96	Celery, outer stalk (1)	114	1,900
Pear halves, dried (10)	932	459	Romaine lettuce, chopped (1 c)	162	1,800
Sirloin steak, lean (8 oz)	928	480	Parsley, chopped fresh (1 c)	322	1,610
Potato, microwaved w/skin (1)	903	212	Zucchini squash, cooked (1 c)	455	1,569
Pinto beans, cooked (1 c)	882	265	Red radishes (10)	104	1,486
Baked potato, whole (1)	844	220	Looseleaf lettuce (1 c)	148	1,480
Spinach, cooked (1 c)	838	41	Mushrooms, raw sliced (1 c)	260	1,444
Cantaloupe melon (½)	825	94	Cauliflower, cooked (1 c)	400	1,333
Kidney beans, canned (1 c)	673	230	Asparagus, cooked (1 c)	558	1,268
Bok choy cabbage, cooked (1 c)	630	20	Tomatoes, whole canned (1 c)	529	1,126
Prunes, dried (10)	626	201	Winter squash, baked (1 c)	1,071	1,116
Peas, dry split, cooked (1 c)	592	230	Cabbage, raw shredded (1 c)	172	1,075
Butternut squash, baked (1 c)	583	83	Tomato, whole raw (1)	255	1,063
Blackeyed peas, cooked (1 c)	573	190	Beets, cooked (1 c)	532	1,023
Watermelon (1 sl)	560	152	Summer squash, cooked (1 c)	346	961
Asparagus, cooked (1 c)	558	44	Cantaloupe melon (½)	825	878
Beets, cooked (1 c)	532	52	Green beans, cooked (1 c)	373	848
Tomatoes, whole canned (1 c)	529	47	Green peppers, whole (1)	144	800
Orange juice, fresh (1 c)	496	111	Carrot, whole fresh (1)	233	752
Apricot halves, dried (10)	482	83	Butternut squash, baked (1 c)	583	702
Zucchini squash, cooked (1 c)	455	29	Apricots, fresh pitted (3)	313	614
Banana, peeled (1)	451	105	Brewers yeast (1 tbsp)	152	608
Nonfat milk or yogurt (1 c)	406	86	Apricot halves, dried (10)	482	581
Cauliflower, cooked (1 c)	400	30	Broccoli, cooked (1 c)	254	552
Green beans, cooked (1 c)	373	44	Wheat bran (¼ c)	103	542
Whole milk (1 c)	370	150	Nonfat milk or yogurt (1 c)	406	472
Summer squash, cooked (1 c)	346	36·	Peach, fresh medium (1)	171	462
Parsley, chopped fresh (1 c)	322	20	Orange juice, fresh (1 c)	496	447
Apricots, fresh pitted (3)	313	51	Lima beans, cooked (1 c)	1,163	447
Sole/flounder, baked (3 oz)	272	120	Banana, peeled (1)	451	430
Mushrooms, raw sliced (1 c)	260	18	Potato, microwaved w/skin (1)	903	426
Tomato, whole raw (1)	255	24	Peach halves, dried (10)	1,295	416
Broccoli, cooked (1 c)	254	46	Orange, fresh medium (1)	237	395
Orange, fresh medium (1)	237	60	Baked potato, whole (1)	844	384
Carrot, whole fresh (1)	233	31	Watermelon (1 sl)	560	368
Chicken breast, roasted (½)	220	142	Pinto beans, cooked (1 c)	882	333
Peanuts, dried unsalted (1 oz)	204	161	Prunes, dried (10)	626	311
Cabbage, raw shredded (1 c)	172	16	Blackeyed peas, cooked (1 c)	573	302
Peach, fresh medium (1)	171	37	Kidney beans, canned (1 c)	673	293
Romaine lettuce, chopped (1 c)	162	9	Peas, dry split, cooked (1 c)	592	257
Apple, fresh medium (1)	159	80	Whole milk (1 c)	370	247
Brewers yeast (1 tbsp)	152	25	Sole/flounder, baked (3 oz)	272	227
Looseleaf lettuce (1 c)	148	10	Pear halves, dried (10)	932	203
Green peppers, whole (1)	144	18	Apple, fresh medium (1)	159	199
Celery, outer stalk (1)	114	6	Sirloin steak, lean (8 oz)	928	193
Red radishes (10)	104	7	Chicken breast, roasted (½)	220	155
Wheat bran (¼ c)	103	19	Peanuts, dried unsalted (1 oz)	204	127
Whole wheat bread (1 sl)	50	70	Whole wheat bread (1 sl)	50	71
Cheddar cheese (1 oz)	28	114	Cheddar cheese (1 oz)	17	25

If you say "potassium" to the average Joe and Jane on the street, they will say back to you "bananas." Everyone knows that bananas contain potassium. But Table 11–8 shows that their potassium content is not notable compared with that of other foods, either on a per-kcalorie or on a per-serving basis. Why did bananas get such a reputation for being high in potassium? Many other fruits have comparable or greater potassium contents, and vegetables have more potassium still, especially on a per-kcalorie basis. People who have just run a marathon tend to think they must run home and eat bananas afterward, but perhaps they should run home and eat potatoes instead.

It is hardly ever necessary to take potassium supplements, even with diuretic use, because food sources are so rich in potassium. Among healthy people, only two groups risk depletion. One group is people who eat diets composed of heavily processed, heavily salted foods. Those people might fail to get enough potassium, but of course, rather than take supplements, they need to change their eating habits. Their nutritional health would be bound to benefit in many other ways. The other group is people who ingest fewer than 800 kcalories a day—for example, people on semifasts to lose weight. A physician must monitor the potassium status of these people and order supplements commensurate with the degree of depletion.[28]

Potassium toxicity is a greater concern than potassium deficiency. The body protects itself from this eventuality as best it can. If you consume more than you need, the kidneys accelerate their excretion and so maintain control. Should their limit be exceeded (if you ingest too much potassium too fast), a vomiting reflex is triggered. However, if the GI tract is bypassed, and potassium is injected into a vein at a high rate, it can stop the heart.

Body-builders might take note that fruit, because of the potassium it contains, may do more for their muscles than meat.

Sulfur

Sulfur is present in all proteins and plays its most important role in determining the contour of protein molecules. Sulfur helps the strands of protein to assume a particular shape and hold it—and so to do their specific jobs, such as enzyme work. Some of the amino acids contain sulfur in their side chains, and once built into a protein strand, one of these amino acids can link to another by way of sulfur-sulfur bridges. The bridges stabilize the protein structure. Skin, hair, and nails contain some of the body's more rigid proteins, and these have a high sulfur content.

There is no recommended intake for sulfur, and no deficiencies are known. Only if a person lacks protein to the point of severe deficiency will she lack the sulfur-containing amino acids.

Amino acids containing sulfur are methionine and cysteine. Cysteine in one part of a protein chain can bind to cysteine in another part of the chain by way of a sulfur-sulfur bridge (see p. 137). Two cysteine molecules linked this way are called cystine (see Appendix C).

Magnesium

Magnesium barely qualifies as a major mineral. Only about 1 ¾ ounces of magnesium are present in the body of a 130-pound person, most of it in the bones. Bone magnesium seems to be a reservoir to ensure that some will be on hand for vital reactions regardless of recent dietary intake. The kidney acts to conserve magnesium; the magnesium not absorbed is excreted in the feces.

Magnesium also acts in all the cells of the soft tissues, where it forms part of the protein-making machinery, and where it is necessary for the release of energy. A major role seems to be as a catalyst in the reaction that adds the last high-energy phosphate bond to ATP. Magnesium also helps relax muscles after contraction and promotes resistance to tooth decay by holding calcium in tooth enamel.

Assessment of magnesium: serum magnesium.

A dietary deficiency of magnesium does not seem likely, but deficiency may occur as a result of vomiting, diarrhea, alcohol abuse, or protein malnutrition; in postsurgical clients who have been fed incomplete fluids into a vein for too long; or in people using diuretics. A severe deficiency causes tetany, an extreme and prolonged contraction of the muscles very much like the reaction of the muscles when calcium levels fall. Magnesium deficit is also thought to cause the hallucinations experienced by people withdrawing from alcohol overdoses.

Recommended intakes of magnesium:
U.S. men's RDA: 350 mg.
women's RDA: 300 mg.
Canadian RNI: 3.4 mg/kg body weight per day.
or for men: 230 to 250 mg.
women: 200 to 220 mg.

Food sources are shown in Table 11−9. Like all the other nutrients discussed so far, magnesium has its own pattern of distribution in foods when they are considered on a per-serving basis, but on a per-kcalorie basis, vegetables are the best source.

TABLE 11–9

Magnesium In Foods

Foods Ranked by Magnesium Per Serving	Magnesium Per Serving (mg)	Energy Per Serving (kCal)	Foods Ranked by Magnesium Per 100 kCalories	Magnesium Per Serving (mg)	Magnesium Per 100 kCal (mg)
Spinach, cooked (1 c)	157	41	Spinach, cooked (1 c)	157	383
Tofu soybean curd (1 block)	133	86	Seaweed, kelp, raw (1 oz)	34	283
Sesame seeds, dry (¼ c)	130	221	Beet greens, cooked (1 c)	97	243
Sunflower seeds, dry (¼ c)	128	205	Wheat bran (¼ c)	46	242
Blackeyed peas, cooked (1 c)	117	190	Broccoli, cooked (1 c)	94	204
Garbanzo beans, cooked (1 c)	115	270	Tofu soybean curd (1 block)	133	155
Shrimp, boiled (3.5 oz)	110	109	Zucchini squash, cooked (1 c)	40	138
Beet greens, cooked (1 c)	97	40	Parsley, chopped fresh (1 c)	26	130
Broccoli, cooked (1 c)	94	46	Summer squash, cooked (1 c)	44	122
Navy beans, cooked dry (1 c)	89	225	Beets, cooked (1 c)	62	119
Lima beans, cooked (1 c)	79	260	Turnip greens, cooked (1 c)	32	110
Kidney beans, canned (1 c)	75	230	Shrimp, boiled (3.5 oz)	110	101
Cashew nuts, roasted (1 oz)	74	163	Mustard greens, cooked (1 c)	21	100
Sirloin steak, lean (8 oz)	67	480	Wheat germ, raw (¼ c)	63	93
Wheat germ, raw (¼ c)	63	68	Bok choy cabbage, cooked (1 c)	18	90
Beets, cooked (1 c)	62	52	Celery, outer stalk (1)	5	83
Figs, dried (5)	56	239	Asparagus, cooked (1 c)	34	77
Baked potato, whole (1)	55	220	Popcorn, air popped (1 c)	23	77
Peach halves, dried (10)	54	311	Green beans, cooked (1 c)	32	73
Oysters, raw (1 c)	54	160	Brewers yeast (1 tbsp)	18	72
Peanuts, dried unsalted (1 oz)	51	161	Bean sprouts, fresh (1 c)	22	69
Wheat bran (¼ c)	46	19	Cabbage, raw shredded (1 c)	10	63
Summer squash, cooked (1 c)	44	36	Sunflower seeds, dry (¼ c)	128	62
Zucchini squash, cooked (1 c)	40	29	Blackeyed peas, cooked (1 c)	117	62
Asparagus, cooked (1 c)	34	44	Looseleaf lettuce (1 c)	6	60
Seaweed, kelp, raw (1 oz)	34	12	Sesame seeds, dry (¼ c)	130	59
Whole milk (1 c)	33	150	Tomato, whole raw (1)	14	58
Turnip greens, cooked (1 c)	32	29	Green peppers, whole (1)	10	56
Green beans, cooked (1 c)	32	44	Clams, raw meat only (3 oz)	31	48
Clams, raw meat only (3 oz)	31	65	Popcorn, oil salted (1 c)	25	45
Nonfat milk or yogurt (1 c)	28	86	Cashew nuts, roasted (1 oz)	74	45
Whole wheat bread (1 sl)	26	70	Mushroom pieces, cooked (1 c)	18	43
Parsley, chopped fresh (1 c)	26	20	Garbanzo beans, cooked (1 c)	115	43
Popcorn, oil salted (1 c)	25	55	Navy beans, cooked dry (1 c)	89	40
Chicken breast, roasted (½)	25	142	Whole wheat bread (1 sl)	26	37
Popcorn, air popped (1 c)	23	30	Oysters, raw (1 c)	54	34
Bean sprouts, fresh (1 c)	22	32	Kidney beans, canned (1 c)	75	33
Mustard greens, cooked (1 c)	21	21	Nonfat milk or yogurt (1 c)	28	33
Sole/flounder, baked (3 oz)	19	120	Peanuts, dried unsalted (1 oz)	51	32
Cantaloupe melon (½)	19	94	Lima beans, cooked (1 c)	79	30
Brewers yeast (1 tbsp)	18	25	Baked potato, whole (1)	55	25
Bok choy cabbage, cooked (1 c)	18	20	Figs, dried (5)	56	23
Mushroom pieces, cooked (1 c)	18	42	Whole milk (1 c)	33	22
Tomato, whole raw (1)	14	24	Orange, fresh medium (1)	13	22
Orange, fresh medium (1)	13	60	Cantaloupe melon (½)	19	20
Green peppers, whole (1)	10	18	Chicken breast, roasted (½)	25	18
Cabbage, raw shredded (1 c)	10	16	Peach halves, dried (10)	54	17
Cheddar cheese (1 oz)	8	114	Sole/flounder, baked (3 oz)	19	16
Looseleaf lettuce (1 c)	6	10	Sirloin steak, lean (8 oz)	67	14
Apple, fresh medium (1)	6	80	Apple, fresh medium (1)	6	8
Celery, outer stalk (1)	5	6	Cheddar cheese (1 oz)	8	7

Study Questions

1. List three properties of water that make it physiologically important. By what routes is water lost from the body?
2. Name the organs, hormones, and major minerals responsible for regulating the constancy of body salts and water balance.
3. What is the major function of sodium in the body? Describe the role of the kidney in regulating blood sodium.
4. Discuss the dietary factors that may affect blood pressure and describe the lifestyle changes recommended for reducing it.
5. List the roles of calcium in the body. How does the body maintain a constant blood level of calcium regardless of dietary intake?
6. When would a calcium supplement be recommended? How would you go about choosing one?
7. List the roles of phosphorus in the body. Discuss the relationships between calcium and phosphorus.
8. State the major functions of chlorine, potassium, magnesium, and sulfur in the body. Are deficiencies of these nutrients likely to occur in your own diet? Why?

Notes

1. A. S. Truswell, Diet and hypertension, *British Medical Journal* 291 (1985): 125–127.
2. Institute of Food Technologists' Expert Panel on Food Safety and Nutrition, Dietary salt, *Food Technology,* January 1980, pp. 85–91.
3. Joint National Committee on Detection, Evaluation, and Treatment of High Blood Pressure, *1980 Report,* NIH publication no. 81–1088 (Washington, D.C.: Government Printing Office, 1980).
4. Institute, 1980; A. M. Altschul and J. K. Grommet, Sodium intake and sodium sensitivity, *Nutrition Reviews* 38 (1980): 393–402.
5. G. Kolata, Value of low-sodium diets questioned (Research News), *Science* 216 (1982): 38–39.
6. D. A. McCarron, Low serum concentrations of ionized calcium in patients with hypertension, *New England Journal of Medicine* 307 (1982): 226–228; D. A. McCarron and coauthors, Blood pressure and nutrient intake in the United States, *Science* 224 (1984): 1392–1398.
7. S. J. Kopp and coauthors, Cardiovascular actions of cadmium at environmental exposure levels, *Science* 217 (1982): 837–839; R. Masironi and A. G. Shaper, Epidemiological studies of health effects of water from different sources, *Annual Review of Nutrition* 1 (1981): 375–400.
8. L. Newman, More "salt" talks: Diet and hypertension (medical news), *Journal of the American Medical Association* 248 (1982): 2949–2951; Truswell, 1985.
9. N. M. Kaplan, Non-drug treatment of hypertension, *Annals of Internal Medicine* 102 (1985): 359–373.
10. M. Biertino, G. K. Beauchamp, and K. Engelman, Long-term reduction in dietary sodium alters the taste of salt, *American Journal of Clinical Nutrition* 36 (1982): 1134–1144.
11. H. Rasmussen, Cellular calcium metabolism, *Annals of Internal Medicine* 98 (1983): 809–816.
12. L. H. Allen, Calcium bioavailability and absorption: A review, *American Journal of Clinical Nutrition* 35 (1982): 783–808.
13. Oxalate content of common foods, *Nutrition and the MD,* September 1979.
14. Allen, 1982.
15. Allen, 1982.
16. N. W. Solomons, An update on lactose intolerance, *Nutrition News,* February 1986.
17. Solomons, 1986.
18. R. R. Recker, Calcium absorption and achlorhydria, *New England Journal of Medicine* 313 (1985): 70–73.
19. M. J. Fregly, Sodium and potassium, Chapter 31 in *Present Knowledge in Nutrition,* 5th ed. (New York: Nutrition Foundation, 1984), pp. 439–458.
20. Dietary potassium and hypertension, *Lancet,* 8 June 1985, pp. 1308–1309.
21. A. W. Voors and coauthors, Relation between ingested potassium and sodium balance in young blacks and whites, *American Journal of Clinical Nutrition* 37 (1983): 583–594.
22. O. Ophir and coauthors, Low blood pressure in vegetarians: The possible role of potassium, *American Journal of Clinical Nutrition* 37 (1983): 755–762.
23. J. A. Wilber, The role of diet in the treatment of high blood pressure, *Journal of the American Dietetic Association* 80 (1982): 25–29.
24. H. W. Lane and J. J. Cerda, Potassium requirements and exercise, *Journal of the American Dietetic Association* 73 (1978): 64–65.
25. D. L. Costill, R. Cote, and W. J. Fink, Dietary potassium and heavy exercise: Effects on muscle water and electrolytes, *American Journal of Clinical Nutrition* 36 (1982): 266–271.
26. N. Akaike, Sodium pump in skeletal muscle: Central nervous system–induced suppression by alpha-adrenoreceptors, *Science* 213 (1981): 1252–1254.
27. Fregly, 1984.
28. P. G. Lindner, Caution: All potassium supplements are not the same! *Obesity and Bariatric Medicine* 10 (1981): 87, 89, 92.

These exercises make use of the information you recorded on Form 2 in Appendix K.

1. Look up and record your recommended intake of calcium. Also record your actual intake, from the average derived on Form 2 (Self-Study 1). What percentage of your recommended intake did you consume? Was this enough? What foods contribute the greatest amount of calcium to your diet? If you consumed more than the recommendation, was this too much? Why or why not? In what ways would you change your diet to improve it in this respect?

2. To estimate sodium intake, it is necessary either to add no salt at the table or to measure the amount you do add. The easiest way to measure salt used is to weigh the salt shaker on a gram balance at the start of the day, use only that salt shaker all day and only for yourself, and weigh it again at the end of the day. The number of grams of salt used, times .40, is the number of grams of sodium used.

SELF-STUDY

Evaluate Your Intakes of Major Minerals

Estimate your sodium intake by totaling the sodium in the foods you consumed with that added at the table. Be careful to note whether the foods were home-prepared, with or without added salt, or whether they were pre-prepared. Read labels if you use processed foods. Be aware that sodium contents of foods are more difficult to estimate, because they are more variable, than other nutrient contents of foods.

Now compare your estimated intake with recommendations described in the chapter—not more than 5 grams (5,000 milligrams) of added salt per day. This means 2 grams (2,000 milligrams) of sodium in the added salt. (By "added salt," we mean salt added in processing or by you in cooking or at the table. It is assumed that foods you eat already contain about 3 grams of naturally occurring salt. So in comparing with recommendations, count only the sodium you find in processed foods and in the salt shaker.) If your typical intake is below this amount, congratulations. If it is not, evaluate the significance to you by taking the Heart Health Quiz presented in Highlight 4B. What was your score on that quiz? Based on the score, will it be important for you to reduce your sodium intakes? If so, how can you realistically do so?

3. Calculate your intakes of magnesium and potassium and compare them with the recommended intakes. If you need to improve your diet with respect to these minerals, how will you go about doing so?

The Trace Minerals

12

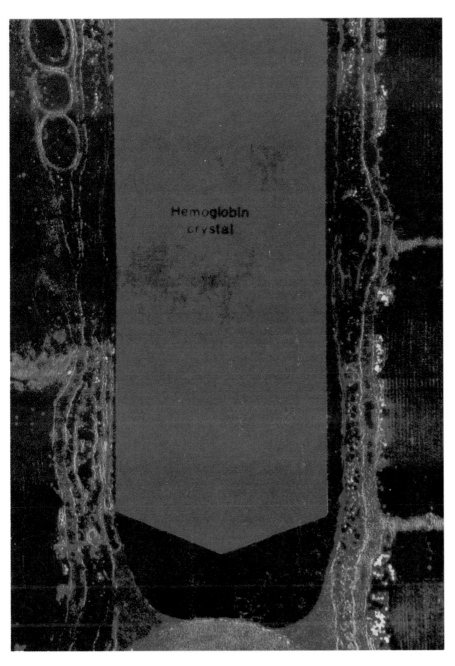

Contents

The red pigment of the blood cells is the protein hemoglobin, which contains iron. Hemoglobin is normally dispersed in the cell fluid, but here, due to an accident in preparation in the laboratory, the hemoglobin has crystallized, showing how abundant it is in the red blood cell. The cell is flanked by the walls of the capillary.

The trace elements (minerals):

- Iron
- Zinc   } RDA nutrients
- Iodine

- Copper
- Manganese
- Fluoride   } Safe and adequate
- Chromium   } doses established
- Selenium
- Molybdenum

- Nickel
- Silicon
- Tin   } Known essential;
- Cobalt   } under study
- Arsenic

At the start of the last chapter, Figure 11−1 showed how tiny are the quantities of trace minerals in the human body. If you could remove them all, you would have only a bit of dust, hardly enough to fill a teaspoon. Yet each of the trace minerals performs some vital role for which no substitute will do. A deficiency of any of them may be fatal, and an excess of many is equally deadly. Remarkably, the way you eat and the way your body handles what you eat normally supplies you with just enough of these minerals to maintain your health.

The contributions of the best-known trace elements—iron, zinc, and iodine—to human nutrition have been thoroughly studied, and the Committee on RDA has established recommended daily allowances for them. For six others, the Committee on RDA published tentative ranges for safe and adequate daily intakes for the first time in 1980. Still others are known to be essential nutrients, but the amounts needed are so tiny that they have not yet been measured. Many others are presently under study to determine whether they too perform indispensable roles in the body.

Iron

Iron is vital to cellular respiration—the processes by which cells generate energy. Every human cell, and in fact every living cell of every kind, contains iron. It is not rare in nature—but it has many hurdles to jump before assuming its duties in the body, and oftentimes, people simply don't maintain sufficient stores to support their health optimally. In fact, iron is a problem nutrient for millions of people, rich and poor, old and young, male and female, at home and abroad.

Iron's two ionic states:

Ferrous iron (reduced): Fe^{++}.
Ferric iron (oxidized): Fe^{+++}.

For details about these ions, oxidation, and reduction, see Appendix B.

The iron-containing proteins at the end of the metabolic pathway include several TCA cycle enzymes and the electron carriers of the electron transport system—known as **cytochromes.** See Appendix C for these pathways.

hemoglobin: the oxygen-carrying protein of the red blood cells.
hemo = blood
globin = globular protein

myoglobin: the oxygen-carrying protein of the muscle cells.
myo = muscle

Iron in the Body

Iron has the knack of switching back and forth between two ionic states. In the reduced state, it carries two positive charges and is known as ferrous iron. In the oxidized state, it carries three positive charges and is known as ferric iron. Thanks to this versatility, it is the ideal mineral to work with proteins involved in oxidation-reduction reactions. Iron is therefore found in several of the proteins at the end of the energy metabolic pathways, where the hydrogens from energy nutrients are finally donated to oxygen.

Iron is also found in many enzymes that oxidize compounds, reactions so widespread in metabolism that they seem to occur everywhere. Iron is thus required for the making of new cells, of amino acids, of hormones, and of neurotransmitters. It is also involved in carrying oxygen from place to place, as part of the protein hemoglobin; and for holding oxygen ready for use in muscle energy metabolism, as part of the protein myoglobin.

Most of the iron in the body is part of hemoglobin. Smaller amounts occur in myoglobin, in other iron-containing proteins, and in the body's stores. Hemoglobin is the oxygen carrier in the red blood cells, and myoglobin is the oxygen-

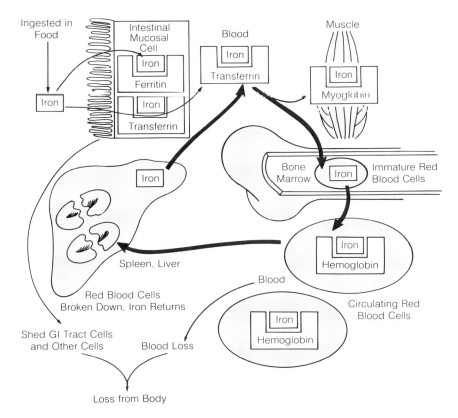

FIGURE 12–1

Iron routes in the body Most iron is recycled. Some is lost with body tissues and must be replaced by eating iron-containing food.

Source: Adapted from L. Hallberg, Iron absorption and iron deficiency, *Human Nutrition: Clinical Nutrition* 36C (1982): 259–278.

Model of hemoglobin. The hundred-odd stacked planes represent the contours of the coiled protein chains. The flat disks represent their heme portions (see later in this chapter), to which oxygen binds.

The two proteins in the mucosal cells are (1) **mucosal transferrin** (trans-FERR-in), which passes the iron on to **blood transferrin,** and (2) **mucosal ferritin** (FERR-ih-tin), which holds it in the cell.

holding reservoir in the muscle cells.* Oxygen keeps the energy-yielding pathway open so that the muscles can remain active. As the muscles use up and expel their oxygen (combined with carbons and hydrogens), the red blood cells shuttle between muscles and lungs to maintain fresh supplies.

Iron clearly is the body's gold, a precious mineral to hoard and guard closely. The number of special provisions for its handling, depicted in Figure 12–1, show how vital it is. To obtain iron, the body provides special proteins in the intestinal mucosal cells to help absorb it from food. Two proteins accomplish this. One transfers it to a carrier in the blood for transport; the other holds some iron in reserve in the mucosal cell. If that iron is needed, it is released into the body; if it is not needed, it is shed from the body in the feces when the cell is shed. Intestinal mucosal cells are born, live, and die over about a three-week period, so this reserve provides a buffer against short-term changes in iron need or supply.

Iron absorbed through the intestinal cells from food is captured by the blood protein transferrin, which carries it to the bone marrow and other blood-manufacturing sites. Each tissue takes up the amount of iron that it needs. The bone marrow and liver take large quantities, which they use to make new red blood cells; other tissues take less. In a pregnant woman, the placenta is avid for iron,

---

*The muscle cells use this oxygen as the receiver for used-up carbon and hydrogen atoms flowing down the glucose-to-energy pathway. These atoms combine to make carbon dioxide and water, the final waste products of metabolism.

The storage proteins are **ferritin** (FERR-ih-tin) and **hemosiderin** (heem-oh-SID-er-in).

Assessment of iron status: red blood cell count, red blood cell volume, measurements of hemoglobin, transferrin, hemoglobin precursors, and iron stores.

Technically, the method of measuring blood transferrin and the iron bound to it is known as measuring the **total iron-binding capacity (TIBC)** and the **transferrin saturation.** The hemoglobin precursor is **erythrocyte protoporphyrin.** The direct test of stores is **leukocyte ferritin.**
erythro = red
proto = precursor
porphyrin = the heme structure
leuco = white

delivering large quantities to the fetus even if this means depriving the mother's tissues of iron. Should there be a surplus, special storage proteins in the bone marrow and other organs store it.

The average red blood cell lives about four months. When it has aged and is no longer useful, it is removed from the blood by the spleen and liver cells, which take it apart and prepare many of the degradation products for excretion. The liver saves its iron, however, and attaches it to the blood carrier transferrin, which transports it back to the bone marrow. There, it is reused to make new red blood cells. Thus, although red blood cells are born, live, and die within a four-month cycle, the iron in the body is recycled through each new generation. Only tiny amounts of iron are lost, principally in urine, sweat, shed skin, and (if bleeding occurs), in blood.

Normally only about 10 percent of dietary iron is absorbed. But if the body's supply is diminished or if the need increases for any reason, absorption increases. More mucosal and blood transferrin is produced so as to pick up more iron from the intestines, and absorb more into the body.

The Iron Requirement and Iron Deficiency

About 80 percent of the iron in the body is in the blood, so iron losses are greatest whenever blood is lost. For this reason, women need more iron, as a well-known television commercial proclaims. Menstruation incurs losses that make a woman's iron needs twice as great as a man's, but anyone who loses blood loses iron.

If absorption cannot compensate for a reduced supply and stores are used up, the red cells become depleted of their hemoglobin. Then iron-deficiency anemia sets in. The most common tests for iron deficiency are measures of the number and size of the red blood cells and of their hemoglobin contents. But before these levels fall, at the very beginning of an iron deficiency, the transferrin concentration *rises*. A sensitive test that will detect a developing iron deficiency

Women need more iron.

Women in general are said to need more iron, yet many women find, when they have their blood cell count or hemoglobin level checked, that it is normal. Does this mean that they don't need more iron? Not necessarily. The difference between women and men is a difference in the body stores of iron, which doesn't show up in these tests. Most men eat more food than women do, because they are bigger, and so their iron intakes are higher. Besides, women menstruate, and so their iron losses are greater. These two factors—lower intakes and higher losses—may put women much closer to the borderline of deficiency. Even though a woman may never have been diagnosed as iron deficient, she is likely to be deficiency-prone. Should she lose blood for any reason (even by giving a blood donation) or become pregnant (so that her blood volume would need to increase), she would need to pay special attention to her diet in an effort to maintain her iron stores. The information about iron in foods, which appears later in this chapter, is especially important for women.

before it is full-blown measures the amount of transferrin in the blood and the amount of iron it is carrying. Simultaneously, the concentration of a hemoglobin precursor rises, because without iron, it can't be converted into hemoglobin. This precursor can be measured in the red blood cells. The determination of the blood cells' ferritin levels is also a sensitive measure of developing iron deficiency, because their ferritin contents parallel those of other body cells.

About 20 percent of all women in the United States and Canada, and 3 percent of men, have no iron in their body stores; some 8 percent of women and 1 percent of men have the outward symptoms of anemia. If iron stores are exhausted, the body cannot make enough hemoglobin to fill its new red blood cells. Without enough hemoglobin, the cells are small. Since hemoglobin is the bright red pigment of the blood, the skin of a fair person who is anemic may become noticeably pale. A sample of iron-deficient blood examined under the microscope shows smaller cells that are a lighter red than normal (Figure 12–2). The undersized cells can't carry enough oxygen from the lungs to the tissues, so energy release in the cells is hindered. Every cell of the body feels this effect; the result is fatigue, weakness, headaches, and apathy. Table 12–1 lists these and other iron-deficiency symptoms.

Long before the mass of the red blood cells is affected, however, a developing iron deficiency may affect behavior. Even at slightly lowered iron levels, the complete oxidation of pyruvate is impaired, reducing physical work capacity

In dark-skinned person, this symptom can be observed by looking in the corner of the eye. The eye lining, normally pink, will be very pale, even white.

Iron-deficiency anemia is a **microcytic** (my-cro-SIT-ic) **hypochromic** (high-po-KROME-ic) **anemia.**
micro = small
cytic = cells
hypo = too little
chrom = color

FIGURE 12–2

Normal and anemic cells.

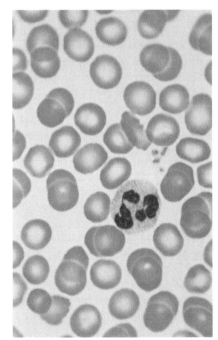

Normal blood cells. Both size and color are normal. The one large, purple cell is a normal "white" blood cell, stained purple.

Blood cells in iron-deficiency anemia (microcytic, hypochromic). The cells are small and pale because they contain less hemoglobin.

Blood cells in pernicious anemia (megaloblastic). The large cells are red blood cells, arrested at an immature stage of development. When they mature, they lose their nuclei.

TABLE 12–1

Iron Deficiency

Effects on muscular work:

- Reduced work productivity
- Reduced tolerance to work
- Reduced voluntary work

Reduced physical fitness; weakness, fatigue

Reduced resistance to cold, inability to regulate body temperature

Reduced resistance to infection (lowered immunity)

Itching of skin

Pale nailbeds, eye membranes, palm creases; concave nails

Pica (clay eating, ice eating)

Lactose intolerance, and possibly intolerance to other sugars

Impaired wound healing

Increased risk of lead and cadmium poisoning

Impaired cognitive function (children):

- Reduced learning ability
- Impaired visual discrimination
- Increased distractibility (inability to pay attention)

Impaired reactivity and coordination (infants)

Source: Adapted from L. Hallberg, Iron absorption and iron deficiency, *Human Nutrition: Clinical Nutrition* 36C (1982): 259–278; N. S. Scrimshaw, Functional consequences of iron deficiency in human populations, *Journal of Nutrition Science and Vitaminology* 30 (1984): 47–63.

There's more on the effects of iron deficiency on children's behavior in Highlight 14.

pica (PIE-ka): a craving for nonfood substances. Also known as **geophagia** (gee-oh-FAY-gee-uh) when referring to clay eating and **pagophagia** (pag-oh-FAY-gee-uh) when referring to ice craving.
picus = woodpecker or magpie
geo = earth
phagein = to eat
pago = frost

and productivity. Children deprived of iron become irritable and restless, due to abnormal levels of the stress hormones in their systems. These symptoms are among the first to appear when the body's iron level begins to fall and among the first to disappear when iron intake is increased again.[1]

A curious symptom seen in some iron-deficient subjects is an appetite for ice, clay, paste, and other unusual substances that do not contain iron and so do not remedy the deficiency. Such people have been known to eat as many as eight trays of ice in a day, for example. This behavior has been observed for years, especially in women and children of low-income groups who are deficient in either iron or zinc, and it has been given the name *pica*. When caused by iron deficiency, pica clears up dramatically within days after iron is given, even if anemia is present and the red blood cells haven't yet responded.

It is difficult to convey the extent and severity of iron deficiency among the world's people. The incidence of full-blown anemia can be stated, but people begin to feel the impact of iron deficiency, without knowing it, long before anemia is diagnosed. Iron deficiency occurs in as many as *half* of all persons in some settings, even in developed countries—most predictably in inner-city and rural poor. With reduced energy available to work, plan, think, play, sing, or learn, people simply do these things less. They don't appear to have an obvious deficiency disease; they just appear unmotivated and apathetic. Because they work and play less, they are less physically fit. The incidence in developed countries of iron-deficiency anemia ranges from 10 to 20 percent. It is higher in the developing countries; therefore the incidence of iron deficiency not severe

Many of the symptoms associated with iron deficiency are easily mistaken for "mental" symptoms. A restless child who fails to pay attention in class might be thought contrary. An apathetic homemaker who has let her housework pile up might be thought lazy. But the possibility is real that both these persons' problems are nutritional.

No responsible nutritionist would ever claim that all mental problems are caused by nutrient deficiencies. But poor nutrition is always a possible cause or contributor to problems like these. When you are seeking the solution to a behavioral problem, it makes sense to check the adequacy of the diet and to have a routine physical examination before undertaking more expensive and involved diagnostic and treatment options.

enough to cause anemia must be higher still.[2] If this one worldwide malnutrition problem could be alleviated, the whole world's morale would improve. True, it is only one of many problems, but it is a major one.

The cause of iron deficiency is usually nutrition—that is, inadequate intake, from ignorance of what foods to choose, sheer lack of food altogether, or from high consumption of the wrong foods. In the Western world, high sugar and fat intakes are often responsible for low iron intakes. Among nonnutritional causes, blood loss is the primary one, caused in many countries by parasitic infections of the GI tract. In some countries, people go through their entire lives losing blood daily and do not know what it is like to feel energetic.

It is conventional to measure the body's iron status by measuring the amount of hemoglobin (in grams per 100 milliliters of blood). The normal level is considered 14 to 15 grams per 100 milliliters for adult men, 13 to 14 for women. Yet many people who have values lower than this have no obvious symptoms; apparently the hemoglobin level at which symptoms of deficiency begin to make themselves felt is an individual matter.

When hemoglobin begins to fall, it is a sign that a long period of depletion of body stores has already occurred. In view of this fact, and in light of the debilitating effects of iron deficiency, it seems reasonable to try to achieve and maintain normal hemoglobin levels, as defined here, for the general population.

Hemoglobin norms for adults:
Men: 14–15 g/100 ml.
Women: 13–14 g/100 ml.

Norms for children:
Ages 2 to 5: 11 g/100 ml.
Ages 6 to 12: 11.5 g/100 ml.

Note that hemoglobin is measured in grams per 100 ml, but we often just use the number alone in speaking of it: "Hemoglobin, 14."

Another standard measure of iron status is the **hematocrit** (he-MAT-oh-crit) a measure of the volume of the red blood cells in a given volume of blood obtained by spinning them in a tube so that they settle to the bottom and then measuring the height of the packed mass.

iron overload: toxicity from iron overdose.

Iron Overload

The body absorbs less iron if its stores are full, but iron toxicity can occur; it is rare, but not unknown. Two kinds of iron overload are known. One is caused by a hereditary defect, the other by the ingestion of too much iron.* Tissue damage, especially to the liver, occurs in both, and infections are likely, because bacteria thrive on iron-rich blood. Effects are most severe in those who also drink large quantities of alcohol, because alcohol not only damages the liver, but also damages the intestine, breaking down its defenses against the absorption

---

Hemochromatosis (heem-oh-crome-a-TOCE-iss) is a hereditary defect in iron metabolism characterized by deposits of iron-containing pigment in many tissues, with tissue damage. *Hemosiderosis* (heem-oh-sid-er-OH-sis) is iron overload characterized by excessive iron deposits in hemosiderin, the normal iron-storage protein.

Iron tablets should be kept out of the reach of children.

Recommended intakes of iron:
U.S. adults' RDA:
- for women during childbearing years:
  18 mg.
- for women after menopause: 10 mg.
  for men: 10 mg.

Canadian RNI:
- for women during childbearing years:
  14 mg.
- for women after menopause: 7 mg.
- for men: 8 mg.

How the recommended daily intake for iron is calculated (for example, for an adolescent girl):
- Losses from urine and shed skin:
  0.5 to 1.0 mg.
- Losses through menstruation (about 15 mg total averaged over 30 days): 0.5 mg.
- Net for growth: 0.5 mg.
- Average daily need (total): 1.5 to 2.0 mg.

Only 10% of ingested iron is absorbed, so this girl must ingest 15 to 20 mg per day. The RDA is therefore set at 18 mg.

About 10% of all women need more than 22 mg of iron a day, 30 days a month, to balance menstrual losses. Other alterations of need: oral contraceptives reduce it by 50%; intrauterine devices (IUDs) increase it by 50%—both by way of effects on menstrual flow.

of excess iron. Certain wines (especially red wines) contain substantial amounts of iron, as well as sugars that enhance iron absorption; so the overconsumption of wine is particularly risky.

Iron overload is more common in men than in women. An argument against the fortification of foods with iron to protect women is that it might put more men at risk of overload. Indeed, there is some evidence from Sweden, where foods are generously fortified with iron, that this measure has increased the incidence of iron overload in men. It is too bad that a measure meant to promote the health of one sex might put the other at risk.

The ingestion of massive amounts of iron can cause sudden death. The second most common cause (after aspirin) of accidental poisoning in small children is ingestion of iron supplements or vitamins with iron. As few as 6 to 12 tablets have caused death in a child. A child suspected of iron poisoning should be rushed to the hospital to have his stomach pumped; 30 minutes may make a crucial difference.

Iron in Foods and Its Absorption

The usual Western mixed diet provides only about 5 to 6 milligrams of iron in every 1,000 kcalories. The recommended daily intake for an adult man is 10 milligrams, and most men easily eat more than 2,000 kcalories; so a man can meet his iron needs without special effort. The recommendation for a woman, however, is 14 to 18 milligrams per day, and 10 percent of all women need 22 milligrams.[3] To get this much iron from the *average* American diet, a woman would have to eat 4,000 kcalories a day. Because women typically consume fewer than 2,000 kcalories per day, some of them understandably have trouble achieving adequate iron intakes. A woman who wants to meet her iron needs from foods must increase the iron-to-kcalorie ratio of her diet so that she will receive about double the average amount of iron—at least 10 milligrams per 1,000 kcalories. This means she must emphasize the most iron-rich foods in every food group.

Table 12–2 shows the amounts of iron in foods ranked by iron per kcalorie, and also by iron per serving. As you can see, meats, fish, and poultry are superior sources on a per-serving basis, but vegetables compare favorably with all other foods on a per-kcalorie basis.

Foods in the milk group are notoriously poor iron sources— as poor in iron as they are rich in calcium. Although these foods are an indispensable part of the diet, they should not be overemphasized. In considering the grain foods, remember that iron is one of the enrichment nutrients. Whole-grain or enriched breads and cereals—not refined, unenriched pastry products—are the best choices (see Chapter 2), and the more of them you eat, the more iron you receive. Finally, among other plant foods, the legume family, the dark greens, and some fruits are the most iron rich.

For most people—especially people whose energy outputs are limited, and most especially women during their menstrual years—it is not enough to eat high-iron foods. You also have to scheme to absorb it maximally—which necessitates learning a few facts about the body's way of receiving it.

Iron occurs in two forms in foods: as heme iron, bound into the iron-carrying proteins hemoglobin and myoglobin in meats, poultry, and fish; and as iron in other forms (nonheme iron). (Another form of iron that may occur

TABLE 12–2

Iron In Foods

Foods Ranked by Iron Per Serving	Iron Per Serving (mg)	Energy Per Serving (kCal)	Foods Ranked by Iron Per 100 kCalories	Iron Per Serving (mg)	Iron Per 100 kCal (mg)
Oysters, raw (1 c)	16.80	160	Parsley, chopped fresh (1 c)	3.72	18.60
Sirloin steak, lean (8 oz)	7.68	480	Spinach, cooked (1 c)	6.42	15.66
Spinach, cooked (1 c)	6.42	41	Oysters, raw (1 c)	16.80	10.50
Lima beans, cooked (1 c)	5.90	260	Bok choy cabbage, cooked (1 c)	1.77	8.85
Braunschweiger sausage (2 pcs)	5.32	205	Sauerkraut, canned (1 c)	3.47	7.89
Beef liver, fried (3 oz)	5.30	185	Looseleaf lettuce (1 c)	0.78	7.80
Peach halves, dried (10)	5.28	311	Beet greens, cooked (1 c)	2.74	6.85
Navy beans, cooked dry (1 c)	5.10	225	Seaweed, kelp, raw (1 oz)	0.81	6.75
Soy beans, cooked dry (1 c)	4.90	235	Brewers yeast (1 tbsp)	1.39	5.56
Hamburger patty, bun (4 oz)	4.84	445	Dandelion greens, cooked (1 c)	1.89	5.40
Kidney beans, canned (1 c)	4.60	230	Wheat bran (1/4 c)	0.98	5.16
Parsley, chopped fresh (1 c)	3.72	20	Mushrooms, raw sliced (1 c)	0.86	4.78
Sauerkraut, canned (1 c)	3.47	44	Green peas, cooked (1 c)	3.15	4.70
Peas, dry split, cooked (1 c)	3.40	230	Clams, raw meat only (3 oz)	2.60	4.00
Blackeyed peas, cooked (1 c)	3.30	190	Broccoli, cooked (1 c)	1.78	3.87
Green peas, cooked (1 c)	3.15	67	Green beans, cooked (1 c)	1.60	3.64
Beef pot roast, lean (3 oz)	3.14	232	Beef liver, fried (3 oz)	5.30	2.86
Prune juice, bottled (1 c)	3.02	181	Asparagus, cooked (1 c)	1.18	2.68
Baked potato, whole (1)	2.75	220	Braunschweiger sausage (2 pcs)	5.32	2.60
Beet greens, cooked (1 c)	2.74	40	Tofu soybean curd (1 block)	2.23	2.59
Sardines, canned (3 oz)	2.60	175	Cabbage, raw shredded (1 c)	0.40	2.50
Clams, raw meat only (3 oz)	2.60	65	Tomato, whole raw (1)	0.59	2.46
Tofu soybean curd (1 block)	2.23	86	Cauliflower, raw (1 c)	0.58	2.42
Shrimp, boiled (3.5 oz)	2.20	109	Navy beans, cooked dry (1 c)	5.10	2.27
Dandelion greens, cooked (1 c)	1.89	35	Lima beans, cooked (1 c)	5.90	2.27
Broccoli, cooked (1 c)	1.78	46	Soy beans, cooked dry (1 c)	4.90	2.09
Bok choy cabbage, cooked (1 c)	1.77	20	Shrimp, boiled (3.5 oz)	2.20	2.02
Apricot halves, dried (10)	1.65	83	Kidney beans, canned (1 c)	4.60	2.00
Green beans, cooked (1 c)	1.60	44	Apricot halves, dried (10)	1.65	1.99
Oatmeal, cooked (1 c)	1.59	145	Summer squash, cooked (1 c)	0.64	1.78
Brewers yeast (1 tbsp)	1.39	25	Blackeyed peas, cooked (1 c)	3.30	1.74
Butternut squash, baked (1 c)	1.23	83	Peach halves, dried (10)	5.28	1.70
Asparagus, cooked (1 c)	1.18	44	Prune juice, bottled (1 c)	3.02	1.67
Wheat germ, raw (1/4 c)	1.13	68	Wheat germ, raw (1/4 c)	1.13	1.66
Wheat bran (1/4 c)	0.99	19	Sirloin steak, lean (8 oz)	7.68	1.60
Whole wheat bread (1 sl)	0.96	70	Sardines, canned (3 oz)	2.60	1.49
Peanuts, dried unsalted (1 oz)	0.92	161	Peas, dry split, cooked (1 c)	3.40	1.48
Chicken breast, roasted (1/2)	0.89	142	Butternut squash, baked (1 c)	1.23	1.48
Mushrooms, raw sliced (1 c)	0.86	18	Whole wheat bread (1 sl)	0.96	1.37
Seaweed, kelp, raw (1 oz)	0.81	12	Beef pot roast, lean (3 oz)	3.14	1.36
Looseleaf lettuce (1 c)	0.78	10	Baked potato, whole (1)	2.75	1.25
Summer squash, cooked (1 c)	0.64	36	Oatmeal, cooked (1 c)	1.59	1.10
Tomato, whole raw (1)	0.59	24	Hamburger patty, bun (4 oz)	4.84	1.09
Cauliflower, raw (1 c)	0.58	24	Cheddar cheese (1 oz)	0.20	0.18
Cantaloupe melon (1/2)	0.56	94	Chicken breast, roasted (1/2)	0.89	0.63
Cabbage, raw shredded (1 c)	0.40	16	Cantaloupe melon (1/2)	0.56	0.60
Sole/flounder, baked (3 oz)	0.30	120	Peanuts, dried unsalted (1 oz)	0.92	0.57
Apple, fresh medium (1)	0.25	80	Apple, fresh medium (1)	0.25	0.31
Cheddar cheese (1 oz)	0.20	114	Sole/flounder, baked (3 oz)	0.30	0.25
Orange, fresh medium (1)	0.14	60	Orange, fresh medium (1)	0.14	0.23
Nonfat milk or yogurt (1 c)	0.10	86	Nonfat milk or yogurt (1 c)	0.10	0.12

contamination iron: iron found in foods as the result of contamination by inorganic iron salts from iron cookware, iron-containing soils, and the like.

heme (HEEM): the iron-holding part of the hemoglobin and myoglobin proteins (Appendix C shows heme's structure). About 40% of the iron in meat, fish, and poultry is bound into heme. Meat, fish, and poultry also contain a factor (**"MFP factor"**) other than heme that promotes the absorption of iron, even of the iron from other foods eaten at the same time as the meat.

Factors that enhance iron absorption:
• Vitamin C.
• Other organic acids.
• Sugars (including the sugars in wine).
• MFP factor.

Factors that reduce iron absorption:
• Phytates; fibers.
• Soy, soy protein, and soy fiber.
• Other legumes.
• Tea (tannic acid); coffee.

in foods is contamination iron—inorganic salts, which are very poorly absorbed, perhaps only 1 to 2 percent at best.) Heme iron contributes only 1 to 2 of the 10 to 20 milligrams of iron the average person consumes in a day; the majority of dietary iron is nonheme iron. Heme iron is absorbed at a relatively constant rate of about 23 percent over a wide range of meat intakes, but nonheme iron's absorption is affected by many factors. By manipulating the factors affecting nonheme iron absorption, consumers can double or triple the amount of iron their bodies actually derive from foods—an advantage for the person whose energy, and therefore iron, intakes are limited. A system of calculating the iron absorbed from a meal has been worked out by Dr. E. R. Monsen and her coworkers and reveals some of the factors worthy of attention (see box).[4]

This calculation does not predict perfectly the amounts of iron that will be absorbed from meals. One flaw is that it gives credit to vitamin C for enhancing nonheme iron absorption only up to a point. Actually, the absorption-enhancing effect of vitamin C continues to rise as the amount of vitamin C in the meal rises, up to a much higher vitamin C dose than 75 milligrams.* Still, the implications of Monsen's calculation are valid in a general way. Even small amounts of meat, fish, poultry, or vitamin C help you absorb iron. For maximum iron absorption, use one or both of these enhancing factors at every meal, and the more vitamin C-rich foods, the better.

Table 12–3 shows that profound differences in actual iron absorbed result from different combinations of foods at meals. The table also makes clear that other, unknown factors must be involved.

The comparison of breakfasts in Table 12–3 reveals the effects of different beverages on absorption. The three breakfasts contained about the same amount of iron, but the amounts absorbed varied severalfold (column 3 of the table). Tea inhibits iron absorption; coffee inhibits it somewhat less; and orange juice greatly enhances it. Even when the iron absorption is measured against the juice's extra kcalories (column 4), the contribution of juice is highly significant. That is, the kcalories orange juice adds are "worth it," since the enhancement of iron absorption is proportionately so much greater.

The comparison of lunches illustrates this theme in another way. The beef and pork-and-bean meals contributed more iron overall than did the sauerkraut-sausage meal (you have to add columns 1 and 2 to see this). Much more iron was absorbed from the sauerkraut-sausage meal, though (column 3), and this meal stacks up especially well against the others when its kcalories are counted (column 4).

The comparison of the two vegetarian meals is also instructive. Both contained exactly the same amount of iron, but only 0.13 milligrams was absorbed from one of them, while all of 0.98 milligrams was absorbed from the other—and the second was lower in kcalories. Clearly, vegetarians can get enough iron from their diets—especially with the help of vitamin C.

The four dinners contributed similar amounts of kcalories, but widely different amounts of iron. The two spaghetti meals show this especially clearly and suggest that the pizza probably could have been helped by the addition of an orange, and perhaps wine instead of beer.

*Vitamin C increases iron absorption linearly up to a vitamin C dose of 1,000 mg. J. D. Cook and E. R. Monsen, Vitamin C, the common cold, and iron absorption, *American Journal of Clinical Nutrition* 30 (1977): 235–241.

Calculation of Iron Absorbed from Meals

Three factors go into the calculation of the amount of iron absorbed from a meal: first, how much of the iron in the meal was heme and how much was nonheme iron; second, how much vitamin C was in the meal; and third, how much total meat, fish, and poultry (MFP) was consumed. (It is assumed your iron stores are moderate; otherwise, you'd have to take this into consideration, too.) Answer these six questions:

1. How much iron was from animal tissues (MFP)? _____ mg
2. Forty percent of this, on the average, is heme iron. _____ mg heme iron
3. How much iron was from other sources? _____ mg
4. This, plus 60 percent of (1), is nonheme iron. _____ mg + .60 × _____ mg = _____ mg nonheme iron
5. How much vitamin C was in the meal? Less than 25 milligrams is low; 25 to 75 milligrams is medium; more than 75 milligrams is high.
6. How much MFP was in the meal? Less than 1 ounce lean MFP is low; 1 to 3 ounces is medium; more than 3 ounces is high.*

Now calculate:

You absorbed 23 percent of the heme iron (2), or _____ mg.

Now, take your best score from (5) and (6). If either vitamin C or MFP was high or if both were medium, the availability of your nonheme iron was high. If neither was high but one was medium, the availability of your nonheme iron was medium. If both were low, your nonheme iron had poor availability. You absorbed:

High availability: 8 percent of the nonheme iron.
Medium availability: 5 percent.
Poor availability: 3 percent.
    Your total: _____ mg nonheme iron absorbed

Add the two together:

        _____ mg heme iron absorbed
        _____ mg nonheme iron absorbed
Total = _____ mg iron absorbed

The RDA assumes you will absorb 10 percent of the iron you ingest. Thus, if you are a man of any age or a woman over 50 years old (RDA 10 milligrams), you need to absorb 1 milligram per day; if you are a woman 11 to 50 years old (RDA 18 milligrams), you need to absorb 1.8 milligrams. If you have higher menstrual losses than the average woman, you may still need more.

---

*Note on #6: We have adapted the calculation of Monsen and coauthors, stating it in ounces. Her actual numbers are less than 23 grams cooked meat, low; 23 to 46 grams, medium; and 69 grams or more, high.

"Although erythrocytes occupy less than fifty percent of the volume of the blood fluid, they can absorb seventy-five times more oxygen than can possibly be dissolved in the plasma itself."
"[Hemoglobin] must be a tricky substance," said Mr. Tompkins thoughtfully.
George Gamow and Martynas Ycas,

Mr. Tompkins inside Himself

TABLE 12–3

Iron Absorption from Different Meals

Meal Composition	Iron Content		Total Iron Absorbed (mg)[a]	Iron Absorbed per 1,000 kCal (mg/1,000 kcal)[b]
	Heme Iron (mg)	Nonheme Iron (mg)		
Continental breakfast[c]				
With coffee (320 kcal)	0.0	2.8	0.16	0.50
With coffee and orange juice (390 kcal)	0.0	3.1	0.40	1.03
With tea (320 kcal)	0.0	2.8	0.07	0.22
Single lunches/dinners				
Hamburger, mashed potatoes, string beans (450 kcal)	0.5	3.0	0.50	1.11
Brown beans, pork, milk (750 kcal)	0.3	5.4	0.51	0.68
Roast beef, green beans, potatoes (480 kcal)	1.0	3.1	0.83	1.73
Sauerkraut with sausage (470 kcal)	0.6	2.0	1.05	2.23
Vegetarian I (7 mg vitamin C)				
Navy beans, rice, corn bread, apple (730 kcal)	0.0	5.8	0.13	0.18
Vegetarian II (74 mg vitamin C)				
Red kidney beans, cauliflower, white bread, cottage cheese, pineapple (620 kcal)	0.0	5.8	0.98	1.58
Complete meals				
Pizza with olives, anchovies, cheese, beer (1,040 kcal)	0.0	4.2	0.33	0.32
Hamburger, french fries, milk shake (1,030 kcal)	1.15	3.9	0.77	0.75
Spaghetti, cheese, catsup, water (1,020 kcal)	0.0	4.9	0.59	0.58
Spaghetti, meat sauce, orange, wine (1,150 kcal)	0.6	7.8	1.95	1.70

[a]Goal for the day is 1.0 mg for a man, 1.8 mg for a woman.
[b]This measure is termed the bioavailable nutrient density of the meal.
[c]Sweet rolls.
Source: Adapted from L. Hallberg, Bioavailable nutrient density: A new concept applied in the interpretation of food iron absorption data, *American Journal of Clinical Nutrition* 34 (1981): 2242–2247.

The differences in iron absorption are so great that to present a table of the iron contents of foods without putting them in this context would be misleading. (This is often the case when nutrition theory is compared with reality. The reality is more complex.) Table 12–2 permits you to select servings of foods that are high in iron, or foods that are high in iron compared with their kcalorie amounts, but the usefulness of these foods can only be fully realized if they are combined artfully into absorption-enhancing meals.

Small amounts of meat and vitamin C help you absorb the iron from other foods.

Contamination, Supplement, and Fortification Iron

Contamination iron may increase the diet's iron. In fact, in populations where an unusually high iron status is found, contamination iron from soil or cookware usually accounts for it. The knowledge that iron salts can contribute to iron intakes has led people to recommend that consumers cook their foods in iron cookware. For example, the iron content of a half cup of spaghetti sauce simmered in a glass dish is 3 milligrams, but it's 87 milligrams when the sauce is cooked in an iron skillet. Even in the short time it takes to scramble eggs, you can triple their iron content by cooking them in an iron pan. Admittedly, the absorption of this iron may be poor (depending on what else is in the meal), but every little bit helps.

Even after taking all the precautions discussed so far, a woman may not accumulate enough storage iron to prepare her for the increased demands of pregnancy and childbirth. The Committee on RDA acknowledges that pregnant women might need supplemental iron. The Canadian RNI also includes this statement. Some supplements are better absorbed than others. If similar to contamination iron, their iron is far less well absorbed than that from food, so the doses have to be as high as 50 milligrams per day. Absorption of iron from iron sulfate, or when taken as an iron chelate, is better. Absorption of iron from supplements is also improved when they are taken with meat or with vitamin C–rich foods or juices. Look for the ferrous form, too; it is better absorbed than the ferric form.

The use of enriched or fortified foods is another option. Iron added to foods is similar to contamination iron, though; it may boost apparent intakes, but its absorption may be poor. It can be so poorly absorbed, in fact, that even prolonged use of enriched foods often seems to do little or nothing to improve people's iron status. In the right food carrier, though, perhaps it can make a difference. At present, 25 percent of all the iron consumed in the United States derives from foods to which iron has been added, including the familiar enriched breads and cereals, and fortified breakfast cereals that boast that they contain 100 percent of the RDA for iron. These food sources may not be "good" in the sense that single servings convey much iron into the body, but they may be "important," because people eat so much of them that they derive significant iron from the total.

enriched, fortified foods: see Chapter 2.

A number of proposals have been made for further fortification—of milk, fish, rice, infant foods, coffee, snack foods, salt, sugar, and soy sauce. Fortification of soy sauce could improve the iron status of a third of the world's people. A proposal to increase the iron level in enriched bread above that now prescribed by FDA regulations has been defeated; that level of fortification is used in Sweden and is believed to account for that country's better iron status than the

United States'. Whatever the iron in the food supply, though, it is clearly the responsibility of consumers themselves to see that they get enough iron. Of all the strategies suggested here, the most effective, least expensive one is not to take supplements, but to eat abundant vegetables, and the accompanying nutritional benefits would be greatest.

In case any reader should be left in doubt about whether foods are a better source of iron than fortification or supplements, this discussion of iron closes with two stories—one that took place in the United States, the other in West Java. The first was a study of over 200 adults in Boston who had hemoglobin levels below 13. Two-thirds were given iron-fortified foods for 6 to 8 months; the others were given the same foods without added iron. At the end of the study, the hemoglobin levels of *all* had increased equally. Foods of the right kinds made the difference, with or without added iron.[5]

The study in West Java involved rubber plantation workers with iron-deficiency anemia. The more anemic they were, the less work they could do, and the more often they got sick with infections. Half were given an iron supplement, the other half a placebo—and unexpectedly, both experienced recovery from their anemia and improved markedly in work output. At first glance, it would seem that all the improvement in both groups must have been due to the placebo effect—and clearly the placebo effect did improve both sets of workers' outputs at first. But placebo effects don't usually last beyond a few weeks, and this effect lasted longer. On close inspection, it turned out that the increased work output in both groups had led to increased pay, and they spent the added pay on food. The food supplied 3 to 5 extra milligrams of iron a day, together with vitamin C. Careful analysis of all the circumstances revealed that it was neither the placebo effect nor the iron supplement, but increased iron intakes from food, that accounted for relief of the anemia and its symptoms.[6]

A placebo is a dummy medication, used for its psychological effect, as described on p. 337.

cofactor: see p. 390.

Zinc

Zinc is active everywhere in the body, as the cofactor for more than 70 enzymes that perform specific tasks in the eyes, liver, kidneys, muscles, skin, bones, and male reproductive organs. Much can be understood about its importance and uses by simply reflecting on its close ties to protein. Wherever protein is, there zinc is, and it helps with whatever jobs proteins do. It is so tightly tied up in the body's tissues that it can be made available, in the case of deficiency, only by breaking them down. A regular dietary supply is therefore important.

Zinc in the Body

Among the enzymes zinc assists are many whose actions have been mentioned in earlier chapters:

- The enzyme that frees the vitamin folacin from its conjugated form so that it can move across cell membranes.

- An enzyme that helps make the molecular units that form parts of DNA and RNA—the genetic material.
- An enzyme that manufactures heme from its precursor in the red blood cells.
- An enzyme involved in essential fatty acid metabolism and the making of prostaglandins.
- The enzyme that releases vitamin A from its storage place in the liver.
- An enzyme that removes hydrogens from alcohols, converting them to aldehydes. This enzyme works in the liver to dispose of the alcohol a person consumes in alcoholic beverages; it also works in the retina of the eye to convert the vitamin A compound retinol to its active form, retinal.

Rather than adding some 60-odd additional specific functions to this list, this discussion simply goes on to say that zinc is "also important" in many other roles—but you can see from this list just how important it is. If space permitted, the details would overwhelm the reader with the sense that zinc is one of the most important of all the nutrients—although, of course, life is equally impossible without any one of them.

Zinc is, then, also important in these functions:

- Tooth development. A deficiency during a woman's pregnancy leads to her infant's teeth's susceptibility to decay later.[7]
- The function of white blood cells in immune protection.
- Protein metabolism and amino acid metabolism.
- Chylomicron formation and release from intestinal cells.

Zinc also forms part of the hormone insulin (although it may not be necessary for insulin's action), interacts with platelets in blood clotting, affects thyroid hormone function, and affects behavior and learning performance. It is essential to normal salt-taste perception, wound healing, the making of sperm, and the development of the fetus. Zinc deficiency impairs all these and other functions, while toxicity has other, unexpected effects, as a later section shows.

Zinc, like iron, helps protect the body from heavy metal poisoning—for example, poisoning by lead and cadmium. This is especially important during development of the fetus and during other times of growth. A later discussion (Chapter 13) reveals the damage these heavy metals can do, and shows the importance of dietary adequacy of zinc and iron in helping ward it off.

No one knows exactly how body proteins distinguish among different metal ions. Iron, zinc, lead, and cadmium all form ions with two positive charges. They can occupy the same sites on some proteins; for example, the carrier transferrin probably cannot distinguish among them, and carries them all. This has advantages; for example, it makes transferrin useful as a carrier of more than one essential trace element. For another example, in a rare disease in which too much copper accumulates in the system, zinc supplements can be used to displace the excess copper.* It also has disadvantages: transferrin is defenseless in that it must carry unwanted intruders. Faced with too much iron, transferrin fails to pick up enough zinc.

---

*Wilson's disease.

Other proteins seem better able to make the distinction between cations. Zinc has its own intracellular storage protein, analogous to iron's ferritin, to hold it inside cells.

The body handles zinc somewhat differently from iron, but with interesting similarities. In the intestine, the mucosal cells provide a two-way passage for zinc from the intestine to the blood and back again. That is, they can secrete zinc out into the intestine, as well as take it up for transfer into the blood.

After zinc has entered a cell lining the intestine, it may become involved in the metabolic functions of the cell itself or pass through the far side of the cell into the blood going to the liver. The absorbed zinc may also become trapped within the cell by a special binding protein similar to the one described earlier for iron.

A homeostatic mechanism seems to be at work to regulate the amount of zinc entering the body. Extra zinc (like iron) is held within the intestinal cell, and only the amount needed is released into the bloodstream. The zinc status of the individual influences the percentage of zinc absorbed from the diet; if more is needed, more is absorbed. Cells are shed daily from the intestinal lining and excreted in the feces; if the zinc trapped in them hasn't been released into the blood by that time, it is shed with them.

Figure 12–3 shows the probable body pathways for zinc. Zinc circulating within the body is taken up by liver cells and becomes bound to a protein inside them (liver metallothioneine). The amount bound depends on the amount of circulating zinc. Zinc circulates in the body until the concentration in and around liver cells reaches a certain threshold. Then any additional zinc is packaged with liver metallothioneine.

Zinc's two main transport vehicles in the blood are albumin and transferrin—the same transferrin that carries iron in the blood. This accounts for the observation that zinc absorption is impaired in several states. Pregnancy and malnutrition, which lower plasma albumin levels, lower plasma zinc levels as well. Anything that binds transferrin might also hinder zinc absorption. In normal individuals, transferrin is usually less than 50 percent saturated with iron, but in cases of iron overload, it is more saturated. Iron excess thus leaves too few binding sites available, thereby causing an impairment of zinc absorption.

The pancreas uses zinc to make some of its digestive enzymes, which it then squirts into the intestine at mealtimes. The intestine thus receives two doses of zinc with each meal—one from ingested foods, and the other from the zinc-rich pancreatic secretions. Thus even zinc that has already entered the body is rescreened periodically by the intestine and can be refused entry or tied up in intestinal cells on any of its times around (see Figure 12–3). Zinc exits the body in feces; urine; and shed tissues, including skin, mucosal cells, menstrual fluids, and semen.

Zinc Deficiency and Toxicity

No nationwide survey has yet been undertaken to assess the extent of zinc deficiency in the United States or Canada, but indications are that it does occur, especially where certain predisposing factors are present. A deficiency of zinc in human beings was first reported in the 1960s from studies with growing children and adolescent males in Egypt, Iran, and Turkey. The native diets were typically low in animal meats and high in whole grains and beans; consequently, they

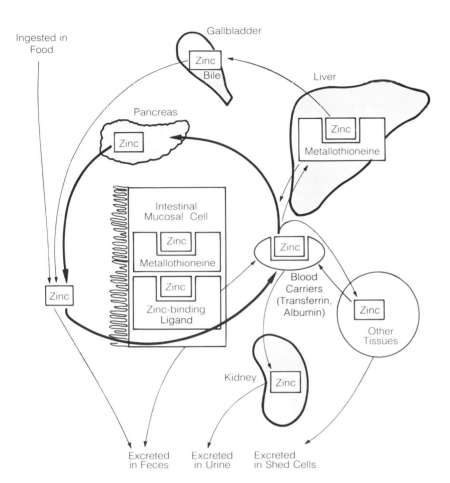

FIGURE 12–3

Zinc's routes in the body. The bold arrows show the enteropancreatic circulation of zinc.

The Egyptian boy in the picture is 17 years old but is only 4 feet tall, like a 7-year-old in the United States. His genitalia are like those of a 6-year-old. The retardation, known as **dwarfism,** is rightly ascribed to zinc deficiency, because it is partially reversible when zinc is restored to the diet.

were high in fiber and phytates. Furthermore, the bread they ate was unleavened; the phytates had not been broken down by yeast in the process of fermentation. The zinc deficiency was marked by severe growth retardation and arrested sexual maturation—symptoms that were responsive to zinc supplementation. The World Health Organization has recommended that for populations that use unleavened whole-grain bread as their staple grain product, the recommended intake of zinc be based on a sliding scale according to its availability.[8]

Since then, zinc deficiency has been recognized elsewhere, and it is known to affect much more than just growth. It alters digestive function profoundly by creating deficits in pancreas function, abnormalities in chylomicron formation, and defects in the GI tract lining. It causes diarrhea, which worsens the malnutrition already present, with respect to not only zinc, but all nutrients. It drastically impairs the immune response, making infections more likely—among them infections of the intestinal tract, which worsen malnutrition, including zinc malnutrition (a classic evil cycle). Zinc deficiency directly interferes with folacin absorption, and it impairs vitamin A metabolism, so the symptoms of those vitamin deficiencies often appear. It disturbs thyroid function and metabolic rate. It alters taste, causes anorexia, slows wound healing—in fact, its symptoms are so all-pervasive that generalized malnutrition and sickness are more likely to be the diagnosis than simple zinc deficiency. Many of the symptoms are similar to those of aspirin toxicity, perhaps because zinc, like aspirin, interacts with the hormonelike prostaglandin system. Table 12–4 lists the symptoms of zinc deficiency, and Table 12–5 itemizes predisposing factors.

Cases of zinc deficiency have occurred in U.S. schoolchildren.[9] A number of Denver children had low hair zinc levels, poor growth, poor appetite, and decreased taste sensitivity. The children were described as "picky eaters" and ate less than an ounce of meat per day. When pediatricians or other health workers evaluating children's health note poor growth accompanied by poor appetite, they should think zinc.

Zinc is a relatively nontoxic element. However, it can be toxic if consumed in large enough quantities. Figure 12–4 shows that zinc doses only a few milligrams above the RDA lower the body's copper content—an effect that, in animals, leads to degeneration of the heart muscle. Higher doses affect choles-

Assessment of zinc status: No single satisfactory test exists, but a combination of these indicators would be present: low zinc in plasma, red blood cells, urine, and plasma enzymes; raised blood ammonia. Hair zinc is a useful assessment measure for populations, but not for individuals, because it is subject to contamination; it is also affected by water hardness.

FIGURE 12–4

Zinc toxicity at different levels of intake.

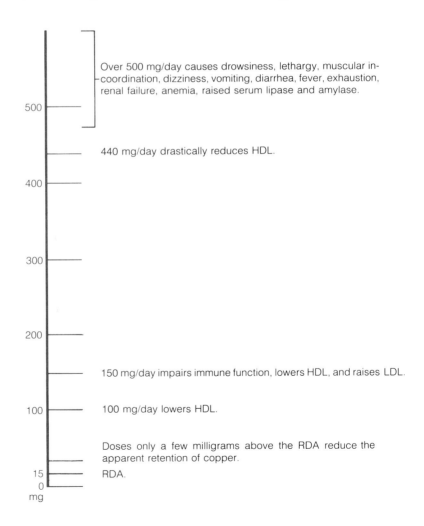

Over 500 mg/day causes drowsiness, lethargy, muscular in-coordination, dizziness, vomiting, diarrhea, fever, exhaustion, renal failure, anemia, raised serum lipase and amylase.

440 mg/day drastically reduces HDL.

150 mg/day impairs immune function, lowers HDL, and raises LDL.

100 mg/day lowers HDL.

Doses only a few milligrams above the RDA reduce the apparent retention of copper.

RDA.

TABLE 12–4

Zinc Deficiency

Disease	Area Affected	Main Effects
(No name)	Blood	Tendency to atherosclerosis; elevated ammonia levels; decreased alkaline phosphatase; decreased insulin concentration
	Bones	Growth retardation; abnormal collagen synthesis
	Cells (all)	Decreased DNA synthesis; impaired cell division and protein synthesis
	Digestive system	Lowered smell acuity; reduced sensitivity to the taste of salt; weight loss; delayed glucose absorption; diarrhea; impaired folacin absorption
	Eyes	Night blindness
	Glandular system	Delayed onset of puberty; small gonads in males; decreased synthesis and release of testosterone; abnormal glucose tolerance; decreased synthesis of adrenocortical hormones; altered thyroid function
	Immune system	Altered skin test responses; reduced cell number in lymph tissue; thymus atrophy; decreased number of antibody-forming cells; altered white blood cell counts; increased susceptibility to infection.
	Liver	Enlargement
	Nervous system	Anorexia (poor appetite); mental lethargy; irritability
	Reproductive system	Impaired reproductive function (rats); low sperm counts; fetal alcohol syndrome
	Skin	Generalized hair loss; lesions; rough, dry appearance; slow healing of wounds and burns
	Spleen	Enlargement
Acrodermatitis enteropathica (rare inherited disease)	Bones	Retarded growth
	Digestive system	Chronic diarrhea; malabsorption
	Eyes	Inflammation in the corners of the eyes (conjunctivitis); hypersensitivity to light (photophobia); scars on the cornea (corneal opacities)
	Glandular system	Small gonads in males
	Immune system	Frequent infections simultaneous with other diseases
	Nervous system	Emotional disorders; irritability; tremors; inability to coordinate muscular movements (cerebellar ataxia)
	Skin	Loss of hair (alopecia); dermatitis of extremities and of oral, anal, and genital areas, with pus

TABLE 12–5

Factors Making Zinc Deficiency Likely

Diseases of the GI tract:
  Diseases causing inflammation of the colon
  Diseases causing malabsorption
Disease of the kidneys
Diseases of the liver:
  Cirrhosis caused by alcohol abuse
  Hepatitis
Genetic predisposition
Hospital-associated disease:
  From drugs that bind zinc
  From prolonged feeding of formulas low in zinc
Increased need of zinc:
  During rapid growth (infancy, adolescence)
  During pregnancy
Injury; inflammation; stress
Intestinal parasites causing diarrhea
Iron supplements
Malnutrition:
  Alcohol caused
  Pica (clay eating)
  Protein-kcalorie malnutrition
Nutrition—diets high in fiber and phytates:
  Middle Eastern diet (high in unleavened bread)
  Vegetarian diet (if high in fiber and phytates)

Source: Adapted from H. H. Sandstead and G. W. Evans, Zinc, in *Present Knowledge in Nutrition*, 5th ed., (Washington, D.C.: Nutrition Foundation, 1984), pp. 479–505; Table 1, p. 488.

Clay eating (pica or geophagia) occurs among the poor in rural areas of the Middle East, and has also been noted in the rural South in the United States. The clay acts to bind zinc (as well as iron) by attracting these positively charged ions, making them unabsorbable in the intestine.

galvanized: term referring to metal containers that have been treated with a zinc-containing coating to prevent rust.

Recommended intake of zinc:
  U.S. adults' RDA: 15 mg/day.
  Canadian RNI for men: 9 mg.
         women: 8 mg.

terol metabolism, alter lipoprotein levels, and appear to accelerate the development of atherosclerosis. Accidental consumption of high levels of zinc may cause vomiting, diarrhea, fever, exhaustion, and a host of other symptoms (Table 12–6). Large doses can even be fatal.

Toxicity from ingestion of zinc can occur from misuse of supplements. Also, acidic foods or drinks that have been allowed to stand for long periods of time in galvanized containers may contain toxic levels of this trace mineral. Galvanized cooking pots, in earlier times, contributed zinc to foods, especially to acid foods, but with the increased use of stainless steel and plastic utensils to prepare and store food, this source of zinc is no longer significant. Galvanized pipes, used in plumbing, may contribute zinc to people's intakes.

Zinc in Foods

The daily recommended intake of zinc is about 10 to 15 milligrams, assuming that 40 percent of dietary zinc is available to the body. The RDA for all age groups are given inside the front cover. Requirements for infants and children are relatively high, due to the role of zinc in normal growth and development; the RDA for older people are not higher than for young adults.

Table 12–7 shows zinc amounts in foods per serving and per 100 kcalories. An average 1,500-kcalorie diet provides about 6.3 milligrams of zinc per day, or about 40 percent of the RDA. Zinc is highest in foods of high protein content, such as shellfish (especially oysters), meats, and liver. As a rule of thumb,

TABLE 12–6

Zinc Toxicity Symptoms

Area Affected	Main Effects
Blood	Anemia: reduced hemoglobin production
Bone	Growth in length, but without normal zinc content
Cardiovascular system	Heart muscle degeneration
Digestive system	Diarrhea; vomiting; decreased calcium and copper absorption
Immune system	Fever; elevated white blood cell count
Kidney	Renal failure
Metabolism	Raised LDL; lowered HDL
Muscle	Muscular pain and incoordination
Nervous system	Nausea; exhaustion; dizziness; drowsiness
Reproductive system	Reproductive failure

two ordinary servings a day of animal protein will provide most of the zinc a healthy person needs. Eggs and whole-grain products are good sources of zinc if large quantities are eaten; the phytate in grains does not inhibit the absorption of zinc in people consuming ordinary diets. Cow's milk protein (casein) binds zinc avidly and seems to prevent its absorption somewhat; infants absorb zinc better from human breast milk. Vegetables, fresh or canned, vary in zinc content depending on the soil in which they are grown. The zinc content of cooking water also varies from region to region.

Foods rich in zinc.

Zinc does not seem to be sensitive in the same ways as iron is to the effects of many dietary factors on its availability. Its absorption is not enhanced by vitamin C, for example—although it does seem to be enhanced by wine, with or without the alcohol present.

Zinc supplements are appropriate in only two instances: when used to remedy an accurately diagnosed zinc deficiency, and when used as a drug to displace other ions in unusual medical circumstances. Otherwise, it should be possible to obtain enough zinc from the diet without resorting to the use of supplements, except for brief periods of time when a balanced vitamin-mineral supplement is necessary (see Highlight 10). Ideally, as already mentioned, people will also obtain their iron from foods, not from supplements—for iron supplements have been seen to impair the absorption of zinc.

Iodine

Iodine occurs in the body in an infinitesimally small quantity, but its principal role in human nutrition is well known, and the amount needed is well established. Iodine is part of the thyroid hormones, which regulate body temperature,

TABLE 12–7

Zinc In Foods

Foods Ranked by Zinc Per Serving	Zinc Per Serving (mg)	Energy Per Serving (kCal)	Foods Ranked by Zinc Per 100 kCalories	Zinc Per Serving (mg)	Zinc Per 100 kCal (mg)
Oysters, raw (1 c)	74.40	160	Wheat bran (¼ c)	1.17	6.16
Sirloin steak, lean (8 oz)	13.38	480	Oysters, raw (1 c)	74.40	4.65
Crab meat, canned (1 c)	5.13	135	Collards, cooked (1 c)	0.93	4.65
Beef pot roast, lean (3 oz)	5.09	231	Wheat germ, raw (¼ c)	2.75	4.04
Hamburger patty, bun (4 oz)	5.01	445	Crab meat, canned (1 c)	5.13	3.80
Beef liver, fried (3 oz)	4.34	185	Miso (3 tbsp)	3.19	3.63
Lamb chop, braised (3 oz)	3.99	238	Shrimp, boiled (3.5 oz)	3.70	3.39
Ground beef, 10% fat (3 oz)	3.74	230	Spinach, cooked (1 c)	1.37	3.34
Corned beef, canned (3 oz)	3.70	185	Mushrooms, raw sliced (1 c)	0.60	3.33
Shrimp, boiled (3.5 oz)	3.70	109	Alfalfa seeds, sprouted (1 c)	0.30	3.00
Blackeyed peas, cooked (1 c)	3.22	190	Sirloin steak, lean (8 oz)	13.38	2.79
Miso (3 tbsp)	3.19	88	Brewer's yeast (1 tbsp)	0.63	2.52
Wheat germ, raw (¼ c)	2.75	68	Beef liver, fried (3 oz)	4.34	2.35
Turkey (3 oz)	2.64	145	Dandelion greens, cooked (1 c)	0.80	2.29
Pinto beans, cooked (1 c)	2.40	265	Beef pot roast, lean (3 oz)	5.08	2.20
Sardines, canned (3 oz)	2.21	175	Parsley, chopped fresh (1 c)	0.44	2.20
Kidney beans, canned (1 c)	2.00	230	Clams, raw meat only (3 oz)	1.40	2.15
Clams, raw meat only (3 oz)	1.40	65	Bok choy cabbage, cooked (1 c)	0.43	2.15
Spinach, cooked (1 c)	1.37	41	Corned beef, canned (3 oz)	3.70	2.00
Wheat bran (¼ c)	1.17	19	Romaine lettuce, chopped (1 c)	0.18	2.00
Swiss cheese (1 oz)	1.10	107	Summer squash, cooked (1 c)	0.71	1.97
Buttermilk (1 c)	1.03	99	Asparagus, cooked (1 c)	0.86	1.95
Whole milk (1 c)	0.94	150	Turkey (3 oz)	2.64	1.82
Collards, cooked (1 c)	0.93	20	Beet greens, cooked (1 c)	0.72	1.80
Peanuts, dried unsalted (1 oz)	0.93	161	Looseleaf lettuce (1 c)	0.18	1.80
Nonfat milk or yogurt (1 c)	0.92	86	Blackeyed peas, cooked (1 c)	3.22	1.69
Cheddar cheese (1 oz)	0.92	114	Lamb chop, braised (3 oz)	3.99	1.68
Tofu soybean curd (1 block)	0.88	86	Ground beef, 10% fat (3 oz)	3.74	1.63
Asparagus, cooked (1 c)	0.86	44	Mustard greens, cooked (1 c)	0.30	1.43
Chicken breast, roasted (½)	0.86	142	Bean sprouts, fresh (1 c)	0.43	1.34
Dandelion greens, cooked (1 c)	0.80	35	Sardines, canned (3 oz)	2.21	1.26
Beet greens, cooked (1 c)	0.72	40	Hamburger patty, bun (4 oz)	5.01	1.13
Sole/flounder, baked (3 oz)	0.72	120	Nonfat milk or yogurt (1 c)	0.92	1.07
Summer squash, cooked (1 c)	0.71	36	Buttermilk (1 c)	1.03	1.04
Brewer's yeast (1 tbsp)	0.63	25	Swiss cheese (1 oz)	1.10	1.03
Green peas, cooked (1 c)	0.60	67	Green beans, cooked (1 c)	0.45	1.02
Mushrooms, raw sliced (1 c)	0.60	18	Tofu soybean curd (1 block)	0.88	1.02
Whole wheat bread (1 sl)	0.50	70	Cauliflower, cooked (1 c)	0.30	1.00
Green beans, cooked (1 c)	0.45	44	Pinto beans, cooked (1 c)	2.40	0.91
Parsley, chopped fresh (1 c)	0.44	20	Green peas, cooked (1 c)	0.60	0.90
Bok choy cabbage, cooked (1 c)	0.43	20	Kidney beans, canned (1 c)	2.00	0.87
Bean sprouts, fresh (1 c)	0.43	32	Cheddar cheese (1 oz)	0.92	0.81
Cantaloupe melon (½)	0.43	94	Whole wheat bread (1 sl)	0.50	0.71
Mustard greens, cooked (1 c)	0.30	21	Whole milk (1 c)	0.94	0.63
Cauliflower, cooked (1 c)	0.30	30	Chicken breast, roasted (½)	0.86	0.61
Alfalfa seeds, sprouted (1 c)	0.30	10	Sole/flounder, baked (3 oz)	0.72	0.60
Broccoli, cooked (1 c)	0.23	46	Peanuts, dried unsalted (1 oz)	0.93	0.58
Romaine lettuce, chopped (1 c)	0.18	9	Broccoli, cooked (1 c)	0.23	0.50
Looseleaf lettuce (1 c)	0.18	10	Cantaloupe melon (½)	0.43	0.46
Orange, fresh medium (1)	0.09	60	Orange, fresh medium (1)	0.09	0.15
Apple, fresh medium (1)	0.05	80	Apple, fresh medium (1)	0.05	0.06

metabolic rate, reproduction, growth, the making of blood cells, nerve and muscle function, and more. These hormones enter every cell of the body to control the rate at which the cells use oxygen. This is the same as saying that thyroxin controls the rate at which energy is released.

Iodine must be available for thyroid hormones to be synthesized. The amount in the diet is variable and generally reflects the amount present in the soil in which plants are grown or on which animals graze. Iodine is plentiful in the ocean, so seafood is a dependable source. Land masses that have been under the ocean have soils rich in iodine; those that have not have iodine-poor soils. In the United States and Canada, the soil is iodine poor in the area around the Great Lakes and the inland valleys of Oregon. In these regions, the use of iodized salt has largely wiped out the iodine deficiency that once was widespread.

The iodization of salt in the Great Lakes region eliminated the widespread misery caused by goiter and cretinism in the local people during the 1930s. Once these scourges had disappeared, a new generation of children grew up who never saw the problem and so had no appreciation of the importance of iodine. Rejecting iodized salt out of ignorance, they allowed iodine deficiencies to creep back into their lives. It is hoped that education is now keeping them informed of the need to continue using iodized salt.

When the iodine level of the blood is low, the cells of the thyroid gland enlarge in an attempt to trap as many particles of iodine as possible. If the gland enlarges until it is visible (Figure 12–5), it is called a simple goiter. Goiter afflicts about 200 million people the world over, many of them in Africa. In all but 4 percent of these cases, the cause is iodine deficiency. As for the 4 percent (8 million), who are mostly in Africa, they have goiter because they overconsume plants of the cabbage family and others that contain an antithyroid substance

Assessment of iodine: Serum protein-bound iodine (thyroxine).

goiter (GOY-ter): an iodine-deficiency disease. Goiter caused by iodine deficiency is **simple goiter.**

goitrogen (GOY-troh-jen): a thyroid antagonist found in food; causes **toxic goiter.**

FIGURE 12–5

Goiter.

cretinism (CREE-tin-ism): an iodine-deficiency disease characterized by mental and physical retardation.

Laura Drake, age 38, a cretin.

Recommended intakes of iodine:
 U.S. adults' RDA: 150 μg.
 Canadian RNI: 160 μg.

(goitrogen) whose effect is not counteracted by dietary iodine. The goitrogens present in plants serve notice that even natural components of foods can cause harm when taken in excess, a theme developed further in Chapter 13.

In addition to causing sluggishness and weight gain, an iodine deficiency may have serious effects on the development of a fetus in the uterus. Severe thyroid undersecretion during pregnancy causes the extreme and irreversible mental and physical retardation known as cretinism. A cretin has an IQ as low as 20 and a face and body with many abnormalities. Much of the mental retardation associated with cretinism can be averted by diagnosis of iodine deficiency and treatment early in pregnancy.

The recommended intake of iodine for adults in 100 to 150 micrograms a day, a minuscule amount. Like chlorine gas, iodine gas is poisonous; however, the iodide ion, which occurs in foods, is far less toxic, and traces of it are indispensable to life. The need for iodine is easy to meet by consuming seafood, vegetables grown in iodine-rich soil, and (in iodine-poor areas) iodized salt. In the United States, you have to read the label to find out whether salt is iodized; in Canada all table salt is iodized.

Excessive intakes of iodine can also cause an enlargement of the thyroid gland resembling goiter, which in infants can be so severe as to block the airways and cause suffocation. A dramatic increase in iodine intakes in the United States concerns observers. Average consumption rose from 150 micrograms per day in 1960 to over 450 in 1970, and reached an all-time high of over 800 micrograms per day in 1974; since then it has declined somewhat but still is several times the RDA. The toxic level at which detectable harm results is thought to be over 2,000 micrograms per day for an adult—only a few times higher than current average consumption levels.[10]

Some of the excess iodine seems to be coming from fast foods, in which iodized salt is liberally used. Some comes from iodates—dough conditioners used in the baking industry—and from milk produced by cows exposed to iodine-containing medications and disinfectants. Now that the problem has been identified, both industries have reduced their use of these compounds, but the sudden emergence of this problem points to a need for continued surveillance of the food supply. In some local areas, overuse of the seaweed kelp and powders made from it has caused iodine toxicity.

Copper

The body contains about 75 to 100 milligrams of copper, which performs several vital roles. It is a part of several enzymes. As a catalyst in the formation of hemoglobin, it helps to make red blood cells. It is involved in the manufacture of collagen and the healing of wounds, and it helps to maintain the sheath around nerve fibers. Most of what is known about copper comes from animal research, which has provided clues about its possible roles in humans. Copper's critical roles seem to have to do with helping iron shift back and forth between its ferrous and ferric states. This means that copper is needed in many of the reactions related to respiration and the release of energy.

Copper deficiency is rare, but not unknown. It has been seen in children with kwashiorkor and iron-deficiency anemia and can severely disturb growth and metabolism. Excess zinc, as mentioned, interferes with copper absorption and can cause deficiency.

The best food sources of copper include grains, shellfish, organ meats, legumes, dried fruits, fresh fruits, and vegetables—a long list showing that copper is available from almost all foods. About a third of the copper taken in food is absorbed, and the rest is eliminated in the feces.

Recommended intakes of copper:
    U.S. suggestion for a safe and adequate intake: 2.0 to 3.0 mg. Do not exceed 3.0 mg.
    Canadian suggestion (tentative): 1.0 to 2.0 mg.

Manganese

The human body contains a tiny 20 milligrams of manganese, mostly in the bones and glands. Still, this represents billions on billions of molecules. Animal studies suggest that manganese cooperates with many enzymes, helping to facilitate dozens of different metabolic processes. Manganese deficiency in animals deranges many systems, including the bones, reproduction, the nervous system, and fat metabolism.

Deficiencies of manganese have not been seen in humans, but toxicity may be severe. Miners who inhale large quantities of manganese dust on the job over prolonged periods show many of the symptoms of a brain disease, with frightening abnormalities of appearance and behavior. "Facial expression is mask-like, the voice monotonous; and intention-tremor, muscle rigidity and spastic gait appear."[11]

Recommended intakes of manganese:
    U.S. suggestion for a safe and adequate intake: 2.5 to 5.0 mg. Do not exceed 5.0 mg.
    Canadian RNI (tentative): 2.0 to 4.1 mg.

The example of manganese underlines the fact that toxicity of the trace elements occurs at a level not far above the estimated requirement. Thus it is as important not to overdose as it is to have an adequate intake. The Committee on RDA underscores this point by adding the special warning to its trace-mineral table "not to exceed the upper end of the range of recommended intakes." The National Nutrition Consortium, too, worries that, now that more trace minerals are known, they will be added to vitamin-mineral pills, making toxic overdoses more likely. The FDA is not permitted to enforce limits on the amounts of trace minerals added to supplements, because some consumers have insisted they must have the freedom to choose their own doses of nutrients; thus this is an area in which buyers must beware. In fact, we suggest avoiding supplements that contain trace minerals, especially in larger than trace amounts. It is safer to consume a diet that provides foods from a variety of sources than to try to put together, without causing toxicity, a combination of pills that will meet all your needs.

Fluoride

Only a trace of fluoride occurs in the human body, but studies have demonstrated that where diets are high in fluoride, the crystalline deposits in bones and teeth are larger and more perfectly formed. When bones and teeth become calcified, first a crystal called hydroxyapatite is formed from calcium and phosphorus. Then fluoride replaces the hydroxy (OH) portions of the crystal, rendering it insoluble in water and resistant to decay.

Drinking water is the usual source of fluoride, although fish and tea may supply substantial amounts. Where fluoride is lacking in the water supply, the incidence of dental decay is very high. Dental problems can cause a multitude of health problems, affecting the whole body. Fluoridation of community water where needed, to raise its fluoride concentration to 1 part per million, is thus an important public health measure. Fluoridation of community water is presently practiced in more than 5,000 communities across the United States, and about 100 million people are drinking it (see Figure 12–6).

The outer two layers of the teeth, enamel and dentin, are composed largely of calcium compounds, including hydroxyapatite and fluorapatite. See p. 66.

hydroxyapatite (high-drox-ee-APP-uh-tite): the major calcium-containing crystal of bones and teeth.

fluorapatite (floor-APP-uh-tite): the stabilized form of bone and tooth crystal, in which fluoride has replaced the hydroxy groups of hydroxyapatite.

FIGURE 12–6

Fluoridation in the United States.

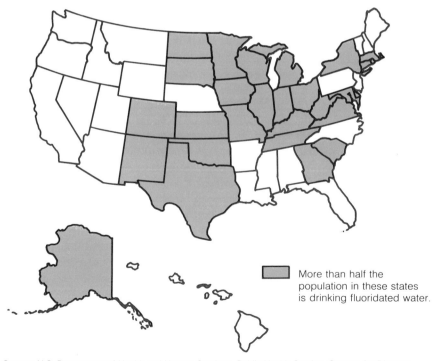

More than half the population in these states is drinking fluoridated water.

Source: U.S. Department of Health and Human Services, Public Health Service, Centers for Disease Control, Dental Disease Prevention Activity, Fluoridation Census, 1980, Figure 1.

In some communities the natural fluoride concentration in water is high—2 to 8 parts per million—and children's teeth develop with mottled enamel (Figure 12–7), a condition called fluorosis. Overzealous parents, who provide their children with too much fluoride in supplement form, can also produce fluorosis in their children's teeth. This condition may not be harmful (in fact, these children's teeth may be extraordinarily decay resistant), but it violates the prejudice that teeth should be white. Fluorosis does not occur in communities where fluoride is added to the water supply.

Not only does fluoride protect children's teeth from decay, but it makes the bones of older people resistant to adult bone loss (osteoporosis). Fluoride is also required for growth in animals and is an essential nutrient for humans; in fact, the continuous presence of fluoride in body fluids is desirable.

Fluoride is toxic in excess, but toxicity symptoms appear only with very high doses or after chronic intakes of 20 to 80 milligrams a day over many years. They include nausea, diarrhea, chest pain, itching, and vomiting. The amount consumed from fluoridated water is typically about 1 milligram a day. Despite its value, violent disagreement often surrounds the introduction of fluoride to a community's water supply.

People whose water supplies do not contain adequate fluoride need to find alternative means of protecting their children's teeth. The best temporary solution seems to be to use fluoride toothpastes and/or to have children obtain a fluoride treatment of the surfaces of their teeth every year. Fluoride tablets are also available. For infants there are vitamin drops with fluoride in them, but their effectiveness is limited.

Chromium

Experiments on animals have shown that chromium works closely with the hormone insulin, facilitating the uptake of glucose into cells and the release of energy. When chromium is lacking, the effectiveness of insulin is impaired, and a diabeteslike condition results.

Like iron, chromium can have different charges. In the case of chromium, the +6 ion seems to be the best absorbed and most effective in living systems. Chromium also occurs in association with several different complexes in foods. The one that is best absorbed and most active is a small organic compound named the glucose tolerance factor (GTF). This compound has been purified from brewer's yeast and pork kidney and is present in many other foods.

Depleted tissue concentrations of chromium in human beings have been linked to adult-onset diabetes and to growth failure in children with protein-kcalorie malnutrition. Chromium has also been shown to remedy impaired carbohydrate metabolism in several groups of older people in the United States. The more refined foods are eaten, the less chromium people obtain from their diets; whole foods are the best sources. Older people are most susceptible to deficiency. Toxicity from eating foods is unknown.

FIGURE 12–7

Fluorosis.

fluorosis (fleur-OH-sis): mottling of the tooth enamel; due to ingestion of too much fluoride during tooth development. *osis* = too much

Osteoporosis: see p. 391.

Recommended intakes of fluoride:
U.S. suggestion for a safe and adequate intake: 1.5 to 4.0 mg. Do not exceed 4.0 mg.
Canadian RNI (tentative): 2.0 to 5.0 mg.

glucose tolerance factor (GTF): a small organic compound containing chromium.

Recommended intakes of chromium:
U.S. suggestion for a safe and adequate intake: 0.05 to 0.2 mg. Do not exceed 0.2 mg.
Canadian RNI (tentative—based on actual intakes): 50 to 100 µg.

Selenium

Selenium is a trace element that functions as part of an enzyme. The enzyme acts as an antioxidant and can prevent oxidation of PUFA, providing an alternative to vitamin E as a source of protection for them.

Selenium deficiency affects the heart. A severe deficiency can cause heart failure; a chronic, mild deficiency enlarges the heart and impairs its function. In some parts of China, selenium deficiency affects hundreds of thousands of children; not until the 1970s, however, was the cause of their heart trouble confirmed and remedied with selenium supplements. The conclusive study of over 36,000 subjects was published in 1980.[12]

The region of China in which Keshan disease is prevalent is a region where the soil and foods are selenium poor. In other parts of the world, selenium-poor soil has been found to correlate with certain kinds of cancer. The question of whether selenium protects against cancer has stimulated research with both animal and human subjects, and it seems possible that dietary selenium adequacy may be one of the many health factors that defend against cancer. Results of research to date have not been clear, however. For example, an attempt was made to show a relationship between blood selenium and breast cancer incidence in women in a selenium-poor area in Oregon, but no such relationship was found. The authors were forced to conclude that there was "no justification at this time for the use of selenium supplements by the people living in this low selenium area."[13]

High doses of selenium are toxic, causing loss of hair and nails, lesions of the skin and nervous system, and possibly damage to the teeth. An outbreak of selenium poisoning arose in China in the 1960s, when a local rice crop failed and inhabitants of five villages consumed vegetables from a region where selenium-rich coal contaminated the soil in which the vegetables were grown. Some 50 percent of the villagers became seriously ill before the cause was discovered.[14]

Molybdenum

Finally, molybdenum has also been recognized as an important mineral in human and animal physiology. It functions as a working part of several metalloenzymes, some of which are giant proteins. One, for example, contains two atoms of molybdenum and eight of iron. Deficiencies of molybdenum are unknown in animals and humans, because the amounts needed are minuscule—as little as 0.1 part per million parts of body tissue. Excess molybdenum causes goutlike symptoms in human beings.

Other Trace Minerals

The trace minerals have been known for decades, but their role as nutrients is a recent surprise. Nickel is now recognized as important for the health of many body tissues; deficiencies harm the liver and other organs. Silicon is known to be involved in bone calcification, at least in animals. Tin is necessary for growth in animals, and probably in human beings. Vanadium, too, is necessary for growth and bone development, and also for normal reproduction; human intakes of vanadium may be close to the minimum needed for health. Cobalt is recognized as the mineral in the large vitamin B_{12} molecule; the alternative name for vitamin B_{12}, cobalamin, reflects the presence of cobalt. In the future we may discover that many other trace minerals also play key roles: silver, mercury, lead, barium, and cadmium. Even arsenic—famous as the poisonous instrument of death in many murder mysteries and known to be a carcinogen—may turn out to be an essential nutrient in tiny quantities.

As research on the trace minerals continues, many interactions between them are also coming to light. An excess of one may cause a deficiency of another. (A slight manganese overload, for example, may aggravate an iron deficiency.) A deficiency of one may open the way for another to cause a toxic reaction. (Iron deficiency, for example, makes the body much more susceptible than normal to lead poisoning.) Good food sources of one are poor food sources of another, and factors that cooperate with some trace elements oppose others. (Vitamin C, for example, enhances the absorption of iron and depresses that of copper.[15]) The continuous outpouring of new information about the trace minerals is a sign that we have much more to learn.

The intricate vitamin B_{12} molecule contains one atom of cobalt.

Study Questions

1. What are the symptoms of iron deficiency anemia? What other nutrition factors besides iron are related to anemia?
2. Differentiate between heme and non-heme iron. Discuss the factors that enhance iron absorption.
3. Discuss possible reasons for a low intake of zinc. What factors affect the bioavailability of zinc?
4. Describe the principal functions of iodine, copper, fluorine, chromium, and selenium in the body.
5. What public health measure has been used in preventing simple goiter? What measure has been recommended for protection against tooth decay?
6. Discuss the importance of a balanced and varied diet in obtaining all the essential trace minerals and avoiding toxicities.

Notes

1. L. Hallberg, Iron, in *Present Knowledge in Nutrition,* 5th ed. (New York: Nutrition Foundation, 1984), pp. 459–478.
2. N. S. Scrimshaw, Functional consequences of iron deficiency in human populations, *Journal of Nutrition Science and Vitaminology* 30 (1984): 47–63.
3. L. Hallberg, Iron absorption and iron deficiency, *Human Nutrition: Clinical Nutrition* 36C (1982): 259–278.
4. E. R. Monsen and coauthors, Estimation of available dietary iron, *American Journal of Clinical Nutrition* 31 (1978): 134–141.
5. S. N. Gershoff and coauthors, Studies of the elderly in Boston: 1. The effects of iron fortification on moderately anemic people, *American Journal of Clinical Nutrition* 30 (1977): 226–234.

Several of these exercises use the information you recorded on the forms in Appendix K.

1. Look up and record your recommended intake of iron. Also record your actual intake. What percentage of your recommended intake did you consume? Was this enough?

2. Which of the foods you eat supply the most iron? Rank your top five iron contributors. How many were meats? Legumes? Greens? Did any of them fall outside these classes? If so, what were they? How much of a contribution does enriched or whole-grain bread or cereal make to your iron intake? Are there refined bread/cereal products in your diet, such as pastries, that you could replace with enriched or whole-grain products to increase your iron intake?

3. Compute your iron absorption from a meal of your choosing, using the Monsen method (p. 417). The RDA assumes you will absorb 10 percent of

SELF-STUDY

Evaluate Your Intakes of Trace Minerals

the iron you ingest. What percentage did you absorb? If you are a man of any age or a woman over 50 years old, you need to absorb about 1 milligram per day; if a woman 11 to 50 years, 1.8 milligrams. How could you eat differently to improve your iron absorption?

4. Are you in an area of the country where the soil is iodine-poor? If so, do you use iodized salt?

5. Record your recommended zinc intake and the amount you actually consumed. What percentage of your recommended intake did you obtain from your diet? Which were your best food sources? What guidelines do you need to follow to be sure of obtaining

enough zinc from the foods you eat?

6. Repeat exercise 5, using magnesium as the subject.

7. Is the water in your county fluoridated? (Call the County Health Department.) If not, how do you and your family ensure that your intakes of fluoride are optimal?

8. Review your three-day food record (Self-Study 1) and separate the foods you ate into two categories: predominantly natural, unprocessed foods like those on the exchange lists and highly processed foods, such as TV dinners, pastries, and instant gravies. Beside each food, record its kcalorie value. How many total kcalories did you consume in three days? Of these, what percentage came from highly processed foods? In light of the discussion of trace elements in this chapter, what implications do you suppose this estimate has for the nutritional adequacy of your diet?

6. Scrimshaw, 1984.

7. Increased dental caries in young rats suckled by zinc-deficient dams, *Nutrition Review* 37 (1979): 232–233.

8. World Health Organization, *Trace Elements in Human Nutrition,* technical report series no. 532 (Geneva: WHO, 1973), pp. 9–15.

9. K. M. Hambidge and coauthors, Low levels of zinc in hair, anorexia, poor growth, and hypogeusia in children, *Pediatric Research* 6 (1972): 868–874.

10. F. Taylor, Iodine: Going from hypo to hyper, *FDA Consumer,* April 1981, pp. 15–18.

11. T. K. Li and B. L. Vallee, Trace elements: B. The biochemical and nutritional role of trace elements, in *Modern Nutrition in Health and Disease,* 5th ed., eds. R. S. Goodhart

and M. E. Shils (Philadelphia: Lea and Febiger, 1973), pp. 372–399.

12. M. H. N. Golden, Trace elements in human nutrition, *Human Nutrition: Clinical Nutrition* 36C (1982): 185–202.

13. T. D. Schultz and J. E. Leklem, Selenium status of vegetarians, nonvegetarians, and hormone-dependent cancer subjects, *American Journal of Clinical Nutrition* 37 (1983): 114–118.

14. G. Yang, S. Wang, R. Zhou, and S. Sun, Endemic selenium intoxication of humans in China, *American Journal of Clinical Nutrition* 37 (1983): 872–881.

15. W. Mertz, The essential trace elements, *Science* 213 (1981): 1332–1338.

Foods and Food Safety

13

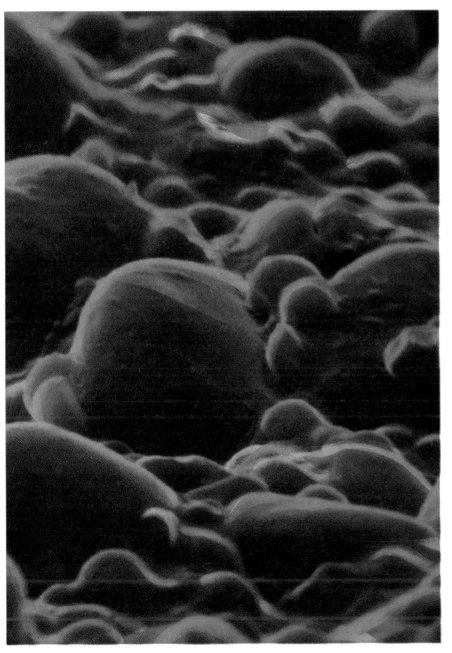

People seldom realize that the foods they eat are often as complex in structure as their own bodies' tissues. Shown here is a sample of dough; the large spheres are starch granules, and the coating is a film of gluten (protein).

To this point, this book has dealt primarily with the nutrients and how your body handles them. Along the way, it has offered some practical pointers about foods. Chapter 2 showed how to plan balanced and varied diets, using food group plans and exchange systems. Highlight 5 dealt with diet planning for the vegetarian. Chapter 8 showed how to plan weight-loss and weight-gain diets, and Chapter 9 made suggestions on cooking to preserve vitamins. Each chapter on nutrients has also contained tables showing the nutrient contents of foods—but no chapter has focused on foods themselves. What are they made of—besides nutrients? What sorts of additives do they contain, and what are the effects of those additives? Are they ever contaminated? If so, with what, and how seriously? How can the consumer prepare foods safely? This chapter deals with these questions.

The first question people ask about what's in foods usually has to do with additives. What are they, why are they there, and are they dangerous in any way? The safety of food additives is not first, or even third, on the FDA's list of priority concerns; it is sixth. In order of concern, hazards within the FDA's areas of responsibility are:

- Food-borne infection, which is increasing because of large-scale operations and multiple transfers involving handling.
- Nutrition, which requires close attention as more and more artificially constituted foods appear on the market.
- Environmental contaminants, which are increasing yearly in number and concentration, and whose consequences are difficult to foresee and forestall.
- Naturally occurring toxicants in foods, which occur randomly in arbitrary levels and constitute a hazard whenever people turn to consuming single foods either by choice (fad diets) or by necessity (famine).
- Pesticide residues, which have established tolerance limits and are regulated, but which require vigilant monitoring.
- Intentional food additives, listed last "because so much is known about them, and all are now, and surely will continue to be, well regulated."[1]

This chapter deals with all these concerns in reverse order—additives first, food poisoning last.

Food Additives

additive: a substance not normally consumed as a food by itself but added to food either intentionally or by accident.

intentional food additive: an additive intentionally added to food, such as nutrients or colors.

indirect (incidental) additive: a substance that can get into food not through intentional introduction, but as a result of contact with the food during growing, processing, packaging, storing, or some other stage before the food is consumed.

It is appropriate to begin with some definitions. Intentional additives are substances put into foods on purpose, while incidental additives are those that may get in by accident before or during processing. This discussion begins with the intentional additives, and after taking them up class by class, goes on to the incidental or indirect additives.

Intentional food additives are substances put into foods to give them some desirable characteristic: color, flavor, texture, stability, or resistance to spoilage. Some additives are nutrients added to foods to increase their nutritive value,

---

Miniglossary of Intentional Food Additives

emulsifiers, stabilizers, thickeners: to give texture, smoothness, or other desired consistencies.

nutrients: to improve nutritive value.

flavoring agents: to add or enhance flavor.

leavening (neutralizing) agents: to control acidity or alkalinity.

preservatives, antioxidants, sequestrants, antimyotic agents: to prevent spoilage, rancidity of fats, and microbial growth.

coloring agents: to increase attractiveness.

bleaches: to whiten foods such as flour and cheese and to speed up the maturing of cheese.

humectants, anticaking agents: to retain moisture in some foods and to keep others (such as salts and powders) free-flowing.

---

such as vitamin C added to fruit drinks or potassium iodide added to salt. The most common ones, roughly in order of the quantities used, are listed in the accompanying miniglossary. In addition, numerous additives are used in still smaller quantities for miscellaneous other purposes.

Regulations Governing Additives

The agency charged with the responsibility of deciding what additives shall be in foods is the FDA. The FDA's authority over additives hinges primarily on their safety. A manufacturer has to go through a special procedure to get permission to use a new additive in food products. The procedure puts the burden on the manufacturer to prove that the additive is safe, and it may take several years to do so. First the manufacturer has to test it chemically to satisfy the FDA that:

safety: the practical certainty that injury will not result from the use of a substance.

- It is effective (it does what it is supposed to do).
- It can be detected and measured in the final food product.

Then the manufacturer has to feed it in large doses to animals, to prove that:

- It is safe (it causes no cancer, birth defects, or other injury).

The manufacturer can't do just any animal tests. The doses have to be large, because animals usually metabolize chemicals faster than people do, and because the times of exposure are necessarily short compared to the human life span. Two kinds of animals (usually rodents and dogs) must be used, and the exposure times are specified. Finally, the manufacturer must submit all test results to the FDA.[2]

The FDA responds to the manufacturer's petition by announcing a public hearing. Consumers are invited to participate at these hearings, where experts present testimony for and against the acceptance of the additive for the proposed uses. Thus the consumer's rights and responsibilities are written into the provisions for deeming additives safe.

If the FDA approves the additive's use, that doesn't mean the manufacturer can add it in any amount to any food. On the contrary: the FDA writes a regulation stating in what amounts, and in what foods, the additive may be used. No additives are permanently approved; all are periodically reviewed.

Many substances were exempted from complying with this procedure in 1958 when the law on additives came into being, because there were no known hazards in their use. These substances, some 700 in all, were put on the GRAS list. However, any time substantial scientific evidence or public outcry has questioned the safety of any of the substances on the GRAS list, a special reevaluation has been made. Meanwhile, the entire GRAS list has been systematically and intensively reevaluated, and all substances about which any legitimate question was raised have been removed or reclassified. A set of 2,100 flavoring agents has similarly been reviewed, as well as some 200 coloring agents.[3]

An exception to the law regards permissibility of additives that may cause cancer. No threshold dose is recognized. To remain on the GRAS list, an additive must not have been found to be a carcinogen in any test on animals or human beings. The Delaney Clause (the part of the law that states this criterion) is uncompromising in addressing carcinogens in foods and drugs and has been under fire in recent years for being too strict and inflexible. Highlight 13A discusses the problems surrounding application of the Delaney clause.

An important distinction that governs determinations of additives' safety is the distinction between *toxic* and *hazardous* substances. "Toxicity—the capacity of a chemical substance to harm living organisms—is a general property of matter; hazard is the capacity of a chemical to produce injury under conditions of use. All substances are potentially toxic, but are hazardous only if consumed in sufficiently large quantities."[4] An additive is not considered to be a hazard if some immense amount that people never consume is toxic. The additive is a hazard only if it is toxic under the conditions of its actual use. Food additives are supposed to be allowed in foods only with a wide margin of safety.

GRAS (generally recognized as safe) list: a list, established by the FDA in 1958, of food additives that had long been in use and were believed safe. The list is subject to revision as new facts become known.

Delaney Clause: a clause in the 1958 Food Additive Amendment to the Food, Drug, and Cosmetic Act (of 1938) that states that no substance that is known to cause cancer in animals or human beings at any dose level shall be added to foods.

toxicity: the ability of a substance to harm living organisms. All substances are toxic if high enough concentrations are used.

hazard: state of danger; used to refer to any circumstance in which toxicity is possible under normal conditions of use.

Food Safety Regulation in the United States

1906   The Pure Food and Drug Act defined pure and adulterated food and specified that only pure food could be sold.

1916   The court permitted addition of caffeine to soft drinks, stating that although it could be harmful, its use in this way would not be. This marked the first legal distinction between theoretical and actual harm (toxicity and hazard).

1938   The Food, Drug, and Cosmetic Act set limits on toxic substances allowable in foods—including both intentional and indirect additives and pesticide residues.

1958   The Delaney Clause was added to the Food, Drug, and Cosmetic Act and the GRAS list was established. The legal definition of the term *food additive* was tightened to exclude pesticide residues, color additives, new animal drugs, and GRAS substances. The Delaney Clause applies only to food additives.

Source: *The U.S. Food Safety Laws: Time for a Change?* a booklet (1982) available from the American Council on Science and Health, 1995 Broadway, New York, NY 10023.

Most additives that involve risk are allowed in foods only at levels 100 times below those at which the risk is still known to be zero; their margin of safety is $\frac{1}{100}$. Experiments to determine the extent of risk involve feeding test animals the substance at different concentrations throughout their lifetimes. The additive is then permitted in foods at $\frac{1}{100}$ the level that can be fed under these conditions without causing any harmful effect whatever. In many foods, naturally occurring substances appear at levels that bring their margins of safety closer to $\frac{1}{10}$. Even nutrients, as you have seen, involve risks at high dose levels. The margin of safety for vitamins A and D is $\frac{1}{25}$ to $\frac{1}{40}$; it may be less than $\frac{1}{10}$ in infants.[5] For some trace elements, it is about $\frac{1}{5}$. People consume common table salt daily in amounts only five times less than those that cause serious toxicity.[6]

Additives are in foods for a reason. They offer benefits, in comparison with which any risks are deemed either small enough to ignore or worth taking. When the benefit to be gained from an additive is small, as in the case of color additives that only enhance the appearance of foods but do not improve their health value or safety, then the risks may be deemed not worth taking. Only 33 of 200 color additives that have been used in the past are now approved for use by the FDA.

It is also the manufacturers' responsibility not to use more of an additive than they have to, to get the needed effect. Additives should also *not* be used:

- To disguise faulty or inferior products.
- To deceive the consumer.
- Where they significantly destroy nutrients.
- Where their effects can be achieved by economical, sound manufacturing processes.[7]

With these distinctions in mind, let's look at a few individual food additives. The focus will be on those that have received the most negative publicity, because people ask questions about them most often.

Artificial Colors

As just mentioned, many coloring agents have been removed from the GRAS list. Only 33 remain, a highly select group that has survived considerable screening. Coloring agents are among the most intensively investigated of all additives. In fact, they are much better known than the *natural* pigments of plants, and we can state the limits on the safety of their use with greater certainty.[8]

Still, the food colors have been more heavily criticized than almost any other group of additives. This is because they are dispensable: simply stated, they only make foods pretty, whereas other additives such as preservatives make foods safe. Hence with food colors we can afford to require that their use entail no risk, whereas with other additives we may have to compromise between the risks of using them and the risks of *not* using them.

An infamous food-coloring agent of an earlier time was red dye number 2, which came under suspicion as a carcinogen in 1970 on the basis of two studies conducted in the U.S.S.R. It was never shown to cause cancer, but it proved impossible to demonstrate that it did *not* cause cancer, either, and so it was banned in the United States in 1976. On the same evidence, Canada concluded that it was not likely to cause cancer, and continued to permit its use.[9]

margin of safety: as used when speaking of food additives, a zone between the concentration normally used and that at which a hazard exists. For common table salt, for example, the margin of safety is $\frac{1}{5}$ (five times the concentration commonly used would be hazardous).

Some people think food colors are dispensable because they only make foods look pretty.

Foods containing tartrazine:
- Orange drinks (Tang, Daybreak, Awake).
- Gatorade (lime flavored).
- Gelatin desserts (Jello, Royal).
- Golden Blend Italian dressing (Kraft).
- Some cake mixes and icings (Duncan Hines, Pillsbury, Cake Mate).
- Imitation banana or pineapple extract (McCormick).
- Seasoning salt (French's).
- Macaroni and cheese dinner (Kraft).
- "Cheez" curls and balls (Planter's).
- Fruit chews (Skittles).
- Butterscotch squares and candy corn (Brock's).

Source: Tartrazine, *Nutrition and the MD*, January 1983.

Highlight 14 discusses the Feingold diet and other nutrition-centered approaches to hyperactivity in children.

More recently, the food color tartrazine has received a lot of publicity because it causes an allergic reaction in susceptible people. Symptoms include hives, itching, and nasal congestion, sometimes severe enough to require medical treatment. People who are allergic to aspirin are especially likely to be affected, but tartrazine sensitivity also occurs in people without aspirin allergy. It is not a common problem; only 1 or 2 in 10,000 individuals may have the reaction, but still, that is over 20,000 individuals in the nation as a whole, and these people rightly demand to know where the dye is in foods so that they can avoid it. It isn't enough to avoid yellow-colored foods, because tartrazine is used to confer turquoise, green, and maroon colors on foods and drugs as well.[10]

Tartrazine was for a while blamed for causing many (some people said most) cases of hyperactivity in children, and a special diet (the Feingold diet), composed entirely of additive-free foods, was recommended for these children. By 1980 it was clear that the majority of cases of hyperactivity are not caused by tartrazine or other additives, but legislation is now in force requiring that tartrazine must be mentioned on all labels of foods that contain it so that consumers can avoid it if they wish.

Artificial Flavors and Flavor Enhancers

While only 33 colors are currently permitted in foods, there are close to 2,000 flavoring agents, making them the largest single group of food additives. One of the best-known members of this group is monosodium glutamate, or MSG (trade name, Accent)—the monosodium salt of the amino acid glutamic acid. MSG is used widely in restaurants, especially Asian restaurants. It is a flavor enhancer; it has no flavor of its own, but increases the perception of flavor from the other substances present in food with it.[11] MSG has received publicity because it may produce an adverse reaction in some individuals—the so-called Chinese restaurant syndrome (already described in Highlight 9A). It has been investigated extensively enough to be deemed safe for adults to use (except people who react adversely to it), but is kept out of foods for infants because very large doses have been shown to destroy brain cells in developing mice.

Artificial Sweeteners

Artificial flavors have been less criticized than colors, perhaps because consumers understand the need for them better. Still, some consumers have challenged

The case of Chinese restaurant syndrome illustrates human suggestibility. No one really knows how common it is. First reported less than 20 years ago, it was at that time thought to be quite rare, but as more and more people have learned of it, more and more people have developed the impression that they suffer from it. Meanwhile, research of the 1980s seems to be demonstrating that MSG is not the only cause of the syndrome, and that most people who don't know they are eating MSG don't have the symptoms. Some skepticism is in order as to just how extensive the syndrome is, just what causes it, and just who has it or what else they might have.[12]

Miniglossary of Artificial Sweeteners

aspartame: a dipeptide (see p. 135) that tastes like the sugar sucrose but is 200 times sweeter. Being composed of amino acids, it has 4 kcal/g, as does protein, but because so little is used, it is virtually kcalorie-free. In powdered form it is mixed with lactose, however, so a 1-g packet contains 4 kcal. It is used in both the United States and Canada.

cyclamate: a 0-kcal sweetener used in Canada, but banned in the United States.

saccharin: a 0-kcal sweetener used in the United States but banned in Canada.

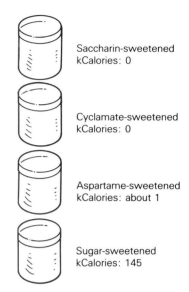

Saccharin-sweetened
kCalories: 0

Cyclamate-sweetened
kCalories: 0

Aspartame-sweetened
kCalories: about 1

Sugar-sweetened
kCalories: 145

Artificial sweeteners save kcalories, but are they safe?

The sugar alcohols (alternative sweeteners), which are caloric, are in a miniglossary on p. 77.

them, preferring that all artificial substances be omitted from foods. Among the most controversial of the artificial flavors are the sweeteners.

The big three synthetic sweeteners are saccharin, cyclamate, and aspartame. Saccharin has been around since before 1900, and dominated the market except for a brief two decades, the 1950s and 1960s, when cyclamate was in wide use. Aspartame was approved by the FDA in 1981, and rapidly began gaining the ascendancy over saccharin.[13]

The cases of saccharin and cyclamate illustrate some general points about additives and food safety that are worth a moment's attention here. Saccharin, used for nearly 100 years in the United States, is presently used by some 50 million Americans, primarily in soft drinks, and secondarily as a tabletop sweetener. Questions about its safety surfaced in 1977, when experiments suggested it caused bladder tumors in rats, and the FDA proposed banning it as a result. The public outcry in favor of retaining it was so loud, however, that Congress placed a moratorium on any action, and the moratorium has since been repeatedly renewed. Products containing saccharin are required to carry the warning label, now familiar to all consumers of diet beverages, that "use of this product may be hazardous to your health. This product contains saccharin, which has been determined to cause cancer in laboratory animals."

Does saccharin really cause cancer? The evidence that it does so in animals is as follows. When male and female rats are fed diets containing saccharin from the time of weaning to adulthood and then mated, and their offspring are also fed saccharin throughout life, the offspring have a higher tendency to develop bladder tumors than comparable animals not fed saccharin. The question was raised for a while whether an impurity in the saccharin used in the tests might be causing the tumors, but was resolved: the saccharin itself was responsible. It wasn't clear whether the tumors were cancerous. On the basis of these findings and in the face of public outcry as loud as that in the United States, Canada banned all uses of saccharin except as a tabletop sweetener to be sold in pharmacies, and permits those sales only with a warning label.

Saccharin has not been shown to cause cancer in human beings. Three large-scale population studies were completed in 1980. One, involving 9,000 people, showed a distinctly greater risk of cancers in some groups, such as women who drank two or more diet sodas a day and people who both smoked heavily and used artificial sweeteners heavily. Another study involving over 1,000 people showed little or no excess risk of bladder cancers, but of course could not conclude that there was no risk at all. As of now, two alternative conclusions are possible:

1. Saccharin causes tumors, possibly cancerous, in rats but not in people.
2. Saccharin is a weak carcinogen in people, and its effects will take more years of exposure to become apparent.

A 1985 review of the experimental and epidemiological evidence related to saccharin's potential to cause cancer concluded that alternative 1 was the more likely. Saccharin appears to cause cancers specifically in rats, and only in their bladders, and is not associated with an increased risk of bladder cancer in human beings.[14]

Cyclamate has had a shorter life than saccharin, dominating the artificial sweetener market for only 20 years. The 1970 ban on its use, although repeatedly appealed, has been continued even though, like saccharin, cyclamate has never been conclusively proven guilty of causing cancer in human beings. In Canada, on the other hand, where saccharin is banned, cyclamate is still in legal use.

As for aspartame, within only a few years of receiving the FDA's approval, it has appeared in dozens of familiar food products and in some totally new ones as well. Worldwide, people have gratefully accepted aspartame as NutraSweet in diet drinks, chewing gum, presweetened cereal, and pudding, and as Equal, a powder to use at home in place of sugar. By 1987, aspartame sales had already surpassed the sales of saccharin, and were also encroaching on sugar sales in some markets.

This amazing popularity is mostly due to aspartame's flavor, which is almost identical to that of sugar. Another lure drawing us to aspartame: the hope that it may be completely harmless, unlike the other sweeteners whose laboratory records are tarnished. Too, aspartame is touted as safe for children, so families wishing to limit sugar are turning to it. Finally, as a sweet-toothed, overweight population, we perceive sugar substitutes as our only way to cheat the scales.

Aspartame is a simple chemical compound: a dipeptide, consisting of the two amino acids, phenylalanine and aspartic acid, joined together with a methyl group attached to the acid end. In the digestive tract, the two amino acids are split apart, absorbed, and used to build protein or burned for energy, just as they would be if they had come from protein in food. The flavors of the components give no clue to the combined effect; one of the amino acids tastes bitter, and the other is tasteless. But aspartame is incredibly sweet—200 times sweeter than sucrose.

The FDA has approved aspartame based on the assumption that no one will consume more than 34 milligrams per kilogram of their body weight in a day. People with PKU have a special warning to limit their intakes.

Years ago, all babies born with PKU were condemned to suffer severe mental retardation caused by phenylalanine buildup, which prevented normal brain development. Today, almost all infants born in developed countries undergo a simple blood test for PKU. If found to have the condition, an infant is raised on a diet free of excess phenylalanine and so develops normally. Since phenylalanine is one of the essential amino acids, the child still needs to take in a little, just enough to cover the need for building new body proteins. Although complicated, the diet is absolutely necessary in the control of PKU, and the consequences of noncompliance are devastating. Luckily, the special diet need only

Structure of aspartame.

Aspartic Acid   Phenylalanine   Methyl Group

PKU (phenylketonuria): the hereditary inability to dispose of the amino acid phenylalanine when it is eaten in excess of the need for building proteins.

continue until the brain and nervous system have reached full maturity. At that time, phenylalanine still builds up in the body, but can do no damage. About 1 in every 10,000 children is born with PKU; 2 more in 10,000 carry a gene that can convey PKU to their children.

This condition poses problems with regard to aspartame. First, and most obviously, children with PKU cannot use unlimited amounts of the sweetener. They can use some, because they need phenylalanine, but there is a compelling reason why they should not get their phenylalanine from this source. Phenylalanine occurs in such protein-rich and nutrient-rich foods as milk and meat, and the PKU child is allowed only a limited amount of these foods. Such a child can obtain only with difficulty the many essential nutrients—such as calcium, iron, and the B vitamins—found along with phenylalanine in these foods. To suggest that this child squander any of the limited phenylalanine allowance on the purified phenylalanine of aspartame, with none of the associated vitamins or minerals essential for good health and normal growth, would be to invite risk of malnutrition.

The woman with PKU who becomes pregnant must, once again, avoid excess phenylalanine in her diet. If an excess should build up in her body, it will also cause an excess to build up in the developing fetus, causing brain damage whether or not the baby has PKU. This requirement to limit phenylalanine puts the pregnant woman in a serious bind, for her need for nutrients peaks to the highest known in adult human beings. She cannot afford to eat "empty" phenylalanine, that is, phenylalanine without the nutrients that accompany it in protein-rich foods. People with PKU need to know which old, familiar products now contain aspartame, and how to avoid them.

Another concern about aspartame's safety has to do with the methyl group it carries on its acid end. Hydrolyzed from the dipeptide during metabolism in the body, the methyl group becomes methyl alcohol (methanol) momentarily—a toxic compound. Then it is oxidized to formaldehyde, another toxic compound, and finally to carbon dioxide. The quantities generated from normal use of aspartame are below the threshold at which these compounds cause harm, but in the testing of aspartame, that threshold had to be determined and its acceptability evaluated.

Still another concern is about the product aspartame breaks down to—diketopiperazine, or DKP for short. Long-term studies using animals have directly tested this product and eliminated it as a source of concern. Still another concern was over the effect changed amino acid concentrations might have on the levels of neurotransmitters in the brain. Experiments with rats, monkeys, and human beings were performed, and none showed any cause for concern. The monkey study involved infant monkeys given up to 3,000 milligrams of aspartame per kilogram of body weight for nine months and showed no ill effects on growth, development, health, or behavior either during the test or on withdrawal of aspartame.[15] The conclusion reached was that aspartame is safe except for people with PKU. Some 500 individual complaints received after its approval were reviewed by the Centers for Disease Control, which concluded that some individuals may exhibit vague, but not dangerous symptoms due to unusual sensitivity to aspartame, but that the product can still be considered generally safe.[16]

The maximum intake of 34 milligrams per kilogram of body weight, assumed by the FDA, is a lot. For a 132-pound person, it adds up to 60 packets of Equal.

What becomes of the methyl group of aspartame.

diketopiperazine (dye-KEY-toe-pie-PER-a-zeen): a product to which aspartame breaks down during metabolism.

About 11 soft drinks sweetened only with aspartame provide this maximum amount. G. D. Searle and Company estimates that if all the sugar and saccharin in the U.S. diet were replaced with aspartame, 1 percent of the population would be consuming the FDA maximum.[17] Some people actually do consume this amount, however. A child who drinks a quart of artificially sweetened fruit-flavored beverage on a hot day, and who has pudding, chewing gum, cereal, and other products with aspartame that day, too, packs in more than the FDA maximum level.

In an attempt to give a guideline for a safe level of aspartame intake, an advisory group to the World Health Organization has recommended a maximum of 40 milligrams per kilogram of body weight per day for adults.[18] A much more conservative limit of three to four packets of Equal per day is suggested by the Canadian Diabetes Association as a safe and useful level.[19] The newsletter for physicians *Nutrition and the MD* states that it is not known if aspartame is safe for children under two years old, and points out that there are "very few if any reasons to use a sugar substitute in infants and young children."[20] Until aspartame has been around for a longer time, it would be best not to let infants be unwitting "testers" of its safety.

Artificial sweeteners whose use may become more common in the future are the so-called left-handed sugars, or L-sugars. A sugar is an asymmetrical molecule (as a hand is an asymmetrical body part), and so it can theoretically occur in two shapes that are mirror-images of each other (as the right and left hands are). Those found naturally in plants are the right-handed, or D-sugars, and the body's enzymes and absorptive machinery are equipped to handle them. L-sugars are just as sweet as D-sugars, and they mix well into baked goods, but they pass through the body unchanged, offering no kcalories. The most promising of the L-sugars appears to be L-fructose, shown in the margin.

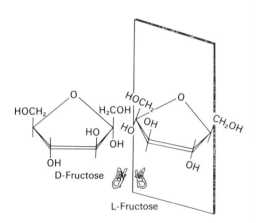

L-sugar: a mirror-image of natural sugar, unutilizable by the body. The L version of naturally occurring D-glucose (dextrose) is L-glucose; the L version of fructose (D-fructose) is L-fructose (levulose).
dextro = right
levulo = left

Antimicrobial Agents

Foods can go bad in two ways: one dangerous, one not. The dangerous way is by becoming hazardous to health; the other way is by losing their attractiveness. An example of the former: molds, bacteria, fungi, and yeasts growing in foods can cause food poisoning either by producing infections or by producing deadly toxins. Preservatives known as antimicrobial agents protect foods from these microbes.

The best-known, most widely used antimicrobial agents are the two common substances salt and sugar. Salt has been used since before recorded history to preserve meat and fish; sugar serves the same purpose in canned and frozen fruits, as well as jams and jellies. (Any jam or jelly that toots its "no preservatives" horn is lying.) Both salt and sugar work by withdrawing water from the food; microbes can't grow without water. Today, other additives such as potassium sorbate and sodium propionate are also used to extend the shelf life of baked goods, cheese, beverages, mayonnaise, margarine, and many other products.

Another preservative is sodium nitrite, added to foods for three main purposes: to preserve their color (especially the pink color of hot dogs and other cured meats), to enhance their flavor by inhibiting rancidity (especially in cured meats), and to protect against bacterial growth. In particular, nitrite prevents the growth of the bacteria that produce the deadly botulinum toxin, the most potent biological poison known. An amount of this toxin as tiny as a single

Two long-used preservatives.

nitrite: a salt added to food to prevent botulism.

botulinum (bot-you-LINE-um) **toxin:** a toxin produced by bacteria that grow in meat, which causes **botulism** (bott-you-lism), a form of food poisoning.

crystal of salt can kill several people within an hour, and in survivors, troublesome aftereffects linger for months.

Nitrites are important additives, and it seems that no others, at present can do the precise combination of jobs they do; but they have been the object of much controversy, because they can be converted in the human body to nitrosamines, and nitrosamines cause cancer in animals. The dilemma is not resolved as yet, but is the subject of continuing controversy. Strategies for avoiding food poisoning by botulinum toxin are offered in the last section of this chapter.

Antioxidants

The other way in which food can go bad is by undergoing changes in color and flavor caused by exposure to air (oxidation). Oftentimes, these changes involve no hazard to health, but they damage the food's quality. Familiar examples of these changes are the ways sliced apples or potatoes turn brown, or oil goes rancid. Preservatives known as antioxidants protect food from this kind of spoilage.

A total of 27 antioxidants are approved for use in foods. Vitamin C (ascorbate) and vitamin E (tocopherol) are among them. Another group of preservatives is the sulfites, cheaper than the vitamins and used in many foods and drugs to prevent oxidation. Until recently, they were especially popular on salad bars, because they could keep raw fruits and vegetables looking fresh. Unfortunately, in the process of freshening, sulfiting agents destroy an appreciable amount of the vitamin thiamin in foods. Also, they cause adverse reactions in people who have asthma or allergies—reactions that can sometimes be dangerous. The FDA has taken a number of steps to protect people who are allergic to sulfites. It has also removed six sulfiting agents from the GRAS list; restaurants are no longer allowed to use them on their salads; and fruit and vegetable suppliers many not use sulfiting agents on the wares they display. Sulfites are still used in beer, wine, and packaged foods, however, and full-disclosure labeling is not required.

Two other antioxidants in wide use are the well-known BHA and BHT,* which prevent rancidity in baked goods and snack foods. BHT provides a refreshing contrast with the negative reputations of many of the other additives. Among the many tests that were performed on BHT were several showing that animals fed large amounts of this substance developed *less* cancer when exposed to carcinogens and lived *longer* than controls. BHT apparently protects against

Nitrosamines (nigh-TROHS-uh-meens) are derivatives of nitrites that may be formed in the stomach when nitrites combine with amines; and nitrosamines are carcinogenic.

$$H^+ + NO_2^- \longrightarrow HNO_2$$

From acid   Nitrite   Nitrous acid

In an acid environment such as the stomach, nitrite salts form nitrous acid. One nitrite salt is sodium nitrite, used to preserve meats.

$$O=N-O-H + H-\overset{|}{N}- \longrightarrow O=N-\overset{|}{N}-$$

Nitrous acid   Amine   Nitrosamine

Nitrous acid reacts with amines to form nitrosamines. Amines are numerous in foods. (Water, H-O-H, is a byproduct.)

> This story provides the opportunity to mention an important point about additives. No two additives are alike, and therefore generalizations about them are meaningless. No valid statement can be made that applies to all of the 3,000-odd different substances commonly added to foods. Questions about which additives are safe, under what conditions of use, have to be asked and answered on an item-by-item basis.

*Butylhydroxyanisole and butylhydroxytoluene.

cancer in two ways. It prevents carcinogens from binding to DNA, and it induces the liver to produce enzymes that destroy carcinogens. The effects occur at a concentration similar to that actually used for BHT in food.[21]

Nutrient Additives

Another class of additives is nutrients added to improve or maintain the nutritional value of foods. Included among these are the four nutrients added to refined grains to enrich them (see p. 27), the iodine added to salt, vitamins A and D added to dairy products, and the nutrients added to fortified breakfast cereals. Nutrients are sometimes also added for other purposes. Vitamins C and E are examples: both are antioxidants and are added to foods to help keep them from spoiling. Vitamin E may be added to bacon to prevent nitrosamine formation while not interfering with the antibotulinal activity of nitrite.

Irradiation

A certain kind of radiation is an additive, too. It has long been known that radiation will kill living cells; and a practical application of this is to use it in food processing. It kills microorganisms and insect pests, inhibits the growth of sprouts on potatoes and onions, and delays ripening in some fruits. The type of radiation used is called ionizing radiation, and it can be generated in several ways.*

Irradiating does not make foods radioactive; it takes stronger doses of radiation to do that. It is easier on foods than heat-sterilizing, leaving them attractive with their texture undisturbed and their flavor altered very little, if at all. Many different kinds of testing have revealed that there is no hazard to the consumer in foods that have been irradiated. It is economically feasible and has been judged promising by both national and international organizations.

Radiation works by destroying parts of the cells' machinery (DNA and RNA) that are involved in reproduction and growth. In the process, it produces other substances that remain in the food after the treatment is over. These are not unlike the substances that are found in food anyway, but a few are unique, and these have been carefully studied. Realistically, they too appear to present no hazard.[22] The unique radiolytic products (URPs) are the same, regardless of what food is being irradiated, so the results of tests that have been done on a few foods apply to other foods as well.

The FDA approves irradiation as a food-processing method and has published regulations to govern its use.[23] As of 1986, legislation was in place establishing limits on the amounts of radiation to be used for various purposes and requiring retail foods that had been irradiated to identify themselves with a logo and the statement that they had been "picowaved."[24] Before long, irradiation may well be an important part of our food-preserving techniques.

URP (unique radiolytic product): a product formed during the irradiation of food.

A food bearing the statement that it has been **picowaved** (PYE-coh-waved) is an irradiated food.

---

*Ionizing rays include X rays, gamma rays, and beta rays (electrons). Radiation sources include gamma ray emitters and electron accelerators. *Irradiated Foods,* a report by the American Council on Science and Health, October 1982, available from the council at 1995 Broadway, New York, NY 10023.

All that has been said so far has indicated that, on the whole, the use of food additives seems to be justified by the benefits they offer, and that the risks associated with their use are small. All intentional additives are closely regulated and monitored. There are questions about their approval and regulation, though, especially with respect to additives suspected of causing cancer, and Highlight 13A pursues the matter further.

Incidental Food Additives

Classed as incidental, accidental, or indirect additives are all substances that find their way into food as the result of some phase of production, processing, storage, or packaging. For example, packaging materials may become indirect additives when small amounts drift into the food. Among indirect additives are tiny bits of plastic, glass, paper, tin, and other substances from packages, as well as chemicals from processing, such as the solvent used to decaffeinate coffee.

Incidental additives are well regulated, just as intentional additives are. All food packagers are required to perform specific tests to discover whether materials from production, processing, storage, or packaging are migrating into foods; if they are, their safety must be confirmed by strict procedures similar to those governing intentional additives. Contamination sometimes occurs, but adverse effects are very rare.

Incidental additives are substances that find their way into food as a result of production, processing, storage, or packaging.

Pesticides and Other Agricultural Chemicals

Pesticides are in a class by themselves. They are chosen for use specifically because they are biological poisons, but they are like food additives in that they are used intentionally. Ideally, each pesticide is used in such a way that it is maximally effective against the insect or other crop pest it is aimed at, and then "disappears." That is, by the time the food is used, no residue remains that will be harmful to the user. In reality, pesticide use can seldom be so selective or well controlled, and there is reason for concern that unwanted, sometimes hazardous pesticide residues drift onto other crops, pollute the water, contaminate the soil, and accumulate in the tissues of animals. The largest contributor of pesticides to the environment is commercial agriculture, but individual homeowners and gardeners add significantly to the total. Table 13–1 lists a sampling of pesticides and their biological effects.

When pesticides were first used, it was considered desirable to use persistent ones—that is, those that would not get washed away or chemically altered—because they would control pests the longest. One of the most satisfactory pesticides from this point of view was DDT. Then it became apparent that DDT's persistence created problems. It began to show up in high concentrations in the fatty tissues of animals. It was shown to be a threat to the survival of the American eagle, whose eggs became too fragile to protect new chicks as a result of DDT poisoning. It turned up in big fish, in carnivorous animals, and in

Grouped with pesticides as agricultural chemicals are:
• Herbicides.
• Insecticides.
• Fungicides.
• Rodenticides.
• Growth regulators.
• Fruiting agents.
• Defoliants.

TABLE 13-1

A Sampling of Pesticides and Their Biological Effects

Type of use	Common names (examples)	Biological effects
Insecticides	Parathion, Malathion	Toxic to nerves; acute poisoning causes respiratory failure.
	Aldicarb, Zectran	Toxic to nerves.
	DDT, Dieldrin, Heptachlor, Chlordane, Mirex	Accumulate in fatty tissues, inhibit electrolyte transport, impair reproduction in birds.
	Ethylene dibromide (EDB)	A carcinogen.
Herbicides	2, 4, 5-T	Toxic generally and to nerves.
	Paraquat	Toxic generally, causes edema in the lungs.
	Prophan	Allergenic.
	Simazine	Carcinogenic.
Fungicides	Captan	Causes birth defects.
	Pentachlorophenol (PCP)	Toxic generally.
Rodenticides	Warfarin	An anticoagulant.
	Red squill	Causes heart failure.
	Compounds 1080, 1081	Inhibit TCA cycle.
	ANTU	Causes edema in the lungs.

Source: Adapted from M. G. Mustafa, Agricultural chemicals, in *Adverse Effects of Foods,* by E. F. P. Jelliffe and D. B. Jelliffe (New York: Plenum Press, 1982), Table 1, pp. 112–113.

human beings, including human breast milk. Finally, in 1972, its widescale agricultural use was banned, and since then the search for less hazardous, less persistent, but still effective pesticides has been intense.

Since the 1960's, both national and international agencies have adopted regulations and standards intended to regulate pesticide use. Chief among these are the Food and Agricultural Organization (FAO), the World Health Organization (WHO), and domestically, the Environmental Protection Agency (EPA) and the FDA. Pesticide use worldwide is increasing and is not well monitored; the hazards may be considerable and are unknown.

In the United States, EPA and other agencies are supposed to establish residue tolerances for pesticides, based on lifetime exposure. Most have margins of safety as do additives. Monitoring activities include sampling of residue concentrations in tissues of fish, birds, and mammals, water, air, foods, and human beings.[25] Pesticides always appear, but appear to be within the limits established by FAO and WHO. There are loopholes and flaws in the law, however. Maximum residues allowed in a commodity assume people will eat moderate quantities of each commodity; they don't always do so.[26] The tests used do not necessarily detect residues of all the pesticides currently in use. When one pesticide is banned, another quickly takes its place, sometimes before regulations and monitoring procedures are firmly in place. Furthermore, toxicity to nerves does not always make itself known right away; sometimes it lies in wait and then causes symptoms long after the initial exposure.[27] The concern that hazards from pesticide use, especially in the developing countries, are growing is a valid concern. It is hoped that sufficient resources will be dedicated to the control of this problem in the future.

On occasion, there are episodes of gross contamination such as spills, accidental mixing of poisons into animal or human feed, illegal overuse, and the like. Then pesticides, like other toxins, become deadly contaminants; and the discussion in the later section, "Contaminants," applies (see p. 461).

Natural Toxicants in Foods

Many commonly used plants and plant products contain naturally occurring toxicants. Poisonous mushrooms are a familiar example; but did you know that a number of common foods have been observed to cause toxic effects?

- Cabbage, mustard, and other plants contain goitrogens, which can enlarge the thyroid gland.
- Potatoes contain solanine, a powerful inhibitor of nerve impulses; the margin of safety, assuming ordinary consumption of potatoes, is $1/10$.
- Spinach and rhubarb contain oxalates, tolerable as usually consumed; but one normal serving of rhubarb contains one-fifth the toxic dose for humans.
- Honey can be a host to the botulinum organism and can accumulate enough toxin to kill an infant.[28]

There are 700 other examples of plants that—as used—have caused serious illnesses or deaths in the Western hemisphere.[29] In contrast, no case of a death or illness has been reported from the use of an additive at levels permitted legally in food.[30]

Some fish are also naturally toxic, presenting a range of hazards from mild illness to instant death. A well-known environmental scientist has said, "One can predict that if the standards used to test manmade chemicals were applied to 'natural' foods, fully half of the human food supply would have to be banned."[31]

Nutrition

How well do we eat? We who live in the United States and Canada are among the richest people in the world: are we also the best nourished? Or are we, as some people say, malnourished under a cloak of fat—overfed, underexercised, and beset with nutrient deficiencies?

Two scientific ways to ask that question are available. One is to determine what foods we eat, calculate or measure the nutrients in them, and compare the amounts of nutrients consumed with a standard such as the RDA—a food

food consumption survey: a survey in which the amounts and kinds of foods people consume are measured, the nutrients calculated, and the nutrient intakes compared with a standard such as the RDA.

nutrition status survey: a survey in which the nutrition status of people is evaluated using diet histories, anthropometric measures, physical examinations, and laboratory tests.

consumption survey. The other way is to assess the nutrition status of the people themselves, using diet histories, anthropometric measures, physical examinations, and laboratory tests as described in Chapter 1—a nutrition status survey. Both kinds of surveys have been conducted many times since before World War Two. The picture has been mixed, from the beginning: yes, we are well nourished; and yes, we are fat, underexercised, and perhaps even beset to some extent with nutrient deficiencies. The picture has also been changing, with major trends taking place. People eat out, now, much more often then they did 50 years ago. They eat far more processed and convenience foods, and they eat fewer whole, farm-type foods. This brief section on nutrition status first reviews the major survey findings from the past 50 years, then attempts to apply them to individuals and suggest some strategies for obtaining optimal nutrition in today's world.

Surveys of Nutrition Status

Before World War Two, a food-consumption survey suggested that as many as a third of the U.S. population might be poorly fed. During the 1940s, 1950s, and 1960s, many further surveys confirmed this impression. Nutrients found lacking in subgroups of the population were the minerals calcium and iron, the B vitamins thiamin and riboflavin, vitamin A, and occasionally vitamin C. Most vulnerable to nutrient deficiencies were girls, women, and elderly men; but no group was without some cases of iron deficiency. Other nutrients now known to be important—vitamin B_6, folacin, magnesium, and zinc, for example—were not studied in the early surveys.

During the 1970s, hunger and malnutrition in the United States came to the public's awareness from the Ten-State (National Nutrition) Survey, conducted in the late 1960s (1968 to 1970). The ten states surveyed were California, Kentucky, Louisiana, Massachusetts, Michigan, South Carolina, Texas, Washington, New York, and West Virginia. The areas within the states were chosen to represent geographic, ethnic, and other features of the whole United States, but to over-represent poverty, so as to be sure to detect nutrition problems associated with it. More than 60,000 people were included.

The survey included diet histories, physical examinations, and laboratory tests of nutrition status. The physical examinations revealed few severe deficiencies, but iron nutrition was a problem in all groups, especially among blacks; and vitamin A status was a major concern, especially among teenagers and Hispanics. Riboflavin deficiency appeared to be a potential problem, especially among blacks, Hispanics, and young people of all ethnic groups. Protein deficiency was not widespread but was seen in the poor; pregnant women and those who were breastfeeding their babies had lower protein intakes and lower blood levels of protein than most other groups. Many nutrients were not studied, including vitamin B_6, folacin, magnesium, and zinc.

Indicators of nutrient deficiencies tended to cluster together. A person deficient in iron was likely to lack vitamin A as well, for example. Generally, blacks and Hispanics had a higher incidence of multiple deficiencies; a higher incidence also occurred in the low-income states. An important finding was that in families in which the homemaker had completed fewer years of school, there were more multiple low values in the family members. Importantly, too, trends seen among the children were also seen in adults in the same families.

Anthropometric measures revealed that people who were less economically deprived had greater height, weight, fatness, skeletal weight, and other indicators of earlier and greater physical development. Blacks were taller than whites and were more advanced in skeletal and dental development, probably reflecting their genetic endowment, not socioeconomic status. Obesity was more prominent in adult women, especially in black women.

Sugar intakes were high in most groups, and high sugar intakes were often seen together with dental decay, especially in adolescents. Low income accompanied dental decay in all groups. The identification of vulnerable groups confirmed the need for programs of many kinds to decrease the risk and incidence of nutrient deficiencies, as well as the need for continued surveillance of the U.S. population's nutrition status.

The Ten-State Survey had a built-in bias: it oversampled among the poor. Still, it provided a disturbing answer to the question, How well do we eat? Clearly, not as well as might be expected in the most prosperous nation in the world.

During the early 1970s, Canada conducted a major survey of its people. Over 19,000 people of all ages and all economic levels had medical, dental, and anthropometric examinations and a dietary interview; most also provided blood and urine samples for analysis. Among the findings were:

- A high incidence of problems with nutrition status in lower-income middle-aged women and older men.
- A negative effect of low economic status on blood levels of certain nutrients, especially vitamin C and folacin.
- Evidence of iron-deficiency anemia in young and middle-aged women and elderly men.
- Evidence of low thiamin intakes in adolescents and middle-aged adults, with some associated biochemical evidence of deficiency.
- Considerable obesity, especially in middle-aged adults.
- A greater risk of deficiency of many nutrients among Indian and Inuit people than among the general population surveyed.

Obesity is widespread, both in Canada and in the United States.

These findings resembled those of the U.S. surveys in the extent of malnutrition, if not in the details. They illustrate that poor nutrition is indeed a problem in the developed countries.

At about the same time (1971 to 1974), the U.S. National Center for Health Statistics conducted a study of over 20,000 people at 65 sampling sites in the United States. This study, known as the HANES (Health and Nutrition Examination Survey), avoided the bias of the Ten-State Survey by adjusting for the effects of oversampling among vulnerable groups. Careful efforts were also made to evaluate protein and energy intakes in relation to height, sex, and age on an individual basis.

The investigators studied intakes of the same seven nutrients as in the Ten-State Survey, and niacin and food energy intakes in addition. Nutrient deficiencies were found for protein, calcium, vitamin A, and iron. As expected, these were more extensive among people below the poverty line than among those above, and they were generally more extensive in blacks than in whites. Among generalizations that emerged:

- Calcium intakes were low for adult black women of all income groups.
- Vitamin A intakes were low for adolescent black girls of all income groups.

■ Iron intakes were low for all women and for infant boys regardless of income.

HANES II, undertaken in 1977 as a follow-up to the HANES, was designed to collect biochemical and other data with the question in mind; Are the low nutrient intakes found earlier reflected in the physical condition of the subjects? Particularly, the investigators wondered whether lab test results would reflect the extensive low iron intakes known to exist in the population. Indeed, malnutrition was found:

■ Low blood values for protein and vitamin A in up to 3 percent of subjects.
■ Low values for thiamin in up to 14 percent of white and 29 percent of black subjects.
■ Low values for riboflavin in up to 3 percent of white and 8 percent of black subjects.
■ Low iron values, by three measures, in 5 to 15 percent of white and 18 to 27 percent of black subjects.

Not everyone with low intakes of a nutrient had low lab values, and the investigators suggested that some of those with low intakes were at the very beginning stages of deficiency—"at risk" for malnutrition.

In measuring the heights and weights of people, the HANES researchers observed a continuing trend toward higher amounts of body fat among fatter Americans. The trend toward higher weights in Americans reflects overnutrition, not "good" nutrition.

Caution has to be exercised in interpreting the HANES study. On the one hand, when average nutrient intakes are looked at, severe deficiencies in individuals can be missed. On the other hand, findings based on a single day's intake—as the HANES findings were—can overestimate the extent of undernutrition. These two limitations of the HANES tend to cancel each other out. The survey's principal usefulness is in identifying the population subgroups most at risk of deficiency and the nutrients most in need of attention.

Further study is needed. In particular, the choice of indicator nutrients should be reexamined. Inadequate intakes may be more prevalent for vitamin B_6, zinc, magnesium, and folacin than for many of the nutrients usually covered in earlier surveys.

Following HANES, another survey—the Nationwide Food Consumption Survey—was conducted by the United States Department of Agriculture (USDA) in 1977 to 1978, to see how much and what kind of food people were eating at home and outside the home. Both surveys, as well as the Canadian survey, confirmed a dawning suspicion: that in spite of widespread obesity, people are not eating large amounts of kcalories. They are fat and getting fatter, but their food intakes are quite modest. This must mean that they are extraordinarily inactive. The average woman consuming the foods typically available to her, who stays within the kcalorie allowance that will maintain her weight, will fail to obtain recommended amounts of several nutrients. Figure 13–1 compares the energy intakes found with those recommended.

The USDA Nationwide Food Consumption Survey, like the Ten-State Survey, showed dietary adequacy related to income. Table 13–2 shows the results for six nutrients. People with lower incomes had lower intakes of five of them. Since 19 million people in the United States are now living at or below the poverty line, these nutrition problems are quite widespread.

FIGURE 13–1

Energy intakes found in the HANES Survey, compared with the recommended intakes.

Source: D. M. Hegsted, Agricultural potentials, in *Plasma Lipids: Optimal Levels for Health,* ed. American Health Foundation (New York: Academic Press, 1980), pp. 143–153; Table 1, p. 144.

Folacin and zinc intakes were not assessed in the Nationwide Food Consumption Survey; insufficient data are available on food contents of these nutrients and on the factors in food that affect their assimilation and use by the body. When further research makes it possible to include these two nutrients in a survey, it will be highly desirable to do so, because deficiencies of both nutrients are suspected in our population.

The survey data were analyzed not only with respect to nutrient intakes but also—in light of the modern concern with overnutrition—with respect to sodium, fat, sugar, and cholesterol intakes. Sodium intakes were not accurately determined, but the following findings were of interest:

■ Very few of those surveyed had fat intakes below the recommended maximum of 30 percent of kcalories.

TABLE 13-2

Persons with Nutrient Intakes At or Below 70 Percent of RDA

Nutrient	Income to $6,000	Income $6,000 to $9,999	Income $10,000 to $15,999	Income $16,000 and Over
Vitamin A	36%	33%	32%	29%
Vitamin B₆[a]	59	51	49	48
Vitamin C	30	29	27	23
Calcium	49	43	39	39
Iron	29	31	33	33
Magnesium	48	40	36	35

Data represent percentage of persons in each income group with intakes at or below 70% of RDA. Example: 36% of all those surveyed whose incomes were at or below $6,000 per year had vitamin A intakes at or below 70% of the RDA.

[a]Vitamin B₆ intakes may not be as deficient as they appear. People who get along on minimal protein intakes need less than the RDA of vitamin B₆ to handle the amount of protein they consume.

Source: USDA Nationwide Food Consumption Survey, 1977–1978.

- Sugar constituted 10 to 15 percent of the kcalorie intakes of most children. (It should probably not exceed 10 percent.)
- Cholesterol intakes ranged up to 450 to 500 milligrams per day in boys and men. (A suggested upper limit is 300 milligrams.)

These findings provide a base of information about our people's food choices that was not available before.

The Nationwide Food Consumption Survey also revealed that all our citizens seemed to be eating from a common table. In other words, most people are eating similar kinds and amounts of food. Probably, therefore, guidelines stated in terms of these foods would benefit everyone.

Most recently, the USDA Household Survey was conducted to determine how people's eating patterns changed between 1950 and 1980. Apparently, people are much more aware than they once were of the health values of certain foods. Three out of five households changed their eating habits within a three-year period during the survey as the result of their new health consciousness, making decisions to:

- Eat more poultry, low-fat milk, and fresh fruits and vegetables.
- Eat fewer eggs.
- Drink less coffee and whole milk.
- Avoid foods containing cholesterol and some additives, particularly salt.

Ironically, though, people are simultaneously eating more sweets and drinking more soft drinks than ever before. In fact, soft drinks have become America's number one beverage, and 80 percent of them are the sugar-containing kind. Only 20 percent are artificially sweetened.[32]

Information is still rolling in from ongoing analyses of the data from the most recent surveys and the same general impressions are being confirmed. People are overconsuming kcalories, under expending energy, or both. The majority are adequately nourished with respect to most individual nutrients, but deficiencies and marginal intakes of nutrients do exist. The remedy for these nutrition problems can be stated in a single sentence: consume less fat, sugar, and salt; choose more foods high in fiber and nutrients relative to their kcalories; and exercise regularly so as to afford a food energy intake sufficient to convey the needed nutrients.

This advice is easy to understand, but a modern trend makes it harder to follow than might be expected. Many of the foods available today are processed, convenience, and fast foods, whose nutrient contributions are not obvious at first sight. The next section develops a nutrition strategy that offers perspective on these foods.

Personal Nutrition Strategy

In Chapter 2, two imaginary people's food choices were introduced and used to illustrate some differences in the nutritional value of meals (see Figure 2–5). Among other differences, one person ate three meat-centered meals (these were called the "Poor Choice" meals), the other ate according to the Four Food Group Plan but added large amounts of vegetables (these were called the "Preferred Choice" meals). Both days' meals presented about 1,800 kcalories, both had approximately equal amounts of protein, and both offered a brownie for

The "Poor Choice" meals

dessert, but that is where the resemblance ended. The meat-centered meals derived about 50 percent of their food energy from fat; the vegetable-eater's meals had less than half that much fat. The meat-centered person ate eggs for breakfast, beef for lunch, and beef for dinner—all animal-protein foods laden with saturated fat. The vegetable-minded person ate no animal-protein food for breakfast except milk, used a modest 2 ounces of cheese for lunch, and chose fish for dinner—a source of polyunsaturated fat.

The meat-centered person thought of meals as consisting of "meat-starch-vegetable/fruit." All three meals followed that pattern. Breakfast was eggs-toast-orange juice; lunch was hamburger-bun-french fries; dinner was steak-potato-lettuce. The vegetable person thought in terms of the Four Food Group Plan and met or exceeded all of its recommendations as follows:

- 2 or more cups milk: 2 ½ cups nonfat milk.
- 2 servings meat: 2 ounces cheese (lunch), 3 ounces fish (dinner).
- 4 or more servings vegetables or fruits: The day's food portions included 4 fruits and 7 half-cup portions of vegetables.
- 4 or more servings whole-grain or enriched breads and cereals: 2 cups of whole grains and a brownie.

The meat-centered person probably was able to consume the meals in only a few bites with very little chewing. This is not a scientific estimate, but a hearty eater might be able to put away the breakfast in 15 bites, the lunch in 15, and the dinner in 35 bites. Only the steak required any serious chewing. The vegetable-minded person might have managed breakfast in 15 bites also, but would doubt-less have required four times that many—with considerable chewing—to put away the 4 cups of food on the luncheon menu, and would have needed at least as many at dinner as well. The contrast points up a major difference between the two sets of meals: the meat-centered meals occupied little space and took little time to eat, while the vegetable-eater's meals were high in bulk and took considerable time to eat.

The "Preferred Choice" meals also took time to prepare. To ease the vegetable eater's task on a busy day, we permitted the use of frozen vegetables, but often a person who chooses to eat this way also spends time cleaning, peeling, and slicing the vegetables that go into such meals. The fruits were fresh; the straw-berries took time to prepare. (The cantaloupe, however, was as fast a food as any milkshake). All in all, the vegetable eater invested more time and energy preparing and eating the day's meals than did the meat-centered person.

It remains to ask how well the two people fared, nutritionally—aside from the protein/fat/carbohydrate comparisons already made. A comparison of the nutrient contributions made by the two people's meals is shown in Table 13–3 and reveals that the vegetable eater's meals were superior in many respects. Take vitamins, for example. Compared with the meat-centered person, the vegetable eater had about the same number of kcalories, but more of almost every vitamin:

- Thiamin, thanks to the larger number of servings of nutritious foods.
- Riboflavin, thanks to the superior intakes of milk and vegetables.
- Vitamins A and C, thanks to the multitude of vegetables and fruits.

Both had equal amounts of niacin and vitamin B_6, because they had equal amounts of protein, although from different sources, and these vitamins tend to accompany protein in foods. The niacin intakes were actually 90 percent of

The "Preferred Choice" meals

TABLE 13-3

Comparison of Preferred versus Poor Choice Meals

	"Poor Choices" (Meat-Centered Meals)	"Preferred Choices" (Four Food Group plus added Vegetables)	Standard for Comparison (U.S. RDA)[a]
Thiamin	1.1 mg	1.5 mg	1.5 mg
Riboflavin	1.6 mg	2.1 mg	1.7 mg
Niacin	18.4 mg	18.1 mg	20 mg
Vitamin B_6	1.6 mg	1.7 mg	2.0 mg
Folacin	253 μg	294 μg	400 μg
Vitamin A	520 RE	4,295 RE	1,000 RE
Vitamin C	93 mg	195 mg	60 mg
Calcium	357 mg	1,459 mg	1,000 mg
Iron	15 mg	11 mg	18 mg[b]
Magnesium	384 mg	411 mg	400 mg
Potassium	2,652 mg	3,785 mg	1,875-5,625[a]
Zinc	15 mg	11 mg	15 mg
Fiber	10 g	48 g	20-30 g[a]
Cholesterol	761 mg	191 mg	<300 mg[a]

Meals were those described and illustrated in Figure 2-5 of Chapter 2.

[a]Standard for comparison in the case of potassium is the recommended safe and adequate daily dietary intake. In the case of fiber, it is a suggested intake. In the case of cholesterol, it is a *Dietary Guideline* (see Chapter 2).

[b]The menstruating woman's RDA is 18 mg, the man's is 10 mg. Thus, this person, if a man, has ample iron; if a woman, may need to take iron supplements or exercise more to earn more kcalories and then spend them on more good iron sources.

the RDA, but the protein intakes from these meals were more than adequate, so additional niacin was derived from the extra protein (see p. 308). Both had equal amounts of folacin: the meat-centered person, thanks to the ¼-head lettuce eaten for dinner; the vegetable eater from all sources.

Next, consider minerals. The vegetable eater received less iron from the day's foods, again because of the lack of meat, but would absorb the iron well, thanks to the abundant vitamin C that accompanied it in the meals. The vegetable eater's zinc intakes also fell a little short, relative to the meat eater's intakes. Magnesium intakes were about the same for both, but the vegetable eater had far superior calcium intakes—1,459 milligrams, in fact, nearly twice the RDA, the amount recommended for women to prevent osteoporosis. Of these 1,459 milligrams, 1,162 came from the 2 ½ cups of nonfat milk and the 2 ounces of cheddar cheese, the rest from the plant foods. Clearly, the vegetable eater's attention to milk and cheese and the meat-centered person's neglect of them made a dramatic contrast in their calcium intakes.

Both people would have received about the same amount of sodium from their foods, had the foods not been salted. However, the meat-centered person's foods probably had considerably more salt added to them (impossible to calculate), especially the fast-food lunch. The vegetable eater had more potassium, and thus a better potassium-to-sodium ratio. This, together with the high calcium intakes, presents a strong nutritional defense against high blood pressure.

As for other constituents of the two days' intakes, the vegetable person fell a little short in vitamin B_6 (85 percent of the RDA) and zinc (73 percent of the RDA), as so should choose better sources of these nutrients on other days. On the other hand, the vegetable person fared markedly better than the meat-centered person in terms of fiber (5 times as much) and cholesterol (about ¼ as much). The two people's protein, carbohydrate, and fat intakes were compared in earlier chapters and they, too, for the most part, reflected creditably on the vegetable eater.

The meat-centered person should not be dismissed with a frown of disapproval, though. It was not possible for this person to cook at home at lunchtime, and it may not have been possible to eat elsewhere than at a steakhouse at dinner. Can such people improve their nutrient intakes other than by completely overhauling their lifestyles? The question is important, because fast foods and convenience foods are a major part of many people's lives today. A Gallup survey taken over a three-year period recently revealed that 30 to 42 percent of those polled had eaten out the day before, 28 percent at a fast food place for lunch.[33] The accompanying box, "Defensive Dining," suggests pointers for people who eat convenience foods, fast foods, airline meals and the like regularly—that is, almost all of us. The person's chief needs for that particular day seem to have been to reduce fat and cholesterol and to add fiber, calcium, and vitamin A. Those needs could have been met, that day, by the substitution of one or more of the meals with other meals con-

Defensive Dining

To avoid defeating your nutrition strategy when eating convenience foods:
- Appreciate airline meals for the fresh, wholesome foods you *can* get from them. Eat selectively. You don't have to eat everything they serve.
- Enjoy frozen meals and "lite" meals for the wholesome ingredients they offer. Supplement with items they do not supply (such as additional vegetables, nonfat milk, fresh fruits).
- Be aware that fortified foods whose labels list the U.S. RDA nutrients have had these nutrients *added* to them. Therefore they may not contain the nutrients that were not in the 1968 RDA table (inside back cover) from which the U.S. RDA were taken. That is, fortified foods may not contain vitamin B_6, folacin, zinc, magnesium, and other nutrients. Use these foods sparingly.
- In fast food places, cut kcalories by ordering diet soft drinks and smaller hamburgers. To cut fat, take the hamburger without the mayonnaise. Cut sodium by having them hold the pickle, ketchup, and mustard. Ask them not to salt your fries.
- Whenever possible, go to the salad bar. Then choose wisely. Salad bar meals can be high in fat and salt, too.
- Don't be fooled by "soda with (selected) vitamins." Drink soda, if you like, but get your vitamins from foods where they all are present, and where minerals and fiber are present, too.
- Remember, it's not the component itself that is harmful, but the dose and frequency of consumption. Enjoy treats and convenience foods at intervals—and make the intervals reasonable.

tributing a greater variety and abundance of vegetables and by the addition of two or more cups of milk or the equivalent in milk products. This would have added kcalories, so kcalories from other foods would need to be reduced; the obvious choices would be those contributing the most fat and cholesterol—the butter, cream, meat, and salad dressing.

This comparison brings to a conclusion the discussion of food sources of nutrients based on the series of tables that began in Chapter 9. Every table presented its information in two ways—ranked by nutrients per serving on the left, and by nutrients per 100 kcalories on the right. The rankings by nutrients-per-serving have long been familiar; people have tended to seek single servings of foods that would deliver large amounts of single nutrients. Examples are a cup of milk for calcium, a hamburger for iron, an orange for vitamin C, and so forth. The approach works, as far as obtaining the nutrients is concerned, but it fails to control kcalories. If you eat this way, you are stuck with the kcalories in those servings of foods, no matter what total they add up to.

The alternative approach, implicit in the rankings on the right sides of the tables, is to select foods that are highest in nutrients per kcalorie, and then eat as much of these foods as you can. In effect, that's what the vegetable eater did on the day of meals shown. Priority 1 was to eat the Four Food Groups, but Priority 2 was to fill in with extra servings of vegetables, and more vegetables, until capacity was reached. (Then came Priority 3: the butter, sugar, and brownie, because room was still left in the kcalorie allowance.) The vegetables weren't notable for their nutrient contributions per traditional half-cup serving, but so many of them were eaten that they became significant sources of nutrients.

The brownie in the vegetable eater's day makes a statement: you *can* enjoy your favorite treats while eating right. The person enjoyed that brownie at the end of a day in which virtually all nutrient needs had been met.

The comparison does not weigh all in favor of either set of meals. Both are extremes. The meat-centered set is too high in fat, cholesterol, and salt, and delivers too little calcium, for its kcalories—but the meals are easy to eat and available everywhere. The vegetable-laden set is higher in nutrients and fiber, but is time-consuming to prepare and too high in bulk for most people to consider eating. (Even so, it was necessary to add butter and sugar to bring the kcalories up to match those in the other meals, without increasing bulk or protein further.) Still, in naming one set "preferred," we have identified the direction most people should probably pursue: eat more vegetables. Eat them in relatively unprocessed form, as far as possible. Eat more fruits—also in relatively unprocessed form. These are only two of the dietary guidelines outlined in Chapter 2: apply all of them.

Finally, exercise, to earn the privilege of eating enough food to deliver the nutrients you need. Energy expenditure, the output side of the energy budget, is the opposite of money expenditure: it is not desirable to *save* energy. The more you spend (within reason, of course), the more food you can afford to eat—both food delivering nutrients and food delivering pleasure. It has been suggested that when the next edition of the RDA are published, a "recommended daily energy output" be included.

Contaminants

The placement of contaminants after nutrition in this chapter reflects the order of FDA's areas of concern. Nutrition was of concern because people need help in choosing, from among the vast array of products available, foods that will deliver the nutrients they need. Contaminants are of concern because, increasingly, they are present in the environment and inevitably, they find their way into foods at times.

Pesticides have already been discussed. They are poisonous by definition, but they are intentionally put on, in, or around foods during growth or storage processes; tolerance levels are set; and their use is regulated and monitored. When they exceed tolerance levels—that is, when accidents happen, they become members of the larger group of substances, contaminants. What are contaminants, and why are they considered so dangerous? A few examples will help to answer this question.

In 1953 a number of people in Minamata, Japan, became ill with a disease no one had seen before. By 1960, 121 cases had been reported, including 23 in infants. Mortality was high; 46 died, and in the survivors the symptoms were ugly: "progressive blindness, deafness, incoordination, and intellectual deterioration."[34] The cause was ultimately revealed to be methylmercury contamination of fish from the bay these people lived on. The infants who contracted the disease had not eaten any fish, but their mothers had, and even though the mothers exhibited no symptoms during their pregnancies, the poison had been affecting their unborn babies. Manufacturing plants in the region were discharging mercury into the waters of the bay, the mercury was turning to methyl mercury on leaving the factories, and the fish in the bay were accumulating this poison in their bodies. Some of the families who were affected were eating fish from the bay every day.[35]

In 1910, Dr. Alice Hamilton of the United States began documenting her observations of the toxicity to humans of another environmentally derived heavy metal, lead. Factory workers intoxicated with lead poisoning exhibited a wide variety of symptoms, she said, including anemia, constipation, loss of appetite, abnormal kidney function, jaundice due to liver damage, "wrist drop" (loss of muscular control of the hand), irritability, drowsiness, stupor, and coma. Mothers exposed to lead had abortions and stillbirths more often, and their children were more often sick.[36] Lead also finds its way into food, as will be shown.

In 1973, in Michigan, half a ton of polybrominated biphenyl (PBB), a toxic chemical, was accidentally mixed into some livestock feed that was distributed throughout the state. The chemical found its way into millions of animals and then into people. The seriousness of the accident began to come to light when dairy farmers reported their cows going dry, aborting their calves, and developing abnormal growths on their hooves. Although more than 30,000 cattle, sheep, and swine and more than a million chickens were destroyed, effects on

heavy metal: any of a number of mineral ions such as mercury and lead, so called because they are of relatively high atomic weight. Many heavy metals are poisonous.

people were not prevented. By 1982 it was estimated that 97 percent of Michigan's residents had become contaminated with PBB. Nervous system aberrations and alterations in the liver and immune systems were among the effects in exposed farm residents.[37]

Mercury and lead are both heavy metals, and PBB is an organic halogen. These two classes of chemicals are among the most toxic and widespread in our environment. A list of the chemical contaminants of greatest concern is presented in Table 13–4, and Figure 13–2 shows how they find their way into foods.

organic halogen: an organic compound containing one or more atoms of a **halogen**—fluorine, chlorine, iodine, or bromine.

TABLE 13–4

Chemical Contaminants of Concern in Foods, U.S., 1970 to 1980

Heavy Metals	Halogenated Compounds	Others
Lead	Chlorine	Asbestos
Mercury	Iodine	Dioxins
Cadmium	Vinyl chloride	Acrilonitrile
Selenium	Ethylene dichloride	Lysinoalanine
Arsenic	Trichloroethylene	Diethylstilbestrol
	Polychlorinated biphenyls (PCBs)	Heat-induced mutagens
	Polybrominated biphenyls (PBBs)	Antibiotics (in animal feed)

Source: E. M. Foster, How safe are our foods? *Nutrition Reviews* (supplement), January 1982, pp. 28–34.

FIGURE 13–2

How contaminants find their way into foods.

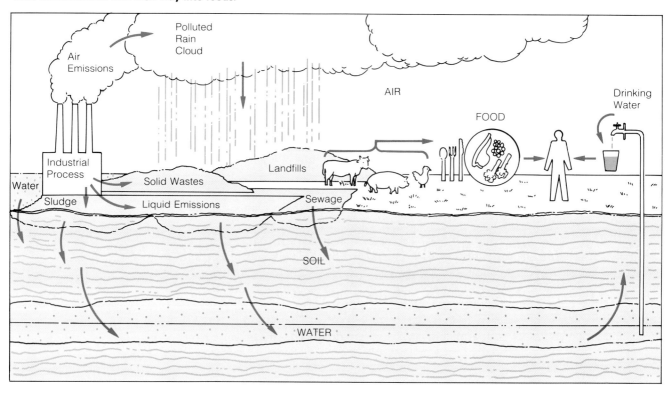

On first studying this subject, a reader is likely to want the question answered, How serious is all this—how dangerous is it for *me*? Yet no one who has pursued the subject realistically expects to have that question answered in any simple way. Contamination may be a negligible problem in your particular area today, but tomorrow it may become a severe one if there is a major spill or other accident. A general answer, then, is that the hazard is probably small, because we are generally well protected, but that in the event of an accident, the risk of toxicity can suddenly become very great. (Recall the meaning of *hazard* as opposed to *toxicity*.)

The number of contaminants we could discuss here, and the amount of information available about them, is far beyond our scope. Instead of dealing superficially with many of them, our choice is to illustrate some principles by discussing only four: the three heavy metals lead, cadmium, and mercury, and the best known organic halogen, PCB.

Lead

Lead is a chemical element, and so is indestructible. It is a metal ion with two positive charges, similar in some ways to nutrient minerals like iron, calcium, and zinc. In fact, it competes with them for some of the slots they normally occupy in the body, but then is unable to fulfill their roles. Thus it interferes with many of the body's systems. The most vulnerable tissues are the nervous system, kidney, and bone marrow. Lead is readily transferred across the placenta, and its most severe effects on the fetus are on the developing nervous system. Absorption of lead is five to eight times greater in children than it is in adults, and it tends to stay in their bodies.[38]

This brings us to the first of several points to be made about contamination. A factor in the potential harmfulness of a contaminant is its persistence—the extent to which it lingers in the body. If a contaminant enters the body and then is rapidly metabolized to some harmless compound, then its ingestion may not give cause for concern. (Vitamin C seems to fall into the category of rapidly metabolized substances, and this accounts for its relative lack of toxicity in most people.) If the contaminant is rapidly and preferentially excreted, then too the body may be able to survive a brief exposure time. But if it enters the body, interacts with the body's systems, is not metabolized or excreted, and fools the cells' protein machinery into accepting it as part of its structure, then the contaminant is dangerous. Additional doses will be piled on top of the first ones, and it will accumulate. All these things are true of lead, and that's why it's so deadly.

Organic halogens like PBB are, as the term *organic* says, molecules like vitamin C that could in theory be metabolized and disposed of—but their deadliness is related to the same factors that make lead so dangerous. They are resistant to metabolism either inside the body (by the body's enzymes) or outside (by microorganisms), and furthermore, they accumulate from one species to the next, with a consequent buildup in the food chain (Figure 13–3).

The anemia caused by lead poisoning is the result of many effects lead has on blood. Besides competing with iron for absorption, lead interferes with several enzymes that synthesize heme, the iron-containing portion of hemoglobin. Lead also deranges the structure of the red blood cell membrane, making it leaky and fragile. Lead interacts with white blood cells, too, impairing their

Factors that determine a chemical's persistence in the environment:
- Resistance to destruction by heat.
- Stability to radiation (example: sunlight).
- Low solubility in water (so that it tends to stick to soil).
- Resistance to acid and alkali.

A factor that determines a chemical's persistence in the food chain is its tendency to concentrate in a body tissue such as bone or (usually) fat. Concentration in fat favors accumulation at the top of the food chain and makes these foods particularly susceptible to contamination:
- Meat.
- Dairy products.
- Fish.
See Figure 13–3.

Cautions about Seafood

So far we have emphasized bacterial contamination of foods. Viruses can also cause food-borne illness transmitted from sick people to well ones through seafood. In order to get nourishment from the surrounding water, filter feeders such as clams and oysters filter the water, collecting tiny particles in their bodies to serve as food. If they happen to be growing in water that has become contaminated with animal or human waste products, the seafood can collect viruses from that waste. For example, waste can contain the virus that causes hepatitis. If the clams or oysters have filtered the virus out of the water, and have it in their bodies, there is a good possibility that a consumer of those shellfish will contract hepatitis.

Another possible seafood hazard is shellfish collected from areas of the algae bloom known as red tide. The shellfish filter the toxin produced by red tide, and concentrate it in their bodies (it's highly toxic to people, but not to shellfish).

This section is not intended to frighten the reader away from eating seafood. Most seafood that is commercially harvested is safe, because it is harvested from uncontaminated water that is tested for these hazards. The message is that extra caution should be used when shellfish are taken from an area not used for commercial harvesting. Local health departments can give information about safe places to collect seafoods.

Finally, if serious food-borne illness is suspected:

1. Call your physician.
2. Wrap and label the remainder of the suspected food, along with its container, so that it can't be mistakenly used; place it in the refrigerator; and hold it for possible inspection by health authorities. Ask your physician whether the food should be saved for bacteriological examination.
3. Notify the Health Hazard Evaluation Board of the U.S. FDA's Bureau of Foods. The sole purpose of this panel of scientists and health experts is to assess how serious a threat to health the food may be.*

The person who follows the suggestions here regarding the selection, storage, and preparation of food will, over a lifetime, reap many benefits. Nutrition knowledge applied in the home has arrived where it belongs.

We have come a long way from the introduction of the term *nutrient* in Chapter 1 to the conclusion of this chapter on foods and food safety. Readers who have followed the path through all its turnings should consider themselves well grounded in the basics of nutrition. To apply these basics to individuals requires still another framework of knowledge: the framework supplied by facts about people's changing nutrition concerns at different ages and stages of life. The next chapters are devoted to nutrition through the life cycle, from conception to old age.

---

*For more information about how the FDA assesses reported hazards in foods, read Determining when a food poses a hazard, *FDA Consumer,* June 1983, pp. 25–28.

Study Questions

1. List the six potential hazards to food within the FDA's areas of responsibility in priority order of concern.
2. What is the difference between a GRAS substance and a regulated food additive? Give examples of each.
3. What are the three most popular artificial sweeteners used today? What are the risks associated with each?
4. What arguments would you use to support or refute the Delaney Clause?
5. How do pesticides and agricultural chemicals become a hazard to the food supply and how are they monitored?
6. Give examples of natural toxicants that occur in foods. What are their toxic effects?
7. Which nutrients were studied in the HANES and Ten-State Surveys? What nutrition-related generalizations were made from these surveys? What criticisms have been made about them?
8. Describe the findings of the National Food Consumption Survey in terms of overnutrition—with respect to energy, fat, sugar, and cholesterol intakes.
9. Give an argument in favor of continued nutrition surveillance in both the developed and developing countries.
10. Describe how contaminants find their way into foods and how a contaminant buildup occurs in the food chain.
11. Describe several measures that help prevent food poisoning. In whom are these conditions most likely to be severe?

Notes

1. A. M. Schmidt, Food and drug law: A 200-year perspective, *Nutrition Today* 10, no. 4 (1975): 29–32.
2. P. Lehman, More than you ever thought you would know about food additives, *FDA Consumer*, April 1979 (reprint).
3. Lehman, 1979.
4. F. M. Strong, Toxicants occurring naturally in foods, in *Nutrition Reviews' Present Knowledge in Nutrition*, 4th ed. (Washington, D.C.: Nutrition Foundation, 1976), pp. 516–527.
5. J. M. Coon, Natural food toxicants: A perspective, in *Nutrition Reviews' Present Knowledge in Nutrition*, 4th ed. (Washington, D.C.: Nutrition Foundation, 1976), pp. 528–546.
6. Strong, 1976.
7. The use of chemicals in food production, processing, storage and distribution, *Nutrition Reviews* 31 (1973): 191–198.
8. T. M. Parkinson and J. P. Brown, Metabolic fate of food colorants, *Annual Review of Nutrition* 1 (1981): 175–205.
9. E. Corwin and W. L. Pines, Why FDA banned red no. 2, *FDA Consumer*, April 1976, pp. 18–23.
10. Tartrazine, *Nutrition and the MD*, January 1983.
11. Lehman, 1979.
12. M. Gore, The Chinese restaurant syndrome, in *Adverse Effects of Foods*, eds. E. F. P. Jelliffe and D. B. Jelliffe (New York: Plenum Press, 1982), pp. 211–223.
13. C. Lecos, The sweet and sour history of saccharin, cyclamate, aspartame, *FDA Consumer*, September 1981, pp. 8–11.
14. Council on Scientific Affairs, American Medical Association, Saccharin: Review of safety issues, *Journal of the American Medical Association* 254 (1985): 2622–2624.
15. Council on Scientific Affairs, Aspartame, review of safety issues, *Journal of the American Medical Association* 254 (1985): 400–402.
16. Council on Scientific Affairs, Aspartame, 1985.
17. *NutraSweet Brand Sweetener, Reference Guide to Aspartame Scientific Research*, a booklet available (© 1985) from Searle Food Resources, Inc., P.O. Box 1111, Skokie, IL 60076.
18. Joint FAO/WHO Expert Committee on Food Additives, International Programme on Chemical Safety, Toxicological evaluation of certain food additives, WHO technical report series no. 669 (Geneva: World Health Organization, 1981), pp. 25–32.
19. G. S. Wong, Aspartame and its safe use, *Diabetes Dialog* 29 (1982): 3.
20. Questions readers ask, *Nutrition and the MD*, January 1984.
21. L. W. Wattenberg, Inhibitors of carcinogenesis, in *Carcinogens: Identification and Mechanisms of Action*, eds. A. C. Griffin and C. R. Shaw (New York: Raven Press, 1978), pp. 229–316.
22. Select Committee on Health Aspects of Irradiated Beef, *Evaluation of the Health Aspects of Certain Compounds Found in Irradiated Beef* (Bethesda, Md.: Life Sciences Research Office, Federation of American Societies for Experimental Biology, 1977, 1979), as cited in Irradiated foods, a report by the American Council on Science and Health, October 1982, available from the council at 1995 Broadway, New York, NY 10023.
23. *Federal Register*, 27 March 1981, as cited in Food irradiation: Ready for a comeback, *Food Engineering*, April 1982, pp. 71–80.
24. New rules and term for irradiation, *Science News*, 18 January 1986, p. 43.
25. M. G. Mustafa, Agricultural chemicals, in *Adverse Effects of Foods* by E. F. P. Jelliffe and D. B. Jelliffe (New York: Plenum Press, 1982), pp. 111–128.
26. Mustafa, 1982.
27. Delayed neurotoxicity, in *Pesticide Residues in Foods*, Report

SELF-STUDY

Study Your Own Diet

Now that you have analyzed the entire array of nutrients in your diet, it's time to reach some conclusions.
1. Review your findings and summarize the strong points and weak points of the way you eat at present. How is your diet presently successful in delivering the nutrients you need within an appropriate number of kcalories? In what respects does it have room for improvement? Describe specific steps you might take to set about improving it with respect to:
■ Balance of meals.
■ Number and regularity of meals.
■ Specific food choices.
2. Having completed all the exercises to this point, you are in a position to decide whether you really need your vitamin-mineral supplement or other supplements. For each nutrient you've studied, compare your RDA or RNI, the amount you consume, and the amount contributed by your supplement. Does the supplement make up for a deficit in your intake, or is it an unnecessary extra? Perhaps, with the appropriate food choices, you can dispense with it.

of the 1975 Joint FAO/WHO meeting, Technical Report Series no. 592 (Geneva: World Health Organization, 1976), pp. 11–13.

28. R. W. Miller, Honey: Making sure it's pure, *FDA Consumer,* September 1979, pp. 12–13; I. B. Vyhmeister, What about honey? *Life and Health,* August 1980, pp. 5–7.

29. A. Brynjolfsson, Food irradiation and nutrition, *Professional Nutritionist,* Fall 1979, pp. 7–10.

30. M. W. Pariza, Food safety from the eye of a hurricane, *Professional Nutritionist,* Fall 1979, pp. 11–14.

31. R. Dubos, The intellectual basis of nutrition science and practice. Paper presented at the NIH conference on the biomedical and behavioral basis of clinical nutrition, 19 June 1978, in Bethesda, Maryland, and reprinted in *Nutrition Today,* July–August 1979, pp. 31–34.

32. R. W. Miller, America's changing diet, *FDA Consumer,* October 1985, pp. 4–5; R. W. Miller, Soft Drinks and six-packs quench our national thirst, *FDA Consumer,* October 1985, pp. 23–25.

33. C. Lecos, What about nutrients in fast foods? *FDA Consumer,* May 1983, pp. 10–15.

34. W. A. Krehl, Mercury, the slippery metal, *Nutrition Today,* November–December 1972, pp. 4–15.

35. Krehl, 1972.

36. M. A. Wessel and A. Dominski, Our children's daily lead, *American Scientist* 65 (1977): 294–298.

37. 97% of Michigan population contaminated by 1973 spills, *Tallahassee Democrat,* 16 April 1982.

38. Metabolism of vitamin D in lead poisoning, *Nutrition Reviews* 39 (1981): 372–373.

39. Wessel and Dominski, 1977; D. Pincus and C. V. Saccar, Lead poisoning, *American Family Physician* 19 (1979): 120–124; Nutritional influences on lead absorption in man, *Nutrition Reviews* 39 (1981): 363–365.

40. K. R. Mahaffey, Nutritional factors in lead poisoning, *Nutrition Reviews* 39 (1981): 353–362.

41. M. B. Rabinowitz, J. D. Kopple, and G. W. Wetherill, Effect of food intake and fasting on gastrointestinal lead absorption in humans, *American Journal of Clinical Nutrition* 33 (1980): 1784–1788.

42. Update: Childhood lead poisoning, *Journal of the American Dietetic Association* 80 (1982): 592, 594.

43. D. G. Lindsay and J. C. Sherlock, Environmental contaminants, in Jelliffe and Jelliffe, 1982, pp. 85–110.

44. Lindsay and Sherlock, 1982.

45. Lindsay and Sherlock, 1982.

46. Lindsay and Sherlock, 1982.

47. Parts of this discussion are adapted from *Foodborne Illness: The Consumer's Role in Its Prevention,* a leaflet available (1976) from The American Medical Association, 535 North Dearborn Street, Chicago, IL 60610.

Questions about Additives and Cancer

Of all the questions consumers have about their foods, the ones that seem to cause the most alarm relate to cancer. Can additives that cause cancer be allowed in foods? The answer is supposed to be no, but some substances that have been suspected to cause cancer are still allowed in foods. What's going on?

What's going on is a controversy in which many of the issues are unclear in consumers' minds. Those issues can't be resolved here, but perhaps they can be made clear.

Brief mention was made in Chapter 13 of the Delaney Clause, a part of the law first signed in 1958, that states that no additive may be allowed in foods that has been shown to cause cancer in animals or human beings. The intention of the Delaney Clause was, of course, to protect the public, like all food safety laws, but it has been a troublesome part of the law for many reasons. Questions it has provoked include the following:

- Why focus on cancer? Is cancer different from other diseases that food additives might cause? What about birth defects, allergic reactions, and others?
- Where should the line on amount of additives be drawn? Could a threshold be set, such that "safe" amounts could be permitted below that threshold? Or, in the case of cancer, is there no such thing as "safe"? Is it true that even a single molecule can cause cancer?
- How should it be determined whether an additive causes cancer? If it causes cancer in animals, does that prove it will cause cancer in human beings?

On each of these questions there are arguments.

Why Focus on Cancer?

Cancer is a serious and dreaded disease, but other diseases are serious too. By focusing on cancer, we tend to neglect other important potential hazards in food such as bacterial poisoning, lead poisoning, and nervous system damage.[1] Some people question the usefulness of the Delaney Clause, because they think it is unnecessary. Other provisions of the law, they say, deal with protection from harmful substances, and carcinogens are implicitly included under those provisions. Those who support the Delaney Clause argue that cancer is different, because, they say, there is no threshold at which carcinogens are safe. Even one molecule can cause cancer, so substances that can cause cancer have to be excluded from the food supply altogether. That brings us to the second question.

Where Should the Line Be Drawn?

Is there a threshold below which the risk from a carcinogen is negligible? Those who say there is no threshold base their argument on the fact that even one molecule of a carcinogen can cause cancer. They fail to realize, though, that vast numbers of molecules have to be present before one of them *will* cause a cancer. To understand why this is so, it is necessary to look inside the cell. The initiating step in cancer formation involves a single molecule altering the genetic material, DNA—

that is, causing a mutation. A simple view of what happens next is that the altered DNA puts out an altered message, the cell makes an altered protein, and a tumor begins to grow. In short, yes: a single molecule can start a cancer; in fact, cancers always start from such single events; and that makes carcinogens unique among hazardous chemicals. The same thing is not true of toxins—for example, neurotoxins or inhibitors of cellular respiration. It takes a certain threshold concentration of the toxin to stop nerve transmission or shut down cellular respiration. Below that threshold, impairment is seen, and some distance below it, there is no detectable effect. A single molecule has no effect at all.

The difference between carcinogens and other toxins would seem to make carcinogens unique, then, and justify their being treated with special dread. However, it is also true that there is a threshold below which the presence of a carcinogen presents a negligible threat. One argument puts it this way: "There are many thousands of 'carcinogenic' molecules present in every cell, and the intrusion of a single molecule would be lost against this background. A homely analogy is that spitting in the ocean won't cause a flood."[2]

As explained in Highlight 4A, cancer develops in several steps, each of which is reversible. The first step is alteration of the DNA, as described, by a single molecule of the carcinogen. DNA is a double-stranded molecule, in which each strand complements the other. The information in DNA thus exists in two copies (analogous to a photograph and its negative). Molecules and particles of radiation constantly bombard the DNA and cause breaks in it, but as long as the breaks are in only one strand, the cell can promptly repair them, using the other strand as a guide. Special enzymes exist for the purpose, known as excision and repair enzymes. These enzymes detect areas of the DNA molecule where the one strand is damaged; they scissor it out of its context; and then, using the other strand as a guide, they resynthesize a corrected strand. An alteration in DNA can thus occur without causing any detectable effect, because it is promptly corrected. In fact, this happens all the time. In other words, single molecules can alter DNA, yes, but even after they have done so, this does not inevitably lead to cancer or even to mutations of any kind. In fact, the alterations will inevitably be corrected as fast as they are made until the rate at which the alterations take place exceeds the rate at which they are corrected—that is, at the threshold concentration of carcinogen.

Sometimes changes in DNA take place and are *not* corrected. If a lesion in DNA occurs as the two strands are separating prior to the making of a new cell, then the opportunity for repair is lost. A new strand will be made to match the damaged DNA; the mistake will be passed on to the daughter cell and will be self-perpetuating. The new cell may, as a result, be a cancer cell, and so will its daughters be. Still, the outcome is not necessarily a tumor because the body's immune system is equipped to recognize and eliminate strange cells. Potential cancers are believed to arise constantly, this way, and in healthy individuals they are constantly extinguished. This view, too, would seem to make it apparent that there need be no concern about single molecules causing cancer. Not only must many molecules be present before one causes the episode that initiates a tumor, but many such episodes have to take place before one finally results in cancer.

Population statistics also support the view that there is a threshold below which carcinogens pose no significant threat. First, enough research has to have been done to prove that the chemical in question is carcinogenic. Second, it has to be possible to state the probability of that chemical's causing cancer in an individual over a lifetime under the conditions of use. Once those two conditions are met, a statement like this is possible: "Substance X, as used, is likely to cause one cancer over the lifetime of 100,000 individuals." Several assumptions have to be applied (Does the risk increase and decrease linearly as the dose increases and decreases?* Is everyone's exposure equal? Is everyone's susceptibility equal?) but these can be identified and agreed on. Then, it becomes possible to make decisions based on that statement. For example, it may be agreed that the probability of a case of cancer from that chemical as used is 1 in 100,000 over a lifetime. Since 4 million individuals are born each year in the United States, a 1 in 100,000 risk would be considered too high; at that risk level, 40 of these people might contract cancer from that chemical in their lifetimes if they didn't die of something else first. A one in a million risk level would also be unacceptable, because four people might contract cancer, but a one in 10 million or one in 100 million level might be deemed acceptable. This is the

---

*Linear extrapolation may not be valid for any carcinogen. Their dose-response curves may all be sigmoid, such that if the dose decreases by a factor of five, the tumor risk decreases by a factor of 25 or more. Such a relationship appears likely for many suspected carcinogens and reduces further the likelihood that they pose a significant risk. This and other challenges to the Delaney Clause assumptions are presented in *Of Mice and Men: The Benefits and Limitations of Animal Cancer Tests,* a report (1984) available from the American Council on Science and Health, 47 Maple Street, Summit, NJ 07901.

kind of thinking done by those concerned with regulating carcinogenic additives; it is called "quantitative risk assessment."[3] This thinking leads to the conclusion that some additives with the potential to cause cancer would not have to be banned altogether; they could be tolerated at an acceptable risk level, perhaps with warning labels to the public.

The question whether to accept the idea that threshold doses of carcinogens are acceptable in foods has become pressing. It relates not only to intentional additives but also to indirect additives, because new technology has made it possible to detect much lower levels of substances in food than the past. Incidental additives may migrate into foods from packaging materials, for example, and if they are carcinogenic, approval for their use can only be given if no detectable residue is present in the food as sold or served. Some were approved in the past because manufacturers appeared able to show them to be altogether absent from the foods with which they had been in contact. But any chemist knows there is really no way to prove the total absence of a substance. Absence of a substance is defined by the sensitivity of the method used to detect its presence. That is, the chemist can't say there is zero substance present, but can only say zero substance was found at a detection level of (for example) one part per million. That only proves there is less than 1 ppm of the substance, not that there is zero.

New analytical techniques have made it possible to detect substances at levels of one part per *billion* (1 ppb) where, ten years ago, only detection of 1 ppm would have been possible. As a result, it has seemed to the public that carcinogenic contaminants were suddenly appearing in foods that hadn't been there before. Actually, they had been there all along, but were first detected only recently. Their detection doesn't necessarily signify an unacceptable risk, because the amounts are so small. But the new sensitivity of analytical techniques, combined with the inflexibility of a law like the Delaney Clause, makes regulations difficult to come up with. Some experts have come to the conclusion that the law on each additive or contaminant should include a statement of the required sensitivity of the detection method. If no residue was found at the designated level, the undetected presence of a residue at a lower level would be legally defined as presenting no significant risk. This reasoning is proposed to apply to incidental additives, but FDA has indicated an interest in broadening it to apply to all compounds covered by the Food, Drug, and Cosmetic Act.[4]

These are some of the complexities surrounding the question whether threshold tolerance levels for carcinogenic substances in foods can be established. The next question is, how can we know whether an additive causes cancer?

How Should Carcinogens Be Identified?

How can it be determined whether an additive causes cancer? Another way to state that question is to ask how applicable the results of experiments using animals are to human beings. Several kinds of tests are used, most commonly involving bacteria, rodents, or both. Each has advantages and limitations, and their interpretation involves applying principles from genetics and physiology, as well as statistics.

An important distinction to begin with is that between *mutagenesis* and *carcinogenesis*. A mutation is any change in DNA that is copied from a cell to its daughter cell. A carcinogenic mutation is one that leads to cancer. A mutagen is any chemical or physical agent that causes mutations. A carcinogen is a mutagen that causes cancer. All

carcinogens are mutagens, but not all mutagens are carcinogens. This distinction offers perspective on one of the tests used to screen material to see if they are carcinogenic. The test, named the Ames test after the scientist who developed it, uses bacteria as the test population, and it screens for mutagens.

Bacteria are excellent subjects for screening compounds for mutagenesis. Their generation time is short, an hour or less in many cases, and millions of them can be grown in a single flask in the lab. A chemical that might cause only one mutation in one billion organisms can be detected overnight using bacteria, and its effects characterized within a few weeks. Bacteria are single-celled and so they can't, of course, get cancer, but they can mutate—and fast. The Ames test involves exposing bacterial cells to test compounds and measuring the rate at which those compounds give rise to certain kinds of mutations.

When a chemical is found mutagenic by the Ames test, it is still a far cry from being proven to be carcinogenic, however. Two major drawbacks beset the Ames test as a carcinogen detector. One is that the kinds of mutations it detects are so-called point mutations, changes at single points along the DNA strands analogous to simple typographical errors in sentences such as leaving a letter out of a word. The kinds of mutations that lead to cancer, though, are translocations—analogous to transpositions of whole words or sentences from one paragraph to another.[5] To detect changes such as this a different test animal would have to be used—one in which rearrangement of the chromosomes could be seen under the microscope.

The other drawback to using bacteria is that they are not physiologically complex, as mammals are. One of the ways cancer arises in multicellular animals is that a substance gets metabolized to another substance—and

then that substance causes cancer. An example is the already familiar nitrite-to-nitrosamine conversion described in Chapter 13. The Ames test has been adapted to take this into account by running test compounds through mammals first, then testing their urine on bacteria using the Ames test. Several substances not found to be mutagenic when tested directly have proven to give rise to mutagens that appear in the urine of animals or people who eat them. Another modification of the Ames test involves mixing enzymes from mouse liver with the bacterial system to permit metabolic reactions to occur that might occur in the mammalian body. By this test, more mutagens turn up than are seen without the liver enzymes.[6] Still, a mutagen is not necessarily a carcinogen, and bacteria don't get tumors, so suspected compounds still have to be tested using animals. The animals of choice are usually rats or mice.

Tests Using Animals

The first question that comes to mind in this connection is "Suppose a chemical does cause cancers in rats. Does that mean it will cause cancer in human beings as well?" Fortunately for researchers, the answer is "Yes, usually." All living cells contain DNA, and a compound that will cause mutations in the DNA of one species will have the same effect in others. Differences can and do arise in the way the compound is metabolized by a given species, though, and these differences can be reflected in differing cancer probabilities.

Rats are much smaller than human beings and they live shorter lives. How can experiments using rats be designed to have maximum applicability to human beings? The FDA's answer to this is as follows.[7]

An experiment with rats can show that there is a dose-response relationship between the substance and the incidence of cancers. That is, the higher the dose, the more cancers. This is stronger evidence of a direct cause-and-effect relationship than the simple appearance of cancers in a group of animals exposed to the substance.

An FDA experiment using rats involves 100 animals exposed to the substance at a high dose, 100 at a low dose, and 100 control animals. Each group includes 50 males and 50 females. They are maintained in a climate-controlled, clean environment; their feed is measured out automatically; and daily observations on their physical characteristics, blood chemistry, food consumption, doses of the test substance, and other data are recorded in a computer. When an animal dies, 28 separate observations on 48 organs are also recorded. Each 100 animals represent the U.S. population of over 200 million people.

The sensitivity of the test is such that a 5 percent excess cancer rate is about the minimum that can be detected. This poses a problem, because an excess cancer rate over controls of 5 percent would represent a disastrous 10 million cases of human cancer in the U.S. population assuming everyone were exposed to the chemical in comparable fashion.

The problem has two possible solutions—to use more animals, or to increase the dose. If FDA used 3 million animals in one experiment, for example, it could detect a probable excess cancer rate, in people, of 2 cases per million (with 99.9 percent confidence, which is taken as certainty). Obviously this wouldn't be practical, since a 600-rat experiment already costs upwards of $600,000. Therefore FDA increases the dose. Assuming the dose-response test has already shown that the risk is proportional to the dose, the demonstration of cancers at a high dose in a small number of animals is equivalent to demonstrating that cancers would be found at a low dose if a larger number of animals were tested.

Better yet, the demonstration that *no* cancers occur at a high dose level establishes the practical absence of risk in a predicted population size of human beings for a lower dose.

Many chemicals can kill, but even at massive dose levels, only a few cause cancer. A specific interaction has to take place between the chemical and the cell,* and the potential for this interaction can be detected using animal experiments. Of 18 substances known to cause cancer in human beings, all but two also cause cancer in animals.[8] Presumably, the reverse is also true, although the important exception of saccharin has to be noted. A 1985 review of all the experimental and epidemiological evidence indicates that saccharin appears to cause cancer only in rats and only in their bladders, and is not associated with an increased risk of bladder cancer in human beings.[9] The correspondence between animal and human responses to possible carcinogens is not perfect, but it is close.

The validity of animal testing has been challenged in a number of ways. For example, it is argued that the high doses of chemicals fed to animals put them under stress; as a result, their immune systems are weakened; and they therefore succumb to cancer not because of the chemical but because of the stress. If this is true, though, it leads to overly conservative interpretation of the test results—an error on the side that protects the public. It is also argued that additives are tested on animals only one by one and not in combination; combinations could cause far greater likelihoods of cancer. For example, heavy drinking superimposed on moderate smoking increases the risk of cancer of the

---

*All of these carcinogens seem to interact with DNA by way of oxygen radicals. B. N. Ames, Dietary carcinogens and anticarcinogens, *Science* 221 (1983): 1256–1265.

ARE YOU RELEVANT?

esophagus 25-fold over the risk caused by smoking alone. Risks caused by additives might be underestimated for real people in the real world of exposure to multiple substances; this is a valid criticism.

Still, animal testing is, to most people's way of thinking, the only way to evaluate the cancer risk associated with new additives with any validity. Epidemiological studies, for ethical reasons, are the only kind that can be performed using human beings, and they can only be performed *after* large numbers of people have been exposed to a substance for a long time. Animal tests may not be perfect, but they are the best available alternative.

The Questions Summed Up

In summary, the regulation of additives suspected of causing cancer is controversial. It is debatable whether they should be altogether forbidden in foods with no threshold level allowed, or whether they should be treated like other harmful food constituents. If thresholds should be permitted, there is a question how to establish them. And the question how they should be identified also draws argument: bacterial screening and animal tests are useful, but their interpretation is difficult. The need to resolve these questions is becoming more pressing, as

Miniglossary

Ames test: a screening test used to determine whether a test substance causes mutations in bacteria.

carcinogenesis: the production of mutations that cause cancer.

dose-response relationship: a relationship between a substance and a test animal's response to it such that the greater the dose, the greater the response—persuasive evidence that the substance causes the response.

excision and repair enzymes: enzymes that cut out damaged sections of DNA and resynthesize corrected segments to replace them.

mutagenesis: the production of mutations.

mutation: an alteration in DNA. Some mutations cause cancer; most do not. A **point mutation** is the simplest kind of mutation—an alteration at one point in a DNA strand. Other mutations are more complex: a **translocation** is one in which a segment is removed from one place and relocated in another place along the DNA, or even moved to a different DNA molecule.

quantitative risk assessment: the assessment of risk, not as all or none, but in quantitative terms.

lower and lower levels of carcinogenic materials become detectable in foods using new analytical techniques.

At present, the Delaney Clause is still in force. It prohibits the addition to foods of any substance that has been shown to cause cancer in animals at any dose level. No threshold level is considered safe, and quantitative risk assessment is not permitted. Specified animal experiments are required to be performed and their results dictate the laws that will follow. It has been proposed that the law be changed to base safety decisions related to additives more on the assessment of real risk to human beings; to allow FDA more latitude in creating regulations; and to allow consumers more freedom of choice in their use of low-risk additives. As of this writing, however, the Delaney Clause is still firmly in place.

NOTES

1. *The U.S. Food Safety Laws: Time for a Change?* a booklet (1982) available from the American Council on Science and Health, 1995 Broadway, New York, NY 10023.
2. G. Clause, I. Krisko, and K. Bolander, Chemical carcinogens in the environment and in the human diet: Can a threshold be established? *Food and Cosmetics Toxicology* 12 (1975): 737–746.
3. P. B. Hutt, Regulating carcinogenic food contaminants, *Cereal Foods World* 26 (1981): 81–83.
4. Hutt, 1981.
5. J. Cairns, as cited by W. Bennett, Cancer—a new idea, *Harvard Magazine*, May–June 1981, pp. 16–18.
6. B. N. Ames, J. McCann, and E. Yamasaki, Methods for detecting carcinogens and mutagens with the Salmonella/microsome mutagenicity test, *Mutation Research* 31 (1975): 347–364.
7. D. Kennedy, What animal research says about cancer, *Human Nature*, May 1978, pp. 84–89.
8. Kennedy, 1978.
9. Council on Scientific Affairs, American Medical Association, Saccharin: Review of safety issues, *Journal of the American Medical Association* 254 (1985): 2622–2624.

HIGHLIGHT THIRTEEN B

World Hunger

Hunger wastes the most precious of all the world's resources—the human being. Despite numerous development programs, malnutrition is not disappearing; the tragic number of malnourished people continues to grow. Nutrition planners are rightly concerned with increased food production, better storage facilities, access to markets, more stable supplies, better nutritional quality of foodstuffs, and ultimately food consumption itself. In addition, these fundamental questions have to be asked: What is restricting the poor's access to food? How can these restrictions be removed? Adequate nutrition can be achieved only when the economic, political, and social structures that hinder food consumption become the targets of change.

Prevalence of Malnutrition

The United Nations Food and Agriculture Organization (FAO) estimates that there are at least a half-billion undernourished people in the world today. These people lack the nutrients to support healthy, active lives. The marks of undernutrition include blind eyes, swollen bellies, skin irritations, general listlessness, and stunted physical growth. Table H13B–1 lists the countries identified by the United Nations as most seriously affected.

Of all population groups, children are most seriously affected by malnutrition. The United Nations World Health Organization (WHO) reports that there are 10 million severely malnourished children under the age of five; these children are below 60 percent of the standard body weight for their age. Another 240 million preschoolers are also estimated to be suffering from malnutrition. Additional millions of children die yearly from the indirect effects of marginal malnutrition—parasites and infectious diseases with accompanying diarrhea, which interact with poor nutrition in a vicious cycle. For example, measles, a relatively mild disease in industrialized countries, has a high mortality rate in Africa. Among poorly nourished children, the mortality rate for measles may be several hundred times the rate among well-nourished children.[2] Chronic diarrhea, whooping cough, tuberculosis, malaria, and parasites also aggravate sickness and mortality in malnourished children.

The light of curiosity absent from children's eyes. Twelve-year-olds with the physical stature of eight-year-olds. Youngsters who lack the energy to brush aside flies collecting about the sores on their faces. Agonizingly slow reflexes of adults crossing traffic. Thirty-year-old mothers who look sixty. All are common images in developing countries; all reflect inadequate nutrition; all have societal consequences.

—Alan Berg

"Leila is a girl of seven in the urban slums of Dacca, Bangladesh. During the last two years her eyes have been growing dim. Today she is stone blind not by accident or birth defect but because of a lack of vitamin A in her daily diet. For this malady there is no cure. Now sightless, Leila is looked upon by her parents as a sign of the curse of Allah. She is kept in the back room and no longer plays with other children. In her isolation from her past playmates and from the lost sights of the world around her, she cries."[1]

TABLE H13B–1

Countries Most Seriously Affected by Hunger

Afghanistan	Guatemala	Niger
Bangladesh	Guinea	Pakistan
Benin	Guinea-Bissau	Rwanda
Burma	Guyana	Samoa
Burundi	Haiti	Senegal
Cameroon	Honduras	Sierra Leone
Cape Verde	India	Somalia
Central African Empire	Ivory Coast	Sri Lanka
Chad	Kenya	Sudan
People's Democratic	Laos	Tanzania
Republic of Yemen	Lesotho	
Egypt	Madagascar	Uganda
El Salvador	Mali	Upper Volta
Ethiopia	Mauritania	Yemen Arab Republic
Gambia	Mozambique	
Ghana	Nepal	

Protein deficiency.

The most widespread form of malnutrition among children in the developing world today is protein-kcalorie malnutrition, or PCM. Children who are thin for their height may be suffering from acute PCM or recent severe food restriction, whereas children who are short for their age have experienced long-term chronic PCM. Stunted growth due to PCM, rather than symptoms of vitamin and mineral deficiency diseases, may be the most common sign of malnutrition in developing countries.[3] Breastfeeding permits infants in many developing countries to achieve weight and height gains equal to children in developed countries until about six months of age, but then the majority of these children, too, fall behind in weight and height. Failure of children to grow is a warning that one of the extreme forms of PCM, marasmus or kwashiorkor, may soon follow (see Chapter 5).

Mother-Child Malnutrition

Pregnant or lactating women, together with their small children, have a greater need for nutrients for their size than other groups because of the higher demand for nutrients during periods of rapid growth (see Chapter 14). When family food is limited, these women and their children are the first to show the signs of undernutrition.

Maternal weight gain during pregnancy is necessary for normal fetal growth and development. Women in developed countries gain an average of 12.5 kilograms (about 27 pounds). Studies among poor women show a weight gain often limited to 5 to 7 kilograms (11 to 15 pounds).[4] Women with lower weight gains in pregnancy more often have low-birthweight babies. Infection, congenital defects, and death are often seen in low-birthweight infants.

In India, several studies show that a significant number of pregnant women are underweight and experience a deficit of 500 to 600 kcalories a day.[5] Women in developing countries are responsible, even during their pregnancies, for most of the physical labor required to procure food for their families. The poor nutrition of these women is also the result of the distribution of food in the family. A mother will feed her husband, children, and other family members first, eating only whatever is left. Cultural and social beliefs also limit food intake.

"Ishmael, age four, was taken by his parents during the terrible drought last year from their two acres of parched farmland to a refugee camp in Wollo Province of Ethiopia in order to get food, medicine, and shelter. Because his mother had a sparse diet when she was carrying Ishmael in her womb, and because he was not fed enough nutritious food for his first four years, Ishmael acts deranged at times, apathetic at others. He grunts instead of talking. His parents will never know that his mother's deficient diet four years ago and his subsequent lack of enough food in his early years have damaged his brain permanently. If Ishmael lives through the current famine, he will never learn to read or write. He will be destined to become the village idiot."[6]

In the Indian Punjab, Dr. Carl Dyer, director of the Johns Hopkins Narangwal Program aimed at reducing malnutrition in local villages, found that a malnutrition rate of 10 to 15% persisted even after a major effort to provide supplementary foods. The majority of those affected were very young females, least able to demand their share and least recognized by other family members as deserving a fair share. In other areas of India, a child may be forbidden to eat curds and fruit because they are "cold," and bananas because they "cause convulsions."[7]

Other instances of malnutrition can be traced to inappropriate "modernization," such as replacing breast milk with formula feeding in environments and economic circumstances that make it impossible to formula feed safely. Breast milk, the recommended food for infants, is sterile and contains antibodies that enhance an infant's resistance to disease. Formula in bottles, however, in the absence of sterilization and refrigeration, is an ideal breeding ground for bacteria. More than 1,300 million people in developing countries do not have access to safe drinking water.[8] Mixing contaminated water with milk powder and feeding this to infants often causes infections leading to diarrhea, dehydration, and decreased absorption of nutrients from the foods the children are given. Malnourished children cannot fight these infections effectively, and many die.

The infant mortality rate ranges from about 50 (Sri Lanka) to over 200 (Afghanistan) in the poorest of the developing countries, as compared with an average of 13 to 20 in the developed countries. The death rate for children from one to four years old is no more favorable; it ranges from 20 to 30 times higher in developing countries than in developed countries.[9] This age span includes the weaning period, one of the most dangerous periods for all children in developing countries. Infection, delayed at first by breastfeeding, appears inevitable after weaning. Causes include ingesting infected water, gruel, or other materials.

In developing countries, the diet's basis is formed by bulky grains such as wheat, rice, millet, sorghum, and corn, and by starchy root crops such as cassava, sweet potatoes, plantain, and bananas. These may be supplemented with legumes (peas or beans) and, rarely, with animal proteins. Infants have small stomachs and can't eat enough of these staples (grains or root crops) to meet their daily energy and protein requirements. A great need exists to develop more adequate and inexpensive weaning foods in the developing countries. The most promising weaning foods are usually concentrated mixtures of grain and locally available peas or beans.[10] Mothers are advised to continue breastfeeding while they introduce weaning foods.

Limited Success in Local Efforts

Infants and children need not be raised in middle-class homes to be protected from PCM. Slight modifications of the children's diets can be immensely beneficial. Encouraging examples are provided by recent experiences in Sierra Leone, Nepal, and Southeast Asia.

In Sierra Leone, Bennimix was developed from subsistence crops and introduced as a supplement to infants' diets. Rice, sesame (benni) seed, and ground nuts were hand pounded to make a flour meal and then cooked. The local children found it tasty—and, whereas they had been malnourished before, they thrived when Bennimix was added to their diets. The village women formed a cooperative to reduce the household drudgery of preparation, and they rotated the work on a weekly or monthly basis.[11] The government also established a manufacturing plant to produce and market the mixture at subsidized prices. The success of the

venture appeared to lie in involving the local people in the process of identifying the problem and devising its solution. It was not considered enough only to accomplish the goals of an agency; the needs of the people were remembered.

A similar success was achieved in Nepal by maximizing the use of local resources and facilities to prepare a supplementary food. Ingredients for the food were soybeans, corn, and wheat, mixed in a 2:1:1 proportion, and yielding a concentrated "superflour" of high biological value suitable for infants and children. A nutrition rehabilitation center tested this superflour by giving the undernourished children and their mothers two cereal-based meals a day, and giving the children three additional small meals of superflour porridge daily. Within ten days the undernourished children had gained weight, lost their edema, and recovered their appetites and social alertness. The mothers, who saw with their own eyes the remarkable recoveries of their children, were motivated to learn how to make the tasty supplementary food and incorporate it into their local foodstuffs and customs.[12]

Another success story is the research surrounding the winged bean plant, cultivated in Southeast Asia for years, but only recently studied by the National Academy of Sciences. The

TABLE H13B–2

The Realities of Hunger

The United Nations reports that there are 520 million malnourished people in the world.

Each year, 15 to 20 million people die of hunger-related causes, including diseases brought on by lowered resistance due to malnutrition. Of every four of these, three are children.

Over 40% of all deaths in poor countries occur among children under five years old.

The United Nations (UNICEF) states that 17 million children died last year from preventable diseases—one every two seconds, 40,000 a day. (A vaccination immunizing one child against a major disease costs 7 cents.) At least 50 million children are permanently blinded each year simply through lack of vitamin A.

More than 500 million people in poor countries suffer from chronic anemia due to inadequate diet.

Every day, the world produces 2 lb of grain for every man, woman, and child on earth. This is enough to provide everyone with 3,000 kcal day, well above the average need of 2,300 kcal.

A person born in the rich world will consume 30 times as much food as a person born in the poor world.

The poor countries have nearly 75% of the world's population, but consume only about 15% of the world's available energy.

Almost half the world's people earn less than $200 a year—many use 80 to 90% of that income to obtain food.

Of the nearly 5 billion people on earth, more than 1 billion drink contaminated water. Water-related disease claims 25 million lives a year. Of these, 15 million are under five years of age.

There are 800 million illiterates. In many countries, half of the population over 15 is illiterate. Two-thirds of these are women.

Sources: *World Hunger: Facts,* available from Oxfam America, 115 Broadway, Boston, MA 02116; Office on Global Education, Church World Service, 2115 N Charles St., Baltimore, MD 21218.

plant is easily cultivated, even in sandy soil and tropical climates, needs no fertilizer, and is completely edible. The winged bean is similar to the soybean, but is much easier to grow. Complemented with corn, it can be made into a weaning food with the protein quality of milk and a high vitamin A content.[13]

These three examples offer hope that the world food situation can be improved by simple means, but they do not fully address the issue of poverty. One-shot intervention programs—offering nutrition education, food distribution, food fortification, and the like—are not enough. It is difficult to describe the misery a mother feels when she has received education about nutrition but is unable to purchase the foods her family needs. She now knows *why* her child is sick and dying but is helpless in *applying* her new knowledge.

Major Problems Still to Solve

The discussion thus far illustrates a major fact that many people are unaware of. World hunger is *not* the result of a world food shortage. The rest of this highlight will show you the realities underlying world hunger and will invite you to become personally involved in bringing about the end of hunger in our lifetime. An understanding of what causes hunger in the world is basic to deciding what must be done.

The world food problem is many things. It is an economic problem, because supply and demand for food are not balanced. It is a technological and environmental problem. It is a demographic problem, as well as a moral scandal in which there are unequal access to resources, extremes of dietary patterns, and an unjust economic system. The world food situation is poignant even when presented statistically (see Table H13B–2). Some of the causes of the problem are shown in Table H13B–3. Two

TABLE H13B–3

Causes of the World Food Problem

Worldwide Problems	Problems of the Developing World
1. Natural catastrophes—drought, heavy rains and flooding, crop failures.	1. Underdevelopment.
2. Environmental degradation—soil erosion and inadequate water resources.	2. Excessive population growth.
3. Food supply-and-demand imbalances.	3. Lack of economic incentives—farmers using inappropriate methods and laboring on land they may lose or can never hope to own.
4. Inadequate food reserves.	4. Parents lacking knowledge of basic nutrition for their children.
5. Warfare and civil disturbances.	5. Insufficient government attention to the rural sector.
6. Migration—refugees.	
7. Culturally based food prejudices.	
8. Declining ecological conditions in agricultural regions.	

Problems of the Industrialized World	Problems Linking Industrial and Developing Worlds
1. Excessive use of natural resources.	1. Unequal access to resources.
2. Pollution.	2. Inadequate transfer of research and technology.
3. Inefficient, animal-protein diets.	3. Lack of development planning.
4. Inadequate research in science and technology.	4. Insufficient food aid.
5. Excessive government bureaucracy.	5. Excessive food aid.
6. Loss of farmland to competing uses.	6. Politics of food aid and nutrition education.
	7. Inappropriate technological research.
	8. Inappropriate role of multinational corporations.
	9. Insufficient emphasis on agricultural development for self-sufficiency.

Source: Adapted from C. G. Knight and R. P. Wilcox, *Triumph or Triage? The World Food Problem in Geographical Perspective,* resource paper no. 75–3 (Washington, D.C.: Association of American Geographers, 1976), p. 4.

generalizations and an important question are suggested by these tables:
1. The underlying causes of global hunger and poverty are complex and interrelated.
2. Hunger is a product of poverty resulting from the ways in which governments and businesses manage national and international economies.
3. The question "Why are people hungry?" has been answered: "Because they are poor." The question that remains to be answered is "Why are people poor?" A diagram of the poverty-hunger web is presented in Figure H13B–1.

Solutions and Alternatives

Experts assure us that we possess the knowledge, technology, and resources to end hunger. As individuals,

FIGURE H13B–1.

Behind hunger stands poverty.

"Fernando is a child of 5 in Bolivia. His father, a hardworking copper miner, and his mother care for him and his six brothers and sisters. Fernando has rickets, is anemic, is small in stature and weak in body. Because of the lack of clean water in his village, he and other members of his family suffer from continual diarrhea. If Fernando is lucky enough to become an adult, he will remain small in stature and weak in body. If Fernando dies soon, his parents will feel impelled to bring another child into the world in the hope that a new child will live to adulthood and be able to care for the parents in old age."[14]

therefore, we can take action to respond to this human suffering. Hunger and poverty in a world that has the means to alleviate them are intolerable and unacceptable—even for one more day. The rest of this highlight will discuss some of the changes necessary, on the international, national, and personal levels, to end world hunger. The issues to be addressed in more detail are:

- *Birth rates.* The importance of realizing that overpopulation is caused not by food abundance, but by hunger.
- *Land reform.* The need for aggressive redistribution of resources.
- *Multinational corporations.* The need for a change in their role in the developing countries.
- *Lifestyle.* How *we* can influence world hunger.

- *Agenda for action.* How *you* can become part of the solution to the world food problem.

Overpopulation and Hunger

The current world population is approximately 5 billion, and for the year 2000 the projected United Nations figure is 6 billion. These facts justify concern over the world's capacity to produce adequate food in the future. It does not necessarily follow, however, that "too many people" is the cause of the world food problem. Actually, poverty seems to be at the root of the problem, and both hunger and overpopulation are caused by poverty. Three factors affect population growth: birthrates, death rates, and standards of living. Low-income countries have high birthrates and death rates and a low standard of living. When a people's

standard of living rises, giving them better access to health care, family planning, and education, the death rate falls first, but then the birthrate also falls. As the standard of living continues to improve, the family earns sufficient income to risk having smaller numbers of children. A family depends on its children to cultivate the land, to secure food and water, and to make the adults secure in their old age. If a family is confronted with ongoing poverty, parents will choose to have many children to ensure that some will survive to adulthood. Therefore, the improvement of poor people's economic status is a most effective means of contraception.

Evidence supports the idea that we first have to reduce the infant mortality rate if we want to reduce the birthrate. Families will only choose to have fewer children if they feel sure their children will *live*. Table H13B–4 shows the relationships between infant mortality rate and population growth rate. These statistics reveal that hunger and poverty in a nation reflect not only the level of national development, but also the people's sense of security.

In many countries where economic growth has occurred and resources have been distributed relatively equally among all groups, the rates of population growth have decreased.

TABLE H13B–4

Infant Mortality Rate and Birthrate in Hungry and Nonhungry Countries

	Hungry Countries	Nonhungry Countries
Average infant mortality rate	113	35
Total infant deaths per year	10.6 million	1.4 million
Size of population	2.3 billion	2.3 billion
Average rate of increase	2.4%	1.0%
Total births per year	86.4 million	38.6 million

Source: Adapted from *The Ending Hunger Briefing Workbook* (available from The Hunger Project, 2015 Steiner St, San Francisco, CA 94115), 1982, pp. 26, 30.

Examples include China, Costa Rica, South Korea, Sri Lanka, Taiwan, and West Malaysia. In countries where economic growth has occurred but the resources have been unevenly distributed, population growth has remained high. Examples are Brazil, Mexico, the Philippines, and Thailand, where a large family continues to be a major economic asset for the poor.[15]

Distribution of Resources/Land Reform

Land reform—giving people a more meaningful stake in food production, development, and the benefits of society—can combine with population control to increase everyone's assets. To introduce this section, a few facts must be presented:

- Much of the world's agriculture is very primitive. More than 50 percent of all food consumed in the world is still hand-produced.
- In many countries, up to 90 percent of the population lives on rural land.
- Of the more than 150 nations of the world, fewer than 24 are democracies. Most governments dictate the day-to-day lives of their people.
- Securing enough food on a day-to-day basis is a problem for as many as a billion human beings.
- The land in many parts of the world does not support the growing of food, even by the wealthy. Furthermore, the poor are often crowded onto mountainous slopes that are even less arable.[16]

The problem of unequal distribution of resources exists not only between rich and poor nations, but also between rich and poor people within nations. The FAO estimates that world food production averages about 3,000 kcalories per person per day, but that food is distributed unequally. Huge amounts of grains are fed to livestock to produce protein foods the poor cannot afford to purchase. Also, by some estimates, at least 20 percent of the total food produced is lost to pests and spoilage.[17]

Again, the problem is poverty; the symptom is inability to purchase basic food for sustenance. But the wealthy nations cannot simply give to the poor; it weakens them further not to fend for themselves. The question of policymakers and nutrition planners is, How do we increase the productivity and self-reliance of the rural poor in a nonpaternalistic fashion? Much is involved, but four things are basic and are required simultaneously. The poor must have greater opportunities for access to land, capital, technology, and knowledge.[18] International food aid is also required during the development period.

Governments have learned from recent history the importance of developing local agricultural technology. A major effort made in the 1960s—the Green Revolution—failed because it

The stark contrasts between rich and poor within a single developing country are depicted here in the homes of the people. The ruler maintains a palace, while the majority of the population lives in city tenements or rural huts.

was not in harmony with local realities. It was an effort to bring the genetic-engineered, petroleum-demanding agricultural technology of the industrial world to the developing countries, but the high-yielding strains of wheat and rice that were selected required irrigation, chemical fertilizers, and pesticides—all costly, and beyond the economic means of too many of the farmers in the developing world.

Instead of transplanting industrial technology into the developing countries, there is a need to develop small, efficient farms and local structures for marketing, credit, transportation, food storage, and agricultural education. International research centers need to examine the conditions of tropical countries and orient their research toward labor-intensive, rather than energy-intensive, agricultural methods.

Environmental concerns must be taken more seriously as well. As important as the amount of land available for crop production is the condition of the soil. Soil erosion is now accelerating on every continent, at a rate that threatens the world's ability to continue feeding itself. Erosion of soil has always occurred; it is a natural process—but in the past it has been compensated for by processes that build the soil up. Farmers should alternate soil-building crops with soil-devouring crops, a practice known as crop rotation. An acre of soil planted one year in corn, the next in wheat, and the next in clover loses 2.7 tons of topsoil each year, but if it is planted only in corn, it loses 19.7 tons a year.[19] When farmers must choose whether to make three times as much money planting corn year after year or to rotate crops and go bankrupt, naturally they choose the profits. Ruin may not follow immediately, but it will follow.[20]

Multinational Corporations: Coordinators of World Hunger?

Businesspeople, economists, and some development specialists often extol the benefits to Third World countries deemed to result from the investments of multinational corporations, especially in fostering economic growth. Other observers, however, are convinced that the multinationals have done more harm than good. Because the negative effects have included malnutrition, a topic of this highlight, they are emphasized here.[21]

The opponents of multinational corporations suggest that hunger is the result of political and economic systems that exploit the poor. A multinational corporation's primary concern is profit.

Agribusiness is now buying or renting more and more arable land. Decisions on what to plant and where to distribute the harvest are made with the balance sheet in mind. Thus it is profitable in poor countries to use land for exportable luxuries even while the people are suffering severe malnutrition because it does not grow enough grain.[22]

The classic example of the subtle exploitation of the poor, related to nutrition, is the competition for farmland between cash crops and food crops. The tragic scenario unfolds this way: Large landowners and multinational corporations control the best farmlands, and they use them mainly to grow crops that can be exported at considerable profit. Native persons work for below-subsistence wages and are forced onto marginal lands to do their own farming. The poor work hard, but they are cultivating crops for other people, rather than for themselves. The money they earn is not enough even to buy the products they help produce. The poor never acquire their share of the profits realized from the marketing of their products. The results: in the United States, imported foods—bananas, beef, cocoa, coconut, coffee, pineapple, sugar, tea, winter tomatoes, and others—fill *our* grocery stores, while the poor who grow these foods have even less food and fewer resources than before. Additional cropland is diverted for nonfood cash crops—tobacco, rubber, cotton, and other agricultural products.

Export-oriented agriculture thus uses the labor, land, capital, and technology that is needed to help local families produce their own food. For example, the effort required to produce bananas for export could be reallocated to provide food for the local people. It has been suggested that one solution to the world food problem is not that the developed countries should *give* more food aid, but that they should *take* less food away from the poor countries.[23] Truly, imported foods raised on land from which thousands of small farmers have been displaced symbolizes the exploitation of the poor as vividly as does a bottle of contaminated formula in the mouth of a dying infant.

Countless examples can be cited to illustrate how natural resources are diverted from producing food for domestic consumption to producing luxury crops for those who can afford them. A few such examples are included here:

- Africa is a net *exporter* of barley, beans, peanuts, fresh vegetables, and cattle (not to mention luxury-crop exports such as coffee and cocoa), yet it has a higher incidence of PCM among young children than any other continent.
- Mexico now supplies the United States with over half its supply of several winter and early spring vegetables, while infant deaths associated with poor nutrition are common.
- Half of Central America's agricultural land produces food for export, while in several of its countries the poorest 50 percent of the population eats only half the protein it needs. (The richest 5 percent, on the other hand, consume two to three times more than they need.)[24]

Besides diverting acreage away from the traditional staples of the diet, multinationals may also contribute to hunger by way of their marketing techniques. Their advertisements lead many consumers with limited incomes to associate products like cola beverage, cigarettes, infant formula, and snack foods with good health and prosperity. These promotions are tragically inappropriate for these people. A poor family's nutrition status suffers when its tight budget is pinched further by purchase of such goods.

The United Nations has commissioned several studies in the hopes of establishing an international code of conduct for the multinational corporations.[25] These powerful organizations can have an immense impact on national economies, for good or for ill. They can, if they choose, increase the credit and capital available to the developing world; and these resources, if properly used, can help to eliminate hunger. The multinationals also possess the scientific knowledge and organizational skills needed to help develop improved food and agricultural systems. However, experience reveals that wise control of these corporations is mandatory to ensure that human needs do not become subordinate to political and financial gains.

Lifestyle: Influencing World Hunger
How we choose to live our individual lives is ultimately a personal matter; however, our choices have an impact on the way the rest of the world's people live and die. Our nation, with 6 percent of the world's population, consumes about 40 percent of the world's food and energy resources. The food problem depends partly on the demands we place on the world's finite natural resources. In a sense, we therefore contribute to the world food problem. People in affluent nations have the freedom and means to choose their lifestyles; people in poor nations do not. We can find ways to reduce our consumption of the world's nonrenewable resources; we can use only what is absolutely required. The admonition, so familiar in childhood, to "clean your plate," as if that would alleviate the suffering of some starving stranger, could well be replaced with the mandate simply to "consume less food." Choosing a diet at the level of necessity, rather than excess, would decrease the resource demands made by our industrial agriculture. Humanitarian

and economic benefits could be achieved, as well.

One major way to reduce the demands we make on world resources is to depend less on animal-based protein and to use more plant-based proteins. Even one meal a week per person would make a difference. Meat does not necessarily have to be eliminated totally from the diet, because ruminants (cattle, sheep, and goats) can use forage crops and crop residues

produced on land not suitable to other crops.[26] In so doing, these animals convert plants indigestible by humans into high-quality animal protein. To understand some of the inefficiency in the consumption of protein and kcalories from animal rather than plant sources, we need to examine the dynamics of the food chain, as shown in Figure H13B–2.

A second way in which the developed world can foster betterment

FIGURE H13B–2

The food chain It takes 3,011 kcalories to bring to a consumer a 1-pound can of sweet corn that has a food value of 375 kcalories. It takes 29,497 kcalories to supply 140 grams of beef, also worth 375 kcalories.

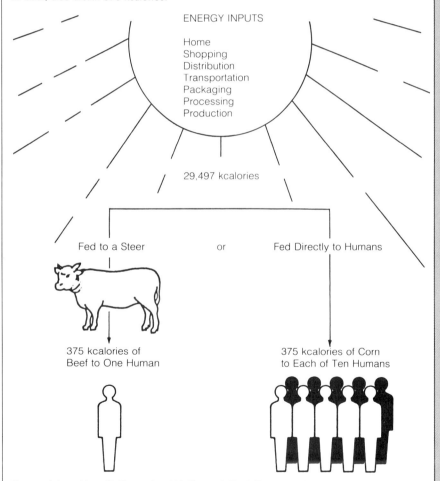

Source: Adapted from D. Pimentel and M. Pimentel, *Food, Energy and Society* (New York: Wiley, 1979).

TABLE H13B–5

Lifestyle: Reducing Energy Consumption

1. Choose to eat lower on the food chain. Learn the basis of plant-protein complementarity.

2. If you eat beef, look for sources of forage-fed or grass-fed, rather than grain-fed, cattle.

3. Grow your own fruits and vegetables whenever possible. This reduces energy needed in commercial transport of these products. Use organic fertilizer and biological pesticides to further reduce energy consumption.

4. Choose an adequate, not an excessive, diet. Avoid having to throw food away after meals.

5. Reduce use of heavily processed foods—frozen specialty and convenience foods.

6. Avoid nonreturnable beverage containers. Recycle glass, aluminum, paper, and other goods.

7. Whenever possible, purchase staple goods in bulk containers. Join or start a food cooperative.

Source: Adapted from D. Katz and M. T. Goodwin, *Food: Where Nutrition, Politics, and Culture Meet* (Washington, D.C.: Center for Science in the Public Interest, 1976), p. 155

of the quality of life in the developing countries is to shift to a less energy dependent lifestyle. This type of private commitment stems from the realization that hunger can be eliminated. Table H13B–5 lists several suggestions for reducing our energy consumption, and the last section of this highlight offers more ways to become further involved in ending world hunger.

This highlight has suggested that the availability of food is dependent on many interrelated factors: population, lifestyle, available arable land, water, fertilizer, energy supply, and others. The present food and energy resources will not meet the needs of the future. A world planning objective might therefore be to balance food supply, energy expenditures, and population growth. Two steps we might take toward achieving this objective might be to use more plant foods in the diet and, as already mentioned, to reduce our energy use. These measures, by themselves, would do nothing to solve the world hunger problem, but they would help create the potential for a solution.

The primary reason to alter our food and energy consumption patterns is not to redistribute our food to underdeveloped countries, but to reduce the demand we make on their resources. This would make those resources available to them for their own self-development.

It follows, of course, that careful planning is required so that the poor themselves realize the potential benefits being suggested here. Guidelines must be developed to divert to needy markets the resources this country would make available, and these guidelines must be reflected in the policies of our government. In the words of an author who has devoted intensive study to world hunger:

We somehow have failed to recognize that doing good for the sake of doing good is self-interest. To most people, ethical concerns are of value. Compassion and human decency may not lend themselves neatly to cost-benefit analysis, but the desire for sound moral values is a legitimate rationale for government action. Somehow, affluent societies must learn to accept this kind of self-interest as a basis for public policy.[27]

Agenda for Action

To summarize what is known about the world food situation, let us examine the conclusions of the Presidential Commission on World Hunger. The members of the commission believe that the 1980s must be a decade of concern for human life. They are convinced that worldwide efforts to overcome hunger and malnutrition and to foster self-reliant development must be intensive. Their major conclusions are listed in Table H13B–6.

Reducing personal consumption, eliminating food waste, and more equitably distributing existing food sources are immediate short-range solutions to end hunger. Long-range solutions are necessary as well, and you may use the resource list in Appendix F to find the organizations that will provide you not only with food for thought, but also with the will to chart your course of action.

Now is an opportune time to exercise our global citizenship on behalf of the poor. One of the most important steps individuals can take is to urge government and corporate policymakers to make hunger a priority item, just as the issues of energy, inflation, and nuclear arms are. Three of the most powerful social movements of this century began with moral outrage against dehumanized situations—sex discrimination, racial discrimination, and the war in Vietnam. Vigorous voices are needed to influence the policies of our governments and corporations, since their present policies of food trade, aid, and investment appear to be keeping the Third World *underdeveloped*. To remain silent is to render support to the status quo. To urge change is to make it known that the way to achieve food adequacy for everyone in a sensible time span is with a detailed, monitored, aggressive policy of redistribution, both at the international and national levels. Further suggestions for your personal contribution to the solution are listed here:

- Read more about national and international food issues. Discuss these issues with a group of friends or co-workers. Be able to articulate them to others.

TABLE H13B–6

Presidential Commission on World Hunger: Conclusions

- The major world hunger problem today is the prevalence of chronic undernutrition—which calls for a political, as well as a technical, solution.
- The world hunger problem is getting worse rather than better.
- A major crisis of global food supply—of even more serious dimensions than the present energy crisis—appears likely by the year 2000, unless steps are taken now to facilitate a significant increase in food production in the developing nations.
- Rising global demand for food must be met within resource limits—of land, water, energy, and agricultural inputs.
- There is no ideal food, no perfect diet, no universally acceptable agricultural system waiting to be transplanted from one geographic, climatic, or cultural setting to another. Assistance programs must focus on self-reliance and respond to the needs of each country. Needs and requirements cannot be generalized.
- In addition to action by the industrialized nations, decisive steps to build more effective national food systems must be taken by the developing countries.
- The outcome of the war on hunger, by the year 2000 and beyond, will be determined not by forces beyond human control, but by decisions and actions well within the capability of nations and people working individually and together.

Source: Adapted from Presidential Commission on World Hunger, *Overcoming World Hunger: The Challenge Ahead* (Washington, D.C.: Government Printing Office, 1980), pp. 180-185.

Hunger and Food Policy Agencies

You may want to learn more about organizations dealing with food policy issues. Agencies willing to help you get the facts include:

- Bread for the World
  6411 Chillum Pl. NW
  Washington, D.C. 20012
- Oxfam America
  115 Broadway
  Boston, MA 02116
- The Hunger Project
  2015 Steiner St.
  San Francisco, CA 94115
- Institute for Food and Development Policy
  1885 Mission St.
  San Francisco, CA 94103
- Interreligious Taskforce on U.S. Food Policy
  110 Maryland Ave. NE
  Washington, D.C. 20002

- Help raise money for volunteer agencies working abroad. Their projects directly affect some portion of the poor at the grassroots level, and are more likely to get food and funds into the hands of the poor than are those of top-heavy bureaucracies.
- Examine the sources of foods and products you buy. You may decide to join in boycotting products imported from developing countries as cash crops, or products of companies that market goods inappropriately in the Third World. What we choose to eat affects not only our lives, but also the lives of those who produce it.
- Attend or organize an event to raise your community's awareness of world food issues. World Food Day occurs annually on October 16, commemorating the founding of FAO, the United Nations agency responsible for improving global access to food. Oxfam America sponsors the Fast for a World Harvest each year in November.
- Support local groups such as food banks and soup kitchens. Donate time, funding, or food.
- Write letters, as often as possible. Ask your government legislators what they are doing to end world hunger. Share your knowledge with them. Write to local newspapers—provide them with information on hunger issues to be shared with their readers. Oxfam America and Bread for the World have guidelines to help you write effectively to these people.

How may we move closer to the ideal of an adequate diet every day for all men, women, and children? Many avenues are open. People can make a difference in the world food problem. We have the technology and resources available to feed everyone on earth. All that is needed is the will to do so.

"Hunger exists not because we can't end it, but simply because we haven't."

—World Runners

Miniglossary

arable: capable of being plowed.
arare = to plow
hunger: the term as used here means a continuous lack of the nutrients necessary to achieve and maintain optimum health, well-being, and protection from disease.
infant mortality rate: the number of deaths during the first year of life per 1,000 live births.
low-birthweight baby: one that weighs less than 2,500 g (5.5 lb) at birth.
multinational corporations: international organizations with direct investments and/or operative facilities in more than one country. The U.S. oil companies are an example.
Third World: the underdeveloped nations of the world that are aligned with neither the communist nor the noncommunist blocs.

NOTES

1. The stories of the children are from D. Burgess, The future of hungry children abroad, *Journal of Current Social Issues,* Summer 1975, p. 36.

2. D. Morley, *Pediatric Priorities in the Developing World* (London: Butterworth, 1973), p. 207.

3. S. N. Gershoff, Science: Neglected ingredient of nutrition policy, *Journal of the American Dietetic Association* 70 (1977): 471.

4. M. Cameron and Y. Hofvander, *Manual on Feeding Infants and Young Children,* 2nd ed. (Protein Advisory Board of the United Nations, 1976), p. 1.

5. S. Ghosh, *The Feeding and Care of Infants and Young Children,* 2nd ed. (New Delhi: Voluntary Health Association of India, 1976), pp. 3–4.

6. Burgess, 1975.

7. Dr. Carl Dyer's findings related to social and cultural beliefs about food in India are from A. Berg, *The Nutrition Factor* (Washington, D.C.: Brookings Institute, 1973), p. 46.

8. I. Rozov, The decade: Not just pumps and pipes, *World Health,* April–May 1983, p. 29.

9. World Bank, *World Development Report 1981,* Table 21.

10. P. Pellet, The role of food mixtures in combating childhood malnutrition, in *Nutrition in the Community,* ed. D. McLaren (New York: Wiley, 1978), pp. 185–202.

11. J. M. Steckle, Improving food utilization in developing countries, *Canadian Home Economics Journal* 27 (1977): 34–39.

12. *National Conference on Primary Health Care,* (Kathmandu: Ministry of Health, Health Services Coordination Committee, WHO, UNICEF, 1977), pp. 9, 25, as cited by M. E. Frantz, Nutrition problems and programs in Nepal, *Hunger Notes* 2 (1980): 5–8.

13. The Hunger Project, *A Shift in the Wind* 13 (1982): 3. A new report, *The Winged Bean: A High Protein Crop for the Tropics,* is available from the Commission on International Relations, National Research Council, 2101 Constitution Ave., Washington, D.C. 24018.

14. Burgess, 1975.

15. J. Kocher, Not too many but too little, in *The Feeding Web: Issues in Nutritional Ecology,* by J. D. Gussow (Palo Alto, Calif.: Bull Publishing, 1978), pp. 81–83.

16. R. R. Spitzer, *No Need for Hunger* (Danville, Ill.: Interstate Printers and Publishers, 1981), pp. 20–23.

17. *Nutrition Week* 13 (1983): 4–5.

18. M. R. Langham, L. Polopolus, and M. L. Upchurch, *World Food Issues* (Gainesville, Fla.: University of Florida Press, 1982), pp. 18–20.

19. National Agricultural Lands Study, *Soil Degradation: Effects on Agricultural Productivity, Interim Report No. 4* (Washington, D.C.: USDA, November 1980), as cited by L. R. Brown, World population growth, soil erosion, and food security, *Science* 214 (1981): 995–1002.

20. Brown, 1981.

21. For the other side of the argument—offering multinationals as part of the solution rather than the problem—see M. L. Kastens, Harvest of hunger: How government meddling threatens the world's food supply, *Futurist* 15, no. 5 (1981): 5–10.

22. R. J. Barnet, Multinationals: A dissenting view, *Saturday Review* 3 (1976): 11, 58.

23. G. Kent, Food trade: The poor feed the rich, *Food and Nutrition Bulletin* 4 (1982): 25–33.

24. F. M. Lappe and J. Collins, *Food First: Beyond the Myth of Scarcity* (Boston: Houghton Mifflin, 1978), p. 15.

25. Interreligious Taskforce on U.S. Food Policy, *Identifying a Food Policy Agenda for the 1980s: A Working Paper* (Washington, D.C.: January 1980), p. 30.

26. The argument in favor of maintaining animal agriculture is discussed in Spitzer, 1981, pp. 183–202.

27. A. Berg, The trouble with triage, *New York Times Magazine,* 15 June 1975, pp. 26–35.

Mother and Infant

14

All that is needed to form a new human being is a single, fertilized egg cell containing instructions (in DNA) to make proteins. The rest will follow. This is a human embryo, three days old; the single egg cell has divided five times, producing 32 cells.

We normally think of nutrition as affecting us here and now. You feel good this afternoon because you ate a good breakfast this morning; your friend feels sleepy because she had a sweet dessert after lunch. But the effects of nutrition also extend over years. The woman who is expecting a baby and the health professional advising such a woman will be strongly motivated to attend to the pregnant woman's nutrition needs if they understand how critical the nutrients are to the normal course of events in prenatal development.

All women should be attending to their nutrition before they become pregnant. If nutrient supplementation is needed, the family-planning period is a good time to get it started. The underweight woman should try to gain weight before she becomes pregnant, to maximize her chance of having a healthy baby.

Pregnancy: The Impact of Nutrition on the Future

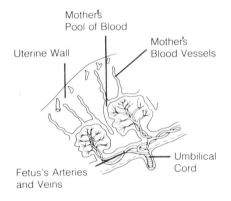

Mother's Pool of Blood

Uterine Wall

Mother's Blood Vessels

Umbilical Cord

Fetus's Arteries and Veins

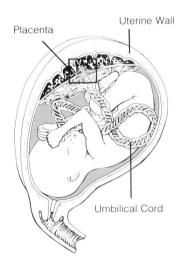

Placenta

Uterine Wall

Umbilical Cord

The only way nutrients can reach the developing infant in the uterus is through the mother's bloodstream. To convey these nutrients, the mother grows a whole new organ, the placenta, a sort of cushion in which the mother's and baby's blood vessels intertwine and exchange materials—nutrients and oxygen going into the baby's system, wastes leaving it to be excreted by the mother. If the mother's nutrient stores are inadequate early in pregnancy, when the placenta is developing, then the early development of her infant will be adversely affected. No matter how well the mother eats later, her unborn baby will not receive optimum nourishment. The infant will be born small and may be unable to attain the full size and health that would otherwise have been possible. After getting such a poor start on life, a girl child may be ill equipped, in her turn, to store sufficient nutrients, and so may also bear a poorly developed infant. Thus the poor nutrition of a woman during her early pregnancy can theoretically have an impact on the health of her *grandchild*, even after that child has become an *adult*.[1]

Critical Periods

Conditions in the uterus at the time of conception determine whether the fertilized egg will successfully implant itself in the uterine wall and begin development as it should. During the two weeks following fertilization, in the implantation stage, the egg cell divides into many cells, and these cells sort themselves into three layers. Very little growth in size takes place at this time; it is a critical period that precedes growth. Adverse influences at this time lead to failure to implant or to other disturbances so severe as to cause loss of the fertilized egg, possibly even before the woman knows she is pregnant. Many drugs affect the earliest intrauterine events and later cross the placenta freely. Most health professionals agree that, if possible, a potential mother should take no drugs at all, even familiar over-the-counter drugs. Nutrition should be, and should have been, continuously optimal.

The next five weeks, the period of embryonic development, register astonishing physical changes (see Figure 14–1). From the outermost layer of cells, the nervous system and skin begin to develop; from the middle layer, the muscles and internal organ systems; and from the innermost layer, the glands and linings of the digestive, respiratory, and excretory systems. At eight weeks, the 3-centimeter-long embryo has a complete central nervous system, a beating heart, a fully formed digestive system, and the beginnings of facial features. Already, an embryonic tail has formed and almost completely disappeared again, and the fingers and toes are well defined.

The growth of each organ and tissue type has its own characteristic pattern and timing. In the fetus, for example, the heart and brain are well developed at 16 weeks, even though the lungs are still nonfunctional 10 weeks later. During the first year after birth, the brain doubles in weight, but it increases only about 20 percent thereafter. In contrast, the muscles will be more than 30 times heavier at maturity than at birth.

Each organ and tissue, then, has its own unique periods of intensive growth. Each organ needs the growth nutrients most during its own intensive growth period. Thus a nutrient deficiency during one stage of development might affect the heart, and at another might affect the developing limbs.

The cells of a single developing organ also follow a schedule unique to them. Each organ has its own specific time for cell division. This time may not be obvious, because it often precedes the period of growth in size. An interesting case is that of the brain. During development of the fetal brain, there is an early period when the cells are increasing dramatically in *number*. Each time a cell divides, it produces two that are half its size. These two do not grow, but divide again, producing four cells that are still smaller. During this time of rapid cell division, the size of the brain hardly changes at all. Later, the cells begin to

placenta (pla-SEN-tuh): the organ inside the uterus in which the mother's and fetus's circulatory systems intertwine and in which exchange of materials between maternal and fetal blood takes place. The fetus receives nutrients and oxygen across the placenta; the mother's blood picks up carbon dioxide and other waste materials to be excreted via her lungs and kidneys.

implantation: the stage of development in which the fertilized egg embeds itself in the wall of the uterus and begins to develop, during the first two weeks after conception.

critical period: a finite period during development in which certain events may occur that will have irreversible, determining effects on later developmental stages. A critical period is usually a period of cell division in a body organ.

embryo (EM-bree-oh): the developing infant during its second to eighth week after conception. Before the second week, it is called an **ovum** (OH-vum) **or zygote** (ZYE-goat).

The brain and central nervous system are first to reach maturity.

FIGURE 14–1

Stages of fetal development.

Very young fetus in amniotic sac (specific age unknown).

Eight-week old fetus showing the beginnings of facial features.

Stages in organ growth:
1. **Hyperplasia** (high-per-PLAY-zee-uh): an increase in cell number.
2. Simultaneous hyperplasia and **hypertrophy** (high-PER-tro-fee): hyperplasia accompanied by an increase in cell size.
3. Hypertrophy (except for the liver).

The brain also goes through a fourth period, multiplication of cell contacts, which depends on both nutrition and social stimulation (learning).

grow and also continue dividing, so that their *size* and *number* increase simultaneously. It is during these first two periods that the total number of cells to be found in the brain is determined for life. Later still, cell division ceases; thereafter, the total number of cells is fixed, but the cells continue to increase in *size*. During this last period, the brain's growth in size is obvious. The development of almost every organ in the body follows a similar pattern, but the timing is different for each.

The third period, during which increase in size is taking place, is the time when the most intensive growth appears to be going on. But actually, the most important events are already over. This fact has important implications for nutrition. The period of cell division is a critical period—critical in the sense that the cell division taking place during that time can occur at only that time, and at no other. Whatever nutrients and other environmental conditions are needed in this period must be supplied on time if the organ is to reach its full potential. If cell division and the final cell number achieved are limited during a critical period, recovery is impossible. Thus early malnutrition can have irreversible effects, although they may not become fully apparent until the person reaches maturity.

The effect of malnutrition during critical periods is seen in the shorter height of people who were undernourished in their early years; in the delayed sexual development of those undernourished during early adolescence; in the poor dental health of children whose mothers were malnourished during pregnancy; and in the smaller brain cell number of children who have suffered from episodes of marasmus. The irreversibility of these effects is obvious when abundant, nourishing food fed after the critical time fails to remedy the growth deficit. Among the many Korean orphans adopted by U.S. families after the Korean War, for example, several years of catch-up growth occurred but did not completely make up for the effects of early malnutrition.

An area of active recent research points strongly to the probability that malnutrition in the prenatal and early postnatal periods also affects learning ability and behavior. Much of the severe mental retardation seen in developed countries such as the United States is of unknown cause, but many cases are thought to be due to protein deficiency during pregnancy. Clearly, then, it is most critical to provide the best nutrition at early stages of life.

Maternal Physiological Adjustments

The last seven months of pregnancy, the fetal period, bring about a tremendous increase in the size of the fetus. Intensive periods of cell division occur in organ after organ.

fetus (FEET-us): the developing infant from the eighth week after conception until its birth.

amniotic (am-nee-OTT-ic) **sac**: the "bag of waters" in the uterus, in which the fetus floats.

uterus (YOO-ter-us): the womb, the muscular organ within which the infant develops before birth.

Meanwhile, the mother's body has been undergoing changes. As already mentioned, she has grown the placenta, which transfers nutrients and oxygen to the fetus and carbon dioxide and other wastes to the mother's bloodstream for excretion by way of her lungs and kidneys. The amniotic sac has filled with fluid to cushion the infant. The mother's uterus and its supporting muscles have increased greatly in size, her breasts have changed and grown in preparation for lactation, and her blood volume has increased by half to accommodate the added load of materials to be carried. The normal gain in weight of mother and child during pregnancy amounts to about 25 to 30 pounds (see Table 14–1).

A mother's physiology changes so much during pregnancy that a naive observer might think that she is ill. She develops an apparent anemia, she may have edema, and her glucose tolerance changes as if she were diabetic. These and other changes are normal for her altered state, however.

The "physiological anemia of pregnancy" results from the great increase in the mother's blood volume. The red blood cells do not increase as much as the blood fluid, so the number of cells per milliliter is low compared with the nonpregnant state. Values for protein, iron, folacin, and other nutrients are correspondingly lowered, while other values rise (cholesterol and fat-soluble vitamins are examples). The clinician who assesses a pregnant woman's nutrition status therefore uses a set of standards specific for pregnancy.

The edema of pregnancy is also "physiological" (that is, expected and normal)—provided that it is not accompanied by indicators of kidney disease such as high blood pressure or protein in the urine. This normal edema results from the raised secretion of the hormone estrogen toward the end of pregnancy, which helps to ready the uterus for delivery.

The altered glucose tolerance of pregnancy is also normal, but an untrained observer could easily confuse it with diabetes. These examples are intended to caution the reader who is unfamiliar with the special standards applicable to pregnancy not to jump to conclusions regarding out-of-line lab test values. The treatment of truly abnormal conditions is the subject of a later section ("Troubleshooting").

TABLE 14-1

Weight Gain during Pregnancy

Development	Weight Gain (lb)
Infant at birth	7½
Placenta	1
Increase in mother's blood volume to supply placenta	4
Increase in size of mother's uterus and muscles to support it	2½
Increase in size of mother's breasts	3
Fluid to surround infant in amniotic sac	2
Mother's fat stores	5–10
Total	25–30

Nutrient Needs

Nutrient needs during periods of intensive growth are greater than at any other time and are greater for certain nutrients than for others, as shown in Figure 14-2. A study of the figure reveals some of the key needs.

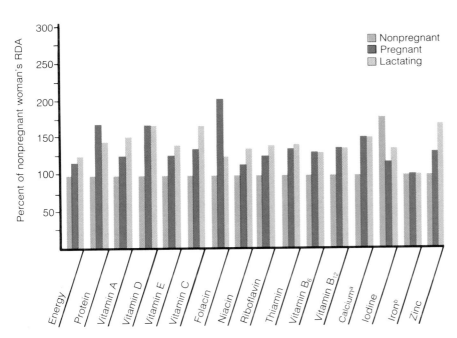

FIGURE 14-2

Comparison of recommended nutrient intakes of nonpregnant, pregnant, and lactating women. The nonpregnant woman's nutrient recommendations are set at 100 percent.

[a]Recommended intakes of phosphorus and magnesium change similarly.
[b]The pregnant woman may need to take an iron supplement.

Recommended energy intake during pregnancy: 40 kcal/kg (18 kcal/lb). Minimum energy intake: 36 kcal/kg (17 kcal/lb).

For a 120–lb woman, this represents at least 2,000 kcal/day, and preferably 2,200 kcal/day.

Recommended protein intake: 75 to 100 g/day.

Recommended carbohydrate intake: about 50% of energy intake. In a 2,000 kcal/day intake, this represents 1,000 kcal of carbohydrate, or about 250 g. Four cups of milk a day will contribute about 50 g carbohydrate. An apple provides 10 g carbohydrate, and a slice of bread provides 15 g, so this recommendation implies generous intakes of fruit and bread exchanges.

Foods containing folacin:
• Green, leafy vegetables.
• Legumes.
• Liver.
• Orange juice and cantaloupe.
• Other vegetables.
• Whole-wheat products.

Foods containing calcium:
Four cups of milk a day will supply 1.2 g calcium. For other food sources, see Chapter 11. The milk should be fortified with vitamin D; if it is not, a vitamin D supplement may be needed.

One of the smallest increases apparent is in kcalories; an increase of only 15 percent (mostly in the latter half of pregnancy) is recommended, but many individual women may need much more. In each case, enough kcalories are needed to spare protein for its all-important tissue-building work. A recommended average intake is 40 kcalories per kilogram of body weight, and energy intake should never fall below 36 kcalories per kilogram. The increased recommendation for protein is more dramatic—from about 56 grams in a nonpregnant woman to about 75 grams per day or more for a pregnant woman—and generous amounts of carbohydrate are needed to spare the protein. There is no harm in a pregnant woman's taking up to 100 grams of protein; in fact, if she has been poorly nourished prior to pregnancy, this may be an ideal intake. There is a limit, though, to the benefits of added protein. If added energy is needed, it is best obtained from carbohydrate.

The extraordinary need for folacin in the pregnant woman is due to the great increase in her blood volume. Folacin-deficiency anemia is more often seen in pregnant women than even iron-deficiency anemia, and it is often advisable for the physician to prescribe folacin as a supplement. As you might expect, the vitamin needed in the next highest amount is the B vitamin that assists folacin in the manufacture of red blood cells—vitamin B_{12}.

Among the minerals, those involved in building the skeleton—calcium, phosphorus, and magnesium—are in great demand during pregnancy, and increases of about 50 percent are recommended. Intestinal absorption of calcium doubles early in pregnancy, and the mineral is stored in the mother's bones. Later, as the fetal bones begin to calcify, there is a dramatic shift of calcium across the placenta, and the mother's bone stores are drawn upon. Most mothers' intakes have to be increased well above their prepregnancy levels. If the mother's intake is less than 1.2 grams per day, she will pay by losing more calcium from her bones than she has stored for this purpose.[2]

The body conserves iron even more than usual during pregnancy: menstruation ceases; and absorption of iron increases up to threefold. (The blood protein responsible for iron absorption, transferrin, increases.) However, iron stores dwindle during pregnancy and at the time of birth. The developing fetus draws on its mother's iron stores to create stores of its own to carry it through the first three to six months of life. This drain on the mother's supply may precipitate a deficiency; furthermore, the mother loses blood as she gives birth. Few women enter pregnancy with adequate stores to meet these demands, so the RDA committee recommends an iron supplement throughout pregnancy and for two to three months after delivery.[3]

Eating Pattern and Weight Gain

If the woman's dietary pattern is already adequate at the start of pregnancy, she can simply increase her servings of nutritious foods to meet her increasing nutrient needs. The nutrients she needs the most are best provided by foods in the milk, meat/meat alternative, and vegetable categories.

Because kcalorie needs increase less than nutrient needs, the pregnant woman must select foods of high nutrient density. For most women, appropriate choices include foods like nonfat milk, cottage cheese, lean meats, legumes, eggs, liver, dark green vegetables, and whole-grain breads and cereals. Vitamin C-rich foods

TABLE 14–2

Daily Food Guide for Pregnant or Lactating Women

Food	Number of Servings		
	Nonpregnant Woman	Pregnant Woman	Lactating Woman
Protein foods			
Animal (2-oz serving)	2	2	2
Vegetable (at least one serving of legumes)	2	2	2
Milk and milk products	2	4	5
Enriched or whole-grain breads and cereals	4	4	4
Vitamin C–rich fruits and vegetables	1	1	1
Dark green vegetables	1	1	1
Other fruits and vegetables	1	1	1

Source: California Department of Health, as cited in Nutrition and the pregnant obese woman, *Nutrition and the MD,* January 1978.

in generous quantities should be present at every meal. A suggested food pattern is shown in Table 14–2.

The pregnant woman must gain weight. Ideally, she will have begun her pregnancy at the appropriate weight for her height and will gain about 25 pounds, most of it in the second half of pregnancy. The ideal pattern is thought to be about 2 to 4 pounds during the first three months and a pound per week thereafter. The teenager needs to gain more. A woman who is underweight to begin with should also gain more—perhaps 30 pounds—and a woman who is obese at the start of pregnancy could perhaps gain less, but still should gain between 16 and 24 pounds.[4]

The weight the pregnant woman puts on is nearly all lean tissue: placenta, uterus, blood, and milk-producing glands, to say nothing of the baby itself. There is thus little place in her diet for empty kcalories such as sugar, fat, and alcohol, which provide no nutrients to support the growth of these tissues and only contribute to excessive fat accumulation. Some of the weight she gains is lost at delivery; the remainder is generally lost within a few weeks or months, as her blood volume returns to normal and she loses the fluids she has accumulated.

If a woman has gained more than the expected amount of weight early in pregnancy, she should not try to diet in the last weeks. Women have been known to gain up to 60 pounds in pregnancy without ill effects. (A *sudden* large weight gain, however, is a danger signal that may indicate the onset of pregnancy-induced hypertension; see "Troubleshooting.")

If the mother does not gain the full amount of weight recommended, she may give birth to an underweight baby. To the uninitiated, this may seem like no catastrophe, and in some instances it is not. A small mother may give birth to a small, normal, alert, and healthy baby. Nothing is wrong with that. On the other hand, a low-birthweight baby may be a malnourished baby, one who is more likely to get sick. Such a baby also is likely to be unable to do its job of obtaining nourishment by sucking and to win its mother's attention by energetic,

Ordinarily, a hemoglobin level below 13 g/100 ml is considered low for a woman (see Chapter 12). In pregnancy, values of 12 g are not unusual, and 11 g is where the line defining "too low" is often drawn. It is usually desirable to use more sensitive measures than hemoglobin if questions about the woman's iron status arise. See Chapter 12.

Food sources of iron:
- Liver and oysters.
- Red meat, fish, and other meat.
- Dried fruits.
- Legumes (dried beans, peas, and lima beans).
- Dark green vegetables.

vigorous cries and other healthy behavior. It can therefore become an apathetic, neglected baby, and this compounds the original malnutrition problem. Thus, for many reasons, babies of normal weight are usually more healthy.

Researchers seeking to find a measure by which they can evaluate the outcome of pregnancy have found that birthweight is the most potent single indicator of the infant's future health status. A low-birthweight baby, defined as one who weighs less than 5 1/2 pounds (2,500 grams), has a statistically greater chance of contracting diseases and of dying early in life. Its birth is more likely to be complicated by problems during delivery than that of a normal baby (defined as weighing a minimum of 6 1/2 pounds, or 3,000 grams). Nutritional deficiency, coupled with low birthweight, is the underlying or associated cause of more than half of all the deaths, worldwide, of children under five years old.[5]

Practices to Avoid

Some substances and practices have an undeserved bad reputation. One or two cups of coffee or tea a day or the equivalent are well within safe limits. Small quantities of artificial sweeteners and sugar are all right. A general guideline can be offered: eat a normal, healthy diet and use all substances in moderation. But some substances are truly harmful and their potential impact is too great to risk.

One such harmful practice is smoking. Smoking restricts the blood supply to the growing fetus and so limits the delivery of nutrients and removal of wastes. It stunts growth, thus increasing the risk of retarded development and complications at birth. Drugs taken during pregnancy can cause birth defects.

Dieting, even for short periods, is hazardous. Low-carbohydrate diets or fasts that cause ketosis deprive the growing brain of needed glucose and cause congenital deformity. Most serious may be the invisible effects. For example, carbohydrate metabolism may be rendered permanently defective, or the infant's brain may be permanently damaged.[6]

The consequences of protein deprivation can be severe. This has been observed most frequently in the underdeveloped countries, but it has also been seen among food faddists who adopted an untested vegetarian diet. Their children's height and head circumference were markedly and irreversibly diminished. Iron deficiency during pregnancy in animals has been seen to give rise to offspring whose brain cells could never store the needed iron thereafter.[7]

Most importantly, excessive alcohol consumption can cause irreversible brain damage and mental and physical retardation in the fetus (fetal alcohol syndrome). The damage can occur with as few as two drinks a day, and its most severe impact is likely to be in the first month, before the woman even is sure she is pregnant. About 1 in every 750 children born in the United States is a victim of this preventable damage.[8]

Oxygen is indispensable, on a minute-to-minute basis, to the development of the fetus's central nervous system, and a sudden dose of alcohol can halt the delivery of oxygen through the umbilical cord. During the first month of pregnancy, the fetal brain is growing at the rate of 100,000 new brain cells a minute, so even a few minutes of such exposure can have a major effect.

Clearly three ounces of alcohol a day is too much to risk, even if the woman stops drinking immediately after she learns that she is pregnant.[9] Birth defects have been observed in the children of some women who drank only two ounces of alcohol daily during pregnancy. Decreased birthweight (often

low birthweight (LBW): a birthweight of 5 1/2 lb (2,500 g) or less, used as a predictor of poor health in the newborn and as a probable indicator of poor nutrition status of the mother during and/or before pregnancy. Normal birthweight is 6 1/2 lb (3,000 g) or more. Low-birthweight infants are of two different types. Some are **premature**; they are born early and are the right size for their gestational age. Others have suffered growth failure in the uterus; they may or may not be born early, but they are **small for gestational age (small for date)**.

A table of the caffeine amounts in beverages and medications is provided in Chapter 16.

fetal alcohol syndrome: the cluster of symptoms seen in an infant or child whose mother consumed excess alcohol during her pregnancy; includes mental and physical retardation with facial and other body deformities.

These facial traits reflect fetal alcohol syndrome, caused by drinking early in pregnancy. Irreversible abnormalities of the brain and internal organs accompany these surface features.

| 1 day | 8 months | 4½ years | 8 years |

associated with increased risk to the newborn) has also been observed among the children of some women who drank two drinks (one ounce of pure alcohol) per day during pregnancy, and at the same level of alcohol intake a sizeable and significant increase occurs in the rate of spontaneous abortions.[10] Also, in a study of 12,000 women, an intake of two drinks a day was found to be significantly associated with detachment of the placenta.[11] One study presents evidence of an association between two drinks a *week* and miscarriages.[12] The accumulating evidence has led the *Journal of the American Medical Association* to take the conservative position that women should stop drinking as soon as they *plan* to become pregnant.[13]

There are probably even more subtle effects, too. Accumulating evidence suggests profound and long-lasting effects of alcohol exposure. An individual exposed before birth to alcohol may respond differently to it in adulthood than if no exposure had occurred—and also to drugs for which alcohol causes cross-tolerance.[14] Research using animals shows that one-fifth of the level of alcohol needed to produce major, outwardly-visible defects will surely produce learning impairment in the offspring. No sign of this impairment will be apparent on the outside, but the damage will be there on the inside.[15] Experiments using animals have even shown that alcohol in the female *before fertilization* may damage the outcome of pregnancy.[16]

As a result of findings like these, the popular magazine *Nutrition Today* takes the position that:

- The pregnant woman who drinks is more likely to give birth to a baby with FAS defects.
- The woman who is pregnant should not drink.
- The woman who is addicted to alcohol should be advised to avoid pregnancy at all costs.
- If, however, a woman addicted to alcohol becomes pregnant, she should be urged to have a preventive abortion.[17]

We might add that, for a woman who drinks heavily during the first two-thirds of her pregnancy, it is important to know that she can still prevent some damage by stopping heavy drinking during the third trimester.[18]

In opposition to that position, the American Council on Science and Health earlier took the position that women who drink only a little during pregnancy should not be hassled with overly conservative advice or made to feel guilty for a health habit that is insignificant in comparison with most others. Recently, however, ACSH has modified its statements. It now says, "Undoubtedly, there is a level of alcohol intake, as yet undetermined, that is not hazardous during pregnancy. Probably an occasional glass of beer or wine is tolerable in pregnancy, just as in the case of driving an automobile, provided that one drink does not lead to another. Total prohibition of drinking is an unacceptable rule for many people. Nevertheless, we believe that many pregnant women will prefer to give up drinking 'for the duration.' "[19] It's a personal choice, but if we had it to make, we'd opt for the healthy baby. We'd give up the pleasures, even of wine with meals, for the duration of pregnancy, and celebrate with champagne (once) after the baby's birth.

Troubleshooting

To avoid the most common problems encountered during pregnancy, some additional measures are helpful. Pregnancy precipitates the onset of diabetes in some women; it is recommended that all pregnant women be screened for diabetes at about the sixth month. Thereafter, at every checkup, a woman's urine should be tested for ketone bodies. Ketonuria may be a clue to diabetes or may warn of the starvation ketosis of ill-advised dieting.

A certain degree of edema is to be expected in late pregnancy, as mentioned, but in a poorly nourished woman, it is often part of a larger problem known as pregnancy-induced hypertension (PIH). Preexisting hypertension and PIH are the most common medical complications of pregnancy. They can cause maternal death, infant death, retarded growth, lung problems, and other birth defects. It is important to keep track of maternal blood pressure throughout pregnancy; and should it indicate PIH, to initiate treatment promptly.* Treatment is medical, and salt restriction is not a part of treatment until and unless the kidneys prove unable to handle a normal sodium load. A normal salt intake is necessary for health.[20]

The nausea of "morning" (actually, anytime) sickness seems unavoidable, because it arises from the hormonal changes taking place early in pregnancy, but it can often be alleviated. A strategy some expectant mothers have found effective in quelling nausea is to start the day with a few sips of water and a few nibbles of a soda cracker or other bland carbohydrate food, to get something in their stomachs before getting out of bed. Carbonated beverages also may help.

Later, as the hormones of pregnancy alter her muscle tone and the thriving infant crowds her intestinal organs, an expectant mother may complain of con-

pregnancy-induced hypertension (PIH), formerly known as toxemia (tox- EEM-ee-uh): a cluster of symptoms seen in pregnancy, including edema, hypertension, and kidney complications. A variety of terms are associated with PIH. Most common is eclampsia; its symptoms include convulsions and coma, associated with high blood pressure, edema, and protein in the urine. Eclampsia may be preceded by preeclampsia, from mild to severe.

The normal edema of pregnancy responds to gravity; blood pools in the ankles. The edema of toxemia is a generalized edema. The distinction helps with diagnosis.

Most severe risk factors for malnutrition in pregnancy:
- Age 15 or under.
- Unwanted pregnancy.
- Many pregnancies close together.
- History of poor outcome.
- Poverty.
- Food faddism.
- Heavy smoking.
- Drug addiction.
- Alcohol abuse.
- Chronic disease requiring special diet.
- More than 15% underweight.
- More than 15% overweight.
These factors at the start of pregnancy indicate that poor nutrition is very likely to be present and to affect the pregnancy adversely.

---

*Blood pressure of 140/90 mm mercury during the second half of pregnancy in a woman who has not previously exhibited hypertension indicates PIH. So does a rise in systolic blood pressure of 30 mm or in diastolic blood pressure of 15 mm on at least two occasions more than six hours apart. R. J. Worley, Pathophysiology of pregnancy-induced hypertension, *Clinical Obstetrics and Gynecology* 27 (1984): 821–835.

stipation. A high-fiber diet and a plentiful water intake will help to relieve this condition. Laxatives should be used only if the doctor orders them, and the type of laxative should be determined by the doctor.

Calcification of the baby teeth begins in the fifth month after conception; 32 teeth are well along in development before birth. For these teeth and for the bones, fluoride may be needed. It is not clear from research whether supplemental fluoride crosses the placenta, but some evidence suggests that it does. Children whose mothers received 1 milligram of flouride daily in addition to using fluoridated water have been observed to have more decay-free teeth at 5 to 9 years of age comparable to children whose mothers only used fluoridated water.[21] If the water is not ever fluoridated, then a prescribed supplement may be desirable.

What a lot for a woman to remember! And this is only the briefest summary of the nutrient needs in pregnancy. With all of this to worry about, can a woman relax and enjoy expecting her baby?

Pregnancy for many women is a time of adjustment to major changes. The woman who is expecting to bear a baby is a growing person in more ways than one. Not only physically, but also emotionally, her needs are changing. If it is her first baby, she senses that her lifestyle will have to change as she takes on the new responsibility of caring for a child. Ideally, she will be encouraged to develop this sense of responsibility by caring for herself during pregnancy. The expectant mother needs support in thinking of herself as a thoroughly worthwhile and important person with a new and challenging task that she can and will perform well. Oftentimes, as a young adult, she is still working out her relationship with her mate; and they both know that the coming of a first baby will affect that relationship profoundly. There is a need for sensitive communication and understanding on both parts in this time of transition.

Women's cravings during pregnancy do not seem to reflect real physiologic needs. Yet women going through this major experience should not be laughed at, and the validity of their feelings should be recognized. If a woman begs her mate, at 2 o'clock in the morning, to go to the nearest all-night grocery to buy her some pickles and chocolate sauce, it is probably not because she lacks a combination of nutrients uniquely supplied by these foods. She is expressing a need, however, as real and as important as her need for nutrients—for support, understanding, and love.

A pregnant woman may crave and eat clay, ice, cornstarch, and other nonnutritious substances. This is pica (recall Chapter 12) and may reflect a need for iron or zinc. The behavior is not adaptive; the substances she craves do not deliver the nutrients she needs.

Preparing for Breastfeeding

Toward the end of her pregnancy, a woman who plans to breastfeed her baby should begin to prepare. No elaborate or expensive procedures are necessary, but breastfeeding in humans involves many behaviors and attitudes that require learning, and it usually goes more smoothly for the mother who prepares than for the one who expects it to happen automatically. More is involved than can be discussed in detail here; it is recommended that the expectant mother read at least one of the many handbooks available on breastfeeding. Talking with women who have breastfed their babies successfully is also helpful, as is having a family and medical team support system.

As far as possible, the mother should discuss her plans in advance with the members of that support system, whoever they may be—her husband, her mother, her other children, the doctor, the midwife, or a nurse. Ideally, there will be classes that she and her husband can attend together before the baby is born. Before the birth time, if possible, she should acquire two or more nursing bras—the kind that give good support and that have drop-flaps so that either breast can be freed for nursing. Also, if her nipples are tender, she should prepare them so that they will become tougher. One book says that human nipples tend to be "overprotected" by the clothing we wear and can be toughened by the following means:

- Stop using soap on the breasts for the last three months of pregnancy so that the skin's own protective secretions can make the nipple area strong and resistant to irritation.
- Let the nipples rub against the outer clothing (wear the nursing bra open, or cut holes in an older bra for each nipple) so that they will be chafed.

A woman with flat or inverted nipples may want to manipulate her breasts by hand to help correct this condition or obtain a nipple shield that will help the nipple evert.

Breastfeeding

If a mother chooses to breastfeed, her nutrient supplies will continue to support the infant's development, as well as her own, even after birth. Adequate nutrition of the mother makes a highly significant contribution to successful lactation; without it, lactation is likely to falter or fail. She should continue to eat high-quality foods to the end of her pregnancy, not attempt to restrict her weight gain unduly, and plan to enjoy ample food and fluid at frequent intervals after she has given birth and until lactation is established.

Nutrient Needs and Eating Pattern

A nursing mother produces 30 ounces of milk a day, on the average, with wide variations possible. At 20 kcalories per ounce, this milk output amounts to 600 kcalories per day. In addition, energy is needed to produce this milk; so the energy allowance for a lactating woman is a generous 750 kcalories a day above her ordinary need. The RDA table suggests that 500 kcalories come from added food, and the rest from the stores of fat her body accumulated during pregnancy for that purpose. As during pregnancy, these kcalories should carry with them abundant nutrients—especially those needed to make milk, such as calcium, protein, magnesium, zinc, and plenty of fluid. Figure 14–2 showed the differences between a lactating woman's nutrient needs and those of a nonpregnant woman, and Table 14–2 showed a food pattern that would meet them.

Logically, the food best suited to support the mother's making of milk is milk, or something that resembles it in composition. The obvious choice is cow's milk. The nursing mother who can't drink milk needs to find nutritionally similar foods such as cheese, calcium-fortified soy milk, or the milk substitutes mentioned in Chapter 11. As during pregnancy, nutritious foods should make up the remainder of the needed kcalorie increase.

The question is often raised whether a mother's milk may lack a nutrient if she is not getting enough in her diet. The answer differs from one nutrient to the next, but in general, the effect of nutritional deprivation of the mother is to reduce the quantity, not the quality, of her milk. For the energy nutrients and most vitamins and minerals, the milk has a constant composition. In severe malnutrition, when nutrients are in short supply, correspondingly less milk will be produced, but it still will have the proper composition. The mother's diet may make her blood cholesterol higher or lower to some extent but seems not to affect her breast milk cholesterol. For some of the water-soluble vitamins and trace minerals, the composition may be more variable. Vitamin C will be low in the milk if it is low in the mother's diet. For most of the vitamins and minerals, though, the breast milk concentrations are nearly constant. Even the taking of a vitamin-mineral supplement seems not to raise nutrient concentrations in the breast milk of an otherwise well-nourished mother. It is best to avoid megadoses of vitamins or other nutrients, of course. And to repeat: water is the major ingredient of milk; a new mother should remember to drink plenty of fluids, no matter how busy she is.

The period of lactation is the natural time for a woman to lose the extra body fat she accumulated during pregnancy. If her choice of foods is judicious, she can tolerate a kcalorie deficit and a gradual loss of weight (1 pound per week) without any effect on her milk output. Fat can only be mobilized slowly, however, and too large a kcalorie deficit will inhibit lactation. On the other hand, if a mother does not breastfeed, she may not as easily lose the fat she gained during pregnancy.

Advantages of Breastfeeding

Emotional bonding is facilitated by many events and behaviors of mother and infant during the early months and years; one of the first can be breastfeeding, beginning right after birth. A critical event in bonding, thought to be mediated by chemical messengers in breast milk, may occur in the first 45 minutes after birth, so this may be an especially important feeding time.[22]

Thereafter, during the first two or three days of lactation, the breasts produce colostrum, a premilk substance containing antibodies and white cells from the mother's blood. Colostrum is sterile as it leaves the breast, and the baby cannot contract a bacterial infection from it even if his mother has one. Thus colostrum helps protect the newborn infant from those infections against which the mother has developed immunity. These diseases are the ones in her environment, and precisely those against which the infant needs protection. Entering the infant's body with the milk, these antibodies inactivate bacteria within the digestive tract, where they would otherwise cause harm. Some of the antibodies also "leak" into the bloodstream, because the infant's immature digestive tract cannot completely exclude whole proteins. These antibodies provide additional protection against such diseases as polio.

Breast milk also contains antibodies, although not as many as colostrum. Colostrum and breast milk also contain a factor (the bifidus factor) that favors the growth of the "friendly" bacteria *Lactobacillus bifidus* in the infant's digestive tract, so that other, harmful bacteria cannot grow there. Another factor

bonding: the forming of a bond between mother and infant.

colostrum (co-LAHS-trum): a milklike secretion from the breast, rich in protective factors, present during the first day or so after delivery, before milk appears.

bifidus (BIFF-id-us, by-FEED-us) **factor**: a factor in colostrum and breast milk that favors the growth, in the infant's intestinal tract, of the "friendly" bacteria *Lactobacillus* (lack-toh-ba-SILL-us) *bifidus*, so that other, less desirable intestinal inhabitants will not flourish.

lactalbumin (lact-AL-byoo-min): the chief protein in human breast milk, as opposed to **casein** (CAY-seen), the chief protein in cow's milk.

lactoferrin (lak- toe-FERR-in): a factor in breast milk that binds iron and keeps it from supporting the growth of the infant's intestinal bacteria.

present in colostrum and breast milk stimulates the development of the infant's GI tract.[23]

Breast milk is also tailor-made to meet the nutrient needs of the human infant. It offers its carbohydrate as lactose; its fat as a mixture with a generous proportion of the essential fatty acid, linoleic acid; and its protein largely as lactalbumin, a protein the human infant can easily digest. Its vitamin contents are ample. Even vitamin C, for which cow's milk is not a good source, is supplied generously by breast milk.

As for minerals, the calcium-to-phosphorus ratio (2:1) is ideal for the absorption of calcium, and both of these minerals and magnesium are present in amounts appropriate for the rate of growth expected in a human infant. Breast milk is also low in sodium. In addition, it contains factors that favor absorption of the iron it contains. Zinc, too, is better absorbed from breast milk, which contains a zinc-binding protein necessary for absorption of zinc by the newborn.

Powerful agents against bacterial infection also occur in breast milk. Among them is lactoferrin, an iron-grabbing compound, which keeps bacteria from getting the iron they need to grow on, helps absorb iron into the infant's bloodstream, and also works directly to kill some bacteria. Another factor favors the infant's absorption of folacin.

Other factors in breast milk include several enzymes; several hormones (including thyroid hormone and prostaglandins); lipids that protect the infant against infection;[24] and a morphine-like compound, for which there are corresponding receptors in the infant's brain.[25] Much remains to be learned about the composition and characteristics of human milk, but clearly it is a very special substance.

In addition, there are indications that breastfeeding provides other benefits. It protects against allergy development during the vulnerable first few weeks; the act of suckling favors normal tooth and jaw alignment; and breastfeeding is unlikely to produce an obese child. It may have other advantages, too; some studies suggest that mothers who breastfeed are less likely to develop breast cancer and to form unwanted clots in the bloodstream after delivery. A woman who wants to breastfeed can derive justification and satisfaction from all these advantages.

When Breastfeeding Is Preferred

Under most circumstances, a woman can freely choose to feed breast milk or formula, knowing that the two modes of feeding are equally beneficial to the infant. However, if the infant is premature, if the family is poor, or if other factors act to the baby's disadvantage, then breastfeeding becomes the preferred choice.

Some authorities feel that a premature baby should be fed breast milk even if the mother can't nurse. That is, if the baby is being kept sealed away in an incubator in the intensive care unit, the mother should express her milk with her hands or a breast pump and carry the milk to the intensive care unit to be fed to the baby. Her own milk is thought to be better for the baby than that of a full-term mother, because its composition is better suited to a premature infant's needs. Breastfeeding manuals show how to use manual massage or breast pumps to obtain milk.

Some communities maintain breast milk "banks"—storage and delivery facilities for breast milk. Mothers who have milk to spare donate it to the bank; others can purchase it when it is needed. Success and safety in milk banking requires use of aseptic technique by the donor and prompt freezing of the milk. Breast milk normally contains bacteria and viruses from the mother's skin and nipple ducts—acceptable for her own baby, but not for someone else's. Freezing is necessary to prevent spoilage while preserving the milk's antibodies and other protective factors, which would be destroyed by pasteurization. The current recommendation is that a premature or ill baby's own mother collect, freeze, and transport her milk daily to the hospital and that banked milk only be used temporarily, if there is no better alternative. Breast milk can be stored safely in the freezer for up to six months, provided that it stays solidly frozen (below 0° F).[26]

A premature baby receiving breast milk may be given a supplement of special formula for premature infants, depending on the philosophy of the clinic responsible for its care. Babies not receiving breast milk can be successfully nourished on this formula alone, and even on total parenteral nutrition (nutrients delivered directly into a central vein).

When Not to Breastfeed

If a woman has a communicable disease such as tuberculosis or hepatitis that could threaten the infant's health, then they have to be separated. Breastfeeding would be possible only by pumping her breasts several times a day, and not worth the struggle. Similarly, if she must take medication that is secreted in breast milk and that is known to affect the infant, she must not breastfeed. Drug addicts, including alcohol abusers, are capable of taking such high doses that their infants can become addicts by way of breast milk; in these cases, too, breastfeeding is contraindicated.

Most prescription drugs, however, do not reach nursing infants in sufficiently large quantities to affect them adversely. Moderate use of alcohol is compatible with breastfeeding. Smoking between feedings is permissible, although it is desirable not to expose the infant to secondhand smoke in the air he breathes. Coffee drinking is fine, in moderation, as is the eating of foods such as garlic and spices. A particular food may affect the baby's liking for the mother's milk; this is a matter that requires individual detective work. (Examples are chocolate in some cases, excess caffeine in others, and foods that cause gas to the mother in others.) If a woman has an ordinary cold, she can go on nursing without worry. The infant will catch it from her anyway, if she is susceptible, and she may be less susceptible than a bottle-fed baby would be, thanks to immunologic protection.

A woman sometimes hesitates to breastfeed because she has heard that environmental contaminants may enter her milk and harm her baby. The decision whether to breastfeed on this basis might best be made after consultation with a physician or dietitian familiar with the local circumstances.

An environmental contaminant that has caused concern is the PCBs, which are found in rivers and waterways polluted by industry. PCBs are stored in body fat and remain in the body; they are excreted only in the fat of breast milk. According to the Committee on Environmental Hazards of the American Academy of Pediatrics, women need not fear contamination of their breast milk with PCBs unless they have eaten large amounts of fish caught in PCB-contaminated rivers, such as the Saint Lawrence Seaway, or have been directly exposed because of their occupations.

aseptic technique: the technique of working in a sterile fashion—that is, in an area free of all bacteria, and kept free of contamination.
a = without
sepsis = infection

For more about contaminants and nutrition, turn to Chapter 13.

Another contaminant of concern is dioxin, which has contaminated some mothers' milk in the south-central states to an extent incompatabile with breastfeeding. Should a woman have any question about PCBs, dioxin, or other contaminants in her breast milk, she should ask the advice of the local state health department.[27]

Vitamin-Mineral Supplements for the Breastfed Infant

It is unnecessary to give vitamin-mineral supplements to a newborn infant. If he is breastfed, breast milk and his own internal stores will meet most of his nutrient needs until he is well into the second half of his first year, and then the introduction of intelligently chosen juices and foods will keep up with his changing requirements. The only exceptions to this statement have to do with vitamin D, fluoride, and possibly iron.

Breast milk does not provide enough vitamin D for the infant who has little exposure to sunlight. This is not a problem in the South, but in northern, smoggy, or fogbound cities, vitamin D deficiency in breastfed babies can cause rickets. The preferred preventive is sunlight, not supplements, but broadly applicable guidelines for exposure can't be given; too many variables are involved. Among the relevant factors are:

- Latitude (how far from the sun).
- Season (winter versus summer).
- Area of skin exposed (winter versus summer clothes).
- Color of skin (light versus dark).
- City versus country (smog filters out the vitamin D-producing ultraviolet rays of the sun).

A light-skinned baby wearing just a diaper in strong summer sun and clear air might make enough vitamin D in a few minutes to meet her daily need. A dark-skinned baby wrapped up for cold weather in a smoggy city might not make enough even if he were outside for several hours.[28] For most babies in most circumstances, some exposure of a small amount of skin to the sun at midday each day will provide a protective dose of vitamin D.[29]

If the baby's only source of fluoride is breast milk, then the pediatrician is likely to prescribe appropriate supplementation. Fluoride does not appear to be secreted into breast milk even if the mother's fluoride supply is ample.[30] As for iron, it may be desirable to begin iron supplements for the breastfed infant at about four months.[31]

Formula Feeding

The substitution of formula feeding for breastfeeding involves copying nature as closely as possible. Human and cow's milk differ; cow's milk is significantly higher in protein, calcium, and phosphorus, for example, to support the calf's faster growth rate. But a formula can be prepared from cow's milk that does not differ significantly from human milk in these respects; the formula makers first dilute the milk and then add carbohydrate and nutrients to make it nutritionally comparable to human milk.

The antibodies in cow's milk do not protect the human baby from disease (they protect the calf from cattle diseases), but the high level of preventive medical care (vaccinations) and public health measures achieved in the developed countries, especially in the United States and Canada, make this consideration less important than it was in the past. Safety and sanitation can be achieved with either mode of feeding by the educated mother whose water supply is reliable.

Like the breastfeeding mother, the mother who feeds formula should be supported in her choice. Bearing and nurturing a baby involves much more than merely pouring nutrients in, in whatever form. The mother who offers formula to her baby has valid reasons for making her choice, and her feelings should be honored. She and the baby can benefit in many ways from the supportive approval of those around them.

Advantages of Feeding Formula

One of the major advantages of formula feeding is that gained by the mother whose attempts at breastfeeding have met with frustration. If she truly doesn't want to breastfeed or, worse, if she earnestly does want to and can't, continuing to try is an agonizing course, as hard on the baby as on the mother. When the mother finally accepts the necessity of formula feeding and weans the baby to the bottle, a period of anguish for both may be followed by the onset of peace and the first real opportunity to develop the all-important mother-child love. Other advantages:

- The mother can be sure the baby is getting enough milk; there is no limit to the supply.
- She can offer the same closeness, warmth, and stimulation during feedings as the breastfeeding mother does.
- Other family members can get close to the baby and develop a warm relationship in feeding sessions.
- The mother will be free, sooner, to give time to her other children or to contribute to the family's income by returning to work.

The attendant who is asked to advise on breastfeeding versus bottle-feeding should remember the advantages of both. In fact, when addressing any audience, you should remember that some members of that audience will be women who bottle-fed their babies. To praise breastfeeding out of proportion or without qualification can only make them feel guilty or angry.

Many mothers choose to breastfeed at first but wean within the first one to six months. This is a nice compromise. Even a few weeks of breastfeeding will significantly reduce the likelihood of the baby's developing an allergy to cow's milk, and this advantage alone is important if such an allergy is likely. Furthermore, the baby gets the immunological protection and all the special advantages of breastfeeding during the most critical first few weeks or months. Then the mother can choose to shift to the bottle and can know she has already given the baby those benefits. But it is imperative that she wean the baby onto *formula*, not onto plain milk of any kind—whole, low-fat, or skim. Only formula contains enough iron (to name but one of many, many factors) to support normal development in the baby's first year.

The Choice of Formula

National and international standards have been set for the nutrient contents of infant formulas. The Infant Formula Act of 1980 requires that formulas meet nutrient standards based on the American Academy of Pediatrics (AAP) recommendations, and in 1982 the FDA adopted quality control procedures to be sure that they do. Formulas that meet the standard are nutritionally similar; small differences in nutrient content are sometimes confusing, but not usually important.

Table 14–3 shows characteristics of human, cow's, and goat's milk, along with those of a formula prepared from modified cow's milk. The animal milks clearly differ significantly from human milk in many respects; you can see that the formula is similar to the animal milks in some ways, and to human milk in others. The formula resembles cow's milk in type and ratio of proteins, total fat, and calcium-to-phosphorus ratio, but has been adjusted to resemble human milk in total protein, carbohydrate, linoleic acid, major minerals, and renal solute load. While obviously not identical to human milk, formula presents the same nutrients in roughly the same proportions for the most part.

Table 14–4 shows the AAP standard for the bulk ingredients of infant formulas and permits you to compare it with human milk and with typical formulas. As you can see, the AAP standard recommends higher protein than is in human milk; this is because the cow's milk protein does not present as perfect a balance of amino acids for the human infant. You can also see that the formulas meet the AAP standard for the nutrients listed. The rest of the AAP recommendations for vitamins and minerals are shown in Table 14–5 to facilitate comparison with any formula of your choice.

For infants with special problems, formulas can be adapted to make them closer in composition to human milk (adjusted protein ratio, lower linoleic acid, lower sodium and other minerals). For premature babies, special premature formulas are available. Special formulas based on soy protein are available for infants allergic to milk protein, and formulas with the lactose replaced can be used for infants with lactose intolerance. For infants with other special needs, many other variations are available.

Replacing the Formula

As soon as the baby's nutrient needs are being met mostly by solid food—at any time after six months—a less complete follow-up formula can be used. As long as formula is the baby's major food, however, it should not be replaced by ordinary milk— primarily because the milk provides insufficient vitamin C and iron.

Once the baby is obtaining at least a third of the total daily kcalories from a balanced mixture of cereal, vegetables, fruits, and other foods, then whole cow's milk in any form, fortified with vitamins A and D, is acceptable as an accompanying beverage.[32] The AAP recommends that it be introduced at six months. Don't offer plain, unmodified cow's milk before six months, though, because the infant's GI tract may be sensitive to its protein, and if so, may bleed.

renal solute load: a measure of the concentration of all dissolved substances in the urine resulting from feeding a milk, formula, or diet. As the kidneys mature, they can handle higher solute loads; the low solute load of breast milk is ideal for the infant, especially the premature infant. A formula with too high a renal solute load can cause dehydration, a life-threatening condition in the infant, by incurring too great an obligatory water excretion.

TABLE 14–3

Major Characteristics of Human Milk, Cow's Milk, Goat's Milk, and Infant Formula

Characteristic	Human Milk	Cow's Milk	Goat's Milk	Formula[a]
Carbohydrate (g/100 ml)	7.2	5.0	4.7	7.0–7.2
Energy (kcal/100 ml)	74	67	76	68
Fat (g/100 ml)	2.7–4.6	3.5	4.1	3.6–3.7
Linoleic acid (% of total fatty acids)	10–15	4	—	13–23
Minerals				
Calcium (mg/l)	340	1,200	1,300	510–550
Calcium-to-phosphorus ratio	2.4	1.3	1.2	1.2—1.3
Iron (mg/l)	0.2–1.0	0.5	0.5	12 or 1.5[b]
Phosphorus (mg/l)	140	955	1,060	390–460
Potassium (mEq/l)	13	35	46	18–20
Sodium (mEq/l)	7	25	18	11–12
Protein (g/100 ml)	1.1	3.5	3.3	1.5–1.6
Renal solute load (mOsm/l)[c]	74	220	—	105–108
Vitamins (per 100 ml)				
Folacin (μg)	2–5	0.3	0.2	5–11
Niacin (mg)	0.15–0.18	0.09	0.2	0.7–1.3
Pantothenic acid (mg)	0.18–0.23	0.4	0.3	0.30–0.32
Riboflavin (μg)	36–37	175	184	63–100
Thiamin (μg)	14–16	44	40	53–65
Vitamin A (IU)	190–250	103 or 190[d]	207	169–250
Vitamin B_6 (μg)	10–11	64	7	40
Vitamin B_{12} (μg)	0.03–0.05	0.4	0.06	0.15–0.21
Vitamin C (mg)	4.3–5.2	1.1	1.5	5.5
Vitamin D (IU)	2.2	1.3 or 38[d]	2.4	40–42

[a]These numbers represent two formulas, Similac and Enfamil.

[b]These formulas are available unfortified or with iron fortification.

[c]The ability of solutes to cause osmosis is measured in terms of *osmols*; the osmol is a measure of the total number of particles. A *milliosmol* equals 1/1,000 of an osmol. Renal solute load is measured in osmols per liter of solution ((mOsm/l).

[d]The higher value represents fortified milk, which should contain 2,000 IU vitamin A and 400 IU vitamin D per quart (1,900 and 375 IU per liter, respectively).

Source: Adapted from K. Brostrom, Human milk and infant formulas: Nutritional and immunological characteristics, in *Textbook of Pediatric Nutrition*, ed. R. M. Suskind (New York: Raven Press, 1981); *Milk-based and Soy-based Formulations Used for Feeding Newborns in the Hospital* (an information sheet from Ross Laboratories, Columbus, OH 43216), January 1979. Data on goat's milk and on vitamins for all milk are adapted from S. J. Fomon, Milks and milk-based formulas, *Infant Nutrition* (Philadelphia: Saunders, 1967), pp. 195–224.

TABLE 14–4

AAP Standard Compared with Human Milk and Infant Formula

Content	Mature Human Milk	AAP Standard	Infant Formula[a]
Energy (kcal/100 ml)	67–75	60–80	67
Protein (% of kcal)	5.2	7–18	9
Fat (% of kcal)	35–58	30–55	47–50
Carbohydrate (% of kcal)	35–44	35–50	41–43

[a]Five formulas were used to generate these data: Similac (Ross), Similac 60/40 (Ross), Enfamil (Mead Johnson), SMA (Wyeth), and Nan (Nestle).

Source: Adapted from K. Brostrom, Human milk and infant formulas: Nutritional and immunological characteristics, in *Textbook of Pediatric Nutrition*, ed. R. M. Suskind (New York: Raven Press, 1981).

TABLE 14-5

AAP Recommendations for Nutrient Levels in Formulas

Nutrient	Recommended per 100 kCal	Recommended per 100 Ml[a]
Protein (g)	1.8–4.5	1.3–3.2
Fat (g)	3.3–6.0	2.3–4.2
Essential fatty acids (linoleic acid) (mg)	300	210
Vitamins		
Vitamin A (IU)	250–750[b]	175–525
Vitamin D (IU)	40–100	28–70
Vitamin K (μg)	4	3
Vitamin E (IU)	0.3 (with 0.7 IU/g linoleic acid)	2.1
Vitamin C (mg)	8	5.6
Thiamin (μg)	40	28
Riboflavin (μg)	60	42
Vitamin B_6 (μg)	35 (with 15 μg/g of protein in formula)	25
Vitamin B_{12} (μg)	0.15	0.11
Niacin (μg equivalent)	250	175
Folacin (μg)	4	2.8
Pantothenic acid (μg)	300	210
Biotin (μg)	1.5	1.1
Choline (mg)	7.0	4.9
Inositol (mg)	4.0	2.8
Minerals		
Calcium (mg)	50	35
Phosphorus (mg)	25	18
Calcium-to-phosphorus ratio	1.1–2.0	1.1–2.0
Magnesium (mg)	6	4
Iron (mg)	0.15	0.11
Iodine (μg)	5	3.5
Zinc (mg)	0.5	0.4
Copper (μg)	60	40
Manganese (μg)	5.0	3.5
Sodium (mg)	20 (6 mEq[c])	(6 mEq[c])
Potassium (mg)	80 (14 mEq[c])	(14 mEq[c])
Chloride (mg)	55 (11 mEq[c])	(11 mEq[c])

[a]Assuming 70 kcal/100 ml. If the formula contains 80 kcal/100 ml, multiply amount in "Recommended per 100 kCal" column by 0.8; if it contains 60 kcal/100 ml, multiply by 0.6; and so forth.

[b]250 to 750 IU would be 75 to 225 μg or RE (retinol equivalents).

[c] Milliequivalents per liter of formula.

Source: Adapted from Committee on Nutrition, American Academy of Pediatrics, Commentary on breast feeding and infant formulas, including proposed standards for formulas, *Pediatric Nutrition Handbook* (Evanston, Ill.: American Academy of Pediatrics, 1979), pp. 119–138.

Cow's milk comes in many forms: pasteurized, homogenized, evaporated, powdered, and others. (The terms are defined in the Miniglossary of Milks.) Any pasteurized milk that has nutritional value equivalent or superior to whole cow's milk is acceptable, but low-fat or skim milk should not be used routinely

Miniglossary of Milks

casein or sodium caseinate: the principal protein of cow's milk. Other milk proteins, found in a higher percentage in human milk, are **whey** and **lactalbumin**.

condensed milk: evaporated milk to which sugar (sucrose) is added before processing, as a preservative. The percentages of kcalories from protein, fat, and carbohydrate in condensed milk are 10, 24.5, and 65.5, respectively. Condensed milk contains 321 kcal/100 ml and is more than twice as concentrated as evaporated milk (146 kcal/100 ml). Accidental use of condensed milk in preparation of infant formula can cause dehydration.

evaporated milk: milk concentrated by evaporation. The milk is preheated (for example, at 120° C, or 248° F, for three minutes) and then run aseptically into cans. The ratio of fat to nonfat solids is the same as in the original milk. By adding water, you derive standard milk; the taste, however, is altered by this process. Whole or skim milk from any species (cow, goat, or other) can be evaporated.

evaporated milk formula: formula made at home from evaporated milk, sugar, and water—seldom used today.

fortified (with respect to milk): milk to which vitamins A and D have been added so that a quart contains 2,000 IU vitamin A and 400 IU vitamin D.

homogenized milk: milk treated to mix the fat evenly with the watery part (fat ordinarily floats to the top as cream). Heated milk is forced under high pressure through small openings to break up the fat into small particles, which then remain dispersed throughout the milk. Whole or partially skimmed milk from any species (cow, goat, or other) can be homogenized.

pasteurized milk: milk that is heat treated to reduce its bacterial count to an acceptable level. Methods vary; a common one is to heat the milk to at least 72° C (161° F), hold it at or above this temperature for 15 seconds, and then cool it rapidly to 50° C (148° F) or lower. Whole or skim milk from any species (cow, goat, or other) can be pasteurized.

powdered milk: completely dehydrated milk solids produced by a variety of processes. Some powdered milks are processed to rehydrate easily (instant milk); others require extensive blending. Both whole and skim milks can be powdered.

whole milk: cow's milk from which the fat has not been removed. The standard of identity for whole milk in most states requires that milk labeled *whole* must contain not less than 3.25% milk fat and not less than 8.25% nonfat milk solids.

See also the milks and milk substitutes defined in Chapter 11.

with infants under a year old; they need the fat of regular milk. Powdered milk is usually skimmed, but fat-containing varieties are available. Most people use either vitamin A and D-fortified whole or evaporated milk.

In a baby's first six months, the choice of formula is important, because whatever is chosen must supply the nutrients of human milk in similar forms and proportions. After the first year, the exact formulation of the milk selected is not so critical, but the choice is still important, because milk or its substitute occupies a place in the diet that no other type of food can fill.

Supplements for the Formula-fed Infant

For the formula-fed infant, the makeup of the formula determines what further supplementation may be necessary. The pediatrician is the expert to consult on local needs.

Formula preparation:
- Liquid concentrate (inexpensive, relatively easy)—mix with equal part water.
- Powdered formula (cheapest, lightest for travel)—read label directions.
- Ready-to-feed (easiest, most expensive)—pour directly into clean bottles.
- Evaporated milk or whole milk—ask nutritionist or nurse; use *both* vitamins and minerals in addition.
- Whole milk—do not use before 6 months.

Nutrition of the Infant

A baby grows faster during the first year than ever again, as Figure 14–3 shows. The growth of infants and children directly reflects their nutritional well-being and is the most important parameter used in assessing their nutrition status. The birthweight doubles in four months, from 7 to 14 pounds, and another 7 pounds is added in the next eight months. (If a ten-year-old child were to do this, the child's weight would increase from 70 to 210 pounds in a single year.) By the end of the first year, the growth rate has slowed down, and the weight gained between the first and second birthdays amounts to only about 5 pounds. This tremendous growth is a composite of the differing growth patterns of all the internal organs. The generalization that many critical periods occur early still holds true.

Changes in body organs during the first year affect the baby's readiness to accept solid foods. At first, all he can do is suck (and he can do that powerfully), but he can only swallow liquids that are well back in his throat. Later (at two months or so) he can move his tongue against his palate to swallow semisolid food. Still later, the first teeth erupt, but it is not until sometime during the second year that a baby can begin to handle chewy food. The stomach and intestines are immature at first; they can digest milk sugar (lactose) but can't manufacture significant quantities of the starch-digesting enzyme, amylase, until somewhat later. Thus they can't digest starch until about three months, with some variation depending on the individual baby.

FIGURE 14–3

Weight gain of human infants (boys) in the first five years.

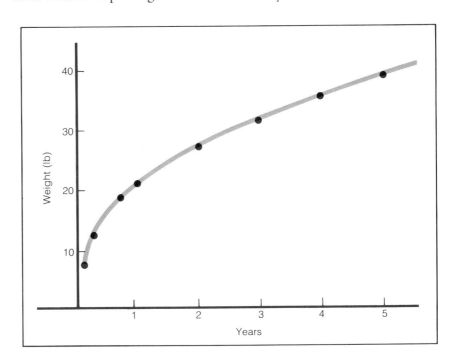

The baby's kidneys are unable to concentrate waste efficiently, so a baby must excrete relatively more water than an adult to carry off a comparable amount of waste. This means that dehydration, which can be dangerous, can occur more easily in an infant than in an adult. Because infants can communicate their needs only by crying, it is important to remember that they may be crying for fluid. A baby's metabolism is fast, so his energy needs are high.

Baby's metabolism:
• Heart rate: 120 to 140 beats/minute.
• Respiration rate: 20 per minute.

Adult's metabolism:
• Heart rate: 70 to 80 beats/minute.
• Respiration rate: 12 to 14 per minute.

Nutrient Needs and First Foods

The rapid growth and metabolism of the infant demand ample supplies of the growth and energy nutrients. Babies, because they are small, need smaller total amounts of these nutrients than adults do; but as a percentage of body weight, babies need over twice as much of most nutrients. Figure 14–4 compares a three-month-old baby's needs with those of an adult man; as you can see, some of the differences are extraordinary. After six months, energy needs increase less rapidly as the growth rate begins to slow down, but some of the kcalories saved by slower growth are spent in increased activity.

The most important nutrient of all, for infants as for everyone, is the one easiest to forget: water. The younger a child, the greater the percentage of the body weight is water, and the more rapid the turnover. Proportionately, more of the infant's body water than the adult's is between the cells and in the vascular space, so this water is easy to lose. Conditions that cause fluid loss, such as vomiting, diarrhea, sweating, or obligatory urinary loss without replacement can rapidly propel an infant into life-threatening dehydration. Fluid and electrolyte imbalances, caused by infection, kill more of the world's children than any other disease or disaster. Because infants can only cry and cannot tell you what they are crying for, it is important to remember that they may need fluid and to let them drink it until their thirst is quenched.

kCalories saved by slower growth are spent in increased activity.

FIGURE 14–4

Nutrient needs of three-month-old infant and adult male compared on the basis of body weight. The adult male's needs are set at 100 percent.

Source: Calculated from the RDA table—inside front cover.

Adult Male
Infant

By weight
% RDA Infant/Adult

2,000

1,500

1,000

500

100

Energy
Protein
Vitamin A
Vitamin D
Vitamin E
Vitamin C
Folacin
Niacin
Riboflavin
Thiamin
Vitamin B$_6$
Vitamin B$_{12}$
Calcium
Phosphorus
Magnesium
Iodine
Iron
Zinc

Iron is the nutrient hardest to provide for infants after weaning from breast milk or formula, because it doesn't occur in adequate amounts in ordinary milk. By the end of the first year, half or more of all infants are receiving less than the RDA for iron, and one-fourth are receiving less than two-thirds of the RDA. Iron may be the nutrient most needing attention in infant nutrition.[33]

The timing for adding solid foods to a baby's diet depends on several factors. If the baby is breastfed, additions to the diet should wait until about six months, but babies not fed solid foods before the end of the first year suffer delayed growth.[34] If the baby is formula-fed, foods might be started gradually beginning at 3 to 4 months, depending on readiness. Indications of readiness are:

- When the infant has doubled its birth weight, or
- When the infant can consume 8 ounces of formula and still is hungry in less than 4 hours, or
- When the infant is consuming 32 ounces a day and wanting more, or
- At 6 months.

Solids should not be introduced too early, because infants are more likely to develop allergies to them in the early months. But all babies are different, and the program of additions should depend on the individual baby, not on any rigid schedule. Table 14–6 presents a suggested sequence.

The addition of foods to a baby's diet should be governed by three considerations: the baby's nutrient needs, the baby's physical readiness to handle different forms of foods, and the need to detect and control allergic reactions. With respect to nutrient needs, nutrients needed early, especially by the formula-fed baby, are iron and vitamin C. Juices and fruits that contain vitamin C are usually among the first foods introduced. A baby's stored iron supply from before birth runs out after the birthweight doubles, so formula with iron, iron-fortified cereals, and later, meat, are recommended.

A term used by many authorities to mean supplemental or weaning foods is **beikost** (BYE-cost).

TABLE 14–6

First Foods for the Infant

Age (Months)	Addition
1 to 4	Diluted juice (for vitamin C)[a]
4 to 6	Iron-fortified rice cereal, followed by other cereals (for iron; baby can swallow and can digest starch now)[b]
5 to 7	Strained vegetables and/or fruits and their juices, one by one (perhaps vegetables before fruits, so the baby will learn to like their less sweet flavors)
6 to 8	Protein foods (cheese, yogurt, cooked beans, meat, fish, chicken, egg yolk)
9	Finely chopped meat (baby can chew now), toast, teething crackers (for emerging teeth)
10 to 12	Whole egg (allergies less likely now)

[a]All baby juices are fortified with vitamin C. Orange juice causes allergies in some babies; apple juice is often recommended as the first juice to feed.

[b]Later you can change cereals, but don't forget to keep on using the iron-fortified varieties. According to *Nutrition and the MD*, April 1981, the iron in cereal specially prepared for babies is so bioavailable that three level tablespoons a day is all they need.

Source: Adapted from the 1979 *Recommendations for Infant Feeding Practices of the California Department of Health Services*, as presented in Current infant feeding practices, *Nutrition and the MD*, January 1980.

It has been suggested that the early introduction of sweet fruits to babies' diets might favor their developing a preference for sweets and lessen their liking for vegetables introduced later. To prevent this, the order should perhaps be vegetables first, fruits later. This practice now has a wide following. As for sweets of any other kind, they have no place in a baby's life. The added kcalories they contribute can promote obesity and perhaps the irreversible multiplication of fat cells, but they convey no nutrients to support growth.

Physical readiness develops in many small steps. For example, the ability to swallow solid food develops at around four to six months, and experience with solid food at that time helps to develop swallowing ability by desensitizing the gag reflex. Later still, a baby can sit up, can handle finger foods, and is teething; then hard crackers and other hard finger foods should be introduced. These promote the development of manual dexterity and control of the jaw muscles.

Some parents want to feed solids at an earlier age, on the theory that "stuffing the baby" at bedtime will make him (or her) more likely to sleep through the night. There is no proof for this theory. On the average, babies start to sleep through the night at about the same age, regardless of when solid foods are introduced, and by three months, 75 percent are sleeping through the night whether or not they are receiving any solid foods.[35]

New foods should be introduced singly, so that allergies can be detected. For example, when cereals are introduced, try rice cereal first for several days; it causes allergy least often. Try wheat cereal last; it is the most common offender. If a cereal causes an allergic reaction (irritability due to skin rash, GI upset or respiratory discomfort), discontinue its use before going on to the next food. About nine times out of ten, the allergy won't be evident immediately, but will manifest itself in vague symptoms occurring up to five days after the offending food is eaten, so it isn't easy to detect. If parents detect allergies in their infant's early life, they can spare the whole family much grief. (Highlight 14 offers more information on allergies.)

As for the choice of foods, baby foods commercially prepared in the United States and Canada are generally safe, nutritious, and of high quality. In response to consumer demand, baby food companies have removed much of the added salt and sugar their products contained in the past, and baby foods also contain few or no additives. They generally have high nutrient density, except for mixed dinners (which contain little meat) and desserts (which are heavily sweetened). An alternative for the parent who wants the baby to have family foods is to "blenderize" a small portion of the table food at each meal. This necessitates cooking without salt, though. Foods adults prepare for themselves often contain much more salt than even commercial baby foods. The adults can salt their own food after the baby's portion has been taken. And babies should never be fed canned vegetables; not only is the sodium content too high, but also the risk of lead contamination is present. It is also important to take precautions against food poisoning and to avoid the use of vegetables in which nitrites are likely to form—notably, home-prepared carrots, beets, and spinach. Honey should never be fed to infants because of the risk of botulism.

At a year of age, the obvious food to supply most of the nutrients the baby needs is still milk; 2 to 3 1/2 cups a day are now sufficient. More milk than this would displace foods necessary to provide iron and would cause the iron-deficiency anemia known as milk anemia. The other foods—meat, iron-fortified cereal, enriched or whole-grain bread, fruit, and vegetables—should be supplied in

milk anemia: iron deficiency anemia caused by drinking so much milk that iron-rich foods are displaced from the diet.

Meal Plan for a One-Year-Old

Breakfast	Snack
1 c milk	½ c milk
3 tbsp cereal	Teething crackers
2 to 3 tbsp strained fruit	
Teething crackers	

Lunch	Supper
1 c milk	1 c milk
2 to 3 tbsp vegetables	1 egg
Chopped meat	2 tbsp cereal or potato
2 to 3 tbsp pudding	2 to 3 tbsp cooked fruit
	Teething crackers

Babies develop sensitivity to their own satiety (see p. 256) at about ten months, another example of developmental readiness.

For more about the prudent diet, turn to Highlight 4B.

Nursing bottle syndrome, an extreme example of tooth decay. This child was frequently put to bed sucking on a baby bottle filled with apple juice, so that the teeth were bathed in carbohydrate for long periods of time—a perfect medium for bacterial growth. The upper teeth have decayed all the way to the gum line.

variety and in amounts sufficient to round out total kcalorie needs. The one-year-old should be sitting at the table and eating many of the same foods everyone else eats. A meal plan that meets the requirements for the one-year-old is shown in Table 14–7.

Looking Ahead

The first year of a baby's life is the time to lay the foundation for future health. From the nutrition standpoint, the relevant problems most common in later years are obesity and dental disease. Prevention of obesity should also help prevent the development of the obesity-related diseases—atherosclerosis, diabetes, and cancer.

Infant obesity should be avoided. Probably the most important single measure to undertake during the first year is to encourage eating habits that will support continued normal weight as the child grows. Primarily, this means introducing nutritious foods in an inviting way, not forcing the baby to finish the bottle or the baby food jar; avoiding concentrated sweets and empty-kcalorie foods; and encouraging vigorous physical activity.

To discourage development of the behaviors and attitudes that plague the obese, parents should avoid teaching babies to seek food as a reward, to expect food as comfort for unhappiness, or to associate food deprivation with punishment. If they cry for thirst, they should be given water, not milk or juice. Babies seem to have no internal "kcalorie counter," and they stop eating when their stomachs are full, so low-kcalorie foods will satisfy as long as they provide bulk.

Beyond these recommendations, some thought is being given to the idea that infants should be started on a "prudent diet" like that recommended for heart patients: restrict fat, increase the ratio of polyunsaturated to saturated fat, and reduce cholesterol intake. To do this demands taking care, of course, not to restrict fat so severely as to deprive them of essential fatty acids needed for growth and nervous system development. Such a diet has been tried with infants up to three years of age. It seems to have done them no harm, while lowering their serum cholesterol. However, this kind of program is only experimental. Babies need the kcalories and fat of normal milk, and most experts agree that they should be fed whole or at least low-fat—not skim—milk until after they are a year old. The only exception might be the seriously obese baby, who should perhaps be started on a prudent diet as early as three months of age.[36] Tampering with the amount of protein in a baby's diet could be especially undesirable, because altered amounts of protein affect the baby's body composition, with unpredictable consequences.[37]

Normal dental development is promoted by the same strategies outlined above: supplying nutritious foods, avoiding sweets, and discouraging the association of food with reward or comfort. In addition, the practice of giving a baby a bottle as a pacifier is strongly discouraged by dentists on the grounds that sucking for long periods of time pushes the normal jawline out of shape and causes the bucktooth profile: protruding upper and receding lower teeth. Further, prolonged sucking on a bottle of milk or juice bathes the upper teeth in a carbohydrate-rich fluid that favors the growth of decay-producing bacteria. Babies permitted to do this are sometimes seen with their upper teeth decayed all the way to the gum line.

Mealtimes

The wise parent of a one-year-old offers nutrition and love together. Both promote growth. It is literally true that "feeding with love" produces better growth in both weight and height of children than feeding the same food in an emotionally negative climate.[38] It also promotes better brain development. The formation of nerve-to-nerve connections in the brain depends both on nutrients and on environmental stimulation.[38]

The person feeding a one-year-old has to be aware that this is a period in the child's life when exploring and experimenting are normal and desirable behaviors. The child is developing a sense of autonomy that, if allowed to flower, will provide the foundation for later confidence and effectiveness as an individual. The child's impulses, if consistently denied, can turn to shame and self-doubt. In light of the developmental and nutrient needs of one-year-olds, and in the face of their often contrary and willful behavior, a few feeding guidelines may be helpful. Following are several problem situations with suggestions for handling them:

■ He stands and plays at the table instead of eating. Don't let him. This is unacceptable behavior and should be firmly discouraged. Put him down, and let him wait until the next feeding to eat again. Be consistent and firm, not punitive. If he is really hungry, he will soon learn to sit still while eating. A baby's appetite is less keen at a year than at eight months, and his kcalorie needs are relatively lower. A one-year-old will get enough to eat if he lets his own hunger be his guide.

■ She wants to poke her fingers into her food. Let her. She has much to learn from feeling the texture of her food. When she knows all about it, she'll naturally graduate to the use of a spoon.

■ He wants to manage the spoon himself, but can't handle it. Let him try. As he masters it, withdraw gradually until he is feeding himself competently. This is the age at which a baby can learn to feed himself and is most strongly motivated to do so. He will spill, of course, but he'll grow out of it soon enough.

■ She refuses food that her mother knows is good for her. This way of demonstrating autonomy, one of the few available to the one-year-old, is most satisfying. Don't force. It is in the one- to two-year-old stage that most of the feeding problems develop that can last throughout life. As long as she is getting enough milk and is offered a variety of nutritious foods to choose from, she will gradually acquire a taste for different foods—provided that she feels she is making the choice. This year is the most important year of a child's life in establishing future food preferences. If a baby refuses milk, an alternative source of the bone- and muscle-building nutrients it supplies must be provided. Milk-based puddings, custards, and cheese are often successful substitutes. For the baby who is allergic to milk, soy milk and other formulas are available.

■ He prefers sweets—candy and sugary confections—to foods containing more nutrients. Human beings of all races and cultures have a natural inborn preference for sweet-tasting foods. Limit them strictly. There is no room in a baby's daily 1,000 kcalories for the kcalories from sweets, except occasionally. The meal plan shown in Table 14−7 provides more than 500 kcalories from milk; one or two servings of each of the other types of food provide the other 500. If a candy bar were substituted for any of these foods, the baby would lose out on valuable nutrients; if it were added daily, he would gradually become obese.

Study Questions

1. Discuss the special problems and energy needs of the different periods of pregnancy. Describe the currently recommended pattern and extent of weight gain during pregnancy.
2. What are the advantages and disadvantages of breastfeeding? How does the recommended diet for a nursing mother differ from that of a pregnant woman?
3. What are the advantages of formula feeding? What criteria would you use in selecting an infant formula?
4. Why are solid foods not recommended for an infant during the first few months of life? Name the indicators of readiness for adding solid foods to an infant's diet.

Notes

1. E. Hackman and coauthors, Maternal birth weight and subsequent pregnancy outcome, *Journal of the American Medical Association* 250 (1983): 2016–2019.
2. R. Kumar, W. R. Cohen, and F. H. Epstein, Vitamin D and calcium hormones in pregnancy, *New England Journal of Medicine* 302 (1980): 1143–1145.
3. Committee on Dietary Allowances, *Recommended Dietary Allowances*, 9th ed. (Washington, D.C.: National Academy of Sciences, 1980), p. 138.
4. Maternal weight gain and the outcome of pregnancy, *Nutrition Reviews* 37 (1979): 318–321; California Department of Health, as cited in Nutrition and the pregnant obese woman, *Nutrition and the MD*, January 1978. Appendix E presents a weight gain grid for use in evaluating the pregnant woman's progress.
5. A. Petros-Barvazian and M. Béhar, Low birth weight: What should be done to deal with this global problem? *WHO Chronicle* 32 (June 1978): 231–232; *New Trends and Approaches in the Delivery of Maternal and Child Care in Health Services* (sixth report of the WHO Expert Committee on Maternal and Child Health), as cited in *Journal of the American Dietetic Association* 71 (1977): 357.
6. R. M. Pitkin, ed., Nutrition in pregnancy, *Dietetic Currents, Ross Timesaver*, January/February 1977; C. S. Mahan, Revolution in obstetrics: Pregnancy nutrition, *Journal of the Florida Medical Association*, April 1979, pp. 367–372.
7. R. L. Leibel, Behavioral and biochemical correlations of iron deficiency: A review, *Journal of the American Dietetic Association* 71 (1977): 399–404.
8. K. K. Sulik, M. C. Johnston, and M. A. Webb, Fetal alcohol syndrome: Embryogenesis in a mouse model, *Science* 214 (1981): 936–938.
9. Alcohol and pregnancy, *Nutrition and the MD*, August 1984.
10. Pregnancy and alcohol warning, *FDA Consumer*, October 1981, p. 2.
11. M. C. Marbury and coauthors, The association of alcohol consumption with outcome of pregnancy, *American Journal of Public Health* 73 (1983): 1165–1168.
12. J. Kline and coauthors, Drinking during pregnancy and spontaneous abortion, *Lancet* 2 (1980): 176–180.
13. Even moderate drinking may be hazardous to maturing fetus (medical news), *Journal of the American Medical Association* 237 (1977): 2535–2536.
14. E. L. Abel, R. Bush, and B. A. Dintcheff, Exposure of rats to alcohol in utero alters drug sensitivity in adulthood, *Science* 212 (1981): 1531–1533.
15. F. L. Iber, Fetal alcohol syndrome, *Nutrition Today*, September/October 1980, pp. 4–11.
16. M. H. Kaufman, Ethanol-induced chromosomal abnormalities at conception, *Nature* 302 (1983): 258–260.
17. *Nutrition Today* letter, 8 April 1981.
18. H. L. Rosett, L. Weiner, and K. C. Edelin, Treatment experience with pregnant problem drinkers, *Journal of the American Medical Association* 249 (1983): 2029–33.
19. *Alcohol Use During Pregnancy*, a booklet from the American Council on Science and Health, 47 Maple Street, Summit, NJ 07901, December 1981.
20. F. P. Zuspan, Chronic hypertension in pregnancy, *Clinical Olstetrics and Gynecology* 27 (1984): 854–873.
21. F. B. Glenn, W. D. Glenn, and R. C. Duncan, Fluoride tablet supplementation during pregnancy for caries immunity: A study of the offspring produced, *American Journal of Obstetrics and Gynecology* 143 (1982): 560–564.
22. B. J. Myers, Mother-infant bonding: Rejoinder to Kennell and Klaus, *Developmental Review* 4 (1984): 283–288.
23. M. Winick, Infant nutrition: Formula or breast feeding? *Professional Nutritionist*, Spring 1980, pp. 1–3.
24. K. M. Shahani, A. J. Kwan, and B. A. Friend, Role and significance of enzymes in human milk, *American Journal of Clinical Nutrition* 33 (1980): 1861–1868; Thyroid hormones in human milk, *Nutrition Reviews* 37 (1979): 140–141; Prostaglandins in human milk, *Nutrition Reviews* 39 (1981): 302–303; J. J. Kabara, Lipids as host-resistance factors of

human milk, *Nutrition Reviews* 38 (1980): 65–73.

25. E. Hazum and coauthors, Morphine in cow and human milk: Could dietary morphine constitute a ligand for specific morphine (mu) receptors? *Science* 213 (1981): 1010–1012.

26. Questions readers ask, *Nutrition and the MD*, December 1981.

27. Committee on Environmental Hazards, American Academy of Pediatrics, PCBs in breast milk, *Pediatrics* 62 (1978): 407.

28. At particular risk are inner-city Black Muslim infants who are breastfed. Not all milks are kind, *Nutrition and the MD*, May 1980; W. F. Loomis, Skin-pigment regulation of vitamin-D biosynthesis in man, *Science* 157 (1967): 501–506; R. M. Neer, The evolutionary significance of vitamin D, skin pigment, and ultraviolet light, *American Journal of Physical Anthropology* 43 (1975): 409–416.

29. P. M. Fleiss, J. Gordon, and J. Douglass, The vitamin D activity of milk (letter to the editor), *Nutrition Reviews* 40 (1982): 286.

30. J. Ekstrand, No evidence of transfer of fluoride from plasma to breast milk, *British Medical Journal* 283 (1981): 761–764.

31. Dr. James C. Penrod, pediatrician, Tallahassee, Florida (personal communication, June 1983).

32. American Academy of Pediatrics, Committee on Nutrition, The use of whole cow's milk in infancy, *Pediatrics* 72 (1983): 253–255.

33. G. II. Johnson, G. A. Purvis, and R. D. Wallace, What nutrients do our infants really get? *Nutrition Today*, July–August 1981, pp. 4–10, 23–26.

34. Winick, 1980.

35. L. L. Clark and V. A. Beal, Age at introduction of solid foods to infants in Manitoba, *Journal of the Canadian Dietetic Association* 42 (1981): 72–78.

36. The prudent diet in pediatric practice, *Nutrition and the MD*, November 1979.

37. L. E. Holt, Jr., Protein economy in the growing child, *Postgraduate Medicine* 27 (1960): 783–798.

38. E. M. Widdowson, Mental contentment and physical growth, *Lancet* 1 (1951): 1316–1318.

39. J. Cravioto, Nutrition, stimulation, mental development and learning, *Nutrition Today*, September–October 1981, pp. 4–8, 10–15.

HIGHLIGHT FOURTEEN

Nutrition and Behavior

Parents often become interested in the effects of nutrition, not only on their children's physical health, but also on their children's behavior. "Will sugar make my child hyperactive?" they wonder. "Might food allergies make my child perform poorly in school?" Questions like these have interested many people, and much information has been generated—some reliable, some not. Popular books inform parents that, yes, sugar does cause hyperactivity and food allergies do affect performance; but research into the effects of nutrition on behavior has tended to yield mostly negative findings along those lines. On the other hand, research has turned up some interesting and important findings about the effects of nutrient deficiencies on children's behavior—deficiencies mild enough so that some are, in fact, seen among significant numbers of children, even in well-to-do families. This highlight takes up the question of adverse reactions caused by substances *in* foods, and also asks what effects on behavior are seen when substances are *not* in foods— that is, when there are nutrient deficiencies.[1]

Food Allergies, Sensitivities, and Intolerances

Mrs. Frantic is at her wits' end with little five-year-old Freddie. He never sits still. He eats erratically. His kindergarten teacher says he is disruptive in the classroom. A neighbor suggests he must be allergic to all the junk foods he is eating. Mrs. Frantic is offended at the idea that Freddie eats junk foods, but would like to believe that he has an allergy, because she feels that such a diagnosis would give her something concrete to do for Freddie. She and Freddie's father agree that she should pursue the possibility, so she visits a local, highly respected allergist. Here's what she learns.

Food allergies are frequently blamed for physical and behavioral abnormalities in both children and adults. However, true food allergies are rare, and are often wrongly blamed for problems with health, mood, and behavior. A true food allergy occurs only when the body's immune system reacts to a food protein or other large molecule as it does to an antigen—by producing antibodies, histamines, or other defensive agents. Normally, true allergic reactions do not occur, because proteins and other large molecules of food are promptly taken apart in the digestive tract. When a food protein or other antigen does leak into the system, though, it elicits the immune reaction. A food antigen invades by way of the digestive tract; other types of antigens often penetrate the system through the skin or the linings of the lungs. An allergic reaction always involves antibody formation, but other immune reactions can occur when cells of the immune system simply produce histamines in response to antigens. Some authorities call these reactions *sensitivities*.

The term *allergy* has two components—sensitization (the presence of antibodies) and the presence or absence of symptoms. An allergic person may produce antibodies without having any symptoms, or may produce antibodies *and* have symptoms. These two conditions are known as *asymptomatic allergy* and *symptomatic allergy*, respectively. Symptoms without antibody production are *not* caused by allergy.

When elicited by way of the digestive tract, the allergic reaction causes nausea and sometimes vomiting. (In the skin, it causes a variety of rashes; and in the nasal passages and lungs, it may cause inflammation or asthma. A generalized, all-systems shock reaction can also occur.) Neurological problems, including behavioral disturbances and depression, have *not* been conclusively demonstrated to result from food allergy.[2]

Allergic reactions to foods can occur with several different timings. A simple classification divides them into "immediate" and "delayed" categories (Table H14–1). In both, the interaction of the antigen with the immune system is immediate, but the appearance of symptoms may come within minutes or after several (up to 24) hours.[3] Diagnosis of an immediate allergic reaction is easy, because symptoms correlate closely with the eating of the offending food, but diagnosis of delayed reactions is

TABLE H14–1

Four Types of Allergies

Type I. Causes immediate hypersensitivity; also known as anaphylactic hypersensitivity; antibody mediated (immediate).

Types II and III. Not included, as they are not known to occur in response to food ingestion.

Type IV. Causes delayed or cellular hypersensitivity; cell mediated (6 to 24 hours).

difficult, because the symptoms may not appear until a day after the food is eaten. This has led to confusion among doctors and clients, who don't know whether the clients' complaints after eating represent true immune-system allergic reactions, intolerances, psychosomatic reactions, or what.

Allergy specialists don't all agree on the terminology used here, nor do they agree on how to test for allergy. They also disagree on the incidence of food allergy. One reviewer reports that it occurs in from 0.3 to 7.5 percent of children;[4] another cites estimates ranging from 0.3 to 60 percent, but concludes that the range is probably somewhere between 0.3 and 25 percent.[5] Immediate hypersensitivity (type I food allergy) is known not to occur in more than 1 percent.

Testing for immediate hypersensitivity can be attempted by any of about 14 different methods, including histories, diaries, challenges with the offending food, skin tests, blood tests, and tests of other tissue samples. Some of these tests are less reliable than others, but many can lead to accurate diagnosis. The foods that most often cause immediate hypersensitivity reactions are listed in Table H14–2. According to one investigator, 91 percent of adverse reactions are caused by only four major foods: nuts (43 percent), eggs (21 percent), milk (18 percent), and soybeans (9 percent).[6] Sensitivity or allergic reactions to single foods are common. Reactions to multiple foods are the exception, not the rule.

On learning these facts, Mrs. Frantic is certain that Freddie doesn't have a type I allergy. He eats all these foods; if he had ever had such a dramatic immediate reaction, she would have noticed—and the symptoms that worry her are not at all like those the doctor has described. She asks how delayed allergies are diagnosed, and receives the following answer.

One way to obtain a valid diagnosis of delayed hypersensitivity is to take the time to do a double-blind challenge study. In such a study, the suspected food or foods are eliminated from the diet until all symptoms have subsided. Then coded capsules are given containing either the suspected food (usually in concentrated, dehydrated form) or a placebo, and records of reactions are kept. Under these circumstances, parents are often surprised to see that their children do *not* react to suspected foods about half the time or more, and are forced to conclude that the suspected allergy is really something else, like a psychosomatic reaction to food.[7]

Another means of testing for food allergies is to initiate an elimination diet (Table H14–3). This is a time-consuming, troublesome process. First, you have to feed a restricted diet, then introduce groups of suspected foods until symptoms appear. Removal of the suspected foods should correlate consistently with relief from symptoms, and reintroduction, with their reappearance. Any group of foods proving to cause symptoms by this method can be split into subgroups for further testing until the individual offending food or foods have been identified.

Allergies are not always diagnosed by these time-consuming, laborious methods, however. In fact, the term *food allergy* is used loosely, even by many physicians, as a kind of catchall term for any circumstance in which an adverse reaction to foods seems to have occurred and a clear diagnosis hasn't been obtained. Among reactions to foods that are confused with true food allergies are:

- Allergic reactions to molds, antibiotics, and other contaminants of foods.
- Chinese restaurant syndrome, a reaction specific to the flavor enhancer MSG (trade name, Accent), described in Highlight 9A. Incidence: one in several hundred.
- Reactions to bacterial toxins such as botulinal toxin and other food poisoning.
- Reactions to chemicals in foods, such as the natural laxative in prunes.
- Symptoms of digestive diseases such as hernias and ulcers, aggravated by eating any food.
- Enzyme deficiencies, such as lactose intolerance, which cause symptoms superficially indistinguishable from those of food allergy.
- Psychological reactions based on the belief that certain foods cause certain symptoms.[8]

Thus a person who has any kind of discomfort after eating— stomachache,

---

TABLE H14–2

Foods That Most Often Cause Immediate Hypersensitivity Reactions (Type I Allergy)

Nuts	Peanuts
Eggs	Chicken
Milk	Fish
Soybeans	Shellfish
Wheat	Mollusks

Source: F. M. Atkins, The basis of immediate hypersensitivity reactions to foods, *Nutrition Reviews* 41 (1983): 229–234.

TABLE H14–3

Elimination Diets

Infant (below three months): milk substitute (not containing soy).

Infant (three to six months): milk substitute (not containing soy) and rice cereal.

Infant (six months to two years): milk substitute (not containing soy) with rice cereal, vitamin supplement, applesauce, pears, carrots, squash, and lamb.

Children over two and adults: lamb and rice. No oral or topical medicines, including aspirin, vitamins, laxatives, or toothpastes.

Source: Adapted from R. H. Buckley and D. Metcalfe, Food allergy, *Journal of the American Medical Association* 248 (1982): 2627–2631.

headache, pain, rapid pulse rate, nausea, wheezing, hives, bronchial irritation, cough, or any other—may conclude that an allergy is responsible, when in fact it is something else entirely. Only careful, skilled testing can distinguish the many possibilities, and such testing is very seldom done.

After learning these facts, Mrs. Frantic is even more disappointed. The situation is more complicated than she wanted to believe at first. If she and the doctor pursue these possibilities, they'll have to investigate all kinds of allergies, not just food allergies. They'll have to consider the possibility of physical problems such as enzyme deficiencies. She had hoped that Freddie's problems could be easily solved by simply eliminating an offending food from the diet, but such is not the case.

Mrs. Frantic now sees, too, that food allergies are not likely to account for Freddie's aberrant behavior. Documented immune system-mediated allergic reactions to foods do not include any instances of behavioral change such as Freddie's hyperactivity. The only abnormal behavior seen in allergic children is the general misery that goes with feeling sick, and this misery is always accompanied by physical allergy symptoms. The doctor agrees that Mrs. Frantic should pursue other possibilities, but warns her that she should watch for any signs of food dislikes on Freddie's part and take them seriously.[9] Real allergies do exist, so be prepared to test for them.

Hyperactivity and Food Additives

Mrs. Frantic decides, next, to visit the pediatrician and ask if Freddie has hyperactivity. Hyperactivity occurs in 5 to 10 percent of young school-age children—that is, in 1 or 2 in every classroom of 20 children. It can lead to academic failure and major behavior problems.[10]

The pediatrician agrees that Freddie is, indeed, very active and distractible,

but says he cannot diagnose hyperactivity on the basis of observations alone. He suggests a trial with stimulant drugs. If Freddie responds to the drugs by calming down, then the behavior problems can be kept under control until Freddie is older—at which time they usually clear up with no residual ill effects. He sums up the evidence: "Of the available methods, by far the most effective and the best documented is the use of the stimulant drugs, [to] suppress overactivity and impulsivity and lengthen attention span."[11] In other words, it seems that prescription medication should at least be considered as the treatment of choice.

But Mrs. Frantic's neighbor is strongly opposed to the use of these drugs. Mrs. Frantic apologizes to the pediatrician for refusing to try this course of action right away, and says she'll be back if she can't find a better alternative. She is considering trying the Feingold diet.

The idea that hyperactivity in children might be caused by the way they eat became popular in 1973, when Dr. Benjamin Feingold put forth his theory that hyperactive children suffer adverse reactions to the artificial flavors and colors in foods. Dr. Feingold suggested that adverse reactions to food-borne compounds—salicylates—related chemically to aspirin are responsible for behavioral problems in children.* He said that hyperactive children should be placed on a diet of natural foods totally free of additives—and he announced that when they are

---

*Aspirinlike compounds (salicylates), to which some people are allergic, include yellow dye no. 5, tartrazine. Incidence: perhaps 1 in 100 cases of allergy. (The *FDA Consumer*, September 1979, p. 29, reports that 100,000 people in the United States may be allergic to yellow dye no. 5. That's 1 in every 2,000 people. If 5 percent of every 2,000 people have allergies, then 1 in every 100 allergic people are allergic to salicylates.)

placed on such a diet, 50 percent calm down, two-thirds of them "dramatically."[12] By 1978, Dr. Feingold's theory was famous, and more than 20,000 children were being fed the Feingold diet.[13]

To see what might be involved in adopting the diet, Mrs. Frantic next consults a dietitian. The dietitian, too, presents discouraging news. She points out that Dr. Feingold's approach to the problem of hyperactivity has not been scientifically validated. His enthusiastic endorsement of his method is striking, but his book provides no evidence of true allergic reactions.[14] Instead, it presents many loose, anecdotal stories of misbehaviors associated with processed foods and alleviated by natural foods. The lack of hard evidence does not mean his theory should be rejected—especially because so many families swear by his diet—but it can't be accepted as proven, either. Furthermore, to impose a Feingold diet on Freddie would involve changing the entire family's lifestyle—a process at least as time-consuming and troublesome as allergy testing. Surprisingly, the dietitian suggests that Freddie might benefit more from the change in lifestyle than from the diet! Here's what she tells Mrs. Frantic.

Efforts to resolve the question of whether the Feingold diet is effective in the treatment of childhood hyperactivity began in 1976, when an expert committee of the Institute of Food Technologists undertook a review of the evidence. They concluded that no controlled studies had confirmed Feingold's claim; his diet had not been evaluated for its long-term effects; and it might not fully meet the nutritional needs of children. They pointed out that, when individual children are singled out for study of the effects of diet on their behavior, diet is not the only thing in their lives that changes. They receive special attention, too, and this may well have beneficial effects on their behavior (the placebo effect). Both the children and their parents and teachers are likely to be influenced by the hope that the experiment will work—and by suggestibility, a factor that is difficult to rule out.[16]

The committee designed a double-blind study to avert these problems, and it was conducted over an eight-month period at the University of Wisconsin. The outcome was not conclusive. Some children seemed to have improved while on the additive-free diet, but an equal number had worsened. In general, Feingold's hypothesis was not borne out by the findings, but the possibility remained that some individual children might have benefited from the diet. Further investigation was recommended. Following this study, several others were conducted with similar results; over a million dollars was spent, but little new evidence in favor of Feingold's theory surfaced. Although a few individual cases of true salicylate allergy are known, and a few individual children seem to have benefited from the Feingold diet, the dietary approach to hyperactivity seems to work mostly by suggestion, if it works at all.[16]

The power of suggestion associated with the Feingold diet is considerable, however. A child who has been deemed hyperactive "learns" that the food she eats has made her that way, and that from now on she and her family are going to eat differently. There will be no more junk foods, no more processed convenience foods, no more casual snacks. Foods will be prepared from scratch at home and eaten together. The whole family's lifestyle will change, and the child's behavior is expected to improve. It does improve—but in response to what? Not only is the family eating differently; they are living differently, and the child is receiving more attention, more of her parents' energy, and more structure than before.

When controlled, double-blind experiments with additive-containing and additive-free foods are conducted, the benefits of the Feingold diet do not materialize as they do in individual family situations. The panels of experts who have reviewed the evidence have concluded that it is indeed not the additive-free nature of the diet that works, but the changed lifestyle that the diet demands.[17] A physician has offered the opinion that the diet "has much appeal, particularly to those who react against modern technology." He quotes the Nutrition Foundation, which sees "no reason to discourage those families who wish to pursue this type of treatment so long as they continue to follow other therapy which is helpful."[18]

Without any answers, parents still have to deal with excitable, rambunctious, and unruly children. Common sense says that all children at times get wild and "hyper." There are many normal, everyday causes of such behavior:

- Attention getting.
- Lack of sleep.
- Overstimulation.
- Too much TV.
- Lack of exercise.

Together, these produce the tension-fatigue syndrome, which can be relieved by giving more consistent care to the child's welfare. It helps especially to insist on regular hours of sleep, regular mealtimes, and regular outdoor exercise.

Mrs. Frantic now sees that Dr. Feingold's approach is unlikely to help Freddie physically, but she has learned that a change in lifestyle might benefit him. She and Freddie's father decide to make a concerted effort to manage Freddie's problems by all the means they have within their own control at home. They start feeding him breakfast daily without fail. They clamp down on his between-meal snacking on sugary foods, and insist that he eat a regular lunch and dinner with them. They insist on his going to bed at a reasonable time. They cut down his TV watching, and make sure that he engages in active play outdoors for at least an hour or two each day. In the process, they find themselves giving him much more positive attention, and having fewer occasions to scold and punish him.

The results are pleasing. Freddie remains a highly energetic child, but his behavior becomes less disruptive. He seems happier. The teacher notices the change. He sits up and takes notice in school. He sleeps better, and eats with a better appetite at mealtimes. He hardly gets sick at all any more. He looks healthier than he did before—as if he had recovered from a physical illness.

No one knows exactly what accounts for the change, but everyone is pleased about it. The allergist is not surprised to find that allergy testing never proved necessary. The pediatrician thinks the parents have effectively, if unknowingly, applied behavior-modification techniques. The neighbor is quite sure that the elimination of the junk foods Freddie was eating before has brought relief, because his diet is now much lower in additives and sugar than it was previously. The dietitian is sure that the addition of structure to Freddie's life has done him good, but privately suspects that the improvement in his diet has also made an important contribution. We agree with the dietitian. It is possible, of course, that something *present* in Freddie's former diet caused his "bad" behavior, but it is also possible that something *missing* from his diet may have been responsible.

Regularity of Meals

Freddie used to skip breakfast quite often. Now he doesn't. Has this helped? The importance of breakfast to children in school has been established by research. Children who eat no breakfast perform poorly in tasks of concentration, their attention spans are shorter, and they even show lower IQs on testing than their well-fed peers.[19] Common sense tells us that it is unreasonable to expect anyone to learn and perform work when no fuel has been provided. By the late morning, discomfort from hunger may become distracting even if a child has eaten breakfast.

The problem that arises for children who attempt morning schoolwork on an empty stomach appears to be at least partly due to hypoglycemia. The average child up to the age of ten or so needs to eat every four to six hours to maintain a blood glucose concentration high enough to support the activity of the brain and nervous system. A child's brain is as big as an adult's, and the brain is the body's chief glucose consumer. A child's liver is considerably smaller—and the liver is the organ responsible for storing glucose (as glycogen) and releasing it into the blood as needed. A child's liver can't store more than about four hours' worth of glycogen; hence the need to eat fairly often. Teachers aware of the late-morning slump in their classrooms wisely request that a midmorning snack be provided; it improves classroom performance all the way to lunchtime. But for the child who hasn't had breakfast, the morning is lost altogether.

Nutrient-poor Diet

Careful food selection is essential to ensure adequate nutrition. To demonstrate this point, we can look at a sample day's menus for one of Freddie's better days before his mother changed his diet. Freddie didn't eat an unusually poor diet, especially for a child who has never learned to like vegetables.

- *Breakfast:* 1 cup of cornflakes with ½ cup of milk; fresh apple slices.
- *Lunch:* Bologna sandwich with 1 ounce bologna and 2 slices of whole-wheat bread; 1 bag of pretzels; 1 cup of milk.
- *Supper:* 2 fried chicken drumsticks; about 20 french fries; 1 roll; a

carbonated beverage; and 1/2 cup of gelatin with nondairy topping (from a fast-food restaurant).
- *Snack:* 4 chocolate sandwich cookies. The analysis of this diet provides the information shown in Table H14–4.

Even though Freddie ate three meals and a snack on this day, his nutrient intake was marginal. Imagine how much worse the picture was when he had no breakfast, or when more sugary foods took the place of some of the nourishing ones. Chances are, the nutrients missed from a skipped breakfast won't be "made up" at lunch and dinner, but will be completely left out of the child's diet that day.

When the story is told this way, it is easy to see a fallacy in the neighbor's theory that additives or sugar directly caused Freddie's problems. Freddie is now eating fewer additives and less sugar, to be sure, but he is also eating more *food* foods— that is, foods that contain the nutrients he needs to grow and develop normally.

The Effects of Nutrient Deficiencies on Behavior

Freddie's mother knew that he ate a lot of sugary foods before she changed his

diet, but she had yet to discover that his diet was also necessarily low in nutrients, the almost inevitable consequence of "sugar abuse." Moreover, neither she nor her neighbor had any idea that Freddie's behavioral problems might be caused by nutrient deficiencies.

Most people are familiar with the role of iron in carrying oxygen in the blood. A less known, but extremely important, function of iron is transporting that oxygen into the cells, where it can be used in essential processes, as in the production of energy. A lack of iron not only causes an energy crisis, but also directly affects behavior, mood, attention span, and learning ability. Iron is involved in the functioning of many molecules in the brain and nervous system. Deficiencies of iron produced experimentally in animals have caused abnormal synthesis and degradation of neurotransmitters; notably, to the system that regulates the ability to pay attention, crucial to learning.[20]

Iron deficiency is the most common nutrient deficiency in children. It is usually diagnosed by use of iron indicators in the *blood* when it has progressed all the way to overt anemia.

TABLE H14–4

Freddie's Nutrient Intakes[a]

RDA for 5-Year-Old		This Day's Meals Provided	
Protein	30 g	58 g	193% of RDA—higher than necessary
Vitamin A	500 RE	177 RE	35% — too low
Thiamin	0.9 mg	0.7 mg	78% — marginal
Riboflavin	1.0 mg	1.2 mg	120% — adequate
Folacin	200 μg	179 μg	90% — probably adequate
Vitamin C	45 mg	42 mg	93% — probably adequate
Calcium	800 mg	544 mg	68% — too low
Iron	10 mg	7.6 mg	76% — marginal
Zinc	10 mg	5.8 mg	58% — too low

[a] A key point to remember: the nutrients that are noted here are just a representation. This child's diet probably lacks others, too.

A child's *brain,* however, is sensitive to slightly lowered iron levels long before the blood effects appear. While the effects of iron deficiency are hard to distinguish from the effects of other factors in children's lives, it is likely that it manifests itself in a lowering of the "motivation to persist in intellectually challenging tasks," a shortening of the attention span, and a reduction of overall intellectual performance. Anemic children perform less well on tests and have more conduct disturbances than their classmates.[21] This is very like a description of hyperactivity, but neither allergy nor sugar is the cause. Before blaming the presence of additives or sugar for these problems, it makes sense to check for the absence of iron. Either way, the same kinds of diet changes—substitution of nutritious foods for nutrient-poor foods—may bring about improvement, but it is important to know why they are effective.

Another nutrient that is bound to be displaced from any diet high in empty-kcalorie foods is thiamin. A fascinating study that linked a "junk diet" to "neurotic behavior" traced the cause to a deficiency of this B vitamin. Twenty patients were identified who had a set of symptoms suggestive of thiamin deficiency, including pains in the chest and abdomen, sleep disturbances, personality changes (aggressiveness and hostility), fevers, digestive upsets, chronic fatigue, and many more. Of the 20 patients, 12 were found to have a diet high in carbonated and other sweet beverages, candy, and common snack foods. All had abnormally low thiamin levels as identified by a blood test (an enzyme known to depend on thiamin for its activity was found to be working inefficiently). Given thiamin supplements, all 20 "noticed marked symptomatic improvement or lost their symptoms completely after thiamin supplement." The researchers reported that "in all cases diet instruction was given. Some patients lost their craving for sweet tasting foods and beverages,

although in some the process was extremely difficult and the temptation to succumb quite similar to that seen in people who express a wish to stop smoking." In the ten who kept their return appointments, blood tests showed the thiamin-dependent enzyme activity restored to normal.[22]

Thiamin is easily displaced by nonnutritious foods. No single food offers enough to meet the daily need. The only way to meet thiamin needs from food is to eat many servings of nutritious foods, relying on each to make a small contribution. Thus a "junk diet" is especially likely to be low in thiamin.

Iron and thiamin are only two of several dozen nutrients that can be deficient in a nutrient-poor or unbalanced diet. Any of the others may be lacking as well, and the deficiencies may cause behavioral, as well as physical, symptoms:[23]

- Protein-kcalorie deficiency—apathy, fretfulness, lack of energy, and lack of interest in food.
- Thiamin deficiency—confusion, uncoordinated movements, depressed appetite, irritability, insomnia, fatigue, and general misery.[24]
- Riboflavin deficiency—depression, hysteria, psychopathic behavior, lethargy, and hypochondria evident before clinical deficiency is detected.[25]
- Niacin deficiency—irritability, agitated depression, headaches, sleeplessness, memory loss, emotional instability (early signs of pellagra onset), and mental confusion progressing to psychosis or delirium.
- Vitamin B_6 deficiency—irritability, insomnia, weakness, mental depression, abnormal brain wave pattern, convulsions, the mental symptoms of anemia, fatigue, and headache.[26]
- Folacin deficiency—the mental symptoms of anemia, tiredness, apathy, weakness, forgetfulness, mild depression, abnormal nerve function, irritability, headache, disorientation,

confusion, and inability to perform simple calculations.[27]
- Vitamin B_{12} deficiency—degeneration of the peripheral nervous system and anemia.
- Vitamin C deficiency—hysteria, depression, listlessness, lassitude, weakness, aversion to work, hypochondria, social introversion, possible iron anemia, and fatigue.
- Vitamin A deficiency—anemia.
- Iron deficiency—fatigue, weakness, headaches, pallor, listlessness, irritability, and the mental symptoms of anemia.
- Magnesium deficiency—apathy, personality changes, and hyperirritability.
- Copper deficiency—iron-deficiency anemia.
- Zinc deficiency—poor appetite, failure to grow, iron-deficiency anemia, irritability, emotional disorders, and mental lethargy.[28]

Eight of the nutrient deficiencies listed above incur anemia, which produces mental symptoms of its own. These symptoms have to be added to all the others (see Table H14–5).

Imagine a child in class or at home with any of these constellations of symptoms. The child may be irritable, aggressive, disagreeable, or sad and withdrawn. One might label such a child "hyperactive," "depressed," or "unlikable," when in fact she may be suffering from simple, albeit marginal, malnutrition. In any such case, inspection of the child's diet by someone knowledgeable about children's nutrient needs is clearly in order. Should suspicion of dietary inadequacies be raised, *no matter what other causes may be implicated*, the people responsible for feeding the child should take steps to correct those inadequacies promptly. Figure H14–1 shows the many signs that an educated eye would notice in evaluating a child's nutrition status.

To say this is not to imply that malnutrition is always "simple." To give

TABLE H14–5

The Mental Symptoms of Anemia[a]

Anorexia
Apathy, listlessness
Clumsiness
Conduct disturbances
Decreased attentiveness
Hyperactivity
Irritability
Learning disorders
Low scores on latency and associative reactions
Low scores on vocabulary tests
Lowered IQ
Perceptual restriction
Reduced physical work capacity
Repetitive hand and foot movements

[a]These symptoms are not caused by anemia itself, but by iron deficiency in the brain. Children with much more severe anemias from *other* than nutritional causes, such as sickle-cell anemia and thalassemia, show no reduction in IQ when compared with children without anemia.

Miniglossary

allergy: an immune reaction to a foreign substance (such as some components of food) in which antibodies are produced. (An immune reaction not involving antibody production is termed **sensitivity** by some researchers.) Allergies may be **symptomatic** or **asymptomatic**.

antibody: a large protein that is produced in response to an antigen, and which inactivates the antigen.

antigen: a substance foreign to the body that elicits the formation of antibodies or an inflammation reaction from immune system cells. Food antigens are usually glycoproteins (large proteins with glucose molecules attached).

histamine: a substance produced by cells of the immune system as part of a local immune reaction to an antigen; participates in causing inflammation.

hyperactivity syndrome in children: a cluster of symptoms in which "the essential features are signs of developmentally inappropriate inattention, impulsivity, and hyperactivity." Other important features are onset before age seven, duration of six months or more, and proven absence of mental illness or mental retardation. Other names associated with hyperactivity: attention deficit disorder, hyperkinesis, minimal brain damage, minimal brain dysfunction, and minor cerebral dysfunction.

salicylates (sa-LISS-ih-lates): compounds related chemically to aspirin, which cause allergy in some individuals. One such compound is yellow dye no. 5, **tartrazine**.

tension-fatigue syndrome: apparent hyperactivity produced in a child by the combination of lack of sleep and overstimulation with anxiety.

FIGURE H14–1

The well-nourished versus the malnourished child.

Normal eyes: bright, clear, pink membranes, adjust easily to darkness.
Malnourished eyes: pale membranes, spots, redness, slow adjustment to dark.

Normal face: good complexion.
Malnourished face: off color; scaly, flaky, cracked skin.

Normal lips: smooth, good color.
Malnourished lips: red, swollen; cracks at corners of mouth.

Normal glands: no lumps.
Malnourished glands: swollen at front of neck, cheeks.

Normal tongue: red, rough, bumpy.
Malnourished tongue: sore, smooth, purplish, swollen.

Normal skin: smooth, firm, good color.
Malnourished skin: dry, rough, "sandpaper" feel; spots or sores; lack of fat under the skin.

Normal hair: shiny, firm in the scalp.
Malnourished hair: dull, brittle, dry, loose and falling out.

Normal internal systems: heart rate, heart rhythm, and blood pressure normal; normal GI function; reflexes and psychological development normal.
Malnourished internal systems: heart rate, heart rhythm, or blood pressure abnormal; liver and spleen enlarged, GI dysfunction; mental irritability, confusion; burning, tingling of hands and feet; loss of balance, coordination.

Normal teeth and gums: no pain or cavities, gums firm, teeth bright
Malnourished teeth and gums: missing, discolored, decayed teeth; gums bleed easily; gums swollen, and spongy.

Normal nails: firm, pink.
Malnourished nails: spoon shaped, brittle, ridged.

Normal muscles and bones: good muscle tone, good posture, long bones straight.
Malnourished muscles and bones: "wasted" appearance of muscles, swollen bumps on skull or ends of bones, small bumps on ribs, bowed legs or knock-knees, pain.

Normal behavior: alert, attentive, cheerful.
Malnourished behavior: irritable, apathetic, inattentive, hyperactive.

just one example of a possible complicating factor: lead poisoning can cause iron-deficiency anemia, and iron deficiency impairs the body's defenses against absorption of lead. The anemia brought on by lead poisoning may be mistaken for a simple iron deficiency. Lead toxicity symptoms are widespread among children—1 out of every 50 children in rural areas and more than 1 out of every 10 inner-city children are affected with lead poisoning.[29] Such problems are important to identify, but still, even while they are being investigated, the child should be fed properly.

The list presented earlier shows that almost any nutrient deficiency can render behavior abnormal. Interestingly, and not surprisingly once you think about it, many different kinds of malnutrition give rise to similar symptoms: apathy, depression, lassitude, weakness, and withdrawal. These symptoms are natural in anyone who feels ill, and nutrient deficiencies, excesses, and imbalances are forms of illness. Poor nutrition certainly does affect behavior.

While we cannot say exactly what caused Freddie's miseries before his mother changed his diet, and in fact we cannot even say with certainty that nutrition factors were involved, we can point to many plausible explanations based on known effects of nutrient deficiencies. We can certainly say that the change in diet benefited Freddie both physically and mentally—probably because it restored his depleted nutrient supplies to the level at which they could fully support his health.

In a casual conversation with the dietitian sometime after the events of this story, Freddie's mother speaks enthusiastically about the wonderful changes the family's new foodways have brought about in Freddie. "I had no idea," she says, "how terrible those foods were that he was eating before. Now I never let him have any processed foods, and we don't even keep sugar—

in any form—in the house at all. I can't believe I didn't know how bad those foods were for him. Now that I know, I tell all other parents to do as I do. If I had my way, I would enact a federal law prohibiting the use of chemicals and sugar in any foods that anybody eats!"

The dietitian is troubled that Freddie's mother has come to this conclusion. She is delighted that Freddie's behavior problems are solved, but it seems only fair not to let Mrs. Frantic continue thinking that chemicals and sugar were solely responsible for all his earlier trouble.

She broaches the subject cautiously, because she doesn't want to alienate Mrs. Frantic. She congratulates her on having done a wonderful job with Freddie's diet—then she attempts, gently, to help her see that the diet as a whole, not the specific foods in it, is what is important. She quotes the statement that "there is no such thing as a junk food—but there is such a thing as a junk diet." She explains the nutrient density concept and shows why sugary colas, which deliver 180 kcalories with no nutrients, have no place in Freddie's diet. Treats like oatmeal cookies or ice cream, however, supply needed nutrients, and so can be included in small amounts; she suggests using sugar artfully to enhance his pleasure in eating nutritious foods.

NOTES
1. This highlight was adapted from Controversies 13 and 14 in E. M. N. Hamilton, E. N. Whitney, and F. S. Sizer, *Nutrition: Concepts and Controversies*, 3rd ed. (St. Paul, Minn.: West, 1985), pp. 404–409, 438–443.
2. R. H. Buckley and D. Metcalfe, Food allergy, *Journal of the American Medical Association* 248 (1982): 2627–2631.
3. S. L. Taylor, Food allergy: The enigma and some potential solutions, *Journal of Food Protection* 43 (1980): 300–306.
4. Buckley and Metcalfe, 1982.
5. Taylor, 1980.
6. C. D. May, Food allergy: Perspective, principles, practical management, *Nutrition*

Today, November-December 1980, pp. 28–31.
7. Taylor, 1980.
8. Buckley and Metcalfe, 1982.
9. V. J. Fontana and F. Moreno-Pagan, Allergy and diet, in *Modern Nutrition in Health and Disease*, 6th ed., eds. R. S. Goodhart and M. E. Shils, (Philadelphia: Lea and Febiger, 1980), 1071–1081.
10. L. Eisenberg, The clinical use of stimulant drugs in children, *Pediatrics* 49 (1972): 709–715.
11. Eisenberg, 1972.
12. Institute of Food Technologists' Expert Panel on Food Safety and Nutrition and the Committee on Public Information, Diet and hyperactivity: Any connection? *Food Technology* 30 (April 1976): 29–34; B. F. Feingold, Hyperkinesis and learning disabilities linked to artificial food flavors and colors, *American Journal of Nursing* 75 (1975): 797–803.
13. M. Morrison, The Feingold diet (letter to the editor), *Science* 199 (1978): 840.
14. B. F. Feingold, *Why Your Child Is Hyperactive* (New York: Random House, 1975).
15. National Advisory Committee on Hyperkinesis and Food Additives, *Final Report to the Nutrition Foundation*, October 1980.
16. National Advisory Committee, 1980; National Institutes of Health Consensus Development Panel, National Institutes of Health, Consensus development conference statement: Defined diets and childhood hyperactivity, *American Journal of Clinical Nutrition* 37 (1983): 161–165.
17. Defined diets and childhood hyperactivity, *Journal of the American Medical Association* 248 (1982): 290–292.
18. G. B. Forbes, Nutrition and hyperactivity (editorial), *Journal of the American Medical Association* 248 (1982): 355–356.
19. E. Pollitt, R. Leibel, and D. Greenfield, Brief fasting, stress and cognition in children, *American Journal of Clinical Nutrition* 34 (1981): 1526–1533.
20. D. M. Tucker and H. H. Sandstead, Body iron stores and cortical arousal, in *Iron Deficiency: Brain Biochemistry and Behavior*, eds. E. Pollitt and R. L. Leibel (New York: Raven Press, 1982), pp. 161–182.
21. R. L. Leibel, Behavioral and biochemical correlates of iron deficiency: A review, *Journal of the American Dietetic Association* 71 (1977): 399–404.
22. D. Lonsdale and R. J. Shamberger, Red cell transketolase as an indicator of nutritional deficiency, *American Journal of Clinical Nutrition* 33 (1980): 205–211.

23. Unless otherwise cited, all of the listed symptoms can be found in R. S. Goodhart and M. E. Shils, eds., *Modern Nutrition in Health and Disease,* 6th ed. (Philadelphia: Lea and Febiger, 1980).

24. Marginal vitamin deficiency, *Nutrition and the MD,* July 1983, p. 3.

25. R. Sterner and W. Price, Restricted riboflavin: With subject behavioral effects in humans, *American Journal of Clinical Nutrition* 26 (1973): 150–160.

26. Marginal vitamin deficiency, 1983.

27. J. H. Pincus, E. H. Reynolds, and G. H. Glaser, Subacute combined system degeneration with folate deficiency, *Journal of the American Medical Association* 221 (1972): 496–497; Neurological disease in folic acid deficiency, *Nutrition Reviews* 39 (1981): 337–338.

28. A. S. Prasad, Clinical, biochemical and nutritional spectrum of zinc deficiency in human subjects: An update, *Nutrition Reviews* 7 (1983): 197–206.

29. Update, childhood lead poisoning, *Journal of the American Dietetic Association* 80 (1982): 592, 594.

Child and Teen

15

Centrioles

Spindle Fibers

Chromosomes

Centriole

Growth requires that cells duplicate all their materials and copy their DNA instructions so each daughter will have a set; and then portion out the two sets to the two daughters. This dividing cell is sorting out its genetic material so that one complete copy will be delivered to each daughter cell. Many kcalories and nutrients are needed to support cell division.

*T*he years of life described in this chapter are often called "the growing years," although, as we have seen, the year before birth and the first year after it are the most growing years of all. Still, there is more to come. From age 1 to 20 or thereabouts, height more than triples, and weight increases up to eightfold or tenfold. Optimal nutrition permits development to realize its full potential.

Secular Trends in Nutrition

Not everyone—indeed, not every population—enjoys the benefits of optimal nutrition. Observations of populations during times of change in their foodways have demonstrated that altered nutrition profoundly affects the timing and extent of young people's maturation.

Among the variables affected are age at menarche, skeletal maturity, and ultimate height achieved. Changes in these variables within a population depend on many factors, but nutrition is thought to be highly significant among them. Others are improvements in medical care and sanitation, which help to prevent disease. These facets of improved socioeconomic status together permit children to mature faster and more fully than their parents. Conversely, socioeconomic setbacks such as natural disasters or wars limit the growth and maturation rates of young people.

Ultimately, when all environmental conditions are ideal, the full genetic potential of a people can be realized, but until then it is impossible to know what that potential may be. In 1840 it might have been thought, for example, that women were supposed to have their first periods at 15 years of age. Their great-granddaughters, in 1930, however, had their first periods at 12 to 13 years of age. This secular trend, a decrease in the mean age at menarche of one-third year per decade from 1840 to 1930, paralleled the accumulation of many economic advantages in our society and ceased in 1930—presumably because the limits of genetic possibility had then been reached.

Height, too, increases with improvement in socioeconomic conditions, but the limit has been reached, at least for the middle and upper classes in Western Europe and North America. The ultimate height achieved is also reached at an earlier age today than it was 100 years ago. Today, most females arrive at their full height by the age of 16 or 17, and males by 18 or 19, whereas 50 years ago both sexes reached their full height at 26 years. Figure 15–1 shows that the average heights of ten-year-olds in the United States increased 10 percent from 1870 to 1970—not because they were growing 10 percent taller, but because they had accomplished 10 percent more of their total growth by that age. In the 1960s, ten-year-olds in India and the United Arab Republic were as tall as ten-year-olds in the United States were around the turn of the century, reflecting the fact that conditions in India and the United Arab Republic were not as conducive to rapid growth and early development as conditions here.

All of this is not to say that all people "should" attain the same heights at the same ages or at maturity. Different races have different genetic potentials.

Effects that can be seen over time measured in years are known as **secular trends**.
saecula = age

menarche (MEN-ark): the age at which the first menstrual period occurs.
mens = menstruation
arche = beginning

Skeletal maturity can be measured by x-raying the 31 bones of the hand and wrist to see how completely formed they are. It can also be measured by timing the fusion of the **epiphyses** (eh-PIFF-uh-sees) to the shafts of the long bones. The epiphyses, the end segments of long bones, contain a thin area of active bone growth. This growth eventually stops, after which no further significant growth in height can occur—only a slight elongation of the trunk.
epi = on
phyein = to grow

Bones of the hand or wrist can be used as an indicator of skeletal maturity. Here, eight developing bony centers are shown. They are markedly more fully mineralized in one child's hand than in the other, although both children are six years old.

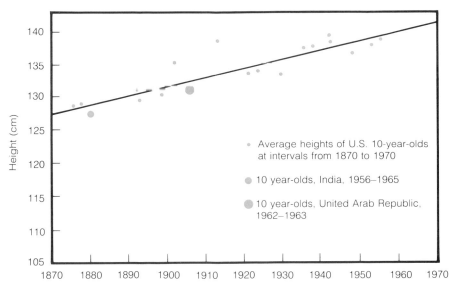

FIGURE 15–1

Children mature earlier today than 100 years ago. The figure shows that ten-year-olds in 1970 were about 140 cm tall, whereas 100 years earlier they were under 130 cm. Indian and U.A.R. children in the 1960s were as tall as U.S. children had been at the turn of the century.

Source: P. V. V. Hamill, F. E. Johnston, and S. Lemeshow, *Height and Weight of Children: Socioeconomic Status, United States*, Vital and Health Statistics series 11, no. 119, DHEW publication no. (HSM) 73–1601 (Washington, D.C.: Government Printing Office, 1972). Data for Indian and U.A.R. children from E. A. Martin and V. A. Beal, *Roberts' Nutrition Work with Children*, 4th ed. (Chicago: University of Chicago Press, 1978), p. 88.

Some are smaller, some taller, because they have inherited different genes for height. Several U.S. surveys have shown that blacks mature earlier and grow taller than whites, all else (including income) being equal. But the example of the Japanese shows that we cannot attribute differences in physical development to differing genetic heritages until we have ruled out the possibility of environmental influences, including differences in adequacy and steady supply of food.

In the case of the Japanese, the adverse effects of times of deprivation, as well as the benefits of improved nutrition, have both been demonstrated in secular trends within this century. The heights of children at each age have steadily increased since 1900, probably mostly as a result of increased protein intakes—except during the Second World War, when food deprivation was severe. The effects are shown in Figure 15–2.

The rest of this chapter describes the growth and development of children in the context of an advanced, industrialized society like the United States, in which even the poor, compared with those of other countries, are not much poorer than the middle class. In other countries, poverty is so much more extreme that many parents' expectations for the physical and mental development of their children cannot realistically be so high as they are here.

Early and Middle Childhood

Nutrient needs change steadily throughout life and vary from individual to individual, depending on the rate of growth, the sex, the previous nutrition and health history, and many other factors. This section takes a general look at preschool and school-age children's needs, and later sections are devoted to the special concerns of teenagers.

FIGURE 15–2

Effect of the war years on heights of Japanese boys. The faster the boys were growing, the more severely they were affected. The figure also shows that boys at each age were taller in 1970 than boys of those ages were in 1900—believed to be an effect of improved protein nutrition, thanks to the availability of more meat after the Second World War. (The same effects were seen in girls.)

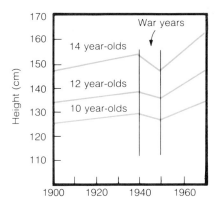

Source: Adapted from E. A. Martin and V. A. Beal, *Roberts' Nutrition Work with Children*, 4th ed. (Chicago: University of Chicago Press, 1978), p. 147, as adapted in turn from Helen S. Mitchell.

One-year-old and two-year-old shown for comparison of body shape.

After the age of one, a child's growth rate slows, but the body continues to change dramatically. At one, babies have just learned to stand and toddle; by two, they can take long strides with solid confidence and are learning to run, jump, and climb. The internal change that makes these new accomplishments possible is the accumulation of a larger mass and greater density of bone and muscle tissue. The changes are obvious in the photos above. The two-year-old has lost much of his baby fat; his muscles (especially in the back, buttocks, and legs) have firmed and strengthened, and his leg bones have lengthened and increased in density.

Thereafter, the same trend—a lengthening of the long bones and an increase in musculature—continues, unevenly and more slowly, until adolescence. Growth comes in spurts; a six-year-old child may wear the same pair of shoes for a year, then need new shoes twice in the next four months.

Just before adolescence, the growth patterns of girls and boys begin to become distinct. In girls, fat becomes a larger percentage of the total body weight, and in boys, the lean body mass—muscle and bone—becomes much greater. Around this time, growth in height may seem to stop altogether for a while. This is the calm before the storm.

Nutrient Needs and Feeding

Healthy growth . . . is dependent on an adequate and continuous supply of energy, protein, and other nutrients to all cells of the body so that they may divide and increase in size to reach their maximum potential.

Ethel Austin Martin and Virginia A. Beal

A one-year-old child needs perhaps 1,000 kcalories a day; a three-year-old needs only 300 to 500 kcalories more. Appetite decreases markedly around the age of one year, in line with the great reduction in growth rate. Thereafter, the appetite fluctuates; a child will need and demand much more food during periods of rapid growth than during slow periods. The nutrients protein and calcium continue to need emphasis, and the food best suited to supply them continues to be milk.

The preadolescent period is the last one in which parental food choices have much influence. As children gather their forces for the adolescent growth spurt, they are accumulating stores of nutrients that will be needed in the coming years. When they take off on that growth spurt, there will be a period during which their nutrient intakes, especially of calcium, cannot meet the demands of rapidly growing bones. Then they will draw on these nutrient stores. The denser their bones are before this occurs, the better prepared they will be.

The gradually increasing needs for all nutrients during the growing years are evident from the RDA table and the RNI for Canadians, which list separate averages for each span of three years. To provide these nutrients, the Four Food Group Plan recommends the following for growing children:

- 3 cups or four ¾ cup servings of milk or milk products.
- 1 egg and two servings of other meat or meat alternates.
- Four or more servings of fruits and vegetables.
- Four or more servings of breads and cereals.

For meat, fruits, and vegetables, a serving is loosely defined as 1 tablespoon per year. Thus at four years of age, a serving of any of these foods would be 4 tablespoons (¼ cup). Because the serving sizes adjust as the child grows older, these recommendations are good from age two to the teen years. Table 15–1 shows details of diet patterns based on this plan.

After the crucial first year, there is still much a parent can do to foster the development of healthy eating habits. The goal is to teach children to like nutritious foods in all four categories.

Experimentation with children's food patterns shows that candy, cola, and other concentrated sweets must be limited in a child's diet if the needed nutrients are to be supplied. If such foods are permitted in large quantities, there are only two possible outcomes: nutrient deficiencies and/or obesity. The child can't be trusted to choose nutritious foods on the basis of taste alone; the preference for sweets is innate. On the other hand, an active child can enjoy the higher-kcalorie nutritious foods in each category: ice cream or pudding in the milk group, cake and cookies (whole-grain or enriched only, however) in the bread group. These foods, made from milk and grain, carry valuable nutrients and encourage a child to learn, appropriately, that eating is fun.

Calcium and riboflavin in a delicious form.

Children sometimes seem to lose their appetites for a while; this is nothing to worry about. The perfection of appetite regulation in children of normal weight guarantees that their kcalorie intakes will be right for each stage of growth. As long as the kcalories they do consume are from nutritious foods, they are well provided for. (One caution, however. Wandering school-age children may be spending pocket money at the nearby candy store.) An overzealous mother, unaware that her one-year-old is supposed to slow down, may begin a lifelong conflict over food by trying to force more food on the child than the child feels like eating.

Nutrition at School

While parents are doing what they can to establish favorable eating behavior during the transition from infancy to childhood, other factors are entering the picture. During preschool or grade school, the child encounters foods prepared and served by outsiders. The U.S. government funds several programs to provide nutritious, high-quality meals for children at school. School lunches are designed to meet certain requirements. They must include specified servings of milk,

TABLE 15–1

Children's Daily Food Pattern for Good Nutrition

Food Group	Servings per Day	Average Size of Serving		
		1 to 3 Years	4 to 5 Years	6 to 12 Years
Milk and cheese (1 oz cheese = 1 c milk)	4	1/2 to 3/4 c	3/4 c	3/4 to 1 c
Meat group (protein foods)	3, more permitted			
Eggs		1	1	1
Lean meat, fish, poultry, legumes (liver once a week)		2 tbsp	4 tbsp	2 to 4 oz
Peanut butter		0 to 1 tbsp	2 tbsp	2 to 3 tbsp
Fruits and vegetables	4, more recommended			
Vitamin C source (citrus fruits, berries, tomato, cabbage, cantaloupe)	1 or more	1/3 to 1/2 c	1/2 c	1 medium orange
Vitamin A source (green or yellow fruits and vegetables) and	1 or more	2 to 3 tbsp	4 tbsp	1/4 to 1/3 c
Other vegetables (including potato) and	2	2 to 3 tbsp	4 tbsp (1/4 c)	1/3 to 1/2 c
Other fruits (apple, banana)		1/4 to 1/3 c	1/2 c	1 medium piece
Cereals (whole grain or enriched)	4, more recommended			
Bread, buns, pizza		1/2 to 1 slice	1 1/2 slices	1 to 2 slices
Ready-to-eat cereals		1/2 to 3/4 oz	1 oz	1 oz
Cooked grains (cereals, macaroni, grits, rice)		1/4 to 1/3 c	1/2 c	1/2 to 3/4 c
Fats and sugars	Optional — These high-kcalorie foods may be included in limited amounts only in addition to the required servings of nutritious foods. Serving sizes listed here are maximum.			
Butter, margarine, mayonnaise, oils		1 tbsp	1 tbsp	2 tbsp
Desserts and sweets (100-kcal portions as follows):		1 to 1 1/2 portions	1 1/2 portions	3 portions

1/3 c pudding or ice cream
2 to 3 cookies, 1 oz cake
1 1/3 oz pie; 2 tbsp jelly, jam, honey, sugar

Source: Adapted from B. B. Alford and M. L. Bogle, *Nutrition during the Life Cycle* (Englewood Cliffs, N.J.: Prentice Hall, 1982), pp. 60–61.

protein-rich food (meat, cheese, eggs, legumes, or peanut butter), vegetables, fruits, bread or other grain foods, and butter or margarine. The design is intended to provide at least a third of the RDA for each of the nutrients. The school lunch pattern was split into several patterns in 1980 to provide for the needs of different ages better than it had done in the past (see Table 15–2).

Parents rely on the school lunch program to meet a significant part of their children's nutrient needs on school days, but children don't always like what they are served. In response to children's differing needs and tastes, the school lunch program has been attempting to do better at feeding children both what they want and what will nourish them. The trend is:

- To increase the variety of offerings and allow children to choose what they are served.
- To vary portion sizes, so that little children may take little servings.
- To involve students (in secondary schools) in the planning of menus.
- To improve the scheduling of lunches so that children can eat when they are hungry and can have enough time to eat well.

A step toward making the lunches more consistent with today's ideals of healthful food has been to drop the requirement for whole milk and to offer low-fat or skim milk instead. Another alteration has been to eliminate the requirement that butter or margarine be served. To help the schools economize,

TABLE 15–2

School Lunch Patterns for Different Ages

Food Group	Preschool		Grades		
	Ages 1 to 2	Ages 3 to 4	K to 3	4 to 6	7 to 12
Meat or meat alternate					
One serving					
Lean meat, poultry, or fish	1 oz	1½ oz	1½ oz	2 oz	3 oz
Cheese	1 oz	1½ oz	1½ oz	2 oz	3 oz
Large egg(s)	1	1½	1½	2	3
Cooked dry beans or peas	½ c	¾ c	¾ c	1 c	1½ c
Peanut butter	2 tbsp	3 tbsp	3 tbsp	4 tbsp	6 tbsp
Vegetable and/or fruit					
Two or more servings, both to total	½ c	½ c	½ c	¾ c	¾ c
Bread or bread alternate					
Servings[a]	5 per week	8 per week	8 per week	8 per week	10 per week
Milk					
A serving of fluid milk	¾ c	¾ c	1 c	1 c	1 c

[a]A serving is 1 slice of whole grain or enriched bread; a whole-grain or enriched biscuit, roll, muffin, and so on; or ½ c cooked pasta or other cereal grain such as bulgur or grits.
Source: School lunch patterns: Ready, set, go! *School Food Service Journal* 34 (August 1980), p. 31.

the program no longer requires that children be served every item, but permits them to select what they will eat, so that there will be less plate waste.

Coincident with the school lunch program is a program of nutrition education and training (NET program) in all the public schools. Originally allocated 50 cents per year per child, this program was cut in 1980 to 9 cents per child, but is reported to be still going strong because program administrators are highly motivated and have been ingenious and creative in accomplishing the program's highest-priority objectives.[1]

One way in which children can learn a lot, sometimes with only small expense to the school, is to take field trips to nearby facilities where nutrition and food operations are going on. Among the possible places to visit are those listed in the margin. At the very least, children can go to the depots where the school food comes in and to the kitchens where it is prepared; and teachers who themselves know something about nutrition can then use the questions that come up as opportunities to do some teaching. Children growing up today need not only to be fed well in the interest of their growth and development, but to learn enough about nutrition to become able to make adaptive food choices when the choices become theirs to make.

Children can learn from:
- Bakeries.
- Mills.
- Dairy farms.
- Milk-bottling plants.
- Farmers markets.
- Vegetable farms and fields.
- Food-processing plants.
- Fast-food places.
- Institutional kitchens.
- Supermarkets.
- Convenience stores.
- Neighborhood gardens.
- Natural-food stores.
- Food salvage banks.

Television and Vending Machines

For the most part, children learn nutrition from parents or teachers who know very little about it. Meanwhile, they hear a great deal about foods from the television set. Many authorities are concerned that television commercials may have a less-than-desirable impact. It is estimated that the average child sees more than 10,000 commercials a year, of which many more than half are for sugary foods. Hundreds of millions of dollars are spent in the effort to sell these foods to children. Most of the concern centers on the issue of sugar. You may recall that not all the public disapproval of sugar is based on scientific findings. However, there is widespread agreement on one point: sticky, sugary foods left on the teeth provide an ideal environment for the growth of mouth bacteria and the formation of cavities. No regulations to prevent the promotion of sticky, sugary foods are in force, however.

It thus remains up to us to determine which food commercials we will believe and which we will not. Dentists, especially, have the obligation to educate their clients individually as long as misleading claims continue to appear on national television. A model eating plan that favors dental health is shown in Table 15–3.

Television is not the only environmental force affecting children's food choices. Another is vending machines, especially in schools. The American Dental Association (ADA) would like to eliminate the sale of confections as snacks in schools, but so far has met with little success. Most progress has been made by way of individual, voluntary initiatives. Experiments have shown that children choose more nutritious snacks if they are offered side by side with the sugary foods. When apples are made available in vending machines, children choose chocolate bars less often. When milk is made available, soft drink use drops considerably.

Soft drinks contain not only sugar, but also caffeine, which is a matter of some concern to pediatricians. A cup of hot chocolate or a 12–ounce cola beverage may contain as much as 50 milligrams of caffeine; two or more such beverages are equivalent in the body of a 60–pound child to the caffeine in 8

When given a choice, children prefer the more nutritious snacks.

TABLE 15–3

Eating Habits to Favor Good Dental Health

Food Group	Foods to Eat	Foods to Avoid
Milk and milk products	Milk Cheese Plain yogurt	All dairy products with added sugar
Fruit	Fresh fruit Water-packed canned fruit	Dried fruit Sugar-packed canned fruit Jams and jellies
Juice	Unsweetened juices	Sweetened juices
Vegetables	Most vegetables	Candied sweet potatoes Glazed carrots
Grains	Most grain products	Grain products with added sugar

Notice that granola bars are among the "bad guys" singled out by dentists. They are a grain food, but so sticky that dentists consider them akin to candy bars. Similarly, dentists see fruit yogurt as the equivalent of ice cream.

Source: L. P. DiOrio, What should we eat? A dentist's perspective. Address presented at the American Dental Association annual meeting, 11 October 1977.

cups of coffee for a 175–pound man. Chocolate bars also contribute caffeine. Children and young adults who are troubled by irregular heartbeats or difficulty in sleeping may need to control their caffeine consumption. (A table of caffeine contents of beverages and medications appears in the next chapter.) As long as such undeniably attractive temptations as cola beverages and candy bars surround children, barriers against their abuse have to be provided by parents and other concerned adults and by teaching the children themselves.

Looking Ahead

In children, as in infants, eating habits help determine whether development takes place in a positive or negative direction. To avoid obesity, the preschool child should be trained to "eat thin." Mealtimes should be relaxed and leisurely. Children should learn to eat slowly, pause and enjoy their table companions, and stop eating when they are full. The "clean your plate" dictum should be stamped out for all time, and in its place parents who wish to avoid waste should learn to serve smaller portions or teach their children to serve themselves as much as they truly want to eat. Physical activity should be encouraged on a daily basis to promote strong skeletal and muscular development and to establish habits that will undergird good health throughout life.

The child who has already become obese needs careful handling. As in pregnancy, weight loss may easily have a harmful effect on growth in children. J. L. Knittle, who has worked with obese children, recommends that they be fed so as to maintain a constant weight while they grow. The object is to restrict the multiplication of fat cells while promoting normal lean body development. Thus the child can grow out of his obesity.

Of all nutritional disorders other than obesity found in U.S. children, the most common is iron-deficiency anemia. It is most prevalent in low-birthweight

The "clean your plate" dictum should be stamped out for all time.

infants, babies from six months to two years of age, and children and adolescents from low-income families.[2]

Dr. S. J. Fomon, pediatrician and specialist in children's nutrition, recommends supplementing the diet of infants to ensure an iron intake of 7 milligrams a day, and modifying their food intakes as they grow older so that they will receive 5.5 milligrams of iron or more per 1,000 kcalories. To achieve this latter goal, milk must not be overemphasized in the diet, because it is a poor iron source; dairy products should be consumed only in the amounts needed to ensure adequate calcium and riboflavin intakes. If skim or low-fat milk is used instead of whole milk, there will be kcalories left for investment in such iron-rich foods as lean meats, fish, poultry, eggs, and legumes. Grain products should be whole-grain or enriched only, and children should learn to avoid bakery goods unfortified with iron, candies, and soft drinks.

Cardiovascular disease is another condition to prevent, and many experts seem to agree that early childhood is the time to put practices into effect that until recently were recommended only for adults. Snacking on high-fat, high-sugar, and high-salt foods should be discouraged, because it sets a pattern that favors the development of atherosclerosis and hypertension. Instead, recommendations like those of the *Dietary Guidelines*, emphasizing foods with a high nutrient density, should be followed.

The *Guidelines* might also help to prevent or retard the onset of diabetes in children who have the genetic tendency toward it. Those who have been studying the effect of nutrition on cancer have suggested that children should follow a "prudent diet." The diet was originally developed for heart patients, but its outlines are the same as those recommended by nutritionists interested in the prevention of cancer.

The prudent diet is described in Chapter 4.

Not everyone agrees that all children should be placed on diets strictly limited in sugar, salt, and fat and high in fruits, vegetables, and whole-grain cereals. However, even those who do not go this far recommend that children be screened early with an eye to determining what conditions each of them might be likely to develop and then paying appropriate attention to diet in each special case. (Figure 15–3 outlines the screening process.) Thus the child of a parent with high blood pressure should be raised on a diet relatively low in salt; the child of a diabetic parent should avoid sugar and be encouraged to eat foods high in complex carbohydrate; and the child of a parent with coronary artery disease should eat foods low in fat—especially saturated fat—and possibly low in cholesterol. In all these situations, the greatest success is likely to be achieved if the whole family, and not just the child, follows the recommended dietary guidelines.

Poor dental health is another preventable condition. The measures recommended for its prevention center around two objectives. First, adequate nutrition is needed to help the mouth and teeth develop properly. This means providing an adequate diet, especially in terms of protein; calcium; vitamins A, C, and D; and fluoride. Where local water supplies are not fluoridated, direct application of fluoride to the teeth at intervals may be necessary. Second, it is important to restrict the supply of carbohydrate foods to the bacteria that cause tooth decay. This means brushing the teeth or washing the mouth after meals (especially meals high in carbohydrate), avoiding snacks that contain sticky carbohydrate, and dislodging persistent particles with dental floss or other devices.

FIGURE 15–3

Nutritional screening of children.

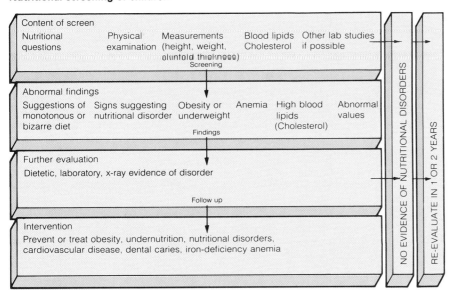

Source: S. J. Fomon, T. A. Anderson, H. Y. W. Stephen, and E. E. Ziegler, *Nutritional Disorders of Children: Prevention, Screening, and Followup,* DHEW publication no. (HSA) 76–5612 (Washington, D.C.: Government Printing Office, 1976), inside front cover.

Mealtimes with Children

It is desirable for children to learn to like nutritious foods in all of the food groups. With one exception, this liking usually develops naturally. The exception is vegetables, which young children frequently dislike and refuse. Even a tiny serving of spinach, cooked carrots, or squash may elicit an expression that registers the utmost in negative feelings (as well as great pride in the ability to make an ugly face). Since most youngsters need to eat more vegetables, the next few paragraphs are addressed to this problem.

Do you remember how you felt when first offered a cup of vegetable soup, a serving of runny spinach, or a pile of peas and carrots? If the soup burned your tongue, it may have been years before you were willing to try it again. As for the spinach, it was suspiciously murky looking. (Who could tell what might be lurking in that dark, ugly liquid?) The peas and carrots troubled your sense of order. Before you could eat them, you felt compelled to sort the peas onto one side of the plate and the carrots onto the other. Then you had to separate, into a reject pile, all those that got mashed in the process or contaminated with gravy from the mashed potatoes. Only then might you be willing to eat the intact, clean peas and carrots one by one—perhaps with your fingers, since the peas, especially, kept rolling off the fork.

Why children respond in this way to foods that look "off" or "messy" to them is a matter for conjecture. Parents need only be aware that this is how many children feel and then honor those feelings. Children prefer vegetables

Children prefer vegetables that are crunchy, attractive in color and shape, and easy to eat.

that are slightly undercooked and crunchy, attractive in color and shape, and easy to eat. They should be warm, not hot, because a child's mouth is much more sensitive than an adult's. The flavor should be mild (a child has more taste buds), and smooth foods such as mashed potatoes or pea soup should have no lumps in them (a child wonders, with some disgust, what the lumps might be). Irrational as the fear of strangeness may seem, the parent must realize that it is practically universal among children and may even have a built-in biological basis.

Little children like to eat at little tables and to be served little portions of food. They also love to eat with other children and have been observed to stay at the table longer and eat much more when in the company of their peers. A bright, unhurried atmosphere free of conflict is also conducive to good appetite. Parents who serve the food in a relaxed and casual manner, without anxiety, provide the emotional climate in which a child's negative emotions will be minimized.

Ideally, each meal is preceded, not followed, by the activity the child looks forward to the most. In a number of schools, it has been discovered that children eat a much better lunch if recess occurs before, rather than after, the meal. With recess after, they are likely to hurry out to play, leaving food on their plates that they were hungry for and would otherwise have eaten. Before sitting down to eat, small children should be helped to wash their hands and faces, so that they can enjoy their meal with "that clean feeling."

Many little children, both boys and girls, enjoy helping in the kitchen. Their participation provides many opportunities to encourage good food habits. Vegetables are pretty, especially when fresh, and provide opportunities to learn about color, about growing things and their seeds, about shapes and textures—all of which are fascinating to young children. Measuring, stirring, decorating, cutting, and arranging vegetables are skills even a very small child can practice with enjoyment and pride.

When introducing new foods at the table, parents are advised to offer them one at a time—and only a small amount at first. Whenever possible, the new food should be presented at the beginning of the meal, when the child is hungry. If the child is cross, irritable, or feeling sick, don't insist, but withdraw the new food and try it again a few days later. Remember, parents have inclinations and dislikes to which they feel entitled; children should be accorded the same privilege. Never make an issue of food acceptance; a power struggle almost invariably results in a confirmed pattern of resistance and a permanently closed mind on the child's part.

The key word, at one year, is *trust;* the parental behavior best suited to promote it is affectionate holding. At two years, the word is *autonomy;* parents should allow children to help make family choices, including sometimes giving them the right to say their favorite word (No!)—at the same time, of course, sensibly preventing the children from dominating the family. At four, when the development of *initiative* is their proudest achievement, children can be encouraged to participate in the planning and preparation of meals. At each age, food can be given and enjoyed in the context of encouraging emotional as well as physical growth. If the beginnings are right, children will grow without the kind of conflict and confusion over food that can lead to nutrition problems.

At every age, there is a negative counterpart—distrust, shame, guilt, inferiority—to the desired development. These, too, can be promoted by unaware parents, even if they have the best of intentions. Mealtimes can be nightmarish for the child who is struggling with these issues. If, as she sits down to the table, she is confronted with a barrage of accusations—"Susie, your hands are filthy . . . your report card . . . and clean your plate! Your mother cooked that food!"—mealtimes may be unbearable. Her stomach may recoil, because her body as well as her mind reacts to stress of this kind.

In the interest of promoting both a positive self-concept and a positive attitude toward good food, it is important for parents to help their children remember that they are good kids. What they *do* may sometimes be unacceptable; but what they *are*, on the inside, are normal, healthy, growing, fine human beings.

The Teen Years

Teenagers are not fed; they eat. For the first time in their lives, they assume responsibility for their own food intakes. At the same time, they are intensely involved in day-to-day life with their peers and preparation for their future lives as adults. Social pressures thrust choices at them: to drink or not to drink, to smoke or not to smoke, to develop their bodies to meet sometimes extreme ideals of slimness or athletic prowess. Few become interested in foods and nutrition except as part of the effort to define themselves by way of vegetarianism, crash dieting, or other efforts. The next few sections emphasize the factors that affect their health for good or for ill, and the information they need to develop and maintain food habits conducive to good health throughout adulthood.

Growth and Nutrient Needs

The adolescent growth spurt begins in girls at 10 or 11 and reaches its peak at 12, being completed at about 15. In boys, it begins at 12 or 13 and peaks at 14, ending at about 19. This intensive growth period brings not only a dramatic increase in height, but also hormonal changes that profoundly affect every organ of the body (including the brain) and that culminate in the emergence of physically mature adults within two or three years. The same nutrition principles apply to this period as to the growth periods previously discussed. The growth nutrients are needed in increased quantities, and there is an added need for iron, caused by the onset of menstruation in girls and by the great increase in lean body mass in boys. These changes, which are taking place in nearly adult-size people, may increase total nutrient needs at adolescence more than at any other time in life. A rapidly growing, active boy of 15 may need 4,000 kcalories or more a day just to maintain his weight.

At the same time, an inactive girl of the same age, whose growth is nearly at a standstill, may need fewer than 2,000 kcalories if she is to avoid becoming obese. Thus there is tremendous variation in the nutrient needs of adolescents.

There is also tremendous variation in the rates and patterns of their growth. Growth charts used for children cannot be used any longer when the signs of

Rule of thumb for teen girls:
- For 5 ft, consider 100 lb a reasonable weight.
- For each inch over 5 ft, add 5 lb.
- For each year under 25 (down to 18), subtract 1 lb.
- For teen boys, see inside back cover.

Teenagers are notorious for eating on the run.

The nutritive value of selected fast foods is presented in Appendix H.

TABLE 15–4

Nutrients in a Hamburger, Chocolate Shake, and Fries

Nutrient	% of RDA
Calcium	47
Iron	21
Protein	42
Riboflavin	57
Thiamin	25
Vitamin A	3
Vitamin C	21

Source: Calculated from the RDA for a teenage male.

puberty begin to appear. The only way to be sure teenagers are growing normally is to compare their heights and weights with previous measures taken at intervals and note whether reasonably smooth progress is being made. Teenagers who want to know what they should weigh should be reassured that any of a wide range of weights is considered normal at this time in life. The rule of thumb on the inside back cover can be modified for teenage girls down to age 18 (see margin) and considered a weight to aim at; but weights well in excess of these are normal, too. Teenage boys can be told that when they have finished growing, they should expect to weigh what the adult charts show, but that while they are growing, it is not unusual for their weights to be quite different from the adult standards.

Teenagers as a group do have nutritional problems, however. Nearly every nutrient can be found lacking in one or another group: iron in young women, kcalories in young men (especially blacks), vitamin A in young women (especially Hispanics), calcium, riboflavin, vitamin C, and even protein. The insidious problem of obesity becomes more apparent, mostly in girls, and especially in black girls. Serious nutrient deficiencies often arise in pregnant teenage girls.

Eating Patterns

Teenagers come and go as they choose and eat what they want when they have time. With a multitude of after-school, social, and job activities, they almost inevitably fall into irregular eating habits. The adult becomes a gatekeeper, controlling the availability, but not the consumption, of food in the teenager's environment. The adult can't nag, scold, or pressure teenagers into eating as they should, because teens typically turn a deaf ear to coercion, and often to persuasion. To "feed" effectively, the gatekeeper must make every effort to allow these young people independence while providing a physical environment that favors healthy development and an emotional climate that encourages adaptive choices.

In the home, a wise maneuver is to provide access to nutritious and economical energy foods that are low in sugar and fat and discouraging to tooth decay. The snacker—and a well-established characteristic of teenagers is that they are snackers—who finds only nutritious foods around the house is well provided for.

Inevitably, teenagers will do a lot of eating away from home. There, as well as at home, their nutritional welfare can be favored or hindered by the choices they make. A lunch of a hamburger, a chocolate shake, and french fries supplies nutrients in the amounts shown in Table 15–4, at a kcalorie cost of 780. Except for vitamin A, these are substantial percentages of recommended intakes at a kcalorie cost many teenagers can afford. Depending on how they adjust their breakfast and dinner choices, teenagers may meet their nutritional needs more than adequately with this sort of lunch. They need only select fruits and vegetables (for vitamins A and C), good fiber sources, and more good iron sources at their other meals.

On the average, about a fourth of teenagers' total daily kcalorie intake comes from snacks. Their irregular schedules may worry adults who think they are feeding themselves poorly, but usually the kcalories they eat are far from empty. They receive substantial amounts of protein, thiamin, riboflavin, vitamin B$_6$, iron, magnesium, zinc, and even calcium (if they snack on dairy products). The nutrients they most often fail to obtain are vitamin A and folacin. Protein usually need not be stressed, but some teenagers should be encouraged to recognize and consume more dairy products (for calcium) and more good vitamin A and folacin sources. (Wherever vitamin A is lacking, folacin is, too, because both are found in green vegetables.)

The teenager's iron needs are a special problem, caused by several factors. Two already mentioned are the teenager's burgeoning iron need and the lack of iron in traditional snack foods. Other factors are the overemphasis on dairy products by some teenagers, vegetarianism, and the low contribution made by fast foods to iron intakes. A National Academy of Sciences committee, writing on this special problem, finds it doubtful that long-term administration of iron tablets is practical and advises against the measure of fortifying snacks and other foods with iron. Instead, the committee recommends that physicians and clinics screen all teenagers for low levels of iron in the blood. Their report stresses the fact that the best dietary source of absorbable iron is meats of all varieties, a point that should in turn be stressed in the nutrition education of teenagers.[3] No doubt they should learn as well to enjoy iron-rich plant foods such as legumes and whole grains. A later section addresses the problem of teaching teens about nutrition.

The Pregnant Teenage Girl

A special case is that of the pregnant teenage girl. Even if she were not pregnant, she would be hard put to meet her own nutrient needs at this time of maximal growth. Nourishing the baby doubles her burden. Figure 15–4 shows that her needs for many nutrients double, although her kcalorie allowance increases by only a few percent. In the case of a girl who begins pregnancy with inadequate nutrient stores or who lacks the education, resources, and support she needs, these problems are compounded.

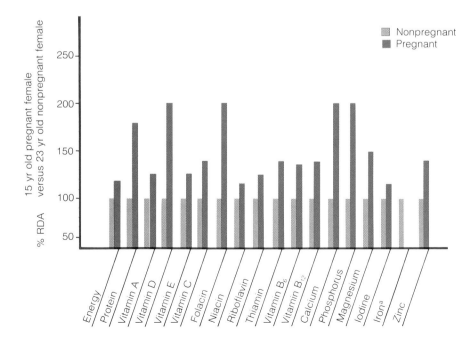

FIGURE 15–4

Comparison of the nutrient needs of a 15–year-old pregnant female with those of a 23–year-old nonpregnant female.

[a]The pregnant woman may need to take an iron supplement.

The complications of pregnancy were discussed in Chapter 14, where it was shown that the consequences of poor nutrition are acute and long-lasting. Complications are common in pregnant teenagers, with toxemia occurring in about one out of every five girls under the age of 15. If one pregnancy is followed by another, the stage is set for kidney damage and pregnancy-induced hypertension that may be irreversible.

Teenage pregnancy has become common. About one out of every five babies is born to a teenager, and more than a tenth of these mothers are 15 or younger. Emphasis on preparing young girls for future pregnancy is needed in public schools and public health programs. Faced with her parents' and classmates' often insensitive reactions, a pregnant girl is likely to wind up alone, with little or no money to buy food and no motivation to seek prenatal care. She urgently needs programs addressed to all her problems, including medical attention, nutrition guidance, emotional support, and continued schooling. A model program for giving nutritional help to teenage mothers, among others, is the WIC (Women's, Infants' and Children's) program, a federally funded program that provides nutrition information and low-cost nutritious foods to low-income pregnant women and their children.

Alcohol and Drugs

The teen years bring exposure to experiences not encountered before. Some complicate the nutrition picture: the use and abuse of alcohol, prolonged use of prescription medications, drug use (and abuse), use of caffeine, and many more.

The nutrition implications of alcohol use and the consequences of its abuse were described in highlight 7B. To sum them all up, alcohol is an empty-kcalorie beverage and can displace needed nutrients from the diet while simultaneously altering metabolism so that even good nutrition cannot normalize it. Those who are unable to use alcohol with moderation must abstain completely from its use if they are to maintain good health.

Many myths and misconceptions are found in the public's picture of alcohol use, and teenagers often cherish incorrect beliefs that lead them to alcohol abuse and addiction if they are susceptible. Being susceptible to alcohol addiction, like being potentially diabetic, is probably an inherited trait and is therefore nothing to be ashamed of. The teenager, however, is apt to be exposed to peer pressure that favors everyone's drinking, and those who can't do so safely are in an unfortunate predicament.

Among mistaken beliefs especially common among teenagers is the notion that a beer drinker can never become an addict. On the contrary, because beer contains alcohol, it is just as capable of contributing to alcoholism as is wine or hard liquor (whiskey, gin, vodka, and the like). It is not the beverage, but the constitution of the consumer, that determines whether he will become addicted to alcohol.

Some beer drinkers maintain that beer has some redeeming features. It makes people drunk less quickly, and it provides valuable nutrients. True, because the alcohol in beer is diluted, it will reach the bloodstream more slowly from the stomach than the same amount of alcohol taken straight. But the carbonation in beer stimulates the stomach, hastening the entry of alcohol into the intestine, where it will immediately be absorbed. As for the nutrient content of beer, an adult male would have to drink at least a six-pack of 12–ounce cans to meet one day's niacin needs and nine six-packs to meet one day's protein needs.

Some young people choose to abstain from alcohol consumption because they know or suspect they are prone to an alcohol problem. Others make the same choice for other reasons. Such people have a hard time in some social settings, because drinking is often not only accepted, but even demanded. It is hoped that highlight 7B shows why it is desirable not to pressure others to drink. Considerate hosts or social groups will welcome the nondrinker and provide nonalcoholic beverages for her enjoyment, just as they would provide nonmeat food for a guest who is a vegetarian.

Not only alcohol, but also many medicines, affect the body's need for and use of nutrients. Prescription medications can affect nutrition status by:

- Increasing or decreasing appetite.
- Causing nausea, vomiting, or an altered sense of taste.
- Inhibiting the synthesis of nutrients.
- Reducing the absorption or increasing the excretion of nutrients.
- Altering the transport, use, or storage of nutrients.

Foods and nutrients can also affect the drugs in the body. Known interactions between drugs and nutrition number several hundred by now; a few were described in Chapter 9.

Users of abusable drugs face multiple nutrition problems:

- They spend their money for drugs rather than for food.
- They lose interest in food during "high" periods.
- Some drugs (for example, amphetamines) induce at least a temporary depression of appetite.
- Their lifestyle lacks the regularity and routine that would promote good eating habits.
- They often have hepatitis, a liver disease transmitted from person to person by the use of contaminated needles, which causes taste changes and loss of appetite.
- They often depend on alcohol, especially when withdrawing from drug use.
- They often become ill with infectious diseases, which increase their need for nutrients.

hepatitis (hep-uh-TIGHT-us): a severe viral liver disease transmitted from person to person either through contaminated water or (as in the case of drug addicts) by way of contaminated needles.

During withdrawal from drugs, one of the most important aspects of treatment is to identify and correct these nutrition problems while teaching and supporting adaptive eating habits.

Teenagers' Food Choices

The teen years are well known as a time of rebellion. This rebellion extends to foods, as well as to all other aspects of lifestyle. Teens decide for themselves what to eat. Access points already mentioned include the refrigerator, the school lunch, and vending machines; but other than controlling the contents of these, adults can expect to have little impact on the nutrient intakes of adolescents—especially by such conventional means as education. Still, most young adults in this country are well fed, for reasons perceptively stated by Dr. Ruth M. Leverton: they get hungry; they like to eat; they want energy, vigor, and the means to compete and excel in whatever they do; and they have many good habits, which are just as hard to break as the bad ones.[4]

Nutrition educators who wish to reach the teenager and young adult with nutrition information must find out and pay attention to two factors: why they sometimes are poorly nourished or develop poor food habits, and what means of communicating reaches them effectively.

The young person with poor food habits and a negative attitude toward food is likely to have at least one of the following characteristics:

- He thinks nutrition means eating what you don't like because it's good for you.
- She has been criticized for her eating pattern but feels fine and sees no ill effects.
- He is uninterested in food, and it plays a negligible role in his very busy life.
- The people she is most likely to listen to are not knowledgeable about nutrition.[5]

The parent or teacher concerned about a teenager's food habits should be aware of what teenagers feel about themselves (some reflection into your own past may recall painful memories in this connection). They crave acceptance, especially from their peers. They need to fit in. In many cases they are greatly dissatisfied with themselves. One of the most important aspects of their image is the body image. Young men want larger biceps, shoulders, chest, and forearms; young women want smaller hips, thighs, and waists. Words to the effect that "you look fine as you are" fall on deaf ears. (The same can be said of adults in some cases, up to the age of about 99.) To be conveyed effectively, nutrition information can be sold as part of a package that will bring about these desired changes. Fortunately, it happens to be true that nutrient-dense, low-kcalorie foods favor the development of strong biceps in men and a trim figure in women.

When the young person who is the target of your campaign possesses and cherishes nutrition misinformation, one of the first questions to ask is whether the practice is beneficial, neutral, or harmful. Opposing a loved ideal is more likely to polarize than to convert the opposition. A practice such as vegetarianism, dieting, or consuming a "muscle-building diet" can be encouraged—with modifications—rather than condemned. Only the most hazardous nutrition practices should be singled out for attention; silence is an option in dealing with the others.

One of the most effective ways to teach nutrition is by example. When nutrition teachers are moralists who fail to practice what they preach, their words fall on deaf ears. The coach and gym teacher, the friendly young French teacher, the admired city recreation director—those who enthusiastically maintain their own health—can have a great impact on teenagers. Remember, this is the period of identity formation, the time of seeking and emulating models.

When communicating nutrition information, above all be sure that you have it straight. We make fools of ourselves when we (for example) admonish our students to follow restrictive patterns when their own choices are already as good as ours or better. There may be no harm in using candy bars to meet part of the kcalorie allowance for an active young adult. It may not be necessary to drink milk if calcium, vitamin D, and riboflavin needs are being met by cheese or other food sources. Satisfactory diets can be designed on a great variety of

YOU'LL NEVER GET ME UP IN ONE OF THOSE THINGS.

foundations. It is the nutrient content and balance of foods, not the specific foods consumed, that make the difference between "good" and "bad" diets.

Much of the work of "teaching" nutrition can be delegated to teenagers themselves. Those who are interested and motivated can be guided to reliable sources and allowed to indulge their own desire to benefit their friends and classmates. Among the best materials prepared to teach teenagers the importance of good nutrition are those made by teenagers themselves.

Finally, remember that teenagers have the right to make their own decisions—even if they are ones you violently disagree with. You can set up the environment so that the foods available are those you favor, and you can stand by with reliable nutrition information and advice, but you will have to leave the rest to them. Ultimately, they make the choices.

Study Questions

1. What are secular trends in nutrition? How does nutrition affect the timing and extent of young people's maturation?
2. How do children learn about nutrition outside the home? Discuss the impact of the School Lunch Program, television, and vending machines on the nutrition status of children. How would you encourage children to be more involved in their own nutrition?
3. Discuss the potential benefits and disadvantages of snacking during the teen years. What nutrition problems are common among teenagers?

Notes

1. H. R. Armstrong and D. B. Root, Managing a lean NET program, *Community Nutritionist* 2 (1983): 8–10.
2. S. J. Fomon, T. A. Anderson, H. Y. W. Stephen, and E. E. Ziegler, *Nutritional Disorders of Children: Prevention, Screening, and Followup*, DHEW publication no. (HSA) 76–5612 (Washington, D.C.: Government Printing Office, 1976), p. 100.
3. Committee on Nutrition of the Mother and Preschool Child, Food and Nutrition Board, National Academy of Sciences, *Iron Nutriture in Adolescence*, DHEW publication no. (HSA) 77–5100 (Washington, D.C.: Government Printing Office, 1977).
4. R. M. Leverton, The paradox of teen-age nutrition, *Journal of the American Dietetic Association* 53 (1968): 13–16.
5. Leverton, 1968.

The Later Years

16

As cells grow old, the "aging pigment," lipofuscin, accumulates. Shown here is a heart muscle fiber (the striped strand at left) surrounded by many mitochondria. The dark, disorganized bodies are lipofuscin.

By the time you are 65 years old, you will have eaten about 100,000 pounds of food. Each bite will have brought with it the nutrients you need, or it will not have. Each meal will have been too high in fat, or just right. The impact of all this eating, together with other lifestyle habits, accumulates over a lifetime, and people who have lived and eaten differently all their lives are in widely different states of health by the time they are 65. Nutrition for the later years, the subject of this chapter, therefore begins at birth, and by the time they are old, different people need to make different adjustments in their ways of life and eating patterns.

In exploring nutrition for older adults, it will be necessary to recognize the wide range of individual situations they represent. It will be helpful to keep three questions in mind:

- What can I do now to prepare myself for the time when I will be an older adult?
- What can I do when I am older (or now that I am older) to keep myself healthy and vigorous so I will enjoy these years?
- How can I, as a relative or a health professional, help those who are in need?

The older person who is healthy and vigorous can enjoy the later years.

The Aging Process

It is easy to get the impression from mortality statistics that people are living longer and longer lives, but this is not true. Two different sets of observations have been made, and we must view them separately to understand what is really happening. On the one hand, fewer people are dying young, so the *average* age at death is greater than it used to be. Infant mortality, especially, has been greatly reduced over the past several decades, so there are fewer deaths at ages one, two, three, and four to pull the average down. On the other hand, however, the *maximum* age at which people die—that is, the *life span*—has changed very little. Most men die at a little past 70; and women, at a little past 75 years of age. Thus it seems that something built into the human organism (we call it aging) cuts off life at a rather fixed point in time.

Why we age as we do, and why we die, no one knows, although many researchers are trying to find out. Among the questions they are asking are:

- To what extent is aging inevitable? Can we retard it through changes in our lifestyle and environment?
- What roles does nutrition play in aging, and what roles can it play in retarding aging?

With respect to the first question, it seems that aging is an inevitable, natural process, programmed into our genes at conception, but that we can adopt lifestyle habits such as exercising and paying attention to our work and recreational environments that will slow the process within the natural limits set by heredity. And with respect to the second question, clearly, good nutrition can retard and ease the aging process in many significant ways. The next sections describe the natural aging of cells and body systems, then examine the roles of nutrition.

Aging of Cells

Cells seem to age in response to outside (environmental) forces, and also to undergo a built-in (genetic) aging process. Environmental stresses that promote aging include extremes of heat and cold, disease, lack of nutrients, the wear and tear of hard physical labor, and the lack of stimulation caused by disuse (for example, of the muscle cells in the legs of a person who can't walk). But even in the most pleasant and supportive of environments, inevitable changes take place in the structure and function of the body's cells.

All theories of aging have one element in common. They agree that at some point, the cells become incapable of replenishing their constituents. When some cells die and their function is lost, other cells dependent on the first ones suffer and also eventually die. Thus whole systems are affected.

A second common element seems to be that aging cells are programmed to stop reproducing after a certain number of cell divisions. Red blood cells multiply only as long as they are in the marrow of the long bones. When they move out of the marrow into the blood, they no longer reproduce; they work for four months and then die. Brain cells all stop reproducing at about 14 months of age. Thus a two-year-old has all the brain cells he will ever have, and has already lost a few. Thereafter, thousands of brain cells die daily, but the daily loss is not noticeable over a few months or years, because so many cells remain. Only the accumulated loss over a lifetime is felt as reflexes are slowed and the brain's direction of other organs gradually becomes impaired. It seems strange that the human species should have evolved such a magnificent instrument for receiving, storing, interpreting, and retrieving information and yet not have evolved a method of repairing it; however, it is not so strange in view of the theory of evolution, because evolution has only provided that we live to reproduce. Natural selection did not operate to confer any advantage on the human organism beyond reproductive age.

The aging process is inevitable, then, and we must live with it as best we can. Fortunately, however, we have inherited magnificent equipment for learning and coping—our brains—and even though they, themselves, age and become less efficient with time, the learning and wisdom we accumulate in life compensate for the unavoidable physical changes.

A third factor in the aging process seems to be that, with the passage of time, cells become cluttered with debris—partially completed proteins and oxidized lipids that are never totally dismantled. This intracellular "sludge" interferes with the efficiency of operations within the cells. The lipid material that accumulates in the cells is known as the pigment of old age.

Another factor may be that cells lose their ability to interpret the DNA genetic code words and so make their proteins incorrectly. As reduced amounts of protein or wrong proteins are produced, cell and organ functions that depend on those proteins also falter. Organs elsewhere in the body may also be adversely affected. A theory somewhat allied to this one is that through some environmental stress, such as radiation, the DNA code itself may become altered. This, too, would lead to the production of wrong proteins.

The aging pigment is **lipofuscin** (lip-oh-FEW-sin).
lipo = lipid
fuscus = brownish gray

If wrong proteins are produced for any reason, another theory states, the body's immune system will react to them as if they were foreign proteins from outside and will produce antibodies to counteract them. Complexes then form between the antibodies and these proteins and accumulate in and among cells as useless debris. This autoimmune theory may account in part for the accumulation of deposits in joints, which causes arthritis.

Finally, another theory of aging suggests that cosmic rays bombard molecules in the cells and split them into highly reactive compounds known as free radicals. These free radicals then bind rigidly to other cellular molecules by way of disulfide bridges. This disrupts the informational content of important molecules and so impairs their function. (Some investigators have suggested that the formation of free radicals might be retarded by the taking of vitamin E supplements.) None of these ideas is more than a theory, but they suggest explanations for the aging of systems described in the next section.

For a picture of the disulfide bridges in insulin, a protein molecule, see the diagram of insulin in Chapter 5. Free-radical formation is explained in Appendix B.

Aging of Systems

The aging of cells is reflected by changes in the organs they are a part of. The most visible changes take place in the skin. As people age, wrinkles increase, partly because of a loss of elasticity and of the fat that lies under the skin. Scars accumulate from many small cuts and roughen the skin's texture. Exposure to sun, wind, and cold hastens wrinkling.

Less visible, but much more important to nutrition, are the changes that take place in the digestive system. The gums deteriorate, causing loss of teeth; gum disease afflicts 90 percent of the population in the decade after age 65. The senses of taste and smell diminish, reducing the pleasure of eating. The stomach's secretions of hydrochloric acid and enzymes decrease, as do the secretions of digestive juices by the pancreas and small intestine, impairing the digestive process. The digestive tract muscles weaken with reduced use, so that pressure in the large intestine causes the outpocketings of diverticulosis. Constipation becomes a problem.

The liver is somewhat different. Liver cells regenerate themselves throughout life, but even with good nutrition, fat gradually infiltrates the liver, reducing its work output. The pancreatic cells become less responsive to high blood glucose levels, and the body's cells become resistant to insulin, so that it takes more to make them respond.

The heart and blood vessels age similarly. All organs and tissues depend on the circulation of nutrients and oxygen, so degenerative changes in the cardiovascular system critically affect all other systems. The decrease in blood flow through the kidneys makes them gradually less efficient at removing wastes and maintaining the blood's normal composition. As the heart pumps blood less forcefully, the capillary trees of the kidneys diminish in size; some kidney cells die. This degenerative process can be retarded by regular exercising, which ensures that an ample volume of blood is pumped into the kidneys, keeping the capillaries open.

The body's systems age at different rates and to different extents. In a lifetime, nerve conduction velocity appears to be affected least and lung function most, with other functions between the extremes:

As the heart pumps less blood into an organ, the capillary trees within that organ recede, leaving some of the cells without nourishment. Exercise promotes maintenance, and even growth, of capillaries.

■ Nerve conduction velocity and cellular enzyme activities decline about 15 percent.

- Cardiac index falls 30 percent.
- Vital capacity and renal blood flow decrease by 50 percent.
- Maximum breathing capacity, maximum work rate, and maximum oxygen uptake fall by 60 to 70 percent.[1]

Like the body's organ systems, the skeletal system is subject to change with the passage of time. Bone-building and bone-dismantling cells are constantly remodeling this structure, but after 40, bone loss becomes more rapid than bone building. The result is osteoporosis—a disease that afflicts close to half of all people over 65. Arthritis, a painful swelling of the joints, is another problem that troubles many people as they grow older. During movement, the bones must rub against each other at the joints. The ends are protected from wear by cartilage and by small sacs of fluid that act as a lubricant. With age, the ends of the bones become pitted or eroded as a result of wear and the loss of cartilage and fluid. The cause of arthritis is unknown, but it afflicts millions around the world and is a major problem of the elderly.

Can Aging Be Prevented?

What can we do to avoid growing old? Is there a magic potion we can drink, a food we can eat, a pill we can swallow? Or, on a more down-to-earth level, are there any lifestyle habits we can adopt to prolong our youth?

As far as potions, foods, and pills go, the answer seems to be no, although the search has gone on since the dawn of human history. We are still looking for the fountain of youth, and quacks who claim to have found it have been selling its waters for centuries. A recent candidate for prevention of aging is superoxide dismutase (SOD).

Another approach to prevention of aging has been to study other cultures in the hope of finding an extremely long-lived race of people and then learning

cardiac index: the cardiac output per square meter of body surface area. The **cardiac output** is the quantity of blood pumped into the aorta each minute. Cardiac output is responsible for transport of substances to and from the tissues; it changes markedly with body size.

vital capacity: the maximum volume of air that can be inhaled into or exhaled from the lungs.

superoxide dismutase (SOD): an antioxidant enzyme. Purified from animal tissues and sold in powder form, it is one of many fraudulent antiaging products on the popular market.

SOD deserves a moment's notice here. It is an enzyme that occurs naturally in the cells of animals, including humans. It acts as an antioxidant, as do vitamin C, vitamin E, and the selenium-containing enzyme described in Chapter 11. Animal species that live the longest, such as human beings, have the highest concentrations of SOD in their tissues, and it has been hoped that the concentration of this enzyme in the human body could be raised and would prolong life.

It doesn't work.[2] Like any other enzyme taken orally, SOD is digested in the stomach and intestine to fragments that the body uses to make its own proteins. If it were injected, it would still be external to cells, and could cause irritation and allergic reactions, but not longer life. The trick would have to be to induce the cells to make more of it themselves (genetic engineering)—and even then, who is to say that higher levels would have a beneficial effect? The body tends to make the right amount of what it needs, as this book has shown in countless examples, and "more" SOD would probably not be "better." Still, many health-food stores and other establishments are doing a brisk business selling it.

If age is venerated, people will claim to be old.

from them the secrets of long life. One scientist traveled far and wide in search of such people, and for a while thought that he had found them in two different geographical areas, because many people in the areas claimed to have lived for over 100 years. Further study revealed, however, that the old-age range in these populations was unremarkable—about 70 to 80, as elsewhere. These people only claimed to be 100 or older, because in their societies age was venerated. The oldsters were remarkably healthy and justifiably proud of it, but not because they ate according to any particular formula. One group ate a lot of meats and sweets; another used large amounts of alcohol and sugar. The secret—the one thing they all seemed to have in common—was that they lived a physically active life. The moral of this story seems to be that people will always lie about their age, but not always in the same direction.

Still another approach has been drastic manipulation of the diet in animals, which has given rise to some interesting and suggestive findings. Rats live longer when their food intake is restricted in the early weeks of their lives, or even when it is restricted during adulthood. The restriction has to be severe, though: to 60 percent of the normal kcalorie intake or even less.

Some of the animals died very young.

You may have heard of these experiments. The first of them were performed long ago, but recent attention to them has inspired articles in the popular press with titles like "Eat Less—Live Longer."

True, the life spans of rats were lengthened by drastic restrictions of their food intakes, and especially their fat intakes, during the time when they would normally be growing. In one experiment, for example, animals allowed to eat freely lived to an average 656 days, while those whose feed was restricted lived to an average 949 days. The experiments were interesting because it was possible to study growth retardation of various organ systems, and to speculate on the cause of the increased length of life of some of the animals—a delay in the onset of certain diseases, for example. But the experiments did *not* suggest any direct applications to human nutrition. One thing often overlooked in discussing them is the disadvantages incurred in the animals given restricted feedings.

For example, half of the restricted animals died *very* early (before 300 days). The average length of life was long because the few survivors lived a very long time. Also, the restriction was severe: "even the shortest period of food restriction in this study was comparable to restriction of the food intake of a human infant kept in an isolated environment for 20 to 25 years to an amount that would permit the infant to grow during that time to about the size of a one-year-old child."[3] Furthermore, the restricted animals that survived were retarded and malformed in a number of ways.

Old people, then, need not conclude on the basis of this evidence that their parents should have starved them when they were younger. Moderation in kcalorie intake is desirable, of course, but extreme starvation, like any extreme, is hardly worth the price.

The food restriction experiments have stimulated much discussion. The views of the experts can best be summed up by saying that disease can *shorten* people's lives, and that poor nutrition practices make diseases more likely or worse. "Good" nutrition, then, by postponing and slowing disease processes, can help to relengthen life back to the maximum life span—but can't extend it further.[4] This brings us to a consideration of the many diseases that seem to come with age, and the relevance of nutrition to them.

Nutrition, Aging, and Disease

Many diseases seem to come with age—heart disease, cancer, diverticulosis, bone disease, brain disease, diabetes, gum disease, and more. To what extent can nutrition prevent or retard the development of these diseases?

Parts of the preceding chapters and highlights have answered this question in part, and Table 16–1 sums up all that has been said. Clearly, an adequate intake of nutrients and fiber from a variety of foods, together with moderate intakes of kcalories and fat, throughout life helps immensely to promote good health in the later years.

Lest Table 16–1 should seem to overstate the case in favor of nutrition, Figure 16–1 puts nutrition (a factor you can control) in perspective with respect to heredity (a factor you can't control). It illustrates the point that some diseases are much more responsive to nutrition than others, and that some are not responsive at all. At one extreme are nutrient-deficiency diseases that can be completely cured by supplying the missing nutrients, and at the other extreme are certain genetic, or inherited, diseases that are completely unaltered by nutrition. Most fall in between, being influenced by inherited susceptibility, but responsive to dietary manipulation that helps to normalize metabolism and counteract the disease process. The potential influence of nutrition is well known in some instances, but in others it remains to be defined. Perhaps the most interesting question to nutritionists studying aging today is: to what extent are the so-called diseases of old age the result of as yet undetected nutrient deficiencies, excesses, or imbalances?

Nutrition quackery is largely based on the notion that certain foods and nutrients have almost miraculous power to promote health. People with cancer, particularly those who feel they can't be helped by therapy, are easy targets for peddlers of nutrition "cures." They may take massive doses of vitamins and/or minerals, some of which may be toxic. Table 16–1 displays an impressive list of health-promoting effects of good nutrition, but there is a difference. It does not advocate the use of specific foods—and certainly not of nutrient supplements—nor does it imply that even the most scrupulous attention to nutrition will guarantee freedom from disease. Taken together, the recommendations of the table simply add up to an adequate, balanced, and varied diet composed of nutritious foods—a quiet, sensible prescription for good nutritional health.

The table does not tell the whole story, however, because it deals only with nutrition. Nutrition shares with other lifestyle factors the responsibility for maintaining health. A complete prescription for good health might read as the list in the margin. Nutrition is represented by three of the six items in this list— one-half of the total. A person who abides by all six practices could expect to be physiologically 30 years younger, by later midlife, than a person who abides

- Get regular sleep.
- Eat regular meals.
- Maintain desirable weight.
- Don't smoke.
- Drink alcohol moderately or not at all.
- Get regular exercise.

TABLE 16–1

Examples of Preventive Effects of Good Nutrition[a]

Adequate intake of protein, kcalories, or essential nutrients helps prevent:

In pregnancy:
Birth defects.
Mental/physical retardation.
Low birthweight.
Poor resistance to disease.

In infancy and childhood:
Growth deficits.
Poor resistance to disease.

In adulthood and old age:
Malnutrition.
Poor resistance to disease.
Brain disease.

Moderation in kcalorie intake helps prevent:
Obesity and related diseases, such as diabetes and hypertension.

Adequate intake of any essential nutrient prevents:
Deficiency diseases such as cretinism, scurvy, and folacin-deficiency anemia.

Adequate calcium intake helps prevent:
Adult bone loss.

Adequate iron intake helps prevent:
Anemia.

Adequate fluoride intake helps prevent:
Dental caries.

Moderation in sodium intake helps prevent:
Hypertension and related disease of the heart and kidney.

Adequate fiber intake helps prevent:
Digestive malfunctions such as constipation and diverticulosis, and possibly colon or other cancers.

Adequate vitamin A intake helps prevent:
Susceptibility to epithelial cancer.

Moderation in fat intake helps prevent:
Hyperlipidemia, susceptibility to some cancers, and atherosclerosis.

Moderation in sugar intake helps prevent:
Dental caries.

Moderation in alcohol intake helps prevent:
Liver disease.
Malnutrition.

Moderation in intake of essential nutrients prevents:
Toxicity states.

[a]Relationships shown are not exclusive; that is, in all but two instances, the nutrition variable does not by itself prevent, but is known to contribute to prevention of, the condition.

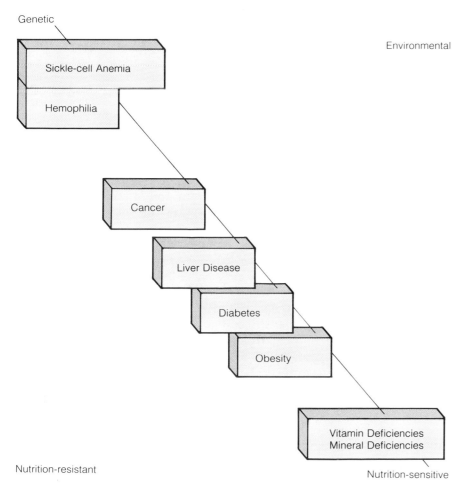

Genetic

Sickle-cell Anemia

Hemophilia

Cancer

Liver Disease

Diabetes

Obesity

Vitamin Deficiencies
Mineral Deficiencies

Nutrition-resistant

Environmental

Nutrition-sensitive

FIGURE 16–1

Nutrition-responsive versus unresponsive diseases. Not all diseases are equally influenced by diet. Some are purely hereditary, like sickle cell anemia. Some may be inherited (or the tendency to them may be inherited) but may be influenced by diet, like some forms of diabetes. Some are purely dietary, like the vitamin and mineral deficiency diseases. Some authorities are concerned that the offering of dietary advice to the public may seem to exaggerate the power of nutrition in preventing disease. Nutrition alone is certainly not enough to prevent many diseases.

Source: Adapted from R. E. Olson, Are professionals jumping the gun in the fight against chronic diseases? *Journal of the American Dietetic Association* 74 (1979): 543–550, Figure 2.

by few or none of them.[5] If you subscribe to the view that your job is to accept the things you can't control and control the things you can, then your nutritional health falls in the second category and deserves your conscientious attention.

Of the degenerative conditions named in Table 16–1, most have been dealt with in earlier chapters. One that has not been mentioned is brain disease—which actually includes many processes that are collectively termed aging of the brain. It isn't clear, yet, to what extent nutrition may play a role in these, but recent evidence suggests that some brain aging may actually be the result of gradual, insidious nutrient deficits. One study revealed that older people whose diets were lower in vitamins C or B_{12} were less able to think clearly, and those whose diets were poorer in riboflavin and folacin had poor memories. The researchers concluded that "subclinical malnutrition may play a small role in the depression of cognitive function in the elderly."[6]

Other studies have implicated other nutrient deficiencies in the aging of the brain. Deficiencies of the vitamins thiamin and niacin are well known to be partly responsible for degenerative changes in the mental function of alcohol abusers. Structural alterations in brain cells accompany these changes, even without alcohol abuse. Recently, attention has focused on deficiencies of two other nutrients: copper and vitamin B_6. Deficiencies of these nutrients have not yet been demonstrated to alter brain cell structures in people, but they do in animals, and they accelerate the aging of the nerve cells.[7]

Another age-related change is seen in the lens of the eye: cataracts—thickenings of the lenses that impair vision and ultimately lead to blindness. Cataracts occur even in well-nourished individuals, due to injury, viral infections, toxic substances, and genetic disorders, but most cataracts are vaguely called "senile cataracts"—meaning "caused by aging." Thoughtful scientists have wondered just what this really means, and have searched for a possible role of nutrient deficiencies, excesses, and imbalances in the causation of cataracts. They have observed several possible (and, it should be emphasized, highly tentative) links: to protein, fat, or sugar (lactose) excess; to kcalorie excess (in diabetics); to deficiencies of the vitamins riboflavin or vitamin E; and to deficiencies of the minerals selenium or zinc.[8] It may be that the formation of some cataracts, at least in persons with diabetes, may be preventable by attention to adequacy and moderation in the diet.[9]

Another major disease that disables the elderly is arthritis. Unlike cataracts, arthritis has for centuries been ascribed to poor diet—wrongly. Although nutrition may bear some relevance to arthritis, as will be shown in a moment, the chief involvement of nutrition with arthritis, to date, has been in the form of quack remedies, including many bizarre diets advertised as arthritis cures. Two or three new popular books on diet for arthritis come out every year, urging people to eat no meat, or drink no milk, or eat all their food raw, or eat only "natural" food, or avoid all additives, or—who knows what will be next? Actually, no known diet prevents, relieves, or cures arthritis,[10] but as long as people keep buying the books that make these claims, the law of supply and demand dictates that such books will keep coming out.

Recently, well researched findings have been reported that link diet to arthritis. Researchers surveyed the diets of 36 people with arthritis and found them marginal with respect to several essential nutrients—especially vitamin E and zinc. These two nutrients, among others, are important to normal function of the body's immune system, and an abnormal immune response may contribute to arthritis. Although no final conclusions can yet be reached, the researchers deem it advisable to obtain adequate, balanced diets.[11] This is an undramatic conclusion, perhaps, but it is honest, good advice.

Weight loss is important for overweight persons with arthritis, because the joints affected are often weight-bearing joints that are stressed and irritated by having to carry excess poundage. Weight-loss diets alone often relieve the worst of the pain in arthritis patients. Weight loss may confer a benefit even on arthritis in the hands, though, for reasons unknown. Perhaps the drastic reduction in fat intake that accompanies the adoption of a kcalorie-restricted diet is in some way beneficial to arthritis sufferers.[12]

These brief discussions of brain disease, cataracts, and arthritis illustrate that nutrition can provide at least some protection against certain diseases of old age. In fact, in general, it is beginning to look as if nutrition may play a greater role than has been realized in preventing many changes once thought to be inevitable consequences of growing older. The next section is devoted to the

Not effective against arthritis:
- Watercress.
- Burdock root.
- Vitamin D.
- Celery juice.
- Calcium.
- Megadoses of vitamins.
- Fasting.
- Fresh fruit.
- Honey.
- Lecithin.
- Yeast.
- Kelp.
- Raw liver.
- Fish liver oil.
- Alfalfa tea.
- *Aloe vera* liquid.
- Superoxide dismutase (SOD).
- 100 others.

food choices of middle-aged and older people, with a view to making needed improvements.

One final word before we leave the subject of nutrition and disease. Illness almost always involves the use of medicines— from over-the- counter types such as aspirins and laxatives to prescription drugs of all kinds. Most of them interact with one or more nutrients in several ways, usually resulting in greater-than-normal needs for these nutrients (see Chapter 9). Older people are especially likely to be using medications, often many at a time, and so they are particularly vulnerable to the negative physical impacts of these drugs. And like the effects of illnesses, the effects of drugs are cumulative over time. To give but one example, arthritis sufferers are often heavy users of aspirin, a superb painkiller and anti-inflammatory agent, but also an agent that prevents the passage of vitamin C from the plasma to the tissues. If plasma vitamin C levels are measured in these patients, then, no deficit is seen, and yet the tissues may be experiencing a deficit. A clinician, observing this effect, recommends "energetic vitamin C therapy" for patients taking large amounts of aspirin—not megadoses, to be sure, but doses of up to 200 milligrams, four times the RDA.[13] Anyone who finds it necessary to take one or several medications on a continuing basis should make special efforts to obtain amounts of nutrients greater than those recommended for healthy people.

Aging affects every body tissue and organ: the brain, the digestive tract, the bones. Many of the changes are inevitable, but a nutrition lifestyle that combines moderation with adequate intakes of all essential nutrients can forestall degeneration and improve the quality of life into the later years.

Nutrition Implications of Aging

Good health habits, including good nutrition throughout life, are the best guarantee of healthy and enjoyable later years. Many of the nutrient needs of the elderly are the same as for younger persons, but some special considerations deserve emphasis. As you read the following discussions about particular elements of the diet, remember that older adults who overemphasize one food group to the exclusion of others are most at risk nutritionally. The familiar maxim holds true throughout the life cycle: the best dietary guideline is to eat a balanced and varied selection of foods.

Energy

Energy needs decrease with advancing age. For one thing, the number of active cells in each organ decreases, bringing about a reduction in the body's overall metabolic rate. For another, older people are less active physically (although they need not be). In 1980, for the first time, the RDA tables presented recommended energy intakes for the older set; these recommendations reflect an estimated reduction of about 5 percent per decade in energy output. The vari-

Older people need not be less active physically than they were when they were younger.

TABLE 16–2

Eating Patterns to Supply the Recommended Energy Amounts for Older People (Exchange System)

Exchange List	Number of Exchanges	
	Woman (1,500 kcal)	Man (2,000 kcal)
Milk (nonfat)	3	3
Vegetable	2	3
Fruit	4	6
Bread	5	8
Meat (lean)	6	7
Fat	5	7

ation is great, so the ranges are wide (see Appendix I), but average figures for people 75 and older are 2,050 kcalories per day for the man and 1,600 for the woman. Table 16–2 shows eating patterns that would supply amounts of kcalories a little lower than the RDA tables show. Because overweight is well recognized as a shortener of the life span, these seem to be life-sustaining recommendations.

Energy intake should be adequate, however. Deficiency can cause PCM, which is common in older people and often goes unnoticed. An observer, seeing the wasted muscle, weakness, and sometimes swelling of protein deficiency, may think, "That person looks old," when in fact he should recognize the symptoms of PCM. Older people who have been trying to lose weight or who have been eating monotonous or bizarre diets are most likely to be affected.[14]

On one side of the energy budget, kcalories are taken in; on the other side, they are spent. If you are motivated to maintain your good health into the later years, you should plan regular exercise into your days. People responsible for the care of older adults should encourage more activity of all kinds and shorter recuperation periods in bed following illnesses.

Ideally, the exercise should be intense enough to increase the heartbeat and respiration rate, and to prevent the atrophy of all muscles (not only the heart) that otherwise takes place. A good flow of blood requires a strong heartbeat and strongly flexing muscles to press expelled lymph back into the bloodstream for recirculation. Many older persons believe that they can't participate in strenuous exercise, but studies have shown that they can do more than they think they can. Any exercise—even a ten-minute walk a day—is better than none, and with persistence, great improvement can be achieved. Modest endurance training can improve cardiovascular and respiratory function and promote good muscle tone while controlling the accumulation of body fat. The older person who has never worked out hard before may be encouraged to learn that the trainability of older people does not depend on their physical prowess in their youth. Improvement during training is due not only to improvement in muscles, but also to the increased blood flow to the brain engendered by the exercise. A major benefit is that, with an increased energy output, you can afford to eat more food and so obtain more nutrients.

Nutrients

The need for *protein* is the same for older adults as it is for younger adults. However, as you grow older, you have to get this protein from less food, so you must seek out low-kcalorie sources of high-quality protein. To protect the protein from being used for energy, you have to include ample complex carbohydrates in your diet along with it.

Low hemoglobin levels have been shown to correlate with protein (as well as iron) content of the diet, and may be the cause of the fatigue and apathy so often mentioned as a problem by older persons. The National Academy of Sciences recommends that older persons consume 12 percent of their kcalories as protein, which works out to be an amount slightly above the RDA for most people. Food patterns that restrict fat and offer abundant carbohydrate of necessity often supply up to 20 percent of the kcalories as protein, and this may be an ideal intake, especially for people whose protein needs are increased by illness.

Fat should be limited in the older person's diet, for many reasons. Cutting fat helps cut kcalories (recall that fat delivers two and a half times as many kcalories per unit of weight as the other energy nutrients) and may also help retard the development of atherosclerosis, cancer, arthritis, and other degenerative diseases. An appropriate intake might be 20 percent of the kcalories from fat. Of those, about half should perhaps be from polyunsaturated fat to contribute the essential fatty acids and to displace the saturated fat thought to contribute to high blood cholesterol.

Complex carbohydrate foods in great varieties should be emphasized in the older person's diet. Any educational campaign conducted to improve the diets of the elderly should emphasize the generous array of vitamins, minerals, and fiber contributed by complex carbohydrate foods.

The *fiber* recommendations for the general population should be stressed as well: increase the use of fruits, vegetables, and whole-grain cereals. The fiber content of these foods is important to prevent constipation and diverticulosis and to bind cholesterol and carry it out of the body.

Adequate *vitamin* intakes can be ensured by including foods from all food groups. Studies have shown that the one food group omitted most often by the elderly is the vegetable group. About 18 percent of older people are reported to eat no vegetables at all. Fruit is lacking in many diets, and up to one of every three older people report never eating fruit. Some men and women do not eat whole-grain breads and cereals, and so lose a significant source of many B vitamins and several minerals. Many do not drink milk and so risk vitamin D deficiency. The risk is greatest for older people who are homebound or who live in smoggy cities; some authorities suggest that the RDA for vitamin D for older people should be set at 15 to 20 micrograms per day, rather than at the present 10 micrograms.[15] The destruction of vitamin E by heat processing and oxidation is well known, and the processed and convenience foods so often used by the elderly and by nursing homes are thought to contribute to a vitamin E deficiency if their use continues over several years.[16]

Not only the omission of certain food groups, but also other conditions, contribute to vitamin deficiency in the elderly. Many take laxatives regularly, and this causes such a rapid transit time through the intestine that many vitamins

After the attainment of middle age, the body becomes more and more subject to the diseases resulting from the regime followed during the first half. . . . Nevertheless, the importance of the diet during the latter half of life must be of nearly the same order as during the first half.

Clive McCay

Fiber is discussed in more detail in Chapter 3.

do not get absorbed. The use of mineral oil as a laxative especially robs the person of the fat-soluble vitamins. Prescription and over-the-counter medications regularly taken by older adults cause vitamin deficiencies. For example, some antibiotics kill intestinal bacteria that produce vitamin K; and many drugs produce a folacin deficiency.

Among the *minerals,* iron deserves first mention. Iron-deficiency anemia is not as common in older adults as in the past, but it still occurs in some, especially in those with low kcalorie intakes.[17] Low hemoglobin can result from a diet low in protein, as already mentioned; but diets low in iron are the usual cause. Heavy reliance on a "tea and toast" diet is cited as a double risk in this connection; what little iron the toast provides is poorly absorbable, while the tannins in tea inhibit iron absorption. (Actually, something in coffee inhibits iron absorption, too, although we don't know yet what it is.[18]) The best insurance for an adequate iron intake is a colorful selection of foods that includes iron-containing red meats as well as fruits and vegetables rich in vitamin C to aid in iron absorption.

Aside from diet, other factors in many older people's lives increase the likelihood of iron deficiency:

- Chronic blood loss from ulcers, hemorrhoids, or other disease conditions.
- Poor iron absorption due to reduced stomach acid secretion.
- Antacid use, which interferes with iron absorption.
- Use of medicines that cause blood loss, including anticoagulants, aspirin, and other arthritis medicines.

Anyone concerned with the nutrition status of an older person should not forget these possibilities.

Zinc deficiencies are probably common in older people. They may affect several functions. Most often associated with zinc deficiencies are loss of taste and slowed wound healing. Loss of taste, however, is often not responsive to zinc supplementation, and it may often arise from some other factor associated with aging. When wounds—for example, bedsores in the sick—are slow to heal, however, a zinc deficiency should be suspected, as these often do respond to zinc therapy.

Another mineral often lacking in older people's diets is calcium, the need for which increases with advancing age. Bone loss occurs insidiously, and may be alarmingly extensive and severe before a person realizes there is any problem at all. The recommendation of 5 cups of milk a day for older adults is difficult to meet, especially for the person who is unaccustomed to using much milk at all. However, there are many alternative strategies for obtaining the needed calcium. If fresh milk causes gas, as some older people report, then cheese should be included. Dry skim milk can be incorporated into many foods. Soup stock made from bones can be used daily.

The use of some medications impairs calcium absorption severely. So does the use of alcohol and caffeine. Older people who use all of these are especially prone to calcium deficiency.

Some authorities hold that all older people should limit their salt intakes. This is hard for people who rely on convenience foods and processed foods extensively, but it is suggested that they eat fresh foods instead, whenever they can.

To obtain the needed minerals, the older person should follow the same recommendation as for vitamins. Every food group—milk and milk products, meat and meat alternates, fruits and vegetables, and grains—should be represented in the diet every day.

Perhaps the most important nutrient of all is *water*. The elderly need to be reminded to drink fluids, because they are likely to be somewhat insensitive to their own thirst signals. They should drink six to eight glasses a day, enough to bring their urine output to about 6 cups per day. A large percentage of nursing home operators note that one of the biggest problems with their elderly clients is getting them to use more water and fruit juices.

You can tell from the color of your urine if you're getting enough water. Bright or dark yellow urine is too concentrated; you need more water. Pale yellow, almost colorless urine is dilute enough; your water intake is ample.

Caffeine

Older people often find they cannot tolerate caffeine as well as they could when they were younger. Caffeine is a true stimulant drug, increasing the respiration rate, heart rate, blood pressure, and the secretion of the stress and other hormones. Its "wake-up" effect is maximal within an hour after the dose. In moderate amounts (50 to 200 milligrams a day), caffeine seems to be relatively harmless.

Caffeine is not addictive, but it is habit forming, and the body adapts to its use to some extent. Sudden abstinence from the drug after long use, even if use has been moderate, causes a characteristic withdrawal reaction. If a person has adapted to a much higher dose level than 50 to 200 milligrams (see Table 16–3), then dropping back to this level may cause the same withdrawal reaction.

An overdose of caffeine produces reactions in the body that are indistinguishable from those of an anxiety attack. People who drink between 8 and 15 cups of coffee a day, for example, have been known to seek help from doctors for complaints such as dizziness, agitation, restlessness, recurring headaches, and sleep difficulties. Before prescribing a tranquilizer,

TABLE 16–3

Caffeine Sources

Source	Caffeine (mg)
Brewed coffee (1 c)	85
Instant coffee (1 c)	60
Brewed black tea (1 c)	50
Brewed green tea (1 c)	30
Instant tea (1 c)	30
Decaffeinated coffee (1 c)	3
Cola beverage (12 oz)	32 to 65
Cocoa (1 c)	6 to 42
Aspirin compound (pill containing aspirin, phenacetin, and caffeine)	32
Cope, Midol, and so on	32
Excedrin, Anacin (tablet)	60
Pre-Mens	66
Many cold preparations	30
Many stimulants	100
No Doz (tablet) or Vivarin	100 to 200

Source: Adapted from Food allergy, *Nutrition and the MD*, July 1978; and P. E. Stephenson, Physiologic and psychotropic effects of caffeine on man, *Journal of the American Dietetic Association* 71(1977):240–247.

the doctor would do well to inquire about the caffeine consumption of such patients.

A large dose of caffeine can also cause extra heartbeats and is believed to have caused heart attacks in people whose hearts were already damaged by degenerative disease. However, neither caffeine nor one of its vehicles, coffee, can be considered a risk factor for the development of atherosclerosis. Still, moderation in the use of caffeine-containing foods and beverages is advisable for all ages, and older people should be alert to the need to reduce their customary doses.

Alcohol

A recent estimate sets the incidence of alcoholism in people over 60 in our society at 2 to 10 percent. Alcohol use has its most profound effects on the vitamins thiamin and folacin and on the minerals calcium and zinc, but it affects nearly every nutrient to some extent. Where it is a problem in elderly people, it must be recognized before it can be dealt with.

Vitamin-Mineral Supplements

The recommended intakes of many of the vitamins and minerals are thought by some nutritionists to be too low for the over-65 group. They recommend supplements, particularly for the water-soluble vitamins, because large amounts pose no great threat of toxicity. However, other nutritionists feel that recommending vitamin supplements is a cop-out, laying the elderly open to exploitation by quacks. Money is better spent, they say, on food of higher quality.

Surveys designed to find out what kinds of nutrient supplements older people are using tend to support the view that in many cases they are wasting their money. A study in a southern California retirement community, for example, showed that 72 percent of the subjects were taking nutrient supplements—mostly of vitamins C and E—but that these choices were not related to the users' dietary intakes; that is, they were not appropriate.[19] Another study, in upper New York State, showed that 10 percent of an elderly population who needed vitamin and mineral supplements either were not taking any, or were taking the wrong ones, and in fact that their doctors had prescribed the wrong ones.[20] Advertising of supplements to the elderly muddies the waters further. Tonics that promise rejuvenation and renewed youth and vigor either hold out false hopes, are incomplete, or are laced with so much alcohol that the lift they seem to provide may be in fact an illusion with a negative effect, if any, on nutrient status.

For the formulations of these supplements, see the tables in Appendix J.

How to choose a vitamin-mineral supplement: see Highlight 10.

The older person would probably be wise to follow the rule of thumb that if the energy intake is below about 1,500 kcalories, then a vitamin-mineral supplement is recommended—not a megavitamin, but just a once-daily type of supplement. This means that many older persons, all except those who are so active that their kcalorie allowances have remained high, should take this precaution.

Practical Pointers

All of the objectives outlined for the older person's diet may seem worthwhile, but they may be hard to achieve, especially for the person living alone who has difficulty buying groceries and preparing meals. Packages of meat and vegetables are often prewrapped in quantities suitable for a family of four or more, and even a head of lettuce can perish before one person can use it all. A large package of meat is often a good buy, but defrosting it enough to get a portion from it for dinner is time-consuming; futhermore, the rest tends to thaw, too. Small packets get lost in the freezer and ruined by freezer burn. For the person who has little or no freezer space, the problem of storage is further compounded. Following is a collection of ideas gathered from single people who are doing a good job of solving these problems and getting nourishing food:

- Buy only three pieces of each kind of fresh fruit: a ripe one, a medium one, and a green one. Eat the first right away and the second soon, and let the last one ripen on your windowsill.
- Buy the small cans of vegetables, even though they are more expensive. Remember, it is also expensive to buy a regular-size can and let the unused portion spoil in the refrigerator.
- Buy only what you will use. Don't be timid about asking the grocer to break open a package of wrapped meat or fresh vegetables.

- Think up a variety of ways to use a vegetable when you must buy it in a quantity larger than you can use right away. For example, you can divide a head of cauliflower into thirds. Cook one-third and eat it as a hot vegetable. Put the other two-thirds into a vinegar-and-oil marinade for use as an appetizer or in a salad. You can keep half a package of frozen vegetables with other vegetables to be used in soup or stew.
- Make mixtures, using what you have on hand. A thick stew prepared from leftover green beans, carrots, cauliflower, broccoli, and any meat, with some added onion, pepper, celery, and potatoes, makes a complete and balanced meal—except for milk. But see the uses of powdered milk that follow: you could add some to your stew.
- Buy fresh milk in the size best suited for you. If your grocer doesn't carry pints or half-pints, try a nearby service station or convenience store.
- Buy a half-dozen eggs at a time. The carton of a dozen can usually be broken in half. However, eggs keep for long periods in the refrigerator and are such a good source of high-quality protein that you will probably use a dozen before they lose their freshness.

- Set aside a place in your kitchen for rows of glass jars containing shelf staple items that you can't buy in single-serving quantities—rice, tapioca, lentils or other dry beans, flour, cornmeal, dry skim milk, macaroni, cereal, or coconut, to name only a few possibilities. Place each jar, tightly sealed, in the freezer for one night to kill any eggs or contaminants before storing it on the shelf. Then the jars will keep the bugs out of the foods indefinitely.

They make an attractive display and will remind you of possibilities for variety in your menus. Cut the directions-for-use labels from the packages and store them in the jars.

- Learn to use dry skim milk. It is the greatest convenience food there is. Not only does it offer much more calcium than any other food, it also is fortified with vitamins A and D. Dry milk can be stored on the shelf for several months at room temperature. It can be mixed with water to make fluid milk in as small a quantity as you like—but once it is mixed, it will sour just like fresh milk. One person says he keeps a jar of dry skim milk next to his stove and "dumps it into everything": hamburgers, gravies, soups, casseroles, sauces, even beverages such as iced coffee. The taste is negligible, but five "dumpings" of a heaping tablespoon each would be the equivalent of a cup of fresh milk. Ask a friend who is a member of Weight Watchers to give you some recipes for delicious milk shakes and ice cream using dry skim milk. Their recipes are for single servings.

- Make soup stock from leftover pork and chicken bones soaked in vinegar. The bones release their calcium into the acid medium, and the vinegar boils off when the stock is boiled. One *tablespoon* of such stock may contain over 100 milligrams of calcium.[21] Then cook something in this stock every day: vegetables, rice, stew—and of course, make soups with it.

- Cook for several meals at a time. For example, boil three potatoes with skins. Eat one hot with margarine and chives. When the others have cooled, use one to make a potato-cheese casserole ready to be put into the oven for the next evening's meal. Slice the third one into a covered bowl, and pour over it the juice from pickles. The pickled potato will keep several days in the refrigerator and can be used in a salad.

- Experiment with stir-fried foods. Use a frying pan if you don't have a wok. Ask your Chinese friends for some recipes. A variety of vegetables and meat can be enjoyed this way; inexpensive vegetables such as cabbage and celery are delicious when crisp-cooked in a little oil with soy or lemon added. Cooked, leftover vegetables can be dropped in at the last minute. There are frozen mixtures of Chinese or Polynesian vegetables available in the larger grocery stores. Bonus: only one pan to wash.

- Depending on your freezer space, make double or even six times as much as you need of a dish that takes time to prepare: a casserole, vegetable pie, or meat loaf. Save the little aluminum trays from frozen foods, and store the extra servings, labeled, in the trays in the freezer. Be sure to date these so you will use the oldest first. Somehow, the work seems worthwhile when you prepare several meals at once.

- Buy a loaf of bread, and immediately store half, well wrapped, in the freezer. The freezer keeps it fresher than the refrigerator.

- If you have space in your freezing compartment, buy frozen vegetables in the very large bags rather than in the small cartons. You can take out the exact amount you need and close the bag tightly with a rubber band. If you return the package quickly to the freezer each time, the vegetables will stay fresh for a long time.

- If you have ample freezing space, you can buy large packages of meat such as pork chops, ground meat, or chicken when they are on special sale. Immediately divide the package into individual servings. Wrap in aluminum foil, not freezer paper; the foil can become the liner for the pan in which you bake or broil the meat, thus saving work over the sink. Don't label these individually, but put them all in a brown bag marked "hamburger" or "chicken thighs" or whatever the meat is, along with the date. The bag is easy to locate in the freezer, and you'll know when your supply is running low.

Although these suggestions will help the older person with the mechanics of food preparation and storage, they meet only a part of the need. Loneliness, too, needs to be dealt with if single life in the later years is to be enjoyed. Even for nutrition's sake, it is important to attend to this problem.

Mealtimes Alone

Old age is a time of losses. This fact has to be faced. Many people who arrive at this time of life don't comprehend the universality of the aging experience. They have made no mental preparations for it. Then, when faced with sorrow, loss, and depression, they turn inward for the explanation and conclude that there must be something wrong with them. This reasoning compounds the distress of the original problem.

Losses can occur in several areas. Old friends are lost when they die or move away; offspring move away also and are too busy to write; there is loss of income on retirement and loss of status in the community. There is loss of control of the environment, such as finding that the home that was to be a haven in retirement now sits in the middle of a high-crime area so that one can no longer walk the streets or visit with neighbors. Familiar shops and fruit stands, where a person knows the owners and is known by them, may close. The aging person develops a feeling of deep loneliness as the familiar environment constantly shifts. But what place, you may well ask, does such a discussion have in a book on nutrition?

Many authorities believe that malnutrition among the elderly is most often due to loneliness. For the 6 million adults over 65 who live alone, the pressing need seems to be for companionship first, then for food. Without companionship, appetite decreases. The association of food with human companionship is built into our genes, and our very first experience with food was combined with human body contact. The social life of the adult is built around food. Most invitations into adults' homes are accompanied by an offer of food or drink. We must admit that feeding is, for human beings, as much a social and psychological event as a biological one.

Having spent a lifetime internalizing the concept of food as part of a social activity, the older adult, alone all day every day, must exert a wrenching effort to place enough importance on the nutrient content of food to prepare it and to eat it alone. Purchasing, storing, and preparing food, as well as cleaning the kitchen, take a tremendous amount of energy. The lonely, depressed person, looking at the task, may forget about the body's needs and say, "What's the use?"

Dr. Jack Weinberg, professor of psychiatry at the University of Illinois, wrote perceptively of this problem:

> In our efforts to provide the aged with a proper diet, we often fail to perceive it is not *what* the older person eats but *with whom* that will be the deciding factor in proper care for him. The oft-repeated complaint of the older patient that he has little incentive to prepare food for only himself is not merely a statement of fact but also a rebuke to the questioner for failing to perceive his isolation and aloneness and to realize that food . . . for one's self lacks the condiment of another's presence which can transform the simplest fare to the ceremonial act with all its shared meaning.[22]

Loneliness is no respecter of income. It affects everyone— the financially secure and the poverty-stricken alike. Newspapers occasionally carry stories of wealthy older persons' being discovered in their mansions, alone and without food. The stories are newsworthy because people wonder why such victims did not ask for help or make arrangements for someone to take care of them—after all, they had plenty of money. The reason is simple. Apathy evolves from loneliness; apathy is expressed in inaction. A victim may sit for long hours in a chair without the energy even to lift her arms. There is no energy to eat, even when food is just a phone call away. Without adequate food, nutrient deficiencies develop that increase the apathy and depression and eventually result in mental confusion. The downward spiral continues, unless intervention by neighbors or friends breaks it at some point.

Let's look at what happens when a person receives too little food. In the first place, the body can't tell why it is receiving too few nutrients or kcalories. The effects are the same on a child dying in a famine in Bangladesh as on a wealthy solitary person who is depressed and refusing food. The water-soluble vitamins are quickly depleted, because they are excreted daily. If they are not restored, mental confusion that resembles senility will be manifested and may even progress to hallucinations and insanity. If the confusion of vitamin deficiency is diagnosed as senility, the elderly person may be wrongly confined to a nursing home.

The story is told of a woman who took her mother-in-law to live with her while the older woman waited for a place in a nursing home. The mother-in-law had exhibited the classic signs of senility—mental confusion, inability to make decisions, forgetting to perform important tasks such as turning off a stove burner—so the family had decided she needed institutional care. After several weeks in the daughter-in-law's home—eating good meals and enjoying

Lonely people:
Become apathetic.
Have no energy to seek food.
Become tired.
Become more apathetic.
Don't reach out to others.
Become more lonely.
Do not eat.
Become malnourished.
Become mentally confused.
Become more isolated.
Become more lonely.

The symptoms of B vitamin deficiencies are listed in Chapter 9, Table 9–2.

The warmth of good company at mealtimes stimulates the older person's appetite.

To avert the devastating effects of loneliness on nutrition, then, the person who is living alone must learn to connect food with socializing. Cook for yourself with the idea that you are also preparing for guests you might want to invite. Or turn this suggestion around: invite guests, and make enough food so that you will have some left for yourself at a later meal. With a wide variety of leftovers on hand, you can invite one or another single friend on the spur of the moment to "Come over and share my frozen dinners with me tonight."

social stimulation—she became her old self again and returned to her home. This story has been repeated with many variations and serves to remind us to seek a careful medical diagnosis before concluding that a person is senile and needs institutional care. What harm could there be in first trying good, balanced meals served with plenty of tender, loving care?

Assistance Programs

To add anxiety to their problems, most retired persons have a loss of real income that occurs because the retirement check is fixed while all other expenses are increasing. This has a direct effect on the amount of money spent on food, because food (and clothing) purchases are among the few flexible items in the budget. Costs of shelter, utilities, and medical care must be paid and then the amount left over stretched to cover food and other needs.

Forced to practice economy, the older person usually first eliminates so-called luxury items such as fresh fruit, vegetables, and milk. In some cases, transportation to and from the market is both expensive and difficult, so that use is made of a nearby convenience store. The foods offered there are limited in variety and are, for the most part, more expensive than the same items in the larger markets. The amount of food that can be purchased is thus curtailed even further, and eating, which should be a pleasure, becomes another reminder of reduced status.

Sometimes older persons fall prey to food fads and fallacies. Led by false claims to believe that health can be improved, aging forestalled, and illness cured by magical food and nutrient preparations, they spend money needlessly on fraudulent health-food products, thus depleting their already limited funds.

Two programs are helpful with older people's money problems, although they are not designed specifically for older people, but for the poor of all ages. The Food Stamp program enables people who qualify to obtain stamps with which to buy food. The Supplemental Security Income (SSI) program is aimed at directly improving the financial plight of the very poor, by increasing a person's or family's income to the defined poverty level. This sometimes helps older people retain their independence.

A self-help effort aimed at enabling older people on limited incomes to buy good food for less money is the establishment of food banks in several areas. A food bank project buys industry's "irregulars"—products that have been mislabeled, underweighted, redesigned, or mispackaged and would ordinarily therefore be thrown away. Nothing is wrong with this food; the industry can credit it as a donation, and the buyer (often a food-preparing site) can buy the food for a small handling fee (10 cents a pound) and make it available for a greatly reduced price. A 1981 observation on this effort was: "This kind of activity becomes even more important as we begin to realize that we're not going to get any additional federal money in the future. We have to find other ways to provide the same services."[23]

A major political move to benefit the elderly was the Older Americans Act of 1965. Title III C (formerly title VII) of this act is the "Nutrition Program for the Elderly." The major goals of this program are to provide:

- Low-cost, nutritious meals.
- Opportunity for social interaction.
- Auxiliary nutrition, homemaker education, and shopping assistance.
- Counseling and referral to other social and rehabilitation services.
- Transportation services.

The program is intended to improve older people's nutrition status and enable them to avoid medical problems, continue living in communities of their own choice, and stay out of institutions. The program was not designed as charity, but during its first years it was found that 80 percent of the participants had incomes less than $200 a month, and 34 percent had incomes under $100 a month.

Sites chosen for congregate meals under this program must be accessible to most of the target population. Volunteers may also deliver meals to those who are homebound either permanently or temporarily. By 1980 there were several hundred home-delivered-meals programs in the United States. Every effort is made to persuade the elderly person to come to the congregate meal site, as the social atmosphere at the sites is as valuable as the nutrition.

Meals on Wheels.

Nursing Homes

Sometimes assistance programs are not enough to meet the needs of older people. They require institutional care. A variety of options exist; a familiar alternative is the nursing home. A nursing home is a medical solution to what, in many cases, is a social problem, but may be necessary for people who need constant medical care.

The relative inquiring into nursing homes should ask the director or dietitian some questions about the food service. Is a choice given the resident in the selection of food? How often are the menus repeated (is the cycle monotonous)? How often are fresh fruits and vegetables served? Is the food fresh and tasty when served? Is a plate check conducted regularly, at least once a week, to discover what the resident is consuming? Does the staff keep track of each person's weight? Is there good communication between the nursing staff and the dietitian so that the dietitian will know if someone is not eating? Is the resident encouraged and helped to go to the dining room to eat so that some socializing will occur? Is the dining room attractive? Does someone help those who can't manage feeding themselves? Are minced meats offered to those who have problems with their dentures? Are religious dietary restrictions honored? How high a proportion of the foods are prepackaged? (No guide can be given for what proportion is desirable, but it should be remembered that processed foods are low in vitamin content and high in salt.) Other questions that the investigator will want to ask have to do with the general atmosphere of the nursing home, in recognition of the effect of social climate on a person's appetite. A nursing home that views residents as persons, not as patients, gets a mark in its favor.

In the nursing home, the dietitian, nutritionist, or nurse responsible for the residents' care should keep in mind the special needs associated with their time in life. The average age of a nursing home resident is 81, and many have problems that can affect nutrition status:

Eating with others improves appetite, and thereby nutrition.

- At least one chronic disease.
- Constipation or incontinence.
- Confusion due to change in environment.
- Poor eyesight or hearing.
- Ill-fitting or missing dentures.
- Inability to feed themselves because of arthritis or stroke.
- Psychological problems, especially depression.
- Anorexia and loss of interest in eating.
- Lack of opportunity to socialize at mealtimes.
- Long-established food preferences.
- Slowed reactions (seeing, holding utensils, chewing, or swallowing).[24]

On admission, their nutrition status should be assessed immediately, and the person responsible for their nutrition care should make every effort to rectify any problems promptly. Thereafter they should be reassessed at regular, frequent intervals and adjustments made as needed.

Opinions differ on the philosophy to adopt for nursing home menus. A multitude of different special diets is difficult and expensive to manage, and one authority recommends a "liberalized geriatric diet" for most cases, rather than modified diets. Based on the assumption that older people "should have the right to choose the food they eat," this general, liberal approach provides in one package the key characteristics of several special diets:

- 1,500 to 2,000 kcalories per day, mostly from nutrient-dense foods, with simple desserts not too high in kcalories.
- Minimal salt used in preparation.
- 65 to 70 grams protein per day from 2 cups milk and 4 to 6 ounces meat or meat alternate.
- At least 6 milligrams iron per day (the RDA for older people is 10 milligrams per day).
- Generous amounts of natural fiber, and fluid intake of 64 ounces per day.[25]

Further modifications can be made available for people with severe disease conditions.

Preparing For the Later Years

The very best help we could give our elderly citizens would be a change of attitude. As a nation, we value the future more than the present, putting off enjoying today so that tomorrow we will have money or prestige or time to have fun. The elderly feel this loss of future. The present is their time for leisure and enjoyment, but they have no experience in the use of leisure time.

Our culture also values the doers, those concerned with action and achievement. The Spanish mother may enjoy her child because he is sitting in her lap and laughing in her face; however, the Anglo-American mother is more likely preoccupied with how well her child is preparing for tomorrow. The elderly are aware of the status given those who are doing something, and of the disrespect given those who lead a contemplative life in retirement.

It would take a near miracle to change the attitude of a nation, but there is a change in attitude that individual persons can make toward themselves as they age. Preparation for this period should, of course, include financial planning, but other lifelong habits should be developed as well. Each adult needs to learn to reach out to others, to forestall the loneliness that will otherwise ensue. Each needs to learn some skills or activities that can continue into the later years—volunteer work with organizations, reading, games, hobbies, or intellectual pursuits—which will give meaning to the activities of the days. Each needs to develop the habit of adjusting to change, especially when it comes without consent, so that it will not be seen as a loss of control over life. The goal is to arrive at maturity with as healthy a mind and body as it is possible to have, and this means cultivating good nutrition status and maintaining a program of daily exercise, too.

Preparation for the later years begins early in life, both psychologically and nutritionally. Everyone knows older people who have gathered around themselves many contacts—through relatives, church, synagogue, or fraternal orders—and have not allowed themselves to drift into isolation. Upon analysis, you will see that their favorable environment came through a lifetime of effort. They spent their entire lives reaching out to others and practicing the art of weaving themselves into other people's lives. Likewise, a lifetime of effort is required for good nutrition status in the later years. A person who has eaten a wide variety of foods, has stayed trim, and has remained physically active will be most able to withstand the assaults of change.

Study Questions

1. What are some of the physiological changes that occur in the body's systems with aging? Can aging be prevented?
2. What roles does nutrition play in aging, and what roles can it play in retarding aging?
3. Discuss the nutrient needs of the elderly. Which nutrients need special consideration? Explain why.
4. What are some physical, psychological, and financial conditions that may contribute to malnutrition in older people?

Notes

1. D. M. Watkin, The physiology of aging, *American Journal of Clinical Nutrition* (supplement) 36 (October 1982): 750–758.

2. S. Zidenberg-Cherr, C. L. Keen, B. Lonnerdal, and L. S. Hurley, Dietary superoxide dismutase does not affect tissue levels, *American Journal of Clinical Nutrition* 37 (1983): 5–7.

3. A. E. Harper, Nutrition, aging, and longevity, *American Journal of Clinical Nutrition* (supplement) 36 (October 1982): 737–749.

4. Harper, 1982.

5. N. B. Belloc and L. Breslow, Relationship of physical health status and health practices, *Preventive Medicine* 1 (1972): 409–421.

6. J. S. Goodwin, J. M. Goodwin, and P. J. Garry, Association between nutritional status and cognitive functioning in a healthy elderly population, *Journal of the American Medical Association* 249 (1983): 2917–2921.

7. E. J. Root and J. B. Longenecker, Brain cell alterations suggesting premature aging induced by dietary deficiency of vitamin B$_6$ and/or copper, *American Journal of Clinical Nutrition* 37 (1983): 540–552.

8. G. E. Bunce, Nutrition and cataract, *Nutrition Reviews* 37 (1979): 337–343.

9. D. R. Davis, Nutritional prevention of cataracts (correspondence), *New England Journal of Medicine* 298 (1978): 55.

10. The items shown in the margin were listed by K. A. Meister, Can diet cure arthritis? *ACSH News and Views,* September–October 1980, p. 10; and in Morsels and tidbits, *Nutrition and the MD,* January 1982.

11. B. Kowsari and coauthors, Assessment of the diet of patients with rheumatoid arthritis and osteoarthritis, *Journal of the American Dietetic Association* 82 (1983): 657–659. Zinc has also been used successfully to relieve some symptoms in rheumatoid arthritis: P. A. Simkin, Oral zinc sulphate in rheumatoid arthritis, *Lancet,* 11 September 1976, pp. 539–542.

12. Dr. Charles P. Lucas, internist at Wayne State University School of Medicine, has observed a low-fat diet, adequate in all essential nutrients and emphasizing fruits, vegetables, and whole grains, to relieve the symptoms of rheumatoid arthritis in a few clients (personal communication, February 1984).

13. M. D. Altschule, *Nutritional Factors in General Medicine: Effects of Stress and Distorted Diets* (Springfield, Ill.: Charles C. Thomas, 1978), pp. 140–141.

14. S. R. Gambert and A. R. Guansing, Protein-calorie malnutrition in the elderly, *Journal of the American Geriatrics Society* 28 (1980): 272–275.

15. A. M. Parfitt and coauthors, Vitamin D and bone health in the elderly, *American Journal of Clinical Nutrition* (supplement) 36 (November 1982): 1014–1031.

16. H. H. Koehler, H. C. Lee, and M. Jacobson, Tocopherols in canned entrees and vended sandwiches, *Journal of the American Dietetic Association* 70 (1977): 616–620.

17. S. R. Lynch and coauthors, Iron status of elderly Americans, *American Journal of Clinical Nutrition* (supplement) 36 (November 1982): 1032–1045.

18. T. A. Morck, S. R. Lynch, and J. D. Cook, Inhibition of food iron absorption by coffee, *American Journal of Clinical Nutrition* 37 (1983): 416–420.

19. G. E. Gray, A. Paganini-Hill, and R. K. Ross, Dietary intake and nutrient supplement use in a Southern California retirement community, *American Journal of Clinical Nutrition* 38 (1983): 122–128.

20. A. A. Sorensen, D. I. Sorenson, and J. G. Zimmer, Appropriateness of vitamin and mineral prescription orders for residents of health related facilities, *Journal of the American Geriatrics Society* 27 (1979): 425–430.

21. A. Rosanoff and D. H. Calloway, Calcium source in Indochinese immigrants (correspondence), *New England Journal of Medicine* 306 (1982): 239–240.

22. J. Weinberg, Psychologic implications of the nutritional needs of the elderly, *Journal of the American Dietetic Association* 60 (1972): 293–296.

23. C. Schuster, Feeding at life's end, *Food Management* 16 (December 1981): 41, 68–71, 76.

24. E. Luros, A rational approach to geriatric nutrition, *Dietetic Currents, Ross Timesaver* 8 (November–December 1981).

25. Luros, 1981.

Nutrition
Assessment and
Care Strategies

17

Contents

We may view water as fairly unremarkable—a liquid that is without color, smell, or flavor. Yet it is the essence of life. This photograph illustrates the vitality and beauty that the simple addition of water gives to an innate object—a laser disc. Likewise, the actions of health care professionals may seem unremarkable as they routinely provide clients with advice, medications, and food. But effective client care has a profound and wonderful effect in easing anxieties and speeding recovery.

Throughout the earlier parts of this book you have developed a basic understanding of nutrition and of how you can apply nutrition principles in your everyday life. You also saw how nutrient needs continue to change throughout life. Now the focus of the chapters shifts from you to your clients.

The knowledge and skills you have gained from earlier chapters certainly can be applied to your clients, but you also need special information. The next few chapters provide some general guidelines for working with clients. They help you identify people's nutrient and nutrition education needs, and show you how to communicate effectively with clients, how people are fed in the hospital, and how commonly used drugs interact with nutrients. What you learn in this and the next two chapters will help you work with people in all health care settings. Nutrition for people with particular medical disorders is the subject of Chapters 20 through 27.

As you shift your focus from yourself to others, keep in mind some of the special needs of clients. They are either sick or are trying to prevent or control diseases. Therefore, they are in different states of health, have different nutrient needs, prefer different foods, and react differently to medical procedures and care. To support their health by way of diet is a complex and difficult task. Health care providers who know the great difference that optimum nutrition makes, however, offer the maximum effort to deliver nutrition care tailored to the needs of each individual.

Nutrition in the Nursing Process

nursing process: an organized approach to problem solving that consists of five steps (assessing, analyzing, planning, implementing, and evaluating).

The nursing process can be used to provide nutrition intervention.

nutrition care plan: a strategy for translating nutrition assessment data into a plan for meeting the client's nutrient and nutrition education needs.

In consideration of the unique needs of each individual, how can successful nutrition intervention be effectively provided? To do so, a systematic and logical approach must be used. The nursing process is such an approach. Although it is beyond the scope of this book to discuss the nursing process in detail, it is important to realize that this process can be used to deliver nutrition care. To identify and solve nutrition problems, follow these five steps:

■ Assess nutrition status.
■ Interpret assessment data to determine nutrient requirements.
■ Develop a plan of action, including client education, for meeting nutrition needs.
■ Implement the nutrition care plan.
■ Evaluate the effectiveness of the nutrition care plan through ongoing assessment, and make appropriate changes.

Responsibility for developing and implementing nutrition care plans is shared by all members of the health care team, although the dietitian, physician, nurse, and client assume the primary roles. The social worker, pharmacist, and physical therapist also can make valuable contributions to nutrition assessment and care (see Highlight 18A). Generally, the greater the participation of team members, the more realistic and attainable the care plan will be. Although the emphasis of this chapter is on people in the hospital, the same principles apply to people seen in outpatient clinics, community centers, nursing homes, private practice, or their own homes.

Nutrition Assessment in Health Care Facilities

Nutrition assessment techniques are useful for determining the nutrition status of people who are ill as well as those who are healthy. Skills in performing nutrition assessments are put to the test when used in the hospital environment. A person may enter the hospital in good nutrition status only to become malnourished. Nutrition status often deteriorates during the course of hospitalization. Serious illness can affect a person's nutrition status in many ways (see Figure 17–1). An illness can:

- Lead to a loss of appetite.
- Interfere with a person's ability to chew and/or swallow food.
- Alter the way food is digested or in other ways interfere with the way nutrients are absorbed.
- Alter the way nutrients are metabolized.
- Alter the way nutrients are excreted.

One, all, or a combination of any of these effects can occur during illness and alter nutrition status.

A person's nutrition status can be assessed by a skilled technician. The first step in the nursing process, nutrition assessment, evaluates a person's health with nutrition in mind. Many factors influence or reflect nutrition status. Consequently, information from many sources must be gathered to make a nutrition assessment. These sources include anthropometric measurements, laboratory tests, physical examinations, and historical data.

Most of the information required for a nutrition assessment can be obtained routinely. For example, hospital admitting forms contain data such as sex, age, height, weight, medical history, medications, diet, allergies, and complaints.

Nutrition assessments include:
- Historical information.
- Anthropometric measures.
- Physical findings.
- Biochemical data.

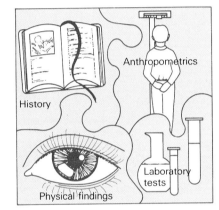

Taken as a whole, the pieces of nutrition assessment fit together to form a complete picture of the person's nutrition status.

FIGURE 17–1

The interrelationships between disease and malnutrition. It should be clear that any illness that contributes to malnutrition can set in motion a vicious cycle. Malnutrition can worsen the host's condition, which makes malnutrition worse.

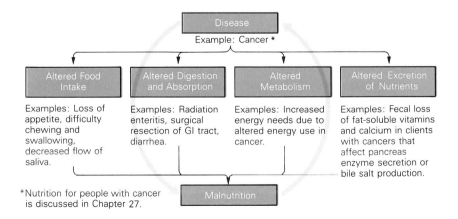

Disease
Example: Cancer *

Altered Food Intake
Examples: Loss of appetite, difficulty chewing and swallowing, decreased flow of saliva.

Altered Digestion and Absorption
Examples: Radiation enteritis, surgical resection of GI tract, diarrhea.

Altered Metabolism
Examples: Increased energy needs due to altered energy use in cancer.

Altered Excretion of Nutrients
Examples: Fecal loss of fat-soluble vitamins and calcium in clients with cancers that affect pancreas enzyme secretion or bile salt production.

Malnutrition

*Nutrition for people with cancer is discussed in Chapter 27.

Furthermore, some lab tests and a physical examination are routinely administered on admission to the hospital. These data can then be organized and expanded to describe an individual's nutrition status. Thus, the client's medical record is a good place to start obtaining information. Additional information can be obtained by talking with the client, the family, and other health care providers; by using the drug record; and by observing what the client eats.

An understanding of the community environment is also important in assessing nutrition status. For example, it is useful to know something about the food habits of the major ethnic groups within the locale, regional food preferences, and nutrition resources and programs available in the community. Local health departments and social agencies often can provide such information.

The more information gathered about a person, the more accurate the assessment will be. Gathering information is a time-consuming process, and time is often a rare commodity in the health care setting. Nutrition care is only one part of total care. It may not be practical or essential to collect detailed information on each person.

A strategic compromise is to screen clients by collecting preliminary data. Data such as height-weight and hematocrit are easy to obtain and can alert health care workers to potential problems. Nutrition screening identifies clients who will require additional nutrition assessment. (See the section on Preventing Protein-kCalorie Malnutrition.)

The following sections describe the principles of nutrition assessment and identify the tests used to collect data. The purpose is to provide a sense of the "what" and "why," but not to teach the actual procedures themselves. Details of the "how to" are presented in Appendix E, and references to this appendix are made wherever they are relevant.

Anthropometric Data

Anthropometrics are physical measurements that provide an indirect assessment of body composition (see Table 17–1). Measurements taken on an individual are compared with standards specific for sex and age. These standards are derived from measurements taken on large numbers of people to indicate the degree of depletion. Anthropometrics are particularly useful when taken periodically and

nutrition screening: the use of preliminary nutrition assessment techniques to identify people who are malnourished or who are at risk for malnutrition.

anthropometric: relating to measurement of the physical characteristics of the body, such as height and weight.
anthropos = human
metric = measuring

Appendix E provides a description of procedures used in taking anthropometric measurements and tables of standards used in the interpretation of them.

TABLE 17–1

Anthropometric Measures Used in Standard Nutrition Assessments[a]

Measurement	Reflects
Height-weight	Overnutrition and undernutrition Growth in children
%IBW, %UBW, Recent weight change	Overnutrition and undernutrition
Midarm circumference	Muscle mass and subcutaneous fat
Fatfold	Subcutaneous fat and total body fat
Midarm muscle circumference	Muscle mass (i.e., protein status)
Head circumference	Brain growth and development in children

[a] Appendix E provides a more detailed description of anthropometric measures.

compared with previous measurements. Such repeated measurements indicate changes in an individual's status.

Anthropometric measurements are easy to take, and little equipment is required. However, their accuracy and value are limited by the skills of the measurer. Mastering the correct techniques requires proper instruction and practice to ensure reliability. Furthermore, significant changes in measurements are slow to occur in adults. When changes do occur, they represent prolonged changes in nutrient intake.

Height-Weight. Height and weight are the most commonly used measurements. The height measurement may not be critical in itself, but it is used to estimate desirable weight and to interpret other assessment data. Once adult height has been reached, changes in body weight are useful in assessing overnutrition and undernutrition.

Weight measurements can be compared with desirable weight tables (see inside back cover), which are specific for height, sex, and frame size. (The limitations of these tables are discussed in Chapter 8.) The height and weight tables use a weight range, rather than pinpointing one weight. This is a good reminder that we cannot determine a "perfect" weight for anyone.

A comparison of a person's actual weight with the ideal weight is used to calculate the *percent ideal body weight* (%IBW). This provides a rough estimation of the degree of overnutrition or undernutrition. A %IBW greater than 115–120 is indicative of obesity; less than 90 is indicative of undernutrition (see Appendix E).

A more valuable parameter for assessing weight measurements is the *percent usual body weight* (%UBW), which considers what is normal for a particular individual. The client, family, or friends and older medical records are sources of information regarding usual weight. Malnutrition can be easily overlooked in an obese subject when using %IBW rather than %UBW (see Appendix E).

Any *recent weight change* can be determined by relating the %UBW to the time period over which a change, if any, has occurred. A five percent weight loss might be significant if it occurred within a month, yet might not be significant if it occurred over five months. Always ask the client about the weight change. Was the change intentional? Why does the client feel his or her weight has changed? Keep in mind that weight measurements are difficult to evaluate in hospitalized clients. Diseases or therapy can cause fluid retention and mask significant weight loss. In fact, starvation itself is accompanied by an increase in extracellular fluid volume.

Growth retardation in infants and young children is an important sign of poor nutrition status. Health professionals generally evaluate growth in infants and children by monitoring the rate of growth (height and weight) and comparing this rate to standard growth charts. (See Appendix E for growth charts.) Again, weight must be considered in relation to height—height and weight should be in approximately the same percentile. Although individual growth measurements may vary, in general, growth should be maintained along the same percentile throughout childhood (see Appendix E). In growth-retarded children, it is desirable that height and weight reach a higher percentile. In overweight children, weight should remain relatively stable as height increases, until weight becomes appropriate for height.

Height and weight are well recognized anthropometrics. Others include the midarm circumference, various fatfold measurements, and head circumference.

Weigh each client regularly.

B.J. is a 45-year-old male of medium frame size with a height of 5'8". He currently weighs 115 pounds. He has lost 15 pounds in the last month.

$$\%IBW = \frac{\text{Actual weight}}{\text{Ideal weight*}} \times 100$$

*Use the midpoint of the ideal weight range.

$$\%IBW = \frac{115 \text{ lbs}}{145 \text{ lbs}} \times 100 = 79\%$$

$$\%UBW = \frac{\text{Actual weight}}{\text{Usual weight}} \times 100$$

$$\%UBW = \frac{115 \text{ lbs}}{130 \text{ lbs}} \times 100 = 89\%$$

Recent weight change—weight loss is significant (almost 4 lb/week).

Midarm Circumference and Fatfolds. Midarm circumference is measured with a nonstretchable tape measure around the arm midway between the shoulder and the elbow. The midarm circumference measures muscle mass and subcutaneous fat. This measurement decreases with both acute and chronic undernutrition and increases in obesity.

Approximately half the fat in the body is directly beneath the skin. In some parts of the body, this fat is more loosely attached, and can be pulled up between the thumb and forefinger. These sites are used for measuring fatfold thickness. By estimating subcutaneous fat, the assessor can approximate total body fat. Since fat stores decrease very slowly with inadequate energy intake, short-term depletion of subcutaneous fat cannot be detected this way. Detectable depletion reflects either long-term undernutrition or intentional weight loss.

The most commonly used site for measuring fatfold thickness is the upper midarm, in the same area as the midarm circumference. A measurement of the triceps fatfold is widely used because the upper midarm is easily accessible. Together with the midarm circumference, it can be used to calculate the derived midarm muscle circumference.

The midarm muscle circumference is derived indirectly, because it cannot be measured. Rather, it is obtained mathematically. The arm is assumed to be circular and the fatfold circumference measure is subtracted from the midarm circumference (see Appendix E). The derived midarm muscle circumference permits an estimate of muscle mass and, thus, is used as an indicator of protein nutriture.

Another method of assessing skeletal muscle function that is gaining popularity is measurement of hand grip strength. An instrument called the dynamometer is used to see how tightly a person can grip. Low grip strength indicates that the person is at risk for poor nutrition status. At least one study has shown that hand grip strength can be used as a simple and inexpensive tool for screening people at risk for poor nutrition status.[1]

Fatfold measurements, midarm circumference, and the derived midarm muscle circumference are reproducible measurements if standard procedures are followed. (Procedures are described in Appendix E.) Accurately following standard procedure requires practice, however. Generally, the same person should measure the same subject routinely for best results. These measurements are then compared with percentile standards. (Standards are shown in Appendix E.)

Head Circumference. Head circumference is generally measured in children under three years of age. Since the brain is rapidly growing during this time, it is believed that malnourished children will have fewer brain cells and a smaller head circumference. As with height and weight, the measured head circumference is plotted on a percentile growth chart (see Appendix E). Head circumference percentile should be similar to weight and height percentiles.

Laboratory Tests

Anthropometrics are used for measuring and assessing observable changes in the body, while lab tests help determine what is happening inside the body (see Table 17–2). Blood and urine samples are used to directly measure a nutrient or a metabolite (end product or enzyme) that is affected by that nutrient.

Detecting subclinical deficiencies is difficult and is complicated because many deficiencies generally occur simultaneously. One of the goals of nutrition as-

Serum is the watery portion of the blood that remains after the cells and clot-forming material is removed; **plasma** is unclotted blood. In most cases, serum and plasma concentrations are similar. Serum samples usually are preferred because plasma samples occasionally clog mechanical blood analyzers.

TABLE 17–2

Laboratory Tests Used in Standard Nutrition Assessments[a]

Lab Test	Reflects
Urinary creatinine excretion	Skeletal muscle mass (i.e., malnutrition) and a standard for other measures
Albumin	Protein status
Transferrin	Protein and iron status
Total lymphocyte count	Protein status
Nitrogen balance	Protein status
Vitamin and mineral tests	Vitamin and mineral status

[a] Appendix E provides a more detailed description of laboratory tests.

Blood samples offer valuable clues in assessing nutrient status.

sessment is to uncover early signs of malnutrition long before a classical deficiency disease develops. Biochemical measurements often can be used to detect subclinical malnutrition. The most common lab tests used in hospitals today for nutrition assessment help uncover PCM. These tests include urinary creatinine excretion, albumin, transferrin, total lymphocyte count, and nitrogen balance.

Laboratory tests and physical findings are useful in assessing vitamin, mineral, and trace element status (see Appendix E). Vitamin and mineral levels present in the blood and urine sometimes represent recent intake rather than long-term intake. This makes detecting a subclinical deficiency difficult. Furthermore, many nutrients interact; a lab value for one nutrient can be affected by the amounts of other nutrients in the body.

Urinary Creatinine Excretion. Creatinine is a breakdown product of an energy source that is present specifically in skeletal muscle. It is excreted at a constant rate determined by the amount of skeletal muscle. Its excretion, therefore, reflects skeletal muscle mass. As skeletal muscle atrophies during malnutrition, creatinine excretion decreases. Standards for creatinine excretion have been developed based on sex and height (see Appendix E). They are used along with the measured creatinine to derive the creatinine-height index (CHI):

$$\frac{\text{Measure urinary creatinine (24 hr sample)}}{\text{Standard creatinine for height and sex}} \times 100$$

Creatinine excretion is also used to determine whether other urinary lab test results are appropriate relative to the size of the individual's skeletal muscle mass. The measurement of urinary creatinine requires a 24-hour urine collection, which may be difficult to obtain. The test is invalid if the subject shows signs of kidney disease, since the disease might reduce the body's ability to excrete creatinine.

Albumin. Albumin accounts for over 50 percent of the total serum proteins. It helps to maintain fluid and electrolyte balance and to transport many nutrients, hormones, drugs, and other compounds. Albumin synthesis depends on the existence of functioning liver cells as well as on an appropriate supply of amino acids. Because there is so much albumin in the body and because it is not broken down quickly, albumin concentrations change slowly. Therefore, albumin is a useful indicator of prolonged protein depletion (see Appendix E). Unlike creatinine, albumin levels can reflect the protein status of the blood and internal organs.

Several measurements are often taken during a blood test. This practice is referred to as SMA (**simultaneous multiple analysis**). SMA is followed by a number (for example, SMA-12) that indicates how many tests will be run.

B.J.'s urinary creatinine excretion was 1,090 mg/24 hr.

$$CHI = \frac{1,090 \text{ mg}}{1,557 \text{ mg}} \times 100 = 70\%$$

Interpretation: Based on the creatinine-height index, B.J.'s skeletal muscle mass is approximately 70% of that which would be expected in a man his size.

B.J. had a serum albumin of 2.4 g/100 ml.

Interpretation: B.J.'s serum albumin is moderately depleted (see Appendix E).

Skin tests provide an index of nutrition status.

Total lymphocyte count (mm³)
= WBC (mm³) × % lymphoctyes

B.J.'s WBC count was 7,500 with 15% lymphocytes.

Total lymphocyte count (mm³)
= 7,500 mm³ × 0.15 = 1,125 mm³

Interpretation: By this standard, too, B.J.'s nutrition status is moderately depleted.

induration: a raised, hardened area of skin.
durus = hard

Nitrogen (N) balance:
N intake = N output

Positive N balance:
N intake > N output

Negative N balance:
N intake < N output

Many other conditions besides malnutrition can depress albumin concentration, including liver disease, advanced kidney disease (nephrotic syndrome), infection, cancer, and burns. Therefore, as is true for *all* parameters used in nutrition assessment, albumin cannot be used alone to determine protein status, but rather as one indicator among many.

Transferrin.   Transferrin is a protein that transports iron between the intestine and sites of hemoglobin synthesis and degradation. It is considered a more sensitive indicator of protein malnutrition than albumin, because it responds more promptly to changes in protein intake and has a smaller body pool.

Most transferrin is synthesized in the liver. Its concentration is inversely related to iron stores; transferrin levels are high in iron deficiency and low when iron storage is excessive. Therefore, the presence of abnormal iron nutriture makes interpretation of the transferrin level as an indicator of protein status difficult. Liver disease, nephrotic syndrome, and burns also cause decreases in transferrin levels.

Immune Status.   Various forms of PCM as well as individual nutrient deficiencies have been associated with depression of the immune system (see Highlight 19). The total number of lymphocytes appears to decrease as protein depletion occurs; so the total lymphocyte count is one index useful in nutrition assessment.

Another test of immune function is antigen skin testing. Organisms (usually three or four kinds) to which most people are immune are injected just under the skin. After 48 hours, the sites of the injections are inspected for raised, hardened areas (induration). Such areas will be apparent in the well-nourished person, but in the malnourished person, hardened areas will not appear or will be very small.

Many factors other than nutrition can interfere with the immune response, and the value of skin testing as an index of nutrition status has been questioned.[2] No studies to date have considered all of the factors that might affect skin test results. Among these factors are age, certain allergies, and chemotherapy.

Nitrogen Balance.   Nitrogen balance studies are useful in estimating the degree to which protein is being depleted or repleted in the body. A simple approach to measuring nitrogen is to measure urine urea nitrogen (UUN) in a 24–hour urine collection. During the same 24–hour period, an accurate record of the subject's protein (nitrogen) intake must be kept to complete the balance study.

Nitrogen intake is calculated by dividing protein intake (in grams) by 6.25 (grams of nitrogen per gram of protein). Nitrogen output per day equals the UUN plus a factor of 4 grams to account for nitrogen lost through the lungs, hair, skin, and nails as well as nonurea nitrogen losses in the urine. The equation for nitrogen balance is:

$$\text{N balance} = \frac{\text{Protein (g)}}{6.25} - (\text{UUN g} + 4\text{ g})$$

As with creatinine excretion, the kidneys must be functioning properly for measurement to be accurate. Additionally, abnormally high nitrogen losses (as seen in clients with severe burns) must be considered if this test is to be valid.

Nitrogen balance studies provide a prime example of the need for communication and cooperation between various health care providers and departments. A nitrogen balance study would be invalid if even one urine specimen were thrown away or if one meal's food intake was not recorded; and the whole procedure would have to be repeated at great inconvenience to the client and staff.

Laboratory tests add a dimension to nutrition assessment. However, as emphasized earlier, many factors influence lab tests; therefore, a single test cannot be relied on to assess nutrition status. When many laboratory tests are combined and are viewed together with anthropometric measures, the whole picture becomes clearer.

Physical Findings

Clues to a person's nutrition status can be identified by examining the person for clinical signs of malnutrition (see Table 17–3). However, many of these signs are nonspecific; they can be associated with many nutrient deficiencies or can be unrelated to nutrition. So, again, physical findings can only be interpreted in light of other assessment findings.

Physical signs of malnutrition appear most rapidly in parts of the body where cells are being replaced at a high rate, such as in the hair, skin, and GI tract. Some of the easily detectible signs of malnutrition and the nutrient deficiencies to which they are related are listed in Appendix E.

Historical Data

Historical data are an extremely important part of nutrition assessment (see Table 17–4). Although such data are often subjective, they reveal many important facts about a person. Furthermore, thorough history taking provides a good sense of the whole person. An adept history taker uses the initial interview not only to gather facts but also to establish rapport.

TABLE 17–3

Physical Findings Used in Standard Nutrition Assessments[a]

Anatomical Sites	Reflects
Hair	PCM
Face	PCM, vitamin A, and iron status
Eyes	Vitamin A, B vitamin, zinc, and iron status
Lips	B vitamin status
Tongue	B vitamin status
Teeth	Mineral status
Gums	Vitamin C status
Glands	PCM and iodine status
Skin	PCM, vitamin A, B vitamin and vitamin C status
Nails	Iron status
Subcutaneous tissue	PCM and obesity

[a] Findings are listed in their approximate physical order on the body to help the care taker remember to look for physical signs from "head to toe." Appendix E provides a more detailed description of physical signs of malnutrition.

TABLE 17–4

Historical Data Used in Standard Nutrition Assessments[a]

Histories	Identifies
Medical	Diseases that affect nutrition status

Diet
    24–hour recall
    food diary
    food frequency record
	Nutrient intake excesses or deficiencies

Drug	Medications that affect nutrition status

[a] Appendix E provides a more detailed description of historical data.

In this section, we will only briefly review major points to be covered in collecting historical data. Later in the chapter, we will discuss the communication tools required to be an effective history taker.

Medical History.   Most often, the medical record or chart contains the person's complete medical history. However, conversations with the person can uncover valuable medical information which was not recorded because "no one asked" or because the client was too upset on admission to think clearly.

The purpose of establishing a sound medical history when assessing nutrition status is to uncover any conditions which place a client at risk for nutrient deficiencies. Important risk factors in the medical and diet histories are listed in Appendix E. Remember that disease can have either long- or short-term effects on nutrition status by interfering with ingestion, digestion, absorption, metabolism, or excretion of nutrients.

Diet History.   A complete diet history includes general information about a person's intake, socioeconomic factors affecting intake, and specific food intake data. Food choices are a very important part of lifestyle and often represent an expression of personal philosophy. Questions asked regarding food intake must always be nonjudgmental to elicit accurate information.

There are several methods for obtaining food intake data, including the 24-hour recall, food diary, and food frequency records. Like anthropometrics and biochemical data, food intakes should be compared with "standards." In this case, the standards are recommended nutrient intakes. The question to be answered is how closely the person's diet meets the recommendations. Are any nutrients excessive or deficient?

A quick assessment can be made by comparing food intake with the Four Food Group Plan (see Chapter 2). When you need detailed information about specific nutrients, the foods can be looked up in food composition tables (such as Appendix H) and the final values compared with standards such as the RDA (see inside front cover). In some facilities, computer programs are available for easily determining nutrient intakes and comparing intakes with standards. Remember, though, that these standards were developed for healthy people. Nutrient needs often change in disease, and these needs should be met by the diet (Chapters 20–27).

What and how a person eats are valuable clues as to how that person will accept diet changes, should they be necessary. This information can be used to provide realistic and attainable goals for the person's nutrition care.

Drug History.   The important interactions of foods and drugs have been increasingly recognized in recent years. Some general classifications of drugs which may influence nutrition status include antibiotics, anticonvulsants, antihypertensive agents, antineoplastic agents (used in chemotherapy), catabolic steroids, oral contraceptives, and vitamin and other nutrient preparations.

If a client is taking any of these types of drugs, the amount and the length of time the drugs have been taken should be noted. Signs of any adverse effects also should be recorded. Nutrient-drug interactions are discussed in more detail in Chapter 19.

The section you have just read has described the components of nutrition assessment (anthropometric measures, laboratory tests, physical findings, and historical data). These can be combined to detect the most probable nutrition problems that clients face. Left undetected and untreated, nutrition problems can hamper recovery from diseases.

To understand the relationship of protein-kcalorie nutrition to serious illness, think of energy stores and protein status as money in the bank. Illness can be compared to a major expense that arises unexpectedly. The person who has saved enough money can pay off the expense without too much difficulty. However, if more and more expenses arise, there may not be enough money to pay all of the bills. The person with little or no savings faces the same problem, but is unable to pay even a small expense.

It is technically incorrect to speak of body protein stores, because proteins (amino acids) are not stored in the body. All protein is functional; that is, it is being used in some capacity (as a part of cell structure, as skeletal muscle, as enzymes or immune factors, or as other body protein components).

Protein-kCalorie Malnutrition and Illness

Why is PCM of particular concern during serious illness? To understand the answer to this question, you must have a basic knowledge of how the body responds to the stress of serious illness.

A person's ability to respond to stress depends, to a large extent, on available energy reserves and protein status, since the body's requirements for protein and energy increase remarkably in stress. When energy is not supplied in adequate amounts from the diet over a period of time, the body uses protein to meet energy needs. When this adaptation occurs, functional protein is lost from skeletal muscle, from organs (liver, gut, and lungs), and from circulating pools of protein (albumin and immune factors).

For the well-nourished person, loss of *some* protein is not critical, since adequate protein remains to support vital functions. However, in prolonged stress or in malnutrition, the protein loss can be serious. For example, loss of protein in a malnourished person following surgery oftentimes results in pneumonia. The loss of a critical number of functioning lung cells combined with a decreased synthesis of immune factors leads to deterioration of lung function and depression of the immune system. The result: pneumonia.

Organs where cells are being replaced rapidly are among the first to be affected by PCM. One such organ system is the GI tract. Once a person develops PCM, the intestinal microvilli gradually shrink and become nonfunctional. Up to 90 percent of them can be lost. The person then has serious difficulty absorbing nutrients, and this makes the PCM worse.

Within the cell, PCM affects the synthesis of enzymes and other protein molecules that are necessary for proper metabolism and maintenance of the cells' structure. These protein molecules usually are synthesized and degraded rapidly in the body to help it adapt promptly to changes in the environment. Losing this ability to adapt is critical.

Protein and fat are used to meet energy requirements once glycogen stores are depleted. Thus these body components are of particular concern in nutrition

The immune system, the body's system for defending against viruses, bacteria, and other foreign agents, is described in Highlight 19.

morbidity: unhealthiness; disease.
mortality: death.
Morbidity and mortality rates are often used as indicators of the success of a health care system.

assessment. When they are depleted, the individual's defenses against disease are threatened. PCM interferes with the body's ability to heal wounds, mount an immune response, and maintain the function of vital organs and skeletal muscle. Furthermore, malnutrition can result in higher morbidity and mortality rates, a greater incidence of postoperative complications, and longer hospital stays; all of these increase health care costs.[3]

Unfortunately, PCM in the hospital is a serious problem, even in the United States. A recent study of people in a hospital found that 55 percent were likely to be malnourished.[4] Furthermore, only 1 in 20 of these people received nutrition therapy either prior to developing complications or early in their hospitalization. You may well wonder how something as basic as sound nutrition can be neglected in hospitals where the latest technology abounds. Part of the problem may be a basic failure of health care professionals, including physicians, to recognize the prevalence of PCM and to fully appreciate its consequences to a person who is battling an illness.

People in the hospital may be deprived of food for days at a time while they undergo medical tests and diagnostic procedures. During the very time when their nutrient needs may be high due to illness, they are not given adequate amounts of nutrients; as a result PCM quickly develops.

Lack of understanding of the role of nutrition in recovery from disease may explain why weight loss often goes unnoticed, diets often are inadequate, and people in the hospital are allowed to reach an advanced stage of depletion (which may be irreversible). Poor communication among various health care providers probably makes a major contribution to PCM. PCM is preventable and occurs partly because of the treatment prescribed to remedy the disease for which the person was hospitalized. PCM is more likely to occur when a physician orders that a person receive nothing by mouth, or orders drugs that interfere with nutrition status, or orders procedures that interfere with nutrient intake. Because PCM results not only from another disease but from the treatment of that disease as well, it is often referred to as *physician-induced malnutrition.*

Physician-induced malnutrition, technically, is **iatrogenic** (eye-AT-ro-GEN-ic) **malnutrition.** This term includes malnutrition caused by prescription medication (see Chapter 19).
iatros = physician
genic = arising from

Take a moment to imagine you are in a foreign country—a country where you do not understand the language. As you walk down the street, you see signs that describe and direct. But they are meaningless to you, for you have yet to learn how to think, speak, or read this new language. Many health care providers travel through hospitals looking at signs of malnutrition without recognizing them. They look at a person's pale complexion and lack of appetite and see only that she has a disease; they see a person's poor posture and lethargic attitude and attribute that to his old age. They have yet to learn to think "nutrition." Malnutrition is easy to miss if you are not looking for it. Caring for people requires that you at least consider the *possibility* that ill health may be due not just to a disease but perhaps to nutrient deficiencies. To overlook nutrition is to provide less than adequate care. The signs of malnutrition are there if you know where to look and how to read them.

Appropriate nutrition assessment can detect the development of PCM. Medical staff who are alert to the signs of PCM can then act to prevent, retard, or reverse its progress. A combination of the tests described earlier can reveal the presence of PCM.

Preventing Protein-kCalorie Malnutrition

Fortunately, many of the problems just discussed can be avoided by taking appropriate measures. You can have an important impact on preventing PCM in these ways:

- Review the individual's diet, drug, and medical history. Does the person's history reveal risk factors for poor nutrition status?
- Check the lab reports. Do urinary creatinine excretion, serum albumin, transferrin, or total lymphocyte count suggest malnutrition?
- Weigh each person on admission and at regular intervals during their hospital stays. (See Appendix E for instructions on how to measure weight.) Is the person's weight for height adequate, but not excessive? Has the person been losing or gaining weight? How much? How fast? Other anthropometric measurements useful in assessing nutrition status are listed in Table 17–1 and described in more detail in Appendix E.
- Look at the person. Are there obvious signs of malnutrition? Is the client emaciated? Obese? Extremely pale? Table 17–3 lists other physical signs of malnutrition.

In addition to the above nutrition assessment procedures, take the opportunity to:

- Check the client's tray frequently to see if food is being eaten. If the client is NPO and unable to eat, how long has it been since the client has eaten? Is the client expected to be able to eat soon? Are adequate nutrients being delivered by vein? (See the box "How to Calculate the Nutrient Content of IV Solutions" in Chapter 18.)
- Most important, communicate any problems that you discover to someone who can help. The problem may go unnoticed if you do not speak up. A dietitian can perform a more in-depth nutrition assessment. Be persistent if you suspect that a problem is being ignored.

This illustrates how nutrition screening is used to identify clients who are malnourished or those who are at risk for malnutrition. Nutrition screening is vital. A recent study showed that nutrition screening at admission in 33 hospitals identified risk for poor nutrition status in over 50 percent of the clients for whom enough information was available to perform the screening.[5] Always check for signs of malnutrition. A person's nutrition status can deteriorate rapidly during the course of hospitalization. You can find a nutrition assessment form for recording information about PCM in Appendix E.

To prevent PCM:
- Check the client's history for risk factors for poor nutrition status.
- Check lab test results.
- Look for physical signs of malnutrition.

Observe what and how much the client eats.

An order which reads "NPO" means that nothing is to be given to the person orally (including food and medications). **NPO** stands for *nil per os*, which means "nothing by mouth." On the other hand, **PO** stands for *per os*, which means "by mouth" or "orally."

Get help if you suspect a problem.

The Nutrition Care Plan

A nutrition care plan translates assessment data into a strategy for meeting the client's nutrient and nutrition education needs. It concentrates on intervention and the client's response to intervention. For example, a care plan would not only document why a weight reduction diet was given, but also how the client reacted to instruction on the diet.

The care process is continuous. The initial care plan may change frequently during hospitalization as new needs are identified. For example, a person admitted on a medical floor for a diagnostic workup may later become a candidate for surgery. As your client's needs change, adjust the care plan to meet them. Be on the alert for changes in medical status so that nutrition needs are not neglected; try a new plan when original approaches fall short.

Up to this point, we have discussed nutrition in the nursing process. You now understand how nutrition assessment is used to determine nutrition status and to devise a plan of action. You have seen how critical nutrition is to the recovery process and have been given guidelines for preventing malnutrition. But there is an important part of nutrition care that we still need to discuss in more detail—communicating with your clients.

Communication and Nutrition Care

A nutrition assessment is only as good as the information you have obtained to formulate it. If you can communicate clearly with your clients and they feel at ease in talking to you, then you can draw a far better picture of their nutrition health.

Effective Communication

Communication makes the difference in client care.

Communication involves the transfer of information from one person (sender) to another (receiver) for the purpose of eliciting a response. Information can be transferred verbally or nonverbally. Charting information in a client's medical record is verbal communication, as is speaking. Touching, smiling, frowning, and the like are forms of nonverbal communication. Regardless of the communication medium, to be an effective communicator you must formulate and express your ideas clearly, and the receiver must interpret what you say as you intended. As illustrated in Figure 17–2, the relationship is dynamic. The roles of sender and receiver are constantly switching between the parties involved in communication. When a person responds to your communication, you must correctly interpret that response.

Close your eyes, and for a moment, imagine that you are in the hospital. You are frightened because you aren't sure what's wrong with you or what will happen next. All of a sudden you have to rely on many people to do things for you. You repeatedly have to ask someone to bring you the things you want or need. Even worse, you feel you have lost control of *yourself*. You must depend on someone else to find out what's happening inside your body and what the best treatment will be. How terrifying to be putting your health (your life) in someone else's hands (a stranger, yet)! Your body is no longer private—everyone seems to be poking, sticking, and probing it. On top of that, you hurt, and many of the examinations, tests, and procedures you must undergo also cause discomfort. You need time to sort through your feelings, but how can you think when every few minutes someone is coming into your room to check vital signs, draw blood, and ask endless questions that you feel you have already answered over and over?

Now open your eyes, and remember to keep them open. You should be able to see how important communication becomes to the person reduced to a dependent state. Many fears and concerns felt by people in the hospital can be relieved when they feel satisfied that those they depend on listen to, understand, and act on their needs. When the people around them respond in this way, individuals retain some control over their environment, and therefore, themselves. Furthermore, you will obtain more accurate information and be able to motivate the person to follow nutrition (or other) advice if you have gained the person's trust and cooperation.

Messages may not be perceived as intended if the words or actions used by the sender have a different meaning for the receiver. Values, ethnic backgrounds, and social influences affect everyone's perceptions of words and actions. For example, when you say, "How are you doing today?" one person may be thinking, "What a dumb thing to say," while another may think, "He really cares about me." Smiling is generally an expression of friendliness, but a smile also can be inappropriate, for example, at a time of grief.

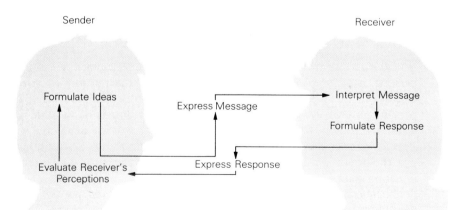

FIGURE 17–2

Communication channels.

Judgmental versus nonjudgmental responses:
- *Helper:* Do you take any type of vitamin or mineral supplements?
- *Client:* I take a vitamin E capsule and 2 grams of vitamin C every day.
- *Judgmental helper response:* You know, of course, that there is no reason for taking these vitamin supplements.
- *Nonjudgmental helper response:* Why do you take these vitamin supplements?

Encourage the person to communicate openly and freely.

Open-versus closed-ended questions:
- *Open-ended*: How do you feel about your new diet?
- *Closed-ended*: You feel fine about your new diet, don't you?

When you and your client communicate, you must assume the role of helper. You can enhance communication by keeping in mind the following points:

- Establish a caring and trusting environment. Let the client know that you care about her as a person and that she can trust you.
- Give each person room to be himself. In other words, accept and value a person for who and what he is. If you react to what a person tells you with advice, criticism, or judgment, he will not feel free to relate important things about himself to you. He may not want to take the chance that you might belittle him either verbally or nonverbally.
- Become an active listener. The client should be the one doing most of the talking.
- Allow the client to control the direction of the discussion. Try not to follow a set form for asking important questions; rather, use such a form as a guide, and ask questions based on what the person is telling you. Effective communication in the health care setting is client centered. After all, the client is the recipient of therapy.
- Avoid using medical terminology or abbreviations that may be confusing to a layperson. For example, a person going to surgery might be needlessly confused and frightened if told that after leaving the OR she would go to the RR and that she should expect to have an IV and an NG tube inserted before she awakens. Always define the medical terms used to explain a person's condition, diagnostic tests, or therapy.

When you talk with a client, it often helps to maintain eye-level contact with your client. This usually means you should sit down so that it is not uncomfortable for the client to look at you. Also, if you stand while your client sits or is lying in bed, you may be nonverbally communicating an unfriendly and overpowering feeling.

Before beginning any type of formal communication with a client, be prepared. Check the chart to get an idea of the past and current history. Arrange for privacy, and adjust the physical environment so that you and your client are comfortable. It is difficult to communicate with anyone in a noisy, poorly lit, or stuffy-hot room.

Verbal Communication

The best verbal communication techniques encourage the person to communicate openly and freely and to provide accurate information. Some of these techniques (in addition to those already discussed) include:

- *Introduction and statement of purpose.* Always introduce yourself, verify the person's name, explain who you are, and define the purpose of your discussion. In so doing, you set the tone for the discussion and let the person know what is expected of him. At this time, it may be valuable to assure the person that all the information he gives you is confidential.
- *Appropriate use of questions.* Open-ended questions are broad questions that give the person a wide choice of answers. They are particularly useful for initiating communication. On the other hand, closed-ended questions and double questions should be avoided. These questions are very narrow, and they limit a person's responses. For example, if you ask a client if she

prefers orange juice or tomato juice, you aren't giving her the chance to tell you she'd really rather have grapefruit juice or even a slice of melon.

■ *Continuous feedback.* Provide the client with continuous feedback to let her know that you are with her and that you understand each other correctly. Table 17–5 lists positive and negative feedback techniques.

■ *Summary of the discussion.* Prior to ending a discussion, be sure that you both agree on what has transpired. Misconceptions or misunderstandings can be identified and clarified immediately. Furthermore, at this time you can arrange for whatever follow-up you may wish to make. For example, "I'll be back tomorrow," or "Let's plan to talk again next week."

As you practice communicating with others, you'll develop techniques that fit your individual style. However, while learning, try out all of the available techniques to discover which ones you use most comfortably and effectively.

Examples of double questions:
• Do you drink orange or tomato juice with breakfast?
• Have you followed a weight-reduction or low-cholesterol diet at home?

TABLE 17–5

Providing Feedback: Do's and Don'ts

Do's	Examples
Encourage the client to continue.	*Helper:* I see. Mm-hm. What else?
Repeat key phrases or ideas.	*Person:* I've been so distraught I've lost 10 pounds.
	Helper: You've lost 10 pounds?
Clarify what the client is saying.	*Helper:* I'm not sure I understand what you mean.
Validate the client's responses.	*Person:* I get so nervous I begin eating like a horse.
	Helper: You eat when you're nervous?
Echo the client's feelings (sometimes called reflecting).	*Person:* After 4 weeks of dieting, I just can't believe that I only lost 2 pounds.
	Helper: You feel frustrated with how slowly you lose weight.
Remain silent, when appropriate, to let the client formulate ideas.	

Don'ts	Examples
Don't talk more than listen.	
Don't interrupt the person's thoughts.	*Person:* I could stay on my diet if . . .
	Helper: If you didn't live alone.
Don't judge or moralize.	*Helper:* You have no excuse for not losing weight
Don't use meaningless expressions.	*Helper:* I know you'll do fine.
Don't demean the person's situation or attitude.	*Helper:* You probably just don't understand how this diet works.
Don't put words into the person's mouth.	*Helper:* What did you have for breakfast today? (Assumes person eats or should eat breakfast.)
Don't give diet advice when seeking information.	*Helper:* You shouldn't eat candy on your diet. (The person may not tell you about other things he "shouldn't" be eating.)

Nonverbal Communication

The use of nonverbal communication techniques is extremely important to the communication process. Your body mannerisms often "speak" as much as your words do. Try to maintain eye contact during the communication process; sit at a close, yet comfortable, distance from the other person; and use appropriate facial expressions and gestures to clarify or emphasize important messages.

One of the most powerful nonverbal communication techniques is silence. During a pause, the other person has a chance to formulate ideas and think. Occasionally, silence indicates that a thought is complete and provides a good time to move on to another topic or to end the discussion.

The Interview

The primary purpose of an interview is to gather information. Almost all health professionals conduct interviews to uncover important clues that affect their clients' health. Often the purpose of the initial interview is to obtain a diet history. Interviews serve as a means of establishing a caring and trusting relationship that will enable the health professional to deliver health care effectively. The information you seek to obtain in the interview generally represents a person's lifelong habits as influenced by complex social, cultural, psychological, religious, and economic factors. No one would share this much without trusting that the interviewer truly cared and would accept the information, whatever it might be. Otherwise, the interviewee might be worried that you would find her strange, think less of her, or be critical of her behavior.

The communication techniques discussed above provide the guidelines by which to conduct an effective diet interview. A checklist of important aspects of the interviewing process is provided in Table 17–6.

Nutrition Counseling

Recently, there has been a tremendous explosion of knowledge regarding the effects of diet on health. However, this knowledge is all but useless if the implications of nutrition research can't be applied successfully by the individual. Nutrition counseling, therefore, must involve much more than simply giving information. When you act as a diet counselor, you must integrate diet changes into your client's lifestyle and provide the motivation the client needs to follow through with your suggestions. In other words, nutrition counseling is only effective if it results in a change in the client's eating habits.

Nutrition counseling is no easy task. You will improve your counseling skills with practice, but always remember that even the best counselor has some failures. After all, it is not you, but your client, who must accept the responsibility for making the necessary diet changes.

You can enhance your counseling skills by following a logical and organized approach. First, you must adequately prepare for the counseling session. Only by thoroughly assessing a person's nutrition, educational, and emotional needs can you hope to make counseling relevant to, and appropriate for, that person. Therefore, your client is your most important resource during the assessment process.

Once you have identified a person's nutrition education needs, you must assess your own knowledge of the subject to be discussed. If you feel insecure

SHE DOESN'T CARE ABOUT THIS.

I NEVER SHOULD HAVE TOLD HER ABOUT THAT!

Body language speaks as loudly as words.

Assess client needs.

TABLE 17–6

Interviewing Checklist

Preparing

- Obtain available background information from medical record and other health care team members.
- Arrange for privacy and improve the physical environment, if necessary.

Initiating the Interview

- Confirm the client's identity.
- Introduce yourself.
- Explain the purpose of the interview.
- Establish rapport.

Conducting the Interview

- Cover one thought at a time.
- Use langauge the client can easily understand.
- Remain objective.
- Look for verbal and nonverbal cues.
- LISTEN.
- Use open-ended questions.
- Provide appropriate feedback.
- Use nonverbal communication techniques.

Closing the Interview

- A few minutes before closing the interview, let the client know that the time is almost over.
- Determine if the client has questions.
- Answer any questions.
- Acknowledge the client's cooperation during the interview.
- Explain the next step for follow-up, if needed.

regarding your knowledge of the diet, medical condition, future treatment plans, and so on, take the time to find out more before counseling begins. However, don't worry about being asked one or two questions you can't answer. You can always check the information and get back to the person. This action is clearly better than giving incorrect advice or ignoring a question.

Assess your own knowledge.

Following an assessment of the person's needs and your own knowledge level, you and your client should jointly develop specific and realistic objectives for meeting the client's nutrition education needs. For example, when planning a low-cholesterol diet instruction, two objectives might be:

Develop objectives.

- The person will be able to explain the rationale for the low-cholesterol diet.
- The person will be able to plan a day's menus using the low-cholesterol diet booklet.

In most cases, a dietitian will be responsible for nutrition counseling. A clinical dietitian is specially trained to provide in-depth counseling. However, in some hospitals, outpatient clinics, and nursing homes, a dietitian may not be available. The nurse or other health care provider may be expected to assume this responsibility. Therefore, it is important for other health care professionals to understand the basic techniques of nutrition counseling.

Assess your own knowledge. Keep abreast of the latest nutrition information.

behavioral objectives: objectives written in such a way that the desired outcome can be either seen or heard.

Determine the content of the session.

Select the teaching method.

Develop a time frame.

Implement your plan.

State your objectives.

Stress personal responsibility.

Use realistic examples.

An unrealistic objective would be to expect the person to know the diet by memory at the end of the first session. By defining objectives in terms of actions (behaviors) that can be observed, you can better evaluate the effectiveness of nutrition counseling.

After developing specific objectives, consider the content of the session (the type and amount of information you will present), as well as the methods you will use (for example, a filmstrip, a diet booklet, food models, practice menus, or a food diary). The person's motivational and educational level will guide your choice of methods and the content of the counseling session. For example, a diet instruction booklet in picture form would be useful for an illiterate adult or for a child. A highly educated and motivated person might benefit by knowing in-depth details about the diet, whereas the same information might overwhelm someone who is already confused.

The final consideration in the preparation step is to develop a tentative time frame for accomplishing objectives. Often (as in the hospital setting), you are limited to a certain number of counseling sessions, and you have to use each session optimally. Your time frame should be flexible and should finally be determined by the client's needs. Some people may move along much faster, and others slower, than originally anticipated.

As you can see, the preparation for a counseling session is as important as the session itself. In reality, these steps can be determined fairly rapidly as you gain experience and sharpen your assessment and planning skills.

The next step in the process is to implement your plan in the actual counseling session. The general communication techniques we discussed previously apply to the counseling session (see also Table 17–7). By the time you begin counseling, you will ideally have seen the person at least once and should have established some rapport. Nevertheless, be sure to confirm the person's identity and diagnosis, restate your identity, and take time to establish a trusting and caring atmosphere. Identify and communicate your objectives clearly. If people know, for example, that they will be asked to explain the rationale for their diet, they may listen more closely to your explanation. Furthermore, this gives the client an opportunity to modify your expectations.

During counseling sessions, you should stress to clients that they are ultimately responsible for their health and for making the necessary diet changes. You will often hear statements such as "You need to talk to my wife; she does the cooking." It does help if the family member who prepares the food is present at the counseling session and understands the diet. However, the client *must* accept that it is he—not his wife and not the counselor—who needs the diet, and that he is responsible for himself. He should be an active participant in the session.

When discussing recommendations for diet changes, be sure that the person can actually apply the changes. For example, the busy executive who frequently eats restaurant meals must know how to make appropriate food choices in restaurants. A person with a low income may need help with incorporating lower-cost food items into the diet, as well as tips on shopping economically. A person who follows a strictly kosher diet must know how to plan meals around the Jewish Dietary Laws.

You can make diet instructions more relevant to individuals by using many examples consistent with their own eating habits. This is more readily done if you are familiar with their diet histories. You can also have them plan personal

TABLE 17–7

Nutrition Counseling Checklist

Preparation
- Assess the client's needs.
- Develop objectives.
- Determine the content of, and methods to be used for, the counseling session.
- Establish a tentative time frame for accomplishing objectives.
- Assess your own knowledge of the subject.
- Arrange for appropriate others to be present at the session.

Implementation
- Establish identity and rapport.
- Improve the physical environment.
- State the objective of the counseling session.
- Discuss the rationale for diet changes.
- Center the session around the client.
- Apply principles of diet to lifestyle.
- Reinforce all positive responses.
- Allow adequate time for counseling.
- Use familiar language.
- Use open-ended questions.
- LISTEN.
- Use nonverbal communication techniques.
- Use appropriate instructional aids.
- Provide accurate information.
- Answer questions.
- Acknowledge the client's cooperation during the session.
- Explain the next step for follow-up, if needed.

Evaluation
- Determine if objectives have been met.
- Determine if the content and methods have been suited to the client's needs.
- Decide if additional counseling is required.
- Evaluate your effectiveness as a counselor.

menus or ask them to tell you what they would select in a restaurant. In some hospitals, clients select foods from the cafeteria line, and you can use this experience to facilitate learning.

Always center diet counseling on the individual. Let her participate actively in the sessions and arrive at conclusions on her own. Stress the positives and successes rather than the negatives and failures in her current diet.

The third step in the process is evaluation. Ask yourself: have the objectives of the counseling session been met? Is a change in the content or the methods of instruction required? Is more time needed for counseling? Have the person's nutrition needs changed? Furthermore, how effective was I as a counselor? What methods worked well, and which were less effective? How can I improve my instructional techniques for further counseling sessions? The answers to these questions will direct your future actions.

Some special considerations should be kept in mind when you counsel a person in the hospital. Unlike the outpatient, the hospitalized individual is a captive audience. It is not necessarily by choice that such a person is discussing diet changes with you. The hospital environment is unlike the home environment. A person who has learned to make proper food selections from the hospital menu may still feel lost about what to eat when outside the hospital. Further-

Provide follow-up.

more, after the immediate danger of illness has passed, the person may soon give up following a special diet. For these reasons, it is advisable to follow up, once the person is at home—through a phone call, home visit, or visit to you by the former client. At the very least, the person should be referred to someone (either you or another agency) who can answer questions regarding the diet.

Professional Communication Networks

There are many opportunities for discussion of clients' concerns among professionals. Keep in mind that to maintain strong professional communication networks is beneficial to both health care professionals and the client.

The Medical Record

medical record: a continuous written account of a client's hospitalization.

diagnosis: the disease a person has or is thought to have.
gnosis = knowing

prognosis: the predicted course and outcome of a disease.
pro = ahead of time, before

One way professionals communicate is through the medical record. The medical record is a compilation of the history, the diagnosis and therapy, and the prognosis for each client. It is an important way of sharing information with the health care team. You can continuously assess your client's condition and response to therapy by reading the medical record regularly. You can use this information to determine how to provide the best possible care.

From the client's perspective, communication channels with health care providers may be frustrating and confusing. One person may be attended by a primary physician, several consulting physicians, residents, interns, three shifts of nurses that change daily, student nurses, nurse's aides, dietitians and dietary aides, and many other health team members (laboratory technicians, physical therapists, social workers, and so on). How exasperating for an individual to communicate a need or concern to one health care provider assuming that the information will be shared, only to have to repeat the request over and over again. In addition, miscommunication between professionals can result in inappropriate therapy and serious consequences to the individual's health.

As a health care provider, you have the responsibility to create effective communication networks between clients and professionals. Closing communication gaps often is a very difficult job. Follow through with information or items you have told the client you would deliver. Otherwise, explain why compliance with some of the requests may be difficult or impossible to handle. Jot down notes to jog your memory, if it helps. When necessary, be sure to forward requests to other departments (for example, a nurse may need to request a certain food item from the dietary department).

Lack of communication creates feelings of helplessness and confusion.

Medical records can be organized in many ways. Learn how to use effectively the record in the facility where you work. Regardless of the type of medical record used, however, you should always record important nutrition information in the client's medical record. Examples of important information are:

- Evaluation of the client's current diet.
- Nutrition assessment data.
- Recommended nutrition therapy.
- The client's acceptance and tolerance of the diet.
- Documentation of diet counseling.
- Any planned follow-up or referral to another person or agency.
- The client's response to nutrition care.

Take time to record important nutrition information in the client's medical record.

In addition to the formal medical record, various health care providers generally keep records of their own. For example, a nurse keeps a nursing care plan, and a dietitian keeps a nutrition care plan. These records contain some of the information contained in the formal medical record. However, they also include plans and notes that are more detailed and pertinent to the individual health team member. For example, a nutrition care plan may have more details regarding a client's reaction to a diet, which will later be considered in preparation for diet counseling. Because nurses are involved with direct client care more often than other team members, it is wise to ensure that the nursing care plan contains information regarding special nutrition needs.

Other Communication Channels

Many opportunities for verbal communication among health team members also exist. Health team members within the hospital can be phoned or paged when problems are identified or questions arise. Physicians who are not in the hospital can be reached in the office, at home, or through an answering service.

Bedside rounds provide an ideal opportunity for professional communication. During rounds, clients are visited and examined as necessary. The health team members discuss the clients' cases either prior to or following the visits. Use these discussions to talk over nutrition problems and to exchange information about the clients' concerns and attitudes.

Nurses also report to one another at the end of each shift. You can use this time to pass along information regarding clients' special nutrition needs or requests.

Professionals can communicate during bedside rounds.

Study Questions

1. What are the five steps in the nursing process that can be used to identify nutrition problems and take corrective measures?
2. Describe the four components of nutrition assessment and what each can reveal.
3. Why is the person who is ill likely to develop malnutrition? How does malnutrition, in turn, affect health?
4. How do energy stores and protein status affect an individual's ability to respond to stress?
5. Think about the problem of PCM in the hospital. Is it widespread? What factors contribute to the problem? What effect can PCM have on the outcome of a hospital stay? What measures can health care providers take to prevent PCM?
6. What is the easiest way to start a conversation with a client in a health care setting? How can you facilitate communication through the use of questions? What types of questions should be used, and what type avoided? What other techniques help to maintain effective

Nutrition Assessment and Care

Mrs. Green, a 38–year-old computer scientist, was admitted to the hospital for testing following a car accident. Her injuries included several broken bones and a collapsed left lung. Her lab report revealed a mildly depleted serum albumin and a moderately depleted total lymphocyte count. After reviewing her medical record, the health care team decided that a complete nutrition assessment was necessary. The following significant information resulted.

- *Anthropometrics*
  Height: 5′7″.
  Weight: 150 lb.
  Frame size: medium.
- *Physical Findings*
  Hair: dull, easily plucked.
  Others: none noted.
- *Medical History*
  Increased nutrient requirements due to the injuries sustained in the car accident.
- *Laboratory Findings*
  Serum albumin: 3 g/dl (mildly depleted).
  Total lymphocyte count: 1,000 mm³ (moderately depleted).

- *Diet History*
  Usual weight: 175 lb.
  Weight loss intentional.
  Very low kcalorie, low-carbohydrate diet over the past six weeks.
- *Drug History*
  One standard multivitamin-mineral daily.
  No other drugs.

1. Determine Mrs. Green's ideal body weight, and calculate percent ideal body weight.
2. Calculate percent usual body weight.
3. Consider Mrs. Green's recent weight change. What is a safe rate of weight loss (see p. 247)? How does Mrs. Green's weight loss compare with the safe rate? Does her recent weight change increase her risk of poor nutrition status?
4. What do Mrs. Green's lab values indicate with respect to her protein status (see Appendix E)?
5. Are there any other factors in Mrs. Green's medical and drug history or physical findings suggestive of malnutrition (see Appendix E)?
6. When conducting an interview to determine a medical, drug, and diet history, what points should you keep in mind to communicate effectively with Mrs. Green?
7. Based on Mrs. Green's nutrition assessment, you determine that she is at a high risk for PCM. Discuss how PCM can affect Mrs. Green's health status. What steps can you take to ensure that Mrs. Green's nutrient needs are being met?
8. Consider opportunities for discussing your concerns about Mrs. Green's nutrition status with other health professionals. What communication networks are available to you?
9. You have consulted other members of the health team, and together you have developed a nutrition care plan. Specifically, the goal is to restore Mrs. Green to optimal nutrition status during hospitalization and provide nutrition counseling regarding a safe weight reduction diet to follow when she is released from the hospital. Discuss the steps necessary to provide effective nutrition counseling.

communication? How should you close a discussion with a client?

7. What is the purpose of an interview? What is the purpose of nutrition counseling? What steps can you take to make nutrition counseling more effective? Discuss each step.
8. What are behavioral objectives? Why are they useful? During a counseling session, how can you encourage the client and make the session relevant?
9. Why is it important to evaluate a nutrition counseling session? What questions should you ask yourself about the session?
10. How can you use the medical record to communicate a client's nutrition needs with other health care professionals? What kinds of information about nutrition should you record? Where else can you find written information about a client's nutrient or nutrition education needs?
11. Discuss some other ways that health care providers can share concerns about a client's nutrition needs.

Notes

1. D. R. Hunt, B. J. Rowlands, and D. Johnston, Hand grip strength—A simple prognostic indicator in surgical patients, *Journal of Enteral and Parenteral Nutrition* 9 (1985): 701–704.
2. P. Twomey, D. Ziegler, and J. Rombeau, Utility of skin testing in nutritional assessment: A critical review, *Journal of Parenteral and Enteral Nutrition* 6 (1982): 50–58.
3. Presented at a Congressional Briefing on the Cost Effectiveness of Nutrition Support hosted by the American Dietetic Association, 23 January 1986. Report based on a study conducted by Arthur Anderson and Company and Ross Laboratories.
4. Congressional Briefing, 1986.
5. S. K. Kamath and coauthors, Hospital malnutrition: A 33-hospital screening study, *Journal of the American Dietetic Association* 86 (1986): 203–206.

HIGHLIGHT SEVENTEEN

Computers in Nutrition: Bits About Bytes

*I*f you have not yet been impressed by the role of computers in our lives, consider the words of Christopher Evans, author of *The Micro Millenium*: "If the automobile industry had developed at the same rate as computers and over the same amount of time, you would be able to buy a Rolls-Royce today for $2.75; it would get 3 million miles to the gallon and would deliver enough power to drive the Queen Elizabeth II oceanliner. And, if you were interested in miniaturization, you could put half a dozen of them on a pinhead." This highlight looks at the computer—one of the tools that assists the health care professional in providing effective nutrition care.

The computer has become an important fixture in the health care setting. Computer programs designed to perform many tasks in health care

Computers are valuable tools for providing effective health care.

facilities are numerous and new programs continue to appear on the market. This highlight cannot teach you how to use a computer or a program, for each has specific instructions. Rather, the purpose of this discussion is to provide an overview of the roles of computers in nutrition.

No doubt about it, the computer is here to stay. The anxiety that many people feel when sitting face to face with a computer terminal needs to be set aside and replaced with an openness to learning how to use this valuable tool to get the job done accurately and efficiently.

In hospitals and other health care settings that use computers, the system generally consists of one computer that is accessed through a network of computer terminals conveniently located at various stations throughout the facility. For example, in the hospital, each nursing station has a terminal. Other terminals are found in various departments, such as the dietary department and the pharmacy. The number of terminals and their locations depends on the needs of the facility. To fully appreciate the workings of a computer, you need to be aware of their capabilities and limitations—their strengths and weaknesses.

Advantages of Computers

The advantages of computers are numerous—they save valuable time and reduce operating costs significantly. As an example, consider the computer billing systems currently in use in most hospitals. Everything that is ordered for a client while in the hospital is ordered via computer. Drugs, IV fluids, x-rays,

physical therapy treatments, as well as other supplies and professional services, are ordered and billed using the computer. In years past, the nurses would have to call in numerous orders for each of many clients to different departments and then ensure that the client was appropriately billed for the supplies or services. You can see how much time this would take, not only for the nurse, but also for the departments receiving orders for supplies and services.

The example described also illustrates another advantage of the computer— reduction of human error. When orders are transmitted verbally, communication errors are more likely to occur. If a nurse is ordering an IV feeding by phone while worried about the client in room 425, and the pharmacist at the other end of the line is in a noisy room, the chances of an unintentional communication error are great. When the communication is printed (as it would be if ordered by computer), the information can be checked and verified.

In addition to fewer communication errors, computers can store large amounts of information which can be retrieved readily when needed. All the information pertaining to the supplies and services for each client is recorded on a daily basis—a lot of information, even if the client has a typical hospital stay. Consider further the total number of clients in the hospital at any one time and you can see how much information the computer can store. Not only can this information be stored, but it can be retrieved in a variety of useful ways. For example, the computer could be asked to calculate the cost of x-rays charged to one client or the number or x-rays taken on all clients in a day. Such information allows hospital administrators to determine what services and supplies are in greatest demand and where operations are not cost-effective.

Many of the functions the computer performs are mundane tasks that have a larger risk of error when performed by human beings. The computer can quickly and accurately calculate solutions to mathematical problems.

Computers can provide confidentiality or accessibility. To maintain confidentiality or security, information can be processed, coded, and stored so that only informed people can access the information. In other instances, information can be easily retrieved by a variety of people at many computer terminals.

These examples provide only a glimpse of how valuable a computer can be in a health care facility. Other applications that relate specifically to nutrition are introduced later in this highlight. When computers are used to their maximum capacity, they can save health care providers time which in turn, can be spent on direct client care.

Limitations of Computers

Our increasing dependence on computers sometimes makes it difficult to keep in mind that computers are only machines. They can only do what they have been programmed to do by human beings. They are not inherently foolproof. Therefore, we must depend on our own knowledge and common sense to interpret the information generated by computers. Nutrient analysis programs are a case in point.

Nutrient analysis programs estimate the amount of various nutrients consumed in a diet and compare that to a standard such as the RDA. Their accuracy depends not only on the record of foods eaten that is presented to the computer, but also on the food composition values that were entered into the data base. Remember that data bases are not perfect; they too are created by human beings. If there are inaccurate values in the data base, then the results of the analysis become meaningless. Furthermore, even with complete and accurate values, the program user must know how to interpret the results appropriately. To adequately interpret the computer analysis, a user must have enough nutrition knowledge to know that nutrient values are only estimates, that food composition varies, and that individual requirements for different nutrients also vary.

Computers also can't be programmed to deal with human elements such as feelings and emotions. A computer program that helps a medical student diagnose a disease and lists possible treatments can't help a physician tell a client he has developed cancer or predict how a client will respond to chemotherapy. In short, computers are tools. They can be most useful, but they cannot replace a thinking human being.

Another problem with computers is that they shut down. When we rely on the computer and the system goes down, chaos results. As an example, computer terminals are used in the hospital to order tests, diets, drugs, and more. When the system is down, each department must be called and given the order (which can easily be miscommunicated). Departments receiving the orders must then process requests. This requires more time because they are being interrupted with phone calls. Times like these require patience; work loads become overwhelming. You may have had a similar experience. You may have heard, "You'll have to call back. Our computer is down, and we can't answer your question now." It may make you wonder how we functioned before computers.

For the most part, the advantages of computers outweigh their limitations. With these considerations in mind, let's take a closer look at the roles of computers in nutrition practice.

Computer Applications in Foodservice

The computer is a valuable tool for communicating information about a client to other health care providers and administrative staff. Admitting information, supplies and equipment used in therapy, drug records, and laboratory results are recorded. This information can then be used to prescribe treatment or to bill clients.

Physicians order diets by computer, which automatically transmits the information to the dietary department. When diet change orders are made, the information is available to the dietary department as soon as it is entered into the computer—again, such a system saves valuable time and reduces errors considerably.

In addition, the dietary department uses the computer as an aid in planning menus. Meals can be planned within budget restrictions; evaluated against standards such as the RDA; and developed according to lab test results or medication schedules. Kitchen management is assisted with food production control by maintaining an inventory of food supplies and accounting for food costs. Labels with client information can be printed by computer and placed on the client's menu for identification when trays are sent to the floors.

Computer Applications in Nutrition Support

More than 200 computer software programs are available in the field of food science and human nutrition.[1] Clinical dietitians are using computers in many day-to-day activities. Among the most commonly used programs in dietetics are nutrient analysis programs that enable the dietitian to estimate the nutrients in a client's diet and compare this intake to a dietary standard such as the RDA. To complete this task without the aid of a computer is tedious and time-consuming. A sample printout from a nutrient analysis program is shown in Figure H17–1.

The analysis of a client's diet is one part of the nutrition assessment process. Computer programs that help with other aspects of the nutrition support process are also available.[2] For example, some programs analyze anthropometric and biochemical data to identify individuals who may be at risk for poor nutrition status. Using a computer to screen clients frees time, allowing many more clients to be screened. Once problems have been identified, corrective measures can be taken.

Computer programs can not only identify nutrient needs, but also can be used to formulate an appropriate feeding program. An example is the selection of a tube-feeding formula.

Much information must be taken into account when choosing a tube-feeding formula and a method of delivery. The decisions can be overwhelming, especially when the person requiring the formula has several medical conditions that affect nutrient needs. A computer program to help manage these many considerations has been developed.[3] Similarly, computer programs are available to help practitioners plan intravenous feeding therapy as well.[4] (Much more information about tube feedings and intravenous nutrition can be found in Chapter 18.) As stated earlier, however, such programs are not foolproof. A qualified practitioner can use these programs as an aid, but they can't substitute for human clinical judgment.

Computer programs can also assist the health care team in monitoring the client's response to therapy. A large volume of data must be considered in determining whether an individual is responding adequately to nutrition support. Computer programs can help integrate this information and save team members' time.

Another computer application in the field of nutrition support is the development of a program to assist dietitians in filling diet prescriptions for clients with phenylketonuria (PKU).[5] PKU is an inherited disorder of metabolism that requires strict adherence to a very restricted diet. To calculate the diet manually is time-consuming and difficult. Again we are reminded, however, the program doesn't eliminate the need for a qualified dietitian. The actual diet prescription, the choice of products, the translation of foods and formula into a suitable diet, and client education rest with a trained professional.

Computer Applications in Nutrition Education

Computers are also useful in nutrition education. In the education of professionals, computer programs are used to teach various aspects of clinical care. Clinical case studies that simulate real-life situations give students practice in dealing with clients and their special needs. The students can work at their own pace, and the instructor has a record of the students' responses. Other programs teach nutrition by giving the students information, and then asking them to answer questions based on the information given.

Likewise, computers can help clients understand the concepts of good nutrition, and the need for special diets. For clients who need special diet advice,

Miniglossary of Computer Terms

bit: short for *binary digit;* the smallest unit of computer information.

byte: a sequence of bits.

data base: the body of information stored by the computer.

diskette: a thin, flexible magnetic disk protected in a jacket; used to store or read computer information.

display screen: the televisionlike monitor, part of the terminal, that allows computer users to see what they are working on.

floppy disk: another name for a diskette.

hard copy: a printed copy of the information stored in the computer.

hardware: mechanical, magnetic, or electronic equipment used to process data. The hardware limits the type of software that can be used (see *software*).

input: the information that is entered into the computer.

mainframe computer: a large computer capable of storing more data than a microcomputer. Mainframe computers can perform multiple functions very rapidly and are used by many large businesses, research centers, and universities.

microcomputer: a smaller computer capable of performing functions similar to mainframe computers. Microcomputers are smaller, less expensive computers frequently found in hospitals and small businesses.

output: the information that the computer prints out on paper or displays on the terminal screen.

program: the set of step-by-step instructions that tell the computer how to perform a task. See also *software*.

software: computer programs which allow the user to perform various functions. Not all software can be used with every computer; hardware and software must be compatible (see *hardware*).

terminal: a keyboard and display screen that allows the user to access and process the information stored in a computer.

FIGURE H17-1

A sample printout from a diet analysis program.

Nutrition summary

QUANTITY	NAME	WGT (G)	CAL	PROT. (G)	FIBER (G)	CARB. (G)	CHOL (MG)	FAT-UN (G)	FAT (G)	VIT A (IU)	B1 (MG)	B2 (MG)	B6 (MG)	B12 (MCG)	FOL. (MCG)
2 ea	Cooked Egg	100	158	12.1	0	1.2	526	5.9	11.1	520	.074	.286	.114	1.31	49
1 cup	2% lowfat milk	244	121	8.12	0	11.7	22	1.62	4.78	500	.095	.403	.105	.888	12
2 pce	Whole Wheat Bread-soft	56	130	5.2	2.8	27.6	0	.8	1.4	2	.18	.060	.076	0	31.2
2 tsp	Butter	9	67.7	.080		.005	21.4	2.5	7.66	289	.000	.003	.000	.000	.291
	TOTALS:	409	477	25.5	2.8	40.5	569	10.8	25.0	1311	.349	.752	.295	2.20	92.4

Nutrition summary

QUANTITY	NAME	WGT (G)	NIAC. (MG)	PANTO (MG)	VIT C (MG)	VIT E (MG)	CA (MG)	CU (MG)	IRON (MG)	MG (MG)	PHOS. (MG)	POTAS. (MG)	SEL. (MCG)	NA (MG)	ZINC (MG)
2 ea	Cooked Egg	100	.060	1.72	0	.77	56	.096	2.08	12.2	180	130	9.56	138	1.44
1 cup	2% lowfat milk	244	.21	.781	2.32	.146	297	.073	.12	33	232	377	5.66	122	.963
2 pce	Whole Wheat Bread-soft	56	1.6	.238	.002	.868	48	.134	1.79	43.6	142	144	26.4	296	1.06
2 tsp	Butter	9	.004			.149	2.25	.002	.015	.166	2.16	2.41	.062	77.9	.004
	TOTALS:	409	1.87	2.74	2.32	1.93	403	.305	4.00	88.9	556	653	41.6	634	3.47

```
Name: Nutrition summary

Items analyzed:

    2    ea  Cooked Egg
    1    cup 2% lowfat milk
    2    pce Whole Wheat Bread-soft
    2    tsp Butter

                    NUTRITIONAL ANALYSIS
                  (Plus % RDA for EXAMPLE)

          Weight:  409  Grams  (14.4 Ounces)

     Calories            477      (22%)**  Carbohydrates   40.5 G   ( 13%)*
     Protein            25.5 G    (54%)    Cholesterol      569 MG  (190%)*
     Dietary Fiber       2.8 G    (13%)*   Fat-unsat.      10.8 G   ( 23%)*
     Vitamin A          1311 IU   (33%)    Fat-total       25.0 G   ( 35%)*
     Thiamin-B1         .349 MG   (32%)    Calcium          403 MG  ( 50%)
     Riboflavin-B2      .752 MG   (58%)    Copper          .305 MG  ( 12%)*
     Pyridoxine-B6      .295 MG   (15%)    Iron            4.00 MG  ( 22%)
     Cobalamin-B12      2.20 MCG  (73%)    Magnesium       88.9 MG  ( 30%)
     Folacin            92.4 MCG  (23%)    Phosphorus       556 MG  ( 70%)
     Niacin-B3          1.87 MG   (13%)    Potassium        653 MG  ( 17%)*
     Pantothenic acid   2.74 MG   (39%)*   Selenium        41.6 MCG ( 33%)*
     Vitamin C          2.32 MG   ( 4%)    Sodium           634 MG  ( 21%)*
     Vitamin E          1.93 MG   (24%)    Zinc            3.47 MG  ( 23%)

            *  No specific RDA; suggested values.
          ** Average value; individual needs may vary.

          Calories from:   Protein          21%
                           Carbohydrates    33%
                           Fats             46%
```

software programs are available to teach the rationale of the diets they need. Such programs are available in the areas of weight control, diabetes, and hyperlipidemias, to name a few. Programs to help clients understand the association of sodium with hypertension and how to identify the sodium content of foods are other examples.

Additional programs are available to educate the public. Some of these are intended to educate consumers about general food and nutrition facts. Others give consumers information about shopping and food costs. These programs may cover such topics as reading labels, using coupons, unit pricing, meal planning, and reducing the amount of food wastage.

Other Applications

Computers have an important role in other areas of nutrition as well. Computer programs can help analyze the data generated in nutrition research studies. They can store this information as it is generated, so that at any time during a study, the researcher can look at any of the variables being studied.

The results of research can then be compiled and reported in written form with the aid of a word-processing program. Word processing is invaluable in many areas of nutrition. In fact, any report, publication, or other written communication that will go through more than one draft (such as this textbook) is much easier to prepare with the help of a word processor.

We have reviewed several applications that computers have in nutrition and discussed a few of the many programs available. No doubt, since this highlight was written, dozens of new programs have been developed. It is not difficult to see that computers will continue to play a greater and greater role in the way we function as health care professionals as well as in other aspects of our lives. Use the computer to your advantage; be aware of the computer programs available in the facility where you work and of others that you might want your facility to purchase. Computer programs will help you do your job more efficiently and save you valuable time.

NOTES
1. R. A. Sager, The software search: A dilemma, *Journal of Dietetic Software* 3 (1986): 8–9.
2. D. A. August and coauthors, Computers and nutritional support, *Nutritional Support Services* 6 (1986): 47–54.
3. J. B. Krasner, A technique for optimization of enteral feeding regimens: Implementation on a microcomputer, *Journal of Parenteral and Enteral Nutrition* 10 (1986): 208–212.
4. F. M. Edwards, Computer assisted planning of parenteral hyperalimentation therapy, *Critical Care Medicine* 10 (1982): 539–543.
5. K. Anderson, B. Kennedy, and P. B. Acosta, Computer-implemented nutrition support of phenylketonuria, *Journal of the American Dietetic Association* 12 (1985): 1623–1625.

Food in the Hospital

18

Contents

The ultimate purpose of hospital food, like all food, is to support the body's functions—all the way down to the individual structures of which cells are composed. These are microvilli on the surfaces of five neighboring cells of the cornea, viewed from the top (the opening art of Chapter 6 shows the microvilli on the surface of the GI tract lining viewed from the side). Like all other cell parts, these intricate structures are made of substances that had to be derived from food.

An RD is a professional trained in nutrition and food science.

registered dietitian (RD): a trained professional with a minimum of a bachelor's degree in nutrition and food science; a year's internship at an ADA approved facility or the equivalent; and a passing score on a national registration exam (a four-hour qualifying exam administered over six competency areas by the ADA). Both administrative and clinical dietitians are often RDs.
Administrative dietitians are primarily concerned with the management of foodservice systems that provide optimal nutrition and quality food, although they sometimes assume some clinical duties as well. **Clinical dietitians** are responsible for direct client care—assessing nutrient needs, developing and implementing nutritional care plans, and evaluating and reporting these results appropriately.

ADA: American Dietetic Association, the professional organization of dietitians in the United States. The Canadian equivalent is the Canadian Dietetic Association, which operates similarly.

dietetic technician: a technically skilled person with an associate's degree which meets ADA educational standards, who works under the guidance of an RD.

"I'd better call in these changes before the lunch deadline."

T he assessment of a client's nutrition status and the development of an appropriate nutrition care plan are important first steps in providing effective client care. The actual delivery of nutrients to the client—by way of food or alternative feeding methods—deserves attention. Health care providers encounter unique problems when clients are fed in hospitals. They need an understanding of the general concepts underlying modified diets and diet therapy.

Foodservice in Health Care Facilities

To prepare and serve food in a health care setting is a challenge. The overall responsibility for foodservice rests with either a chief administrative dietitian or a foodservice manager. These individuals direct all aspects of foodservice—from purchasing to delivery of food to the client.

The clinical dietitian works directly with clients to assess their nutrition status, to plan appropriate diets, and to provide nutrition education. The nurse often reinforces the nutrition education given by the dietitian. In some facilities, dietetic technicians assist the dietitians in both administrative and clinical responsibilities. Other dietary employees include clerks, aides, cooks, porters, and other assistants.

Many hospitals provide menus for clients to select the meals they will receive while hospitalized. This system helps to ensure that clients will receive foods they enjoy and will eat. It also gives clients the feeling of having some control over something in the hospital environment.

In facilities where it is not possible to offer a selective menu, the dietary department serves a balanced diet, altering the basic diet according to dietary orders as necessary. Generally, even these menus are flexible. For example, if the vegetable served at dinner is broccoli, a food the client doesn't like, green beans might be substituted.

You can help your clients greatly, as well as save yourself needless aggravation and time, by learning about the foodservice system in the health care facility where you work. Some of the things you will want to know include:

- The number to call and the procedure to follow to request a diet the physician has ordered, make diet changes, or report problems with the client's tray.
- The number where you can reach the dietitian, in case a client needs special nutrition advice.
- The times when meals are plated, so that you can call in any requests before these times.
- The location of the diet manual—usually available at each nursing station—and its contents.

Once you understand how the dietary department operates, you will know where to turn for help when your client is having problems with food or nutrition.

The hospital is used as an example of a health care facility in this chapter, because it is a setting familiar to most health care providers. Long-term care facilities, such as nursing homes and mental institutions, use similar systems; the information presented in this chapter applies to those settings as well. However, special concerns arise in long-term care facilities.

A person in a short-term care facility may not eat well while hospitalized, but can make up for nutrient deficits by eating well at home. The resident in a long-term care facility eats in the same place continuously and depends on the foodservice department to provide nutritious and acceptable foods. To provide nutritious foods that a person cannot or will not eat does no good. Therefore, the foodservice department must make an extra effort to vary the foods offered in order to avoid monotony. Furthermore, the foodservice department must ensure that clients on special diets receive and eat appropriate foods.

Hospital Foods: The Professional Perspective

The primary goal of diet therapy is to achieve or maintain optimal nutrition status. Optimal status is achieved when the cells are provided appropriate amounts of energy, protein, carbohydrate, fat, vitamins, major minerals, trace elements, and water. These nutrients, in turn, must be provided in a form that is easy for the body to use. For example, if a person's GI tract is not functioning, it will do no good to provide that person with a standard diet.

Each diet prescribed for an individual has its own rationale and purpose. The rationale of a weight reduction diet is to provide less energy from food so that the person will use stored energy and lose weight. The purposes of weight reduction may vary from improving self-image to gaining better control of blood glucose levels.

A person benefits maximally from diet therapy if his nutrition needs have been correctly identified and an appropriate nutrition care plan has been designed. The diet therapy is then selected to meet specific needs and to complement other medical therapy. For example, a diet planned for an individual with insulin dependent diabetes mellitus (IDDM) must be coordinated so that food is available during the times when the body will have insulin.

Standard and Modified Diets

Regular or *standard diets* are typical diets that provide the recommended daily allowances of nutrients and include all foods. Modifying the regular diet is much like tailoring a suit. A tailored suit is the same suit after alterations—only it fits better. So it is with the modified diet. A modified diet is a basic nutritious diet that emphasizes a variety of foods; it is "tailored" by adjusting

modified or therapeutic diet: a regular diet that is adjusted to meet special nutrition needs. Such diets can be adjusted in consistency, in level of energy and nutrients, in amount of fluid, in number of meals, or by the elimination of certain foods.

The diet manual specifies foods excluded or included on various modified diets.

diet order: a physician's written statement in the medical record of what diet a client should receive.

the consistency; by adjusting the level of individual nutrients, energy, or fluid; by altering the number of meals; or by eliminating certain foods. Table 18–1 gives examples of modified diets used to treat diseases involving different organ systems.

It's helpful to think about modified diets in terms of the symptoms or conditions they relieve rather than in terms of the diseases they are used to treat. People are different, and so are the diets they need. Two people with the same disease may need two different diets. Conversely, people in two completely different states of health may benefit from the same diet. Consider two people with cancer and a third who is pregnant. One person with cancer may be nauseated and may need dietary suggestions for controlling nausea. The other person with cancer may be overweight and not experiencing any nausea. The dietary suggestions you make to each cancer client will be different. However, a pregnant woman who is experiencing nausea may benefit from the same recommendations that you make for the nauseated person with cancer.

The exact foods excluded or included on a specific modified diet differ among hospitals, generally in minor ways. These variations reflect different schools of thought regarding diet. You can familiarize yourself with a particular institution's diets by reading the diet manual.

In larger hospitals, diet manuals are compiled by the staff of dietitians and approved by the hospital administrator, several physicians, and representatives of the nursing service. A smaller hospital may adopt the diet manual of another hospital or an organization such as the state dietetic association. The diet manual describes what foods are allowed and not allowed on each diet, the rationale and indications for use of the diets, sample menus, and information regarding the nutritional adequacy of the diets. The diets listed in the manual are those available through the dietary department.

The physician prescribes the client's diet and writes the diet order in the medical record. However, the dietitian or other health care team member may consult with the physician about a diet prescription or make recommendations when changes in the diet orders appear warranted.

Similarly, the dietitian or nurse may make recommendations to physicians when diet orders are unclear. Keep in mind that many employees in the dietary department do not have formal training in nutrition. These employees may have difficulty interpreting vague diet orders. Whenever possible, the health care team jointly recommends the most appropriate diet.

The name given to the diet should be consistent with the name given in the diet manual. To avoid miscommunication, the physician must describe exact modifications, when appropriate. For example, a 1,200-kcalorie diet, rather than a low-kcalorie diet, should be specified. A "low-sodium diet" request should specify the amount of sodium; otherwise, it could be interpreted as containing anything from 500 to 4,000 milligrams of sodium.

When a physician's order for a diet is unclear, ask the physician to clarify the order. In many cases, however, the physician is not available, and the dietitian will determine the exact modification. The dietitian then records the exact diet being requested in the medical record. If a dietitian is not available and the dietary department receives vague orders from the nursing station, a house diet (usually specified in the diet manual) will be sent.

TABLE 18–1

Summary of Modified Diets by Organ System

Disorders	Possible Diet Modifications
Conditions affecting or involving the GI tract, liver, and exocrine pancreas[a]	
Broken jaw	Mechanical soft
Celiac disease	Gluten-restricted
Cirrhosis	Protein-restricted, sodium-restricted, fluid-restricted
Constipation	High-fiber, increased fluids
Cystic fibrosis	Low-fat, high-kcalorie, high-protein
Dental caries	Mechanical soft
Diarrhea	Liquid, low-fiber, regular, fluid and electrolyte replacement
Difficulty swallowing (dysphagia)	Mechanical soft, tube feeding, total parenteral nutrition (TPN)
Diverticulitis	Low-fiber
Diverticulosis	High-fiber
Dry mouth	Mechanical soft
Dumping syndrome	Carbohydrate-restricted; no concentrated sugars; small, frequent feedings; fluid and electrolyte replacement
Gallbladder disease	Low-fat, kcalorie-restricted, regular
Gastritis	Low-fiber, bland
Hepatic coma	Protein-restricted, sodium-restricted, fluid-restricted
Hepatitis	Regular, high-kcalorie, high-protein
Hiatal hernia	Small, frequent feedings; low-fat; bland; kcalorie-restricted
Ill-fitting dentures	Mechanical soft
Indigestion (dyspepsia)	Low-fiber; bland; small, frequent feedings
Inflammatory bowel disease	Low-fiber, low-fat, high-kcalorie, high-protein, fluid and electrolyte replacement, lactose-restricted, tube feeding, TPN
Lactose intolerance	Lactose-restricted
Malabsorption	Low-fat, high-kcalorie, high-protein, fluid and electrolyte replacement
Missing teeth	Mechanical soft
Nausea	Low-fiber; bland; small, frequent feedings
Oral surgery	Mechanical soft
Pancreatitis	Low-fat; regular; small, frequent feedings; tube feeding; TPN
Peptic ulcer	Bland
Periodontal disease	Mechanical soft
Plastic surgery of head or neck	Mechanical soft, tube feeding, TPN
Reflux esophagitis	Small, frequent feedings; low-fat; bland; kcalorie-restricted
Short bowel syndrome	Low-fat, high-kcalorie, high-protein, fluid and electrolyte replacement
Ulcers of mouth or gums	Mechanical soft, bland
Vomiting	Fluid and electrolyte replacement

TABLE 18–1

(continued)

Disorders	Possible Diet Modifications
Conditions of the endocrine pancreas[a]	
Diabetes mellitus	Carbohydrate-controlled, kcalorie-restricted, fat-controlled, high-fiber
Hypoglycemia	No concentrated sweets; small, frequent feedings
Conditions affecting the heart and blood vessels	
Atherosclerosis	Fat-controlled, kcalorie-restricted, sodium-restricted, high-fiber
Congestive heart failure	Sodium-restricted; kcalorie-restricted; low-fiber; bland; small, frequent feedings; fluid-restricted
Coronary heart disease	(See *Atherosclerosis*)
Hyperlipidemias	Fat-controlled, kcalorie-restricted, carbohydrate-controlled
Hypertension	Low-sodium, kcalorie-restricted, high-potassium; fat-controlled
Myocardial infarction	Low-sodium; kcalorie-restricted; low-fiber; bland; small, frequent feedings; moderate-temperature foods; fat-controlled
Conditions affecting the kidneys	
Acute renal disease	Protein-restricted, high-kcalorie, fluid-controlled, sodium-controlled, potassium-controlled, fat-controlled, carbohydrate-controlled
Chronic renal disease	Protein-restricted, low-sodium, fluid-restricted, potassium-restricted, phosphorus-restricted
Kidney stones	Increased fluid intake, calcium-controlled, low-oxalate
Nephrotic syndrome	Sodium-restricted, high-kcalorie, high-protein, potassium-restricted
Urinary tract infections	Increased fluid intake, acid-ash diet
Conditions affecting many organ systems	
Burns	High-kcalorie, high-protein, increased fluid intake
Cancer	High-kcalorie, high-protein (see also specific related conditions: Dry mouth, Indigestion, Malabsorption, Nausea, Plastic surgery of head or neck, Ulcers of mouth or gums, Vomiting, and so on)
Food sensitivities	Elimination of offending substance
Galactosemia	Galactose-restricted
Obesity, overweight	kCalorie-restricted, high-fiber
Phenylketonuria (PKU)	Phenylalanine-restricted
Stroke	Mechanical soft, regular, tube feeding
Surgery	Regular, high-kcalorie, high-protein, increased fluids
Underweight	High-kcalorie, high-protein

[a]The pancreas produces both external (exocrine) and internal (endocrine) secretions. The external secretions (enzymes) play an important role in the digestion of food; the internal secretions (insulin and other hormones) play a primary role in the regulation of glucose metabolism.

Because the physician is ultimately responsible for a client's diet order, it is easy for others to follow the order without further consideration. But all health care providers are responsible for the client's care.

Ideally, a dietitian visits all clients and reviews the charts of every person admitted to the hospital. But often the dietitian is assigned to so many people that this is virtually impossible; therefore, most clinical dietitians see only people on modified diets or people they have been asked to see. Some smaller hospitals may not even employ a full-time clinical dietitian.

Mistakes occur daily because of inappropriate diet orders. For example:

- A grossly overweight individual is described as "well-nourished" and placed on a regular diet. Because the person is not on a modified diet, the dietitian does not see him, and he receives an inappropriate diet and no nutrition advice.
- A physician orders that a person be kept NPO after midnight for a lab test to be run in the morning. Due to a miscommunication, the doctor thinks that the order is changed after the test, but it isn't. The individual is needlessly "starved" for three or more days.
- A person routinely enjoys foods low in sugar and salt. Foods served on the regular diet are too salty for her, so she eats very little food. Furthermore, she feels the hospital has totally neglected its responsibility to provide nutritious foods to its clients.

NPO: see p. 587.

Why isn't the diet ordered correctly in the first place? In cases where many doctors, interns, and residents are seeing a client, miscommunication can easily occur. The individual may communicate needs more clearly and more often to the nurse or other health care provider than to the physician. Furthermore, the client's doctor may not consider nutrition to be a significant part of the client's care. Whatever the reason, you should be aware that written diet orders are not always appropriate. When they are not, contact the dietitian or alert the physician.

Alternative Feeding Methods

The majority of people in the hospital are given oral diets—either regular or modified—to provide for nutrient needs. If a person cannot eat adequate amounts of ordinary foods to meet these needs, however, other methods of feeding can be used. These methods include supplemental feedings, tube feedings, and intravenous nutrition, discussed in more detail later in this chapter. Figure 18–1 summarizes some of the steps involved in deciding how to feed a client.

When a client can't eat enough food from regular meals, the first step is to try to supplement the diet. You can try to give nutritious snacks between meals. Many clients do well with such snacks. For clients who find it easier to drink than to eat, liquid supplements are useful. Psychologically, liquids seem to be

FIGURE 18-1

Selecting the feeding method.

Which would you rather drink?

complete formula: a liquid formula that supplies all the nutrients needed when given in sufficient volume.

less filling, and they are much easier for debilitated, weak, or tired individuals to handle.

Liquid supplements can include common drinks like milk, milkshakes, or instant breakfast drinks. Commercially prepared liquid formulas also are available (some of these formulas are listed in Appendix L). These liquids can be fortified with powdered milk to make them higher in protein. kCalories can be increased by adding a source of carbohydrate such as corn syrup or sugar. Commercial products (also listed in Appendix L) can be used to increase the protein, fat, or carbohydrate content of any liquid supplement.

Even when a person enjoys a liquid supplement, palatability becomes a problem after long-term use. You can help relieve boredom by using more than one type of supplemental feeding. Try adding flavorings such as chocolate, decaffeinated instant coffee, and strawberry or other fruit flavorings to the supplement. Commercially prepared flavor packets are available in a wide variety of flavors; these packets can be conveniently kept at the bedside for use as desired.

Serve liquid feedings attractively. Liquids served from a can are far less appealing than those served in a glass. Remember to serve the formula cold and to provide an ice bath to keep the formula cold so that it can be sipped as desired.

A liquid formula that supplies all the nutrients needed is called a complete formula. A complete formula always should be used when the liquid formula is the sole source of nutrients. However, complete formulas can be (and often are) used as supplemental feedings. When used in this way, they augment the nutrient level of the diet even though they may not be given in quantities large enough to meet all nutrient needs alone.

Hospital Foods: The Client's Perspective

Hospital food—what do you think of when you see or hear these words? What are your own experiences with hospital food, or the experiences of someone close to you?

People in the hospital often look forward to eating. They enjoy the chance to select foods, because it is one of the few experiences in the hospital in which they have a choice. Clients cannot choose when they will get different tests, how much blood they will have drawn, what nurse will care for them, or what time they will have surgery.

To the client, food is also something familiar in an unfamiliar environment. As opposed to the many things imposed on the client, food can be eaten or refused. It is the one aspect of the hospital situation the client can control.

DENNIS the MENACE

"SORRY, SONNY. THIS FOOD IS FOR **SICK** PEOPLE."

"I'M NOT FEELIN' SO HOT!"

Complaints about food are often a way of venting fear, frustration, anger, and physical pain. People who are worried about their health, upset over their progress, disturbed by the way they are being treated, or in pain are likely to complain about food.

Problems with foodservice, unrelated to the client's physical or mental state, can interfere with appetite. For one, hospital food is not cooked as food is at home—a considerable problem when the client must eat three meals a day for many days in the hospital. Food may be served at times when the client just isn't hungry. If a client has just undergone a painful treatment, he'll be too upset to eat. Unfortunately, the food may also be cold by the time it arrives in the room. The client often must eat alone, in bed, which can make mealtimes more of a chore than a pleasurable experience. Food is so important to most people that a bad experience with it in the hospital can make them and those who work with them agitated and angry.

All this is not to say that every person in the hospital has problems with food. The majority of people will eat adequate amounts of food, even if they complain about it. If their intakes decrease somewhat, the deficit will be easy to correct once they are eating familiar foods in their home environments.

The loss of appetite can have a serious effect on the health or recovery of some people, however. These individuals lose their appetites at a time when they can least afford a nutrient deficit. Use the steps discussed in Chapter 17 (p. 587) to identify clients at risk for poor nutrition status. In such cases, it is especially important to improve the appetite and otherwise ensure that adequate nutrients are provided.

Helping the Client Eat

Of all health professionals, nurses and nursing assistants have the closest and most frequent contact with a client. These professionals most often shoulder responsibility for delivering food to the client's room, preparing the client to eat, observing problems the client may be having with food, and communicating the client's needs to the appropriate person or department.

If a client has a poor appetite or is constantly complaining about food, try to get to the root of the problem. You can reassure the client who is frightened, angry, or confused. Simply showing that you care helps improve a client's appetite. Be sure the client understands that nutrition is a part of the recovery process. When it is permissible and possible, a friend or family member can bring favorite foods from outside the hospital if these foods will help the client eat better. This may be especially useful if the client is a child.

You can also ask yourself and your client these questions to help improve appetite:

To get clients to eat well, make them feel comfortable and cared for.

- Does she understand the importance of nutrition to the recovery process?
- If he is on a modified diet, does he understand why? Does he know which foods are allowed and not allowed on the diet?
- Does she understand how to mark her menu correctly so that she receives the foods she wants?

If clients need help in any of these areas, give them the advice they need. Dietitians are the professionals to call if the problem is too big for you to handle alone. The dietitian works closely with the client to find acceptable foods.

Your own attitudes about the hospital's food can affect your client. Try to be positive; never say something like, "I couldn't eat this stuff either." Instead, say, "The dietary department really tries to make foods the way you like them. Let me call the dietitian. I'm sure he can help you." When a dietitian or food-service manager is unavailable, a list of alternative foods available from the dietary department can generally be found at each nursing station.

All clients can benefit from a few steps that help make mealtimes more enjoyable. Encourage the client to wash her face and hands and to brush her teeth or rinse her mouth before eating. Be sure she is comfortable, either in bed or sitting in a chair. Make sure the extension table is placed at a comfortable height and distance, and that the table is clean. A clean, odor-free room also helps. These steps should be taken before the tray arrives so that the client can enjoy her meal while foods are still at the right temperature.

When the food cart arrives on the floor, each tray should be checked:

- Verify that the client's name is correct. A client's room number may have been incorrectly recorded, or a new client may have been admitted to a room.
- Check to see that the client is receiving the right diet.
- Look at the tray to see if the client has received the foods that were ordered.
- Scan the tray for overall appearance. The client will eat better if the food is served attractively. Order a new tray if foods are not servable.

Once you have checked the trays, serve them immediately—while warm foods are still warm and cold foods are still cold.

These suggestions may seem a bit overwhelming at first glance. However, when you look at them more closely, you will realize that many of the steps become routine, and they are not as time-consuming as they originally appear. Furthermore, your effort can mean a lot to the client whose illness, fears, and frustrations significantly interfere with the desire to eat.

Confirm that the right meal is delivered, and make sure it is served attractively.

The Sick Child

A sick child often requires special care to ensure that nutrient needs are met. Those who care for children must be sensitive to their needs and feelings. Many of the hints given in Chapter 15 for helping children to eat are useful for working with the ill child as well. Additional pointers from people experienced in working with children are:

- Notice the child's posture. Body language will tell you if a child is frightened, hurting, or uncomfortable.
- Touch the child often and lovingly. Your touch communicates more than your words.
- As with adults, let the child choose what to eat as much as possible. Foods brought from outside the hospital can help, if it is permissible.
- Make sure the child eats the food. Notice if he doesn't. Putting it in front of him is not enough.
- Stay with the child during the meal, or make sure a loved person is there. The child will eat and assimilate food better if her anxiety and loneliness are soothed.

A frightened child may be unable to eat.

Clients sometimes receive nutrient solutions through tubes.

tube feeding: feeding a nutrient solution via a tube into the stomach or intestine.

enteral nutrition: delivering nutrients into the intestines. Oral diets and tube feedings are types of enteral nutrition. However, the term *enteral nutrition* is frequently used interchangeably with *tube feeding*. *enteron* = intestine

FIGURE 18–2

Transnasal feeding tube placement.

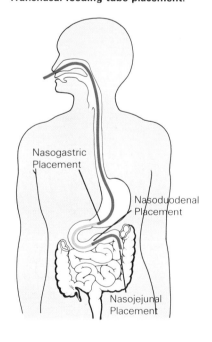

- Encourage the child to eat what he needs most first. This will ensure that nutritious foods get eaten before he gets too full to complete his meal.
- Let her eat with other children if possible. She'll enjoy mealtimes more, accept more food, and eat for a longer period.
- Avoid painful procedures near mealtimes. The stress of pain or fear shuts down digestion and turns off interest in food.

Nutrition care contributes importantly to a child's recovery, even though its effects may not be immediately obvious.

Tube Feedings

An individual who has a functioning GI tract but who is unable to orally ingest enough nutrients to meet present needs is a candidate for a tube feeding. Such a person may have physical problems that make chewing and swallowing difficult, may have no appetite, may be in a coma, or may have very high nutrient requirements. Tube feedings are generally not used for those who have severe vomiting, upper GI bleeding, or complete intestinal obstructions.

Feeding Tube Placement

You may be wondering just how someone is fed by tube. If the thought of being "force fed" seems terrible to you, you may feel better knowing that the administration of tube feedings has improved dramatically in recent years. More importantly, tube feedings have been used effectively to prevent and correct life-threatening diseases such as PCM, thus improving the medical outlook for many people. In this section, we will discuss how tubes are placed and what the implications are for each type of placement. The Miniglossary describes various feeding tube placement sites.

Feeding tubes are most commonly inserted through the nose and passed into the stomach or intestine. This is called transnasal placement (see Figure 18–2). The client is fully alert during the procedure and helps pass the tube by swallowing. Feeding tubes can be passed transnasally with minimal discomfort when the correct size and type of tube are used and the person is emotionally prepared for the procedure. The major disadvantage of transnasal tube placement is that the client who is disoriented or uncooperative can easily pull the tube out. Furthermore, if an inappropriate tube is selected, the nasal passages and esophagus can become irritated.

When a feeding tube cannot be passed through the nose, esophagus, or stomach due to an obstruction, a feeding ostomy may be created (see Figure 18–3). A feeding ostomy is an opening into the esophagus, stomach, or jejunum through which a feeding tube is passed. Usually the openings are surgically formed. However, newer techniques for gastrostomies have been developed that allow the feeding ostomy to be made at bedside without general anesthesia. Feeding ostomies are useful for clients receiving long-term tube feedings, because they are invisible under clothing and they eliminate feeding tube irritation. The most obvious disadvantage of the feeding ostomy is that it often involves surgery.

FIGURE 18–3

Feeding ostomy sites.

Miniglossary of Feeding Tube Placement Sites

transnasal: through the nose. A **transnasal feeding tube** is one that is passed through the nose.

naso — nose

nasogastric (NG): from the nose to the stomach.

nasoenteric: from the nose to the intestine. **Nasoenteric feedings** include both nasoduodenal and nasojejunal feedings.

nasoduodenal (ND): from the nose to the duodenum.

nasojejunal (NJ): from the nose to the jejunum.

feeding ostomy: an opening in the esophagus, stomach, or intestine through which a feeding tube is passed.

ostomy = a surgically formed opening

esophagostomy (ee-soff-uh-GOSS-toe-mee): a surgically made opening in the esophagus through which a feeding tube can be passed.

gastrostomy (gas-TROSS-toe-mee): a surgically made opening in the stomach through which a feeding tube can be passed.

jejunostomy (JEE-ju-NOSS-toe-mee): a surgically made opening in the jejunum through which a feeding tube can be passed.

A **duodenostomy** (DEW-odd-eh-NOSS-toe-mee) is an inconvenient feeding ostomy site, because the duodenum swings toward the back of the body and is not easily accessible.

The advantage of using a nasogastric, esophagostomy, or gastrostomy route for a tube feeding is that the digestive process begins in the stomach. The stomach empties its contents at a controlled rate, giving the intestine time for adequate digestion and absorption. The disadvantage of these feedings is that people sometimes tend to regurgitate them. If the regurgitated fluids are inhaled and reach the lungs, a fatal infection may develop.

Intestinal feedings into the duodenum or jejunum are less likely to cause regurgitation of fluids, because the fluids have to travel farther to come back up. More importantly, two sphincters are working to keep the fluids down: the pylorus and the cardiac sphincter (see p. 169). The major disadvantage of intestinal feedings is that the controlled emptying action of the stomach is lost. Formulas must be carefully selected, and care must be taken to avoid diarrhea and dehydration.

The skin surrounding a feeding ostomy site sometimes becomes irritated from the GI secretions that may leak into the area, and infection can result. Close attention to skin care is usually effective in treating this problem.

Table 18–2 lists the features of the various feeding tube placement sites. As you can see, each is useful in a different set of circumstances.

Feeding Tubes

The safety and comfort of tube feedings have been enhanced greatly through the development of soft, flexible, small-diameter feeding tubes. Traditional feeding tubes, made from stiffer materials (rubber or polyvinyl chloride), were sometimes referred to as "garden hoses." They became even stiffer when exposed

An infection of the lung caused by inhaling fluids regurgitated from the stomach is called **aspiration pneumonia.** Aspiration pneumonia can be a fatal complication of a tube feeding.

TABLE 18–2

Features of Various Feeding Tube Sites

Site	Insertion	Potential Irritations	Risk of Regurgitation[a]	Long-term Tolerance	Chance of Removal by Uncooperative Client
Nasogastric	Nonsurgical	Nasal passages, esophagus	High	Fair[b]	Likely
Nasoduodenal	Nonsurgical	Nasal passages, esophagus	Low	Fair[b]	Likely
Nasojejunal	Nonsurgical	Nasal passages, esophagus	Low	Fair[b]	Likely
Esophagostomy	Surgery required	—	High	Good	Unlikely
Gastrostomy	Surgery required	Skin irritation	Moderate	Good	Unlikely
Jejunostomy	Surgery required	Skin irritation	Low	Good	Unlikely

[a]Relative to the other feeding sites. The absolute risk of regurgitation is small.
[b]When the appropriate type and size of tube are used.

peristalsis: see p. 172.

TABLE 18–3

Guide to Feeding Tube Sizes

Formula	Tube Sizes (French)*
Intact protein formulas (excluding protein isolates)	8 to 12
Protein isolates	7 to 10
Protein hydrolysates	5 to 6

*The smaller sizes can be used when the feeding is delivered by pump.

intact protein formula: a liquid diet that contains a complete protein that has not been altered.

to digestive juices—which was uncomfortable to the client. Furthermore, large-diameter tubes caused the cardiac sphincter to open more, increasing the likelihood of regurgitation.

The newer feeding tubes have gained wide acceptance; they are much smaller in diameter and are made from pliable materials that are less irritating. They do not stiffen when exposed to gastric juices. Indeed, the client on a tube feeding often becomes unaware of the tube's presence within several hours after it has been inserted.

Many newer tubes are designed for placement in the intestine. These tubes are longer and are weighted at one end, to help them pass spontaneously from the stomach into the intestine during normal peristalsis.

Generally, the physician assumes responsibility for ordering the feeding tube; but occasionally, the nurse or dietitian orders it. If you must order the tube, order the smallest size through which the feeding will flow. Table 18–3 gives some general guidelines regarding the proper tube sizes for various types of formulas.

Formula Characteristics

The number of formulas available to feed people either orally or by tube is staggering (see Appendix L). Formulas are available to meet many medical and nutrition needs. Formulas can also be modified using other supplements to meet an even wider range of needs.

Two major types of formulas are available. Those that contain proteins, carbohydrates, and fats of higher molecular weights are called *intact formulas.*

These types of formulas are given to people who are able to digest and absorb nutrients without difficulty. Intact formulas can be protein isolate formulas or blenderized formulas. A protein isolate formula contains a purified protein.

Blenderized diets are complete formulas made from table foods that are mixed smoothly into a liquid form. Baby food meats, milk, iron-fortified baby cereals or potatoes, strained vegetables, and strained fruits are typical ingredients. The nutrient contents of these blenderized diets must be checked (usually by the dietitian) to ensure their adequacy. Liquid vitamin-mineral preparations can be added to fortify the formula.

Blenderized diets made as just described are seldom used in institutional settings. Commercially available blenderized formulas are far more convenient to use, their nutrient composition is constant, they flow through feeding tubes more readily, and far less risk of bacterial contamination is associated with their use.

The second type of formula is hydrolyzed formula. These formulas contain smaller molecules of protein (including dipeptides and tripeptides), fat, and carbohydrate. They are, in a sense, "predigested," and therefore only minimal further digestion is needed. People who lack digestive capabilities or who have a smaller than normal area for absorbing nutrients may benefit from these formulas.

Defined-formula diets are the simplest of the hydrolyzed protein formulas. They contain free amino acids, simple carbohydrate, and very little fat. Several recent studies suggest that the dipeptides and tripeptides available from hydrolyzed formulas may actually be better absorbed than the free amino acids from defined-formula diets.

Commercially available formulas are available in ready-to-use liquid form, as a concentrate, or in powdered form, depending on the formula. Standard formulas provide about 1 kcalorie per milliliter. Formulas are also available to meet higher energy and protein needs in a smaller volume; for example, 1.5 kcalories per milliliter. Other formulas meet the specific needs of people with diseases who require different proportions of protein, carbohydrate, and fat. These formulas benefit those with liver, kidney, and lung diseases.

A small number of formulas are termed *modular feedings*. Some are intact, and some are hydrolyzed. They serve only to add certain nutrients or energy to the diet, rather than being complete in themselves (see Appendix L).

protein isolate: a type of intact protein; a protein with high biological value that has been separated from a source containing a variety of proteins. A **protein isolate formula** contains a protein isolate as the source of protein.

blenderized diet: a liquid diet made from a combination of table foods. Blenderized diets usually contain pureed meat, vegetables, fruits, milk, and starches with vitamins and minerals added as necessary. They can be made in a blender or purchased commercially.

hydrolyzed protein: an intact protein treated with acids or enzymes to yield a combination of free amino acids and short peptide chains. A **protein hydrolysate formula** contains hydrolyzed protein as the source of protein.

The term **monomeric** (mon-oh-MERR-ic) is sometimes used to describe formulas that have hydrolyzed protein or free amino acids as the source of protein. **Polymeric** (POLL-ee-MERR-ic) formulas contain an intact protein source.
monomer = single unit
polymer = chain of units

Some hydrolyzed formulas are called **elemental** or **defined-formula diets** because the nutrients are present in the most elemental or simple form. The term *defined-formula diet* is preferable to the term *elemental diet*.

modular feedings: incomplete formulas that contain specific nutrients, used as supplements.

Osmolality

Osmolality is a measurement of the concentration of molecular and ionic particles in a solution. The greater the number of particles in a solution, the greater the osmolality. The important thing to know about osmolality is that water flows from an area of low osmolality to one of higher osmolality (see pp. 376–377).

The osmolality of normal blood serum is about 300 milliosmoles (mOsm) per liter. The osmolality of formulas ranges from about 250 to over 800 milliosmoles. A formula that approximates the osmolality of the serum is referred to as an isotonic formula. A hypertonic formula has a higher osmolality than serum.

A hypertonic formula in the intestine can cause water to be drawn from in and around the body cells into the intestine. If an individual's body has had

osmolality: the number of molecular and ionic particles (measured in osmoles) per kilogram of water in a solution.

isotonic formula: a formula with an osmolality similar to that of blood serum (300 mOsm).
iso = the same
ton = tension

hypertonic formula: a formula with an osmolality higher than that of blood serum.
hyper = greater, more

time to adapt to the hypertonic solution, this is usually not a problem. However, if adaptation has not occurred, diarrhea, vomiting, cramps, or nausea can result. Therefore, the most desirable formulas are those as near isotonic as possible, all else being equal.

A hydrolyzed protein formula may contain exactly the same amount of protein as an intact formula, but it contains many more particles. Hydrolyzed formulas are therefore higher in osmolality than most intact protein formulas and so are more likely to cause the GI symptoms discussed above.

Residue and Fiber

fiber: the portion of food that is found in the colon because we don't have the enzymes to digest it.

residue: the total amount of material in the colon; it includes undigested food, intestinal secretions, bacteria, and the turnover of intestinal cells.

Dietary fiber is the portion of food that cannot be digested by the human digestive tract. Residue is a combination of undigested and unabsorbed food in the colon. Intestinal secretions, bacteria, and the turnover of intestinal cells also contribute residue. The residue content of the diet is largely responsible for fecal bulk. As you will see in later chapters, people with certain GI disorders need diets that are low in residue. Higher-residue diets may help stimulate normal bowel function in people who do not need low-residue diets. Furthermore, recent studies in rats suggest that certain fibers (pectins) may be fermented in the intestine to short-chain fatty acids that may actually provide a fuel source to the lining of the intestine, enabling it to adapt more readily after large portions of the small bowel have been resected (see Chapter 22).[1]

Since hydrolyzed formulas are almost completely absorbed, they leave little residue in the gut. Protein isolate formulas have a low to moderate residue content.

Other Characteristics

Formulas can be made from many different ingredients. For example, some contain lactose, while others are lactose-free. One formula may derive its protein from a source of higher biological value (see p. 149) than another formula. These characteristics of formulas are important when a formula is chosen for a client.

Another characteristic of different formulas that varies widely is their cost. Costs vary greatly for individual products in different parts of the country and for different hospitals. However, as a general rule, hydrolyzed formulas are more costly than intact formulas, because they require more commercial modification.

No formula is perfect. In general, the more digestible the formula, the higher its cost and osmolality, and the lower its palatability. As a rule of thumb, because hydrolyzed formulas are more costly and more likely than other formulas to cause complications, they should be used only for people who can't digest and absorb nutrients adequately.

Steps in Formula Selection

With so many formulas available, how do you select the best formula for the client? The ideal formula for an individual is one that meets nutrient needs with the least risk of complications and at the least cost. A person benefits from a diet only if energy, protein, carbohydrate, fat, vitamin, and mineral needs are met. People receiving liquid formulas often have altered nutrient needs due to illness, so meeting these needs is important. Furthermore, such a person depends on one food source to meet all nutrient needs.

A formula given orally needs to taste good. As a general guide, the more hydrolyzed a formula and the lower its fat content, the less tasty it will be. However, remember that people's likes and dislikes vary greatly, and what might seem quite unpalatable to you or me might be perfectly acceptable to someone else.

Carefully assess each client before selecting a formula (see Figure 18–4). Some factors to consider in formula selection include:

- The client's digestive and absorptive function.
- The placement of the feeding tube (stomach versus intestine).
- Nutrient requirements.
- Individual tolerances (food allergies and sensitivities).

Let's turn our attention to each of these factors.

Digestive and Absorptive Function

You can narrow the choice of formulas considerably just by determining if a person's GI tract is functioning. To provide a person with appropriate amounts of nutrients will do no good if the nutrients cannot be digested and absorbed.

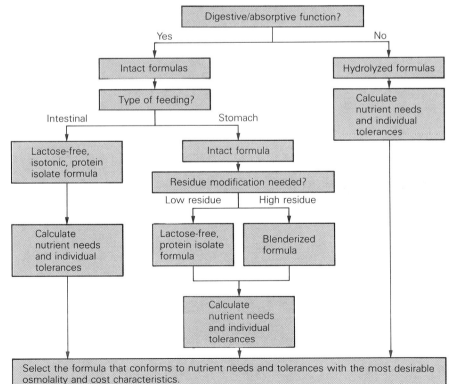

FIGURE 18–4

Narrowing the choice of formulas.

People who don't have a functioning GI tract are not candidates for oral or tube feedings. However, people with minimal GI function may be able to benefit from certain formulas. Therefore, the chemical composition of the formula must be considered.

The next several chapters discuss what diseases cause problems with digestion and absorption. For now, just remember that any person with impaired digestive or absorptive function may need a hydrolyzed formula. If, however, the individual's GI tract is functional, intact formulas are a better choice, since they are generally lower in osmolality, less expensive, and are less likely to cause complications.

Placement of the Feeding Tube

Another factor to consider in formula selection is where the feeding is being delivered. The major concern is for feedings delivered directly into the intestine. These feedings must be easily digested, but they do not have to be hydrolyzed if the GI tract is functional. However, the small intestine is more sensitive than the stomach to hypertonic solutions, so that isotonic feedings are desirable. Isotonic protein isolate formulas work well for intestinal feedings when a hydrolyzed formula is not required.

Nutrient Requirements

A person's energy (carbohydrate and fat), protein, vitamin, major mineral, and trace element requirements will help determine the most appropriate formula. These nutrient needs often are altered considerably in various diseases, as you will see in the chapters that follow.

When you consider nutrients, don't forget water. As a general guideline, adults require from 1,500 to 2,000 milliliters of pure water a day. A person with a high fever may require an additional 500 to 1,500 milliliters a day. Other conditions, such as heavy sweating and some types of kidney disease, may increase water requirements. In other types of kidney disease, as well as in liver and heart disease, the total water may need to be restricted.

The formula itself already contains water. You can figure that formulas that contain 1 kcalorie per milliliter contain about 850 milliliters of water per liter of formula. Any additional water needed can be given between feedings or to rinse out the feeding tube.

A client (J. K.) needs a total of 3,000 ml of a formula per 24 hours to meet her nutrient needs. Therefore, she will need 125 ml every hour to get 3,000 ml for the day.

If a formula contains 850 ml of water per liter of formula and a person is given 3,000 ml of formula, then he will get 2,550 ml water in the feeding solution:

$$\frac{850 \text{ ml}}{1 \text{ l}} \text{ as } \frac{X \text{ ml}}{3 \text{ l}}$$

$$X = 850 \text{ ml} \times 3 = 2,550 \text{ ml}.$$

Many adults who normally tolerate milk become temporarily lactose intolerant following GI surgery or during radiation therapy or chemotherapy. When they are given a formula with lactose, they become bloated and develop cramps and diarrhea. The nurse or dietitian who is alert to this possibility can save such a person much misery and pain by using a formula that is lactose-free.

Individual Tolerances

Individual tolerances must be considered in formula selection. The person with food allergies or food intolerances is given a formula that does not contain the offending substances. Often, lactose-free formulas are desirable. Temporary and permanent lactose intolerances are frequently encountered.

In the final analysis, you really can only make an educated or informed guess about the best formula for an individual. Therefore, it becomes critical to monitor each person's nutrition status and tolerance to the formula to ensure that individual needs are being met. Table 18–4 lists the major steps in monitoring people on tube feedings.

TABLE 18–4

Checklist for Monitoring Clients on Tube Feedings

Before starting a new or intermittent feeding:	Complete a nutrition assessment. Check tube placement. Check residual formula in stomach (if 150 ml, consider possible reasons for delayed gastric emptying).
Every half hour:	Check gravity drip rate, when applicable.
Every hour:	Check pump drip rate, when applicable.
Every two to four hours of continuous feeding:	Check residual.
Every four hours:	Check vital signs, including blood pressure, temperature, pulse, and respiration. Check sugar and acetone in urine; monitoring sugar and acetone can be discontinued after 48 hours if test results are consistently negative in a nondiabetic client. Refill feeding container.
Every eight hours:	Check intake and output. Check specific gravity of urine. Chart client's acceptance of, and tolerance to, tube feeding.
Every day:	Weigh client. Change feeding bag and tubing. Check electrolytes, blood urea nitrogen, and blood glucose daily until stabilized.
Every seven to ten days:	Check all laboratory findings. Reassess nutrition status.
As needed:	Observe client for any undesirable responses to tube feeding; for example, nausea, vomiting, or diarrhea. Check tube placement (for nasogastric placement only). Check nitrogen balance. Check laboratory data. Clean feeding equipment. Chart significant details.

Start the feeding at 50 ml/hour at half strength and then progress the feeding as follows:

- After 8 hours:
  75 ml/hour at half strength.
- After 16 hours:
  100 ml/hour at half strength.
- After 24 hours:
  125 ml/hour at half strength.
- After 36 hours:
  125 ml/hour at full strength.

If our client, J. K., received her formula intermittently six times a day, at each feeding she would need 500 ml of formula.

3,000 ml ÷ 6 feedings = 500 ml/feeding.

If she received the formula only four times a day, she would need 750 ml of formula at each feeding.

3,000 ml ÷ 4 feedings = 750 ml/feeding.

She would probably tolerate this volume of solution very poorly if it were given to her within a few minutes at each feeding.

If J. K. received continuous drip feedings over 24 hours, she would receive 125 ml/hour.

3,000 ml ÷ 24 hours = 125 ml/hour.

If she received the total volume of solution by continuous drip for 16 hours, she would receive 187.5 ml/hour.

3,000 ml ÷ 16 hours = 187.5 ml/hour.

bolus delivery: delivery of a four- to six-hour volume of feeding solution within a few minutes.

intermittent feeding by slow drip: delivery of a four- to six-hour volume of feeding solution over 20 to 30 minutes.

continuous drip administration: delivery of a feeding solution continuously over a 16- to 24-hour period.

Administering a Tube Feeding

People placed on tube feedings often have had surgery or have not eaten for several weeks, and they may not be able to tolerate large volumes or highly concentrated formulas. Therefore, formulas may need to be diluted to one-half or one-third strength (see Figure 18–5) at first. Initially, give the formula slowly, at about 50 milliliters per hour. If the person tolerates the formula, the rate of feeding can be increased by 25 milliliters per hour every 8 to 12 hours. Once the final desired rate has been reached, the strength is increased. If a new rate or strength is not tolerated, you can back up and try increasing it more slowly, giving the person more time to adapt.

In the past, almost all people were placed on diluted formulas when tube feedings were initiated. However, recent studies suggest that in people with normal GI functioning, diluting formula is unnecessary.[2] As a rule of thumb, people who have serum albumin levels that are less than 3.5 grams per 100 milliliters are more likely to have problems tolerating concentrated formulas.[3]

A day's volume of a formula can be given in many ways. For example, a person can be fed four to six times daily. In such a case, the total volume of formula needed for the day is divided by four or six, respectively. Feedings given intermittently allow the client greater freedom of movement between meals. If the amount of formula necessary for each feeding is given within a few minutes, it is called a bolus feeding. Feedings given by this method may be poorly tolerated—they lead to more complaints of abdominal discomfort, nausea, fullness, and cramping. Feedings delivered intermittently (four to six times a day), but allowed to infuse over a longer period (20 to 30 minutes), are often better tolerated. This makes sense. After all, you do not gobble down a meal in just a few minutes, especially when you are not feeling well anyway.

Feedings also can be delivered slowly over a 16- to 24-hour period. This feeding method is called continuous drip. Pumps (similar to those used for delivering intravenous solutions) can be used to ensure that the formula is given slowly. Continuous drip administration is useful for people who have poor tolerance to large volumes of formula. Generally, intestinal feedings (particularly jejunal feedings) are delivered by continuous drip.

Regardless of the method used to deliver a formula, elevate the client's head to at least a 30-degree angle during the feeding and for 30 minutes following an intermittent feeding to minimize the possibility of regurgitation.

Tube Feedings for Infants and Children

Tube feedings are used to nourish children of all ages—from the premature infant to the adolescent. The proper care of a child requires that you remember that a child is not just a small adult. Unlike adults, whose nutrient needs are based on the maintenance of a developed body, children are growing. The infant's GI tract is immature, and intestinal motility is sluggish even in a healthy infant. Therefore, he has a limited capacity to meet nutrient needs. As with all age groups, formula selection and choice of feeding route are determined after a thorough nutrition assessment. The accuracy of the assessment depends on the assessor's knowledge and consideration of the unique characteristics of children.

To work effectively with an infant or child, you must work effectively with the parents or guardians as well. Be sure that loved ones feel comfortable and can communicate openly with you. Parents or guardians are encouraged to participate fully in the child's care. They may be worried about handling the child, fearing that they may cause discomfort or dislodge the feeding tube. Show the parents how to handle the child, and watch them while they try your suggestions. Assure them that their support of the child is important, and allow them to help as much as possible. Stress the importance of their roles in the child's recovery.

Dolls or stuffed toys can be used to explain the tube insertion and feeding procedure to the young child. Usually, very small feeding tubes are used to minimize discomfort. In babies, the use of very small diameter tubes minimizes interference with the baby's airways. The feeding tubes are frequently removed after each feeding in infants. This frees the infant's airways between feedings and reduces the risk that formula will back up into the esophagus and be aspirated into the lungs.

In infants, tubes are often inserted from the mouth to the stomach, rather than through the nose. Babies breathe through their noses, not their mouths. Therefore, tubes inserted through the mouth allow infants to breathe more easily.

Tube feedings for infants are given in very small amounts. The infant's stomach is smaller, and gastric emptying is slower. Aspiration pneumonia, then, can occur more readily if too much formula is in the stomach at one time. In addition, the infant can have difficulty adapting to even minor changes in a

FIGURE 18–5

Formula dilution.

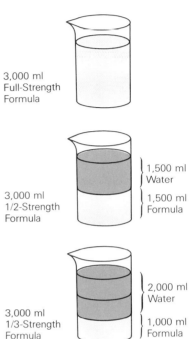

3,000 ml
Full-Strength
Formula

3,000 ml
1/2-Strength
Formula

1,500 ml
Water

1,500 ml
Formula

3,000 ml
1/3-Strength
Formula

2,000 ml
Water

1,000 ml
Formula

A person being fed by tube. This feeding is being delivered by gravity drip.

Tube feedings can also be delivered by pump. A typical setup is shown here.

Parents or guardians actively involved in the care of the hospitalized child feel they are important to a child's recovery.

formula's composition, so the formula's concentration, infusion rate, and volume must be carefully monitored. Changes in any of these formula parameters are made individually, so that the source of any intolerance can be readily identified.

Keep in mind the developmental age of the child at all times. Feeding skills must be mastered at the appropriate age, or it may be difficult for the child to learn the skill at all. When possible, infants are given some of the tube feeding in a bottle or by spoon. The use of a pacifier during a feeding helps maintain an association of sucking and swallowing with eating and fullness. Occupational therapists can help stimulate appropriate development when problems occur in infants who have received long-term tube feedings.

When infusion pumps are used to administer a tube feeding to a young child, special precautions are in order. The bright lights, interesting sounds, and many controls may make the pump seem like a toy.[4] The device should be kept at a safe distance so that the child can't change the flow rate or pull the intravenous pole and infusion device over. The child could be injured, and damage to the pump could result.

The adolescent is more like an adult in tolerating and adapting to a tube feeding. But the teenager's psychological profile can interfere with acceptance of the tube feeding. The teenager may worry about the appearance of the tube and fear that peers will not accept her. These suggestions can help:

- Encourage the teen to be as active as possible.
- Allow teens to dress in their own clothes, when possible. Suggest that favorite things from home be brought to their rooms (posters, stuffed toys, or bulletin boards).
- Explain the tube-feeding procedure and its importance.
- Include the teen in the decision-making process whenever possible. She can help arrange her daily schedule and can help with feedings. In some cases, the teen can rinse out the feeding bag and tubing and refill the feeding bag when necessary.
- Encourage the teen to maintain contact with friends and keep up with hobbies and activities he enjoys.

Above all, be someone the teenager can trust and talk to. This advice, of course, applies to clients of all ages.

Complications Associated with Tube Feedings

The complications most frequently associated with tube feedings often are preventable. People receiving the proper formula, administered correctly, seldom have problems with tube feeding. Major complications can be prevented through careful monitoring. Table 18–5 summarizes problems associated with tube feedings, their causes, and their prevention.

TABLE 18–5

Causes and Prevention of Tube-feeding Complications

Complication	Cause	Prevention
Diarrhea	Bacterial contamination	Take care in preparation, storage, and administration of formula.
	Lactose intolerance	Use lactose-free formula in high-risk clients.
	Hypertonic formula	Dilute formula and increase concentration gradually; use continuous drip administration of formula.
	Low serum albumin	Dilute formula and increase concentration gradually.
	Drug therapy	Use antidiarrheal agents; change drug therapy, if possible.
Dehydration	Excessive diarrhea	See first five items.
	Inadequate fluid intake	Give water.
	Carbohydrate intolerance	Use continuous drip administration of formula; monitor sugar levels in blood and urine; consider administering insulin.
	Excessive protein intake	Monitor blood electrolyte levels.
Aspiration pneumonia	Regurgitation of formula, which is subsequently inhaled into lungs	Use nasoenteric, gastrostomy, or jejunostomy feedings in high-risk clients; use small-diameter transnasal tube; elevate head of bed during feeding; use continuous drip method of delivery.
Vomiting	Obstruction, stomach emptying slowly	Check gastric residual; use continuous drip method of administration.
Nausea, cramps, distension	Obstruction, stomach emptying slowly; intolerance to concentration or volume of formula	Check gastric residual; use continuous drip method of administration; dilute formula, increasing gradually.

Diarrhea

Diarrhea is the most frequently cited complication of tube feedings. Diarrhea can result from a number of causes, including bacterial contamination of the formula, lactose intolerance, hypertonic formulas, low serum albumin, and drug therapy.

Several abbreviations are used to name IV solutions, including:
- D: dextrose.
- W: water.
- NS: normal saline (0.9% sodium chloride solution).

These abbreviations are combined to specify IV solutions as follows:
- D_5W
  Read as: 5% dextrose in water (the subscript following the *D* tells you the percentage of dextrose required).
- $D_{10}W$
  Read as: 10% dextrose in water.
- $D_5$1/2 normal saline
  Read as: 5% dextrose in a 1/2 normal saline solution (0.45% sodium chloride).
- How would you read $D_{50}W$?

peripheral vein: the smaller-diameter veins that bring blood to the extremities (arms and legs).

peripheral total parenteral nutrition (PTPN): the provision of a nutrient solution that meets nutrient needs by peripheral vein.

A typical peripheral TPN solution contains:
- 750 ml of 2.5% amino acid solution.
- 750 ml of 6.25% dextrose solution.
- 1,500 ml of 10% fat emulsion.

maintain fluid and electrolyte, as well as acid-base, balances. For the well-nourished person who is expected to eat within a few days following surgery, simple IV solutions are very useful.

Generally, adults with normally functioning kidneys receive from 2½ to 3½ liters of a 5 percent dextrose solution following a major trauma or surgery. Electrolytes are replaced as needed. Three liters of a 5 percent dextrose solution contribute about 150 grams glucose, or about 510 kcalories per day (see the box, "How to Calculate the Nutrient Content of IV Solutions"). Simple IV solutions are far from complete nutritionally. Given for short periods of time, however, they are not harmful. People who can't eat for long periods of time, those who are malnourished, and those who have high nutrient requirements need more complete solutions.

IV Fat Emulsions and Peripheral Total Parenteral Nutrition

Simple glucose solutions or those solutions containing only amino acids present a major drawback—they fall far short of meeting total nutrient needs. The problem is that the small-diameter peripheral veins become irritated and eventually collapse when highly concentrated nutrient solutions are infused. If less-concentrated solutions were used, it would take 12 to 15 liters of solution a day to deliver all the needed nutrients. This volume is far more than the body can safely handle.

The availability of IV fat emulsions has solved this problem and made it possible to deliver needed nutrients by peripheral vein. An IV fat emulsion makes the difference for two reasons. First, it is a concentrated source of kcalories. Ten percent fat emulsions provide 1.1 kcalories per milliliter, and 20 percent fat emulsions provide 2.0 kcalories per milliliter. Second, IV fat is isotonic to blood and does not irritate the veins the way hypertonic glucose and amino acid solutions do.

IV fat is also important because it provides essential fatty acids, thus preventing deficiencies. IV fat can safely provide up to 60 percent of the total daily energy requirement.

The use of IV fat, amino acids, and dextrose given by peripheral vein to meet all energy needs is called *peripheral total parenteral nutrition (PTPN)*. IV vitamins, minerals, and trace elements can also be given to provide for other nutrient needs.

A typical peripheral TPN solution delivers about 2,500 kcalories per day and provides about 90 grams of amino acids. More than half of the kcalories are contributed by IV fat. Clients who are candidates for peripheral TPN include those who need only short-term nutrition support (about 7 to 14 days), people with normal renal function who do not have excessive energy requirements, people in whom inserting an IV catheter into a central vein might be difficult, and people on oral or tube feedings who may need additional nutrients.

Some people react adversely to IV fat emulsions. Immediate reactions may include fever, warmth, chills, backache, chest pain, allergic reactions, dizziness, blurred vision, and lymphocytosis (excess number of lymph cells). Irritation and inflammation of the vein are also possible. After long-term administration, the most commonly observed adverse effect is the deposition of a brown pigment in certain liver cells. These pigments disappear after parenteral therapy is stopped, and their effect on liver function is unknown. Other effects of long-term administration may include enlarged liver and spleen, and a decreased number of blood platelets and white blood cells.

TPN by Central Vein

Another method used to meet all nutrient needs by vein is called *central total parenteral nutrition (TPN)*. When the term *TPN* is used alone, it refers to TPN by central vein. In central TPN, the IV catheter is surgically placed in a large-diameter central vein (see Figure 18–6). Almost a gallon of blood rushes through one such vein, the superior vena cava, each minute. Here, highly concentrated solutions can be quickly diluted. By the time these solutions reach the peripheral veins, they are not irritating.

The most important advantage of central TPN, then, is that much more concentrated solutions of nutrients can be delivered. People who cannot or should not be fed through the GI tract are candidates for TPN; it is indicated whenever long-term parenteral nutrition will be required, when nutrient requirements are high, or when people are severely malnourished. Some specific conditions that may necessitate its use are listed in Table 18–6. The actual need for TPN must be determined by the individual's medical and nutrition needs.

total parenteral nutrition (TPN): a method of meeting all nutrient needs by using large-diameter central veins. Another word for TPN is **intravenous hyperalimentation (IVH).**
Hyperalimentation means feeding higher-than-normal amounts of nutrients either orally, enterally, or parenterally.
hyper = greater than normal
alimentation = the process of providing nutrients to the body

central veins: the larger-diameter veins located close to the heart (see Figure 18–6).

IV catheter: the thin tube inserted into a vein through which nutrient solutions or medications can be given directly.

FIGURE 18–6

The central veins used for TPN. The superior vena cava is one of the largest-diameter veins and is usually used for giving TPN solutions. When it cannot be used, the internal jugular vein is the next choice, followed by the external jugular vein. Can you see why?

TABLE 18–6

Possible Indications for TPN by Central Vein

Severe protein-kcalorie malnutrition.
Nutritional repletion necessary to improve response to surgical or medical therapy.
Prolonged vomiting.
Prolonged diarrhea.
Anorexia nervosa.
GI tract obstruction.
Prolonged absence of intestinal peristalsis (ileus).
Enterocutaneous fistulas.
Short bowel syndrome.
Inflammatory bowel disease.
Cancer.
Burns.
Trauma.
Pancreatitis.

Note: These indications are not absolute. Occasionally, clients with these indications can be fed successfully by tube or orally.

Ideally, the person should not reach a severely depleted state before TPN is initiated. It is much easier to maintain nutrition status than to try to replenish lost nutrient stores with TPN.

The TPN Solution

One liter of a typical TPN solution contains 25% dextrose and 3.5% amino acids. Often, 3 l of the solution are given daily and provide 3,000 kcal and 105 g protein.

The actual concentrations of amino acids and dextrose that compose the final TPN solution are determined by each person's unique nutrient needs. People who are extremely malnourished or highly stressed (by burns or infection) require higher levels of protein and kcalories than moderately malnourished or mildly stressed individuals.

Traditionally, TPN solutions provide energy needs primarily from dextrose. IV fat is given periodically (two 500–milliliter bottles per week) to meet essential fatty acid requirements. Currently, however, the trend is to use IV fat emulsions more frequently as a kcalorie source.[9] This is particularly true for people in respiratory failure, because oxidation of glucose in the body results in an increased output of carbon dioxide and can lead to respiratory acidosis.

respiratory acidosis: a condition of too much acid in the blood caused by failure of the lungs to ventilate properly. Excess acids are normally released from the lungs during exhalation; diseased lungs, however, are unable to perform this function adequately.

In addition to dextrose, amino acids, and fat, electrolytes and vitamins are added to the TPN solution. The normal ranges of requirements for these nutrients are listed in Table 18–7. Trace elements should also be added to the solution, since deficiencies can otherwise arise. Trace element deficiencies have been reported in people maintained on TPN for long periods of time. Although exact requirements are unknown, Table 18–8 lists suggested trace element additions to the TPN solution. Essential fatty acid requirements are met by giving

TABLE 18–7

Normal Range of Daily Vitamin and Mineral Requirements during TPN

Vitamin[a]	Recommended Amount
Vitamin A (IU)	3,300
Vitamin D (IU)	200
Vitamin E (IU)	10
Vitamin C (mg)	5
Folacin (μg)	400
Niacin (mg)	40
Riboflavin (mg)	3.6
Thiamin (mg)	3.0
Vitamin B_6 (mg)	4.0
Vitamin B_{12} (μg)	5.0
Pantothenic acid (mg)	15
Biotin (μg)	60

Mineral[b]	Normal Range
Sodium (mEq)	60 to 150
Potassium (mEq)	70 to 150
Chloride (mEq)	Equal to sodium
Calcium (mEq)	0.2 to 0.3/kg
Magnesium (mEq)	0.35 to 0.45/kg
Phosphorus (mmol)	7 to 10/1,000 kcal

[a]Data from American Medical Association, Department of Foods and Nutrition, Multivitamin preparations for parenteral use: A statement by the Nutrition Advisory Group, *Journal of Parenteral and Enteral Nutrition* 3 (1979): 258–262.
[b]Data from J. P. Grant, *Handbook of Total Parenteral Nutrition* (Philadelphia: Saunders, 1980), p. 98.

IV fat periodically or by applying corn or safflower oil (10 to 15 milliliters) to the skin three times a day.[10] Other possible additions to the TPN solution include:

- Albumin, to increase serum albumin concentration.
- Heparin, to prevent clots from forming on the IV catheter, which might obstruct the flow of the TPN solution.
- Insulin, to help regulate blood sugar levels.

Adding albumin, heparin, and insulin directly to the TPN solution is a controversial practice. Not all institutions consider these substances TPN additives. Where they are used, only additives needed by each individual are given.

Insertion and Care of the TPN Catheter

The insertion of an IV catheter for TPN requires a surgical procedure. However, a qualified physician may insert the catheter at bedside rather than in an operating room. The client generally is awake but is given a local anesthetic; unnecessary apprehension can be avoided by explaining the procedure to the client.

TABLE 18–8

Guidelines for Trace Element Use in Parenteral Nutrition

Trace Element	Suggested IV Intake	Comments
Zinc	2.5 to 4.0 mg	Add 2.0 mg for adult in acute catabolic state; add 12.2 mg/l of small bowel fluid lost; add 17.1 mg/kg of stool or ileostomy output.
Copper	0.5 to 1.5 mg	
Chromium	10 to 15 μg	Add 20 μg for stable adult with intestinal losses.
Manganese	0.15 to 0.80 mg	

Source: Adapted from American Medical Association, Department of Foods and Nutrition, Guidelines for essential trace element preparations for parenteral use, a statement by an expert panel, *Journal of the American Medical Association* 241 (1979): 2051–2054.

Because of the proximity of the catheter insertion site to the heart, the danger that disease-causing microorganisms will enter the bloodstream and heart is great. The dressing around the catheter site is changed frequently to keep the site clean.

The term used to describe the presence of disease-causing bacteria in the blood is **sepsis**. Sepsis is a major complication of TPN.

Administering the TPN Solution

A TPN feeding is started slowly to give the person time to adapt to the high glucose concentration and osmolality of the TPN solution. During the first 24 hours, 1 or 2 liters of TPN solution are infused by continuous drip. An infusion pump is used to ensure a slow rate of delivery. Electrolytes and blood and urine glucose are monitored periodically. If the blood glucose level is unacceptably high and a high urine glucose level exists, the cause is investigated and treated. After the first 24 hours, the infusion rate is increased by 1 liter a day until the desired volume of solution is given within 24 hours.

Changes in the infusion rate can cause significant hypoglycemia or hyperglycemia, which can lead to coma, convulsions, and even death, so all changes should be made gradually and with caution. When the administration of solution gets behind or ahead of schedule, the drip rate should be adjusted to the correct hourly infusion rate, but no attempt should be made to speed up or slow down the drip rate to meet the originally ordered volume. When a person is being taken off TPN, the infusion rate of the solution must be gradually tapered off; otherwise, hypoglycemia might occur. Table 18–9 lists the many types of complications associated with TPN, and Table 18–10 summarizes how people on TPN are monitored.

cyclic parenteral nutrition: the periodic administration of standard TPN solutions.

Another way of administering TPN is called cyclic parenteral nutrition; this method of periodic administration of standard TPN solutions may help prevent a problem that has been observed when TPN is given continuously. When a person receives a TPN solution by continuous drip, insulin levels stay high. In turn, the individual can't mobilize fat stores for energy, and eventually, fat may be deposited in the liver. Studies are currently being conducted to determine if cyclic infusion of TPN might correct this problem.

A person on cyclic parenteral nutrition receives a standard TPN solution for 14 to 16 hours a day, and then only amino acids and fat for 8 to 10 hours a

TABLE 18-9

Complications Associated with TPN

Complications Related to Catheter Insertion or Care

Fluid in the chest (hydrothorax).
Air or gas in the chest (pneumothorax).
Blood in the chest (hemothorax).
Catheter tip broken off, obstructing blood flow (catheter embolism).
Air leaking into catheter, obstructing blood flow (air embolism).
Hole or tear made in heart by catheter tip (myocardial perforation).
Catheter inadvertently placed in subclavian artery (arterial puncture).
Improperly positioned catheter tip.
Sepsis.
Blood clot (thrombosis).

Metabolic Complications

Elevated blood glucose (hyperglycemia).
Low blood glucose (hypoglycemia).
Dehydration.
Coma from excessive glucose load (hyperosmolar, hyperglycemic, or nonketotic coma).
Low blood magnesium (hypomagnesemia).
Low blood calcium (hypocalcemia).
High blood phosphorus (hyperphosphatemia).
Low blood phosphorus (hypophosphatemia).
Low blood potassium (hypokalemia).
Essential fatty acid deficiency.
Trace element deficiencies.
High blood ammonia levels (hyperammonemia).
Acid-base imbalances.
Elevated liver enzymes.

day. Cyclic administration more closely approximates a normal diet, since during sleep there usually is no nutrient intake. Liver function returns to normal when this form of TPN is used. Additionally, it seems that fewer kcalories are necessary for maintaining nitrogen balance, probably because the person uses body fat for energy.

Parenteral Nutrition in Infants and Children

Earlier we discussed the special concerns that arise when infants and children are fed by tube. Many of these same concerns arise when infants and children

TABLE 18–10

Guidelines for Monitoring People on TPN

Frequency of Monitoring	Clinical or Biochemical Parameter
Every four to six hours	Urinary glucose
	Vital signs (respiration, pulse, temperature)
Daily	Weight
	Strict intake and output
	Urine specific gravity
Daily until stable, and then two to three times weekly	Serum glucose
	Serum electrolytes
	Blood urea nitrogen
Weekly	Nutrition assessment
	Serum protein
	Serum calcium
	Serum phosphorus
	Serum ammonia
	Complete blood count

are fed intravenously. For example, you must work with the child's parents or guardians and actively involve them in the child's care. Again, developmental feeding skills appropriate for age are a concern. Infusion pumps used to deliver IV solutions must be kept at a safe distance from the child. The suggestions given earlier for helping the teenager adapt to a tube feeding apply equally to the teenager fed intravenously.

The infant fed intravenously poses additional problems. The exact nutrient needs of each infant, especially of premature infants, are difficult to determine. To give a synthetic mixture that will adequately promote growth without overloading an immature system is a challenge. Such mixtures may not contain substances that naturally occur in foods that are needed by infants, but have not yet been identified.

The renal system of an infant is immature, and it cannot adjust to changes in the blood as rapidly as an adult's renal system. Furthermore, an infant's body has a much larger percentage of fluid, so changes in the fluid compartment of the infant's body can cause major problems. When a feeding is delivered directly into a vein of an infant, then, it is easy to see that too much or too little of any solution constituent can cause a problem. Too much fluid can quickly stress the infant's immature renal system; too little fluid can quickly cause dehydration. Too much glucose can rapidly lead to hyperglycemia, with severe consequences; if the feeding is discontinued rapidly or if the tube becomes dislodged, hypoglycemia can be quickly precipitated. The list of such possible complications could go on for virtually every substance found in the IV solution. Possible sources of all complications should be considered.

To feed an infant by the IV route is a challenge.

Transitional/Combination Feedings

Once the problem causing the need for tube feedings or IV nutrition has resolved, the client is gradually weaned onto an oral diet while the volume of the special feeding is tapered. Care must be taken to ensure that the individual's nutrient needs will continue to be met. For example, a person on a tube feeding should be eating adequate amounts of food by mouth before the tube feeding is discontinued. The person can eat "around the tube" as the volume of the tube feeding is gradually tapered off. In many cases, the person can drink the same formula that was earlier given by tube.

The transition from IV feeding to an oral diet can be accomplished in different ways. One way is to place the client on a tube feeding. The volume of the IV nutrition solution is decreased as an increased volume of tube feeding is tolerated. If the tube feeding is not tolerated, the person can still rely on TPN to meet nutrient needs. The person can also be weaned from the TPN solution while oral intake is increased, avoiding the use of a tube.

Study Questions

1. What is the difference between an administrative and a clinical dietitian? Which type of dietitian would you call to talk to a client you thought was malnourished?
2. What information should you know about the foodservice system in the facility where you work?
3. What is the primary goal of diet therapy, and how is this goal achieved?
4. What are modified diets? How are they used? Where can you get information about modified diets in the facility where you work?
5. Who is responsible for prescribing a client's diet? How should the diet be ordered?
6. Why are meals and food important to the client in the hospital? Which clients are of particular concern if they are not eating?
7. How can you help prevent problems with food? Where can you turn for help if a client has a problem you are unable to solve?
8. How and why should food trays be checked before they are delivered to a client's room?
9. Describe some things you can do to help a sick child to eat.
10. What can you do to encourage a client to drink liquid supplements? What are complete formulas? What are blenderized formulas? What are intact formulas? What are hydrolyzed formulas and defined formula diets?
11. What are tube feedings? How are feeding tubes placed?
12. What factors are considered in selecting an appropriate formula for a tube feeding? How does the digestive and absorptive function of the client narrow the formula choice? How does the feeding route influence formula selection? How do nutrient needs and individual tolerances affect the choice of formula?
13. Discuss the ways in which tube feedings can be administered to clients.
14. What are the major complications of tube feedings? What are their causes? How are they prevented or corrected?
15. What special characteristics of children must be considered when an infant or child is fed by tube? Why are feeding tubes usually removed after each feeding when an infant is tube fed? How can an adolescent who is being fed by tube be helped to accept the feeding situation?
16. Describe the differences between routine IV solutions, peripheral TPN solutions, and central TPN solutions. When is each type used?
17. How have IV fat emulsions made it possible to meet maintenance nutrient requirements by vein?
18. What are the components of a typical TPN solution? What other additives may be present? How many kcalories are in 1 liter of a TPN solution containing 25 percent dextrose and 5 percent amino acids?
19. How are TPN catheters inserted? How is a TPN feeding initiated? Stopped? Why?
20. Describe some ways in which a person on tube feedings or parenteral nutrition can be weaned to ordinary table foods.

Total Parenteral Nutrition

Mr. Small has been admitted to the hospital for a diagnostic workup. He has been steadily losing weight. He appears emaciated, and states that he can't swallow and has lost his appetite. He was afraid to come to the hospital and has waited a long time before checking in. After a thorough examination, Mr. Small has been found to have an obstruction in his esophagus. The nutrition assessment reveals severe PCM. Surgery will be required as soon as possible. Mr. Small is placed on central TPN prior to surgery. He progresses well, gains weight, and undergoes surgery about two weeks after admission. During surgery, a feeding jejunostomy is made.

1. What factors in Mr. Small's history indicate the need for central TPN?
2. How would you explain the need for TPN to Mr. Small?
3. Is the placement of a feeding jejunostomy during surgery a good idea? Why or why not?

About two days after surgery, Mr. Small begins to receive feedings through the jejunostomy. His digestive and absorptive capacity are intact.
4. Specifically, what type of formula would you recommend for Mr. Small's tube feedings?
5. How does the feeding route influence your selection of formula?
6. How would you begin the tube feeding? How would you progress it? How would you deliver it?
7. When should Mr. Small be taken off central TPN? How should this be accomplished?
8. After several weeks, Mr. Small is ready to take some foods by mouth. How does this affect his tube feeding?

Notes

1. M. J. Koruda and coauthors, The effect of a pectin-supplemented elemental diet on intestinal adaptation to massive small bowel resection, *Journal of Parenteral and Enteral Nutrition* 10 (1986): 343–350.

2. P. P. Keohane and coauthors, Relation between osmolality of diet and gastrointestinal side effects in enteral nutrition, *British Medical Journal* 288 (1984): 678–680.

3. J. L. Rombeau, Advances in enteral feeding, an address presented at the Georgia Dietetic Association Annual Meeting, 17 July 1986.

4. J. S. Paine, Practical aspects of nasogastric feeding in pediatric patients from a ward nursing perspective, *Nutritional Support Services* 6 (1986): 11–14.

5. K. R. Anderson and coauthors, Bacterial contamination of tube-feeding formulas, *Journal of Parenteral and Enteral Nutrition* 8 (1984): 673–678.

6. J. D. Welsh, Diet therapy in adult lactose malabsorption: Present practices, *American Journal of Clinical Nutrition* 31 (1978): 592–596.

7. E. L. Brennan, Albumin: A role in nutritional support? *Nutritional Support Services* 6 (1986): 15.

8. N. Metheny, P. Eisenberg, and M. Spies, Monitoring patients with nasally placed feeding tubes, *Heart Lung* 14 (1985): 285–286.

9. H. Gilder, Parenteral nourishment of patients undergoing surgical or traumatic stress, *Journal of Parenteral and Enteral Nutrition* (1986): 88–99.

10. J. P. Grant, *Handbook of Total Parenteral Nutrition* (Philadelphia: Saunders, 1980), p. 138.

The Nutrition Support Team

Eight o-clock Wednesday morning: nutrition support rounds. The core members of the nutrition support team (a physician, a dietitian, a nurse, and a pharmacist) are discussing all clients who are receiving special nutrition support. Mrs. A is on TPN after surgery; Mr. B has a broken jaw and is on tube feedings; Ms. C is receiving an IV solution. The nutrition support team helps ensure that the hospital staff provides safe and appropriate nutrition support.

The client's nutritional health is the focus of all the team members' efforts. The client is a team member, too; the client's cooperation is necessary to successful implementation of a nutrition care plan.

Functions of a Nutrition Support Team

The nutrition support team performs many important functions. Team members identify people who may be malnourished or at risk nutritionally by using nutrition assessment techniques. Once these individuals have been identified, the team members serve as consultants. Furthermore, team members serve as a nutrition information resource to the hospital staff—answering questions and solving problems as they arise.

Team members also monitor all clients on special nutrition support. They maintain records of each client's progress and review the benefits and complications that arise from the special nutrition support measures taken.

Nutrition support team members also must keep abreast of new developments

The team's goal is safe and effective nutrition support.

in their field. Team members analyze new products and review current research. This enables them to provide optimal care, and to ensure cost control.

Each health professional possesses specialized knowledge. Working as a team permits them to integrate this knowledge, so that the client receives the benefits of their combined expertise. Team members also benefit—their jobs

are made easier, because they learn how each other team member functions, and in so doing can utilize their co-workers maximally, saving themselves time.

The Physician

The director of the nutrition support team is generally a physician. The physician is responsible for:

- Supervising the activities of other team members.
- Developing guidelines for the safe use of nutrition support.
- Monitoring the rate of complications and, when possible, correcting problems that arise.
- Conducting in-hospital educational and training programs for the professional staff.

Additionally, the physician is available as a consultant to other physicians, in which case the physician becomes involved with direct client management. During nutrition support rounds, the physician oversees the discussion and review of each person receiving special support and makes recommendations as appropriate.

The Dietitian

The dietitian has an obvious role as the nutrition expert on the team. The dietitian determines nutrient requirements and translates the physician's diet orders into food or feedings.

Generally, the dietitian is directly responsible for assessing the client's nutrition status. The dietitian often measures, calculates, records, and evaluates nutrition status parameters. Sometimes the dietitian supervises others who gather the data needed to make a nutrition assessment.

The dietitian must have a complete and thorough knowledge of liquid formulas in order to determine which products will best meet the requirements of people who need them. For people who will be fed by tube, the dietitian recommends the correct formula, administration schedule, and appropriate feeding tube. He should be familiar with all enteral feeding equipment so that he can answer questions if they arise. The dietitian recommends alternative formulas and/or administration schedules when the client has trouble tolerating a feeding regimen.

The dietitian helps people on special nutrition support to understand and cope with their unique feeding situations. The dietitian visits the clients daily, continuously assessing their nutrient intakes and nutrition status. The dietitian actively works with the individuals to ease the transition from parenteral nutrition or tube feeding to oral intake. The dietitian also assists in selecting and training clients for home parenteral and enteral nutrition programs. Whenever possible, the dietitian makes home visits to all clients receiving tube feedings or special formulas orally.

The dietitian provides in-service training for other dietitians and nurses on such topics as nutrition assessment, the correct techniques of formula administration and care, and formula selection. The dietitian also acts as a liaison between the dietary department and the nutrition support team.

The Nurse
The nurse on a nutrition support team plays a central role in client care management and client relationships. She explains nutrition support techniques to clients and their families. This includes explaining the need for special nutrition support, as well as describing catheter or transnasal tube insertion. When clients go home on special nutrition support, the nurse assumes the primary responsibility for teaching them how to follow their programs. The nurse also coordinates discharge from the hospital, being sure the person has all the supplies and equipment needed. The nurse makes arrangements for follow-up care, if necessary, and is usually the person available 24 hours a day to answer the questions of people receiving home nutrition support.

For clients on parenteral nutrition, the nurse ensures that the proper techniques of catheter care are followed. In some hospitals, the nutrition support nurse inserts transnasal tubes for people on enteral support. In other facilities, this nurse supervises the staff nurses to answer their questions and prevent complications. Like other members of the nutrition support team, the nurse assists in monitoring clients, looking out for mechanical or metabolic complications. The nurse also administers skin tests and assesses reactions to them.

An important function of the nutrition support nurse is to act as a liaison between the team and the rest of the nursing staff. The nurse teaches the staff nurses, as a group and individually, the rationale for special nutrition support and the techniques needed to administer it. The nurse also assists in training physicians and other concerned health care professionals.

The Pharmacist
The pharmacist on the nutrition support team ensures that IV fluids are prepared correctly and provides training for the hospital staff who will be handling these fluids. The pharmacist must develop a knowledge of available nutrient solutions and should be able to assist in writing IV fluid orders, formulate nutrient infusions that are not commercially available, and detect any stability problems in IV solutions.

The pharmacist plays a key role in pointing out possible nutrient-drug interactions. This team member also shares in the responsibility of monitoring clients, helps train individuals for home parenteral nutrition, and teaches concerned health care professionals about nutrition support techniques.

Other Team Members
Other health care professionals can be an important part of the health care team. The physical therapist can provide an individualized exercise program to enhance skeletal muscle protein synthesis or mineral uptake by bone, and can help the client gain independence by developing muscular strength. The social worker provides practical and emotional support, particularly for people on home nutrition support programs. He helps find funding and social services for individuals who need assistance. Staff, IV, and infection-control nurses may also participate whenever they have problems or suggestions regarding nutrition support.

How the Team Approach Works
The actual members of the nutrition support team and their duties vary considerably in different hospitals. Many times, duties overlap. For example, the dietitian and nurse may both do nutrition assessments, insert nasogastric tubes, or administer skin tests. As pointed out, all team members monitor and visit clients on special nutrition support.

One research study demonstrated the benefits of the team approach to nutrition support. The risk of complications from TPN decreases when a team is used to implement and monitor appropriate TPN techniques.[1] This decrease in complications means that people can be maintained more safely on TPN and that hospital costs will be reduced.

Nutrition support rounds are just about over. The physician reports that Mrs. A is ready to go home tomorrow. She has been weaned from the TPN solution and gradually has increased her oral intake. Thanks to the dietitian's suggestion that Mr. B begin to eat "around the tube," he is now eating a regular diet. Ms. C's problem with an infusion pump was noted by an alert nurse, and this prevented hyperglycemia. The pharmacist described an easy solution to a problem the team was having with fluid orders.

The old adage that "two heads are better than one" is most appropriate to understanding the team approach. Many eyes are available to see a problem, many brains are available to seek a solution. Teamwork works.

NOTES
1. A. E. Nehme, Nutritional support of the hospitalized patient: The team concept, *Journal of the American Medical Association* 243 (1980): 1906–1908.

HIGHLIGHT EIGHTEEN B

Special Nutrition Support at Home

Mrs. Reed has been hospitalized for over 14 months. She suffers from Crohn's disease and has had repeated operations to remove parts of her small intestine. Crohn's disease is an inflammation of the small intestine that frequently leads to malabsorption (see Chapter 22). When Mrs. Reed was first admitted to the hospital she was severely malnourished, and the repeated operations have put a great stress on her body. An abnormal opening, or fistula, has formed between her small intestine and skin. When she takes food by mouth, drainage from the fistula increases, which can cause serious fluid and electrolyte disturbances. Mrs. Reed was placed on central TPN, and since then, her medical condition and nutrition status have steadily improved. At various times during her hospitalization, oral intake has been tried, but each time her condition has worsened, and she has had to go back on TPN.

From a medical standpoint, Mrs. Reed is stable and could probably manage well at home. She is in the hospital primarily to receive TPN. Mrs. Reed is depressed about staying in the hospital, and she and her family are eager to have her go home. The nutrition support team (see Highlight 18A) has been asked to evaluate her for a home parenteral nutrition (HPN) program.

Since the first report of a person sent home successfully on HPN in 1969,[1] the use of HPN has expanded rapidly. The number of people benefitting from these programs continues to grow, and health care professionals who work with home parenteral and enteral nutrition (HPEN) are gaining valuable experience to improve the quality of special nutrition home care. Although the exact number of people on HPEN programs is unknown, it is estimated that from 2,000 to 5,000 people are on HPN, and from 15,000 to 20,000 are on HEN (home enteral nutrition).[2]

Overview of HPEN

The goals of HPEN must be individualized to meet each person's unique requirements. One person may require HPEN for a short time until a medical condition stabilizes. Another may require HPEN permanently.

In any case, one objective of HPEN, as with TPN and tube feedings in the hospital, is to maintain or achieve adequate nutrition status. However, HPEN has an added dimension; it permits a person to get special nutrition support at home in familiar surroundings. If you have ever been in the hospital yourself, or taken a long trip for that matter, you probably remember what comfort and relaxation you experience when you return to your own bed, can get things when you need them, and know where things are. The familiarty of home is comforting.

In some cases, people who require HPEN can resume many activities such as going to work, driving, playing sports, and many more. In general, HPEN allows people the opportunity to lead more normal lives.

An additional benefit of HPEN is cost savings. It is less expensive to maintain a person on parenteral or tube feedings when that person or the family assumes responsibilities formerly performed by hospital staff. On the average, HPN costs about half of what the care would cost in the hospital, whereas in HEN, costs are reduced by 75 percent.[3]

Selection of Candidates for HPEN

Members of the nutrition support team determine which people are candidates for HPEN. In addition to medical considerations, the person's psychological profile and financial resources (particularly for HPN) are considered. Furthermore, the hospital and staff must have the resources to provide appropriate training for the client. Finally, the client must have access to the equipment, supplies, and professional support that are necessary for a successful HPEN program.

The person on HPEN and the people directly involved in the person's care must have stable personalities and be able to rationally handle problems as they arise. Severe consequences could result if a depressed or unstable client on HPN mixed her formula incorrectly or improperly cared for the catheter site.

The HPEN candidate or those who will care for him must be intellectually capable of learning the techniques of HPEN and understanding complications that might arise. Many professionals agree that a partner who is firmly committed, stable, and highly motivated to assist the person in the HPN program is most beneficial.[4]

Although home care may be less costly than hospital care, HPEN, particularly HPN, is still expensive. Many people could not afford such a program without help from private

Recently, interest in the possibility of third party reimbursement for HPEN has increased significantly as more and more hospitals offer HPEN programs and the benefits of such programs become apparent. (Third party reimbursement refers to a party, other than the client or the hospital, that pays for some of the client's expenses. Private insurance, Medicare, and Medicaid are examples.) Such reimbursement is often essential for the client who could otherwise not afford HPEN. Health care professionals share the responsibility for carefully documenting a client's need for HPEN in order for the client to receive reimbursement for some expenses. Areas that each health care professional should deal with in order to increase the likelihood of third party reimbursement include the following:[6]

- The medical justification for the use of TPN or tube feedings must be stated and should make it clear that the client's medical condition precludes the use of the GI tract for nourishment. In the case of tube feedings, a specific reason why nourishment cannot be taken by mouth must be given.
- The reason why special nutrition support will be necessary for at least 90 days must be clearly stated.
- The rationale for the particular course of treatment must be justified. For example, for a client on tube feedings, nutrient needs and the formula necessary to meet these needs should be specified. If additional equipment, such as a feeding pump, is necessary, the justification for its use must be related to the client's specific condition. Rather than stating that a feeding pump is necessary because it delivers formula more accurately, the justification should state that the client was unable to tolerate enteral formula when it was not delivered by pump.
- The physician must recertify the client's continuing need for nutrition support every 90 days.

Although the physician is ultimately responsible for the report of a client's need for special nutrition support at home, all health care professionals involved in home programs need to understand the mechanics behind third party reimbursement. Be prepared to provide the necessary information to the physician to help ensure that clients who qualify for home nutrition support receive as much financial support as possible.

insurance, Medicare, or Medicaid. Reimbursement for medical services from these agencies is more likely for clients receiving HPN as opposed to HEN.[5] Even with such support, the person will still have many expenses. Occasionally, volunteer groups or private donations can help supplement the client's resources.

Training the Individual for HPEN

Not all hospitals, even those with nutrition support teams, are capable of training clients for HPEN. Hospital personnel may not have been trained in the techniques of HPEN or there may not be enough qualified instructors to teach clients and make home visits. The quality and safe use of HPEN depend on the client's complete understanding of the HPEN program.

Clients on HPN must learn how to administer the HPN solution, as well as how to care for the catheter. Some clients also mix their own HPN solutions. If they do, they must be carefully trained in the proper mixing methods and in using aseptic techniques.

During the training period, clients and their families are made aware of catheter-related and metabolic complications and are taught what steps to take if they occur. Health care professionals train clients in the technical aspects of HPN, prepare them psychologically and physically for the transition from hospital to home, and help them work out systems for fitting HPN into their home schedules. In much the same way, candidates for HEN are thoroughly trained in the mixing and administration of tube feedings and in the management of complications.

Candidates for HPEN are trained while they are still in the hospital. The client, or the person who will care for the client, must be able to assume responsibility for the client's care before discharge from the hospital. Practicing in the hospital gives the client a chance to try the system out with help nearby, if needed.

Once at home, the person must be able to return to the training center or the physician for follow-up and be visited regularly by a registered nurse who has received HPEN training. A registered nurse or physician must also be available 24 hours a day to answer questions and to handle emergencies. Ideally, a dietitian will visit the client regularly to assess nutrition status and to recommend adjustments in enteral feeding programs.

The client must have access to the supplies necessary to maintain an HPEN program. Generally, supplies are obtained through the hospital or a pharmacy. Numerous commercial supply services are available to provide supplies and equipment directly to the client's home. If the client travels, supplies can be sent to other locations.

How HPN Works

Different types of HPN programs are in current use. Ideally, clients are given as much responsibility for their own care as they can handle. For example, a client who is capable of mixing the solutions and changing the catheter dressings is trained to do so. Typically, family members also learn the techniques, so that they can assist in the procedures whenever necessary.

A special type of catheter often is inserted for HPN; it enters the subclavian vein but is tunneled under the skin and eventually exits near the middle of the chest (see Figure H18B–1). The use of this technique makes it possible for the client to see the catheter site and to inspect it for changes, as well as to perform dressing changes.

Another method for infusing HPN solutions that is quickly gaining popularity is the subcutaneous port. Unlike a typical catheter that has an outside portion exposed, the port is totally implanted under the skin. Totally implanted devices appear to be associated with a lower infection rate, and they do not require a dressing except when the nutrient infusion is being delivered.[7] The port is cosmetically superior (an advantage for the adolescent), and it results in less restriction of activity (an advantage for young children and other active people). However, disadvantages are also associated with the subcutaneous port. Each use of the port requires a fresh skin puncture, which can be painful. It is also more difficult to surgically implant the port.[8]

The most common method of nutrient administration is for the client

FIGURE H18B–1

Placement of an HPN catheter. In this case, the catheter is tunneled under the skin before going into the subclavian vein; in other cases, the catheter may enter the subclavian directly. The catheter has a Dacron cuff; connective tissue from the person's skin grows into this cuff and helps hold it in place.

to use an infusion pump set at a rate that delivers the total volume of solution needed for the day within 8 to 12 hours. Most people can tolerate solutions delivered this way.[9] The total volume of solution can be placed in large-capacity IV bags so that the client can infuse the solution while sleeping or at any other convenient time. This method of delivery allows freedom of movement during much of the day.

The client starts the solution slowly to avoid hyperglycemia and tapers it at the end of the feeding to avoid hypoglycemia. Each time the client disconnects the IV tubing, heparin is injected into the catheter to prevent clotting.

For people who cannot tolerate an 8- to 12-hour infusion rate, nutrients are infused over 24 hours. Those who are ambulatory can benefit from a

FIGURE H18B–2

Lightweight vest containing a small pump and IV bags so that the individual on a continuous IV infusion is free from machines.

lightweight vest that holds a small pump and IV bags. This system allows the client to move around freely with little inconvenience (see Figure H18B–2).

Some people prepare their own HPN solutions from bottles of IV dextrose and amino acids. Others receive their bottles premixed. Of course, the premixed bottles are more costly, but they are advantageous when the client's (or family member's) ability to correctly mix the solution is questionable.

How Do People on HPN Cope?

Several social and psychological problems accompany the use of HPN.[10] These problems must be recognized and resolved to successfully implement an HPN program. Problems common to people on HPN include depression, delirium, drug dependency, grief, and anxiety.[11] People on HPN must learn to cope with their inability to eat or drink normally and their dependency on a machine for survival.

However, many people in successful HPN programs have a reasonable quality of life.[12] HPN allows people to resume many activities, including employment, sexual activity, recreation, swimming, social activity, and travel. Women on HPN successfully carry and deliver babies. Students return to college. One person on HPN was quoted as saying, "Do I miss the taste of real food? Sure. But you get used to it. Look at the alternative. Ten years ago I would have been dead of starvation."[13]

Home Enteral Nutrition

HEN programs are similar to HPN programs in many ways. HEN is the choice of feeding method for the person who must continue special nutrition support at home.[14] Enteral nutrition preserves normal bowel function, it is simpler to prepare and deliver, it is less expensive, and it has fewer complications than parenteral feedings.

Feeding ostomies often are placed for long-term tube feedings. Some people learn to use a transnasal tube, which they insert at each feeding. When possible, an intermittent feeding schedule is arranged so that the person is free to move between meals. Generally, infusion pumps are used only if necessary; they are expensive to purchase or rent. People who must receive a continuous drip feeding are trained to use the pump. Small pumps, easily concealed in clothing, are available to allow more freedom of

movement for clients on continuous drip feedings.

The person on HEN either makes a tube feeding from blenderized table food or purchases a commercially prepared, premixed formula. Most clients prefer to purchase formula. A premixed formula should be used whenever the person's ability to mix the formula is questionable.

Generally, a nurse visits the person on HEN at home, and the client sees a physician at regular intervals. In some programs, dietitians make home visits also. A qualified nurse, dietitian, or physician must be available to answer questions as they arise.

The tremendous growth of HPEN programs offers new hope for many people who otherwise could have survived only in the hospital. As more and more people begin HPEN programs, health professionals continue to find better methods of helping people help themselves. In the future, more will be learned about the technical, psychological, and social implications of HPEN, and the quality of care will continue to improve.

NOTES
1. M. E. Shils and coauthors, Long term parenteral nutrition through an external arteriovenous shunt, *New England Journal of Medicine* 283 (1970): 341–344.
2. L. Howard and coauthors, A review of the current national status of home parenteral and enteral nutrition from the provider and consumer perspective, *Journal of Parenteral and Enteral Nutrition* 10 (1986): 416–424.

3. Howard and coauthors, 1986.
4. I. L. Mackenzie, Evaluation of the patient for home parenteral nutrition, *Nutritional Support Services*, February 1982, pp. 16–19; S. J. Dudrick and coauthors, Update on ambulatory home hyperalimentation, *Nutritional Support Services*, April 1981, pp. 18–21; M. Perl and coauthors, Psychological aspects of long-term home hyperalimentation, *Journal of Parenteral and Enteral Nutrition* 4 (1980): 554–560.
5. Howard and coauthors, 1986.
6. T. R. VonderBrink, Documentation for home nutritional support, *Nutrition in Clinical Practice* 1 (1986): 173–174.
7. N. K. Naomi and D. S. Richardson, Homecare open forum, *Nutritional Support Services* 6 (1986): 22–23.
8. J. H. Bodzin, Homecare open forum, *Nutritional Support Services* 6 (1986): 23, 25.
9. C. Marein and coauthors, Home parenteral nutrition, *Nutrition in Clinical Practice* 1 (1986): 179–192.
10. M. A. Ryder and B. M. Wolfe, Psychosocial limitations to home parenteral nutrition, *Nutrition in Clinical Practice* 1 (1986): 200–204; A. E. Robinovitch, Home total parenteral nutrition: A psycho-social viewpoint, *Journal of Parenteral and Enteral Nutrition* 5 (1981): 522–525; M. Perl and coauthors, Psychological aspects of long-term home hyperalimentation, *Journal of Parenteral and Enteral Nutrition* 4 (1980): 554–560; B. S. Price and E. L. Levine, Permanent total parenteral nutrition: Psychological and social responses of the early stages, *Journal of Parenteral and Enteral Nutrition* 3 (1979): 48–52.
11. Marein and coauthors, 1986.
12. Marcin and coauthors, 1986; J. R. Wesley, Home parenteral nutrition: Indications, principles, and cost-effectiveness, *Comprehensive Therapy* 4 (1983): 29–36; K. Ladefoged, Quality of life in patients on permanent home parenteral nutrition, *Journal of Parenteral and Enteral Nutrition* 5 (1980): 132–137.
13. D. Ingber, People who never need to eat, *Science Digest*, January 1982, pp. 34–35.
14. J. K. Nelson, P. J. Palumbo, and P. C. O'Brien, Home enteral nutrition: Observations of a newly established program, *Nutrition in Clinical Practice* 1 (1986): 193–199.

Nutrition and Drug Therapy

19

Contents

Drugs work best when their actions against disease agents are highly specific; that is when they do least harm to the body itself. The body's own immune defenses against diseases are like the most effective drugs. Shown here are antibodies (dot shapes) attacking protein molecules (stringy shapes). As you can see, each antibody attaches to a specific location on the protein and renders it incapable of carrying out its normal function.

M ost people are aware that prescription drugs have side effects. Antihistamines can make you sleepy; antibiotics can upset your stomach. Even the nonprescription drug aspirin can lead to blood loss. But not everyone is aware that medicines can profoundly affect nutrition status—and the reverse, that nutrition can affect the way the body responds to drugs. Several hundred interactions among drugs, nutrients, and foods are known.

Not all drug-nutrient interactions occur every time a person takes a drug. The chance that an adverse interaction will result in nutrient deficiencies increases if the drug is taken over a long period of time, if the person is taking several drugs simultaneously, or if the person is in poor nutrition status when drug treatment begins. Understandably, elderly people (who are often malnourished and who frequently take several drugs for long periods of time) and people who have high nutrient requirements are most likely to develop problems.

Nutrients and drugs may interact in many ways, producing one or more of the following effects:

Nutrients and drugs interact in many ways.

- Drugs can alter food intake by depressing or stimulating the appetite.
- Nutrients and foods can change the way a drug is absorbed; drugs can change the way nutrients are absorbed.
- Nutrients can interfere with the intended actions of drugs.
- Nutrients can alter the metabolism and excretion of drugs; drugs can alter the metabolism and excretion of nutrients.

Table 19–1 summarizes the mechanisms by which these interactions occur.

Although some drug-nutrient interactions are produced intentionally, more often than not, these interactions are unintentional. To protect against undesirable interactions, health care professionals must be alert to the effects of drugs and nutrients on one another.

Drugs That Affect Food Intake

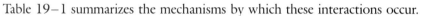

A person's food intake can be affected by any drug that changes the appetite, alters perceptions of taste and smell, causes sores or inflammation of the mouth, or induces nausea or vomiting.

Let's look at some specific examples of such interactions. A kindergarten boy, Tim, has been diagnosed as hyperactive, and an amphetamine has been prescribed for treatment. Although the medication has helped to improve Tim's behavior, it has also caused undesirable side effects: loss of appetite, altered taste sensitivity, dry mouth, and nausea.

Mrs. Kevin provides another example. She has cancer and has been losing weight rapidly. One part of the problem is that the drug therapy causes loss of appetite, taste alterations, mouth sores, nausea, and vomiting.

These examples represent only two of the many drugs that result in a decreased intake of food. Any drug that causes a person to eat less food over time can lead to malnutrition and multiple nutrient deficiencies.

TABLE 19–1

Mechanisms of Food-Drug Interactions

Drugs Can Change Food Intake by:

Altering the appetite.
Interfering with taste or smell.
Inducing nausea or vomiting.
Causing sores or inflammation of the mouth.

Foods Can Change Drug Absorption by:

Changing the acidity of the digestive tract.
Stimulating secretion of digestive juices.
Altering motility of the digestive tract.
Binding to drugs.

Drugs Can Change Nutrient Absorption by:

Changing the acidity of the digestive tract.
Altering digestive juices.
Altering motility of the digestive tract.
Inactivating enzyme systems.
Damaging mucosal cells.

Foods Can Change Drug Metabolism by:

Interfering with a drug's action.
Contributing pharmacologically active substances (example: tyramine).

Drugs Can Change Nutrient Metabolism by:

Acting as structural analogs.
Interfering with metabolic enzyme systems.
Binding to nutrients.

Foods Can Change Drug Excretion by:

Changing the acidity of the urine.

Drugs Can Change Nutrient Excretion by:

Altering reabsorption in the kidneys.
Displacing nutrients from their plasma protein carriers.

Many drugs can cause nausea. Sometimes giving these drugs with meals helps alleviate the nausea; drugs that should be given with foods are listed in Table 19–2.

Absorption and Drug-Nutrient Interactions

A different kind of interaction between foods and drugs involves absorption. The presence of food or a particular nutrient can affect the way a drug is

over-the-counter (OTC) drugs: drugs that can be purchased without a prescription.

Many people believe that drugs available without a prescription (over-the-counter, or OTC, drugs) are harmless. Such is not the case. For example, aspirin (probably the most common OTC drug) can lead to anemia and possibly hemorrhage when it is used over long periods. A further danger in using OTC drugs is that a serious problem can be masked by covering up the symptoms. For example, a person who repeatedly takes antacids for stomach discomfort may be ignoring the signs of an ulcer.

Another problem with OTC drugs is that they may contain hidden ingredients that are undesirable in some cases. For example, some antacids contribute significant amounts of sodium (Alka-Seltzer contains 521 milligrams per tablet) or calcium (Tums has 500 milligrams per tablet). Although these effects may be insignificant in healthy individuals, they can aggravate some medical conditions.

Aluminum hydroxide-containing antacids (such as Amphojel or Digel) can lead to phosphorus depletion. Furthermore, the use of OTC aluminum-containing antacids to control high blood phosphorus levels in people with impaired renal function has been implicated as the primary cause of aluminum intoxication.[1] Aluminum intoxication causes neurological symptoms such as muscle spasms, seizures, and mental dysfunction. Even in people with normal renal function, the chronic use of aluminum-containing antacids has been associated with several cases of osteomalacia.[2]

All drugs—prescription and nonprescription alike—should be taken with caution. The mistaken belief that all nonprescription drugs are harmless can be dangerous.

A variety of drugs is available without prescription.

absorbed, and the reverse is also true: the presence of a drug can affect the way a nutrient is absorbed.

Effects of Food on Drug Digestion and Absorption

Food can enhance, delay, or reduce the absorption of a drug. Let's look at how this works. Food in the stomach triggers the secretion of gastric acid, which lowers the pH of the stomach. Therefore, drugs that are negatively affected by increased acidity should be taken on an empty stomach.

For example, Mary was told to take a prescribed antibiotic on an empty stomach (one hour before, or two to three hours after, meals), because the drug she is taking is degraded by high acidity. Sam, on the other hand, has been prescribed a capsule with specific instructions not to drink milk at the same time he takes the capsule. Why? The capsules Sam is taking are specially coated to dissolve in the low acidity of the intestine, and milk alters the acidity of the stomach so that the capsule dissolves there instead. This is undesirable, because the drug can irritate the stomach lining and cause discomfort.

The presence of food in the stomach also stimulates the secretion of bile acids into the intestine, which enhances fat digestion and absorption. Some medications dissolve in, and are better absorbed along with, fat. These drugs

Some drugs work better when taken with food.

TABLE 19–2

Recommended Timing of Drug Administration with Meals

Drugs	Give on Empty Stomach (1 hour before or 2 to 3 hours after meals)	Give ½ Hour before Meals	Give with Food or Milk	Don't Give with Milk or Dairy Products	Don't Give with Fruit Juices	Can Give with or without Meals
Acetosulfone sodium			X			
Adrenocorticosteroids		X				
Allopurinol			X			
Ambenonium chloride		X				
Aminophylline			X			
Aminosalicylic acid	X					
Amoxicillin	X					X
Ampicillin	X				X	
Anisotropine methylbromide	X					
Aspirin			X			
Atropine sulfate		X				
Belladonna		X				
Bethanechol chloride	X					
Bisacodyl				X		
Busulfan			X			
Carbamazepine			X			
Carbenicillin indanyl sodium	X					
Carisoprodol			X			
Cephalexin						X
Cephradine	X					
Chloral hydrate			X			
Chlordiazepoxide		X				
Chlorothiazide			X			
Chlorpromazine			X			
Chlorpropamide			X			
Chlorthalidone			X			
Cimetidine			X			
Cloxacillin sodium	X				X	
Colchicine			X			
Co-trimoxazole	X					
Cyclacillin	X					
Cyclandelate						X
Cyclophosphamide						X
Demeclocycline	X					
Dicloxacillin sodium	X					
Digoxin				X		
Dipyridamole	X					
Doxycycline hyclate				X		X
Erythromycin	X					
Erythromycin, enteric coated						X

Drug administration terms:
- **ac:** *ante cibes*; before meals.
- **bid:** *bis in die*; twice daily.
- **c:** *cum*; with.
- **hs:** *hora somni*; at bedtime.
- **pc:** *post cibum*; after meals.
- **qid:** *quater in die*; four times daily.
- **tid:** *ter in die*; three times daily.

(continued)

TABLE 19–2

(continued)

Drugs	Give on Empty Stomach (1 hour before or 2 to 3 hours after meals)	Give ½ Hour before Meals	Give with Food or Milk	Don't Give with Milk or Dairy Products	Don't Give with Fruit Juices	Can Give with or without Meals
Erythromycin estolate or succinate						X
Erythromycin stearate	X					
Estradiol			X			
Estrogen			X			
Ethacrynic acid			X			
Fenoprofen calcium	X					
Ferrous sulfate, fumarate, lactate, or gluconate				X		
Furosemide			X			
Glycopyrrolate		X				
Griseofulvin			X			
Hydralazine hydrochloride			X			
Hydrochlorothiazide			X			
Hydroflumethiazide			X			
Hydroxyurea			X			
Ibuprofen	X					
Indomethacin			X			
Isoniazid			X			
Isoxsuprine			X			
Levodopa hydrochloride			X			
Lincomycin	X					
Lithium carbonate			X			
Lomustine	X					
Magnesium oxide			X			
Meclofenamate sodium						X
Mefenamic acid			X			
Melphalan	X					
Mepenzolate bromide	X					
Methylthiouracil			X			
Methysergide maleate			X			
Metoprolol tartrate			X			
Metronidazole			X			
Minocycline						X
Mitotane			X			
Nafcillin sodium	X					
Nalidixic acid						X
Naproxen	X					
Nitrofurantoin			X			
Oral contraceptives			X			
Oxacillin sodium	X					
Oxyphenbutazone			X			
Oxytetracycline	X			X		
Penicillin G	X					
Penicillin K						X

TABLE 19–2

(continued)

Drugs	Give on Empty Stomach (1 hour before or 2 to 3 hours after meals)	Give ½ Hour before Meals	Give with Food or Milk	Don't Give with Milk or Dairy Products	Don't Give with Fruit Juices	Can Give with or without Meals
Phenformin hydrochloride			X			
Phenmetrazine hydrochloride		X				
Phenobarbital	X					
Phentolamine			X			
Phenylbutazone			X			
Potassium salts			X			
Prednisolone			X			
Prednisone			X			
Procainamide hydrochloride						X
Promethazine hydrochloride			X			
Propantheline bromide		X				
Propoxyphene hydrochloride			X			
Propranolol hydrochloride			X			
Quinidine sulfate			X			
Rauwolfia serpentina			X			
Reserpine			X			
Rifampin	X					
Salicylamide			X			
Spironolactone			X			
Sulfinpyrazone			X			
Sulfonamide	X					
Tetracycline	X			X		
Theophylline			X			
Thioguanine			X			
Tolbutamide			X			
Triamterene			X			
Trihexyphenidyl hydrochloride			X			
Trimeprazine tartrate			X			
Uracil mustard			X			
Valproic acid			X			
Warfarin			X			
Zinc sulfate			X			

should be given with food. The antifungal drug griseofulvin, for example, is better absorbed with fat.

Food delays the rate at which the stomach empties. Therefore, when you want a drug to work rapidly, you should take it on an empty stomach. For example, aspirin given on an empty stomach works faster than when it is given

In some cases food and drug intake must be coordinated to achieve the desired drug actions.

Miniglossary of Drug Actions

amphetamines: stimulate the central nervous system; used in the treatment of obesity and of hyperactivity in children.

analgesics: relieve pain.

anesthetics: block sensations of pain or touch.

antacids: neutralize the acidity of the stomach.

antibiotics: kill microorganisms or interfere with their growth.

anticoagulants: prevent or slow down blood clotting.

anticonvulsants: prevent or reduce the occurrence of seizures.

antidepressants: help alleviate severe depression.

antidiabetic agents: reduce blood sugar levels.

antifungal agents: kill fungus or prevent its growth.

antihistamines: counteract inflammation; used to treat allergies.

antihypertensive agents: reduce blood pressure.

anti-infective agents: kill microorganisms or interfere with their growth.

anti-inflammatory agents: reduce tissue inflammation.

antilipemics: counteract or prevent accumulation of fats in the blood; cholesterol-lowering agents are antilipemics.

antimicrobials: kill microorganisms or interfere with their growth.

antineoplastic agents: prevent or inhibit the growth of malignant tumor cells.

antitubercular agents: inhibit growth of the bacteria that cause tuberculosis.

cardiac glycosides: increase the force of heart muscle contractions.

cathartics: cause rapid expulsion of intestinal contents, usually in semiliquid form; very strong laxatives.

chelating agents: bind to toxic heavy metals (lead, arsenic, gold, and mercury) to promote their excretion.

corticosteroids: can be used as anti-inflammatory agents, to suppress undesirable immune responses, or as replacement therapy for people who can't synthesize corticosteroids.

diuretics: increase the excretion of urine.

hypocholesterolemics: reduce blood cholesterol levels.

hypoglycemic agents: reduce blood sugar levels; same as *antidiabetic agents*.

laxatives: cause intestinal contents to be rapidly expelled.

oral contraceptives: prevent pregnancy.

Some drugs should not be taken with milk or dairy products.

on a full stomach. However, aspirin also can be irritating to the GI tract. The presence of food can act as a buffer and reduce this irritation. As a guideline, then, if rapid action is not essential, food taken simultaneously with aspirin (or other drugs that irritate the GI tract) can help reduce nausea, lessen irritation, and prevent damage to the lining of the GI tract.

Additionally, there are instances in which the desired action of a drug must be timed with food intake. For example, some drugs used to treat ulcers decrease gastric acid secretion and gastric motility. The person should take the drug just before a meal so that it will be effective while gastric acid secretion is stimulated.

Specific nutrients in food also can have a negative effect on drug absorption. A classic example is the interactions of tetracycline, calcium, and iron. Clients are instructed not to take tetracycline with milk or dairy products. The calcium from dairy products binds to the drug and reduces the amount that is absorbed. Other minerals can also bind tetracycline so that it is unavailable for absorption. Antacids that contain calcium carbonate (such as Tums) also can reduce the absorption of tetracycline. In addition, iron supplements should not be taken

Mrs. O'Connor visited her physician after she began noticing pain on urination and a general rundown feeling. The results of blood tests and urinalysis confirmed a diagnosis of a urinary tract infection and iron-deficiency anemia. The doctor prescribed tetracycline (250 milligrams four times a day) for the urinary tract infection and 300 milligrams of ferrous sulfate (an iron supplement) three times a day. On Mrs. O'Connor's return visit two weeks later, the physician discovered that both her urinary tract infection and her anemia persisted. The doctor checked her drug and meal history and found that she had been taking her medications as follows:

| 7:00 A.M. | Tetracycline |
| | Iron tablet |

(Soon after Mrs. O'Connor took these medications, she often felt nauseated, so she took two antacids containing calcium carbonate.)

CASE STUDY

Food and Drug Interactions

8:00 A.M.	Breakfast
12:00 P.M.	Tetracycline
	Iron tablet

(She felt nauseated and took two more antacids.)

1:00 P.M.	Lunch
5:00 P.M.	Tetracycline
6:00 P.M.	Supper
10:00 P.M.	Tetracycline
	Iron tablet

(She felt nauseated and took two more antacids.)

| 11:00 P.M. | Bed |

1. Can you spot any possible drug-nutrient interactions in Mrs. O'Connor's drug and diet history? (See Tables 19–2 and 19–3.)
2. What could be causing Mrs. O'Connor's nausea? Can anything be done to correct the problem? What recommendations would you make? The doctor told Mrs. O'Connor to stop taking the tetracycline and iron at the same time and to discontinue the antacids altogether. He recommended that she eat a small amount of food (but no dairy products or foods high in calcium) when she took her medications.
3. Was the doctor's advice sound? Why or why not?
4. Try working out a new schedule for Mrs. O'Connor so that the iron is given either three hours before or two hours after the tetracycline. Remember that the tetracycline should preferably be given one hour before or two hours after meals.

at the same time as tetracycline; the absorption of each is reduced by the other when they are taken simultaneously.

Effects of Drugs on Food Digestion and Absorption

Drugs can act similarly to food in altering pH, digestive secretions, and GI motility. These drug effects influence the digestion and absorption of nutrients. Some drugs can interfere with the enzyme systems necessary for the absorption of some nutrients. Others actually alter the mucosal cells that absorb nutrients. The antibiotic neomycin, for example, causes structural changes in the intestinal villi. This may explain the malabsorption of carbohydrate that is associated with neomycin use.[3] Still other drugs bind to specific nutrients so that they can't be absorbed. Table 19–3 summarizes the effects of many drugs on the absorption, metabolism, and excretion of nutrients.

Nutrient absorption can be affected when a drug alters GI acidity. Antacids raise the pH of the stomach and in so doing can decrease iron absorption. A lower pH enhances the formation of ferrous iron (Fe^{++}), which is the absorbable form of iron. Potassium chloride (used as a potassium supplement) decreases the pH of the small intestine, interfering with the absorption of vitamin B_{12}.

Several drugs increase the absorption of nutrients. For example, enzyme replacements are pancreatic enzymes given specifically to increase the absorption

When drugs cause a change in the intestinal environment by changing motility, altering pH, or interfering with bile acids, the change is called a **luminal effect**.

Drugs that interfere with a nutrient's ability to be absorbed across the intestinal mucosa are said to exert a **mucosal effect**. Mucosal effects include actual damage to the mucosal cells and inactivation of enzyme systems.

Selected Drug-Nutrient Interactions[a]

Drug	Nutrient	Effect on Nutrition
Alcohol	Energy	↓ intake
	Protein	↓ intake
	Fat	↑ buildup in liver
		↓ absorption
	Thiamin	↓ absorption
		↓ storage
	Vitamin B$_6$	↓ activation
	Folacin	↓ absorption
		↓ utilization
	Vitamin B$_{12}$	↓ absorption
	Magnesium	↑ urinary excretion
	Zinc	↑ urinary excretion
Amphetamines	Many nutrients affected	↓ intake
		Anorexia, dry mouth, metallic taste, nausea, vomiting
Analgesics		
Aspirin	Folacin	↓ serum levels
		Altered transport
	Vitamin C	↑ urinary excretion
	Thiamin	↑ urinary excretion
	Vitamin K	↑ urinary excretion
	Iron	May cause blood loss
Antacids		
Aluminum hydroxide	Phosphorus	↓ absorption
Other types	Thiamin	↑ destruction
Anticoagulants	Vitamin K	↓ conversion to active form
Anticonvulsants	Folacin	↓ serum levels
	Vitamin B$_6$	↓ serum levels
	Vitamin B$_{12}$	↓ serum levels
	Vitamin D	↓ conversion to active forms
	Vitamin K	↑ requirement
Antimicrobials (antibiotics)		
Chloramphenicol	Riboflavin	↑ requirement (?)
	Vitamin B$_6$	↑ requirement (?)
	Vitamin B$_{12}$	↑ requirement (?)
Neomycin	Fats	↓ absorption
	Nitrogen	↓ absorption
	Carbohydrates	↓ absorption
	Folacin	↓ absorption
	Vitamin B$_{12}$	↓ absorption
	Fat-soluble vitamins	↓ absorption
	Calcium	↓ absorption
	Iron	↓ absorption
	Potassium	↓ absorption
	Vitamin K	↓ intestinal synthesis
Penicillin	Potassium	↑ urinary excretion
Tetracycline	Fat	↓ absorption
	Amino acids	↓ absorption
	Calcium	↓ absorption

[a] ↑ = increases; ↓ = decreases; (?) = possible effect.

TABLE 19–3

NUTRITION AND DRUG THERAPY   659

(continued)

Drug	Nutrient	Effect on Nutrition
Tetracycline (continued)	Iron	↓ absorption
	Magnesium	↓ absorption
	Zinc	↓ absorption
	Niacin	↑ urinary excretion
	Riboflavin	↑ urinary excretion
	Folacin	↑ urinary excretion
	Vitamin C	↑ urinary excretion
Antineoplastic agents 5-Fluorouracil	Protein	↓ absorption
		↓ synthesis
Methotrexate and pyrimethamine	Folacin	Folacin antagonist
	Vitamin B_{12}	↓ absorption
	Fat	↓ absorption
	Many nutrients affected	↓ intake
		Anorexia, nausea, vomiting, mouth sores
Antitubercular drugs Cycloserine	Vitamin B_6	Vitamin B_6 antagonist
	Protein	↓ synthesis
	Calcium	↓ absorption (?)
	Magnesium	↓ absorption (?)
	Vitamin B_6	↓ serum levels (?)
	Folacin	↓ serum levels (?)
	Vitamin B_{12}	↓ serum levels (?)
Isonicotinic acid hydrazide (INH)	Vitamin B_6	Vitamin B_6 antagonist
		↑ urinary excretion
		Causes deficiency
	Niacin	Causes deficiency
	Vitamin B_{12}	↓ absorption
		↓ serum levels
Para-aminosalicylic acid	Folacin	↓ absorption
	Vitamin B_{12}	↓ absorption
	Fat	↓ absorption
	Iron	↓ absorption
Chelating agents Penicillamine	Vitamin B_6	↑ requirement
		↑ urinary excretion
	Zinc	↑ urinary excretion
	Iron	↑ urinary excretion
	Copper	↑ urinary excretion
	Many nutrients affected	↓ intake
		Alterations in taste; anorexia, nausea, vomiting
Cholesterol-lowering agents Cholestyramine	Fat and cholesterol	↓ absorption
	Fat-soluble vitamins	↓ absorption
	Folacin	↓ absorption
	Iron	↓ absorption
	Vitamin B_{12}	↓ absorption
		↓ blood levels
	Calcium	↑ urinary excretion
		↓ blood levels

(continued)

TABLE 19–3

(continued)

Drug	Nutrient	Effect on Nutrition
Cholesterol-lowering agents (continued)		
Clofibrate	Vitamin B_{12}	↓ absorption
	Iron	↓ absorption
	Many nutrients affected	↓ intake
		Alterations in taste; nausea and GI irritation
Colchicine	Fat	↓ absorption
	Vitamin A	↓ absorption
	Folacin	↓ absorption
	Vitamin B_{12}	↓ absorption
	Sodium	↓ absorption
	Potassium	↓ absorption
Corticosteroids	Vitamin D	↑ metabolism
		↑ requirement
	Vitamin B_6	↑ requirement
	Vitamin C	↑ requirement
		↑ urinary excretion
	Calcium	↓ absorption
		↑ urinary excretion
	Phosphorus	↓ absorption
	Zinc	↑ urinary excretion
		↓ serum levels
	Glucose	↑ serum levels
	Triglycerides	↑ serum levels
	Cholesterol	↑ serum levels
	Potassium	↑ urinary excretion
	Nitrogen	↑ urinary excretion
Diuretics		
Furosemide	Calcium	↑ urinary excretion
	Sodium	↑ urinary excretion
	Potassium	↓ serum levels
	Chloride	↓ serum levels
	Magnesium	↓ serum levels
	Zinc	↑ serum levels
		↓ storage in liver
Mercurials	Thiamin	↑ urinary excretion
	Calcium	↑ urinary excretion
	Sodium	↑ urinary excretion
	Potassium	↑ urinary excretion
	Chloride	↑ urinary excretion
	Magnesium	↑ urinary excretion
Thiazides	Sodium	↑ urinary excretion
	Potassium	↓ blood levels
	Chloride	↓ blood levels
	Calcium	↑ urinary excretion
		↑ blood levels
	Magnesium	↑ urinary excretion
	Phosphorus	↓ blood levels
	Glucose	↑ blood levels (?)

TABLE 19–3

(continued)

Drug	Nutrient	Effect on Nutrition
Diuretics (continued)		
Triamterene	Sodium	▲ urinary excretion
	Folacin	▼ serum levels
	Vitamin B_{12}	▼ serum levels
Glutethimide	Vitamin D	▲ metabolism
Hydralazine hydrochloride	Vitamin B_6	▲ urinary excretion
Hypoglycemics		
Phenformin hydrochloride and metformin	Vitamin$_{12}$	▼ absorption
Laxatives		
Cathartics	Fat	▼ absorption
	Glucose	▼ absorption
	Vitamin D	▼ absorption
	Calcium	▼ absorption
	Potassium	▼ absorption
Mineral oil	Fat-soluble vitamins	▼ absorption
	Carotene	▼ absorption
Levodopa	Amino acids	▲ requirement
	Vitamin B_6	▲ requirement
	Vitamin C	▲ requirement
	Sodium	▼ urinary excretion
	Potassium	▼ urinary excretion
Oral contraceptives	Vitamin B_6	▲ requirement
		▼ blood levels
	Riboflavin	▲ requirement
		▼ blood levels
	Folacin	▼ absorption
		▼ blood levels
	Vitamin B_{12}	▼ blood levels
	Vitamin C	▼ blood levels
	Vitamin A	▲ blood levels
	Calcium	▲ absorption
	Iron	▲ serum levels
	Copper	▲ serum levels
	Magnesium	▼ blood levels (?)
	Zinc	▼ blood levels (?)
Potassium salts	Vitamin B_{12}	▼ absorption
Sulfonamides		
Salicylazosulfapyridine	Folacin	▼ absorption
		▼ blood levels
	Iron	▼ blood levels
Others	Folacin	▼ intestinal synthesis
	Vitamin K	▼ intestinal synthesis
	B vitamins	▼ intestinal synthesis

Adapted from: R. E. Hodges, *Nutrition in Medical Practice* (Philadelphia: Saunders, 1980), pp. 323–331; R. C. Theuer and J. J. Vitale, Drug and nutrient interactions, in *Nutritional Support of Medical Practice*, eds. H. A. Schneider, C. E. Anderson, and D. B. Coursin (Hagerstown, Md.: Harper and Row, 1977); D. A. Roe, *Drug-Induced Nutritional Deficiencies* (Westport, Conn.: AVI, 1985).

of various nutrients. Additionally, lactase enzyme replacements are available to aid in the digestion of lactose in people with a lactase deficiency.

Laxatives—drugs that cause the GI contents to be rapidly expelled—may give nutrients little time for absorption. Taking laxatives regularly can lead to decreased absorption of fat-soluble vitamins, protein, calcium, and glucose. Chronic use of some laxatives damages the structural integrity of the intestinal cells. Mineral oil, another laxative, interferes with the formation of micelles—particles formed in an early step of fat digestion. The fat-soluble vitamins (A, D, E, and K) dissolve in the oil and are lost in the feces rather than absorbed.

The antibiotic neomycin binds bile salts and has been reported to reduce absorption of fat, fat-soluble vitamins, amino acids, vitamin B_{12}, lactose, potassium, calcium, and iron. In addition, neomycin appears to reduce the activity of pancreatic lipase and damage mucosal cells. Furthermore, by destroying the intestinal bacteria that synthesize vitamin K, it may induce a vitamin K deficiency with long-term use. Other antibiotics may cause similar malabsorption problems. Table 19–4 shows some additional nutrients that are affected by various drugs.

Metabolic Food-Drug Interactions

So far this chapter has discussed ways in which foods and drugs interact to cause changes in food intake and nutrient and drug absorption. Food and drugs can also interact to alter metabolism and excretion; a few of many possible examples follow.

Effects of Nutrients and Foods on Drug Metabolism

Two basic types of food-drug interactions affect the way a drug works:

- The presence of certain nutrients can change the way the body uses a drug.
- Certain substances in foods can interact with drugs to alter the drug's action.

pharmacologic dose: a dose of a nutrient that exceeds normal requirements and can produce a druglike effect. The amount of a nutrient the body needs and can use is termed a **physiologic dose.**

pharmaco = drug

When vitamins are given in pharmacologic doses, they can lower blood levels of some drugs and thereby reduce the drugs' effectiveness. For example, Jake has epilepsy and must take an anticonvulsant medication (phenytoin, or Dilantin) to prevent seizures. His body has reacted to the drug by making more drug-metabolizing enzymes, and these enzymes require folacin to work efficiently. On the one hand, given too little folacin, Jake will be unable to metabolize phenytoin and he will develop symptoms of folacin deficiency as well. Given too much folacin, on the other hand, he may experience more seizures and need higher doses of the drug to control them. A balance between the drug and the vitamin must be found that protects him from both seizures and folacin deficiency.

Another example is Mrs. Ferguson, who has had several blood clots in the veins of her leg. To prevent a recurrence, her doctor has prescribed an anticlotting

TABLE 19–4

Nutrients That May Be Affected by Drugs

Nutrients	Agents That Affect Nutrient Status
Protein	5-Fluorouracil, neomycin
Carbohydrates	Metformin, phenformin, corticosteroids, chlorothiazide
Fats and fatty acids	Neomycin, cholestyramine, clofibrate
Thiamin	Antacids, ethanol, carbohydrates
Riboflavin	Boric acid, oral contraceptive steroids
Niacin	Isoniazid, 6-mercaptopurine, 5-fluorouracil
Vitamin B_6	Isoniazid, ethanol, oral contraceptive steroids, penicillamine, hydralazine, cycloserine, levodopa
Folates	Diphenylhydantoin, methotrexate, pyrimethamine, ethanol, oral contraceptive steroids, phenylbutazone
Vitamin B_{12}	Para-aminosalicylic acid, barbiturates, colchicine, cholestyramine, phenformin, oral contraceptive steroids
Vitamin C	Aminopyrine, cigarettes, diphenylhydantoin, oral contraceptive steroids, paraldehyde, salicylates
Vitamin A	Mineral oil (disputed), cholestyramine, oral contraceptive steroids
Vitamin D	Phenobarbital, diphenylhydantoin, cholestyramine, mineral oil
Vitamin E	Mineral oil, iron, polyunsaturated fatty acids, cholestyramine
Vitamin K	Sodium warfarin (Coumadin), barbiturates, ascorbic acid, mineral oil
Essential fatty acids	Continuous infusions of glucose
Sodium	Thiazides, ethacrynic acid, spironolactone (Aldactone)
Potassium	Thiazides, cathartics
Calcium	Oxalates, fatty acids, phytates, phosphates
Phosphorus	Aluminum hydroxide, total parenteral nutrition
Magnesium	Ethanol, ethacrynic acid
Iron	Phytic acid, oxalates, phosphates, ascorbic acid
Zinc	Ethanol, penicillamine, oral contraceptive steroids
Copper	Ethanol, penicillamine, phytates, corticosteroids

Source: R. E. Hodges, *Nutrition in Medical Practice* (Philadelphia: Saunders, 1980), p. 328. Reprinted with permission.

agent, sodium warfarin (Coumadin), which is working well. Mrs. Ferguson is also overweight. Her husband recently persuaded her to embark on a diet with him that involves eating large quantities of green vegetables and lettuce salads every day. At her next checkup, her clotting time has shortened from 20 to 14 seconds. Why?

Her doctor is alert to nutrition problems and deduces the reason: vitamin K from the green vegetables and lettuce is overwhelming the drug, which normally works by interfering with vitamin K's clot-promoting action. The doctor negotiates an agreement with Mrs. Ferguson. She is to continue eating those healthful foods until further notice, and he will adjust the drug dose accordingly.

Occasionally, people with severe depression are treated with drugs called monoamine oxidase (MAO) inhibitors, which block the action of the enzyme monoamine oxidase. Tyramine, a substance found in some foods, normally undergoes conversion in the body to an inactive form through the action of monoamine oxidase. When MAO inhibitors are given, tyramine remains active and causes the release of norepinephrine. As a result, the person can develop severe hypertension and headaches. Blood pressure can rise high enough to be fatal. Table 19–5 lists foods that are major sources of tyramine.

People taking certain types of diuretics that cause loss of potassium may need to be cautioned about eating genuine licorice, which can cause more potassium loss and more retention of water and salt. Most American-made licorice uses synthetic licorice flavoring, which is not a problem. However, imported licorice may contain the natural extract.

TABLE 19–5

Food Sources of Tyramine[a]

Foods Very High in Tyramine	Foods High in Tyramine

Cheeses, aged
  Boursault
  Camembert
  Cheddar
  Stilton
Yeast extracts
	Bologna
	Dried, salted, or pickled cod
	Dried, salted, or pickled herring
	Pepperoni
	Salami

Foods Moderately High in Tyramine	Foods Containing Moderate Amounts of Tyramine

Cheeses
  Blue
  Brick, natural
  Brie
  Gruyère
  Mozzarella
  Parmesan
  Romano
  Roquefort
Chianti wine
Meat tenderizers
	Broad beans (fava, Chinese pea pods)
	Caffeine (in large amounts)
	Chocolate (in large amounts)
	Liver, chicken, and beef
	Pineapple
	Plums
	Raisins
	Soy sauce

Foods Low in Tyramine	

Ale
Avocados
Bananas
Beer
Cheeses
  American, processed
  Cottage
	Cream
	Ricotta
	Figs
	Sherry
	Sour cream
	White wine

[a]The tyramine content of each type of food varies. Data on tyramine content may be based on small sample sizes.

Effects of Drugs on Nutrient Metabolism

Some drugs have a chemical structure similar to that of a vitamin or a metabolite. A drug of this type can displace the vitamin or metabolite from an enzyme and block a normal metabolic pathway. Many types of drugs used to treat cancer are of this type. Cancer cells, like normal cells, need the real vitamin to grow. When the vitamin is not available, they die. Unfortunately, other growing cells in the body also need the vitamin, and vitamin deficiency results. Methotrexate and pyrimethamine, which are structurally similar to folacin, are examples of this type of drug (see Figure 19–1).

Anticonvulsants interfere with vitamin metabolism in a different way. You may recall that once vitamin D has been absorbed, it is converted to 25–hydroxy vitamin D in the liver, and then to its more active form, 1, 25–dihydroxy vitamin D, in the kidney. Anticonvulsants interfere with the conversion of vitamin D in the liver. Less 25–hydroxy vitamin D reaches the kidney, so less of the dihydroxy vitamin is formed.

A drug can also bind to a nutrient, thereby making it unavailable to the body. An example is the drug isonicotinic acid hydrazide (INH), used to treat tuberculosis. INH binds with vitamin B_6, and both are excreted in the urine.

An **antivitamin**, or **vitamin antagonist**, is a substance structurally similar to a vitamin that interferes with the normal activity of the vitamin.
anti = against

An **antimetabolite** is similar to an antivitamin, but it affects the activity of a metabolite. (A **metabolite** is any compound produced during metabolism.) An example is 5–fluorouracil, an antimetabolite of uracil, a base necessary for RNA synthesis.

Food-Drug Interactions and Excretion

When some foods (breads and protein-rich foods) are metabolized, their end products can potentially produce an acid urine. Other foods (fruits, vegetables,

Folacin

Methotrexate

Pyrimethamine

FIGURE 19–1

Two antivitamins. Because methotrexate and pyrimethamine are structurally similar to folacin, they compete for the enzyme that normally activates folacin.

Hypertension

Mr. Coggins is a 72-year-old man who has been treated in an outpatient clinic for hypertension over the past four years. Since his wife died one year ago, he has been eating poorly and has lost 15 pounds. The doctor has prescribed a diuretic (chlorothiazide) for his hypertension and a potassium supplement, because chlorothiazide can lead to potassium depletion.

1. What factors in Mr. Coggins's history suggest that he is at risk for poor nutrition status? What factors in his history suggest that drug-nutrient interactions should be considered in his case?

2. What are the possible side effects of the diuretic and potassium supplement that Mr. Coggins is taking? (See Tables 19–3 and 19–4).

3. Should these prescription medications be given with food or on an empty stomach? Give the reasons for your answer.

4. If Mr. Coggins also were taking prednisone and aspirin for arthritis, how would his risks of drug-nutrient interactions be changed? What other possible nutrient deficiency would you need to be alert to?

---

and milk) potentially produce an alkaline urine. The pH of the urine affects the degree to which some drugs are reabsorbed from the renal tubules back into the blood. A low urinary pH decreases the excretion of acidic drugs like aspirin and phenobarbitol. Thus these drugs remain in the blood for longer periods of time when the urine is acidic. Since bacterial growth is inhibited in a low-pH urine, it is often desirable to lower the urinary pH when antibiotics are given for urinary tract infections. Vitamin C is sometimes given in large doses to acidify the urine.

Drugs can increase or decrease the excretion of nutrients in the urine. For example, some diuretics can increase the excretion of calcium, potassium, magnesium, and zinc. Birth control pills, on the other hand, may decrease the urinary excretion of calcium, phosphorus, magnesium, and zinc.

The excretion of a nutrient may be increased when a drug causes it to be displaced from the plasma protein that normally transports it. When attached to the larger protein, some nutrients would not be filtered by the kidney; however, the much smaller unbound nutrient is readily excreted. An example is aspirin, which may increase folacin excretion by displacing folacin from its carrier protein.

A Word About Alcohol

The interactions between alcohol and nutrition status are so numerous that they deserve special emphasis here (see also Highlight 7B), especially since alcohol is a widely used and abused drug. Alcohol affects the intake, absorption, metabolism, and excretion of nutrients.

Chronic use of alcohol suppresses the appetite and thus interferes with the ingestion of nutrients. Alcohol is directly toxic to the pancreas, liver, and GI tract. Damage to the pancreas leads to insufficient production of digestive enzymes, which may explain why amino acids and fats are malabsorbed in alcohol abusers. (Alcohol also reduces the absorption of thiamin, folacin, and vitamin B_{12}.) The damaged liver may be unable to adequately store nutrients or activate enzyme systems necessary for nutrient metabolism. The metabolism of thiamin, folacin, vitamin A, and vitamin D is affected by liver disease. Zinc, magnesium, and potassium are excreted in increased amounts in the urine. In addition, iron may be stored in excessive amounts in the liver, increasing liver damage.

Alcohol not only affects nutrients, but also interacts with other drugs. Highlight 7B presents some of the reasons why.

The severe thiamin deficiency frequently seen in alcohol abusers is believed to cause **Wernicke's encephalopathy** (VER-nick-ee's en-SEF-ah-LOP-ah-thee). a syndrome characterized by mental disturbances and an inability to coordinate muscular movements.
encephalo = brain
path = disease

Drugs and Modified Diets

A relationship between foods and drugs that often goes unnoticed is the contribution of nutrients from drug sources. For example, many drugs contain considerable sodium, sugar, potassium, and other electrolytes. Keep this in mind when you work with people who are following diets restricted in sodium, electrolytes, or sugar. Many liquid preparations have sugar added to make them taste better. Antibiotics often contain considerable amounts of sodium. Intravenously administered medications may provide sodium or dextrose.

Unpleasant-tasting drugs are sometimes mixed with a food or beverage to make them more palatable. Use this practice cautiously—as previously discussed, pH can have an effect on the absorption and stability of the drug. The same cautions should be exercised when medications are given with tube feedings—which, like foods, vary in pH.

People being fed by tube often are given finely crushed tablets through the tube. However, this practice should be avoided.[4] If the feeding tube becomes clogged, the tube may have to be reinserted. Also, some types of tablets and capsules are intended to release their contents slowly, and they should not be crushed, or the person might be exposed to an excessive dose of the drug at one time. Liquid medications should be used whenever they are available. The feeding tube should be flushed with water before and after medication is delivered through it. This helps ensure that the medicine is delivered to the lower GI tract rather than sticking to the sides of the tube.[5]

The place where the feeding is delivered is also of considerable importance. A drug that dissolves in the acidic environment of the stomach may not be as readily absorbed if delivered directly to the duodenum or jejunum. Similarly, a drug that is absorbed optimally in the duodenum may be poorly absorbed in the jejunum.

A recent case report has pointed out a possible interaction between tube feeding formulas and tetracycline.[6] Certain electrolytes present in formulas can bind tetracycline and cause it to pass unabsorbed through the intestinal tract.

Drugs, foods, and nutrients interact in many ways. The amount of information available is overwhelming; therefore, it would be difficult, if not impossible, to remember all the drugs and nutrients that interact, and to be able

When delivering medications by tube, use liquids whenever available; if not, crushed tablets may be necessary.

Elderly people who frequently take several drugs for long periods of time are at high risk for nutrient deficiencies.

to apply this information in a clinical situation. Try to keep things in perspective by remembering what is most important:

1. Be aware of the groups of people who are at high risk for developing drug-related nutrient deficiencies. These groups include people with high nutrient requirements, those who must take drugs over a long period of time, those who are taking several drugs simultaneously, and those with poor nutrition status.
2. Be alert. Drug-nutrient interactions can and do occur.
3. Be familiar with the nutrient interactions of drugs commonly used by your clients.

Study Questions

1. Describe the conditions that increase the risk of drug-induced nutrient deficiencies. Based on your answer, which groups of people would most likely be at risk?
2. In what ways can drugs and food or nutrients interact?
3. Discuss the possible dangers of OTC drug preparations.
4. Give some examples of how drugs can interfere with food intake.
5. How can the acidity of the stomach affect drugs? How does food affect the acidity of the stomach? Give some examples of how food can change the acidity of the stomach and some examples of how different drugs are affected by these changes.
6. Look up the following drugs in Table 19–2, and describe how they should be administered in relationship to food intake:
   - Digoxin.
   - Erythromycin.
   - Amoxicillin.
   - Ampicillin.
   - Oral contraceptives.
   - Tetracycline.
7. Describe the effect of food on the rate the stomach empties. How can you use this relationship to determine whether a drug can be taken with or without food? What other factors besides the rate of gastric emptying are important to consider in determining whether foods will alter drug availability?
8. Give some examples of drugs that interfere with nutrient digestion and/or absorption. Describe the way these interactions occur.
9. Discuss the ways that nutrients or foods affect drug metabolism, and provide at least one example of such an interaction.
10. How do antivitamins and antimetabolites interfere with normal nutrient metabolism?
11. How do foods affect the acidity of the urine? How does the acidity of the urine affect the body's metabolism of drugs? Provide some examples of how urinary pH alters drug metabolism.
12. Briefly describe the ways in which alcohol can affect the intake, digestion, absorption, and metabolism of nutrients.
13. What additional considerations about drugs should be made when a person is on a modified diet? What considerations should be made when a person receives medications through a feeding tube?

Notes

1. A. Lione, Aluminum intake from non-prescription drugs and sucralfate, *General Pharmacology* 16 (1985): 223–228.
2. Lione, 1985.
3. P. G. Holtzapple and S. E. Schwartz, Drug-induced maldigestion and malabsorption, in *Drugs and Nutrients: The Interactive Effects*, eds. D. A. Roe and T. C. Campbell (New York, NY: Marcel Dekker, Inc., 1984).
4. B. Wright and L. Robinson, Enteral feeding tubes as drug delivery systems, *Nutritional Support Services* 6 (1986): 33–37, 47–48.
5. Wright and Robinson, 1986.
6. K. E. Fagerman, D. McGuigan, and B. Pixley, Potential interaction between enteral feeding solutions and oral tetracycline, *Nutrition in Clinical Practice* 1 (1986): 257–258.

Nutrition and Immunity

Chapter 19 discusses drugs—man-made weapons in the war against disease. Once a disease is contracted, drugs can be important to survival. However, more basic to survival is the body's ability to fight off a disease. The body's natural defense against disease, the immune system, and the effects of nutrition on this system, are the focus of this Highlight.

Each day we confront an environment teeming with disease-causing organisms. Generally, we remain unaware of the legions of cells within us that fight off foreign organisms too small for us to see. The remarkable capacity of people to survive such an environment is a tribute to the immune system.

The immune system has no central organ of control, but rather depends on various organs and white blood cells. Their interactions and secretions defend the body against infectious organisms such as bacteria and viruses. The immune system also eliminates damaged body cells, eliminates malignant cells, and helps rid the lungs of foreign particles. Immunity depends on the ability to recognize foreign materials and destroy or otherwise neutralize them. Table H19–1 describes the major components of the immune system.

Occasionally, our immune systems are fooled; an immune response may be mounted against a harmless protein, such as milk protein, and the immune system triggers an allergic reaction. Sometimes microorganisms manage to penetrate our defenses, and we develop a cold, the flu, an infection, or a more damaging disease. However, it is

TABLE H19–1

Major Components of the Immune System

First line of defense
  Skin
  Mucus
  Tears, sweat, secretions of sebaceous glands
    Digestive enzymes

Second line of defense
  Granulocytes
  Macrophages

Third line of defense
  Sensitized T-lymphocytes
  Antibodies

important to keep in mind that for each successful penetration of the system, thousands of attempts are averted.

External Defenses

The skin provides the most exterior protection against foreign organisms and chemicals for our bodies. Bacteria normally found on the skin are unable to gain access into the body because the skin is a formidable barrier. Additionally, glands associated with the skin secrete chemicals (in sweat, tears, and oily secretions of the sebaceous glands) toxic to some types of bacteria.

Body openings (such as eyes, nose, mouth, lungs, GI tract, and genitourinary tract) are protected by the mucous membrane linings which produce mucus. Mucus secretions contain antimicrobial chemicals and enzymes that are lethal to invading bacteria. More importantly, mucus is

sticky; it can "catch" foreign materials, which can then be disposed of more readily. Mucus from the lungs is eliminated through the cough reflex and spit out or swallowed. If it is swallowed, the acid environment of the stomach, together with digestive enzymes, can destroy many microorganisms. If an invader does gain entry into the body (through a cut in the skin, for example), the organs and cells of the immune system are called into action.

Internal Defenses

The cells that participate in the immune function can be found throughout the body, but they are primarily housed in lymph tissue—the thymus, lymph nodes, spleen, bone marrow, and areas lining the GI tract (see Figure H19–1). Three types of white blood cells—the phagocytes and two types of lymphocytes—are the most important cells in the immune system (see Figure H19–2). You may take comfort in knowing that of the 100 trillion cells that make up the human body, one in every hundred is a white blood cell.[1]

The white blood cells are the mobile components of the immune system. When the body is wounded or invaded by a microorganism, white blood cells transported to that area by way of the circulatory system provide a rapid and potent defense against infection. As mentioned, there are three types of white blood cells, and all three are formed from the same precursor cells.

The Phagocytes
Phagocytes are the scavengers of the immune system and are the first to

FIGURE H19–1

The lymph tissues and bone marrow. Bone marrow is not lymph tissue, but it is the site of production of cells important to the immune response. Not shown: the patches of lymph tissue in the GI tract.

FIGURE H19–2

The immune system.

arrive at the scene if an invader gains entry. They are continuously circulating throughout our bodies, ready to call into action a defense system at the first sign of trouble. When a phagocyte spots a foreign substance, it engulfs (ingests) and digests that substance in a process called phagocytosis (see Figure H19–3). In this way, phagocytes clear the lungs of the residue from cigarette smoke and environmental contaminants.

The principle phagocytes are macrophages and granulocytes. Certain types of phagocytes secrete proteins called monokines, which are important in the immune response. One of the monokines activates certain lymphocytes important to the immune response; another is responsible for the fever and ill feeling that frequently accompany an infection.

In addition to producing a monokine that activates lymphocytes, macrophages also call lymphocytes into action in another way. As the macrophage engulfs an invading organism, it detaches a portion of the invading cell (an antigen) and displays that portion on its own cell surface. The presence of the antigen on the macrophage's surface activates a special group of lymphocytes (see below) into action. Thus, if the

phagocytes cannot work fast enough to rid the body of the invader, lymphocytes will be ready to aid in the body's defense.

Let's look at what we have so far. Invaders enter the body through a cut in the skin. Immediately, phagocytes swarm into the area and destroy many of them. Certain monokines alert the lymphocytes to prepare for action. Macrophages display antigens on their surface for recognition by the lymphocytes. Another monokine that produces fever may also be secreted. This monokine stimulates the brain to raise the body's temperature—fever enhances the activity of the immune system.

The process of phagocytosis must be selective to ensure survival of the body. Phagocytes must be able to distinguish foreign or damaged cells from functional cells so that the body does not digest itself. Still, phagocytosis is a general process; many types of foreign particles can be handled in this way.

The Lymphocytes

The lymphocytes serve a different function in the immune system. All lymphocytes originate from precursors in the bone marrow but are released

from the bone marrow and mature into two distinct types of lymphocytes—T-cells and B-cells. T-cells travel to the thymus and are then housed in the lymph tissues. B-cells migrate to the lymph nodes located throughout the lymphatic system.

Unlike the macrophages and granulocytes, the lymphocytes are important in the body's defense against specific invading organisms. This more specific immune response depends on prior exposure to the invading organism, recognition of it when exposed again, and reaction to it.

T-cells

The T-cells participate in cell-mediated immunity, so named because the T-cells travel directly to the invasion site and battle foreign organisms. Four types of T-cells are important in the immune response. The first type, the helper T-cell, recognizes the antigen displayed by the macrophages and uses this information to send chemical messages to the other T-cells to prepare them for joining the fight.

One such chemical message is sent to a second type of T-cell, the inducer T-cell. Inducer T-cells trigger the maturation of functionally distinct T-cells from precursor cells in the thymus. In this way, more cells are produced to participate in attacking foreign organisms.

Another message is sent to a third type of T-cell, the killer T-cell. Killer T-cells release powerful chemicals that disrupt the cell membranes of infected, foreign, or malignant cells. As the battle draws to a close, a fourth type of T-cell, the suppressor T-cell, begins to slow down the immune response and eventually halts it.

As you can see, the helper T-cells play a pivotal and critical role in the immune response. If they fail to recognize antigens and to alert other T-cells to prepare to fight, the part of immunity conferred by the T-cells is lost. To fully appreciate the importance

FIGURE H19–3

Phagocytosis. During phagocytosis, a foreign substance is engulfed by a white blood cell and eventually surrounded and digested.

of helper T-cells, consider the epidemic disease acquired immune deficiency syndrome (AIDS). People with AIDS suffer from a total collapse of the immune system because the AIDS virus infects helper T-cells.[2] Victims of AIDS frequently die from infections that ordinarily do not cause disease in people with normal immune function.

Unlike the phagocytes, which are capable of inactivating many different types of invaders, T-cells are highly specific. Each T-cell can attack only one type of antigen. This is a remarkable ability when you consider that nature creates millions of antigens. After T-cells have been made to destroy an antigen, some of the lymphocytes serve as memory cells. If a person is exposed to the same invading organism again, the immune system remembers how to produce the right type of T-cell and so can respond much more quickly. T-cells are especially active in defending the body against fungi, viruses, parasites, and a few types of bacteria; they can also destroy cancer cells. T-cells are involved in the rejection of newly transplanted tissues.

B-cells

B-cells are important in a different type of immunity—humoral immunity. Helper T-cells alert B-cells to the presence of foreign invaders and thus prepare B-cells to join in the response to the assault on the body. An invader reaching the lymph tissues triggers the B-cells to rapidly divide and then to produce antibodies. Unlike the T-cells, the B-cells don't travel to the invasion site directly. Instead, they send their secreted antibodies to the site.

When antibodies arrive at the site of invasion, they stick to the surface of the foreign particles and make them easier targets for attack by phagocytes. Antibodies can also kill the invading organism directly.

Antibodies, like T-lymphocytes, react selectively to a specific foreign organism. Some of the B-cells serve as memory cells, so that the next time the foreign organism is encountered, the immune response can occur with greater speed. B-cells play a bigger role in resistance to infection than do T-cells.

In summary, the body's first line of defense against foreign materials is provided by the skin, the mucous membranes, and various body secretions. Should a microorganism gain entrance into the body, phagocytes are called into play. Phagocytes produce chemicals that activate T-cells. Macrophages display antigens from the unwelcome cells on their surfaces, so that the invader can be recognized and destroyed by T-cells. At the same time, the B-cells secrete specific antibodies that can directly kill invading organisms and also make them easier targets for attack by macrophages.

The preceding discussion of the immune system is an oversimplification of a very complex subject. The phagocytes, T-cells, and B-cells were discussed as separate entities but are really interdependent and synergistic; much other information has not been included. However, the purpose has been served: to provide some general background so that you can appreciate the role that nutrition plays in immunology.

The Role of Nutrition

People who suffer from malnutrition develop more infections than well-nourished people. Infection is a significant cause of mortality and morbidity in children with PCM. A vicious cycle develops in which malnutrition reduces resistance to infection, and infection further aggravates malnutrition. Exactly how this happens isn't clear yet. However, it has been shown that nutrition intervention can improve resistance to infection.[3] Researchers continue to uncover bits and pieces of information that are helping to form a more complete picture of the nutrition-immunology interaction. Table H19—2 summarizes some of this information.

As mentioned earlier, the first barriers a foreign material encounters when trying to enter the body are the skin and the mucous membranes. Malnutrition causes changes in these tissues that compromise their function.

TABLE H19—2

Effects of Malnutrition on the Immune System

Immune System Component	Effects of Malnutrition
Skin	Thinner, with less connective tissue and collagen
Mucous membranes	Microvilli flattened; secretory immunoglobulin A reduced
Lymph tissues	Thymus gland atrophied; lymph nodes and spleen smaller; T-cell areas depleted of lymphocytes
Phagocytosis	Kill time delayed
Cell-mediated immunity	Circulating T-cells reduced
Humoral immunity	Circulating immunoglobulin levels normal; antibody response may be impaired

During malnutrition the skin becomes thinner, with less connective tissue and collagen.

The mucous membranes are also affected. The microvilli of the mucous membranes become flattened. PCM causes changes in the mucosa of the GI tract that allow entry of antigens through the intestine that would normally be barred. One type of antibody present in mucous membrane secretions (including those of the lungs and GI tract) is depressed in malnutrition. These findings may help explain why malnourished children have repeated lung and GI tract infections.

Malnutrition does not appear to consistently interfere with phagocytosis once an organism has entered the body. Results of studies in this area have met with mixed results. However, the information gathered from various studies suggests that the activity of phagocytes may be altered by malnutrition, although no single function of phagocytes can consistently account for this alteration.[4]

Cell-mediated immunity, a function of the T-lymphocytes, appears to be markedly affected by malnutrition. People with severe PCM consistently are found to have atrophy of the thymus gland; low levels of circulating lymphocytes; and involution of the thymus, spleen, lymph nodes, and the lymph-associated areas of the intestinal tract.[5] The areas of the lymph tissues that house the T-cells are depleted of lymphocytes. The skin-testing procedure discussed in Chapter 17 is one measurement of cell-mediated immunity. Several studies have shown that malnourished people do not react to skin testing (indicating that cell-mediated immunity is impaired) and that vigorous nutrition support can restore the normal reaction.[6]

Malnutrition seems to affect T-cell function more than B-cell function. Antibodies secreted from B-cells belong to a family of proteins commonly called

The immune system has several lines of defense.

immunoglobulins. In malnourished people, the blood levels of immunoglobulins are not decreased, although as already noted, one type of immunoglobulin found in mucous secretions is depressed. Data support the concept that immunoglobulin production is generally not affected during malnutrition.

Studies in the area of malnutrition and immunity are difficult to conduct. Part of the reason is that malnourished people or animals often have infections, which greatly influence metabolism and the use of nutrients. It is hard to sort out the variables and determine which effects result from infection and which from malnutrition.

The Role of Individual Nutrients

Just as generalized malnutrition has an effect on the immune system, so can deficiencies or excesses of individual

nutrients. A workshop sponsored by the American Medical Association on single-nutrient effects on immunologic functions tied together the available research findings on the subject.[7] Some of the information is presented here; still, the currently available data are far from complete.

Changes in immune function in humans have been associated with deficiencies of folacin, iron, and zinc and with excesses of vitamin E and essential fatty acids. Furthermore, clinical reports suggest that changes in immune function accompany deficiencies of vitamins A, B_6, B_{12} and C; deficiencies of pantothenic acid; and elevated blood cholesterol levels. Studies in animals link the levels of many vitamins, minerals, trace elements, amino acids, fatty acids, and cholesterol with immunologic changes. Table H19–3 lists nutrients reported to

Miniglossary of Immunity Terms

acquired immunity: immunity directed at specific organisms (also called **specific immunity**). The lymphocytes mediate this type of immunity, which depends on prior exposure, recognition, and reaction to invading organisms. Two types of specific immunity are **cell-mediated immunity** and **humoral immunity.**

antibody: a protein produced by the B-cells in response to invasion of the body by a foreign protein (see also pp. 142–143).

antigen: see p. 526.

cell-mediated immunity: immunity conferred by the actual reaction of T-cells to an invading organism.

gamma-interferon (in-ter-FEAR-on): the monokine that is responsible for the fever and malaise that frequently occur during an infection.

helper T-cells: the T-lymphocytes capable of recognizing antigens and alerting other T-cells to prepare to mount a response.

humoral immunity: immunity conferred by antibodies secreted by B-cells and carried to the invaded area by way of the body fluids.

immune system: the body's natural defense system against foreign materials.

immunity: the body's ability to recognize and eliminate foreign materials.

immunoglobulin: a protein which is capable of acting as an antibody.

immunology: the study of the immune system.

inducer T-cells: T-lymphocytes that stimulate precursor cells in the thymus to develop into mature T-cells.

innate immunity: immunity directed at foreign organisms in general (also called **nonspecific immunity**). The skin, mucous membranes, and phagocytes are a part of this type of immunity.

interleukin-1 (in-ter-LOO-kin): the monokine that activates lymphocytes.

involution: reduction in size and loss of function of an organ.

killer T-cells: T-lymphocytes that release chemicals that can destroy an invading organism. Also called **cytotoxic T-cells.**

macrophage: the type of phagocyte that secretes **monokines**.

monokines (MON-oh-kine): various proteins secreted by phagocytes that help mediate the immune response.

mucus: see p. 75.

nonspecific immunity: See *innate immunity*.

phagocytosis (FAG-oh-sigh-TOE-sis): the process by which some cells (phagocytes) engulf and destroy foreign materials.
phagein = to eat
kytos = cell
osis = intensive

precursor cell: a simple cell that matures. Precursor white blood cells are capable of maturing into three different types of cells.

sebaceous (see-BAY-shus) **glands**: glands generally associated with hair follicles that secrete fat droplets which lubricate the skin.

secretory immunoglobulin A: the antibody of the mucous membranes, usually depressed in malnutrition.

specific immunity: See *acquired immunity.*

suppressor T-cells: T-lymphocytes that slow down the immune response and eventually turn it off.

influence immune function, with the effect of each.

A Word about Nutrition and AIDS

Much of the information about the immune system accumulated in recent years has been the result of research on the disease AIDS. So deadly is AIDS that in the United States alone nearly 20 people a day die from it.[8] By late 1985, the number of cases of AIDS in the United States had risen to 14,000.[9]

Due to the many interrelationships between the immune system and nutrition status, it is not surprising that researchers have begun to look at the role of nutrition in AIDS. Severe PCM is a common finding in people with the disease.[10] It has also been shown that blood selenium levels are significantly diminished in people with AIDS.[11] The severe wasting associated with AIDS appears to be related to poor food intake, increased nutrient requirements, and GI malabsorption. Because we know that poor nutrition status can compromise immune function, it seems possible that malnutrition caused by AIDS may further impair immune function and set in motion a vicious cycle of recurrent infections and eventually death.[12]

Obviously, much work in the area of AIDS and nutrition will have to be completed before anyone will know if there are true benefits from maintaining good nutrition status in people with AIDS. One recent report outlined the medical course of a person with AIDS who was able to maintain his weight and visceral protein status on a home TPN program and an unrestricted oral diet.[13] The effectiveness of this therapy on the course of the disease has not yet been determined. However, common sense seems to indicate that careful attention to the nutrition status of the person with AIDS should be attempted.

TABLE H19–3

Effects of Selected Nutrients on the Immune System

Nutrient Deficiency	Effects
Vitamin A	Depletion of T-lymphocytes[a]; increased frequency and severity of some infections[a]; increased incidence of infections (human beings)[b]
Vitamin B_6	Depressed cell-mediated and humoral immunity[a]; reduced antibody responses to vaccines (human beings)
Folacin	Impaired response to skin tests; lymph tissue atrophy[a]; reduced numbers of white blood cells[a]; impaired cell-mediated and humoral immunity[a]
Pantothenic acid	Depressed antibody responses (human beings)
Vitamin B_{12}	Some reduction of phagocytosis by granulocytes (human beings)
Vitamin E[c]	Depressed antibody responses[a]; impaired response to skin tests[a]
Iron	Atrophy of lymph tissue; impaired response to skin tests; defective phagocytosis (human beings)
Zinc	Atrophy of lymph tissues; abnormalities in cell-mediated and humoral immunity (human beings)
Individual amino acids	Impaired humoral immunity[a]

[a]Information is from animal studies
[b]Some reports support this finding, but more information is needed.
[c]Vitamin E excess can cause inhibition of multiple immune functions in human beings.

As you can see, nutrition plays an important role in our ability to defend ourselves against disease-producing organisms. As you read Chapter 20, note that the stress of injuries such as surgery and burns often makes a person vulnerable to infection and that these stresses affect nutrition status. Keep in mind what you have just learned about nutrition and the immune system.

NOTES
1. P. Jaret, Our immune system: The wars within, *National Geographic* 169 (1986): 702–734.
2. Jaret, 1986.
3. J. W. Alexander, Immunity, nutrition and trauma: An overview, *Acta Chirurgica Scandinavica* 522 (1985): 141–150.
4. J. D. Stinnett, Protein-calorie malnutrition and host defense, in *Nutrition and the Immune Response* (Boca Raton, Fla.: 1983), p. 113.
5. Stinnett, 1983, p. 114.
6. R. M. Suskind, Malnutrition and the immune response, in *Nutrition in Clinical Care* (New York: McGraw-Hill, 1982), pp. 403–417.
7. W. R. Beisel and coauthors, Single-nutrient effects on immunologic functions, *Journal of the American Medical Association* 245 (1981): 53–58.
8. Jaret, 1986.
9. J. Laurence, The immune system in AIDS, *Scientific American* 253 (1985): 84–93.
10. P. O'Sullivan, R. A. Linke, and S. Dalton, Evaluation of body weight and nutritional status among AIDS patients, *Journal of the American Dietetic Association* 85 (1985): 1483–1484.
11. B. M. Dworkin and coauthors, Selenium deficiency in the acquired immunodeficiency syndrome, *Journal of Parenteral and Enteral Nutrition* 10 (1986): 405–407.
12. Dworkin and coauthors, 1986.
13. T. L. Domaldo and L. S. Natividad, Nutritional management of patient with AIDS and cryptosporidium infection, *Nutritional Support Services* 6 (1986): 30–31.

Nutrition and Stress: Surgery, Infection, and Burns

20

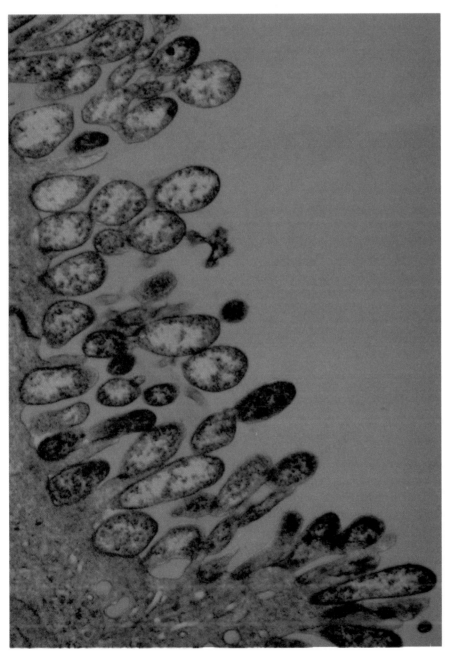

The two cells at left are being attacked by dozens of invasive microorganisms (oval shapes)—a major form of stress. The cells need to build up tremendous defenses against such invasions, defenses to which adequate nutrition is crucial.

homeostasis: see p. 15.

Stress that occurs as part of the body's normal and healthy functioning is known as **physiologic stress**. Stress imposed by disease or an abnormal bodily insult such as surgery, burns, fever, or infection is **pathologic stress**. One type of pathologic stress is **trauma**—a physical injury to the body such as a broken bone, a gunshot wound, or surgery.

Metabolically, **fasting** and **starvation** have the same consequences in the body. In fasting, food intake is voluntarily discontinued, whereas in starvation, lack of food intake is involuntary.

Under normal circumstances, the body is a finely tuned instrument that operates efficiently to maintain an internal balance. Even small changes in the internal environment, such as the influx of nutrients entering the body following a meal, set in motion a series of metabolic events to restore homeostasis—that is, to bring the body back to a state of equilibrium. Occasionally, though, the body is confronted with a more drastic change in the internal environment, such as surgery, a broken bone, an infection, or a burn. Again, the body senses the insult and sets in motion the mechanisms necessary to bring the body back to its normal balance. However, because the stress involved in these cases is greater, the mechanisms required to reestablish balance are more complicated and difficult. The complex changes the body undergoes when confronted with stress are collectively called the stress response. This chapter discusses the more severe stresses imposed on the body by illness or injury. We will look at the effects of nutrition status on the stress response, as well as the effects of the stress response on nutrition status and nutrient needs.

The Response to Stress

The body responds uniquely to each type of stress, as well as to the severity of stress. For example, the response would be different for a well-nourished person undergoing minor elective surgery (a mild stress) than it would be for a person with extensive burns (a severe type of stress). Although the response to each type of stress is unique—mending bones requires a different response than healing a wound or fighting an infection—the general metabolic responses to stress are similar (see Chapter 6, Figure 6-9).

To understand the stress response, it is helpful to understand the metabolic changes that occur as a result of fasting. Fasting is one type of stress. The metabolic changes that occur during fasting present a fairly uncomplicated picture of the stress response. If you can visualize this picture, you can use it to understand the more complex changes that occur when more severe stresses are imposed on the body. Chapter 7 gives a complete description of the metabolic events associated with fasting (pp. 214-216) that you may want to review. A brief summary is provided here.

After a short period of starvation, the body draws on stored carbohydrate, fat, and protein to meet energy needs (see Figure 7-11 on p. 214). Liver glycogen (the stored form of carbohydrate) breaks down to maintain blood glucose levels. Fatty acids are mobilized to provide fuel for many cells in the body. However, the brain requires glucose, and fatty acids cannot be converted into glucose.

Glycogen stores become depleted fairly soon after starvation begins. The body must have another source of glucose, so protein tissues begin to break down to supply those amino acids that can be used to make glucose. Glycerol from fat also can be used to make new glucose, but this process is inefficient. Generally, in the first few days of a fast, amino acids provide about 90 percent of the needed glucose and glycerol, about 10 percent.

Thereafter, the body adapts to a different energy source and so conserves vital protein. As fat continues to break down, the liver begins to synthesize ketones (see pp. 215–216), which the brain and other tissues use as an energy source, reducing the need for glucose. (The brain still needs some glucose, though.) At the same time, the body lowers its energy needs by slowing its metabolic rate. The net effect is that the body conserves its fat and lean tissues more than in the earlier stages of the fast. However, as the fast continues and more of these tissues are used for energy, the starved person is less able to perform work and the functioning of vital organs (including the GI tract, heart, and lungs) is compromised. It has been estimated that, in a person who starts at normal weight, a weight loss of 35 to 40 percent, which represents losses of about one-quarter to one-third of body protein mass, is fatal.[1]

Don't forget that during this whole process, other nutrients have influential roles, too. Vitamins and minerals are important cofactors in the metabolic reactions that are occurring. Their levels are also being drained.

More severe stresses such as surgery or infection cause a similar chain of metabolic events, except they occur more rapidly and to a greater extent (see Figure 20–1). The stress response is mediated by hormonal changes and is characterized by an increase in metabolic activity (hypermetabolism) and an accelerated breakdown of body energy reserves (catabolism) rather than conservation of protein and fat tissues. Table 20-1 lists many of the changes in hormone levels during stress and their effects on metabolism. In the period following injury, the person who is stressed has elevated blood glucose levels (hyperglycemia), negative nitrogen balance, increased retention of fluid and sodium, and increased excretion of potassium.

When several stresses occur at the same time, body tissues break down to a greater degree, amplifying the loss of vital protein. Multiple stresses can easily

hypermetabolism: accelerated metabolic activity.
catabolism: see p. 205.

FIGURE 20–1

Metabolic response to stress. The degree to which the body is affected by stress depends on the severity and duration of insult.

TABLE 20–1

Major Hormonal Changes That Occur during Severe Stress[a]

Hormone	Alteration	Metabolic Effect
Catecholamines	Increase	Glucagon release ↗
		Insulin/glucagon ratio[b] ↘
		Glycogen breakdown ↗
		Glucose production from amino acids ↗
		Mobilization of free fatty acids ↗
Cortisol	Increases	Mobilization of free fatty acids ↗
		Glucose production from amino acids ↗
		Utilization of glucose by many cells except brain ↘
Glucagon	Increases	Glucose production from amino acids ↗
		Glycogen breakdown ↗
Insulin	Decreases	Storage of glucose, amino acids and fatty acids ↘
Antidiuretic hormone	Increases	Retention of water ↗
Aldosterone	Increases	Retention of sodium ↗

[a]These changes are part of the immediate stress response. As adaptation occurs and recovery is in progress, hormone levels gradually return to normal.
[b]Whenever the ratio of insulin to glucagon decreases, the net effect is that catabolism predominates. In the immediate stress response, hormones affect the muscle cells making them unable to use blood glucose even during hyperglycemia. Skeletal muscle breaks down to supply glucose.

occur in one person—for example, a person may not eat following surgery and may develop an infection with a fever.

The metabolic changes that occur during the initial stress response are believed to be positive changes that help support the immune system, repair damaged tissues, and maintain vital organ function. These changes constitute an adaptation that is sustained for as long as necessary (or until exhaustion occurs). Figure 20–2 illustrates the phases of a stress response. When the adaptation is no longer necessary, the rate of catabolism is gradually reduced, blood glucose levels fall, and nitrogen balance is slowly restored. The amount of time it takes for the body to return to normal depends on the degree of stress. A well-nourished person can tolerate a short period of severe stress without adverse effects. However, a severely malnourished person does not have the protein reserves necessary to continue meeting the increased metabolic demands of severe injury. The result is exhaustion which may result in complications such as infection or organ failure. This further compromises the client's physical state and makes recovery more difficult.

The **acute,** or **flow, phase** of the stress response is the catabolic period immediately following the onset of stress. During the **adaptive phase,** the body adjusts to the stress to minimize losses. If adaptation fails, **exhaustion** follows. If adaptation succeeds, **recovery** follows.

Nutrition and Surgery

The body's ability to adapt to the stress of surgery is influenced considerably by a person's nutrition status. If you think about the roles nutrients play, you'll have little difficulty seeing why nutrition status affects a person's ability to recover

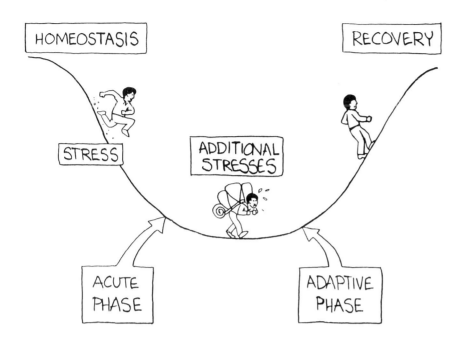

FIGURE 20–2

Phases of a stress response. During the initial stress response, hypermetabolism sends nutrient reserves on a downhill course. As adaptation occurs, nutrient balances are gradually restored. If depleted of nutrients, the person will be unable to make the uphill trip and may not recover (exhaustion). A person who is carrying a heavier load (additional stress) will plunge downhill faster and have a more difficult climb.

from surgery. Consider protein alone: it is the material of antibodies needed to fight infection, of collagen needed to form scars, of all cells needed to rebuild damaged tissue, of plasma proteins that maintain fluid and electrolyte balance, of the matrix on which bones are rebuilt after fractures, and of many more crucial tissue constituents. In addition, amino acids provide glucose when glycogen stores are depleted. The protein-deficient person is handicapped in being inadequately supplied with all these factors and more.

It is no surprise, then, that malnourished people undergoing surgery have been found to have a high incidence of postoperative mortality, morbidity, infections, and delayed wound healing. Furthermore, the surgical procedure itself may directly influence intake, digestion, and absorption of nutrients, which may lead to malnutrition even in a person whose nutrition status before surgery was good. A person who develops complications following surgery is even more likely to become malnourished because of the additional stress placed on the body. The following discussion will concentrate on the nutrition needs of people undergoing general surgery. The next two chapters discuss specific nutrition needs associated with various surgeries of the GI tract.

Surgery may influence nutrient intake, digestion, and absorption.

Nutrition before Surgery

Whenever possible, a person's nutrition status should be optimal prior to surgery. Optimal status may be difficult to achieve, however, since the illness that necessitates the surgery or the psychological stress associated with it may interfere with food intake or nutrient utilization, increasing the likelihood of malnutrition. Additionally, many diagnostic and laboratory tests can be given only after the person to be tested has fasted or has followed a nutritionally inadequate liquid diet, which further taxes nutrition status. On the other hand, obesity also is a risk factor, and excess weight should be reduced before surgery whenever possible.

Check the hospital diet manual to determine what a "regular" and a "high-kcalorie, high-protein" diet contain.

Before surgery, a regular diet is generally adequate for well-nourished people who are expected to have no complications afterward. They can withstand short-term starvation and some degree of protein catabolism without serious consequences. Regular hospital diets provide ample kcalories and generally exceed the RDA for protein.

For people who are malnourished, diets high in kcalories and protein are recommended prior to surgery. A method for calculating energy needs in various types of stress is shown in Table 20-2. In most hospitals these clients receive high-kcalorie and high-protein supplements and snacks between meals. Such diets generally provide about 1,000 kcalories more than a regular diet and 125 grams of protein daily. A closer approximation of specific protein requirements can be made by conducting a nitrogen balance study (see pp. 146-147). For people with functioning GI tracts who cannot consume an adequate intake orally, tube feeding may be indicated. Furthermore, TPN may be initiated before surgery if use of the GI tract is contraindicated (see Chapter 18).

Vitamins, minerals, and trace elements should be provided to meet individual needs. A person with iron-deficiency anemia will be given iron supplementation before elective surgery or a blood transfusion when surgery must be performed immediately. The need for B vitamins increases when kcalorie and protein intakes increase. However, diets higher in kcalories and protein usually contain increased amounts of these nutrients as well; thus the person who is accepting the variety of foods offered needs no supplements.

All foods and fluids are generally withheld for at least eight hours before surgery. This step helps prevent regurgitation and aspiration, which can occur during anesthesia or recovery. For people undergoing GI surgery, liquids or foods low in residue are given for two or three days before surgery to minimize the amount of fecal material in the gut and help prevent distension after surgery.

TABLE 20–2

Stress and Energy Needs

BMR (p. 245) and BEE (here) express the same thing: basal energy need. The equation for BMR is traditionally used in physiology and fitness laboratories; that for BEE, in hospitals. The two equations yield slightly different results, each suitable for the purposes intended.

The increments for activity used in the hospital (here) differ from those on p. 245 for similar reasons. All are approximations; all require judgment in their application.

Basal Energy Expenditure (BEE)[a]
  Women
    $BEE = 655 + [9.6 \times \text{wt in kg}^b] + [1.7 \times \text{ht in cm}^b] + [4.7 \times \text{age in years}]$
  Men
    $BEE = 66 + [13.7 \times \text{wt in kg}] + [5 \times \text{ht in cm}] + [6.8 \times \text{age in years}]$
Add to BEE for activity
    20% Sedentary
    35% Moderately active
    50% Active
Add to BEE for stress
    10–15% Uncomplicated elective surgery
    20–40% Complicated surgery or fractures
    50–100% Major burn
Add to BEE for fever (if present)
    13% per degree centigrade[b]
Add to BEE for growth (if necessary)
    5% Moderate weight loss
    10–15% Severe weight loss

[a]This is the Harris-Benedict equation frequently used to estimate energy needs.
[b]See inside back cover for equations to convert kg, cm, and °C.

Low-residue and residue-free liquid supplements are available to meet all the nutrient needs of people on liquid diets. These supplements can be given either orally or by tube to people who are malnourished or who will be unable to eat for some time after surgery.

Nutrition after Surgery

The immediate nutrition-related concern following surgery is the maintenance of fluid and electrolyte balance. The loss of blood, fluid, and electrolytes from the body during surgery can lead to dehydration and shock. Additional fluids may be lost thereafter, from fever, draining wounds, vomiting, and diarrhea. Fluids and electrolytes are replaced by IV infusion after surgery, because peristalsis in the GI tract is inactive in the immediate postoperative period. The amount of fluid given is determined by such factors as the person's blood pressure, pulse rate, urinary output, level of consciousness, breathing patterns, and body temperature, to name a few. Until peristalsis returns, foods and fluids cannot be given orally.

A standard hospital diet adequate in all nutrients is the diet of choice after uncomplicated elective surgery for the well-nourished person who can tolerate solid foods. People with depleted nutrient stores and people with postsurgical complications need high-kcalorie, high-protein diets. No less than 1.5 grams of protein per kilogram of ideal body weight should be supplied. To increase energy intake, the fats and carbohydrates in the diet also are increased.

People on TPN prior to surgery will most likely be kept on TPN until their oral intake is adequate. Evidence has accumulated to suggest that people on TPN should receive nonprotein kcalories from a combination of IV fat and glucose, rather than the traditional routine of using glucose alone.[2] Intravenous fat does not elevate blood levels of insulin, as glucose does; high insulin levels interfere with the body's use of amino acids to make new protein.

The surgeon who anticipates that a person may have difficulties in resuming oral intake may construct a feeding gastrostomy or jejunostomy during surgery. Tube feedings can then be continued until oral intake is adequate.

The objective of postsurgical nutrition support is to prevent weight loss and the depletion of nutrients. Generally, the diets of people who are not receiving special nutrition support (IV or tube feedings) progress from clear liquids to full liquids and on to a regular diet as tolerated.

A clear liquid diet consists of foods that are clear and liquid or that liquefy at room temperature. The purpose of a clear liquid diet is to provide fluids and electrolytes to prevent dehydration. Clear liquids are easily digested and absorbed and contribute little or no residue in the GI tract. Table 20-3 and the

shock: a sudden drop in the blood volume that disrupts the supply of oxygen to the tissues and the return of blood to the heart. Many events can lead to shock; some include major blood loss, trauma, and dehydration.

She may look as if she has adequate nutrient stores, but looks can be deceiving. Inside an obese person, a malnourished person may be hidden.

The general progression of diets after surgery from clear liquids to full liquids to a low-fiber diet to a regular diet is collectively called a **progressive diet**.

clear liquid diet: a diet consisting of foods that are clear and liquid or that liquefy at room temperature.

full liquid diet: a diet consisting of clear and opaque liquid foods and those which liquefy at room temperature.

> When you think of nutrient-depleted people, don't forget that overweight people can be depleted, too. It is easy to overlook malnutrition in these individuals. Although overweight persons may have adequate fat stores, their bodies may have lost vital protein. The period immediately following a major injury or surgery is *not* the time for a weight reduction diet.

Sample clear liquid diet menu.

Breakfast
Strained orange juice
Flavored gelatin
Ginger ale
Coffee or tea
Sugar

Lunch
Bouillon
Apple juice
Flavored gelatin
Coffee or tea
Sugar

Supper
Bouillon
Cranberry juice
Flavored gelatin
Coffee or tea
Sugar

Between meals
Soft drinks,
gelatin, or fruit
juices as tolerated

TABLE 20–3

Foods Included on Liquid Diets

Clear Liquid Diets

Bouillon
Broth, fat-free
Carbonated beverages
Coffee, regular and decaffeinated
Commercially prepared clear liquid
    formulas
Fruit juices, strained
Gelatin
Popsicles
Tea

Full Liquid Diets

All clear liquids
Any commercially prepared formula
Cooked cereals, strained
Custard
Flavorings
Fruit ices
Honey
Ice cream, plain
Potatoes, mashed and diluted in cream
    soups
Pudding
Sherbet
Soups, strained vegetable, meat, or
    cream
Syrup
Vegetable juices
Vegetable purees, diluted in cream
    soups

---

sample menu show the foods allowed on clear liquid diets. Clear liquid nutrition formulas that meet all nutrient needs are also available. In some hospitals these formulas are routinely used following surgery to prevent the severe kcalorie and protein deficit that occurs when incomplete liquid diets are fed. The use of formulas has other advantages: formulas have a specific osmolality compatible with the client's fluid balance; and they are often lactose-free, which accommodates the loss of lactose tolerance often seen in GI dysfunction. They may be better tolerated by the individual who needs a liquid diet.[3]

A full liquid diet includes both clear and opaque liquid foods and those that liquefy at room temperature. Table 20-3 lists foods allowed on full liquid diets.

Take a close look at the foods allowed on a standard clear liquid diet. You can see why many people find these foods unappetizing and boring. Even more disturbing, consider the nutritional quality of the diet—it is deficient in kcalories and most nutrients. Then consider that a stressed person's nutrient requirements are increased. Care must be taken to ensure that no one is kept on a standard clear liquid diet for any length of time.

Often the postsurgical diet order simply says "diet as tolerated." A nurse or dietitian consults with the client and uses discretion in advancing the diet from liquids to regular. Sometimes someone forgets to advance the diet. Other times a person truly cannot tolerate foods other than clear liquids; in these cases, further steps must be taken. Liquid formulas, tube feedings, or total or supplemental IV nutrition may be necessary.

If you work with people after surgery, remember to check their diets. If they must stay on liquid formulas for several days, alert the dietitian or suggest to the physician that a supplemental formula be considered.

Sample full liquid diet menu.

Breakfast
Orange juice
Strained oatmeal
Eggnog
Milk
Sugar
Margarine

Lunch
Apricot nectar
Creamed soup
Pudding
Milk
Coffee or tea
Sugar

Supper
Apple juice
Creamed soup
Custard
Milk
Coffee or tea
Sugar

Between meals
Milkshakes (made
  with plain ice
  cream), eggnog,
  pudding, custard,
  or gelatin

A sample full liquid menu is shown here. Any liquid nutrition formula can be included on a full liquid diet to meet nutrient needs.

Depending on the type of surgery and the quality of the diet, supplements of some nutrients may be necessary. The need for many of the B vitamins increases when energy and protein intakes are increased. Vitamin C deserves special attention also; it helps form collagen, which plays an important role in wound healing. Vitamin K is important after surgery because of its role in blood clotting. Like vitamin C, zinc is involved in wound healing.

Malnutrition after surgery may be further complicated by anorexia and immobilization. Lack of appetite can be improved by serving foods the person likes, at the correct temperature, in an attractive manner. Some people tolerate frequent, small meals or snacks, whereas others prefer larger meals served less often. Individualizing the diet is very important. Exercise is important, too. Encourage clients to get out of bed and begin minimal exercise (such as walking) as soon as medically safe. Chapter 18 gives additional suggestions to improve a client's appetite.

Nutrition and Infection

In areas of the world where people suffer from malnutrition, the incidence of infection is high. Infection further contributes to malnutrition, and a downward spiral takes its course. The discovery of this association has sparked great interest in how nutrition affects the immune system. In recent years, research in this area has expanded tremendously. A brief look at the role of nutrition in immunity is given in Highlight 19.

During an **infection,** the body is invaded by a disease-causing microorganism or virus that causes illness. **Sepsis** results from the presence of microorganisms or their poisonous products directly in the bloodstream. **Septicemia** (sep-tee-SEE-me-ah) is a synonym for sepsis.

Sally, a 20-year-old prelaw student, went to the emergency room of the university hospital complaining of nausea, fever, and severe pain in the lower right portion of her abdomen. The diagnosis was appendicitis, and Sally was taken to surgery for an appendectomy (removal of the appendix). Sally's height and weight on admission were 5 ft 7 inches and 132 lb, respectively. She had experienced a 5-lb weight loss in the past month, which the dietitian attributed to irregular

CASE STUDY

Surgery

eating habits during a heavy work schedule.

1. From the limited information about Sally's nutrition history presented here, what can you say about Sally's nutrition status? Are there any risk factors for poor nutrition status? What other data would be useful in evaluating her nutrition status?

2. Because Sally had emergency surgery, nothing could be done to improve her nutrition status before surgery. If surgery had been anticipated, what advice could you have given Sally about her diet? Specifically, what kind of a diet would you have recommended?

3. What kind of a diet would be appropriate for Sally after surgery? Consider kcalorie, protein, vitamin, and mineral needs.

4. Consider Sally's nutrition education needs. What type of nutrition advice could Sally benefit from? Who could provide this advice?

The **incubation period** of an infection is the interval between exposure to the infection and development of related symptoms.

A **fever** is an increase of temperature of more than 1° F above normal (98.6° F).

A person who is **febrile** (FEE-brile) has a fever; **afebrile** (AY-fee-brile) means "without fever."

The **convalescent period** of an infection describes the period of recovery from illness; during convalescence the body develops positive nutrient balances.

Once an infection has developed, the metabolic events that follow greatly influence nutrient needs. The response to infection is for the most part similar to the response that occurs with surgery or other injury. However, the body takes longer to adapt to using ketones for energy, so the early protein losses are more severe. Infection often develops in people already stressed by malnutrition, surgery, or other injury. The anorexia, nausea, vomiting, diarrhea, and immobilization that occur in infected persons place further demands on nutrient stores.

The course of an infection goes something like this. Following exposure to an infective agent, a period of time (generally a few days) passes before the first symptoms of the infection appear. Shortly after this period, most infections cause a fever to develop. After the onset of fever, the catabolic changes that characterize the stress response begin. Hyperglycemia develops. The body's losses of nitrogen (from protein catabolism) and intracellular electrolytes (potassium, magnesium, phosphorus, zinc, and sulfur) exceed intake, and negative body balances develop. These negative balances are aggravated by reduced intake of food. If diarrhea and vomiting also occur, the body loses even more nutrients. Because of associated hormonal changes, the infected individual may retain water and sodium.

When an infection lasts for a long time, the person gradually begins to conserve nitrogen. However, this occurs after he has already suffered marked weight loss and muscle wasting. Once the illness has ended, the person generally develops positive balances that restore the body to its normal composition. The time it takes for the body to reach a positive balance and the duration of the positive balance depend on the extent of nutrient deficiencies, as well as the quality and quantity of food intake. During this time, a well-balanced diet is essential to restore vital nutrient reserves. A good diet may also help guard against the development of additional infections.

The overriding concern in the infected person is to identify and eliminate the invading organism. Often, antibiotics are prescribed. Remember that antibiotics may alter nutrient intake or otherwise interfere with nutrition status (see Chapter 19).

Nutrient Needs

Fever is a major factor in determining the energy needs of the infected person. The basal metabolic rate (BMR) increases approximately 13 percent for each 1 degree centigrade (7 percent for each 1 degree Fahrenheit) the temperature rises above normal (98.6 degrees Fahrenheit; 37 degrees centigrade). (The scientific name for the centigrade temperature scale is Celsius. Conversion equations are provided on the inside back cover.) Additional kcalories should be given for activity, particularly for the person who is restless. Weigh the client daily, and monitor changes in body weight. When you assess body weight, keep in mind that the person who is infected may retain sodium and water or, conversely, may be dehydrated. Therefore, the scale weight may not always reflect tissue weight changes.

The immune system functions best when protein status is optimal. The actual protein requirements of the person who is infected depend largely on the total kcalorie consumption. However, at a minimum, the protein intake should be consistent with the RDA for age, weight, and sex. These allowances should be increased by 10 percent per 1 degree centigrade (5.5 percent per 1 degree Fahrenheit) of fever.

Closely monitor the person who is infected to ensure that fluid needs are being met. In some infectious diseases, particularly those that involve vomiting, diarrhea, or considerable sweating, fluid needs may be as high as 3 to 4 liters per day. On the other hand, the infected person may retain water due to the hormonal changes that accompany fever. Excessive fluid in these cases can cause fluid overload. Dehydration is usually not a problem for people with infections that are not accompanied by diarrhea, vomiting, or excessive sweating.

Little information is available regarding increased requirements for specific vitamins and minerals during infection. As mentioned, the need for B vitamins increases with increased intake of kcalories and protein but remains consistent with the RDA. Vitamin supplements should be given in their normal doses throughout the course of illness or, at most, in amounts not more than two times the RDA. This supplementation will cover the possibility that vitamins may be metabolized or excreted in large amounts during hypermetabolic states.[4] Likewise, losses of intracellular electrolytes (which are also in negative balance during an infection) can generally be covered through foods. Sodium may have to be restricted in people who are retaining this electrolyte. The general guidelines for feeding people after surgery also apply to people with infections. People who are nauseated or anorexic may accept liquids more readily than solid foods.

Persons with infections often develop a type of anemia (anemia of infection) that does not respond to iron, folacin, or vitamin B_{12} therapy. At the onset of an infectious illness, blood levels of iron rapidly decline as iron moves into the liver cells for storage. The iron, then, is not available to make new hemoglobin, and anemia results. However, this shift of iron from the blood to the liver helps fight the infection. Once in storage, the iron is unavailable to bacteria, which need it to carry out metabolic functions. Therefore, supplemental iron is not given for this type of anemia.

A. J. is a 22-year-old male who is 5 ft 9 inches tall, weighs 160 lb, and has a temperature of 103° F. To calculate the impact of fever on his energy needs, first determine his BMR (for males: 1 kcal/kg/hr; for females: 0.9 kcal/kg/hr).

$$1 \text{ kcal} \times \frac{160 \text{ lb}}{2.2 \text{ kg}} \times 24 \text{ hr} = 1{,}745 \text{ kcal/day.}$$

A. J.'s temperature is 4.4° F above normal. His BMR increases by:

$$4.4° \text{ F} \times 7\% = 31\%.$$

His energy needs increase by:

$$1{,}745 \text{ kcal} \times 31\% = 541 \text{ kcal.}$$

His energy needs are:

$$1{,}745 \text{ kcal} + 541 \text{ kcal} = 2{,}286 \text{ kcal.}$$

Fever has added more than 500 kcal to A. J.'s energy needs. Additional kcalories must be considered depending on his activity level.

A. J.'s protein needs can be calculated from his RDA for protein:

$$0.8 \text{ g} \times \frac{160 \text{ lb}}{2.2 \text{ kg}} = 58 \text{ g protein.}$$

The fever increases his protein needs as follows:

$$4.4° \text{ F} \times 5.5\% = 24\%.$$
$$58 \text{ g} \times 24\% = 14 \text{ g.}$$

His total protein needs are:

$$58 \text{ g} + 14 \text{ g} = 72 \text{ g.}$$

Nutrition and Burns

A burn is sometimes called a **thermal injury**.

Psychological and emotional concerns of the person who is burned often outweigh interest in food.

The fluid containing plasma proteins and electrolytes that leaks out through the capillaries is called the **exudate** (EX-you-date).
exsudare = to sweat out

An extensive burn represents an extreme state of stress to the body. Figure 20-3 shows the area of the skin affected by burns of different degrees. The metabolic response to a burn results in major shifts in fluid and electrolyte balance, rapid tissue catabolism, and a rapid loss of body mass. The person who is burned quickly uses up the energy and protein reserves necessary for survival. Moreover, most people with burns experience anorexia and depression, leading to poor food intake and further deterioration of nutrition status. Therefore, the nutrition needs of the person with extensive burns are high. The burn injury itself may make eating difficult because of the associated pain or because of its physical location (for example, the hands). Immobilization and lack of exercise further aggravate the situation.

Not all people with burns require aggressive nutrition support. People who are well nourished and whose burns cover less than 20 percent of their body surface area (BSA) can do well on regular diets. People with more extensive burns or those at risk for poor nutrition status should be monitored aggressively to ensure that they receive appropriate nutrition support.

Nutrient Needs

Immediately after a person is burned, dramatic changes take place in the circulatory system. Plasma proteins (mainly albumin) and electrolytes leak through the capillaries into the interstitial space and the burned area. The collection of fluid in the interstitial space causes considerable edema. Plasma volume can be reduced by more than one-half of its normal volume in people with 40 percent BSA burns.[5] During this time, then, the primary consideration of therapy is providing enough fluid and electrolytes to maintain circulatory volume and prevent shock. Fluids are given to maintain urinary output at about 50 milliliters

FIGURE 20–3

Depth of burn wounds.

per hour. Isotonic fluids are given intravenously, because the person who is severely burned experiences a temporary absence of peristalsis and cannot take fluids by mouth. On an average, 3 to 5 liters are needed to replace fluid losses daily. However, in some cases over 10 liters of fluid may be required.

Normal bowel activity usually returns in the period following fluid replacement, and attention to adequate nutrition becomes essential. Hypermetabolism reaches a peak at about the end of the first postburn week and then gradually becomes normal over a period of several weeks. The duration of the hypermetabolic state depends on the severity of the burn. Hypermetabolism is associated with extreme protein catabolism and weight loss. The rate of hypermetabolism also is related to the severity of the burn, reaching a maximum with a 50 percent BSA burn.

Researchers have tried to estimate the kcalorie needs of the person who is burned. Recent studies have suggested that there is an upper limit of kcalories required by the person who is burned.[6] That limit is set close to twice the amount needed to meet the BMR. One commonly used estimation of energy needs is given here.[7]

Adults:

[25 kcal × preburn body wt (kg)] + [40 kcal × %BSA burned].

Children:

[38 to 100 kcal* × preburn body wt (kg)] + [40 kcal × %BSA burned].

Always remember that these equations are used only to provide an estimate of requirements. Adjustments in kcalorie intake should be made as indicated by body weight changes or complications (such as infection), which may change energy needs. Nitrogen balance can generally be achieved by giving 2 to 3 grams of protein per kilogram of body weight per day.[8]

Specific vitamin and mineral requirements for people with burns have not been established. However, in consideration of the high energy and protein requirements, as well as nutrients needed for tissue repair and blood and skin losses, additional B vitamins in amounts up to two times the RDA are often given. Vitamins and minerals that are potentially toxic (such as fat-soluble vitamins and many trace minerals) or those that can alter normal body balances (such as calcium and phosphorus) should only be given in amounts that meet the RDA. Because vitamin C and zinc are known to be essential to wound healing, these nutrients may be provided in amounts that exceed the RDA.

Goals for Meeting Nutrient Needs

As soon as the bowel becomes active, feeding should begin.[9] At the latest, nutrition support should begin by the fourth postburn day. If bowel activity has not resumed by this time, then peripheral or central parenteral nutrition should be started. By the seventh postburn day, kcalorie intake should approximate energy demands. If a person has active bowel motility but cannot eat enough food, then a tube feeding should be initiated.

To encourage the individual with a burn to eat, remember to keep the total person in mind. Emotional support is important. Understandably, food may

---

*The kcalories required depend on the child's age.

B. T. is a 39-year-old female who weighs 130 lb. She recently sustained a 60% BSA burn. Her energy needs can be calculated as follows:

$$[25 \text{ kcal} \times \frac{130 \text{ lb}}{2.2 \text{ kg}} + [40 \text{ kcal} \times 60] = 3{,}877 \text{ kcal}.$$

B. T.'s protein needs range from 118 to 177g protein daily:

$$2 \times \frac{130 \text{lb}}{2.2 \text{ kg}} = 118 \text{ g}.$$

$$3 \times \frac{130 \text{ lb}}{2.2 \text{ kg}} = 177 \text{ g}.$$

D. Z., an 11-month-old baby who weighs 20 lb, recently suffered a 30% BSA burn. His energy needs can be calculated as follows:

$$[100 \text{ kcal} \times \frac{20 \text{ lb}}{2.2 \text{ kg}}] + [40 \text{ kcal} \times 30] = 2{,}109 \text{ kcal}.$$

D. Z.'s protein needs range from 25 to 38 g daily:

$$2 \times 1.4 \text{ g/kg} \times \frac{20 \text{ lb}}{2.2 \text{ kg}} = 25 \text{ g}.$$

$$3 \times 1.4 \text{g/kg} \times \frac{20 \text{ lb}}{2.2 \text{ kg}} = 38 \text{ g}.$$

Occasionally, people with extensive burns develop deep ulcers (usually in the duodenum) called **Curling's ulcers,** which can cause major bleeding. When bleeding is profuse, the person cannot be fed orally. For these individuals, TPN may be indicated.

Dead, burned skin is called **eschar** (ES-car). As the eschar becomes loose, it is removed so that the burn wound can close as soon as possible. The removal of the eschar is called **débridement** (day-breed-MON) [French] or more commonly (dee-BREED-ment).
eschara = scab

Hydrotherapy, sometimes called **tanking,** is used to cleanse the burn wound and help loosen the eschar. The person is placed in a large whirlpool tub, where the wounds are gently cleansed with a special soap that helps prevent infections.

Physical therapy is important for preventing **contractures,** or loss of joint function, in people with burns. As the burn wound heals, the new skin is very tight, and it may pull the area surrounding a joint into a nonfunctional position.

Exercise can help improve the appetite and restore normal nutrient balances.

bedsores: the breakdown of skin and underlying tissues caused by constant pressure on and lack of oxygen to that area of the skin. Bedsores are often called **pressure sores** or **decubitus** (dee-CUE-beh-tus) **ulcers**.
de = down
cumbere = to lie

seem unappealing to the person who faces a lengthy hospital stay, a great deal of pain, and fear of permanent disfigurement. Burn therapy, which generally includes whirlpool baths and the cutting away of dead skin and tissue, is extremely painful. If possible, these treatments should be scheduled so as not to interfere with mealtimes. Pain medications should be given prior to meals so that mealtimes are enjoyable.

People may feel awkward about eating when the location of a burn interferes with self-feeding. An occupational therapist may be able to adapt feeding utensils to assist the client. Encourage the client to get up and walk around and begin physical therapy as soon as possible. This measure helps prevent further catabolism associated with injury, improves morale, and also may help to stimulate the appetite.

Nutrition Care with Other Trauma

Although there are some differences in the nutrition care of people with various types of stress and trauma, for the most part the care is similar. Diets high in kcalories, protein, vitamins, and minerals, with close attention to fluids, are the general rule. The same is true for mechanical types of trauma such as bone fractures.

Immobilization, which commonly occurs during periods of other stress and trauma, itself alters metabolism. During immobilization the body loses nitrogen and calcium. Calcium is lost from bone when the weight bearing and muscle tension produced by normal activity do not occur. In prolonged immobilization, blood and urine levels of calcium may increase, causing calcium stones to form in the kidney and bladder. Restricting dietary calcium does not alleviate the problem. The best treatment is for the client to become active as soon as possible. A high-protein diet helps minimize negative nitrogen balance but may increase the risk of calcium stone formation. High-protein diets are associated with increased urinary excretion of calcium (see p. 156).

Bedsores occur when constant pressure is exerted on the skin, reducing blood flow to the area. Eventually the skin breaks down and dies. The tissues and muscles under the skin, and even the bone, may also be involved in the breakdown. In addition to inadequate oxygen to the area, several nutrition risk factors have been associated with bedsores, including negative nitrogen balance, anemia, vitamin and mineral deficiencies, underweight, and overweight. The best treatment is prevention. Regularly turning and repositioning the person who is bedridden alleviates pressure and minimizes the risk of bedsores.

Screening individuals who are at risk for poor nutrition status is important. Those who are severely underweight have a greater risk of developing bedsores because there is less fat to pad the area between the skin and the bone. Those who are overweight are also at risk; although they have adequate or excessive padding between the bone and the skin, the pressure of excess weight on bony areas makes them more susceptible to bedsores.[10] Special care should be taken to ensure that people with bedsores or those at risk for developing them receive diets that fully meet their nutrient needs.

M r. Sampson, a 48-year-old journalist, has been admitted to the emergency room. He suffered a third-degree, 40 percent BSA burn when he was trapped in a burning building. His height and weight on admission were 6 ft and 175 lb, respectively. The physician ordered lab work, including serum proteins, that has not yet been reported.

1. Identify Mr. Sampson's immediate postinjury needs. Should he be fed orally during this time? Why or why not? If not, how would you determine when Mr. Sampson can begin eating foods orally?

2. Do you have enough information to determine Mr. Sampson's preinjury, preburn nutrition status? If not, what information would be useful? Is information about preburn nutrition status important in this case? Why or why not?

3. Calculate Mr. Sampson's kcalorie and protein needs for burn healing. Discuss what other nutrients must be considered.

4. Discuss some general guidelines for providing all of Mr. Sampson's nutrient needs. What physical and emotional factors must be considered?

5. If Mr. Sampson cannot get adequate nutrients orally by the fourth to seventh postburn day, how should he be fed?

6. Describe the role of physical therapy and exercise in Mr. Sampson's treatment.

Hospitalized or injured people often are afraid and anxious. These feelings stimulate the activity of the stress hormones that intensify stress and suppress GI activity (see Chapter 6). In addition, these feelings can interfere with food intake by causing anorexia or nausea. Therefore, whenever you can relieve someone's anxiety, you also hasten physical recovery.

Nutrition Assessment

Of course, all of the parameters of nutrition assessment discussed in Chapter 17 are applicable to the individual who is stressed or injured. However, some important aspects of the assessment should be emphasized here:

- An accurate assessment of the person's *preinjury* nutrition status is vital for determining nutrient needs and risk of complications.
- Careful and continuous monitoring of nutrition status is critical to ensure that nutrient needs are being met by the diet. Individuals' nutrient stores can become depleted rapidly.
- For people on oral diets, a careful history of food likes and dislikes will be invaluable in encouraging adequate oral intake.
- Anthropometrics must be interpreted cautiously in the period immediately following the injury. Weights may be misleading because people may be retaining or losing water. Also, the location of wounds may make arm anthropometrics impossible.
- In people with burns, low serum albumin and transferrin levels are due to the loss of plasma proteins through the burn wound and into the

interstitial fluid. Low values are to be expected and are not useful as indices of nutrition status immediately following the burn injury.

- In all stressed individuals, serum albumin concentrations may be reduced for a while. Levels that remain depressed for more than seven days following the insult can be evaluated as an indicator of poor protein status.[11]

Because stress taxes the body's nutrient stores, it is critical to be aware of nutrition status in people suffering stress or trauma.

Study Questions

1. What is the stress response, and what is its purpose?
2. How does the stress response differ from the body's response to starvation?
3. Describe the effect of nutrition status on the body's ability to respond to stress.
4. What are some factors that can lead to poor nutrition status prior to surgery? What type of diet should be eaten in the days before surgery? What diet modifications are made right before surgery, and why?
5. What is the purpose of a clear liquid diet? What foods are allowed on this diet? Construct a sample clear liquid diet, and consider the practical limitations of following such a diet.
6. Describe a full liquid diet. How can liquid nutrition formulas be used to improve liquid diets?
7. Discuss the role of tube feedings and parenteral nutrition after surgery. When would these diets be indicated?
8. What is the immediate nutrient concern after surgery? How is this concern dealt with?
9. Think about the effect of malnutrition on the immune system and the effect of infection and disease on nutrition status. What factors influence nutrient needs during an infection? What nutrients are of particular concern?
10. Describe the changes in body fluids that occur immediately after a person suffers an extensive burn. What is the primary concern during this period? How are these needs met?
11. When can a person be fed by mouth after a burn? What metabolic events occur during a burn injury, and how do they affect nutrient needs?
12. Describe the kcalorie and protein needs of an adult and a child with a burn. Calculate your own kcalorie and protein needs based on a 50% BSA burn.
13. Discuss the goals for meeting the nutrient needs of a person with an extensive burn. How are people with burns fed? What factors influence the nutrition status of the person with a burn?
14. What effects does immobilization have on nutrient balances, and how can these effects be minimized?
15. What is a bedsore? How can bedsores be prevented and treated?
16. Discuss some major factors to keep in mind when you assess the nutrition status of a person with severe stress or trauma.

Notes

1. J. J. Reilly and A. L. Gerhardt, Modern surgical nutrition, *Current Problems in Surgery* 22 (1985): 1-81.
2. H. Gilder, Parenteral nourishment of patients undergoing surgical or traumatic stress, *Journal of Parenteral and Enteral Nutrition* 10 (1986): 88-99.
3. D. P. Murray and coauthors, Survey: Use of clear and full liquid diets with or without commercially produced formulas, *Journal of Parenteral and Enteral Nutrition* 9 (1985): 732-734.
4. J. Kirkpatrick and R. Nelson, Preoperative nutritional support: Indications and strategies, *Nutritional Support Services* 1 (1981): 28-29; R. V. Heatley, R. H. Williams, and M. H. Lewis, Pre-operative intravenous feeding: A controlled trial, *Postgraduate Medical Journal* 55 (1979): 541-545.
5. P. R. Rogenes and J. A. Moylan, Restoring fluid balance in the patient with severe burns, *American Journal of Nursing* 76 (1976): 1953-1957.
6. W. W. Turner and coauthors, Predicting energy expenditures in burned patients, *Journal of Trauma* 25 (1985): 11-16; J. R. Saffle and coauthors, Use of indirect calorimetry in the nutritional management of burned patients, *Journal of Trauma* 25 (1985): 32-39.
7. P. W. Curreri, Nutritional replacement modalities, *Journal of Trauma* (supplement) 19 (1979): 906-908.
8. S. J. Bell and J. Wyatt, Nutrition guidelines for burned patients, *Journal of the American Dietetic Association* 86 (1986): 648-653.
9. T. G. Jensen and coauthors, Nutritional assessment indications of postburn complications, *Journal of the American Dietetic Association* 85 (1985): 68-72.
10. E. D. Durr, Nutritional intervention for patients with pressure sores, *Nutritional Support Services* 6 (1986): 28-29.
11. J. P. Grant, P. B. Custer, and J. Thurlow, Current techniques of nutritional assessment, *Surgical Clinics of North America* 61 (1981): 437-463.

HIGHLIGHT TWENTY

Ethical Issues in Clinical Nutrition

Chapter 20 described how stresses on the body can drastically alter nutrient needs, and why meeting these needs is vital to recovery in some cases. It is only in recent years that we have at our disposal the capability of providing these nutrients for people who cannot take food by mouth. The technical advances made in the areas of enteral and parenteral nutrition have been lifesaving for many. However, as is true with many new technologies, the availability of special nutrition support forces health care professionals to deal with ethical dilemmas—specifically, when it is morally and legally appropriate to use special nutrition support techniques, and when these techniques should be discontinued.

The purpose of this highlight is to discuss some of the ethical questions that have been raised regarding the use of enteral and parenteral nutrition. You will find that we do not draw conclusions or solve the problem; we present the facts for you to consider and form your own opinions.

A Look at the Problems

Under most circumstances, the decision to feed a person by tube feeding or TPN is clear-cut. The person who is expected to recover from a disease and sustain an acceptable quality of life is given whatever form of nutrition support is necessary. Unfortunately, some clients have not received adequate nutrition support due to poor judgement or negligence. If a person were to die because nourishment was withheld, the care takers would be held responsible. In all likelihood, a malpractice lawsuit would result. In one case, an out-of-court settlement of $400,000 was negotiated by a hospital charged with failure to provide needed care, including nutrition support, to a person with Crohn's disease.[1] In another case, murder charges were brought against a corporation that owns a nursing home in Texas. An 87-year-old resident had been maintained on a diet of only 636 kcalories for 41 days.[2] (At the time of this writing, the latter case has not been decided.)

The decision becomes less clear when the person is not expected to recover. How aggressively do we support the person who is terminally ill or permanently comatose? How do we respond to elderly or physically disabled people who refuse special nutrition support because they feel the quality of their lives is so poor that they do not wish to be sustained? Do we allow such a choice? Are health care professionals morally and legally obligated to comply with or to deny such requests? Furthermore, when people are incompetent and unable to speak for themselves, who, if anyone, should be

When is it morally and legally appropriate to use special nutrition support techniques?

Miniglossary

artificial feeding: parenteral and enteral nutrition. Feeding by a route other than the normal ingestion of food.

brain dead: having an irreversible loss of the brain function necessary to sustain life.

cerebral palsy: a loss of sensation and ability to control movement that results from defects in the brain or trauma at birth.

comatose: in a state of deep unconsciousness from which the person cannot be aroused.

gangrene: death of tissue.

homicide: murder.

living will: a document signed by a competent adult that specifically states that the person does not wish any heroic measures to be taken in the event of terminal illness or irreversible coma from which the person is not expected to recover.

organic brain syndrome: a group of mental disorders associated with brain damage or impaired brain function.

allowed to make such life-and-death decisions? These questions are but a few of the unanswered concerns that have evolved along with the technology of special feeding techniques.

Individual Rights

Individuals have a legal right to refuse medical treatment, even if that treatment is considered to be necessary to sustain life. From a legal standpoint, refusal of treatment is not considered suicide as long as the person's eventual death results from the underlying disease and not from the person's own doing.

However, the situation changes when the person is comatose, incompetent, or otherwise unable to refuse or accept medical treatment. How can his wishes regarding treatment be made known? To address this concern, many states have enacted laws that authorize living wills.[3] A living will allows competent people to specify that no "extraordinary treatments" be administered to them in the event that they are diagnosed as

A living will gives competent adults a chance to make known their wishes that no heroic efforts be made to revive them in the event that they become terminally ill or comatose and they are unable to authorize or refuse medical treatments.

terminally ill and are unable to make the necessary decisions at that time.

Advances in modern technology, particularly respirators, prompted the development of living wills. Considered a major medical breakthrough, respirators can literally breathe for a person who is unable to breathe. Many people who are otherwise brain dead are put on respirators and kept alive.

The much-touted case of Karen Ann Quinlan heightened public awareness to the use of modern technology to maintain life when death was thought to be inevitable and when such measures were refused. Quinlan lapsed unexpectedly into a coma and was placed on a respirator. When her physicians determined her brain injuries were irreversible, and that only the machine kept her alive, her parents requested that the respirator be disconnected. The hospital and physicians were unable to comply with this request, and the case went to court. A year later, the parents won the right to have the respirator disconnected, but only after a great deal of hardship and expense. Quinlan continued to receive antibiotics and high-nutrient feedings until she died of pneumonia 9 years later.

This case sparked many debates on death with dignity. People worry that they will be in similar circumstances and fear they will become a financial and emotional burden to those who care for them. Some people feel that the new technology interferes with their natural right to die. Others feel that God, not a machine, should determine how and when an individual dies.

What does death with dignity and living wills have to do with tube feedings and parenteral nutrition? As technology has improved to the extent that a person can be fed totally by parenteral and enteral nutrition, questions regarding the use of these feedings to sustain an individual who is terminally ill or in an irreversible coma have surfaced.

On the one hand, it is argued that nourishment and hydration do not constitute "extraordinary treatment." Indeed, nourishment is so basic to life that feeding a person, even through mechanical means, should not be considered extraordinary. Furthermore, feeding a person has traditionally not been considered to be painful or obtrusive. Those who argue this side of the case find it totally unacceptable that food or water would be withheld or withdrawn from a living being for any reason.

On the other hand, it is argued that using parenteral and enteral nutrition to replace the normal process of eating is not different from using a respirator to replace the process of breathing. These individuals feel that the placement of a feeding tube or TPN catheter *is* obtrusive and uncomfortable. They feel that withholding and withdrawing nutrition support is morally and legally justified for individuals who request that no heroic measures be made to sustain their lives in the event of terminal illness or irreversible coma.

Often, it is unclear which of these positions the individual with the terminal illness supports. Even those who have signed living wills may not have considered whether nutrition support is an extraordinary treatment. Basically living wills state that only measures that will preserve the person's comfort and dignity should be taken. It is unclear whether the individual who signs the living will intends to include or exclude the use of parenteral or enteral nutrition as such a measure. Several states with living will legislation specifically *exclude* the right to withhold or withdraw nourishment or hydration.[4]

To date, the number of court cases that specifically involve withholding or withdrawing nutrition support is relatively small. This suggests that many cases are being resolved among the people involved in the individual's care—the person, her family, and the health care team.

Court Cases and Their Outcomes

Over the years, court cases have been useful in establishing legal guidelines for withholding and withdrawing nutrition support. The cases have involved both competent and incompetent individuals. The details of some of the cases are presented here to help you see some of the problems that have been encountered and how the courts handled them.

In one of the first cases that involved artificial feeding, two physicians were charged with criminal homicide in the death of a 55-year-old man who suffered a cardiac arrest while undergoing GI surgery.[5] The man was revived, placed on a respirator, and determined to be in a vegetative state that was believed to be irreversible. The man's family requested that the respirator be discontinued, and later agreed that IV feeding tubes also be removed. The family members felt that they were complying with what the man would have directed had he been able to do so. A nurse who disagreed with the decision to remove the IV tubes complained to authorities, and the case was heard in court.

Some important precedents resulted from the case. For one, the court ruled that the physicians were not required to continue treatment that would not improve the client's chances for recovery. The court also ruled that a spouse may make the decision regarding medical treatments for a person who is unable to make the decision himself. (Be sure to note that a member of the health care team, the nurse, was instrumental in bringing the case to court, because she objected to the treatment.)

In another case, the nephew of an 84-year-old woman with organic brain syndrome and several other chronic diseases requested that her nasogastric (NG) feeding tube be removed.[6] The nephew had refused permission for amputation of a gangrenous leg, and

the woman had unexpectedly survived the gangrene. The testimony given regarding the woman's mental and neurological brain status was inconclusive.

The court initially ordered the removal of the NG tube, but the decision was appealed and eventually reversed. The court ruled that discontinuing the NG feeding would result in death—death that was not from the woman's underlying medical condition, and thus would constitute homicide. During the legal process, the woman died with the feeding tube in place. Later, the state supreme court reversed the lower court's decision. This court ruled that life-sustaining equipment could be withheld or withdrawn from nursing home residents under the following circumstances:

- If there is clear and reliable evidence (such as a living will) that the person would not choose to have the treatment if she were able to give directions.
- If there is some general evidence that the person would not want the lifesaving measures, and the suffering and pain the treatment would involve does not outweigh the benefits and enjoyment the person would gain from the procedure.

When there is no indication of the person's wishes regarding life-sustaining measures, they can be discontinued only if the burden of providing these measures clearly and markedly outweighs the benefits to the individual. The pain caused by withdrawing the treatment is also to be considered in weighing the benefits versus the negative aspects of treatment.

The court ruled against the use of artificial feeding in the case of an 85-year-old nursing home resident who was depressed over a series of debilitating diseases and chose to hasten his death by fasting.[7] The court ruled that the man could not be force-fed because he was fully competent when he made his decision. This case is

unusual because the person involved would not have died from an underlying condition if he had been refused permission to starve to death.

Conversely, in the highly publicized case of Elizabeth Bouvia, the court initially ordered that a feeding tube be kept in place against Bouvia's objections.[8] Bouvia, who is in her mid-twenties, suffers from a severe case of cerebral palsy. She checked into a hospital, asking to be kept comfortable while she starved herself. The hospital refused, and the case went to court.

The court ruled against Bouvia, supporting the hospital's position that it could not be forced into assisting in an apparent suicide. Subsequently, Bouvia's condition deteriorated markedly. She is bedridden, totally dependent on others to care for her, and in constant pain from a severe form of arthritis that requires morphine for relief. She appealed the court's decision and requested removal of the feeding tube that was initially inserted against her will. She contended that she could take food orally and does not plan to commit suicide by starvation. Again the court denied her request. Bouvia appealed that ruling and requested that the feeding tube be removed until a decision is made on her case.

In April of 1986 the court ruled that until her case is heard, the feeding tube is to be removed. The court stated that given her medical condition, Bouvia has the right to let nature take its course, and that that decision is not the same as a decision to commit suicide.

This is only a brief look at some of the court cases that have been heard throughout the country involving nutrition support techniques. A trend appears to be developing from the rulings in these cases. The court system tends to view nutrition support as a medical treatment procedure rather than routine care.[9] It also appears that the court will most likely authorize withdrawing or withholding nutrition support in cases involving the terminally ill and those with permanent loss of consciousness.

Future Considerations

Many people agree that the decision to withdraw or withhold nutrition support is one best made by the individual, his family, and the health care team rather than the court system. That decision should be based on circumstances that are carefully considered by all parties involved.

One way the feelings of the individual can be made known is through the living will discussed earlier. People who wish to have every effort made to keep them alive in the event of terminal illness or irreversible loss of consciousness should make their wishes known in writing, even if their state does not have a living will provision. Likewise, those who prefer to die with no heroic or special efforts made to keep them alive need to do the same. In any case, the individual's preference should be known to her physicians and family and should be a part of the medical record.

An added advantage of planning ahead for future care in the case of a terminal illness or irreversible state of unconsciousness is that others are freed from the guilt and anxiety of having to make that decision. Imagine the anxiety a spouse, for example, would have to go through in directing the health care team to stop nutrition support, knowing that it would hasten death. That decision would be far easier if the spouse knew that was what the individual would want, or better yet, if a legal document took the decision out of the spouse's hands altogether.

Living wills are not authorized in some states, and in other states specifically exclude withholding nourishment and hydration. People who prefer that these techniques not be used in the event of imminent death or vegetative state may need to take further legal actions to ensure that their wishes be carried out. The durable power of attorney may be an appropriate alternative.[10] A durable power of attorney allows competent adults to designate another competent adult as an agent to make decisions for them in the event they are incapacitated. The durable power of attorney has yet to be tested in court, but it may be a feasible alternative for ensuring that the individual's requests be carried out in states that do not authorize living wills or in states that do not allow nourishment and hydration to be withheld.

The many ethical and legal problems that have evolved with the improved technology for delivering nutrients present tough challenges for individuals, their loved ones, the health care team, and the legal system. It is likely that new questions will arise in the future. One thing is clear: the solutions to these problems are as complex as the problems themselves.

Health care professionals, particularly physicians, can find themselves in awkward and difficult positions regarding aggressive nutrition support. On the one hand, they are obligated to provide optimal care. Negligence could result in a malpractice suit. On the other hand, health care professionals are client advocates. In this role, they must respect the wishes of the people in their care. Again, there is no easy answer to this dilemma. Each case must be carefully decided on its individual circumstances and actions taken as appropriate.

NOTES
1. A. Barrocas, J. Farquharson, and M. Fernandez, Legal considerations in nutritional support: 1986 update, *Nutritional Support Services* 6 (1986): 33.
2. Barrocas, Farquharson, and Fernandez, 1986.
3. All states except Alaska, Hawaii, Kentucky, Massachusetts, Michigan, Minnesota, Nebraska, New Jersey, New York, North Dakota, Ohio, Pennsylvania, Rhode Island, South Carolina, and South Dakota have authorized the use of living wills. B. Mishkin, Withholding and withdrawing nutritional support: Advance planning for hard choices, *Nutrition in Clinical Practice* 1 (1986): 50–52.
4. These states include Arizona, Colorado, Connecticut, Florida, Georgia, Illinois, Iowa, Maine, Maryland, Missouri, New Hampshire, and Oklahoma. Indiana requires only that appropriate nutrition and hydration be provided, a vague statement that could be interpreted in many ways. Mishkin, 1986.
5. Mishkin, Courts entangled in feeding tube controversies, *Nutrition in Clinical Practice* 1 (1986): 209–215; R. Dresser, Discontinuing nutrition support: A review of the case law, *Journal of the American Dietetic Association* 85 (1985): 1289–1292.
6. Mishkin, Courts entangled in feeding tube controversies, 1986; R. Dresser, 1985.
7. Mishkin, Courts entangled in feeding tube controversies, 1986; R. Dresser, 1985.
8. Mishkin, Courts entangled in feeding tube controversies, 1986.
9. Dresser, 1985.
10. Mishkin, Withholding and withdrawing nutritional support, 1986.

Disorders of the Upper GI Tract

21

Contents

This picture, taken through a light microscope, shows a single villus of the small intestine, in which several hundred cells are visible. Each cell's location can be deduced from the presence of a blue-stained nucleus. When magnified even more, these cells turn out to be bristling with surface projections of their own, the microvilli. The opening art of the next chapter provides a close-up look at a few cells with their microvilli. Figure 6–3 on page 178 illustrates these surface features of the small intestine wall.

The GI tract is a remarkable and unique organ. As a conduit from the external world surrounding us to our internal body environment, it discriminates nutrients from substances for which the body has no use. Indeed, a healthy GI tract allows us to ingest, digest, and absorb nutrients—functions essential to life. Conversely, a diseased GI tract can interfere with one or all of these functions and have a significant impact on health. This chapter describes how some upper GI tract disorders affect food intake and vice versa. The next chapter presents disorders of the intestines and their effects on food intake and nutrition status.

Problems of the Upper GI Tract

The upper GI tract begins with the mouth. In the mouth, the teeth and jaw muscles work to reduce food particles to a size that can be easily swallowed and digested. A variety of dental, medical, and surgical conditions can create temporary or permanent problems with chewing or swallowing. Table 21–1 lists some of these conditions. In these cases, the diet must be adjusted, or the person will eat too little, lose weight, and suffer the consequences of a deteriorating nutrition status.

The process of chewing is sometimes called **mastication** (mass-tih-KAY-shun).

A mechanical soft diet is used to minimize the discomfort of chewing and swallowing. Such a diet is a highly individualized, yet simple, modification of a regular diet: it eliminates those foods the person cannot easily chew or swallow. A person with a newly broken jaw may be able to handle only liquids; a person without teeth may be able to eat pieces of baked chicken or fish, ground beef, casseroles, canned fruits, and soft cooked vegetables. The permitted foods may be liquid, chopped, or pureed, or regular foods with a soft consistency. When a mechanical soft diet is ordered, the person usually receives pureed foods until a dietitian or nurse determines which foods can be tolerated.

mechanical soft diet: a diet that excludes all foods that are difficult to chew or swallow; also called a **dental soft diet**.

Each person's tolerance of food consistency varies greatly. Talk to the person about which foods are difficult to handle. Try to provide clients on the mechanical soft diet with foods that are as similar to those of a regular diet as possible. These foods will offer the most variety, increase the person's acceptance of them, and reduce the likelihood of nutrient deficiencies.

TABLE 21–1

Conditions That Interfere with Chewing or Swallowing

Broken jaw	Periodontal disease
Dental caries	Radiation therapy of the head and neck
Dryness of the mouth	Sensitivity to hot or cold
Ill-fitting dentures	Strokes (sometimes)
Missing teeth	Surgery of the head and neck
No teeth	Ulceration of mouth or gums
Oral surgery	

Take a moment to think about a pureed diet. A typical dinner of baked chicken, boiled potatoes, and green beans is now white mush, more white mush, and a green blob. In many hospitals, baby foods routinely replace pureed foods. Baby foods are nutritious, but they often taste bland since they are prepared without salt or spices. Whether pureed or baby foods, the consistency is a psychological block to eating, and malnutrition can result.

Can you improve the situation? The answer is yes. First, be sure your client needs pureed rather than chopped foods. Second, help your client select colorful meals. For example, substitute mashed sweet potatoes for white potatoes in the meal above. Such a change adds appetizing color to a meal. Serve the food attractively and at the right temperature. Lastly, unless the physician has ordered otherwise, suggest spices that will improve the taste of the food. Many people think that because they are on a special diet they are not allowed to have additional seasonings.

Finally, talk to the administrative dietitian or foodservice manager if pureed diets are consistently a problem. Pureed foods should be smooth but thick—not watery or thin. Furthermore, regular foods that have been pureed should be served instead of baby food whenever possible.

Serve colorful pureed meals at the appropriate temperature, seasoned to taste.

All seasonings and types of foods are allowed on a mechanical soft diet. However, highly seasoned or acidic foods (citrus fruits and tomatoes, for example) may be painful to someone with mouth ulcers. In addition, foods that contain nuts or seeds can easily get trapped in the ulcer and cause discomfort.

Dysphagia

The esophagus transports food from the mouth to the stomach and is important in swallowing. Disorders of the esophagus, therefore, can affect the ability to swallow and cause dysphagia. Dysphagia can be the result of psychological problems as well as physiological ones; we will discuss only those causes of dysphagia that can be helped by diet.

One such cause of dysphagia is achalasia. The cause of achalasia is unknown. In achalasia, nerves that control the motility of the esophagus do not function properly, and the muscles of the esophagus are unable to propel the food bolus downward toward the stomach. Additionally, the cardiac sphincter does not relax and open during swallowing to allow the food to pass from the esophagus into the stomach. Foods and fluids accumulate in the esophagus of a person with achalasia, which explains the sensation of food sticking in the throat. Gradually, either the pressure of the food causes the cardiac sphincter to open, or the person regurgitates the food.

At first, the person with achalasia may experience only temporary and mild dysphagia. As the condition worsens, the symptoms become more painful. The esophagus widens as achalasia progresses (see Figure 21–1). The person becomes fearful of eating and gradually reduces food intake. Marked weight loss and nutrient deficiencies are likely to be present by the time the person seeks medical attention. A further danger exists—the person may aspirate food stag-

dysphagia (dis-FAY-gee-ah): difficulty in swallowing.
dys = bad
phagein = to eat

achalasia (ack-ah-LAY-zee-ah): dysfunction of the esophagus. Achalasia is sometimes called **esophageal dyssynergia** (ee-SOF-ah-GEE-al dis-sin-ER-gee-ah) or **cardiospasm.**
a = not
chalasis = relaxation
dys = bad
synergia = cooperation

The **cardiac sphincter** is often called the **lower esophageal sphincter (LES)** or the **gastroesophageal sphincter.** (The passage of food through the GI tract is described on pp. 169-174.)

The fear of eating is called **sitophobia** (SIGH-toe-FOE-bee-ah).
sitos = food
phobos = fear

Achalasia. The muscles of the esophagus do not function properly. The cardiac sphincter does not relax to allow food to pass through to the stomach. The esophagus gradually enlarges.

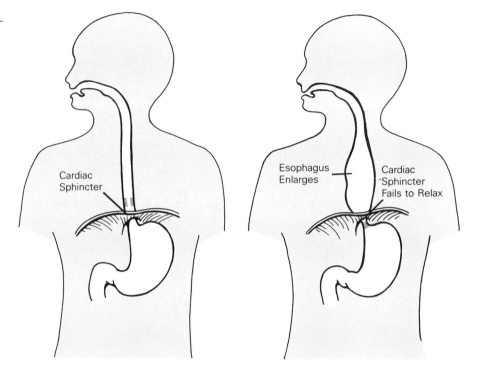

The fear of eating is called **sitophobia** (SIGH-toe-FOE-bee-ah).
sitos = food
phobos = fear

When an organ, such as the esophagus, becomes enlarged beyond normal dimensions, it is said to be **dilated.** To make an organ or vessel larger is called **dilation** or **dilatation.**

reflux esophagitis (ee-sof-ah-JIE-tis): the backflow or regurgitation of gastric contents from the stomach into the esophagus, causing inflammation of the esophagus.
re = back
fluxus = flow

A disease or condition that develops slowly, shows little change, and lasts a long time is said to be **chronic.** The term **acute** describes diseases or conditions that develop rapidly, have severe symptoms, and are of short duration.
chronos = time
acutus = sharp

The continuous reflux of gastric juices may cause scarring of the esophageal mucosa. As scar tissue forms, the diameter of the esophagus narrows, a condition referred to as an **esophageal stricture.**

nating in the esophagus into the lung, and this could lead to a serious lung infection.

The person with achalasia will only be able to tolerate liquid or semiliquid foods in small servings. Suggest liquid supplements to meet nutrient needs. Tube feedings and parenteral nutrition may be indicated, particularly if the person is severely malnourished or unable to consume adequate nutrients orally.

The treatment for achalasia is to either stretch or partially slit the cardiac sphincter so that it is no longer functional. This makes the person more comfortable, but it does not restore motility to the esophageal muscles. Because the cardiac sphincter remains open, reflux esophagitis is a common complication.

Reflux Esophagitis

Reflux esophagitis is an irritation in the lower esophagus. It occurs when the cardiac sphincter does not close tightly enough, allowing the highly acidic gastric contents to splash backward into the esophagus. These acidic fluids irritate the esophageal mucosa.

Reflux esophagitis can occur any time the pressure of the cardiac sphincter is not great enough to keep it closed. You can see why people treated for achalasia often develop esophagitis. When esophagitis becomes chronic, the inner diameter of the esophagus may become narrowed by inflammation and scarring. Dysphagia and the same problems seen in achalasia can result. Chronic esophagitis also can cause ulcers to form in the esophagus. Table 21–2 lists some foods and substances that affect cardiac sphincter pressure.

A burning pain called heartburn occurs when the gastric juices reflux into the esophagus. The pain is severe enough to awaken a sleeping person. Heartburn usually hurts behind the sternum (see Figure 21–2), often spreading into the neck and back of the throat in waves. Heartburn is especially likely when pressure in the stomach exceeds pressure in the esophagus, so it occurs more frequently when a person lies down or bends over.

The best treatment of reflux esophagitis is prevention. Clients are instructed to avoid substances that reduce cardiac sphincter pressure and to avoid any activity that raises pressure in the stomach. A client with active reflux esophagitis should try to reduce gastric acidity and use foods that are least likely to irritate an already inflamed esophagus.

Dietary advice is an important part of the prevention and treatment of reflux esophagitis. Instruct the client to:

■ Eat small, frequent meals and drink liquids one hour before or after meals to avoid distending the stomach.

heartburn: a burning sensation felt behind the sternum caused by stomach acid splashing back up into the esophagus.

TABLE 21–2

Substances That Affect Cardiac Sphincter Pressure

Elevates Pressure	Lowers Pressure
Bethanechol	Alcohol
Metoclopropamide	Anticholinergic agents
Protein	Atropine
	Caffeine-containing beverages
	Chocolate
	Cigarette smoking
	Fat
	Peppermint and spearmint oils

A. Normal.   B. Reflux.

FIGURE 21–2

Effect of gastric pressure on reflux. Whenever the pressure in the stomach is greater than the pressure in the esophagus, the chance of reflux increases. Overeating and overdrinking can cause the stomach to be overdistended, increasing the pressure in the stomach.

- Refrain from lying down or bending over and from wearing tight-fitting garments, particularly after eating, to avoid increasing stomach pressure.
- Lose weight, if necessary.
- Limit fat, alcohol, caffeine, and peppermint and spearmint oil intake, to avoid lowering cardiac sphincter pressure.
- Limit decaffeinated coffee, caffeine-containing foods and beverages, and red pepper, to avoid stimulation of gastic acid secretion.
- Avoid acidic juices such as orange, grapefruit, and tomato juice when experiencing the symptoms of reflux esophagitis, to minimize irritation to the esophagus.

Other measures are also helpful in preventing and treating reflux esophagitis. Advise clients not to smoke cigarettes; cigarette smoking can reduce cardiac sphincter pressure. In addition, antacids or other drugs may be prescribed to neutralize the acidity of gastric juices. Advise the person to sleep with the head of the bed elevated, so that the chest is higher than the stomach, to prevent reflux. Generally, these measures can control esophagitis. However, in some cases surgery may be indicated if medical management fails.

Hiatal Hernia

Normally, the stomach lies completely below the diaphragm. The esophagus passes through the diaphragm by way of an opening, the esophageal hiatus. A hiatal hernia results when the opening in the diaphragm weakens, allowing a portion of the stomach to protrude above the diaphragm (see Figure 21–3). The symptoms of hiatal hernia result from esophagitis caused by the reflux of the acidic gastric juices into the esophagus. The goals of nutrition care for hiatal hernia are the same as those given earlier for esophagitis: that is, to prevent reflux, to neutralize gastric acidity, and to eliminate foods that irritate the esophagus.

Elevate the head of the bed to minimize the likelihood of reflux from the stomach to the esophagus.

diaphragm (DYE-ah-fram): a muscular wall separating the abdomen from the thoracic cavity.

esophageal hiatus (high-AY-tus): the opening in the diaphragm through which the esophagus passes.

hiatal hernia: a protrusion of a portion of the stomach through the esophageal hiatus of the diaphragm. There are several types: sliding (see Figure 21–3), rolling, or short esophagus.
hiatus = to yawn

Disorders of the Stomach

Whenever you turn on the television set, you are likely to see several advertisements touting cures for indigestion, heartburn, and gas. These terms have become so familiar that any GI discomfort may be incorrectly described and treated as one of these disorders.

Indigestion or dyspepsia are vague terms used to describe any discomfort in the GI tract, primarily in the stomach. Indigestion can be a symptom of many disorders, either in the GI tract or in other organs. Oftentimes, indigestion is caused by emotional tension. You may hear a person comment that "I have a nervous stomach" or "I'm so mad my stomach feels like it is tied in a knot." In addition to emotional factors or underlying medical conditions, indigestion can be caused by eating too much, eating too rapidly, or chewing insufficiently.

dyspepsia: vague abdominal discomfort. Dyspepsia is a symptom, not a disease.
dys = bad
peptein = to digest

Hiatal Hernia

Mrs. James is a 49-year-old accountant who recently underwent a complete physical examination. She told her physician that she has been feeling fairly well, except for heartburn that has been occurring with increasing frequency. The attacks are most likely to occur after she has eaten a large meal, particularly if she lies down after eating. She told the doctor she has been under a great deal of pressure, this being the middle of the tax season.

Her past medical history does not reveal any significant health problems,

although she had been advised to stop smoking cigarettes and to lose 20 lb during her last physical. A diet history taken by the nurse shows that Mrs. James skips breakfast, usually eats lunch hurriedly while she continues to work, and eats a large dinner at about 8:00 P.M. She generally enjoys one or two alcoholic beverages in the evening

before going to sleep. She drinks 6 to 8 cups of coffee during the day and has not quit smoking. Her current height and weight are 5'6" and 155 lb, respectively. X-rays of the upper GI tract reveal that Mrs. James has a sliding hiatal hernia.

1. What is a sliding hiatal hernia? How does a hiatal hernia lead to heartburn?

2. Describe a care plan for Mrs. James. What suggestions can you give her to help relieve the symptoms she is having associated with the hernia? What other therapy might be prescribed by her physician?

People with reflux esophagitis tend to become chronic antacid users. Recall from Chapter 19 that nutrient imbalances are likely to develop in people using drugs for long periods of time. It is also important to remember that some antacids contain high amounts of sodium (those containing sodium bicarbonate) and calcium (those containing calcium bicarbonate). People with some disorders such as hypertension, need to avoid sodium and may be unaware of its presence in these products. Calcium must be avoided by people with certain types of kidney stones. The chronic use of a particular antacid may be contraindicated for these people and those with other medical problems.

Generally, no diet modifications are necessary for a temporary bout of indigestion. When indigestion occurs frequently, the cause (whether it be physical, emotional, or dietary) should be identified. Helpful dietary advice to offer:

- Eat slowly, at regular times, and in a relaxed atmosphere.
- Follow a low-fiber diet.
- Avoid excessive amounts of fats, alcohol, and caffeine-containing foods and beverages.
- Avoid any food known to cause indigestion.

A low-fiber diet provides foods that are least likely to cause an obstruction in the intestinal tract. It is the diet frequently recommended when the intestinal tract is narrowed by inflammation or scarring, when GI motility is slowed, or as an intermediate diet after surgery as a person progresses from a liquid diet to a regular diet. Table 21–3 lists foods included in and eliminated from a low-fiber diet. A sample menu is illustrated on p. 705.

FIGURE 21–3

Relation of upper GI tract to diaphragm.

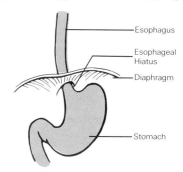

Esophagus
Esophageal Hiatus
Diaphragm
Stomach

A. Normally the stomach lies below the diaphragm, and the esophagus passes through the esophageal hiatus.

B. A *sliding hiatal hernia* is the most common type of hiatal hernia.

Low-fiber diet and **soft** diet are two names for the same diet. A **low-residue** diet is similar, with one exception—milk is restricted on a low-residue diet.

TABLE 21–5

Postgastrectomy Diet

Food Item	Allowed	Excluded	Comments
Meats/meat alternates	X		Any type
Grains/starchy vegetables			
Plain breads, crackers, rolls, unsweetened cereal, rice, pasta, corn, lima beans, parsnips, peas, white potatoes, sweet potatoes, pumpkin, yams, winter squash	X		Limit to 5 servings daily
Sweetened cereal; cereal containing dates, raisins, or brown sugar		X	
Nonstarchy vegetables			
Chicory, Chinese cabbage, endive, escarole, lettuce, parsley, radishes, watercress	X		As desired
Asparagus, bean sprouts, beets, broccoli, brussels sprouts, cabbage, carrots, cauliflower, celery, cucumbers, eggplant, green pepper, greens, mushrooms, okra, onions, rhubarb, sauerkraut, string beans, summer squash, tomatoes, turnips, zucchini	X		Limit to two ½-c servings daily; individual tolerances will vary
Vegetables prepared with sugar		X	
Fruits			
Unsweetened fruits and fruit juices	X		Limit to three servings daily
Sweetened fruits and fruit juices		X	
Fats	X		Any type
Beverages			
Milk (whole milk, nonfat milk, or buttermilk)	X		If tolerated
Coffee, tea, dietetic carbonated beverages	X		
Alcohol, carbonated beverages, sweetened milk, cocoa, fruit drinks		X	
Desserts			
Cakes, cookies, ice cream, sherbet		X	
Other			
Honey, jam, jelly, syrup, sugar		X	

Anemia also can be caused by a deficiency of vitamin B_{12} or folacin. Recall that vitamin B_{12} cannot be absorbed without an intrinsic factor, which is synthesized in the stomach. Depending on the location and extent of the gastric resection, production of this intrinsic factor may be minimal or absent, and vitamin B_{12} absorption correspondingly impaired. Vitamin B_{12} must then be given by injection to correct the deficiency. Supplemental folacin can be given orally.

Absorption of both vitamin B_{12} and folacin can be impaired in the person who develops blind loop syndrome. In some types of gastric resections, a portion of the small intestine is bypassed, so it is nonfunctional. Stasis occurs in the segment of the intestine that is bypassed. Bacteria that would normally not be present in that part of the intestine flourish. The bacteria compete with the host for vitamin B_{12} and folacin, limiting the supply available to the host. The bacteria also partly dismantle the bile salts, so that they become ineffective in fat digestion and absorption or even inhibit these processes (see Figure 21–7). The results are fat malabsorption and vitamin B_{12} and folacin deficiencies. To help correct the problem, parenteral vitamin B_{12} and oral folacin supplements are given along with antibiotics to inhibit bacterial growth. Fat may be restricted to prevent steatorrhea. Sometimes the blind loop must be removed surgically.

General malabsorption is a problem in a person who has had a total gastrectomy or in a person whose stomach has been surgically connected directly to the jejunum. Normally, when food enters the duodenum, the hormones secretin and cholecystokinin are released. In turn, these hormones mediate the release of digestive enzymes and bile, which are then secreted into the duodenum. When the duodenum is bypassed, these normal digestive processes also are bypassed. Additionally, malabsorption can result from the rapid passage of food through the GI tract, a problem when the stomach no longer controls the rate of gastric emptying.

A different type of gastric surgery used in the treatment of morbid obesity is gastric partitioning or gastric stapling. A row of surgical staples is placed in the stomach, which effectively reduces the size of the stomach, making it difficult for the individual to eat large amounts of food. A small opening allows food to slowly pass into the lower portion of the stomach so that it can be digested and absorbed.

blind loop syndrome: the problems of fat malabsorption and vitamin B_{12} depletion that can result from the overgrowth of bacteria in a bypassed segment of the intestine.

stasis (STAY-sis): standing still. Normal actions of the intestines keep a steady stream of secretions flowing through them. Stasis in a blind loop allows bacteria to flourish.

The fatty diarrhea characteristic of fat malabsorption is **steatorrhea** (stee-ah-toe-REE-ah). The stools are foamy, greasy, and malodorous.
steatos = fat
rhea = flow

morbid obesity: twice or more the average desirable weight given in life insurance tables or 100 lb more than desirable weight.

A. Bile has an affinity for fats and water, so it can bring them together.

B. The enzymes now have access to the emulsified fat.

C. In blind loop syndrome, bacteria damage the bile, so that it is ineffective in fat digestion and absorption. The result is fat malabsorption and steatorrhea.

FIGURE 21–7

Steatorrhea is a common symptom of blind loop syndrome.

Water

Fat

Enzyme

Bacteria

Bile

Mrs. Grayson was admitted to the emergency room in serious condition after suffering severe abdominal injuries in a car accident. After her initial examination, a surgeon was consulted, and Mrs. Grayson was taken to surgery immediately. A gastrojejunostomy (see Figure 21–5) was performed. Mrs. Grayson was sent to the intensive care unit following surgery and is recovering as expected. The health care team anticipates that Mrs. Grayson will likely have nutrition-related problems when she begins taking foods by mouth, and they are taking measures to prevent these problems from occurring.

1. Review Figure 21–5 to understand the procedure that Mrs. Grayson underwent. Consider the possibility that she might develop dumping syndrome, blind loop syndrome, and general malabsorption. Describe how these conditions might occur.

2. What diet will Mrs. Grayson be placed on after she begins oral intake? Describe the diet and how the diet is progressed. What advice can you give Mrs. Grayson to prevent dumping syndrome?

3. Discuss the nutrition-related concerns associated with blind loop syndrome. How can these concerns be handled?

---

gastric partitioning: surgery in which a line of surgical staples is placed in such a way as to make the upper portion of the stomach smaller; used to treat morbid obesity. Also called **gastric stapling, gastric plication,** or **gastroplasty.**

Because gastric partitioning is a relatively new procedure, there is little information regarding its long-term safety and effectiveness. The purpose of the discussion here is not to discuss the procedure or its merits, but rather to alert you to the nutrition concerns of people who have undergone gastric partitioning.

A liquid diet is necessary for about eight weeks after oral intake is started.[2] Liquids reduce the risk that the line of surgical staples will be disrupted and will flow easily through the opening to the lower stomach. Only small amounts of liquids can be tolerated at one time because of the reduced size of the stomach; overeating or overdrinking can result in vomiting.

After about two months, the person can gradually try to eat soft foods and then regular foods as tolerated. Again, only small amounts of any food can be taken at one time. Clients must understand that if they drink high-kcalorie liquids or eat small amounts of high-kcalorie foods all the time, they will not lose weight.

Nutrition Assessment

As you have seen in this chapter, disorders of the upper GI tract can have adverse consequences on nutrition status. When you assess the nutrition status of people who have these disorders, you will be wise to keep some special points in mind:

■ Get a thorough diet history. People who have difficulties in chewing or swallowing may have poor intakes of one or several nutrients. Other disorders such as nausea, indigestion, gastritis, or peptic ulcers are often associated with intolerances to certain foods. A good diet history can be useful for pinpointing offending foods so that they can be avoided. For the person who has undergone gastric partitioning, diet histories are useful in assessing kcalorie intake and eating habits.

■ Monitor weight regularly. Disorders of the upper GI tract often lead to weight loss due to either poor food intake or malabsorption of nutrients. Conversely, weight gain can have a negative impact on controlling symptoms of reflux esophagitis and for individuals who have undergone gastric partitioning.

- Assess biochemical parameters with caution in people with severe vomiting or those with dumping syndrome. If the individual is dehydrated, lab values will appear deceptively elevated.

Study Questions

1. Describe some conditions of the mouth that can affect the ingestion of nutrients. What diet can be useful for ensuring that nutrient needs are met in these cases? How should the diet be planned?
2. What is achalasia? How is the disorder managed?
3. What is a hiatal hernia? What causes the symptoms associated with a hiatal hernia? What advice can you give the person with a hiatal hernia to prevent and treat these symptoms?
4. Under what circumstances can indigestion, nausea, and vomiting be a risk to nutrition status?
5. Discuss the therapy for peptic ulcers.
6. Describe the events associated with dumping syndrome. What diet is helpful in preventing these symptoms? Discuss the advice you could give a person with dumping syndrome.
7. What is blind loop syndrome? What are the nutrition consequences? How are these problems avoided or dealt with?
8. Discuss the dietary recommendations and the rationale behind them for a person who undergoes gastric partitioning.

Notes

1. B. H. Yaffe, Stomach disorders can be minimized, *Environmental Nutrition* 8 (1985): 1–3.
2. A. S. Graney, L. B. Smith, and K. A. Hammer, Gastric partitioning for morbid obesity: Postoperative weight loss, technical complications, and protein status, *Journal of the American Dietetic Association* 86 (1986): 630–635.

Disorders of the Intestines

22

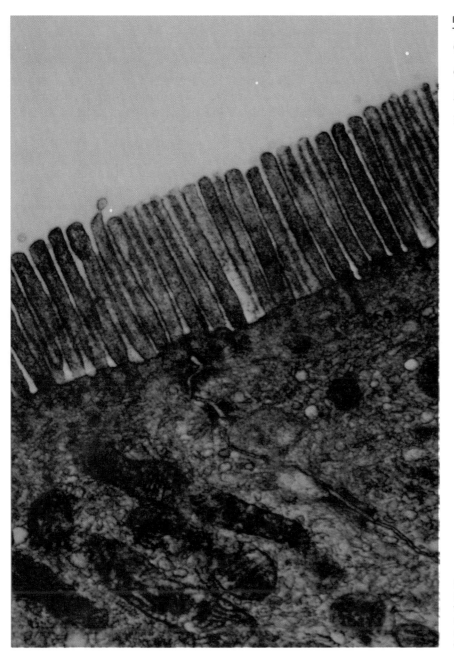

Contents

Gastrointestinal disorders, because they impair digestion and absorption, interfere with the nutrient supply to all other body systems. These delicate microvilli, on the surfaces of intestinal cells, are easily disrupted by digestive disorders.

*T*he intestines absorb nutrients from foods for use by the body. It is easy to see that disorders of the intestines, particularly those that result in malabsorption, have a grave impact on nutrition status. Disorders of the intestines, however, do not always result in malabsorption. Diet plays a role in the prevention and treatment of these disorders.

Common GI Problems

Most of us experience at least one of a variety of GI problems on occasion. In some cases, these problems are symptoms of an underlying disease process. However, they can occur as isolated incidents, and often present no cause for alarm.

Gas

Excessive gas in the GI tract is called **flatulence** (FLAT-you-lens) or **flatus** (FLAY-tus). Flatus describes the expulsion of gas through the mouth (belching) or rectum. The gurgling sound created by the movement of gas through the intestine is called **borborygmy** (BORE-bo-RIG-me).

Another word for belching is **eructation** (eh-ruck-TAY-shun).

Many people complain of problems attributed to excessive gas. For some, belching is the complaint. Others blame intestinal gas for abdominal discomforts such as cramping or distension. Most people feel these problems occur after they have eaten certain foods.

Contrary to popular belief, belching is not caused by gas formed from certain foods in the stomach. Rather, belching occurs when air that has been swallowed or sucked in is expelled. People who excessively belch have acquired a bad habit, usually unconsciously. They suck in or swallow air, often as a result of tension or eating too fast. Occasionally, belching can be a sign of a more serious disorder. People with gallbladder pain, colonic distress, or an impending obstruction of a coronary blood vessel may belch frequently.

Little is known about the production of intestinal gas. It appears that some gas is derived from swallowed air. Other gases appear to be formed by bacteria in the gut. This happens because human beings lack the enzymes necessary to digest and absorb certain types of carbohydrate that are found in some vegetable products, such as beans. The gut bacteria do have the necessary enzymes, and so they metabolize the undigested carbohydrate, producing gas. (One type of gas, methane, is produced in only a third of the population.) It's easy to see why people who absorb carbohydrates poorly (such as those with a lactase deficiency) are likely to complain of excessive gas.

People whose excess gas production results from malabsorption can be treated accordingly. For people who are methane producers, however, diet has little effect. Foods that produce gas usually must be determined individually. Your client can test foods suspected of forming gas by omitting them individually for a trial period and seeing if there is any improvement. Foods that have been associated with intestinal gas are listed in Table 22-1. A diet that excludes foods that produce gas is useful for treating some disorders. For example, a person who survives a heart attack benefits from such a diet immediately after the heart attack, because stomach distension can cause the diaphragm to be pushed up toward the heart, increasing the heart's work load.

TABLE 22–1

Foods That May Cause Intestinal Gas

Apples	Carrots	Pastry
Apricots	Celery	Potatoes
Bagels	Citrus fruits	Pretzels
Bananas	Eggplant	Prune juice
Beans	Milk	Raisins
Bread	Milk products	Wheat germ
Brussels sprouts	Onions	

Source: Adapted from information in L. O. Sutalf and M. D. Levitt, Follow-up of a flatulent patient, *Digestive Diseases and Sciences* 24 (1979): 652–654.

Some foods may cause intestinal gas.

Diarrhea

Diarrhea occurs when bowel movements become more liquid or more frequent than usual (see p. 195). In diarrhea, either fluids are not absorbed as the intestinal contents move quickly through the GI tract or water is drawn from cells lining the intestinal tract and added to the food residue.

Emotional and physiological stress, nervous tension, and overeating can trigger diarrhea, as can some drugs, foods, and spices that irritate the GI tract. Spoiled food and bacterial overgrowth in the gut can also be causes. Malnutrition can be a cause of diarrhea. Recall from Chapter 18 that many people on tube feedings develop diarrhea. Infants and children frequently develop diarrhea when they are ill or given formulas that their immature GI tracts cannot tolerate.

Many times an acute case of diarrhea develops and remits in 24 to 48 hours. Unless it is very severe, this type of diarrhea seldom requires medical treatment. Eliminate food irritants and drink clear liquids to treat this type of diarrhea.

On the other hand, chronic diarrhea is a cause for concern. Chronic diarrhea can result from other disorders (malabsorption or PCM) or medical treatments (radiation therapy or drugs). The person with chronic diarrhea can become dehydrated, having lost large amounts of water and electrolytes.

Oftentimes, the GI tract is rested in cases of severe diarrhea. All foods and beverages may be withheld for 24 to 48 hours. During this time, fluids and electrolytes are replaced intravenously. The person then tries a clear liquid diet and progresses to a full liquid diet; a low-fiber diet; and, finally, a regular diet as tolerated. If the diarrhea is aggravated as the diet is progressed, then the person can be given nothing by mouth (NPO), and IV nutrition must be supplied. A person with severe diarrhea may suffer from weight loss and multiple nutrient deficiencies. Care should be taken to prevent or correct these problems.

Once a person is on an oral diet, applesauce or scraped raw apples are sometimes given every two to four hours. These foods contain pectin, a carbohydrate that attracts water and improves the consistency of the stools. Of course, if a food is known to have irritated the intestine, it should be eliminated. The exact treatment plan depends on the cause of the diarrhea.

Diarrhea that results from an accelerated movement of fluids and electrolytes from the intestinal capillaries into the lumen of the intestine is called **secretory diarrhea.** When unabsorbed water and electrolytes cause diarrhea by increasing the osmolarity of the intestinal contents, then **osmotic diarrhea** exists. Fat that is not absorbed but excreted in the stools results in **steatorrhea,** as previously mentioned. Severe, chronic diarrhea is often called **intractable diarrhea.**

When identifiable injuries to the GI tract result in diarrhea, the diarrhea is called **organic.** On the other hand, in **functional** diarrhea, the cause of the problem is unknown.

Constipation

You may joke about, or be irritated by, the laxative commercials on TV, but many people believe the message the advertisements are sending. For example, Mr. Jones must have a daily bowel movement or else he will be headachy and

Television commercials make laxatives seem harmless, but there are safer remedies.

irritable bowel syndrome: a common GI disorder characterized by spasms of the colon. It is also called **spastic colon, spastic diarrhea,** and **mucous colitis.**

irritable. The screen then shows Mr. Jones the next day, feeling his old jovial self because his pharmacist has persuaded him to take a laxative.

Constipation occurs when the muscles of the colon fail to push the intestinal contents along, resulting in difficult or painful bowel movements. The causes of and recommendations for the treatment of constipation are on pp. 195-197.

Hospitalized or institutionalized people often suffer from constipation. Stress from disease, nervous tension, and inactivity are contributing factors. Constipation also can occur as a result of irregular and excessive contractions of the colon. This disorder, the irritable bowel syndrome, seems to be associated with emotional stress. Because of the spasms, intestinal contents move irregularly along the colon and can result in diarrhea, constipation, or both in alternating sequence.

What can be done about constipation? If discomfort is associated with bowel movements, consult a doctor in order to rule out the presence of organic disease. For example, constipation sometimes warns of an intestinal obstruction, a tumor, or diverticular disease (discussed later). If constipation is found to be functional rather than organic, then it becomes appropriate to institute corrective measures.

Adding fiber to the diet may help to relieve constipation. Some fibers absorb water and so soften stools. Because dietary fiber is not digested, it also adds bulk to the stool. Fiber can be added to the diet by emphasizing whole-grain breads and cereals, fruits and vegetables, dried beans and peas, and nuts. A sample high-fiber diet menu is shown below. Cereal fiber is the preferred fiber for increasing stool weight. Wheat bran can be used to increase the fiber content of the diet significantly. A rounded teaspoon of unprocessed bran contains 2.4 grams of fiber. Bran can be sprinkled on cereal, salads, applesauce, and many other food items or added to beverages. Many breakfast cereals contain a considerable amount of fiber. Appendix H offers dietary fiber contents of foods. Chapter 3 provides additional information about fiber.

Fluids can also help augment stool weight and softness. Prunes and prune juice contain a laxative and may also be useful. Regular exercise and a consistent eating and drinking schedule can help. Occasionally, laxatives may be indicated, but they should only be used after a doctor has been consulted.

Use laxatives only when recommended by a physician.

Breakfast
Orange juice
All-bran cereal
Soft-cooked egg
Whole-wheat toast
Margarine
Milk
Coffee or tea

Lunch
Hamburger on whole-wheat bun with lettuce and tomato
Salad/dressing
Apple
Milk
Coffee or tea

Supper
Baked chicken
Brown rice
Broccoli
Fresh carrots
Pineapple
Whole-wheat roll
Margarine
Milk
Coffee or tea

Sample high-fiber diet menu.

TABLE 22–3

Low-Fat Diet (5

Use:

1. Nonfat milk
   fruit ices.
2. Up to 6 oz
   to three reg
3. Up to six se
   - 1 tsp butt
   - 1 strip cri
   - 1 tbsp he
   - ⅛ avocad
   - 2 tbsp lig
   - 6 small m
   - 5 small o.
   If fat is used
4. All vegetabl
5. All fruits pr
6. Plain white
7. Clear soups
8. Angel food
   meringues.
9. Jelly, jam, h

Do not use:

1. Whole milk.
2. Pastries, cak
3. More than ⊃
   frankfurters)
4. More than s
5. Desserts, ca
6. Creamed so

Suggestions:

1. To make the
2. To increase
3. To improve
   allow that f
   suggestions

- Use veg
  frying.
- Make h
  off the ⊃

You can also s
feature recipe
People wi
from a low-fa
medium-chair
many kcalori
from long-cha
of oil in salad
MCT cannot

---

status. (
such cas
   Mal:
area of
trients a
cussed t
digestive
factors f
   Mal:
sible. M
absorbe⊂
(see Ch:
(steator
   The
loss of f

TABLE 22–

Risk Fact

Decrease
Intake

Abdomin
Anorexia
Bowel res
Emotiona
Food into
Indigestic
Nausea

Los
kca

Ironically, frequent use of laxatives can actually lead to chronic constipation. Laxatives are generally safe when they are used on occasion, but when used for too long, the colon loses its ability to respond to natural stimulation. The lining of the intestine becomes irritated, and muscular reflexes diminish. Thus, a temporary problem can become permanent. Furthermore, as discussed in Chapter 19, nutrient deficiencies can develop when laxatives are used.

Most cases of constipation are harmless, although some may be accompanied by abdominal discomfort. Chronic constipation, however, is believed to be associated with other problems. The constant pressure of straining to defecate may result in hemorrhoids or the formation of diverticula.

Diverticular Disease

Sometimes pouches, or diverticula, form along the large intestine in areas where the intestinal muscles are weak, often at points where blood vessels enter the muscle. (Diverticulosis is introduced and a diagram of diverticula is on p. 72.) Evidence suggests that the pouches result from high pressure in the intestinal lumen. Excessive intestinal contractions cause segments of the intestine to be pinched off. Pressure builds in the segment and forces the membrane of the intestine through the weakened intestinal muscle layer (see Figure 22-1). Diverticulosis is the condition in which diverticula have formed in the intestine.

The person with diverticulosis is symptom-free and may not know the disorder exists. But in some people, fecal material gets trapped in the diverticula, causing inflammation and infection; this condition is called diverticulitis. People with diverticulitis may complain of cramps, alternating periods of diarrhea and constipation, dyspepsia, flatus, and abdominal distension. Occasionally a diverticulum may rupture; this is life-threatening. If the diverticula become inflamed repeatedly, the intestinal wall can thicken, narrowing the intestinal lumen and resulting in an obstruction. An inflamed bowel segment can also stick to other pelvic organs, which can result in fistula formation and obstruction of the intestine—serious medical problems that can be fatal.

defecate: see p. 195.

hemorrhoids (HEM-oh-roids): painful clusters of dilated and twisted veins in the lower rectum and anus.
haima = blood
rhein = to flow

diverticulosis: see p. 72.

fistula (FIS-too-lah): an abnormal opening between two organs or from an organ to the skin.
fistula = pipe

FIGURE 22–1

Intestinal pressure.

A. Pressure inside the intestine normally dissipates along the length of the bowel.

B. When contractions are excessive, a segment of bowel may become pinched off. Pressure in the segment builds because it cannot escape normally, and pouches form.

A

expe
desc
he is
he o
furth
bloa
to th
that
phys
dive

enteric hyper
per-ok-sa-LOC
excess oxalate
about because
oxalate in the
formation.
enteric = inte

water-miscib
soluble vitami
water and car

PLE
ALI
GR

Sample low-f

short-bowel syndrome: a complex of
symptoms that may include diarrhea,
weight loss, malabsorption, hypocalcemia,
hypomagnesemia, and anemia; it can
occur whenever the absorptive surface of
the small bowel is reduced.

proximal: the first part or the part that is
closest to the point of attachment.

FIGURE 22–3

Nutrient absorption in the GI tract. In
the first half of the small intestine,
absorption of 90 to 95% of nutrients takes
place. After a resection, nutrient absorption
is reduced.

Intestinal Surgery

Surgery of the intestine may be necessary for people with inflammatory bowel diseases, cancer of the intestine, obstruction, diverticulitis, or impaired blood supply to the intestine. Generally, up to 50 percent of the small bowel can be resected without serious consequences. The actual absorption of nutrients after a small bowel resection depends on three factors:

- The extent and location of the resection.
- The presence or absence of the ileocecal valve (p. 169).
- The adaptive ability of the remaining bowel.

When a large segment of the small intestine must be resected, the absorptive surface of the small intestine is reduced considerably. The person may experience diarrhea, weight loss, muscle wasting, protein and fat malabsorption, hypocalcemia, hypomagnesemia, and anemia. When several of these conditions occur at the same time, they are collectively called the *short-bowel* or *short-gut syndrome*.

People with short-bowel syndrome generally absorb carbohydrates and most water-soluble vitamins without difficulty. When more than 8 feet of the proximal jejunum have been resected, however, the absorption of fat, protein, fat-soluble vitamins, calcium, and magnesium can be impaired. When the ileum has been resected, vitamin B_{12} must be supplemented parenterally, since the ileum is the site of vitamin B_{12} absorption. Also, bile salts are normally reabsorbed in the ileum. If they are not reabsorbed, there will be a reduced body pool of bile salts available for recycling to aid in fat absorption (see Figure 22-3).

The ileocecal valve controls the rate at which the intestinal contents move from the small to the large bowel. When the valve is absent, transit time through the small intestine is rapid, and the time available for nutrient absorption is limited.

After a small bowel resection, a remarkable adaptive mechanism occurs in the portion of the intestine that remains intact. The bowel gets longer, thicker, and wider. The result is a greater ability of the remaining bowel to absorb

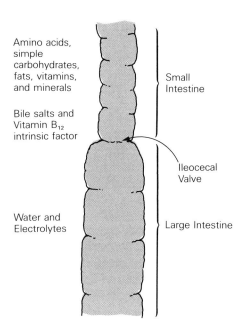

Amino acids,
simple
carbohydrates,
fats, vitamins,
and minerals

Bile salts and
Vitamin B_{12}
intrinsic factor

Water and
Electrolytes

Small
Intestine

Ileocecal
Valve

Large Intestine

nutrients. The presence of nutrients in the remaining gut appears to stimulate this adaptive process. However, if too much bowel has been resected, even this adaptation will be inadequate. People who become malnourished despite all efforts of prevention may require permanent support by parenteral means.

Immediately after surgery, the primary nutrition concern is the replacement of fluids and electrolytes. Parenteral feedings are given immediately after surgery. Oral feeding, tube feeding, or TPN should be initiated as soon as possible to ensure that energy and protein needs are met. The diet is gradually progressed to a high-protein, low-fat, oral diet. Fat restriction reduces steatorrhea and, thus, helps minimize the loss of fat, fat-soluble vitamins, calcium, and magnesium. MCT can be used to provide additional kcalories. Research in animals (rats) suggests that adding pectin to the diet can significantly improve adaptation of the bowel following a resection.[6] Further studies will be needed to see if such an effect will occur in human beings.

Resections of the large intestine are less likely to result in nutrient deficiencies, because absorption of most nutrients occurs before the intestinal contents reach the colon. However, losses of fluids and electrolytes can be a problem, since they are normally reabsorbed in the colon.

An ileostomy involves the removal of the entire colon and rectum; a stoma, or opening, is made from the ileum and brought out through the abdomen to allow for defecation (see Figure 22-4). In a colostomy, only the rectum and anus are removed, and the stoma is formed from the remaining part of the colon. A watery stool will result from an ileostomy, whereas a more formed stool is produced by a colostomy.

After oral intake is initiated following surgery, people who have undergone ileostomies or colostomies are generally placed on bland, low-fiber diets to help promote healing of the stoma and to prevent irritation. However, encourage the client to resume a normal diet as soon as possible. Foods should be added individually and in small amounts so that their effects can be assessed. If a new food causes problems, it can be tried again a few months later.

Ostomates are often concerned about gas, odor, and loose and watery stools. Foods that cause excessively watery stools must be determined individually for each person. Certain raw fruits and vegetables and highly spiced foods cause

stoma (STOH-ma): a surgically formed opening; after an ileostomy or colostomy, a stoma is formed from the cut-off end of the intestine through the abdominal wall, through which excretion of wastes occurs.

ostomate (OSS-toe-mate): a person who has a surgically-formed opening from the bowel to the outside of the body, bypassing the anus. An **ileostomate** (ILL-ee-OSS-toe-mate) has an **ileostomy**; a **colostomate** (ko-LOSS-toe-mate) has a **colostomy.**
stoma = window

FIGURE 22–4

Colostomy and ileostomy.

A. Colostomy. The rectum and anus are removed, and the stoma is formed from the remaining colon.

B. Ileostomy. The entire colon and rectum are removed, and the stoma is formed from the ileum.

Sara was first diagnosed with Crohn's disease when she was 18 years old. At that time, she weighed 120 lb and was 5'7" tall. Her normal weight was 130 lb until she began having the symptoms that eventually were found to be caused by Crohn's disease. Since that time, she has been hospitalized several times and has undergone surgery twice to resect portions of the small bowel. She has an ileostomy. She is now 21, her weight is 123 lb, and she is in the hospital again with a suspected intestinal obstruction. As anticipated from her weight loss

CASE STUDY

Crohn's Disease

history, Sara's nutrition assessment shows that she is suffering from severe PCM. Sara's physician decided to begin TPN, with strict orders that nothing be given by mouth in the hope that surgery could be avoided.

1. Review Sara's weight history. What is her ideal body weight? What measures could have been taken to avoid weight loss?

2. Do you think that Sara will benefit from TPN? Why or why not?

3. Assume that Sara does well on TPN and is able to avoid surgery. What type of diet will she be placed on when oral intake resumes? Are there any dietary precautions made necessary by the ileostomy? What individual nutrients should be considered?

4. Consider Sara's long-term dietary management. What goals for weight gain should be established? How would you monitor results?

A health care professional specially trained to assist ostomates in learning the proper methods of caring for ostomy sites is the **enterostomal** (en-ter-oh-STOME-al) **therapist (E.T.).**

celiac (SEE-lee-ack) **disease:** a sensitivity to gliadin that causes flattening of the intestinal villi and generalized malabsorption; also called **gluten-sensitive enteropathy** (EN-ter-OP-ah-thee) or **celiac sprue.**

gluten (GLUE-ten): a vegetable protein found in wheat, oats, rye, and barley.

gliadin (GLIGH-ah-din): a fraction of the gluten protein.

atrophy: see p. 91.

problems for some ileostomates. Beer and other alcoholic beverages may cause diarrhea and gas. Gas and odors can be precipitated by such foods as beans, onions, green peppers, cabbage, turnips, and beets.

Stress the importance of drinking plenty of fluids to the ostomate. Reassure the individual that excess fluid taken above and beyond the amount lost through the ostomy will be absorbed and excreted by the kidneys and will not make the diarrhea worse.

New ostomates have many adjustments to make after surgery. They may feel they have lost control over a basic and private function. The retraining required to care for the ostomy and maintain bowel function may be difficult. Ostomates may also be worried that loved ones, particularly spouses, may find them unattractive. The health care team must work closely with each person and that person's family to help them make the necessary adjustments and resume normal activities.

Celiac Disease

Celiac disease provides an example of how changes in intestinal mucosal cells can cause malabsorption. Celiac disease is a hereditary disorder with an incidence of about 1 in every 2,000 to 3,000 births. It is characterized by malabsorption resulting from a sensitivity to gluten. Gluten is a protein found in wheat, oats, rye, and barley. A fraction of the gluten protein, gliadin, acts as a toxic substance. It causes the intestinal villi to atrophy, seriously reducing the absorptive surface of the intestinal tract. The disaccharidases and carrier molecules normally found on the villi become deficient. Malabsorption of many nutrients, including fat, protein, carbohydrate, fat-soluble vitamins, iron, calcium, magnesium, zinc, and some water-soluble vitamins, results.

The person with celiac disease often experiences steatorrhea, diarrhea, weight loss, and malnutrition. Anemia may occur as a result of iron, folacin, or vitamin B_{12} deficiency. Because protein is malabsorbed, serum protein levels can fall dramatically, and edema and swelling result. The individual may bleed easily

Normal intestinal villi.

Villi affected by celiac disease.

because of clotting abnormalities precipitated by a vitamin K deficiency. Furthermore, calcium deficiency can result in tetany and bone pain.

Fortunately, the intestinal changes can be reversed almost completely when gluten is removed from the diet. Generally, improvement can be expected within a few weeks if the diet is strictly followed. However, lactase deficiency and lactose intolerance may be permanent. If the person does not follow the diet, symptoms return.

The treatment for celiac disease sounds deceptively simple: eliminate gluten. Unfortunately, gluten is found in many common foods. As you can see from Table 22-4, many foods contain wheat, oats, rye, or barley in some form. Wheat flour is used as an extender in many processed foods (ice cream, salad dressings, and canned foods).

You can help people with celiac disease and those who care for them to understand what foods to avoid. Be sure they understand how to read food labels. Suggest the use of arrowroot, corn, potato, rice, and soybean flours as substitutes for wheat flour in recipes. A low-gluten wheat starch flour is also available as a substitute to be used by people with allergies and intolerances. Families with a member who has celiac disease need a lot of support from the health care team. Books, recipes, and addresses of sources for special food products are available; share them with the family.

An easy way to remember the grains that must be restricted in celiac disease is to remember **WORB** (wheat, oats, rye, and barley).

Disaccharidase Deficiencies

The disaccharidases are the enzymes that split disaccharides (lactose, sucrose, and maltose) to monosaccharides (glucose, galactose, and fructose) so that they can be absorbed. The disaccharidases are normally found along the intestinal villi. A deficiency of any disaccharidase results in carbohydrate malabsorption. The unhydrolyzed disaccharide remains unabsorbed in the intestine, causing the intestinal contents to become hyperosmolar. Large volumes of water are drawn into the gut to equalize the osmolarity, and this results in cramps, distension, and diarrhea. Bacteria present in the intestine metabolize the undigested sugars to irritating acids that further contribute to cramping and diarrhea.

TABLE 22–4

Gluten-restricted Diet

Meat and meat alternates

Any allowed except those that are breaded or those that are prepared with bread crumbs.

Milk and milk products

Any allowed except milk mixed with Ovaltine, commercial chocolate milk with a cereal additive, pudding thickened with wheat flour, ice cream or sherbet containing gluten stabilizers.

Fruits and vegetables

Any allowed except those that are breaded or prepared with bread crumbs.

Grains

Allowed: Bread, cereal, or dessert products made from arrowroot, buckwheat, cornmeal, wheat starch, soybean flour, or gluten-free starch; gluten-free macaroni or porridge; tapioca; cornmeal, cornflakes, popcorn, hominy; rice, cream of rice, puffed rice, rice flakes; potato chips.

Not allowed: Bread, cereal, or dessert products made from wheat, rye, oats, or barley; commercially prepared mixes for biscuits, cornbread, muffins, pancakes, buckwheat pancakes, cakes, cookies, and waffles; bran; pasta, macaroni, and noodles; malt; pretzels; wheat germ; doughnuts; ice-cream cones.

Other (not allowed)

Beer; ale; certain whiskeys (Canadian rye); cereal beverages (Postum); root beer; commercial salad dressings that contain gluten stabilizers; soups containing any ingredient not allowed (barley, noodles, etc.).

A person born with little or no lactase activity has **primary lactose intolerance. Secondary lactose intolerance** is caused by another disease. **Developmental lactose intolerance** describes a lactase deficiency that develops as a person grows older.

Be alert to the presence of lactose in a food whenever the label's ingredient list includes:
• Milk.
• Milk solids.
• Lactose.
• Whey.
• Casein.

Lactase deficiency is the most frequently seen disaccharidase deficiency. In rare cases, a person is simply born with a deficiency of lactase. More often, lactase deficiency develops as a consequence of another disease, or as the person grows older. In some people, normal lactase levels gradually fall as they become adults. Developmental lactose intolerance is more prevalent among black Americans, native Americans, and Asians than among Caucasians.

The intestinal cells that produce lactase are located on the delicate fringe of microvilli that form the brush border of the intestinal villi (see p. 178). Any condition that changes the brush border can lead to lactose intolerance. We have already discussed some disorders and conditions that can result in either temporary or permanent lactose intolerance: inflammatory bowel diseases, celiac disease, PCM, GI tract surgery, and radiation therapy.

A lactose-restricted diet is a highly individualized diet, because people vary widely in the amount of lactose they can tolerate. The person sensitive to even small amounts of lactose must follow a lactose-free diet as shown in Table 22-5. A sample menu is also illustrated. As you can see, this diet can be difficult to follow because lactose is a hidden ingredient in many foods. The person on a lactose-free diet needs to be a label reader. Remind the client to avoid foods that include these ingredients: milk, milk solids, lactose, whey, and casein. Even some drugs contain lactose as fillers; therefore, check all drugs with the pharmacist.

TABLE 22–5

Foods to Avoid on a Lactose-free Diet

Meat and meat alternates

Breaded or creamed meats, fish, or poultry; sausage, cold cuts containing nonfat-milk solids; omelets or soufflés made with milk; some peanut butter.

Milk and milk products

Whole, nonfat, evaporated, condensed, or dried milk; yogurt; cheese; ice cream; sherbet; whey and casein milk treated with lactobacillus/acidophilus culture; custard; pudding.

Fruits and vegetables

Any canned or frozen fruit or vegetable processed with lactose; creamed, breaded, or buttered vegetables.

Grains

Breads and rolls made with milk; prepared muffin, biscuit, waffle, pancake, cake, or cookie mixes; some dry cereals; French toast; pie crusts made with butter or margarine.

Other

Some cocoas, instant coffees, margarines, and dressings; butter; cream; creamed soups; chewing gum; chocolate; toffee; peppermint; butterscotch; caramels; some drugs and vitamin-mineral supplements; monosodium glutamate; some artificial sweeteners, including Equal and Sweet 'N Low.

Fortunately, not all people with lactose intolerance must avoid lactose completely. The amount of lactose allowed depends on the client's tolerance. Many times only milk, milk beverages, creamed foods, and ice cream have to be avoided. Cheese can be tolerated. Some people can also drink buttermilk or eat yogurt, because much of the lactose in these products has been converted to lactic acid

Sample lactose-free diet menu.

Breakfast
½ c grapefruit juice
1 soft-cooked egg
2 slices toasted Italian
   bread
Milk-free margarine
Jelly
Coffee or tea

Lunch
3 oz roasted chicken
1 baked potato
Salad with homemade
   vinegar/oil dressing
Milk-free roll
Milk-free margarine
Coffee or tea

Supper
4 oz roast beef
½ c rice
½ c cooked carrots
Milk-free bread or roll
Fresh fruit
Coffee or tea

An enzyme preparation added to milk splits lactose into glucose and galactose.

by the bacteria used in the fermentation process. Chocolate milk may be better tolerated than regular milk, although the reason for this tolerance is unknown. Many people can use commercially prepared products containing lactose without difficulty. Some may even be able to use milk or ice cream in limited quantities. Others can add an enzyme preparation (Lact-Aid) to milk before they drink it. The enzyme splits much of the lactose in milk to glucose and galactose.

A word of caution: people who consume no milk or too little milk and milk products often have diets that are calcium deficient. Encourage the use of milk and milk products for those who can tolerate them. Others should use calcium-fortified soy milk as a beverage or in cooking. In some cases, a calcium supplement may be indicated.

Nutrition Assessment

As we have seen, diseases of the GI tract can affect nutrition status by interfering with food intake, affecting the absorption of nutrients, or increasing nutrient needs. Remember to keep these points in mind when you interpret nutrition assessment data:

- Obtain a detailed history of weight fluctuations, food tolerances, and chronic drug use. Weight loss commonly occurs in GI tract disorders, and the client is at risk for PCM. Likewise, the chronic drug use often necessary to treat GI tract disorders can contribute to malnutrition. A history of food tolerances is extremely important in planning a diet that will cause the least discomfort.
- Interpret anthropometric measurements cautiously. Anthropometric measurements will be affected by the state of hydration. Keep in mind that anthropometric measurements, including weight, may be deceptive in people who have edema. Remember that people with low serum albumin levels (malabsorption and weight loss) often have edema.
- Consider that biochemical measurements may falsely appear to be high in dehydration. Dehydration is a possibility in anyone who is experiencing severe diarrhea or vomiting.
- Look for signs of individual nutrient deficiencies that can be present in people with long-standing GI tract disorders. You must assess not only their intake, but also note any possible interferences with absorption, such as short-bowel syndrome.

Study Questions

1. Describe the dietary treatment of diarrhea. When is diarrhea a cause for alarm?
2. What is constipation? What changes in diet and lifestyle can help prevent constipation?
3. What theory explains the development of diverticula in the intestine? What dangers are associated with diverticular disease? What diet is useful for treating diverticular disease? What precautions should the person trying a high-fiber diet for the first time take?
4. Discuss various conditions that can lead to malabsorption. Why is fat frequently the biggest problem in people with malabsorption? What are the effects of fat malabsorption?

What dietary modifications can be useful in treating fat malabsorption?

5. Recommend ways to make a low-fat diet palatable and easy to follow.

6. What are inflammatory bowel diseases? Distinguish between Crohn's disease and ulcerative colitis. How can inflammatory bowel diseases lead to malabsorption?

7. Describe the diet therapy for a person with Crohn's disease. Discuss the possible advantages of TPN and hydrolyzed formulas for people with Crohn's disease.

8. What is the recommended diet for the person with ulcerative colitis? What is the primary concern in this disorder?

9. What factors affect absorption after small bowel surgery? Describe short-bowel syndrome and its effect on nutrition status.

10. Describe the adaptive process that occurs in the remaining intestine after a portion of the intestine is resected. What diet is most useful following intestinal resections?

11. What is an ileostomy? What is a colostomy? What diet, if any, can benefit the person who has undergone one of these procedures?

12. What protein and fraction of a protein are of particular concern in the person with celiac disease? What diet is useful in the treatment of celiac disease? Plan a day's menu for a person with celiac disease using Table 22-4 as a guide. Think about and discuss the difficulties involved in following the diet.

13. Describe lactose intolerance. What types of foods are avoided on a lactose-restricted diet? Discuss the variability of lactose-restricted diets, and give suggestions for preventing calcium deficiency in people following these diets.

Notes

1. J. B. Kirsner and R. B. Shorter, Recent developments in "nonspecific" inflammatory bowel disease: Part 1, *New England Journal of Medicine* 306 (1982): 775-785.

2. M. I. Gee and coauthors, Protein-energy malnutrition in gastroenterology outpatients: Increased risk in Crohn's disease, *Journal of the American Dietetic Association* 85 (1985): 1466-1474; P. Hodges and coauthors, Protein-energy intake and malnutrition in Crohn's disease, *Journal of the American Dietetic Association* 84 (1984): 1460-1464.

3. M. I. Gee and coauthors, Nutritional status of gastroenterology outpatients: Comparison of inflammatory bowel disease with functional disorders, *Journal of the American Dietetic Association* 85 (1985): 1591-1599.

4. M. J. Ostro, G. R. Greenberg, and K. N. Jeejeebhoy, Total parenteral nutrition and complete bowel rest in the management of Crohn's disease, *Journal of Parenteral and Enteral Nutrition* 9 (1985): 280-287.

5. R. G. Rees and coauthors, Elemental diet administered nasogastrically without starter regimens to patients with inflammatory bowel disease, *Journal of Parenteral and Enteral Nutrition* 10 (1986): 258-262.

6. M. J. Koruda and coauthors, The effect of a pectin-supplemented elemental diet on intestinal adaptation to massive small bowel resection, *Journal of Parenteral and Enteral Nutrition* 10 (1986): 343-350.

Disorders of the Liver, Exocrine Pancreas, and Gallbladder

23

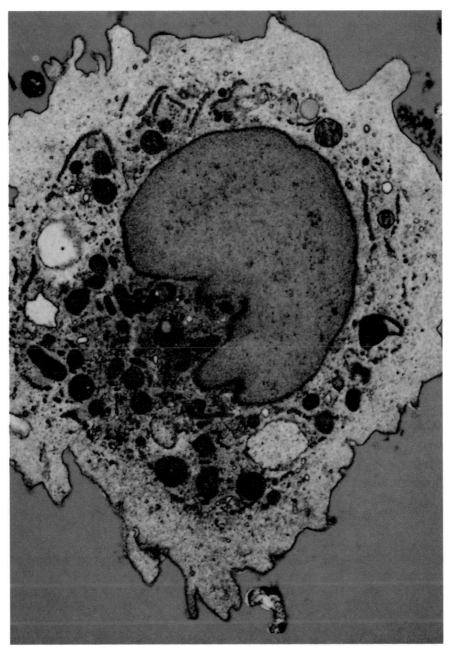

Contents

This giant cell is a macrophage, a cell that devours and digests foreign particles, assisting the body in defending against disease. Normal liver function is important to proper production of the macrophages.

The liver, pancreas, and gallbladder play integral roles in the digestion and absorption of nutrients (see p. 176). Furthermore, the liver serves as a processing plant; nutrients and other metabolites arriving there may be metabolized, packaged, stored, detoxified, or shipped out for the use of other organs.

The pancreas has both endocrine and exocrine functions. In this chapter, we will focus on its exocrine function. As an exocrine gland, the pancreas secretes many digestive enzymes, along with a bicarbonate-rich digestive juice that raises the intestinal pH for optimal enzyme activity. The endocrine function of the pancreas includes the production of the hormones insulin and glucagon, which is discussed in the next chapter.

The gallbladder serves as a storage area for the bile salts produced by the liver. The bile salts are necessary for the digestion of most fats and fat-soluble vitamins.

endocrine, exocrine: see p. 172.

The gallbladder and the duct system that conveys bile from the liver to the intestine is the **biliary** (BILL-ee-air-ee) **tract** (see p. 104).

Disorders of the Liver

The liver's central roles in the digestion, absorption, and metabolism of nutrients cannot be overemphasized (see Figure 6-8 on p. 186). In addition, the liver functions in other ways to maintain the body's well-being; for example, it is the site where many drugs and toxic waste products are prepared for excretion. Table 23-1 summarizes some of the many functions of the liver.

With all these vital tasks to perform, there is little wonder that disorders of the liver can have profound effects on both nutrition and general health status. Liver disease can result from alcohol abuse, congenital disorders, chemicals, infections, biliary tract obstructions, heart disease, and other causes. The rest of this section describes several types of liver diseases. Dietary management of liver disease depends to a large extent on the type and severity of the disease.

Fatty Liver

fatty liver: see p. 237. Also called **hepatic steatosis** (STEE-ah-TOE-sis).

Fatty liver results from a build up of triglycerides in the liver. This occurs when triglycerides are synthesized excessively, not oxidized to fatty acids, received by the liver from the blood in abnormally high amounts, not released back into the blood, or a combination of these factors. Highlight 7B discusses the development of fatty liver in the alcohol abuser.

When triglycerides accumulate in the liver, the liver enlarges. Fatty liver itself is usually not harmful and often can be reversed. However, the accumulation of fat suggests the presence of an underlying primary disease that can be serious. Aside from alcohol abuse, fatty liver can be associated with the use of some drugs (corticosteroids or tetracycline), kwashiorkor, obesity, mismanaged TPN, and small bowel bypass surgery. Fatty liver associated with small bowel bypass surgery can rapidly progress to more serious liver disease and death.

Fatty liver caused by malnutrition can be reversed by correcting nutrient deficits. In alcohol abuse, abstinence from alcohol, in addition to a good diet,

TABLE 23–1

Functions of the Liver

Protein Metabolism

    Conversion of amino acids to energy sources (oxidative deamination)
    Synthesis of nonessential amino acids (transamination)
    Synthesis of nitrogen-containing compounds from amino acids (purines, pyrimidines)
    Urea synthesis
    Plasma protein synthesis

Carbohydrate Metabolism

    Maintenance of normal blood glucose levels
    Glycogen storage
    Conversion of monosaccharides to glucose

Fat Metabolism

    Synthesis of cholesterol, phospholipids, and lipoproteins
    Production of ketone bodies
    Oxidation of fatty acids
    Synthesis of triglycerides

Other

    Synthesis of bile salts
    Synthesis of blood coagulation factors
    Detoxification of alcohol, drugs, wastes, and other foreign substances

is necessary. If drug ingestion is responsible, the drug is discontinued. Otherwise, there is no specific therapy for fatty liver.

Hepatitis

Hepatitis is a more serious liver disease in which liver tissue becomes inflamed. The most common causes are viruses (hepatitis A virus, hepatitis B virus, and non-A, non-B hepatitis virus), alcohol, and drugs. The hepatitis A virus is spread through contaminated water, food, or sewage. The hepatitis B and the non-A, non-B hepatitis viruses are transmitted parenterally (through blood transfusions, dialysis, or use of contaminated needles by drug addicts) and results in a more serious type of hepatitis. It is possible that other causes of hepatitis will be identified in the future. Hepatitis is sometimes a minor illness, but it can be fatal.

In the early stages of hepatitis, the person may suddenly develop anorexia, nausea, vomiting, and fever. Later, as bile pigments spill from the diseased liver into the blood, the person develops jaundice and a dark urine. The liver may also enlarge.

Provide a normal, well-balanced diet to the person with hepatitis who is in good nutrition status. The malnourished person with hepatitis, like any malnourished person, needs a high-kcalorie, high-protein diet. People with alcohol-related hepatitis are at high risk for poor nutrition status. Malnutrition is a common complication of alcohol abuse, and hepatitis puts an additional stress

hepatitis: inflammation of the liver caused by a virus or toxin (also defined on p. 545). Hepatitis can progress to cirrhosis (see below).
hepat = liver
itis = inflammation

jaundice: see pp. 349, 363.

on the body. Nutrients help liver cells to regenerate. When anorexia is severe, IV glucose solution may be given temporarily. Suggest small, frequent meals, liquid supplements, or both for the person who cannot eat. Tube feedings should be considered if nausea or anorexia is severe and if it continues for a long time or if the person is malnourished. Intravenous feedings may be necessary if vomiting becomes a problem. Occasionally, a person with hepatitis develops liver failure and hepatic coma, which will be discussed later.

Cirrhosis

Cirrhosis is the most serious and irreversible type of liver injury. In cirrhosis, liver cells filled with fat or damaged by inflammation die, and scar tissue invades the liver. Chronic alcohol abuse is the most common cause of cirrhosis in the United States. Not all alcohol abusers develop cirrhosis, however; its incidence among alcohol abusers is about 10 to 12 percent. Furthermore, not all people with cirrhosis are alcohol abusers. Cirrhosis can result from several other causes. Either fatty liver or hepatitis can progress to cirrhosis.

Normal liver tissue is soft and flexible, but scars are unyielding. The portal vein and the hepatic artery carry 1½ quarts of blood every minute through the miles of intermeshed capillaries in the liver. This huge volume of blood cannot pulse easily through the mass of scar tissue in the cirrhotic liver, so it backs up into the portal vein. Consequently, blood pressure in the vein increases sharply, causing portal hypertension. A diagram of the liver's circulatory system is shown in Figure 23-1. You may also want to review the vascular system figure on p. 184.

hepatic (he-PAT-ik): of, like, or pertaining to the liver.

cirrhosis (seer-OH-sis): see pp. 154, 237. **Laënnec's cirrhosis** is the type associated with alcohol abuse and malnutrition.

The impact of alcohol abuse on nutrition status is discussed in Highlight 7B.

The **portal vein** carries nutrients from the digestive organs to the liver; the **hepatic artery** brings oxygen-rich blood from the heart to the liver; the **hepatic vein** returns blood from the liver to the heart (also defined on p. 182).

portal hypertension: increased blood pressure in the portal vein caused by obstructed blood flow through the liver.

FIGURE 23–1

The liver's circulatory system. Note that poor circulation in the liver can cause high blood pressure in the portal vein. Back pressure can also enlarge veins surrounding the intestinal system, including the esophagus.

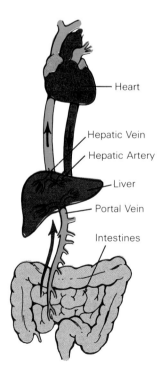

- Heart
- Hepatic Vein
- Hepatic Artery
- Liver
- Portal Vein
- Intestines

As pressure rises, plasma is forced out of the liver's blood vessels into the abdominal cavity, and the belly swells. The accumulation of fluid in the abdominal cavity is the kind of edema called *ascites*, a self-aggravating condition. Because the volume of blood in the circulatory system is now reduced, less blood reaches the kidneys, and they respond by calling for more aldosterone. As a result, the body retains sodium, and edema spreads to all body compartments. To make matters worse, the diseased liver cannot dispose of aldosterone as it normally does, so aldosterone levels remain high.

Normal blood flow through the liver is blocked, so some of the blood takes a detour through smaller vessels around the liver and out to the rest of the body. These shunts, or collaterals, often develop in the area of the esophagus. Frequently, the raised pressure enlarges them so that they bulge into the lumen of the esophagus, like varicose veins in the legs, creating esophageal varices. The lining of the esophagus on top of the varices eventually erodes. Many times the erosion penetrates into the varices themselves, and massive bleeding follows. A person who has bled from esophageal varices will very likely bleed again, and death can occur during any bleeding episode.

Under normal circumstances, the liver removes ammonia from circulation and converts it to urea (see box entitled "Ammonia Production"). A seriously diseased liver can't synthesize urea adequately and so can't remove ammonia from the blood. The problem is further aggravated because some blood carrying ammonia is not even reaching the liver; instead, it is bypassing the liver by way of the collaterals. Elevated blood ammonia levels insult the central nervous system, compounding the risk of hepatic coma.

Hepatic coma is a dangerous complication of liver disease. Typically, the person with impending hepatic coma exhibits mental disturbances such as changes in judgment, personality, or mood. Sometimes sleep patterns change. Such a person may be unable to reproduce a simple shape, such as a star. A sweet, musty, or pungent odor may develop on the breath. Flapping tremor is also seen in the precoma state. Just before passing into coma, the person becomes very difficult to arouse.

The exact mechanisms causing hepatic coma are unknown, but rising blood ammonia levels play an important role. Most people in hepatic coma have elevated blood ammonia levels, although the degree of the elevation does not necessarily correlate with the severity of the coma. This poor correlation may be because blood ammonia levels do not reflect brain ammonia levels. Two substances (glutamine and ketoglutarate), which are produced when brain ammonia levels are high, have a higher correlation with degree of coma. Other nitrogen-containing compounds that appear to be produced from the metabolism of methionine by bacteria in the colon may also be involved.

Blood amino acid patterns also change in hepatic coma. Aromatic amino acids normally are catabolized by the liver, and this catabolism is impaired in liver disease. Consequently, aromatic amino acid levels rise. Hormonal changes that occur in liver disease (specifically, elevated insulin levels) result in the uptake of branched-chain amino acids by muscle cells. Therefore, branched-chain amino acid levels fall. This change may cause the production of unusually high levels of certain substances that act like neurotransmitters, and these substances may, in turn, contribute to hepatic coma. Another consequence of this altered amino acid metabolism is high blood ammonia levels, which, as we've already noted, is associated with hepatic coma.

ascites: see p. 141.

collaterals: small blood vessels developed to divert blood flow away from an obstructed organ. These blood vessels are also called **shunts.**

esophageal varices (ee-SOFF-ah-GEE-al VAIR-ih-seez): tangles of distended blood vessels that protrude into the esophagus.

A high blood level of ammonia is called **hyperammonemia.** Normal blood ammonia levels range from 80-110 μg/dl.

hepatic coma: a state of unconsciousness that results from severe liver disease; also called **portal systemic encephalopathy.**

flapping tremor: uncontrolled movement of the muscle group that causes the outstretched arm and hand to flap like a wing; occurs in hepatic coma and other diseases that cause encephalopathy.

Phenylalanine

Aromatic amino acids are characterized by a ring structure.

Valine

Branched-chain amino acids are characterized by a branched structure.

neurotransmitter: see p. 201.

Ammonia Production

Blood ammonia comes from several sources, but principally from the GI tract. In the GI tract, ammonia is produced by intestinal bacteria and, from protein digestion, by enzymes. Therapy designed to reduce blood ammonia, therefore, is aimed at reducing the amount of protein present in the GI tract, as well as eliminating ammonia-producing bacteria. Figure 23-2 illustrates how ammonia is produced in the body.

An obvious way to meet the aim of therapy is to limit food protein. However, even if no protein is given in the diet, the GI tract will contain protein available for digestion, because it constantly sheds cells into its lumen, which can then be digested. Moreover, the person with liver disease is likely to have GI bleeding from gastritis, ulcers, or esophageal varices; the blood serves as an additional source of protein. These three main protein sources in the GI tract—food, shed mucosal cells, and blood—account for about two-thirds of the ammonia found in the blood.

Another source of ammonia in the GI tract is urea. Most of the blood urea is filtered into the urine for excretion, but about 25 percent of the body's urea finds its way into the GI tract instead, where gut bacteria metabolize it to ammonia. Another small but significant ammonia source is metabolic processes carried on by cells all over the body.

Diagrams on pp. 211-212 show how the liver and kidneys normally cooperate to remove excess nitrogen from the body. The liver performs the first step (converting ammonia to urea); the kidneys, the second (filtering urea into the urine). A diseased liver fails to do its job for two reasons—first, because, as already mentioned, the ammonia isn't flowing into the liver as it should; and second, because the liver's dead and dying cells can't efficiently convert the ammonia they do receive. In fact, the ammonia is directly toxic to them, as it is to all cells of the body.

You can see how this vicious cycle feeds itself: more ammonia is produced, organ function deteriorates, and less can be detoxified. You can also see why, in liver disease, blood ammonia levels are elevated, whereas in kidney disease, blood urea levels rise.

Many drugs used in the treatment of liver disease work on the intestine to disrupt this vicious cycle. At the same time, diet, by supplying just enough, but not too much, protein (with its nitrogen), helps relieve the metabolic load of the liver.

Dietary guidelines in liver disease:
1. 35 to 50 kcal/kg actual body weight.
2. Liver disease: 0.5 to 1.0 g protein/kg body weight. Impending coma: Reduce protein to 20 to 35 g/day; increase in increments of 10 to 15 g/day for 5 to 7 days until individual tolerance or 1.0 g/kg body weight (whichever is lower) is reached. Coma: Give no protein. Gradually increase protein as condition improves.
3. If ascites is present, restrict sodium to 250 to 2,000 mg/day and fluid to 1,500 to 2,000 ml/day. Increase sodium and fluid intake as liver function improves.

A protein-restricted diet is a cornerstone of therapy in cirrhosis. A daily intake of 35 to 50 kcalories per kilogram of actual body weight (about 2,000 to 3,000 kcalories) is recommended to maintain the person in positive nitrogen balance. Enough protein should be given so that liver cells can regenerate, but too much protein will result in more ammonia buildup, which can lead to hepatic coma. In the absence of hepatic coma, the diet should be adequate in kcalories and meet the RDA for protein (0.5 to 1.0 grams per kilogram body weight).

A few studies have suggested that higher protein intakes may be desirable.[1] Yet if coma is likely, the excess protein makes it even more likely (by generating

FIGURE 23–2

Ammonia production in the body.

ammonia). Therefore, it seems wise that protein intake should be moderate, and protein quality high.

A person with signs of impending coma requires additional dietary modifications. Protein intake must be restricted to 20 to 35 grams (or less) of high-quality protein per day. Once coma has set in, the person is given no protein. As improvement becomes evident (the client's neurological status is assessed regularly), protein can gradually be increased in 10- to 15-gram increments per day for five to seven days until the RDA for protein is reached. People should not be kept on zero-protein diets for more than a few days. Such diets cause breakdown of body proteins, which can make matters worse.

Foods that contain preformed ammonia or contain amino acids that readily form ammonia in the body should also be restricted. These foods include cheeses (American, beer, cheddar, domestic blue, and Tilsit), some poultry and meat (chicken, ground beef, ham, and salami), buttermilk, gelatin, Idaho potatoes, onions, and peanut butter.[2]

Vegetable protein may be better tolerated than meat protein, perhaps because vegetable protein has fewer amino acids that readily form ammonia. In addition, diets high in plant foods contain more fiber which prevents constipation, thereby reducing the time available for the production and absorption of ammonia in the gut. Such diets have been shown to reduce both urea nitrogen production and urinary nitrogen excretion.[3]

It has been thought that the cirrhotic liver can't handle fat. Indeed, such a liver exposed to the continued onslaught of alcohol can't manufacture the lipoproteins to rid itself of accumulated lipids. But without alcohol, and with enough protein as new raw material, the cirrhotic liver seems to manage well enough. Fat helps make foods more appetizing to a person whose appetite is poor. In addition, fat delivers kcalories efficiently. Therefore, fat is not restricted unless the cirrhotic person develops steatorrhea, a clear sign that fat absorption has failed. Even then, the diet should probably supply fat for kcalories, but as MCT which is handled by the body differently (see box entitled "How Medium-Chain Triglycerides are Digested and Absorbed" in Chapter 22).

Total abstinence from alcohol is necessary to protect the liver from further injury. The cirrhotic person should never drink alcoholic beverages again.

The diet is usually supplemented with large amounts of water-soluble vitamins (up to five times the RDA). Remember that the B vitamins are coenzymes necessary for the liver's many metabolic reactions and repair work. In malnutrition, the water-soluble vitamins are among the first to be depleted. A person with a prolonged prothrombin time should be offered vitamin K supplements. Otherwise, fat-soluble vitamins are provided only if a deficiency has been identified. Frequently, the RDA amounts of these vitamins are adequate.

prothrombin time: the time it takes for clotting to occur. Both vitamin K deficiency and liver disease can prolong the time it takes for the blood to clot.

For people with ascites, fluids and sodium are also restricted. The level of restriction varies with the severity of the ascites. Sodium amounts may range from 250 to 2,000 milligrams a day; fluids, from 1,500 to 2,000 milliliters a day. Weigh the person *daily*. Weight fluctuations are used to assess changes in fluid balance. If weight gain is rapid, the person is retaining fluid. Sudden weight loss, in contrast, indicates that the person is successfully excreting water. Table 23-2 shows diet patterns used for various sodium-restricted diets. A sample 60-gram protein, low-sodium diet is also shown.

To provide a diet low in sodium that will stimulate the appetite and provide adequate protein is a difficult task. Many high-protein foods (for example, eggs, meat, and milk) also contain significant amounts of sodium. Special low-sodium supplements and milk products are available to circumvent this problem. When

Sample 60-gram protein, low-sodium (1,000 mg) diet menu. Foods on this low-sodium menu are cooked without salt. To increase the sodium, salt is added to foods. To decrease sodium further, unsalted butter and milk is used. The kcalories provided by this menu depend on how much fat is used in cooking. Extra kcalories, if needed, are provided by encouraging the liberal use of fats and sugars from foods that do not contain protein (for example, butter and table sugar).

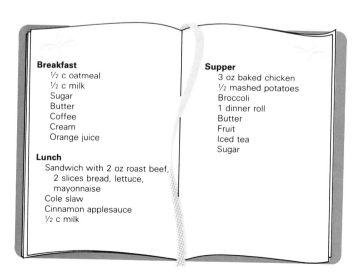

Breakfast
½ c oatmeal
½ c milk
Sugar
Butter
Coffee
Cream
Orange juice

Lunch
Sandwich with 2 oz roast beef, 2 slices bread, lettuce, mayonnaise
Cole slaw
Cinnamon applesauce
½ c milk

Supper
3 oz baked chicken
½ mashed potatoes
Broccoli
1 dinner roll
Butter
Fruit
Iced tea
Sugar

TABLE 23–2

Low-Sodium Diets

Foods	\multicolumn{4}{c}{Number of Servings Allowed on Various Levels of Sodium Restriction}				Serving Size	Sodium per Serving (mg)
	250 Mg	500 Mg	1,000 Mg	2,000 Mg		
Nonfat, whole, and evaporated milk	0	2	2	2	8 oz	120
Low-sodium milk	2	Not restricted	Not restricted	Not restricted	8 oz	7
Meat, fish, poultry, and unsalted cheese	4	4	4	6	1 oz	25
Egg	1	1	1	1	1	60
Bread and allowed ready-to-eat cereal	0	0	2	5	1 slice or ¾ oz	200
Low-sodium bread, cereal, and cereal products	7	7	7	4 or more	Varies	5
Fresh, frozen, or canned without salt: asparagus, bean sprouts, broccoli, brussels sprouts, cabbage, cauliflower, cucumbers, eggplant, endive, escarole, green pepper, collard and turnip greens, lettuce, mushrooms, okra, onions, radishes, rhubarb, rutabaga, string beans, summer squash, tomatoes, watercress, zucchini, and low-sodium tomato and vegetable juices	2	2	2	Not restricted	½ c	9
Fresh, frozen, or canned without salt: corn, lima beans, parsnips, peas, potatoes, pumpkin, sweet potatoes, winter squash, and yams	1	1	1	Not restricted	½ c	5
Canned vegetables and vegetables frozen with salt	0	0	0	1	½ c	200
Salted butter and margarine	0	0	2	6	1 tsp	50
Regular mayonnaise	0	0	2	6	1½ tsp	50

General diet guidelines:

The foods listed below cannot be used unless they have been calculated into the diet; however, allowances can be made, particularly when the higher levels of sodium are allowed. For example, if a person on a 2 g sodium diet does not drink milk, you can allow 240 mg of sodium from any other food source (see Appendix H for the sodium content of foods). With this in mind, avoid the following foods:

1. Salt used in cooking or at the table.
2. Highly salted snacks, such as potato chips, corn chips, tortilla chips, salted popcorn, and pretzels.
3. Barbeque sauce; bouillon cubes (except low sodium); catsup; celery salt, seeds, or leaves; chili sauce; garlic salt; horseradish made with salt; meat extracts, sauces and tenderizers; monosodium glutamate; prepared mustard; olives; onion salt; pickles; relishes; saccharin; soy sauce; and Worcestershire sauce.
4. Commercial foods made with milk: ice cream, sherbet, malted milk, milk mixes, and milk shakes.
5. Artichokes, beets, carrots, Chinese or red cabbage, greens (except those listed with vegetables in table above), sauerkraut, and spinach.
6. Maraschino cherries, crystallized or glazed fruits, and dried fruit with sodium sulfite added.
7. Brains; kidneys; canned, salted, or smoked meats; bacon; luncheon meats; chopped or corned beef; kosher meats; shellfish; regular cheeses; egg substitutes; and regular peanut butter.
8. Salted butter or margarine, salt pork, commercial salad dressing (except low sodium), and salted nuts.
9. Leavening agents, such as baking powder and baking soda; rennet tablets; pudding mixes; and molasses.
10. Fountain beverages; instant cocoa mixes; prepared beverage mixes (including fruit-flavored powders); and commercial candy, cakes, cookies, sweetened gelatin mixes, pastries, puddings, cakes, and biscuit mixes.
11. Most commercial dry cereals or instant hot cereals. Puffed wheat, puffed rice, and shredded wheat are allowed.

Source: Adapted from American Dietetic Association, *Handbook of Clinical Dietetics* (New Haven, Conn.: Yale University Press, 1981).

In our discussion of these diets, try to picture the diet. Consider, for example, what the person on a 30-gram protein diet is actually eating. On such a diet, the total protein allowance would be spent on just one egg, 2 ounces of meat, a half cup of milk, and one serving each of vegetables and bread.

No doubt, you can already see some problems. The amounts allowed from the major food groups are small. The kcalorie content is also low. You can now see why fat is not restricted unless necessary: adding fat wherever possible can help boost kcalorie intake and satiety. Other foods that do not contain protein, such as some types of candy, jelly, and sugar, can also help. But these items obviously lack nutrients.

If the person must follow a sodium or fluid restriction, especially a strict one, it is like adding insult to injury. A person offered such a diet may not want to eat at all. You will need to offer much advice on making foods tasty, and much encouragement.

sodium intake must be severely restricted, it is important to note even the sodium content of the local water supply and of medications.

The person who has bleeding esophageal varices will be unable to consume food by mouth. When there is no bleeding, the person may be advised to follow a low-fiber diet (see Chapter 21) to avoid irritation, painful swallowing, or bleeding.[4] However, this advice is controversial, and its benefits are unclear. The person with anorexia may accept food more willingly in small, frequent meals than in fewer large ones. Diet is vital to recovery from cirrhosis. Therefore, every effort must be made to ensure its acceptance. Work closely with the person and the family to individualize the diet, and serve foods attractively. Try the tactics suggested in Chapter 18 to encourage the client to eat.

If the person with cirrhosis cannot eat enough food by mouth, little time should be wasted in beginning a tube feeding or parenteral nutrition. Both types of special nutrition support have been used successfully in people with cirrhosis. In fact, special TPN and enteral nutrition formulas are available for the person with liver disease. These formulas contain low levels of aromatic amino acids and amino acids that tend to form ammonia easily, and they are enriched with branched-chain amino acids. Although these formulas theoretically should be advantageous for the person with liver disease, their value has not been conclusively verified in clinical tests.[5] Indeed, one study evaluated the effect of two oral formulas—one a standard casein-based formula and the other an enriched branched-chain amino acid formula—in the treatment of cirrhosis.[6] Both formulas proved to be equally effective and safe in maintaining nutrition status when used in the treatment of people with cirrhosis.

Blood ammonia levels can also be reduced with drugs. Neomycin and lactulose are two such drugs. Neomycin kills the intestinal bacteria that produce ammonia. The mechanism of action of lactulose is unknown, but it has been suggested that it works by causing diarrhea (thus loss of ammonia) and by converting ammonia to a form that can't be reabsorbed into the body.

M r. Sloan is a 48-year-old carpenter who has been in the hospital many times. His problem with alcohol abuse was recognized years ago, and since that time he has entered alcohol rehabilitation programs several times. However, as of this time, his problem with alcohol abuse continues. Mr. Sloan was recently admitted to the hospital, and a diagnosis of alcoholic cirrhosis has been confirmed. At 5′7″ tall, Mr. Sloan, who once weighed 150 lb, now weighs 120 lb. He looks thin, although his abdomen is distended with ascites, and his skin is yellow. His liver disease is advanced, and he is showing signs of impending hepatic coma. Laboratory findings include:

- SGOT, 295 units (above normal).
- SGPT, 187 units (above normal).

CASE STUDY

Cirrhosis

- Alkaline phosphatase, 13 Bodansky units (above normal).
- BUN, 8 mg/dl (normal).
- Blood ammonia, 125 μg/dl (above normal).

These findings are consistent with liver disease.

1. What is cirrhosis? Describe the consequences of cirrhosis.
2. From the limited information available, what can you say about Mr. Sloan's nutrition status? What are his %IBW and %UBW? Do you expect his blood albumin levels to be normal? If

not, why not? Describe some specific nutrient deficiencies associated with alcohol abuse (see Highlight 7B).
3. What dietary changes are recommended for the person with cirrhosis? How will Mr. Sloan's diet be altered, now that he is in a precoma state?
4. Why is Mr. Sloan's abdomen distended? Explain the development of ascites in liver disease. How is the diet adjusted for people with ascites?
5. Would you expect Mr. Sloan's blood ammonia levels to be high? Why or why not? Explain why blood ammonia is frequently elevated in people with liver disease.
6. Define portal hypertension, jaundice, and esophageal varices. How would Mr. Sloan's diet be changed if he were found to have esophageal varices?

Disorders of the Exocrine Pancreas

The pancreas produces many enzymes necessary for the digestion of protein, fat, and carbohydrate. It also secretes a bicarbonate-rich juice that provides an optimal pH for activation of these enzymes. Consequently, disorders of the pancreas can have significant impact on absorption and nutrition status.

Fat malabsorption is the biggest concern in pancreatic disorders, because only the pancreas makes lipase, which is necessary for fat digestion. In contrast, the intestine can help somewhat with the digestion of protein and carbohydrate by secreting its own amylase, disaccharidases, and proteases. The two disorders of the pancreas discussed in this section, pancreatitis and cystic fibrosis, both lead to malabsorption. Before reading this section, you may wish to review the section on malabsorption in Chapter 22.

lipase: see p. 138.
amylase: see p. 174.
disaccharidase: see p. 138.
protease: see p. 138.

Pancreatitis

Pancreatitis is an inflammation of the pancreas that is most often caused by biliary tract disease, surgery (often of the stomach or biliary tract), or alcohol abuse. Exactly how these disorders cause pancreatitis is unknown. Blood vessels that supply the pancreas become more permeable and allow fluid and plasma proteins to leak into the space between the pancreatic cells. The result is localized

pancreatitis: inflammation of the pancreas.

People with acute pancreatitis are often in pain—one of the most severe kinds of pain known in any illness. The worst usually subsides in about two to three days. Try to do everything you can to ease your client through this difficult time. Obviously, it will help not to discuss food and diet, even though you want to be sure nutrition needs are met, until the person feels better.

Dietary guidelines in acute pancreatitis:
1. Initial treatment: IV fluids to maintain fluid and electrolyte balance and NG suction. No food by mouth. If severe, or if malnutrition is a problem, use TPN.
2. After pain stops and serum amylase levels fall, progress from a clear liquid diet to a low-fat diet to a regular diet as tolerated.

edema and damage to the pancreas. The damaged pancreas retains pancreatic secretions, including digestive enzymes, and these begin to digest the pancreas itself. The blood picks up some of these enzymes, causing serum amylase and lipase levels to rise. These elevated levels are indicators of pancreatitis.

If the edema compresses blood vessels, the oxygen supply to the cells can be cut off, resulting in cell death. Fat tissue near the pancreas can also die. If the enzymes destroy blood vessels, bleeding can occur.

Typical symptoms of pancreatitis are high serum amylase levels, severe abdominal pain, and oftentimes nausea and vomiting. The goal of therapy is to reduce the stimulation of pancreatic secretions. No food is given by mouth, since food stimulates bicarbonate and enzyme secretions from the pancreas. An NG tube is inserted, but not for feeding. Instead, the tube serves as a straw to suction out the stomach's contents; this further reduces stimulation of the pancreas.

Fluids and electrolytes are given intravenously to maintain normal balance. Edema, losses through NG suction, and the lack of oral food and fluid intake disrupt fluid and electrolyte balance. If pancreatitis is severe or if the person is malnourished, TPN may be indicated. Some studies suggest that TPN does not stimulate pancreatic secretions to the degree an enteral diet would, but results of experiments in this area are unclear.[7] People with milder forms of pancreatitis may benefit from tube feedings of hydrolyzed formulas, although no controlled studies can document the benefits of such feedings.[8]

A person who is free of abdominal pain, has active bowel sounds, and has normal or near-normal serum amylase levels can try an oral diet. Progress the diet from a clear liquid diet (see p. 000) to a low-fat diet (see p. 000) and, finally, a regular diet as tolerated. At the first sign of pain, or if serum amylase levels rise, food is withheld; when these signs and symptoms subside, food can be reintroduced. Six small meals may be better tolerated than larger, less frequent meals.

Sometimes an acute attack of pancreatitis doesn't subside, or reoccurs at frequent intervals. This condition describes chronic pancreatitis, most commonly caused by repeated alcohol abuse. Pancreatic tissue is destroyed and, like nerve tissue, cannot regenerate.

The pancreas normally excretes enzymes far in excess of needs, so even after extensive damage has occurred, digestion may still proceed normally. However, with chronic pancreatitis and extensive degeneration of the pancreas, digestion, especially of fat, is permanently impaired. A special diet is required. Diet therapy during active attacks is the same as already given. Between attacks, the client should follow a bland, low-fat diet.

The goals of diet therapy in chronic pancreatitis are to:

■ Maintain optimal nutrition status.
■ Reduce steatorrhea, if present.

Mrs. Corey is a 52-year-old homemaker admitted to the hospital with severe abdominal pain, nausea, and vomiting. Laboratory tests revealed a very high serum amylase level, a low serum albumin level, and red blood cell indexes consistent with folacin deficiency anemia. Mrs. Corey was diagnosed as having pancreatitis. Her height and weight are 5′3″ and 100 lb, respectively.

Mrs. Corey's family expressed concerns to the physician that Mrs. Corey may have a problem with alcohol abuse. The health care team is

CASE STUDY

Pancreatitis

concerned not only with the diagnosis of pancreatitis, but also with Mrs. Corey's nutrition status and possible alcohol abuse.

1. What is pancreatitis? Why are serum amylase levels elevated in people with pancreatitis? How can pancreatitis lead to poor nutrition status?

2. Discuss factors in Mrs. Corey's

medical history that put her at risk for poor nutrition status. For the purposes of this question, assume that Mrs. Corey is an alcohol abuser.

3. What is the treatment for the person with pancreatitis? Describe both the immediate care and the care after the acute attacks occur.

4. Would TPN or tube feedings be a possibility for Mrs. Corey? Why or why not?

5. If Mrs. Corey developed a problem with chronic pancreatitis, how would her diet be altered? What other measures would be taken to ensure adequate digestion and absorption?

- Minimize pain, if necessary.
- Avoid subsequent attacks of active pancreatitis.

A low-fat, bland diet is recommended. Small meals may be easiest to digest. The person with chronic pancreatitis usually tolerates about 50 to 70 grams of fat per day; restricting fat to less than this amount is unnecessary (see p. 724–725 for a description of a low-fat diet). Enzyme replacements taken with meals aid in the digestion and absorption of protein and fat. Absolutely no alcohol is permitted.

If steatorrhea persists, fat-soluble vitamins are given in supplement form. Vitamin B_{12} absorption may be reduced, so injections of vitamin B_{12} may be required. The person who needs extra kcalories may benefit from products containing MCT.

Pancreatitis also may damage the cells that produce insulin. In such cases, the individual with pancreatitis becomes glucose intolerant, as in diabetes, and must follow a diabetic diet in addition to the restrictions already mentioned (see Chapter 24).

Enzyme replacements are extracts of porcine or bovine pancreatic enzymes that help the person digest protein and fat.

Cystic Fibrosis

Cystic fibrosis (CF) is a hereditary disease that may affect many organs, including the pancreas, lungs, liver, heart, gallbladder, and small intestine. CF affects approximately 20,000 to 30,000 Americans.[9] It is estimated that one in every 20 people is a carrier; that is, approximately 10 million people have the potential to transmit the CF trait to their children. CF is the most common cause of pancreatic insufficiency in children and young adults. People with CF often have three major symptoms: pancreatic insufficiency, chronic lung disease, and abnormal electrolyte levels in the sweat. The pancreas is affected in 80 to 85 percent of people with CF. The airways of the lungs also become plugged with mucus, making it difficult for the person to breathe. Lung infections become likely and are the usual cause of death in CF.

cystic fibrosis: a hereditary disorder that affects many organs, including the pancreas, lungs, liver, heart, gallbladder, and small intestine; often abbreviated **CF.**

fibrous: composed of fibers. The development of excess fibrous tissue is **fibrosis.**

In the person with CF, the airways of the lungs become plugged with thick mucous secretions, which makes it difficult to breathe and increases the likelihood of pulmonary infections. Lung infections are the usual cause of death in CF.

Assessing nutrition status regularly is imperative for the child with CF.

CF is characterized by production of a thick mucus by glands throughout the body. The mucus obstructs the small pancreatic ducts and interferes with the secretion of digestive enzymes and pancreatic juices. Eventually, the enzyme- and bicarbonate-secreting cells are surrounded by the mucus and are gradually replaced by fibrous tissues. Malabsorption results, affecting many nutrients— fat, protein, vitamins, and minerals—and frequently leading to malnutrition. Many young people with CF are short and thin for their ages.

The energy needs of people with CF are about 150 percent of the RDA for their sex and age. Energy needs are high due to the loss of nutrients through malabsorption, frequent infections, and energy required simply to breathe. Children with CF often fail to meet even normal energy requirements, explaining why many of these children fail to grow to their potential.

A high-kcalorie, high-protein, fat-restricted diet that is nutritionally balanced and carefully tailored to the individual's tolerance is recommended. In the past, diets for people with CF were often severely restricted in fat. However, individuals generally know how much fat they can consume before uncomfortable GI symptoms occur. Furthermore, fat is an important source of kcalories and essential fatty acids. Essential fatty acid deficiences are well documented in children with CF. Therefore, the current trend is to prescribe a liberal fat intake for the person with CF who can tolerate it. For individuals who cannot tolerate fat, MCT oil can provide additional kcalories.

An important part of therapy is the use of enzyme replacements. Enzyme replacements help lessen malabsorption considerably, but they do not correct it completely. People who have persistent steatorrhea, gas, flatulence, and abdominal distension may need to have their dosages of enzyme replacements adjusted rather than their fat intakes reduced.[10]

Breastfeeding is recommended for the infant with CF, as it is for any infant. However, infants who are not breastfed can usually tolerate a regular infant formula taken with enzyme replacements. Additional kcalories can be added to the formulas by adding carbohydrate or fat supplements (see Appendix L).

As you read about CF, keep in mind that the person with this condition is usually a child. All of the concerns and suggestions discussed in Chapters 15 and 17 regarding children and how they can be encouraged to eat can be helpful in working with the child with CF.

Another consideration to keep in mind is that CF is a difficult disorder for both the client and the family. The person faces repeated hospitalizations and oftentimes an early death. The child's guardians must deal with many aspects of care important to the child's survival, only one of which is nutrition. The child and the caretakers need your support, encouragement, and advice.

Pay special attention to making the diet as nearly normal as possible. Consider for a moment the social implications of CF. In addition to a restricted diet, the child participates in physical therapy treatments daily, takes enzyme replacements with meals, and may need to take antibiotics to prevent or treat lung infections. An unnecessarily restrictive diet is a burden that will not yield desirable results.

Low-fat infant formulas are used for infants who cannot tolerate the fat of regular formulas. As the child is weaned from breast milk or infant formula, fat is restricted only if steatorrhea cannot be controlled by enzyme replacements.

The best way to ensure that people with CF are eating enough is to assess their nutrition status regularly, with particular attention to monitoring height and weight. Nutrition care plans can then be revised as necessary.

Vitamin supplements are usually given. The fat-soluble vitamins should preferably be given in a water-miscible form, which can be absorbed without fat. Zinc supplements may also be needed.

Maintenance of adequate nutrition status for the person with CF is extremely important; nutrition status and the severity of pulmonary disease appear to be related.[11] Several research centers are experimenting with home parenteral and enteral nutrition programs to help meet the higher nutrient needs imposed by CF.[12] Children eat a regular diet and are fed by tube or parenteral nutrition during the night to help augment nutrient intake. In one study of malnourished children with CF, weight gain was achieved in seven of eight people placed on supplemental tube feedings at night.[13] Although pulmonary function did not improve, there was a reduced incidence of pneumonia and improved feelings of well-being. Such programs are promising, although practical difficulties and demands on people with CF and their caretakers are problems.

Depletion of electrolytes (sodium and chloride) is another nutrition-related concern. Fever, high environmental temperature, or diarrhea can rapidly precipitate electrolyte depletion. During such times, provide the person with extra salt.

Recall that water-miscible fat-soluble vitamins readily mix with water and can be absorbed without fat (see p. 724).

Disorders of the Gallbladder

The gallbladder stores and concentrates the bile produced in the liver. Sometimes the gallbladder becomes inflamed (cholecystitis) or filled with stones (cholelithiasis). If a stone obstructs the outlet of the gallbladder, choledocholithiasis can result.

The symptoms associated with cholecystitis vary. Pain in the area of the gallbladder may occur gradually or suddenly and can be quite severe. Frequently, nausea, vomiting, and flatulence are present.

Many factors are involved in gallstone formation. Hereditary factors, gender (being female), obesity, and some drugs may predispose the individual toward developing gallstones. Diabetes, ileal disease or resection, and diet may also be implicated. Women are more likely to develop gallstones than men, but gallstones do occur in men, and the incidence increases in both sexes with aging.

Gallstones are of two general types: cholesterol gallstones and pigment gallstones. About 85 percent are of the cholesterol type, which form when the cholesterol in the bile gets too concentrated, either from excessive cholesterol synthesis or decreased bile synthesis. The cholesterol becomes insoluble in the bile and precipitates; as more and more cholesterol precipitates, stones form. Restricting cholesterol in the diet does not alter the course of cholesterol stone formation.

cholecystitis (KO-lee-sis-TIE-tis): inflammation of the gallbladder.
chole = bile

cholelithiasis (KO-lee-le-THIGH-ah-sis): stones in the gallbladder. When the stones obstruct the common bile duct leading to the intestine the condition is called **choledocholithiasis** (ko-LED-oh-ko-lee-THIGH-ah-sis).
litho = stone

Low-fat diets have traditionally been prescribed for people with gallbladder diseases. The rationale was that fat in the intestine causes the gallbladder to contract, which can cause pain. However, a recent study showed that the gallbladder contracts and ejects bile at the same rate after either a high- or a low-fat meal.[14]

The best advice for clients with gallbladder ailments seems to be not to avoid fat, necessarily, but to consume a well-balanced diet and avoid foods, or amounts of foods, that cause pain. Some people are truly intolerant to fat or to particular foods, and their diets should be adjusted accordingly. Obese people should be encouraged to lose weight, especially if surgery is being considered. A high-fiber diet is thought to help prevent gallstone formation, but more research is needed to confirm this possibility.

Oftentimes, people with gallstones must have their gallbladders removed (cholecystectomy). Following surgery, the same care as outlined in Chapter 20 for other people after surgery is given. When the person advances to an oral diet after surgery, fat is allowed as tolerated.

cholecystectomy (KO-lee-sis-TEK-toe-me): surgical removal of the gallbladder.
cyst = bladder
ectomy = removal

Nutrition Assessment

When you assess the nutrition status of people with disorders of the liver, pancreas, and gallbladder, keep several points in mind:

- People with diseases of the liver and pancreas (especially those who abuse alcohol) are often malnourished. Obtain an accurate diet history to calculate nutrient requirements and to pinpoint inadequate nutrient intake.

- People who abuse alcohol normally derive much of their daily kcaloric intake from alcohol. If that energy source is eliminated, as it is when the person is hospitalized, special care must be taken to ensure that energy needs are met through an adequate diet. Routinely reassess nutrition status to ensure that energy needs are met.

- When the pancreas or gallbladder is diseased, the diet history also offers the opportunity to estimate the person's tolerance for fat.

- The person with cirrhosis may retain considerable amounts of fluids. This will affect weight measurements and, if generalized edema is present, also arm anthropometrics and laboratory results. Under these circumstances, weight is not a useful indicator of body tissue gains and losses but can be monitored to see if the person is mobilizing fluids. Weight loss, then, is a good sign that some liver function is returning.

- Another strategy useful in people with ascites is to measure abdominal girth. Place a tape measure around the back and over the person's abdomen directly over the umbilicus. Repeat the measurement periodically. A decreasing abdominal girth indicates that fluid is being mobilized. If girth increases, the ascites is becoming worse.

- In people with extensive liver disease, serum albumin levels will be low. Supplying extra amino acids will not help if the liver doesn't function well enough to synthesize albumin. Serum albumin levels may also be low in people with pancreatitis. Usually, people with CF have normal albumin levels.

Attention to nutrition and nutrition assessment parameters is important to the recovery of people with disorders of the liver, exocrine pancreas, and gallbladder.

Notes

1. J. Smith and coauthors, Enteral hyperalimentation in undernourished patients with cirrhosis and ascites, *American Journal of Clinical Nutrition* 35 (1982): 56–72.

2. D. Rudman and coauthors, Ammonia content of foods, *American Journal of Clinical Nutrition* 26 (1973): 487–490.

3. F. L. Weber and coauthors, Effects of vegetable diets on nitrogen metabolism in cirrhotic subjects, *Gastroenterology* 89 (1985): 538–544.

4. B. J. Visocan, Nutritional management of alcoholism, *Journal of the American Dietetic Association* 83 (1983): 693–696.

5. D. R. Antonow and C. J. McClain, Nutritional support in alcoholic liver disease, *Journal of Parenteral and Enteral Nutrition* 9 (1985): 566–567.

6. M. L. Christie and coauthors, Enriched branched-chain amino acid formulas versus a casein-based supplement in the treatment of cirrhosis, *Journal of Parenteral and Enteral Nutrition* 9 (1985): 671–678.

7. D. F. Kirby and R. M. Craig, The value of intensive nutritional support in pancreatitis, *Journal of Parenteral and Enteral Nutrition* 9 (1985): 353–357.

8. Kirby and Craig, 1985.

9. *Cystic Fibrosis,* a pamphlet from the National Institute of Arthritis, Diabetes, Digestive, and Kidney Research Advances, publication no. (NIH) 81-1981 (Washington, D.C.: Government Printing Office, July 1981).

10. V. S. Hubbard and P. J. Mangrum, Energy intake and nutrition counseling in cystic fibrosis, *Journal of the American Dietetic Association* 80 (1982): 127–131.

11. L. A. Lester and coauthors, Supplemental parenteral nutrition in cystic fibrosis, *Journal of Parenteral and Enteral Nutrition* 10 (1985): 289–295.

12. L. D. Levy and coauthors, Effects of long-term nutritional rehabilitation and body composition and clinical status in malnourished children and adolescents with cystic fibrosis, *Journal of Pediatrics* 107 (1985): 225–230; A. L. Mansell and coauthors, Short-term pulmonary effects of total parenteral nutrition in children with cystic fibrosis, *Journal of Pediatrics* 104 (1984): 700–705; R. W. Shepherd and coauthors, Changes in body composition and muscle protein degeneration during nutritional supplementation in nutritionally growth retarded children with cystic fibrosis, *Journal of Pediatric Gastroenterology and Nutrition* 2 (1983): 439–446.

13. E. O'Loughlin and coauthors, Nutritional rehabilitation of malnourished patients with cystic fibrosis, *American Journal of Clinical Nutrition* 43 (1986): 732–737.

14. M. Mogadam and coauthors, Gallbladder dynamics in response to various meals: Is dietary fat restriction necessary in the management of gallstones? *American Journal of Gastroenterology* 79 (1984): 745–747.

Study Questions

1. What is fatty liver, and what causes it? What diet modifications, if any, are useful for the treatment of fatty liver?

2. What is hepatitis, and what nutrition concerns arise in the person suffering from hepatitis?

3. Discuss cirrhosis, and describe how cirrhosis leads to portal hypertension, ascites, formation of collaterals, esophageal varices, and elevated blood ammonia levels.

4. Describe the dietary treatment of the person with cirrhosis and hepatic coma. Consider special dietary concerns of the person with ascites and esophageal varices.

5. What is pancreatitis, and how can it lead to malabsorption of nutrients? Contrast the dietary treatment of a person with acute pancreatitis with the dietary treatment of a person with chronic pancreatitis.

6. What is cystic fibrosis? What are the nutrition needs of the child with CF?

7. How is the infant with CF fed? What is the optimal diet for the child and young adult with CF?

8. What drug therapy is necessary in the prevention of severe malabsorption in the person with CF? What signs and symptoms suggest that this drug therapy needs to be adjusted?

9. Discuss the role of nutrition in the prevention and treatment of gallbladder diseases.

Nutrition and Adaptation

You now have some understanding of the many metabolic reactions that take place in the human body, and of the impact nutrients have on these. We have just discussed disorders of the liver, an important organ in modulating adaptative responses to the changing internal environment. Now is a good time to learn what adaptation means and how it occurs.

Although you may not realize it, you have already learned a lot about nutrition and adaptation. In Chapter 20 you saw how the body adapts to stress and how nutrition impacts this response. In Chapters 21 through 23 you learned how diets are used to help the individual adapt to different disorders.

The term *adaptation* has some meaning to everyone. When you say that you have adapted to a situation, you mean that something inside you has changed so that you can handle the situation better. You might be astonished to learn how literally it is true that adapting means something inside you changes.

In nutrition, adaptation has specific meanings. Understanding these allows the health professional to provide care tailored to a client's needs. When we say, "He hasn't adapted to a standard diet yet; let's build up to it gradually," or "Before we attempt surgery on this person, we had better build her up nutritionally; she isn't equipped to withstand it at this point," we are speaking of physical realities.

Adaptation also explains otherwise incomprehensible everyday happenings. Why is it, for example, that a person can drink large amounts of alcohol on one occasion without getting drunk, while on another he can't? How is it that a woman can absorb 30 percent of the iron she ingests when she is pregnant or iron deficient, but only 10 percent when she is not? Why does a prescription drug work so much more powerfully in the body of a person who hasn't eaten for two days than in the same person when he is well fed?

Nutrition books often make vague statements about the state of the body. They comment that the body's response to stress, or to illness, or to medication, drugs, or nutrients depends on its nutrition, health, or physiologic status. These statements have specific meanings, and this highlight is intended to help you understand that meaning.

For any change to come about, the body's machinery—its proteins—has to be changed, and this can be brought about in two ways. First, the *rate* at which the proteins work can be either sped up or slowed down. Second, the *number* of working protein units can be increased or decreased. The first kind of change, the change in rate of action, makes possible quick responses to short-term needs. The second, the change in number of working protein units, brings about adjustments to longer-term, more gradual changes in demand.

The second kind of change is the subject of this highlight. Whenever a demand is placed on the body such that its ordinary responses (rate changes) are not enough to handle the situation, the body's physical equipment (number of protein molecules) needs to be altered.

In some ways, the body's machinery is similar to the workings in a factory. Of course, the equipment inside a cell is different in a major way from that in a factory. This difference makes the cell much more adaptable to changing circumstances. A factory is built of heavy, permanent equipment, which can turn out a specific number of products—say, cars—per day for as long as it is maintained and operated. Should demand increase, a major renovation would have to take place to enlarge the factory or build a new one. Should demand decrease, some of the equipment could be idled. In either case, however, a certain amount of inefficiency would be inevitable. The factory is inelastic; it is not prepared to shrink or to grow as a cell can. In a cell, the protein machinery is being replaced all the time anyway—every hour—and so to alter its nature or extent is not a demanding undertaking.

How does this replacement take place? Most of the body's machinery is composed of protein—enzymes, transport proteins, "pumps," membrane receptors, and the like. Each type of machinery is represented by a population of identical molecules, each with a certain life expectancy. At any point in time, some of its members are newly made and just beginning to work, others are established and hard at work, and still others are at the end of their useful lives and about to be dismantled and their parts recycled. The making and the taking apart balance so that the number of protein molecules present and working remains constant (see Figure H23−1). These rates may be fast (nine out of every ten protein molecules in the population may be replaced every hour) or slow (one out of every ten may be replaced in a month.)

The rate at which a cell replaces any particular set of proteins determines the *half-life* of the proteins—a term that characterizes the stability of their population size. Some proteins have a short half-life, others a long one. Under constant conditions, the difference between the two kinds is not obvious, but if a disturbance arises, the differing half-lives have a marked effect. For example, suppose protein synthesis suddenly shuts down (perhaps an essential amino acid is missing). The proteins with short half-lives will rapidly disappear from the cell, because they are still being rapidly degraded, whereas those with long half-lives will linger and continue to work, because their degradation is proceeding slowly.

The explanation just given has presented several concepts that biochemists usually express in technical terms. They speak not only of the *half-life* of proteins, but of the *rate of synthesis* and the *rate of degradation*. Using these terms, they devise precise mathematical formulas to quantitatively describe exactly what is going on within a cell or organ system. The description given here of the kinds of changes that take place in the body as it continuously adapts to its changing environmental circumstances is adequate for our purposes. The examples that follow enhance that understanding.

The Body Exposed to Alcohol

The first time a person drinks an alcoholic beverage, it may not be handled well. You may hear the comment that "it went straight to my head," as if there were no way for the body to get rid of the alcohol. However, on repeated drinking, a person finds it easier to tolerate alcohol. In the heavy drinker, a marked adaptation occurs that has an effect on many aspects of the person's health. Ordinarily, everyone possesses a certain number of alcohol-metabolizing

FIGURE H23–1.

Enzyme adaptation. The number of enzymes at work is normally constant (A), not because the same molecules are always there, but because new ones are appearing as fast as the old ones are disappearing. The number can be changed by changing the rate of synthesis (B and C) or by changing the rate of degradation (not shown).
A. Steady state. A constant number of enzymes is present in the cell because the rate of synthesis equals the rate of degradation.
B. The rate of synthesis has been slowed. Now there is a smaller, and declining, number of enzymes working in the cell.
C. The rate of synthesis has been sped up. Now there is a greater, and increasing, number of enzymes working in the cell.

Miniglossary

atrophy: see p. 91. Atrophy of an organ reflects a decreased rate of synthesis or an increased rate of degradation of enzymes and other proteins, cells parts, and even whole cells. See also *hypertrophy.*

degradation: breaking down. Enzymes may break things down, but enzymes and other proteins are also broken down themselves, normally at a constant rate that is characteristic for each protein. By changing the *rate of degradation* of a particular protein, the cell can change the total number of molecules of that protein that will be present at any given time.

half-life: the length of time it takes for half of a population (in this case, of protein molecules) to disappear after synthesis of new members has stopped. Under these circumstances, the half-life depends on the rate of degradation. The term *half-life* is a shorthand way of describing how fast a population of proteins can change in size.

hypertrophy: see p. 156. Hypertrophy of an organ reflects an increased rate of synthesis or a decreased rate of degradation of enzymes and other proteins, cell parts, and sometimes even whole cells. See also *atrophy.*

induction (of enzymes): the process by which an enzyme is made to appear in response to a need for it. A signal (perhaps a hormone, perhaps the substance the enzyme works on) arrives at the portion of DNA, or gene, that codes for that enzyme; the gene's information is copied into molecules of messenger RNA; and these are sent out to the cell's protein-making bodies (ribosomes), where the enzyme is made.

synthesis: making. Enzymes may synthesize substances, but they are also themselves synthesized. The synthesis of proteins proceeds at a rate that is characteristic for each protein. Alteration of the *rate of synthesis* of a particular protein can alter the number of molecules of that protein that are present in the cell.

enzymes in the liver—enough to metabolize about one drink's worth of alcohol every hour and a half. These enzymes are constantly being replaced. In response to repeated heavy drinking, the liver establishes and maintains a larger population of enzymes to metabolize alcohol. After many weeks, months, or years, the heavy drinker is able to handle alcohol almost twice as fast as the first time. This is an adaptive response, and in the sense that alcohol is toxic, it confers an advantage on the body. However, it has some consequences.

The liver's adaptation to alcohol affects its ability to handle certain drugs as well, because some of the alcohol-metabolizing enzymes also work on drugs. With all of these additional enzymes manufactured and inserted into its membranes, the liver can now metabolize *both* alcohol and drugs faster than the unadapted liver can. Now, when the physician prescribes a drug, it is metabolized and excreted from the body faster than the doctor might expect. You can see that a physician prescribing drugs for someone would have to be aware of that person's previous drug and alcohol use in order to prescribe correctly. (See Highlight 7B for more details on the liver's alcohol-metabolizing systems.) Perhaps you can generalize from this to see that many other aspects of the prior "chemical history" of a person will determine what the body is ready for, how much, and at what rate it can be, handled.

The Child with Advanced Protein Deficiency

In the last stages of kwashiorkor, when the disease has become severe, the digestive system shuts down, and the pancreas stops producing digestive enzymes. In this case, adaptation involves making *less* of something. This confers a survival advantage on the child, because energy and building blocks are thereby conserved to serve higher-priority purposes, such as maintaining the brain, heart, and lung tissues and their minimum vital functions. The making of less equipment for the GI tract and pancreas is reflected in the atrophy of those organs. They lose so much protein (and associated supporting lipid and other material) that they become physically smaller. The intestinal villi shrink, and the areas of the pancreas that produce digestive enzymes disappear.

When a child with kwashiorkor is brought to the hospital very near death, the health professional has to take care to restore normal feeding in stages. The child is not equipped—literally does not have the equipment—to digest food. The first choice is simple carbohydrates in small quantities, with only a very little protein—just enough nutrition to engage the available enzymatic machinery. If this little bit of nourishment can be digested, then the body will begin to adapt to eating protein again (make more digestive enzymes, using the newly supplied amino acids and energy). Then, more foods containing protein, and finally fat, can be given. The body will not produce fat-digesting enzymes and the proteins necessary for carrying fat until the many other proteins that are of higher priority for recovery have first been made.

Not all children with kwashiorkor can recover. In some cases, the process of degeneration has gone too far. In the early stages, the body has the resources to adapt, but they can be exhausted.

This example shows that, as far as possible, the body is directly responsive to the tasks it is given to do. The exact enzymes the pancrease produces in malnutrition at each stage have not been studied in the human being. Most likely they are exactly those required to take care of its needs most efficiently. In kwashiorkor, carbohydrate has been present in the diet, so the pancreas has probably maintained production of the enzyme amylase to digest it. Fat has not been present, so production of pancreatic lipase has probably been halted.

Providing kcalories in the usable form—as carbohydrate—lifts the constraints from the making of digestive enzymes. Providing just a little fat at first gives the signal for the pancreas to start making the lipase enzyme again. Step by step, nutritional therapy builds up to a normal diet. If too much is given too soon, the system would be overwhelmed, and the child might die. A diet manual might say, "Avoid whole milk during the first week, because fat is poorly tolerated at the start." However, the person reading with an understanding of enzyme adaptation might see deeply into this simple statement to the underlying reality: the enzymes aren't there at first. (They come back slowly, in response to being presented with the material they work on, a phenomenon biochemists call enzyme *induction*.)

The Person Fed Too Much Protein

In Chapter 5 you read about protein overload and the negative effects it can have on the body: animals fed high-protein diets experience hypertrophy of their livers and kidneys. The reason for this hypertrophy may be obvious after the examples of adaptation given previously. What should jump to mind is, that means proteins. The liver and kidneys must be making additional enzymes to manage all the additional amino acids that are flooding the system. In fact, amino acids are

metabolized in the liver. A large and active group of enzymes is necessary to perform this metabolism. Their presence is reflected in an enlarged liver. The kidneys have also enlarged because they have built additional nitrogen-excreting machinery.

The Vitamin C Megadoser

When a pregnant woman takes megadoses of vitamin C, her body adapts by accelerating its destruction and excretion of the vitamin. So too does the fetus's body. Both mother and fetus produce large amounts of a vitamin C–destroying enzyme. These adaptations are fine—until the baby is born. The baby now has an overdeveloped vitamin C–destroying machinery, but only a normal intake of the vitamin. The result is scurvy, the vitamin C–deficiency disease. The current intake is normal, but the infant's previous intake has brought about an abnormal state of apparent need. What was adaptive in the womb has proved maladaptive after birth. The baby's body will readjust, but it will take time—how long depends on the half-life of the proteins involved.

The High Consumer of Cholesterol

A person who consumes no cholesterol has to maintain enzymes to make it. The person who consumes just enough cholesterol to supply the body's needs maintains fewer cholesterol-making enzymes. And a person who eats excess cholesterol maintains few or no cholesterol-making enzymes; in fact, the liver has to produce enzymes that will destroy the cholesterol brought back from depots around the body, where it has been rejected for lack of need. Thus three apparently similar people with diverse diets may have quite different cellular machinery at work in their bodies. One makes enzymes to

manufacture cholesterol. The second makes few enzymes for either manufacturing or destroying cholesterol. The third makes enzymes to destroy it. (We are not talking here about the person who has inherited a defective gene for the cholesterol-destroying proteins and whose intake has to be carefully controlled.)

This is still another way in which adaptation takes place, and it should emphasize the point of this highlight. Any protein the body can make is a candidate for regulation. A protein can be made or degraded rapidly, slowly, or not at all. Normally, the steady state prevails—a comfortable rate of synthesis accompanied by a matching rate of degradation—but when circumstances change, the responses can be as finely orchestrated as a symphony.

Thus it is that whenever the health professional approaches a person with therapy—whether it be nutrition, drug, exercise, or whatever—it cannot be assumed that the body has a certain fixed set of characteristics. What that person did yesterday or last week or is accustomed to eating, drinking, smoking, breathing or doing, determines the protein equipment, which may be quite different from that of the person in the next bed in the same hospital room. The very number of molecules devoted to serving each of the body's multitude of purposes differs from one individual to the next. It is hoped that this highlight has made you understand these differences so that you have a deeper insight into what is meant by such vague phrases as those quoted at the start: *nutrition, health, and physiologic status*. Seeing the impact of nutrition status on present health will help equip you to practice wise diet therapy. You may even be persuaded that what you eat and drink today will affect your health tomorrow and in the months and years to come.

In contrast, NIDDM usually develops later i with obesity. In NIDDM, insulin secretion is n the cells of the peripheral tissues (muscle and fat Obesity intensifies the insulin resistance. Even enough insulin, it can't use it normally. Type II Type I diabetes, and it progresses more slowly.

There are other, less common classifications of have hyperglycemia without any symptoms of (dition was called *chemical diabetes,* but now it tolerance. Another classification, called *gestational* women who develop hyperglycemia while pregr childbirth. People who develop diabetes during st infection, or pregnancy) but who are normal a having a *previous abnormality of glucose tolerance.* Th closely to ensure that they do not develop diab *normality of glucose tolerance* is another classifica close monitoring; it includes people who have a developing diabetes. This group includes people diabetes and women who have given birth to babi Finally, diabetes can develop secondary to other and cystic fibrosis or through exposure to some (

What Happens in Diabetes?

Diabetes is introduced in Chapter 3 (p. 56–57) constancy of blood glucose level. The basic probl is unable to get into the cells. Instead, glucose bu in hyperglycemia. Normally, the kidneys retain g But when blood glucose levels get too high, the (glucosuria). Glucosuria generally occurs when bl milligrams per milliliter (see Figure 24–1).

People with uncontrolled diabetes also can bec the blood glucose concentration rises, an osmotic (from the cells into the blood. (Remember that w centrated to a more concentrated solution.) Furth the urine, water leaves with it (also an osmotic effec fluid and the extracellular fluid become depleted produces excessive urine (polyuria) and, being deh excessive thirst (polydipsia). Polyuria and polydip of diabetes.

Normally, insulin signals the body that it has activities that favor the storage of protein, carbol hances the uptake of amino acids, glucose, and fatty protein synthesis, glycogen synthesis in the liver ai The net effect is a reduction in blood glucose levels. presence of some insulin prevents energy stores from

When insufficient insulin is produced, or whei respond, they are deprived of the substrates they n and glucose may abound in the cells' fluid environm(access to them and therefore must mobilize their o\

Diabetes and Hypoglycemia

24

Contents

In diabetes, nerves, blood vessels, and kidney structures may all become disrupted. Shown here is one of the delicate structures in the kidney—a glomerulus (diagrammed in Figure 6–7, page 185). The coil of capillaries with blood cells within them (black) lies within the cup-shaped glomerulus (orange); surrounding kidney tissue is shown here as blue.

I

Ov
of the
with n
disord
to attri

Dial

diabetes mellitus (MELL-ih-tus or mell-
EYE-tus): a disorder of energy metabolism
caused by an absolute or relative
deficiency of insulin. (See pp. 56-57 for
additional definitions and introductory
remarks.)
mellitus = honey-sweet (sugar in
the urine)

Another type of diabetes caused by
inadequate secretion of antidiuretic
hormone is called **diabetes insipidus** (in-
SIP-i-dus). It is treated with medication.
insipid = without taste (no sugar in
the urine)

Diabet
diabete
of insul
    Dia
with di
diabetes
and nor
Togethe
diabetes
24–1.
    Gen
play son
93 perc
people)
cases.[1] I
The cell
take inst

TABLE 24—

Features

Other nar

Age of on
Associated
Insulin red
Insulin red

FIGURE 24–1

Overview of diabetes.

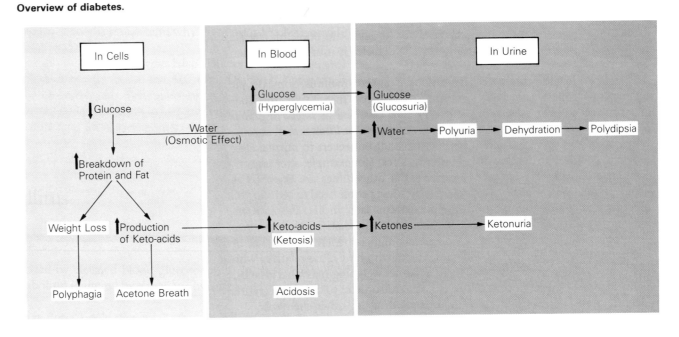

polyphagia (PAUL-ee-FAY-gee-ah):
excessive eating.

ketosis: the accumulation of excessive
ketone bodies in the blood (see p. 215).

acetone breath: a distinctive, fruity odor
that can be detected on the breath of a
person who is experiencing ketosis (see
p. 215).

ketonuria: the presence of ketone bodies
in the urine.

diabetic coma: a complication of
uncontrolled diabetes precipitated by
ketosis.

**hypersosmolar hyperglycemic
nonketotic coma:** a complication of
uncontrolled Type II diabetes precipitated
by the presence of hypertonic blood and
dehydration.

sources. The liver responds to the large amounts of fat being broken down by
making ketone bodies. These ketone bodies accumulate in the blood, compounding the problem of dehydration. The losses of both glucose and ketone
bodies (both energy substrates) in the urine and the breakdown of protein lead
to weight loss. This explains why the person with insulin-dependent diabetes
is likely to be thin, and may eat excessively (polyphagia). (As mentioned earlier,
people with Type II diabetes tend to be obese rather than thin. They overeat
because their cells, lacking energy fuels, are hungry. The insulin they do have
slowly takes effect, storing the excess energy they have consumed as fat.)

If Type I diabetes goes uncontrolled, excessive levels of ketones persist in
the blood (ketosis). The presence of one type of ketone (acetone) can be detected
by a fruity odor on the breath. The ketones are acidic; when they build up in
the blood, they cause the pH of the blood to be lowered. Ketones begin to
appear in the urine (ketonuria). In addition, sodium and potassium become
depleted because they are excreted along with the ketones. The loss of sodium
and potassium, both base formers, worsens the acidosis. When acidosis becomes
severe enough, a potentially fatal coma may follow.

People with Type II diabetes generally are not prone to ketosis, since they have
enough insulin to prevent the excessive buildup of keto-acids. However, they are
in danger of slipping into another kind of coma, hyperosmolar hyperglycemic nonketotic coma. As the name implies, this occurs when blood glucose concentrations
become excessive, resulting in osmotic diuresis and dehydration. Acidosis is not
present.

The metabolic aberrations seen in diabetes can be used to test people for
the presence of diabetes. These tests are described in the box entitled "Biochemical Tests for Diabetes Mellitus."

death in NI
to the limb
must be ar
amputation

Disordt
may also dt
85 percent
Diabetes is

Nerve
which can
Consequer
gress rapid
to them. T
and again

The spe
the goals c

- Mair
- Prevt
- Encc

Diet thera

- Help

The pe
without di
to minimi
complicati

No on
range can
mulating
no harm.

Treatii
Diabei

A diagnos
feel overw
is a comn
ready to p
should be
bring fear
followed.
must be
can be o
IDDM to

Biochemical Tests for Diabetes Mellitus

The diagnosis of diabetes mellitus can be made based on clinical symptoms and the plasma glucose level following an overnight fast. A plasma glucose concentration of greater than 140 mg/100 ml on more than one occasion, establishes a positive diagnosis.

Another method of diagnosing diabetes is the glucose tolerance test. The person follows a high-carbohydrate diet for at least three days before the test, and can not take medication, smoke cigarettes, or exercise during the test. Furthermore, the test may not be valid if the person is emotionally or physiologically stressed.

A glucose tolerance test works like this. First, blood is drawn (after an overnight fast) to obtain the fasting glucose level. The person is then given a measured amount of glucose to drink (in the form of a flavored beverage). Blood is taken again at regular intervals of 30 to 60 minutes (various clinics use different intervals). Table 24–2 lists the upper limits considered normal and the values suggestive of diabetes for each time interval. At least two of the glucose levels should exceed the latter values in order for diabetes to be diagnosed. A person whose glucose levels fall between the upper limits of normal and the values suggestive of diabetes is diagnosed as having impaired glucose tolerance.

Urine tests often provide the first clue that a person may have diabetes. Urine tests for sugar and ketones are often performed during routine examinations. Although positive tests for these substances do not always mean diabetes (for example, ketones may be present in people who are following low-carbohydrate diets or fasting), they suggest the need for blood tests. Urine is tested by dipping indicator paper into the urine sample. The paper changes color, and is then compared with a color chart to determine the approximate concentration of glucose. The results are read as percentages, designating how much glucose is present in the urine.

To use another method of urine testing, a tablet is dropped into the urine sample; the color of the urine is then compared with a color chart. People can check their urine at home using the methods taught by professionals at the hospital or clinic. This enables them to be sure their insulin and diet are appropriate, as well as to keep careful records to review at their next medical appointment.

Urine is checked before meals and at bedtime. The double-void method of urine collection is recommended by some practitioners, although its usefulness has been questioned.[2] (To use this method, the person voids once, voids again one-half hour later, and tests the second sample.) This method ensures that the glucose measurement does not reflect the concentration of urine stored in the bladder for a long time.

Direct monitoring of blood glucose levels at home may help some individuals maintain control of their glucose levels, and more and more people with diabetes are using this system. Blood testing is more sensitive than urine testing, because blood glucose levels must exceed 180 mg/100 ml before glucose spills into the urine. When used properly, home monitoring of blood glucose can help maintain blood glucose levels between

Carbohydrate:

$$2{,}200 \text{ kcal} \times 50\% = 1{,}100 \text{ kcal.} \quad 1{,}100 \text{ kcal} \div 4 \text{ kcal/g} = 275 \text{ g.}$$
$$2{,}200 \text{ kcal} \times 60\% = 1{,}320 \text{ kcal.} \quad 1{,}320 \text{ kcal} \div 4 \text{ kcal/g} = 330 \text{ g.}$$

Fat:

$$2{,}200 \text{ kcal} \times 38\% = \quad 836 \text{ kcal.} \quad \quad 836 \text{ kcal} \div 9 \text{ kcal/g} = 93 \text{ g.}$$

His diet should contain 66 to 110 g protein, 275 to 330 g carbohydrate, and a maximum of 93 g fat.

4. *Translate the diet prescription into a meal plan.* A day's exchanges for a sample 2,200-kcal diabetic diet is given in Table 24–4. Other diet patterns at different kcalorie levels are shown in Table 2–9, p. 43.

5. *Divide the kcalories and carbohydrate into tenths, and determine the distribution of the meals.* For example, let's say our client needs three meals and two snacks (one midmorning and one before bed). A typical distribution might go like this:

$$2{,}200 \text{ kcal} \div 10 = 220 \text{ kcal.}$$
$$281 \text{ g carbohydrate} \div 10 = 28 \text{ g carbohydrate.}$$

Table 24–5 gives an example of how this works out in the daily meal plan in which the distribution of kcalories and carboydrate is to be 2/10, 2/10, 3/10, 3/10, and 1/10.

kCalories from fat should be derived equally from monounsaturated, polyunsaturated, and saturated sources (see Chapters 4 and 25), which may help protect against atherosclerosis (see Highlight 4B). Encourage the use of low-fat and nonfat milks, lean meats, and polyunsaturated margarines to meet this objective.

In Type I diabetes, the timing and composition of meals and snacks must be consistent from day to day, and they must be eaten at about the same time each day. Better blood glucose control can sometimes be maintained by eating

pruritus
vye): se\
genitalia
pruritus
vulva =

TABLE 24–4

A Day's Exchanges for a Sample 2,200-kCalorie Diabetic Diet

Exchange Group	Number of Exchanges	Carbohydrate (g)	Protein (g)	Fat (g)
Starch/bread	11	165	33	trace
Meat, lean	6	—	42	18
Meat, medium-fat	1	—	7	5
Vegetable	3	15	6	—
Fruit	5	75	—	—
Milk, nonfat	2	24	16	trace
Fat	7	—	—	35
Total		279	104	58

TABLE 24–5

Distribution of Energy and Carbohydrate in a Sample Diabetic Diet

	Breakfast (2/10)	Midmorning Snack (1/10)	Lunch (3/10)	Supper (3/10)	Bedtime Snack (1/10)	Total
Energy (kcal)	440	220	660	660	220	2,200
Carbohydrate (g)	56	28	84	84	28	280

These figures are approximations. Chances are that you will not be able to divide meals so that the kcalories and carbohydrate are distributed exactly as you would wish. (See the sample 2,200-kcal diabetic diet menu.)

Sample 2,200 kcal diabetic diet menu.

Breakfast
  1 soft-cooked egg
  ½ c oatmeal
  1 slice whole-wheat toast
  1 tsp margarine
  1 banana
  kcal: 445—CHO: 60 g

Midmorning Snack
  ½ c orange juice
  6 saltine crackers
  ¼ c cottage cheese
  kcal: 195—CHO: 30 g

Lunch
  Ham sandwich with 2 oz boiled ham
    and 2 tsp mayonnaise
  ¼ c baked beans
  Marinated broccoli/tomato salad
  1 small apple
  1 c nonfat milk
  kcal: 685—CHO: 82 g

Supper
  3 oz chicken
  ⅔ c sweet potatoes
  1 tsp margarine
  Salad
  2 tsp salad dressing
  2 whole-wheat rolls
  ⅓ cantaloupe
  Iced tea
  kcal: 660—CHO: 80 g

Bedtime Snack
  1 c nonfat milk
  3 c popcorn
    with 1 tsp margarine
  kcal: 215—CHO: 27 g

CHO = carbohydrate

small meals with two or three snacks. Carbohydrates need to be eaten at every meal and snack, roughly in proportion to total kcalories. Each meal usually contains from 20 to 40 percent of the total kcalories and carbohydrate, and each snack, about 10 percent. The distribution often consists of three meals, a bedtime snack, and sometimes a midafternoon or midmorning snack, depending on the individual's blood glucose levels and insulin schedule. (See Table 24–5 and the sample menu for examples.)

As mentioned, the diet for the person with diabetes is based on the exchange system. Food is divided into groups based on contents of kcalories, carbohydrate, protein, fat, and other nutrients. The person with diabetes learns that foods on any one list can be "exchanged" freely for one another. However, foods from one list cannot be exchanged for foods on another list. Appendix G provides details of the exchange lists.

As discussed previously, the use of CSII systems for delivering insulin could change diet therapy remarkably for people with Type I diabetes. Research regarding the effects of the currently used systems is sorely lacking. Researchers investigating dietary practices of people with diabetes found that control of blood glucose was significantly better in people on insulin pump therapy.[6] However, these individuals also experienced a significant weight gain. These findings

In the past, people with diabetes were often advised to weigh their foods on gram scales so that portion sizes would be exact. This is called a **weighed diet.** It is no longer considered necessary to weigh foods. Instead, foods can be measured with common household measuring utensils. This is referred to as a **measured diet.**

The exchange lists were devised to permit people with diabetes to choose from a wide selection of normal foods and yet stay within a diet plan. They work so well that they have been adopted for many other uses—for example, they are used extensively for weight reduction and fat-controlled diets (see Chapters 8 and 25). Exchange lists can be used to calculate the nutrient composition of any person's diet. It is well worth the time and energy to become familiar with the energy, protein, carbohydrate, and fat content and the foods included on each list.

Exchange lists can be used to tailor a diet to an individual's preferences. However, many dietitians and other practitioners use standard exchange patterns that have already been calculated. Chapter 2 and Table 24–4 contain examples of different diet plans, or standard patterns. The patterns provide such a healthful balance of energy nutrients, and the lists offer such a variety of wholesome foods to choose from, that many authorities believe the diabetic diet is the healthiest diet anyone can follow. This is comforting news to people with diabetes, who can share their diets with their families to everyone's benefit.

Standard patterns do save time, but they should always be adjusted to the individual. For example, the planner can substitute one bread exchange (80 kcalories, 15 grams of carbohydrate) for 1 1/2 fruit exchanges (90 kcalories, 15 grams of carbohydrate). If the client doesn't drink milk (90 kcalories, 12 grams of carbohydrate), the planner can substitute ½ serving of bread and 1 ounce of lean meat (95 kcalories, 8 grams of carbohydrate). The most important thing is to adjust the diet to the client's preferences to help ensure diet compliance.

suggest that dietary education is necessary for pump users. The need for future studies in this area is apparent.

Exercise, Delayed Meals, and Illness

During periods of unusually intense exercise, the person with Type I diabetes will need more food, since exercise has an insulinlike effect. Some physicians recommend a reduction in the insulin dose. This is in addition to, or occasionally, instead of, taking additional foods. People with diabetes are advised to monitor their blood glucose before, during, and after strenuous exercise to make sure they do not become hypoglycemic.[7] As a general guideline, about 10 to 15 grams of additional carbohydrate should be given before exercise of moderate intensity. Allow about 20 to 30 grams of carbohydrate for vigorous activity.[8]

The person with Type I diabetes, like all people, occasionally misses a meal. When this happens, some carbohydrate should be taken to protect against hypoglycemia. Usually 15 to 30 grams of carbohydrate will forestall hypoglycemia for one to two hours.

The person with IDDM who is in the hospital may also have problems with missing meals. The person may be NPO for tests, following surgery, or if GI problems prevent food intake. Standard procedures for dealing with this prob-

6 saltine crackers = 15 g carbohydrate.

lem vary with each hospital. One method is to replace at least half the prescribed carbohydrate and kcalories within three hours after the missed meal. If this cannot be done, the physician is notified and may decide that some other measure is necessary (changing the insulin schedule or giving IV dextrose). Sometimes diet prescriptions are changed so that more simple carbohydrates (which are easy to eat or drink) are included.

Concentrated carbohydrates also may be allowed when the person with diabetes has a poor appetite because of illness. Soft drinks are often given. The main concern is to prevent starvation and vomiting. During stress, however, it may be desirable to reduce intake somewhat, because insulin requirements are high during stress. Reducing total kcalorie and carbohydrate intake helps limit the need for extra insulin.

A source of sugar sometimes overlooked is certain drugs. The person with diabetes should be warned that both OTC and prescription drugs may contain sugar. Members of the health care team, too, should be alert to this possibility.

People with diabetes can receive central TPN or commercial tube feedings that contain considerable amounts of simple sugars. However, extra care must be taken in monitoring people with diabetes so that insulin dosage can be adjusted to meet the higher simple carbohydrate loads. Some people are unable to tolerate the higher levels of carbohydrate in TPN even when additional insulin is given. In these people, the concentration of glucose may have to be reduced and additional kcalories provided by IV fat emulsions (see Chapter 18). For those who cannot tolerate simple carbohydrates from tube feedings, blenderized feedings that do not contain simple sugars can be devised.

Alcohol and Dietetic Foods

A question commonly asked by the person with diabetes is, Can I have alcohol? The person whose blood glucose is well controlled can usually include some alcohol with the consent of the physician. Alcohol can cause hypoglycemia in any person; therefore, the person with diabetes, who is susceptible to hypoglycemia anyway, must be especially careful. Recommend that the person use it only in small quantities and with, or shortly before or after, meals. Remember that hypoglycemia may be overlooked if the person appears to be intoxicated.

Furthermore, alcohol's low nutrient density requires that it be consumed on a limited basis. kCalories from alcohol must be calculated into the daily allowance. Fat kcalories are most often traded for alcohol kcalories. Drinks that contain carbohydrate (drinks made with mixers, sweet wines, and liqueurs) are best avoided. If used, their carbohydrate content must be considered in the diet calculation. Whiskey, gin, vodka, and rum do not contain carbohydrate.

The combination of alcohol and oral hypoglycemic agents may cause flushing of the skin and a rapid heartbeat. Forewarn clients of this possible reaction.

Another common concern of people with diabetes is how to replace sugar, and foods that contain sugar, in the diet. In general, special "dietetic" foods are not necessary. Oftentimes *dietetic* is misinterpreted to mean "no kcalories," but this is not necessarily the case. Some dietetic foods may be low in sodium instead of sugar, or they may have a reduced, but still significant, number of kcalories.

Some dietetic foods may be helpful. These include artificially sweetened soft drinks, artificial sweeteners, and water-packed canned fruits. kCalorie-free soft drinks and beverages (such as artificially sweetened tea) can be used freely and

Sweeteners that are used to take the place of sugar (sucrose) are called **alternative sweeteners. Nonnutritive sweeteners** (aspartame and saccharin) do not contain appreciable kcalories; they are also called **artificial sweeteners. Nutritive sweeteners** (fructose, sorbitol, and xylitol) contain the same number of kcalories as an equivalent amount of sugar.

Some dietetic foods may be helpful.

are often well liked. Artificial sweeteners that do not contain significant kcalories can help make the diet more acceptable. More information about alternative and artificial sweeteners is provided in Chapters 3 and 13.

Special Concerns for the Child with Diabetes

The overall approach to diabetes is the same throughout life, but special problems may become apparent at different stages. Consider some of the problems of the child with diabetes. Growth is sporadic, and it is difficult to predict how many kcalories a child will need at any one point in time. Appetite and activity also vary widely from day to day. A child may be quite active after school when the sun is shining but may be planted in front of the television on a rainy day.

For these reasons, a flexible diet is frequently recommended for the child with diabetes. This is not to say that the diet is unrestricted, however. Meals must be balanced and provide a wide variety of foods. Concentrated sweets are only given at times of vigorous physical activity or to treat hypoglycemia. The child is not forced to finish a meal, but meals should not be skipped, since hypoglycemia can result. If the child finishes a meal and wants more, seconds can be provided. Plan meals for approximately the same time each day, and serve the child the same foods as the rest of the family. Snacks are usually provided two or three times a day.

A particular concern of parents is that their child with diabetes may develop hypoglycemia during the night, which thus would go unrecognized. Snacks before bedtime may be helpful, especially if the child engages in strenuous activity late in the day. Glucose levels can be monitored before bedtime (especially in the newly diagnosed child) to help parents protect against hypoglycemia during the night.

All children frequently develop infections of the GI and respiratory tracts, and the child with diabetes is no exception. Anorexia, vomiting, or both often accompany these infections. For the child with diabetes, care must be taken to prevent hypoglycemia, which can easily occur under these conditions. The principles outlined earlier for illness apply here; hospitalization may be required if a child is unable to maintain adequate glucose levels.

A child's activity varies from day to day. A flexible diet is recommended.

Hypoglycemia that develops during the night is called **nocturnal hypoglycemia**. It is dangerous, because it can go unrecognized in the sleeping person. Adults as well as children can develop nocturnal hypoglycemia.

Treating the Person with Non-Insulin Dependent Diabetes Mellitus

In many ways, the treatment of NIDDM is the same as that of IDDM. The main goals of therapy are the same. Because Type II diabetes results from a resistance to insulin rather than from lack of insulin, there are some important

K athy, a 12-year-old girl, and her parents became worried when she began losing weight, urinating excessively, and always complaining of thirst. She was diagnosed with Type I diabetes about a year ago. Kathy's grandfather also has diabetes. Recently, Kathy was admitted to the emergency room. She complained of nausea, vomiting, and intense thirst. The physician noted that Kathy was confused and breathing hard, and could smell acetone on her breath. Urine tests were positive for glycosuria and ketonuria, and the blood glucose level was 400 mg/100 ml. The diagnosis was diabetic ketoacidosis. Kathy is 5 ft tall and weighs 75 lb.

CASE STUDY

Type I Diabetes

1. Explain the appearance of the symptoms that eventually led to the initial diagnosis of diabetes.
2. How does diabetes lead to ketoacidosis? Were Kathy's physical symptoms and laboratory tests consistent with this diagnosis? How would the ketoacidosis be managed? How can you distinguish between diabetic ketoacidosis and insulin shock?

3. When Kathy recovers, what information will she need in or prevent future incidents of ketoა What dietary advice would you want to reinforce?
4. Assume that Kathy has never been instructed on a diabetic diet. What dietary modifications are important for her to follow?
5. Think about and discuss the influence of Kathy's age on her outlook and ability to cope with diabetes. What problems does her age pose? Consider some ways you might help her deal with these problems.
6. Discuss the possible role of diet in preventing the vascular complications of diabetes.

differences. People with Type II diabetes can frequently control their blood glucose levels by diet alone. In other cases, drugs are given in addition to diet to maintain acceptable blood glucose levels.

The Diet in NIDDM

The primary goal of diet therapy in NIDDM is weight reduction, if it is necessary—and the majority of people with NIDDM are obese. Glucose tolerance may show marked improvement with weight loss. Therefore, weight loss should begin immediately. Investigators report that the blood glucose response to diet therapy in Type II diabetes of long duration (more than five years) is significantly poorer than in Type II diabetes of short duration (two years or less). This difference is noted despite a similar degree of weight loss and duration of diet therapy in the two groups.[9]

In some centers, obese individuals with diabetes who have severe hyperglycemia are initially prescribed fasts or follow diets very low in kcalories (600 kcalories per day) until blood glucose levels are under control. These individuals must be carefully monitored and such a diet should not be continued for long. Weight reduction diets higher in kcalories (1,200 kcalories per day) may then be given until the desired weight is reached.

A moderate exercise program is helpful in many cases. Exercise also helps improve blood glucose control, glucose tolerance, and insulin action in NIDDM.[10] It is widely believed that 80 to 90 percent of all people with NIDDM who are overweight can achieve metabolic control if they follow a low-kcalorie diet combined with an exercise program of moderate intensity.[11]

The timing and distribution of meals for the person with Type II diabetes is not critical, provided that concentrated sweets are avoided and that the total number of kcalories is consistent with the diet plan. Usually, only three meals a day are recommended. This helps prevent excessive snacking and possible

TABLE 24–6

Comparisons of Type I and Type II Diabetic Diets*

Diet Approach	Type I	Type II
Reduce kcalories	Usually not necessary	Yes
Keep ratio of carbohydrate, protein, and fat consistent for each feeding	Yes	No
Eat meals at regular times	Yes	Not necessary
Eat more frequent meals	Yes	No
Use food to treat or prevent hypoglycemia	Yes	No
Replace carbohydrate when appetite is poor or meals are missed	Yes	No
Eat extra food for intense exercise	Yes	No

*Philosophies vary. Not every diet therapist would follow these guidelines in every case.

weight gain. Table 24–6 compares the key components of diet therapy in Type I and Type II diabetes.

The exchange list system provides the basis for the diet in Type II diabetes. If the person is already at ideal weight, a diet excluding concentrated sweets may be recommended. Table 24–7 lists the foods that should be avoided on such a diet.

Oral Hypoglycemic Agents

Some people with Type II diabetes are unable to adequately control their blood glucose levels by diet alone. When control is inadequate because of stress, failure to lose weight, or other factors, oral hypoglycemic agents are often prescribed.

Two groups of oral hypoglycemic agents —the biguanides and the sulfon-ylureas—have been used in the treatment of NIDDM. The biguanides have undesirable side effects and were removed from the market in the United States in 1977. However, they are still used on a limited basis in some countries. No one knows exactly how the sulfonylureas work, although part of their effect is to stimulate the release of insulin from the pancreas.

oral hypoglycemic agents: drugs that can be taken by mouth to lower blood glucose levels. These drugs are ineffective in IDDM.

TABLE 24–7

Foods Avoided on a Diet That Excludes Concentrated Sweets

Cakes	Fruit ices	Milkshakes
Candy	Fruit juices, sweetened	Molasses
Cookies	Gelatin, sweetened	Pastries
Cranberry sauce	Honey	Pies
Doughnuts	Ice cream	Popsicles
Frappés	Jam	Pudding
Frosting	Jelly	Sweet rolls
Fruits, canned, glazed, frozen or cooked with sugar	Marmalade	Sugar
	Milk, chocolate or condensed	Syrup
Fruit drinks		Vegetables, glazed

Mr. Evans was 52 years old when he was first diagnosed with Type II diabetes. He visited his physician after experiencing symptoms of excessive thirst, excessive urination, and excessive appetite. Mr. Evans, who stands 5'11" tall, currently weighs 200 lb. He experienced a 30-lb weight gain over the past 2 years. His fasting blood glucose is 235 mg/dl. The health care team has evaluated Mr. Evans's case, and has decided that the first goal is to bring his blood glucose levels under control. Mr. Evans will begin a one week fast to bring his blood glucose levels down rapidly. The dietitian has provided instructions and tips to help Mr. Evans stay on the fast. The

CASE STUDY

Type II Diabetes

physician and nurse also reinforce the concepts of the fast with him. Mr. Evans is now ready to begin eating again. He is worried about his health, and overwhelmed with all the information he has been given over the past few weeks.

1. How does Type II diabetes differ from Type I diabetes? Which of the two types of diabetes is more prevalent? What factors in Mr. Evans's history might have predisposed him to Type II diabetes?

2. What will be the primary objective of the diet therapy for Mr. Evans? Determine Mr. Evans's ideal body weight, and plan a diet for him. (Use the information in the box entitled, "How to Plan a Diabetic Diet Using Exchange Lists.") What was the rationale for using a fast initially? What other measure might help Mr. Evans bring his blood glucose under control?

3. Can Type II diabetes usually be controlled by diet alone? What alternative treatments are available for the treatment of Type II diabetes?

4. Consider Mr. Evans's emotional state of health. How can the health care team help Mr. Evans during this difficult period?

The use of oral hypoglycemic agents is controversial because of the findings of the University Group Diabetes Program (UGDP) study. This study, conducted by competent professionals over an eight-year period, found that tolbutamide (one type of sulfonylurea) is associated with a significant increase in deaths from heart attacks. However, much criticism surrounds the way the study was conducted. Some physicians refuse to prescribe oral hypoglycemics; if their clients' blood glucose levels cannot be controlled by diet alone, insulin is used. Others try oral hypoglycemics in Type II diabetes when diet therapy alone fails. However, there is agreement that oral hypoglycemics do not replace diet therapy. The diet is continued, even when these drugs are used.

Treating the Pregnant Woman with Diabetes

Diabetes during pregnancy poses special concerns for both the mother and infant. The woman may experience episodes of severe hypoglycemia or hyperglycemia. Hypertension, preeclampsia, and toxemia are prevalent in pregnant women with diabetes. Infants of women who have diabetes may be large at birth, and may develop severe hypoglycemia (which can be fatal). There is also a high incidence of respiratory distress and congenital abnormalities. Perinatal mortality in infants born of pregnant women with diabetes is more than 200 deaths per 1,000 births.[12]

Pregnancy in all women is associated with insulin resistance and elevated blood insulin levels. Insulin levels begin to rise soon after conception, although

Infants with bodies that are large for their gestational age are said to have **macrosomia** (mac-row-SO-me-ah).
macro = large
soma = body

respiratory distress: a disorder of the lung membranes that results in delayed onset of respiration at birth and difficulty in breathing after birth.

perinatal (PERR-ee-NAY-tal): before, during, or shortly after birth.
peri = around
natal = birth

The hormones that antagonize the action of insulin during late pregnancy are placental lactogen, cortisol, prolactin, and progesterone.

during this period, insulin resistance is not a problem. This change in early pregnancy makes sense. Increased insulin promotes increased storage of energy nutrients to provide for the developing fetus. Later in pregnancy, the picture changes. Although insulin levels continue to remain high, the tissues become insulin resistant. Hormones that act antagonistically to insulin reach higher levels. This shift in late pregnancy signals the body to stop storing energy fuels and provides for the fetus to extract energy nutrients rapidly during the mother's fasting.

You can see why these changes can have serious metabolic effects for the woman with diabetes who is pregnant. For the woman with IDDM, insulin dosages must be monitored and adjusted regularly. Hypoglycemia may occur early in pregnancy because of transfer of glucose to the fetus, vomiting, or reduced food intake resulting from nausea. Often, however, insulin dosage must be increased. If hypoglycemia occurs, insulin dosages may be reduced temporarily.

In the last half of pregnancy, insulin requirements increase. The nutrient needs of the pregnant woman with diabetes are the same as those of any other pregnant woman, and the diet is planned accordingly, using the exchange lists. However, the diet should always contain a bedtime snack, for two reasons. For one, it prevents episodes of hypoglycemia that may occur in the early morning. For another, it provides a source of fuel for the developing fetus and prevents the buildup of ketones.

For the pregnant woman with NIDDM, diet is the cornerstone of therapy. Oral hypoglycemic agents are occasionally given, although insulin may be needed in some cases. When oral hypoglycemic agents are used, they are discontinued late in pregnancy and replaced with insulin, because their use is associated with hypoglycemia in the newborn infant.

Gestational diabetes (as mentioned earlier) is the type of diabetes that develops during pregnancy, usually in the later part of gestation when the tissues become insulin resistant. An increased concern for this type of diabetes has arisen because of the frequency with which it occurs. Gestational diabetes may be seen in up to 3 percent of all pregnancies in the United States.[13] The management of gestational diabetes is the same as for the woman with NIDDM.

Blood glucose monitoring is recommended for all pregnant women with any type of diabetes. Careful attention to blood glucose control is essential. In addition to blood glucose monitoring, pregnant women may also monitor urine ketone levels. Ketosis in early pregnancy is associated with congenital malformations, and possibly central nervous system disorders and lower intelligence quotients in the offspring.

Education for the Person with Diabetes

The team approach is most beneficial for educating the person with diabetes. A combination of group and individual counseling can help reinforce education objectives, as well as provide a forum for clients to discuss their concerns and

A typical occurrence in the hospital is this. The dietitian is paged to instruct a person on a diabetic diet. There sits the person, suitcase packed, anxiously waiting to go home. Generally, this dietitian will never see the person again.

The diabetic diet instruction has little chance of success when given under these circumstances. The person is concerned with getting home and may not be able to concentrate. Even if the client is patiently attentive, one counseling session is inadequate for teaching this diet.

How can this situation be prevented? Usually, physicians are responsible for ordering diet instuctions. If they fail to do so, remind them that a person hasn't been instructed yet. The diet advisor should be aware of people on special diets, instruct them throughout their hospitalization, and follow through either with home visits or with referrals to agencies or individuals that can provide continued help.

share ideas with others who have similar medical problems. Education of the person with diabetes must include:

- Diet instruction.
- Instruction in the use of insulin or oral hypoglycemic agents, if necessary.
- Instruction regarding changes in diet and insulin to accomodate exercise or stress.
- Instruction in the complications of diabetes and their prevention and treatment.

As you can see, the person with diabetes has a lot to learn. The teaching and learning process will take time; a person just getting over the shock of being told the diagnosis is diabetes may find all this new information difficult to grasp and accept.

Always plan and adjust therapy with the person's lifestyle in mind. Encourage the client to be active in the planning process. Regularly reassess the person's understanding of the treatment plan. Involve not only the person with diabetes, but also those the person lives with, in the learning process. The best adjustment may occur if the whole family attends live-in training sessions for a week. In the case of a child, a summer camp especially for children with diabetes offers the chance to "live" the lifestyle under supervision.

Hypoglycemia

Like diabetes, hypoglycemia is an imbalance in glucose homeostasis. The two major types of hypoglycemia are fasting and postprandial hypoglycemia. Their major distinguishing characteristics are shown in Table 24–8. Chapter 3 (pp. 54–56) provides important information on hypoglycemia, including its diag-

TABLE 24–8

Characteristics of Fasting and Postprandial Hypoglycemia

	Fasting	Postprandial
Onset of symptoms	Gradual; occurs after fasting	Sudden; occurs 2 to 5 hours after meals
Type of symptoms	Headache, mental dullness, fatigue, confusion, amnesia, seizures, unconsciousness	Anxiety, irritability, sweating, intense heartbeat, hunger, trembling
Duration of symptoms	Persistent	Transient
Possible causes	Hormonal imbalance, drugs, tumors	Early Type II diabetes, gastric surgery, TPN
Clinical course	Can be serious; treat underlying problems	Less serious; treat with diet
Other names	—	Alimentary, reactive, idiopathic, functional

nosis and development. We have also discussed some causes of hypoglycemia in the clinical setting—for example, in the person who has dumping syndrome after gastric surgery or when central TPN solutions are discontinued too quickly. Postprandial hypoglycemia also occurs in some inborn metabolic disorders and sometimes in early Type II diabetes.

In true postprandial hypoglycemia, diet is the mainstay of therapy. The diet is similar to the diabetic diet, and the exchange lists are often used for instruction. The person is advised to avoid all concentrated sweets and to eat four to six small meals a day. kCalories appropriate to achieve or maintain IBW are given. A recent survey of teaching hospitals found that 83 percent of the respondents use either a low-carbohydrate or a moderately restricted carbohydrate diet for people with hypoglycemia, even though the value of this restriction is disputed.[14] Alcohol is omitted or restricted if the person tolerates it poorly.

Nutrition Assessment

A main concern in the nutrition assessment of the person just diagnosed as having diabetes is the accurate assessment of appropriate weight. This is the basis for calculating the total kcalories in the diet. On reassessment, kcalories may need to be readjusted frequently, particularly in the young person who is growing.

Spend as much time as you can in obtaining an accurate diet history from the person with diabetes. This step is instrumental in planning an acceptable diet, as well as noting possible nutrient deficiencies. During reassessment, the diet history is useful to monitor compliance with the treatment plan. In the person with Type I diabetes, the history is important for assessing the individual's knowledge of how to adjust the diet for unusually strenuous exercise, missed meals, or illness, as well as how to prevent or treat hypoglycemia.

Arm anthropometrics may be difficult to obtain and interpret in some people with Type I diabetes. This is true when the midarm area has hypertrophied from repeated insulin injections. Fat measurements can be made using other areas of the body in these cases.

Study Questions

1. What are the two major types of diabetes? What type is more common? Describe some differences between the two types.
2. Describe the basic problem in diabetes, and tell how it leads to these symptoms: hyperglycemia, glucosuria, dehydration, polyuria, polydipsia, weight loss, polyphagia, acetone breath, ketosis, and ketonuria.
3. What is hyperosmolar hyperglycemic nonketotic coma? How is it different from the coma that can be caused by severe hyperglycemia in the person with Type I diabetes?
4. What biochemical tests are used to diagnose diabetes? What methods can the person with diabetes use to monitor glucose levels? What is glycosylated hemoglobin, and what advantage is there in measuring it in the blood?
5. What types of complications can arise as a result of diabetes?
6. What are the goals of therapy for all people with diabetes? Describe the three components that must be coordinated for the person with Type I diabetes?
7. What two types of insulin requirements do our bodies have, and how is commercially available insulin given to simulate these requirements? Why is insulin not taken orally? Describe the advantage of continuous subcutaneous insulin infusion (CSII).
8. What is the recommended distribution of nutrients for the diet in the treatment of Type I diabetes? What types of carbohydrates are recommended in the diet? What type of fat is recommended?
9. Why are the timing and composition of meals important considerations in planning a diet for a person with Type I diabetes? How is the carbohydrate content of the diet adjusted for exercise? How is the diet adjusted if meals are skipped?
10. Describe some general guidelines for the use of alcohol in the diabetic diet. Are dietetic foods always allowed? Why or why not?
11. Consider some of the special needs of children who have diabetes. How is the diet adjusted to meet these needs? What measures can be taken to safeguard against nocturnal hypoglycemia?
12. What is the primary goal of diet therapy in the person with Type II diabetes? How does diet therapy for Type I diabetes differ from Type II diabetes?
13. What events occur in all pregnancies that may interfere with the control of blood glucose levels in the woman with diabetes who is pregnant? How is the pregnant woman with Type I diabetes managed? How is the pregnant woman with Type II diabetes managed?
14. What is gestational diabetes? How is the woman with gestational diabetes managed?
15. Describe the dietary education needs of the person with diabetes, and discuss some ways that the process can be enhanced.
16. What is hypoglycemia? What type of hypoglycemia is treated with diet? For this type of hypoglycemia, what diet is recommended?

Notes

1. J. K. Davison, Non-insulin-dependent diabetes mellitus, in *Clinical Diabetes Mellitus: A Problem Oriented Approach,* ed. J. K. Davison (New York: Thieme, 1986), pp. 11–25.
2. D. W. Guthrie, D. Hinnen, and R. A. Guthrie, Single-voided vs. double-voided urine testing, *Diabetes Care* 2 (1979): 269–271.
3. P. H. Forsham, Diabetes mellitus: A rational plan for management, *Postgraduate Medicine,* March 1982, pp. 139–154.
4. P. Sinnock and R. S. Most, Diabetes mortality and morbidity data, in *Clinical Diabetes Mellitus: A Problem Oriented Approach,* ed. J. K. Davison (New York: Thieme, 1986), pp. 620–622.
5. B. R. B. El-Beheri Burgess, Rationale for changes in the dietary management of diabetes, *Journal of the American Dietetic Association* 81 (1982): 258–261.
6. A. F. Capper, S. W. Headen, and R. M. Bergenstal, Dietary practices of persons with diabetes during insulin pump therapy, *Journal of the American Dietetic Association* 85 (1985): 445–449.
7. J. S. Skyler and M. L. Reeves, Intensive treatment of Type I diabetes, in *Diabetes Mellitus: Management and Complications,* eds. J. M. Olefsky and R. S. Sherman (New York: Churchill, 1985), pp. 31–79.

8. K. M. West, Diabetes mellitus, in *Nutritional Support of Medical Practice*, 2nd ed., eds. H. A. Schneider, C. E. Anderson, and D. B. Coursin (New York: Harper & Row, 1983), pp. 139–154.

9. M. Nagulesparan and coauthors, Diminished effect of caloric restriction on control of hyperglycemia with increasing known duration of type II diabetes mellitus, *Journal of Clinical Endocrinology and Metabolism* 53 (1981): 560–568.

10. M. Trovati and coauthors, Influence of physical training on blood glucose control, glucose tolerance, insulin secretion, and insulin action in non-insulin-dependent diabetic patients, *Diabetes Care* 7 (1984): 416–420.

11. M. Berger, Oral agents in the treatment of diabetes mellitus, in *Clinical Diabetes Mellitus: A Problem Oriented Approach*, ed. J. K. Davison (New York: Thieme, 1986), pp. 262–273.

12. P. Anastasio, New concern over gestational diabetes, *Environmental Nutrition*, February 1986, pp. 1–2.

13. R. K. Kalkhoff, Medical management of diabetes in pregnancy, in *Clinical Diabetes Mellitus: A Problem Oriented Approach*, ed. J. K. Davison (New York: Thieme, 1986), pp. 472–484.

14. L. Schaffer Bell, L. N. Tiglio, and M. M. Fairchild, Dietary strategies in the treatment of reactive hypoglycemia, *Journal of the American Dietetic Association* 85 (1985): 1141–1143.

Inborn Errors of Metabolism

Having read about diabetes, you are now in a position to more fully appreciate how errors of metabolism can have far-reaching effects on the entire body. Even a single defect can result in serious consequences, because organ systems are interrelated and do not function in isolation. The purpose of this highlight is to examine errors of metabolism—errors present in the individual's genetic makeup. You will see that these errors have serious consequences to the body.

Phenylketonuria (PKU)

Imagine a happy pair of parents proudly viewing their beautiful baby in the hospital nursery. The infant looks flawless, and they are thrilled, after waiting so long, to welcome the child into the world. But unknown to them, the newborn has a hidden disorder— phenylketonuria (PKU)—the symptoms of which have not yet emerged.

Before screening for PKU became routine, this story would have become a tragedy. The parents would take their child home, and the behavior would be like any other baby's behavior—for a while. But gradually, signs of retardation would begin to appear. By half a year of age, the baby would be more irritable and active than other babies. By a year, the behavior would be noticeably abnormal: waving arms, grinding teeth, and maybe even having convulsions. The child would become overdependent and immature. Already, irreversible brain damage would have occurred. By two years more symptoms would apppear: the child might be unable to walk; perhaps never learn to talk; and the IQ would probably be below 30, maybe as low as 20. It is hard to believe that a change in diet, early in infancy, could have prevented this, but in the case of PKU and many disorders like it, it is true.

Causes of PKU

PKU results from an enzyme defect. One of several enzymes that normally convert the amino acid phenylalanine to tyrosine malfunctions, with serious consequences (see Figure H24–1). The result is that abnormally high concentrations of phenylalanine build up, and other compounds derived from it accumulate and damage the developing nervous system. At the same time, tyrosine becomes deficient because it is not being made from phenylalanine, as it normally would be. In effect, tyrosine becomes an essential amino acid. Compounds derived from tyrosine are also lacking. One of these is the hormone epinephrine.

Miniglossary

carrier: an individual who possesses one dominant and one recessive gene for a recessive trait, such as an inborn error. Such a person may show no signs of the trait but can pass it on.

dominant: of a mutated gene, one that has an observable effect on an organism even when it is paired with a normal gene; see also *recessive*.

familial hypercholesterolemia: a hereditary disease characterized by inability of the liver cells to remove cholesterol from the blood.
hyper = too much
emia = in the blood

galactosemia (ga-LACK-toc-SEE-me-ah): an inborn error of metabolism in which galactose cannot be metabolized normally to compounds the body can handle. An alternative metabolite accumulates in the tissues, causing damage.

mutant: an organism carrying a mutation that shows up. Often a mutant must carry two copies of the mutation, one in each gene, before the effects are seen.
muta = change

mutation: an alteration in a gene, such that an altered protein is produced.

phenylketonuria (FEN-ill-KEY-toe-NEW-ree-ah) **(PKU):** an inborn error of metabolism in which phenylalanine cannot be converted to tyrosine. Alternative metabolites of phenylalanine (phenylketones) accumulate in the tissues, causing damage, and overflow into the urine.
phenyl = a ring structure found in many important molecules
ketone = (see p. 215)
uria = in the urine

recessive: of a mutated gene, one that has no observable effect on an organism as long as it is paired with a normal gene that can produce a normal product. In this case, the normal gene is said to be *dominant*.

sickle-cell anemia: a hereditary disease caused by an alteration in the hemoglobin molecule. The altered hemoglobin carries oxygen less efficiently and also causes a change in the red blood cells so that they become sickle-shaped.

FIGURE H24-1

The biochemical defect in PKU.

A. Normally, the amino acid phenylalanine encounters two enzymes that convert it to other compounds. One (the major one) adds an OH group to it to form the very similar but distinct amino acid tyrosine. The other enzyme (which can't handle much phenylalanine at a time) removes its amino group to make the compound phenylpyruvic acid. Ather enzymes act on this compound to make other phenyl acids. (Do you see the subtle differences in structure among these three compounds?)

Normal:

Phenylalanine ⟶ Tyrosine

⬇

Phenylpyruvic Acid

⬇

Other Phenyl Acids

PKU:

Phenylalanine ⟶ X · · · (No Tyrosine)
(accumulates)

⬇

Phenylpyruvic Acid
(accumulates)

⬇

Other Phenyl Acids
(accumulate)

B. In PKU, the major enzyme is malfunctioning, so little or no conversion of phenylalanine to tyrosine can take place. The minor enzyme works to capacity, producing abnormal amounts of the phenyl acid products. Phenylalanine itself also accumulates (not all is processed). Abnormally high concentrations of these substances accumulate all over the body and, together with the relative lack of tyrosine, cause irreversible damage to the developing brain.

One of the smallest types of cells ever studied, a bacterial cell, bears genes for at least 1,000 different enzymes. Mutations are possible in all of these genes. Human cells have hundreds of times as many proteins of major importance, and, in theory, any of them can appear in many different mutant forms. Not only the genes for enzymes, but also those for other proteins such as the "pumps" that move nutrients into and out of cells, the carriers that transport them in the blood, and the structural proteins of cell membranes, connective tissue, and the like, can be affected by alterations in genes.

In many cases, a mutation in a gene will produce such catastrophic effects that the organism inheriting that gene will not survive; it will die before birth (a lethal mutation) or before reaching reproductive age. In such a case, the mutation will not be passed on to any offspring; it is "selected out" of the gene pool. But in other cases, a mutant gene can be carried by an individual so long as it is paired with a normal gene that permits production of the needed protein. Only when two mutant genes from two different carriers segregate into the same individual do the effects of the protein's malfunction appear. Such is the case with PKU and most of the other inborn errors of metabolism. They are rare, recessive traits.

PKU has been known for only about 50 years. Following its discovery, a multitude of other inborn errors have been recognized. A familiar one is sickle-cell anemia, in which one of the amino acids of the hemoglobin molecule is replaced by a different amino acid at one of the molecule's dozens of sites. Some 150-odd other mutant forms of hemoglobin are known (most have no observable effects). Another is familial hypercholesterolemia, which may account for about 20 percent of all heart attacks that occur before 60 years of age. The defective protein is one in the liver cell membranes that remove

Breakfast
2 tbsp raisins
5 tbsp cream of rice
2 tsp sugar
8 oz Lofenalac*

Midmorning Snack
4 oz orange juice

Lunch
½ small banana
2 tbsp tomato soup
(without milk)
3 tbsp rice
1½ tsp margarine
8 oz Lofenalac

*Lofenalac is a special formula
that is low in phenylalanine.

Afternoon Snack
4 oz Lofenalac
5 Ritz crackers

Supper
2 tbsp instant potatoes
(without milk)
3 tbsp green beans
4 tbsp vegetable and
beef broth
1½ tsp margarine
¾ c sliced peaches
8 oz Lofenalac

Bedtime Snack
2 tbsp raisins
4 oz Lofenalac

Sample phenylalanine-restricted diet menu for a child with PKU.

cholesterol from the blood.

These examples could be multiplied many times, but they are enough to give you a basic understanding of inborn errors of metabolism. For inborn errors of metabolism in which diet plays a role, that role is often critical.

Diet Therapy for PKU

The effect of diet therapy in the treatment of PKU is so remarkable that it is like magic. In almost every case, the devastating array of symptoms just described can be greatly modified or almost completely prevented. The phenylalanine content of the diet is carefully controlled to prevent it from reaching levels in the body that can damage tissue.

To achieve this, special formulas and foods have been developed that contain normal amounts of all the amino acids except phenylalanine. Phenylalanine is an essential amino acid—that is, the body can't make it—and it is needed to build protein, so it is not completely excluded from the diet. Rather, the goal is to provide just that amount of phenylalanine the child needs without giving too much, so that excess levels

cannot build up. This situation is similar to diet in hepatic coma (see Chapter 23), where the goal is to provide enough protein for the body's need without providing too much, because excess protein can worsen the disorder.

Planning a diet for an infant with PKU is not easy. A dietitian specially trained in working with people with inborn errors of metabolism is generally responsible for planning the diet. To be sure the diet prescription is appropriate, blood phenylalanine levels are carefully monitored, and diet changes made as indicated. The diet must provide ample kcalories, protein, and essential nutrients. Tyrosine is not made from phenylalanine in PKU, so adequate tyrosine is carefully added to the diet. Infants are given special formulas low in phenylalanine, and later, solids are introduced gradually. The diet planner uses special lists of foods to plan the diet. A sample menu for a child with PKU is shown. Take a close look at it. You can understand why the diet is difficult to follow.

Some controversy exists about whether the diet of the child with PKU can be discontinued after the child reaches age 6 to 8. It was previously

believed that the diet could be discontinued after that age with no ill effects. However, recent reports suggest that the diet should be continued into adolescence and early adulthood.[1]

The successful treatment of PKU depends on the people who care for the infant or child. The special care the child requires may be difficult, but the consequences of not following the diet are too great to risk. The support and encouragement of health team members can help the parents cope with the disorder and the effects it has on their own and their child's lifestyles.

Screening for PKU

In nearly every state, hospitals screen newborn infants for PKU before it can damage development. Any of several tests can be administered that will pick up elevated phenylalanine levels in the blood or metabolic products of phenylalanine in the urine. If an abnormality is found, further testing is undertaken to clarify the diagnosis.

An important factor in screening infants for PKU is diet. If the infant is given a screening test before phenylalanine is received from the diet (breast milk or formula), abnormalities will not be apparent. For this reason, many pediatricians repeat the test for PKU when they see infants for the first visits after birth.

About one in every 14,000 babies has classic PKU. Another one in 10,000 has a variation of the disorder. The prognosis for such babies was grim in the past. Approximately one of every 100 to 200 institutionalized mentally retarded individuals had PKU. Today, some fifty years after the disorder was first recognized, there are clinics, teaching programs for parents, commercial products, cookbooks, and ongoing research programs devoted to PKU.

The Carrier of PKU

PKU is a recessive trait; that is, it normally does not appear in a person who carries just one gene for it. Like all genes, the gene for the enzyme that is defective in PKU comes in two copies: one from the mother, the other from the father. The baby who inherits a defect-free gene from one parent will be able to make a functioning enzyme; that is, the normal type is dominant. Only if defective genes from both parents turn up in the child does the defect become apparent. Another way to say this is that only if both parents are carriers can they have a child with PKU; and even then, they may not, because either one or both of them may pass on a defect-free gene to each child (see Figure H24–2). People may not even know that they are carriers—hence the importance of testing all members of a family in which PKU has appeared, and of genetic counseling for carriers (and their spouses) who consider having children.

The Pregnant Woman with PKU

Because the dietary treatment of PKU has been so successful, more and more women with PKU are reaching childbearing age. Infants born of mothers with PKU frequently have congenital abnormalities. Stillbirths and spontaneous abortions are also common. It is not known whether these complications can be averted if the woman strictly adheres to a phenylalanine-restricted, tyrosine-supplemented diet. However, the risk of not following the diet is clear.

This brief discussion of PKU is to give you insight into inborn errors of metabolism and the important role that diet can play in their treatment. Another inborn error of metabolism, galactosemia, involves carbohydrate metabolism rather than protein metabolism.

Galactosemia

Galactosemia is an inherited disorder caused by a deficiency of any of several

FIGURE H24–2

The inheritance of PKU.

A. If both parents possess two copies of the gene for the normal enzyme for processing phenylalanine, their children will, of course, inherit defect-free genes from both.

B. If both parents are carriers (possess one gene for PKU), then they can both pass on the PKU gene by one of their children. For each birth, there is one chance in four that the child will have PKU, two chances that the child will be a carrier, and one chance that the child will be PKU-free.

enzymes that normally convert galactose to glucose in the body. In the more severe case, an infant given milk, which contains a galactose unit in each molecule of lactose, vomits and has diarrhea after the very first feeding. Growth begins to fail within days after birth, and liver damage is apparent within a week. Death may follow soon after. If the child lives, the unmetabolized galactose is shunted along an alternative pathway to form an abnormal product that causes cataracts, damage to the sexual organs, and brain damage to the point of severe mental retardation.

Galactosemia differs from PKU in several ways. First, galactose is not an essential nutrient (as phenylalanine is), so the dietary treatment is simpler. Galactose is simply excluded from the diet. Since galactose occurs only in

lactose (the sugar in milk), milk and milk products are avoided. Second, it is known that dietary compliance must be lifelong for those with galactosemia. Third, *carriers* of galactosemia (those carrying one gene for the trait) are not symptom-free. Their bodies can't manage galactose quite as well as those who have perfect genes; reduced enzyme activity can be detected. Even though they can eat a normal diet, it is thought that during pregnancy they should eliminate galactose to avoid damage to the fetus.

Galactosemia is perhaps two or three times more rare than PKU, but it must be treated immediately if its consequences are to be averted. The diet for galactosemia is basically a lactose-free diet (see Chapter 22) that is instituted soon after birth. In early infancy, the diet can be lifesaving.

Special soy-based formulas that are lactose-free are used instead of standard infant formulas. Breastfeeding is contraindicated, because breast milk contains large amounts of galactose.

Other Inborn Errors

In this highlight, we have discussed the inborn errors of metabolism PKU and galactosemia, because these two metabolic disorders are among the more frequent types encountered. Even at that, they are rare. You may be wondering what other enzymes are subject to defects and what other inborn errors are possible.

Every enzyme the body makes has its code carried by a gene. Any gene can mutate so that the protein it makes differs from the normal protein in some way. In 999 cases out of 1,000, the result of a mutation is a disadvantage or disaster for the organism.

NOTE
1. M. R. Seashore and coauthors, Loss of intellectual function in children with phenylketonuria after relaxation of dietary phenylalanine restriction, *Pediatrics* 75 (1985): 226-232; C. H. Lou, Decreased vigilance and neurotransmitter synthesis after discontinuation of dietary treatment of phenylketonuria in adolescence, *European Journal of Pediatrics* 144 (1985): 17-20.

Disorders of the Heart and Blood Vessels

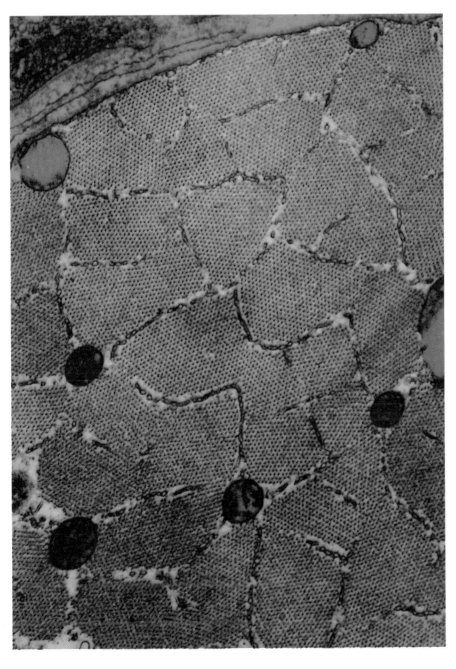

Contents

The fine structure of the heart muscle shows the molecular elements of which it is composed: these are bundles of heart muscle fibers cut crosswise, viewed end-on. Round openings among the fibers are blood vessels, carrying nutrients and oxygen to them and waste products away.

With red lights flashing and siren screaming, the ambulance races toward the hospital. The victim is one of many people who will suffer from a heart attack this year. In 1982 about one-half of all deaths among adults in the United States were due to cardiovascular diseases.[1] Cardiovascular diseases remain the leading cause of adult deaths in the United States.[2] The cost is enormous; over 12 million potential years of life are lost each year from these premature deaths. In terms of dollars and cents, it is estimated that the economy lost $59 billion in productivity due to illness and premature deaths attributed to cardiovascular disorders. Despite these grim statistics, mortality from cardiovascular disease (CVD) has been declining by about 2 percent per year since 1968. Although this news gives us a reason to be optimistic, there is still a good deal to be done.

The most common cardiac disorder is coronary artery disease (CAD), which accounts for as many as 800,000 new heart attacks and another 450,000 recurrent heart attacks every year. Over 5 million people in the United States are affected by CAD.

Diseases of the heart and blood vessels are grouped together and termed **cardiovascular disease (CVD).** When the blood supply to the heart is obstructed, **coronary artery disease (CAD)** or **coronary heart disease (CHD)** results. In **ischemic** (iss-KEE-mic) **heart disease (IHD),** the blood supply to any organ or tissue may be cut off (see p.131 for definitions of related terms).

Atherosclerosis

The most common type of CAD, atherosclerosis, is characterized by an accumulation of lipid plaque within the arterial wall. Since the arteries carry blood away from the heart, they are more responsive than veins to the beat of the heart as it pumps blood outward. They must expand as a large volume of blood rushes by and then contract so that a steady blood pressure is maintained. Highlight 4B provides an overview of nutrition and atherosclerosis and discusses the role of diet in the prevention of the disorder. You may want to review the Miniglossary on p. 131, which defines many terms used in this chapter. The information in this chapter reinforces some of the concepts presented earlier and focuses on the nutrition care of those who already have coronary heart disease (CHD).

As an atherosclerotic plaque invades the artery and enlarges, it narrows the lumen, thus raising the pressure of the blood against the wall. The increased pressure can damage the artery wall, as well as all the organs in the body. The plaque also causes the wall to lose its elasticity so that it cannot expand in response to the beat of the heart; thus the blood pressure rises further.

If the plaque narrows the lumen enough, it can completely block the flow of blood. The result is death to all tissues depending on that artery for nutrients and oxygen. However, before that happens, it is more likely that a clot will form, plugging the artery. If the blood supply to the heart muscle is cut off, a heart attack can result. When a critical supply of blood to the brain is involved, the result is a stroke. The kidneys, lungs, and peripheral arteries can also be affected. Figure 25–1 shows the interrelationships among various cardiovascular disorders. Review Highlight 4B for more information about risk factors for the development of atherosclerosis and dietary factors that may help in its prevention. Tables H4B–3 and H4B–4 on pp. 129–130 summarize information about the effects of different foods and nutrients on blood cholesterol levels.

A general term used to describe thickening and hardening of the arteries is **arteriosclerosis**. When this process is due to the accumulation of lipid plaques within the arterial wall, the condition is **atherosclerosis.**

Three major risk factors in the development of atherosclerosis:
• Smoking.
• High serum cholesterol.
• High blood pressure.

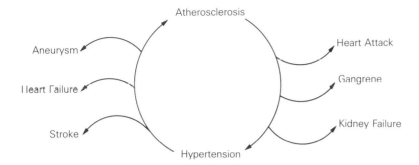

FIGURE 25–1

Interrelationships of various cardiovascular disorders.

Controlling Blood Lipids

The best treatment of atherosclerosis is prevention. All attempts should be made to control the risk factors of atherosclerosis whenever possible. As far as diet is concerned, the American Heart Association (AHA) recommends that all people (regardless of their blood lipid levels) eat less meat, eggs, and dairy products (except those made of nonfat milk); eat more fish and poultry; change the type of fat used; and eat more starches, fruits, and vegetables. Keep in mind that the diet recommended for all people provides approximately 30 percent of the total kcalories from fat, 55 percent from carbohydrate, and 15 percent from protein. Saturated, monosaturated, and polyunsaturated fats should contribute equally to fat kcalories. Cholesterol intake of less than 300 milligrams per day is recommended. Complex carbohydrates are encouraged.

The diet may be difficult for many people to follow, and drastic changes cannot be expected overnight. The development of many new products that fit the prudent diet meal plan (cholesterol-free eggs, special cheeses, and polyunsaturated margarines) can help considerably. The AHA has many pamphlets and recipe booklets available to both professionals and the public to help them make the suggested dietary changes.

The AHA recommendations that all people follow a prudent diet is controversial. However, a growing body of evidence does suggest that lowering serum cholesterol levels in people with elevated serum cholesterol reduces the risk of heart disease. A seven-year, double-blind study of over 3,000 people, the Lipid Research Clinics Coronary Primary Prevention Trial (LRC-CPPT), found a strong association between lowering blood cholesterol levels and reducing the risk of CHD.[3] The study group's serum cholesterol levels were reduced by 9 percent as compared with the placebo group. In addition, that group had a 20 percent reduction in the appearance of angina pectoris, the incidence of abnormal electrocardiograms, and the number of coronary bypass operations. A greater reduction of serum cholesterol was found to be associated with a lowered risk for heart disease. A combination of diet and drugs was used to lower cholesterol in the study group. Therefore, it is not possible to determine whether diet alone could achieve such an effect. However, it seems reasonable that serum cholesterol lowered by any means could be effective, and many experts in the field support the view that lowering serum cholesterol by diet is desirable.[4]

Another recent study of over 356,000 American men showed an increased risk of coronary heart disease associated with elevations in serum cholesterol that were previously regarded as normal.[5] The results were seen over a wide variety of people: nonsmokers without hypertension, smokers without hypertension, nonsmokers with hypertension, and smokers with hypertension. The

The American Heart Association recommends a diet low in fat and high in complex carbohydrates.

risk was found to be continuous and graded; that is, the more elevated the serum cholesterol, the greater the risk of coronary heart disease. This study suggests that many individuals, not just those with elevated lipid levels, can benefit from measures, including diet, that help reduce serum cholesterol levels. For now, let's look at the diet that is recommended to achieve this end.

The fat-controlled diet is used to treat people who have elevated blood lipids, or hyperlipidemia. Cholesterol, triglycerides, or both may be elevated. Since these lipids are carried through the blood in the lipoproteins, different lipoproteins are also elevated. (Lipoproteins are discussed on pp. 105–108.) For example, when cholesterol levels are high, low-density lipoproteins (LDL) are elevated; when triglycerides are high, the very-low-density lipoproteins (VLDL) or chylomicrons are elevated. An elevation of any lipoprotein is called *hyperlipoproteinemia*. Table 25–1 summarizes the dietary modifications useful for controlling various lipid elevations.

One of the most widely used systems for classifying hyperlipidemias is shown in Table 25–2. Using this system, six basic types of hyperlipidemias have been identified. These include types I, IIa, IIb, III, IV, and V. Types II and IV are by far the most common, and they are associated with an increased risk of CHD. Table 25–2 shows which lipoproteins are abnormal in each type of hyperlipidemia. In each case, the abnormalities are different. For our purposes here, however, we are not concerned with specific types of hyperlipidemias as much as with how we can use the diet to change abnormal lipoprotein patterns.

The AHA recommends a gradual reduction of total fat, saturated fat, and cholesterol for the treatment of elevated serum cholesterol and triglyceride levels.[6] Weight reduction is also important for the person who is overweight. Complex carbohydrates are recommended. One study suggests that the use of an oat product along with a fat-controlled diet can help lower serum cholesterol levels.[7] The first phase of treatment is the same diet that is recommended for all people,

fat-controlled diet: a diet in which both the amount and type of fat are limited and defined.

hyperlipidemia (HIGH-per-LIP-ih-DEE-me-ah): elevated blood lipids. This term is often used interchangeably with **hyperlipoproteinemia** (HIGH-per-LIP-oh-PRO-teen-EE-me-ah), or elevated blood lipoproteins.

Elevated serum triglyceride levels is called **hypertriglyceridemia.** Elevated serum cholesterol levels is called **hypercholesterolemia.**

TABLE 25–1

Dietary Approaches to Lowering Blood Lipids*

Elevated Lipid	Major Lipoprotein Involved	Dietary Approach
Dietary triglycerides	Chylomicrons	Total fat restriction
Triglycerides	VLDL	Weight reduction Restriction of total fat to less than 20 to 30%of total kcalories
Cholesterol	LDL	Restriction of saturated fat to 10% of fat kcalories Restriction of cholesterol to 100 to 300 mg/day

*The dietary approach to raising HDL would include weight reduction, correction of elevated triglycerides (see above), and a moderate consumption of alcohol.

TABLE 25–2

The Hyperlipidemias

Type	Lipoprotein abnormality
I	Elevated chylomicrons, triglycerides, and cholesterol
IIa	Elevated LDL and cholesterol
IIb	Elevated LDL, VLDL, cholesterol, and triglycerides
III	Elevated VLDL, cholesterol, and triglycerides
IV	Elevated VLDL; normal or elevated cholesterol and triglycerides
V	Elevated chylomicrons, VLDL, triglycerides, and cholesterol

regardless of blood lipid levels (see above). After this adjustment has been made, the diet is further restricted as follows:

- 25 percent of kcalories from fat, with equal amounts of the three types of fats.
- 60 percent of kcalories from carbohydrate, emphasizing complex carbohydrates.
- 15 percent of kcalories from protein.
- Cholesterol intake of 200 to 250 milligrams per day.

In the final phase, the diet is restricted further, as follows:

- 20 percent of kcalories from fat, with equal amounts of the three types of fat.
- 65 percent of kcalories from carbohydrate.
- 15 percent of kcalories from protein.
- Cholesterol intake of 100 to 150 milligrams per day.

The client's response to the diet in terms of both blood lipid levels and compliance determines which level of restriction is appropriate. Drug therapy is recommended only if diet therapy fails to bring lipids to normal levels, if blood lipid levels are markedly elevated, or if the risk of CHD is especially high due to other risk factors.

Hyperlipidemia often occurs along with other diseases, including diabetes (Chapter 24), hypertension (this chapter), and renal disease (Chapter 26). When these disorders are present in tandem, the diet is adjusted accordingly.

Elevated chylomicrons (as in types I and V hyperlipidemia) are treated with a low-fat diet. Instruct the client to limit the total amount of fat, not the type. This makes sense, since chylomicrons are made to transport dietary fat. MCT oil can be used as a source of fat in type I hyperlipidemia, because MCT are not transported in the chylomicron. However, MCT oil is not used in type V, because it may cause an even greater increase in VLDL, which are elevated already.

Encourage the person with types I or V hyperlipidemia to avoid alcohol. Alcohol may cause elevated serum triglyceride levels. Furthermore, types I and V hyperlipidemia may occur secondary to alcohol abuse or pancreatitis (see Chapter 23), both of which require that alcohol be avoided.

Evidence is mounting that low serum levels of HDL may be a significant risk factor for the development of CHD. Dietary measures aimed at raising HDL levels include weight reduction (if necessary), correction of hyper-

A cluster of symptoms associated with markedly elevated levels of chylomicrons in the blood is called **chylomicronemia** (KYE-lo-MY-crow-NEE-me-ah) **syndrome.** Lipid deposits in the skin and retina, as well as acute pancreatitis, are some characteristics of this syndrome.

There is a big difference between low-fat and fat-controlled diets, although these terms are often confused. A low-fat diet is low in total fat, without particular concern for the type of fat. On the other hand, a fat-controlled diet generally allows more total fat, but prescribes the type of fat to be consumed.

triglyceridemia, and a moderate consumption of alcohol. Additionally, frequent and vigorous exercise and abstinence from cigarette smoking are encouraged.

The diabetic exchange lists can easily be adapted for use by people with hyperlipidemia. Carefully adjust the cholesterol and saturated fats in the diet by limiting the use of medium- and high-fat meats, whole milk, saturated fats, and bread exchanges high in fat. Lists of foods quite similar to the diabetic exchange lists are available from the National Institutes of Health. The AHA also has booklets available.

Other Treatments

Drugs that lower serum lipid levels are called **antilipemic agents.**

As a rule, drugs are not used to treat hyperlipidemia unless diet therapy is unsuccessful. A three month trial period on diet alone is recommended. Drugs that lower serum lipids have two sites of action. Some work in the GI tract to prevent the absorption of cholesterol. Others work in the body after lipids are absorbed by different, and often unknown, mechanisms. A promising new drug, lovastatin, has been reported to lower cholesterol levels by nearly 30 to 40 percent.[8] Although the drug is not currently available, it may surface on the market in the near future. Some drugs are mainly effective in lowering triglycerides; others more effectively lower cholesterol. All of these drugs can adversely affect nutrition status by interfering with food intake (see Chapter 19). These drugs, their effects, and associated nutrition problems are summarized in Table 25−3.

TABLE 25−3

Drug Therapy in Hyperlipidemias

Drug	Lipid Lowered	Nutrition-related Side Effects
Cholestyramine	Cholesterol	Nausea, vomiting, abdominal discomfort, constipation; ☛ vitamin B_{12} absorption; malabsorption of fat-soluble vitamins and calcium
Colestipol	Cholesterol	(Same as above)
Clofibrate	Triglycerides, cholesterol	Nausea, vomiting, abdominal discomfort, loose stools; ☛ absorption of carotene, glucose, iron, vitamin B_{12}, and electrolytes
Gemfibrozil	Triglercerides, cholesterol	Nausea, vomiting, abdominal discomfort
Lovastatin	Cholesterol	Diarrhea, flatulence, altered taste perceptions
Nicotinic acid	Triglycerides, cholesterol	Nausea, vomiting, abdominal discomfort; decreased glucose tolerance
Probucol	Cholesterol	Nausea, vomiting, abdominal discomfort, diarrhea

Many factors other than diet can contribute to elevated blood lipid levels. Therefore, other lifestyle changes must be considered. Exercise may be important, especially for the person who is overweight. The person may be advised to stop smoking cigarettes. People with other medical disorders may be advised to follow a different type of therapy. One such disorder is hypertension. In the next section we will discuss hypertension, its role in coronary heart disease, and its treatment.

Hypertension

Hypertension is the most prevalent CVD, believed to affect some 60 million Americans.[9] It contributes to 500,000 cases of strokes and an estimated 1.25 million coronary events annually.[10] An arterial pressure of 140/90 millimeters of mercury (mm Hg) or greater arbitrarily defines hypertension. Above this level, the incidence of CVD increases more significantly.

Hypertension can occur secondary to kidney diseases and various hormonal imbalances. However, such causes can be identified in only a small number of cases. Most of the time, the cause of hypertension is unknown, that is, it is essential or primary.

Hypertension can result when the diameter of the arteries is reduced (as in atherosclerosis) or when the volume of the blood moving through the arteries is increased. (The first case is like pinching off a garden hose; the second is like turning the water on all the way; both increase pressure.) Increased pressure caused by reduced diameter of the arteries appears to play a greater role in hypertension.

Although we don't know what causes peripheral resistance, most investigators believe that the kidneys are involved. The kidneys play a major role in blood pressure regulation through the enzyme renin and the hormone aldosterone (see p. 383). Norepinephrine, which constricts blood vessels and increases the rate and strength of the heartbeat, also may be involved. Additionally, a predisposition to hypertension appears to be inherited. The enzyme kallikrein and prostaglandins may also be implicated.

Many dietary factors have been studied to determine if they play a role in the development of hypertension, including the minerals sodium, potassium, magnesium, and, more recently, calcium. For a discussion of the roles of these minerals in the development of hypertension, see pp. 384–386.

Whatever the cause of hypertension, eventually peripheral resistance increases. This makes it harder for the left ventricle of the heart to pump blood through the system. If hypertension goes unchecked, eventually the left ventricle becomes enlarged and finally cannot handle the load. The result is heart failure. Hypertension is the major cause of heart failure, either alone or in combination with atherosclerosis. Increased pressure can also lead to a stroke, and the kidneys can be damaged when the heart is unable to adequately pump blood through these vital organs.

People with hypertension may be unaware that they have a problem. A major national effort has been made to identify and treat them. Even mild hypertension

hypertension: see p. 382.

In a blood pressure reading, the first figure is the **systolic** blood pressure and the second, the **diastolic** blood pressure. The systolic pressure represents arterial pressure caused by the contraction of the left ventricle of the heart. The diastolic pressure is the arterial pressure when the heart is between beats (see p. 384).

peripheral resistance: the resistance to the flow of body fluids caused by a reduced diameter of the arteries.

Any substance that helps enlarge the diameter of the arteries is a **vasodilator** (VAS-oh-dye-LAY-tor). A **vasoconstrictor** (VAS-oh-kon-STRIK-tor) reduces the diameter of the arteries.

The enzyme **kallikrein** (kal-ee-KREE-in) splits a specific blood protein to form **kinin** (KYE-nin). Kinins act as vasodilators, inducing hypotension and increasing blood flow in small blood capillaries; in addition, they stimulate the release of a prostaglandin (see p. 98) that helps counteract vasoconstriction.

Health care professionals measure blood pressure to identify and treat people with hypertension.

These foods are high in sodium.

1 tsp of salt contains about 2 g of sodium.

(diastolic pressure of 90 to 104 millimeters of mercury) can be dangerous, and individuals with mild hypertension benefit from treatment.[11] An urgent need to prevent and safely treat hypertension is suggested by these findings.

Diet in Hypertension

The role of diet in the prevention of hypertension has been debated extensively. Most of the controversy centers on whether a high-sodium diet causes hypertension and, conversely, whether a sodium-restricted diet can prevent it (see pp. 381–387). The evidence as to whether a moderately low sodium intake can prevent hypertension is inconclusive. However, many professionals and agencies (including the FDA) believe that enough evidence is available to warrant a recommendation to the general public to moderately restrict sodium intake. They reason that at worst, such a diet cannot be harmful.

The value of incorporating a low-sodium diet in the treatment of established hypertension is far less controversial. Studies have shown that even mild restriction of sodium can produce a modest but definite fall in blood pressure.[12] Weight is also important in the control of hypertension. The overweight hypertensive person can reduce blood pressure simply by losing weight. Beneficial effects are seen even when the person does not achieve ideal body weight. The authors of one study concluded that weight loss could help reduce the dosage of medication needed to control hypertension or eliminate the need for medication altogether.[13] Another study was conducted to see if medication could be withdrawn safely from people who had been maintained on aggressive hypertensive drug therapy for five years.[14] Also examined was the effect of weight loss and sodium restriction in helping these people withdraw from drug therapy. The results of the study showed that normal blood pressure could be attained without drug therapy in 50 percent of the people who were studied. Modest weight loss (about 10 pounds) or a limited intake of sodium (about 1,600 milligrams per day) more than doubled the chance that the person could remain unmedicated.

You can help the person with hypertension most by encouraging weight loss (if necessary) and a sodium-restricted diet. Usually sodium is restricted to 2 to 4 grams per day. Recommend that the individual avoid foods high in salt and that no salt be added to foods at the table. Table 25–4 lists the foods not

TABLE 25–4

No-Added-Salt Diet

- You may lightly salt foods during cooking, but do not add salt at the table.
- Avoid foods high in sodium, including:

Meats—bacon; bologna; cold cuts; chipped or corned beef; frankfurters; smoked meats; sausage; salt pork or codfish; canned, salted, or smoked fish.

Sauces, seasonings, and condiments—regular catsup; celery, garlic, and onion salt; regular chili sauce; commercial meat extracts; meat tenderizers; monosodium glutamate; olives; pickles; prepared mustard; soy and Worcestershire sauce.

Other—regular canned or frozen soups; regular bouillon; soup mixes; pretzels, popcorn, crackers, nuts, potato chips, or other salted snack foods; sauerkraut; regular cheese; regular peanut butter.

- Low-sodium products can be substituted for regular foods.

allowed on a no-added-salt diet. In the past, diets very low in sodium were often recommended for people with hypertension. However, these diets are hard to follow and are of limited value.

When sodium is retained in the body, potassium is excreted. For this reason, many practitioners recommend that good sources of potassium be included in the daily diet. When people with normal blood pressure are fed large quantities of sodium, ultimately their blood pressure rises—and at the same time, their potassium excretion increases. If fed potassium simultaneously with the sodium, they do not have a rise in blood pressure.[15] Additionally, some diuretics used in the treatment of hypertension can lead to a potassium deficiency. People on these drugs must be particularly careful to include good sources of potassium in their daily diets; they may be advised to use potassium supplements. Table 25–5 lists foods high in potassium, Table 11–4 on p. 385 provides the potassium and sodium contents of whole unprocessed foods versus processed foods, and Appendix H lists the potassium and sodium content of foods. Watch for signs of hypokalemia, such as weakness (particularly of the legs), unexplained numbness or tingling sensation, cramps, irregular heartbeat, and excessive thirst and urination. Blood levels of potassium should be monitored regularly to prevent hypokalemia.

In 1944, a diet consisting of rice, sugar, and fruit was found to be effective in the treatment of hypertension. It was later learned that the **Kempner rice diet** worked because it is very low in sodium. The diet is very restrictive, deficient in many nutrients, and no longer in use.

Remind clients that whole foods of all kinds—fruits, vegetables, grains, meats, fish and poultry—are good sources of potassium (see p. 401).

Drugs used to treat hypertension include **diuretics** and **adrenergic blockers.** Diuretics work by increasing fluid loss, thus lowering blood pressure (see pp. 142, 271). Some cause potassium to be excreted in excess. Adrenergic blockers interfere with a neurotransmitter to alter blood pressure.

hypokalemia (HIGH-poe-ka-LEE-me-ah): low levels of potassium in the blood.

TABLE 25–5

Foods High in Potassium

Vegetables

Artichokes*	Rhubarb*
Broccoli	Rutabagas
Brussels sprouts	Tomatoes
Parsnips*	Tomato juice*
Pinto beans	Vegetable juice*
Pumpkins*	Winter squash*
Potatoes, baked* or pared and boiled	Yams

Fruits

Apricots*	Orange juice
Apricot nectar	Oranges
Avocados*	Papayas*
Bananas	Peaches*
Cantaloupes*	Pears
Dates*	Pineapple juice
Figs	Pineapples
Grapefruit juice	Prune juice*
Grapefruits	Prunes*
Honeydew melons*	Raisins*
Nectarines*	Tangerines

Other

Chocolate	Molasses, dark* and light
Cocoa	Peanuts*
Meat*	Walnuts*
Milk*	Wheat germ

*Typical serving contains more than 250 mg potassium.

Sample no-added-salt, fat-controlled, high-potassium diet menu. Foods for this menu are prepared with little or no salt and a minimal amount of fat. The fats used for cooking or for flavor are monounsaturated and polyunsaturated.

Breakfast
¾ c cantaloupe
½ c all-bran cereal
Skim milk
1 slice toast
Special margarine
Coffee or tea
Sugar (optional)

Lunch
Broiled chicken breast
Baked potato
Tossed salad
Hard roll
Special margarine
Allowed dressing
Skim milk
1 small banana

Dinner
Sautéed scallops (use allowed oil)
Brown rice
Broccoli
Hard roll
Special margarine
1 medium orange
Coffee or tea

Foods to enjoy on a sodium-restricted diet.

Hints for the diet advisor:
- Recommend that the client reduce sodium gradually.
- See the client regularly.
- Encourage the client to experiment with spices and flavorings.
- Advise the client to be a label reader: sodium can be found in foods, water, medicines, toothpastes, and mouthwashes.

Many professionals also advise hypertensive clients to follow a fat-controlled prudent diet. This measure is taken because hypertensive people are at greater-than-normal risk for developing CHD. Other dietary measures that may be recommended (although evidence on these factors is inconclusive at present) include the use of foods high in calcium and the elimination of caffeine and alcohol from the diet. A sample no-added-salt, fat-controlled, high-potassium diet menu is shown.

People may find it difficult to drastically change their sodium intake. Foods eaten without salt may taste unpalatable to the person who normally uses it liberally. Diet compliance is most unlikely when a person is handed an instruction sheet without additional encouragement or guidance.

Several things can help. For one, reduce sodium gradually so that the person can adjust to the flavor of unsalted foods. This implies that you will see the person regularly for follow-up, which also is important. Encourage the person to experiment with other spices and herbs to add flavor to foods. Table 11–5 on p. 387 provides a list of these spices and flavorings. Several cookbooks with helpful tips are available.

Teach your clients to read labels and recognize sources of sodium (see p. 387 margin entry). Local water supplies may have a high sodium content.

A person whose blood pressure falls suddenly when she stands up is experiencing **orthostatic hypotension.**

In many cases, people with hypertension are advised not to drink coffee or caffeine-containing foods, because some studies have shown that caffeine may increase blood pressure. Caffeine may be beneficial, however, for people who experience a sudden drop in blood pressure when they stand. In a limited study of 12 people who experienced this type of hypotension after eating, caffeine (250 milligrams, or about the amount in 2 cups of coffee) given after breakfast helped lessen the change in blood pressure.[16]

When this water is used in food products, it may contribute significantly to sodium intake.

Help people to realize that processed foods, milk, and other dairy products are high in sodium. Most people are surprised to learn that a serving of cornflakes contains more sodium than a serving of cocktail peanuts—and that a serving of chocolate pudding contains still more.[17] Medications such as antacids, antibiotics, cough medicines, laxatives, pain relievers, and sedatives may contain sodium. Some toothpastes and mouthwashes also contain large amounts of sodium; recommend that people rinse thoroughly after brushing their teeth or using a mouthwash, as well as that they avoid swallowing these compounds.

Low-Sodium Products

Many low-sodium products are available for use with low-sodium diets. In general, you can plan a palatable diet without using these products. Some people, however, like to use them to add variety. Be aware that many of these products are not sodium-free, so the amount of sodium they do contain must be calculated into the diet.

In salt substitutes, the sodium is generally replaced by potassium. Some people don't like the taste of salt substitutes but may find them acceptable if used sparingly. Don't heat them, though, because they turn bitter. Often people find food more acceptable without any salt at all. The use of a potassium-containing salt substitute serves the dual purpose of increasing potassium intake while reducing sodium. However, salt substitutes containing potassium should not be used by people with renal insufficiency. Some products contain a combination of half regular table salt and half salt substitute. Although these products may be more palatable, they also can contribute a significant amount of sodium to the diet.

People with renal disease should not use potassium-containing salt substitutes.

The **coronary arteries** deliver nutrients and oxygen to the heart.

spasm: an involuntary, convulsive contraction.

rheumatic (roo-MAT-ik) **heart disease:** a general term used to describe heart damage (often affecting the heart valves) that occurs due to rheumatic fever (caused by a bacterial infection).

The enzymes of the heart that are elevated in the blood after a heart attack include serum glutamic-oxalacetic transaminase (SGOT), lactic dehydrogenase (LDH), and creatine phosphokinase (CPK).

Heart Attacks

The heart gets its nutrients and oxygen not from inside its chambers, but from arteries that lie on its surface. A myocardial infarction (MI), or heart attack, occurs when the supply of blood to the heart muscle is cut off, resulting in tissue death. Atherosclerosis is a common contributor to heart attacks; some other contributors are hypertension, abnormal blood clotting, spasms of the coronary arteries, infection of the membrane covering the heart, and rheumatic heart disease. As an area of heart tissue dies, enzymes that are associated with heart cells leak out into the general circulation in much the same way that digestive enzymes leak out of the pancreas in people with pancreatitis. A raised level of these enzymes in the blood is often used in diagnosing heart attacks.

Probably all of us know at least one person who seems destined for a heart attack: an overweight, hard-driving executive with hypertension who only jokes about exercising and dieting. Then one day it happens. When you visit this person in the hospital, you can hardly believe your ears.

Overnight, it seems, your friend's attitude has changed dramatically. Facing mortality, your friend places a new value on life. Suddenly any advice the health care team can offer is respected. The time has arrived to take positive steps toward changing lifestyle habits and improving the chances for survival.

Your friend is a typical MI victim. Like a sponge, any advice that may help is eagerly soaked up. This person is one of the most enjoyable clients to work with, listening carefully to what the health care team says and trying hard to follow advice.

Be sure to seize the opportunity afforded to you by offering sound and useful counsel. The person will benefit from your suggestions, and you will be rewarded by the person's interest and appreciation.

Dietary guidelines after an MI:
1. Offer nothing by mouth until shock resolves; IV fluids if necessary.
2. After several hours, give a 1,000- to 1,200-kcal, 2-g-sodium diet consisting of liquids or soft, bland foods of moderate temperature in small, frequent feedings.
3. After 5 to 10 days, adjust the diet to meet individual needs, generally in 3 mcals a day.

The heart attack victim, like an accident victim, is in shock at first. In shock, fluid leaves the vascular compartment and moves temporarily to the interstitial space. The person experiences this fluid shift as if it came from dehydration and complains of extreme thirst. The body does not need water when this occurs, however, and increasing its fluid load at such a time is unwise.

Do not offer food to an individual immediately after an MI; nausea is common. If, as shock resolves, the person still remains nauseated, IV infusions are started to prevent dehydration.

After several hours of observation, the person can usually begin to eat. At this time, provide foods that minimize the work of the heart. The diet is moderately restricted in sodium (about 2 grams) and is low in kcalories (1,000 to 1,200). Begin with liquid or soft, bland foods given in frequent, small feedings. These foods are easier to eat and may reduce gas formation and abdominal distension. Abdominal distension pushes the diaphragm up toward the heart, thus placing additional stress on the heart muscle. Serve foods neither too hot nor too cold. Temperature extremes can stimulate nerves that slow the heart rate. Many practitioners also restrict caffeinated beverages during the first few days after an MI, but this measure is controversial.

After the person is out of immediate danger (about five to ten days), tailor the diet to meet individual needs—for example, to deal with hyperlipidemia, hypertension, obesity, diabetes, or the like. Oftentimes, a diet to reduce weight, control fat, and moderately restrict sodium is appropriate and can be planned to include only three meals a day.

People who continue to have chest pain after an MI may benefit from eating small, frequent meals. Advise them to eat slowly and not to exercise immediately after meals.

Congestive Heart Failure

Many diseases—CVD, hypertension, and kidney disease—can lead to congestive heart failure (CHF). In CHF, the heart can no longer pump enough blood through the circulatory system. Because the heart is not adequately pumping, blood flow to the kidneys is reduced. This change signals the kidneys to retain fluid. The retained fluid increases the load on the heart and further weakens it. Since blood entering the heart from the veins cannot be pumped out effectively, peripheral, and sometimes pulmonary, edema result. The person becomes "congested" with excess fluids. The heart enlarges and begins to beat more rapidly to try to compensate for its inability to pump. CHF is life threatening, particularly when it is accompanied by pulmonary edema.

Another complication occurs because of the heart's inadequate pumping ability. The supply of nutrients and oxygen normally carried in the blood to the peripheral tissues is disrupted. Malnutrition can result, particularly as the disorder progresses. Other factors intensify the risk of malnutrition, including anorexia, altered taste sensitivity, intolerance to food odors, physical exhaustion precipitated simply by the act of eating, the diet used for treatment (some people find the diet unappealing), and the long-term use of medications that interfere with nutrition status. Undernutrition in these people often goes unnoticed, because edema masks their underweight condition. Malnutrition, in turn, can precipitate or aggravate heart failure.[18]

Diuretics and drugs that increase the strength of heart muscle contractions are important in the treatment of CHF. Bed rest helps to reduce the work load of the heart.

A sodium- and fluid-restricted diet is used to reduce the work required of the damaged heart and to alleviate edema. The level of sodium restriction is determined by the individual's tolerance. Generally, a 2-gram-sodium diet (see Chapter 23, p. 745) and a fluid restriction of about 1½ to 2 liters of fluid are provided daily. Such a diet can help prevent fluid overload and reduce diuretic needs.[19]

The person with CHF is often underweight and malnourished, as described above. However, if the person is overweight, weight reduction is very important in relieving additional stress to the heart.

People suffering from CHF can easily become exhausted when eating and may benefit from small, frequent meals and snacks. As in MI, provide small feedings of foods least likely to form gas, which will reduce the abdominal distension that displaces the diaphragm toward the heart. Liquid formulas of high nutrient density may be useful. Tube feedings of such formulas may be necessary to prevent severe malnutrition when the person cannot take adequate foods by mouth. If a tube feeding is necessary, the feeding should be delivered with the person in a sitting or only slightly reclining position to reduce the risk of aspiration. In some cases, TPN may be required, with particular care taken to ensure that the amount of fluid given will not overload the person.

congestive heart failure (CHF): a syndrome in which the heart can no longer adequately pump blood through the circulatory system.

pulmonary edema: fluid in the lungs.

Enlargement of the heart is **cardiomegaly** (CAR-dee-oh-MEG-ah-lee). A rapid heart rate is **tachycardia** (TACK-ee-CAR-dee-ah). *mega* = big *tachys* = rapid

Heart disease can lead to PCM, usually marasmus; the tissues fail to receive enough nutrients when the heart is weak. This PCM is called **cardiac cachexia** (ka-KEKS-ee-ah).

Drugs frequently used to increase the strength of the heart's contractions are **digitalis** (DIJ-ih-TAL-is) **glycosides**.

Dietary guidelines for CHF:
• Restrict sodium and fluids.
• Lose weight, if necessary.
• Eat small, frequent meals.
• Use foods least likely to cause distension.

CASE STUDY

Hyperlipidemia and Hypertension

Mr. Garrett, age 45, has just been diagnosed to have type IV hyperlipoproteinemia. He is 5′7″ tall and weighs 200 lb. Mr. Garrett has a family history of CHD. His diet is high in kcalories, cholesterol, total fat, saturated fats, and sodium. He smokes a pack of cigarettes a day, and his lifestyle leaves him little room for exercise. Mr. Garrett also has hypertension, for which diuretics have been prescribed. He frequently forgets to take his pills, though, and his blood pressure is often quite high.

1. Name the risk factors for CHD in Mr. Garrett's history. Which of them can he control? Which can be helped by diet? What complications can result from CHD?

2. What type of diet, if any, would you recommend for Mr. Garrett's type of hyperlipidemia? Explain the rationale for each diet change. How will his current diet change? What types of foods should he eat?

3. What type of diet, if any, would you recommend for Mr. Garrett's hypertension? What suggestions might you offer to help him make the necessary diet changes? Are these diet changes consistent with those you would recommend for type IV hyperlipidemia? What blood value should be monitored regularly? Why?

4. Name at least three ways in which Mr. Garrett could benefit from losing weight. How can exercise fit into a weight loss plan? Plan a day's menu for Mr. Garrett based on the diet you would recommend for him.

5. Discuss nutrition considerations if Mr. Garrett should have a heart attack, CHF, or a stroke. Describe the relationships of these disorders to hyperlipidemia and hypertension.

FIGURE 25–2

Special feeding devices.

These cups can be used by people who cannot grasp handles well.

Using a plate with a built-up side allows food to be pushed onto a spoon or fork with one hand.

Utensils with built-up handles or cuffs are also useful for people who cannot grasp well.

Although it is important to provide adequate nutrients to the person with CHF, overfeeding the severely malnourished person is also a concern. Too rapid refeeding may increase the blood volume and metabolic rate and overload the already taxed heart. A gradual return to optimal intake is a wiser course.

Nutrition and the Stroke Victim

When blood flow to the brain is insufficient, or when blood vessels burst and blood flows into the brain, a stroke, or cerebrovascular accident (CVA), results. A stroke is actually a cerebrovascular rather than a cardiovascular disorder. Recovery for some stroke victims is unremarkable. The optimal diets for these people are based on their underlying medical condition (such as hyperlipidemia, hypertension, or obesity).

However, many stroke victims have either temporary or permanent problems with chewing, swallowing, and the physical process of eating. The care of people with difficulties in chewing and swallowing and the mechanical soft diet are discussed in Chapter 21. Tube feedings often are indicated initially. Many people who have problems with the physical aspects of eating can be helped a great deal through the use of special feeding devices. Several of these devices are shown in Figure 25–2.

Many other nutrition-related concerns may arise in people who have suffered strokes. For one, other medical conditions, such as hypertension or atherosclerosis, may require additional diet modifications. They may suffer from temporary or permanent problems that interfere with the ability to communicate. This makes it difficult to tell health care providers about foods they will eat or about problems they may be having with foods. Additionally, kcalories in the diet are a concern. kCalories may need to be limited due to inactivity. Clients who must relearn how to walk or use other muscle groups will be better able to do so if they are not overweight. However, underweight can be a problem for physical rehabilitation also, and care should be taken to ensure that the person does not become malnourished.

Nutrition Assessment

To help pinpoint areas of particular concern in the nutrition assessment of individuals with CVD, consider the following:

- In taking a diet history, pay particular attention to the total kcaloric intake and to the sodium, cholesterol, saturated fat, and polyunsaturated fat content of the diet. This will help you determine how significant recommended diet changes will be if they are necessary. The medical history will alert you to other conditions, such as diabetes, that may alter nutrient needs.
- Generally, anthropometric measurements in most people with CVD do not pose problems. The exception is the person with edema (such as in CHF).
- Standard lab values, such as albumin and transferrin, may be abnormal in people with either hypertension or CHF if they are retaining fluids. The serum cholesterol and triglyceride levels are monitored in people with hyperlipidemia. Monitoring serum potassium levels in people on diuretics is essential.

Regardless of the person you are assessing, look for factors in the history that increase the risk for CHD. Based on this information, you may be able to suggest a prudent diet and other relevant lifestyle changes before the problem of CHD becomes evident.

Study Questions

1. What is atherosclerosis? How can atherosclerosis lead to hypertension, thrombosis, angina, heart attacks, and strokes?
2. What diet does the American Heart Association recommend for all people to reduce the risk of heart disease? How do the recommendations change for the person with definite hyperlipidemias that involve elevated cholesterol and triglyceride levels? What diet is recommended for the person with type I or type V hyperlipidemia?
3. Describe other measures that may be useful for lowering serum lipid levels.
4. What is hypertension? What causes hypertension?
5. Discuss the role of diet in hypertension. What dietary advice would you give the person with hypertension? What suggestions could you give the person with hypertension to make the necessary diet changes easier to incorporate?
6. What is a myocardial infarct, and what events trigger an attack? Describe the diet therapy of the heart attack victim immediately after a heart attack, after several hours, and

after a week. State the rationale for each diet modification you list.

7. What is congestive heart failure? Why is malnutrition common in the person with CHF?

8. Describe the diet recommended for the person with CHF. What is the rationale for each of the recommendations? Discuss some special concerns that must be considered when feeding the person with CHF by tube feeding or TPN.

9. Consider some of the ways in which nutrition can be affected in the victim of a stroke. How can nutrition affect the way a person responds to physical therapy?

Notes

1. W. B. Kannel and T. J. Thom, Incidence, prevalence, and mortality of cardiovascular diseases, in *The Heart,* 6th ed., ed. J. W. Hurst (New York: McGraw-Hill, 1986), pp. 557–565.

2. Centers for Disease Control, Years of life lost from cardiovascular disease, *Journal of the American Medical Association* 256 (1986): 2794.

3. Lipid Research Clinics Program, The Lipid Research Clinics Coronary Primary Prevention Trial results: 1 and 2, *Journal of the American Medical Association* 79 (1984): 351–374.

4. Nutrition Committee and Council on Arteriosclerosis, American Heart Association, Recommendations for treatment of hyperlipidemia in adults, *Circulation* 69 (1984): 1065A–1090A; Consensus Conference: Lowering blood cholesterol to prevent heart disease, *Journal of the American Medical Association* 253 (1984): 363–371; M. E. DeBakey and coauthors, Diet, nutrition, and heart disease, *Journal of the American Dietetic Association* 86 (1986): 729–731.

5. J. Stamler, D. Wentworth, and J. D. Neaton, Is the relationship between serum cholesterol and risk of premature death from coronary heart disease continuous and graded? *Journal of the American Medical Association* 256 (1986): 2823–2828.

6. Nutrition Committee and Council on Arteriosclerosis, American Heart Association, 1984.

7. L. V. Van Horn and coauthors, Serum lipid response to oat product intake with a fat-modified diet, *Journal of the American Dietetic Association* 86 (1986): 759–764.

8. The Lovastatin Study Group II, Therapeutic response to lovastatin (Mevinolin) in nonfamilial hypercholesterolemia, *Journal of the American Medical Association* 256 (1986): 2829–2834.

9. E. D. Frohlich, Physiological observations in essential hypertension, *Journal of the American Dietetic Association* 80 (1982): 18–20.

10. Kannel and Thom, 1986.

11. Hypertension Detection and Follow-up Program Cooperative Group, The effect of treatment on mortality in "mild" hypertension, *New England Journal of Medicine* 307 (1982): 976–980.

12. J. A. Wilber, The role of diet in the treatment of high blood pressure, *Journal of the American Dietetic Association* 80 (1982): 25–29.

13. E. Reisin and coauthors, Effect of weight loss without salt restriction on the reduction of blood pressure in overweight hypertensive patients, *New England Journal of Medicine* 298 (1978): 1–6.

14. H. G. Langford and coauthors, Dietary therapy slows the return of hypertension after stopping prolonged medication, *Journal of the American Medical Association* 253 (1985): 657–664.

15. A. W. Caggiula, R. R. Wing, and R. G. Jacob, An apple a day: The role of potassium in the treatment of mild hypertension, *Behavioral Medicine Abstracts* 4 (Summer 1983): 137.

16. J. Onrot and coauthors, Hemodynamic and humoral effects of caffeine in autonomic failure, *New England Journal of Medicine* 313 (1985): 549–554.

17. Salt and high blood pressure, *Consumer Reports,* March 1979, pp. 147–149.

18. S. M. Poindexter, W. E. Dear, and S. J. Dudrick, Nutrition in congestive heart failure, *Nutrition in Clinical Practice* 1 (1986): 83–88.

19. R. W. Hamilton and V. M. Buckalew, Sodium, water and congestive heart failure, *Annals of Internal Medicine* 100 (1984): 902–903.

Nutrition and the Lungs

The heart and lungs work together to ensure the delivery of oxygen to the cells of the body and to remove wastes generated by metabolic processes in these cells. Although disorders of the heart have received much attention from health care professionals and from the public, nutrition for people with disorders of the lungs is a largely neglected area of clinical nutrition today. This is unfortunate, because mortality from obstructive lung diseases is increasing more rapidly than from cancer. (At the same time, mortality from cardiovascular and cerebrovascular diseases is actually decreasing; see Figure H25–1.) The cost of obstructive lung diseases in terms of health care, wages, and time lost from work exceeds $15 billion per year.[1]

Like heart disease, chronic obstructive pulmonary disease (COPD) appears to be multifactorial. Efforts have been under way to identify the risk factors for COPD and to clarify the disease process itself. One example of such an effort is a recent workshop on nutrition and the respiratory system sponsored by the National Institutes of Health.[2] Researchers are also looking for ways to improve the length and quality of life for people with COPD. Does nutrition play a role? Research in this area is scant, although some information is available.

A Word about COPD

COPD is a persistent obstruction of airflow through the lungs. The two major types of COPD are emphysema and chronic bronchitis. The primary risk factor for COPD is smoking. Other risk factors that may play a role include exposure to environmental pollution (including exposure of nonsmokers to cigarette smoke); alcohol consumption; family history of respiratory disorders; and, possibly, repeated respiratory tract infections in young children.

In emphysema, the small passages and air sacs (alveoli) within the lungs lose their elasticity. The victim has trouble exhaling to remove air taken in during inspiration. Stale air containing an excess of carbon dioxide becomes trapped in the lung, and the lung enlarges to accommodate the increased air volume. As the lung walls expand, they thin out; then they tend to collapse during exhalation. Emphysema is believed to be caused by the destruction of elastin, the major structural protein in the normal lung.

The individual with chronic bronchitis suffers from a different problem. In chronic bronchitis, excessive mucus is produced, which clogs the air passages (bronchioles). These passages also become inflamed, which contributes to the obstruction.

Regardless of the type of COPD, eventually the exchange of gases (oxygen and carbon dioxide) between

FIGURE H25–1

Percent change in death rates, 1970 to 1979. Among these leading causes of death in the United States, COPD is increasing most rapidly. (Data are adjusted for the aging of the population.)

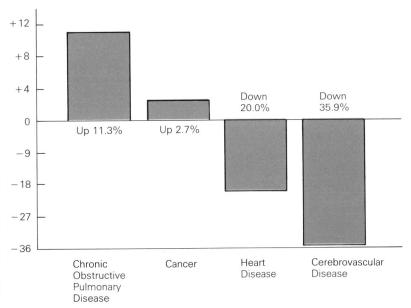

Source: U. S. Department of Health and Human Services, Ninth Report of the National Heart, Lung, and Blood Advisory Council, NIH publication no. 81–2334, 1981.

the atmosphere and the body becomes impaired. It becomes more difficult for the oxygen necessary for metabolism to reach the tissues, and for carbon dioxide (a waste product of metabolism) to be removed. No cure for COPD is available; treatment is aimed at relieving the symptoms.

Nutrition Risk Factors in the Development of COPD

At present, no known risk factors for the development of COPD are directly related to nutrition. However, a possibility that nutrition plays an indirect role clearly exists. For example, poor nutrition status in children has been associated with a high incidence of pulmonary infections (see Highlight 19). Investigators have also noticed a tendency toward emphysemalike changes in starving children and adults.[3] The lungs are constantly exposed to bacteria and viruses. Defense mechanisms in the lungs normally prevent these pathogens from entering the body. Nutrient deficiencies are associated with changes in the numbers and activity of various cells of the immune system in the lungs. In addition, there is reduced movement of the hairlike projections (cilia) in the lungs, that normally help to sweep pathogens out of the system. Thus bacterial adherence to lung cells increases.[4] Since repeated respiratory infections may be a risk factor for COPD, nutrition may have an indirect role in its development.

Nutrition Status and COPD

Once a person has developed COPD, two nutrition-related problems are frequently noted—weight loss and infection. PCM is widespread in people with COPD.[5] One study noted that hospitalized people with cancer and pulmonary diseases have the highest overall prevalence of malnutrition.[6] Measurements of nutrition status and

pulmonary function in these people suggest that nutrition status may be related to the severity of the disease.[7]

As COPD advances, weight loss progresses. The lungs are muscles that lose mass and strength as body weight decreases. This in turn negatively affects lung function. Furthermore, infections are more likely to occur in a client with poor nutrition status and pulmonary disease. The incidences of heart failure and mortality are higher in people with COPD who lose weight.[8]

Some possible explanations as to why many individuals with COPD are at risk for poor nutrition status include:

- Anorexia and poor food intake.
- Increased energy expenditure associated with labored breathing.
- Drug therapy.
- Increased energy needs during periods when mechanical ventilators are used to sustain adequate respiration.
- Repeated infections.

Weight loss in COPD has commonly been attributed to loss of appetite. However, many investigators have concluded that neither poor intake nor impaired absorption alone accounts for the weight loss.[9] Clients with stable COPD who weighed less than 75 percent of standard body weight reported higher kcalorie and protein intakes than COPD clients with body weights closer to standard.[10] The authors of the study concluded that kcalorie needs increase as the disease progresses; it is increased nutrient needs, not poor intake of nutrients, that explains weight loss in people with stable COPD. Still, anorexia and poor food intake may be a problem for the person with advanced COPD. The person may be unable to verbalize feelings of hunger and may not be able to take adequate nourishment.[11] When on a mechanical ventilator, the person may feel weak, uncomfortable and overwhelmed. Food consumption, and therefore protein and kcalorie intake, is frequently poor.[12]

requirements and contribute to poor nutrition status in people with COPD. People who require mechanical ventilation are in a hypermetabolic state, which also increases the risk of poor nutrition status.

The frequent respiratory infections seen in COPD also contribute to malnutrition. As we discussed in Highlight 19 and Chapter 20, infection raises nutrient needs, and nutrient deficiencies, in turn, can increase the likelihood of infection. The severe weight loss that can occur in COPD may create a vicious cycle of malnutrition and infection. Furthermore, if weakened by malnutrition, the lungs cannot expel bacteria as they normally do.

Another possibility is that weight loss in people with COPD may be an adaptive response.[13] People without COPD who lost weight during a period of semistarvation had a reduced metabolic rate and, therefore, a reduced need for respiratory gas exchange. This effect may actually be beneficial for the person with lung disease. Much more research is necessary to clarify this issue. Researchers hope to clearly delineate the exact mechanisms of weight loss in COPD in the near future. With this knowledge, the best approach in helping people with COPD to maintain weight can be defined and used in the clinical setting.

Nutrition and Respiratory Failure

In today's intensive care units, respiratory failure is a frequent cause of illness and death. Respiratory failure can occur as a result of advanced COPD or many other disorders. Respiratory failure occurs when the lungs are no longer able to perform their function in exchanging gases.

Malnutrition can contribute to respiratory failure in several ways. As discussed previously, lung muscle mass can be reduced as a result of malnutrition; this makes it harder for

Miniglossary

alveoli (al-VEE-oh-lie): air sacs in the lungs (one sac is an **alveolus**).

bronchioles (BRON-key-ohls): the small air passages from the trachea to the lungs.

bronchitis (bron-KYE-tis): inflammation of the lung's air passages.

bronchos = wind pipe

itis = inflammation

chronic obstructive pulmonary disease (COPD): diseases that cause blockage of the lung's air passages and thus interfere with the exchange of gases between the air and the body. Also called **chronic obstructive lung disease (COLD)** and **chronic obstructive airways diseases (COAD).**

elastin: a structural protein in the lung.

emphysema (EM-fe-SEE-ma): a type of COPD in which the lungs lose their elasticity and the victim becomes breathless.

intercostal muscles: the muscles between the ribs.

inter = between

costa = rib

mechanical ventilator: a machine that "breathes" for the person who can't.

Pickwickian syndrome: diminished pulmonary function caused by obesity.

pulmonary (PULL-mow-na-ree): concerning or involving the lungs.

respiratory failure: failure of the lungs to perform.

---

the malnourished person to carry on forceful respiratory movements and increases the likelihood of developing pulmonary infections. If serum protein levels fall dramatically, the osmotic pressure exerted by these proteins will be lost, and pulmonary edema can result.[14] When a mechanical ventilator is used, it may take longer to wean the person from the ventilator if the lungs are weak. Therefore, careful attention must be paid to meeting nutrition needs in people under intensive care.

People with respiratory failure spend more energy, especially during attempts to wean them from mechanical ventilation. The type of nutrients used to provide energy appears to be important. These people are often candidates for TPN, and standard TPN solutions are high in glucose. However, glucose generates more carbon dioxide when metabolized than does fat. High-glucose solutions may put additional stress on the lungs to rid the body of excess carbon dioxide. For this reason, many authorities currently recommend that the TPN solution derive half its

nonprotein kcalories from fat and half from glucose.[15] Little information is available regarding the use of tube feedings for nutrition support of the person in respiratory failure. One study addressed this question and reported the successful use of enteral nutrition in a few people.[16]

The Effect of Obesity on Pulmonary Function

The exchange of gases in the lungs is impaired in severe obesity. Obesity interferes with the ability of the intercostal muscles and the diaphragm to ventilate the lungs. The result is that the body can't retain enough oxygen and carbon dioxide levels remain high. This condition, called the Pickwickian syndrome, is characterized by lethargy and an uncontrolled tendency to sleep. The Pickwickian syndrome is the only known disorder in which excess adipose tissue, in the absence of any other contributing factors, can lead to death.[17]

Even in less severe obesity, more work is required of the lungs when extra weight is carried on the chest wall. As a result, obese people may have trouble breathing when they exercise or when they develop respiratory infections.

Much work remains to be done regarding nutrition and the lungs. The presentations here are brief and are only intended to call your attention to these neglected subjects.

NOTES

1. U.S. Department of Health and Human Services, *Ninth Report of the National Heart, Lung, and Blood Advisory Council*, NIH publication no. 81–2334 (Bethesda, Md.: National Heart and Lung Institute, 1981).

2. N. H. Edelman, R. B. Rucker, and H. H. Peavy, Nutrition and the respiratory system, *American Review of Respiratory Diseases* 134 (1986): 347–352.

3. A. Braude-Heller, J. Ratbalsam, and R. Elbinger, Clinique de la famine chez les enfants, as cited in J. Askanazi and coauthors, Nutrition and the respiratory system, *Critical Care Medicine* 10 (1982): 163–172.

4. Edelman, Rucker, and Peavy, 1986.

5. D. P. Murray and J. M. Blaloc, Nutritional status in stable outpatients with chronic obstructive pulmonary disease, *Abstracts in Clinical Research* 31 (1983): 65A.

6. L. Bushman and R. Russell, Malnutrition among patients in an acute-care veterans facility, *Journal of the American Dietetic Association* 77 (1980): 462–465.

7. N. L. Keim and coauthors, Dietary evaluation of outpatients with chronic obstructive pulmonary disease, *Journal of the American Dietetic Association* 86 (1986): 902–906.

8. E. Vandenbergh, K. P. van de Woestijne, and A. Gyselen, Weight changes in the terminal stages of chronic obstructive pulmonary disease: Relation to respiratory function and prognosis, *American Review of Respiratory Disease* 95 (1967): 556–566.

9. P. d'A Semple and co-authors, Diet, absorption and hormone studies in relation to body weight in obstructive airways disease, *Thorax* (1979): 738–788; A. M. Hunter, M. A. Carey, and H. W. Larsh, The nutritional status of patients with chronic obstructive pulmonary disease, *American*

Review of Respiratory Disease 124 (1981): 376–381.

10. Keim and coauthors, 1986.

11. C. N. Noller and S. Mobarhan, Enteral feeding in patients with advanced chronic obstructive pulmonary disease, *Nutritional Support Services* 6 (1986): 37–39.

12. A. G. Driver and M. LeBrun, Iatrogenic malnutrition in patients receiving ventilatory support, *Journal of the American Medical Association* 244 (1980): 2195–2196.

13. H. Bassili and coauthors, Effect of nutritional support on weaning patients off mechanical ventilators, *Journal of Parenteral and Enteral Nutrition* 5 (1981): 161-163.

14. Edelman, Rucker, and Peavy, 1986.

15. Noller and Mobarhan, 1986.

16. J. N. Armstrong, Nutrition and the respiratory patient, *Nutritional Support Services* 6 (1986): 8, 10, 32.

17. E. J. Drenick, Definition and consequences of morbid obesity, *Surgical Clinics of North America* 59 (1979): 963–979.

Disorders of the Kidneys

26

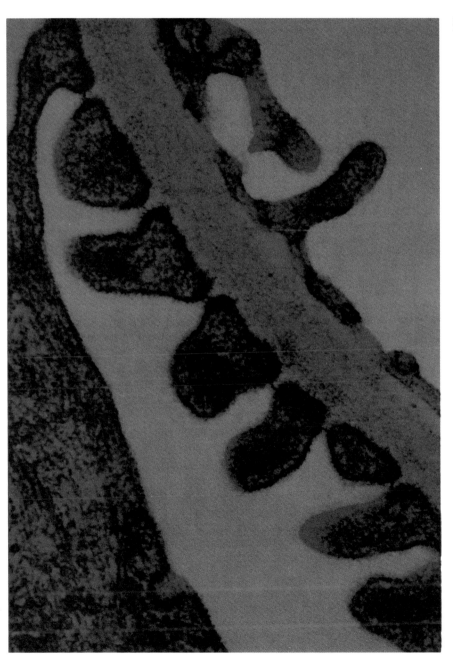

Contents

The art at the start of Chapter 24 showed a kidney glomerulus. Here is another view of kidney fine structure; the pink band is a membrane separating one working compartment from another.

The kidneys certainly illustrate the old adage that good things come in small packages. Although the kidneys are each only about the size of a fist, they are the key organs in the maintenance of chemical homeostasis in the body.

Probably the best way to appreciate the kidneys' vast importance is to learn what happens when they aren't working properly. Kidney failure can be a devastating, and frequently fatal, disease. However, the management of persons with renal disease has improved greatly, and today the prospect of a full, high-quality life is not beyond reach.

What the Kidneys Do

The kidneys are two bean-shaped organs located just above the waist on each side of the spinal column. The working unit of the kidney is the nephron. Figure 26–1 introduced the kidneys in a discussion of the vascular system in Chapter 6. It is presented again to illustrate the filteration of wastes from the blood and the relation of various kidney parts. Each of the approximately one million nephrons (per kidney) consists of a tuft of capillaries enclosed by a cup-shaped membrane called the *glomerulus,* and an associated tubule. The kidneys' job is to filter out substances that the body doesn't need and eliminate them in the urine. In so doing, these organs serve many important homeostatic functions: they maintain fluid, electrolyte, and acid-base balance; and they rid the body of metabolic waste products.

Some 1,200 milliliters of blood passes through the kidneys every minute—about one-quarter of the heart's total output. Blood rushes through the glomeruli at about 650 milliliters per minute, and from this blood, 120 milliliters of fluid filters through the glomeruli and enters the tubules. The fluid that enters the tubules, called the filtrate, is watery looking, because it is devoid of red blood cells. The rate at which filtrate is formed, known as the glomerular filtration rate (GFR), is an index of kidney function.

As the filtrate travels down the tubules, its composition is continually changing. In the end, substances the body needs are returned to the general circulation, and waste products (including excess metabolites) are eliminated in the urine. Thus the kidneys maintain chemical homeostasis.

The work of the kidneys doesn't end here. They help regulate blood pressure by secreting the enzyme renin and by responding to the hormone aldosterone (see Figure 26–2). The kidneys also produce another hormone, erythropoietin, which stimulates red blood cell production. Finally, the kidney is the site where vitamin D is converted to its active form. Active vitamin D plays an essential role in normal calcium absorption, calcium and phosphorus metabolism, and bone maintenance.

The **nephron** (NEF-ron), the working unit of the kidney, consists of the glomerulus and a tubule. The **glomerulus** (glow-MARE-you-lus) is a cup-shaped membrane enclosing a tuft of capillaries. The first part of the **tubule** surrounds the glomerulus. A pressure gradient between the glomerulus and the tubule returns needed materials to the blood and sends wastes to the bladder.

The kidneys:
- Maintain fluid, electrolyte, and acid-base balance.
- Eliminate metabolic waste products.
- Help regulate blood pressure.
- Produce a hormone that stimulates red blood cell production.
- Activate vitamin D.

glomerular filtration rate (GFR): the rate at which filtrate is formed by the nephron. Normally, GFR is between 90 and 120 ml/min.

Blood Vessel Carrying Blood into Glomerulus

Glomerulus

Capillaries of Glomerulus

Blood Vessel Carrying Blood Away from Glomerulus

Tubules

Blood Vessel Carrying Blood Back to Body

Blood Vessel Carrying Blood Alongside Tubule

To the Bladder

FIGURE 26–1

One of the kidney's many functioning nephrons. Blood flows into the glomerulus, and some of its fluid is filtered into the tubules (1). Then the blood passes alongside the tubules, which return fluid and substances needed by the body (2). The waste materials that remain pass from the tubules on to the bladder (3).

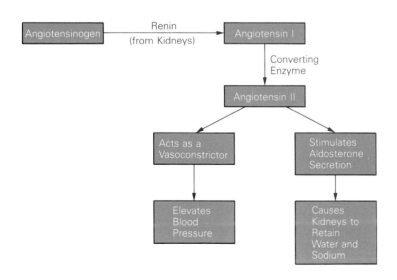

Angiotensinogen

Renin (from Kidneys)

Angiotensin I

Converting Enzyme

Angiotensin II

Acts as a Vasoconstrictor

Stimulates Aldosterone Secretion

Elevates Blood Pressure

Causes Kidneys to Retain Water and Sodium

FIGURE 26–2

The renin-angiotensin mechanism. Renin from the kidney splits the plasma protein angiotensinogen to form angiotensin I; in the presence of another enzyme, angiotensin I is activated to angiotensin II, which acts as a vasoconstrictor and stimulates aldosterone secretion. The net effect is to raise blood pressure.

Renal Failure

renal failure: failure of the nephrons to maintain normal function.

Chronic renal failure [is like] a downhill course for your patient; acute renal failure is like seeing him go over a cliff no one quite knew was there.

                                    J. L. Stark

nephritis (nef-RYE-tis): inflammation of the kidney. **Pyelonephritis** (PIE-eh-low-neh-FRY-tis) is an inflammation of the kidney and bladder, and **glomerulonephritis** (glow-MARE-you-low-neh-FRY-tis) is an inflammation of the glomerular capillaries.

Impairment of renal blood flow because of renal artery damage is called **nephrosclerosis** (NEF-row-skle-ROW-sis). It can be caused by hypertension or atherosclerosis.

uremia (you-REE-me-ah): toxic waste products in the blood, associated with renal insufficiency.

uremic syndrome: a complex of symptoms seen late in renal failure, caused by uremia.

When urea (which can be excreted through sweat) crystallizes and becomes visible on the skin, the condition is called **uremic frost.**

With all these vital functions to perform, it is easy to see why renal failure results in serious consequences. Renal failure can occur suddenly (acute renal failure) or over a period of time (chronic renal failure). It occurs when the nephrons lose sufficient function so that they cannot maintain normal homeostatic and hormonal mechanisms. Oftentimes acute renal failure is only temporary. Chronic renal failure is usually irreversible.

Renal disease may be caused by damage to the kidneys themselves, as in nephritis, renal artery obstruction, nephrotic syndrome (see below), kidney stones (see Highlight 26), and renal tubular disorders. Renal failure can also result from other diseases, such as diabetic nephropathy, hypertension, atherosclerosis, and septic shock.

As the nephrons fail, the composition of the blood and urine changes. Therefore, laboratory tests of these fluids are useful for the evaluation of renal function. Clearance tests measure the GFR, which is reduced as renal failure progresses. Blood urea nitrogen (BUN), creatinine, and uric acid are the body's principal nitrogen-containing metabolic waste products. They accumulate in the blood when renal function is impaired, and high levels of BUN, creatinine, and uric acid are seen in the person with renal failure.

As renal failure progresses to a severe stage, the buildup of toxic waste products in the blood (uremia) precipitates a complex of symptoms called the uremic syndrome. The person with uremia experiences a wide array of symptoms in virtually every body system. Fatigue, weakness, decreased mental alertness, muscular twitches, muscle cramps, anorexia, nausea, vomiting, stomatitis, and an unpleasant taste in the mouth are some of these symptoms. The skin may itch uncomfortably. In later stages, GI ulcers and bleeding are common.

Chronic Renal Disease

The capacity of the kidney to function despite loss of some nephrons is referred to as **renal reserve.**

Abnormal accumulation of nitrogen-containing substances in the blood is called **azotemia** (AZE-oh-TEE-me-ah). Normal BUN levels are 10 to 20 mg/dl. A BUN of 50 to 150 mg/dl indicates serious impairment of renal function. BUN may rise to as high as 150 to 250 mg/dl in end-stage renal disease.

In chronic renal disease, the nephrons are gradually and progressively destroyed. The remaining nephrons get bigger in an attempt to maintain normal functioning. The hypertrophied nephrons work so efficiently that about 80 percent of the nephrons can be destroyed before renal function is seriously affected. The GFR may decrease to one-tenth of the normal rate—10 to 12 milliliters per minute—before symptoms appear. You can see, then, why renal disease may be advanced before it is even detected.

The early stages of renal disease generally involve no dietary restrictions. However, as nitrogen-containing waste products build up in the blood and the GFR is reduced, the person with renal disease benefits from dietary restrictions aimed at preventing hypertension, edema, congestive heart failure, and uremia.

The diet is prescribed and regularly adjusted based on the degree of renal insufficiency.

Eventually, if renal failure progresses far enough, diet alone cannot prevent uremia. At this point, the person must begin dialysis or receive a kidney transplant to survive. (See box entitled "Dialysis and Kidney Transplants.")

The metabolism of nutrients and their end products is significantly affected by renal failure for many reasons. Some of these include:

- Failure to excrete toxic waste products.
- Inability of the renal tubules to reabsorb many needed nutrients.
- Reduced GI absorption of some nutrients.
- Reduced inactivation of many hormones, including insulin, parathyroid hormone, glucagon, and thyrotropin.
- Reduced synthesis of other important substances, such as erythropoietin and active vitamin D.
- Alteration of nutrient needs by other medical therapy (drugs and dialysis).
- Limited food intake because of GI distress, depression, superimposed illnesses, or restrictive or unpalatable diets.

Because of these difficulties, the nutrition status of people with chronic renal disease is often compromised. The child with renal disease often fails to grow normally, and people of any age with renal disease may have reduced muscle mass, fat tissue, and visceral protein levels. These characteristics are frequently called the *wasting syndrome*. Special attention to nutrient needs can help prevent this problem. The objectives of dietary management of chronic renal failure are:

- To achieve or maintain optimal nutrition status and nitrogen balance.
- To prevent the buildup of toxic metabolic products, thus minimizing the risk of uremia.
- To delay progression of renal failure, thus postponing the need for dialysis.
- To foster the client's well-being.
- To prevent complications, such as growth failure, wasting syndrome, bone disease, hypertension, edema, and congestive heart failure.

The severe stage of renal disease in which diet alone is no longer effective in maintaining normal functions is called **end-stage renal disease (ESRD)**.

Normal GFR is between 90 and 120 ml/min. Dialysis is usually initiated when the GFR falls below 4 to 5 ml/min.

The next several sections are written as if they were addressed to the diet planner: " 'You' must reduce protein in this condition, increase kcalories in that." In fact, you, the reader, may not be the diet planner, but it is important for you to understand what that person has to do. As you read the following sections, notice how complex the diet for renal disease is and how critical the control of certain nutrients is. Pay close attention to what those nutrients are, keeping in mind how food choices will be affected by restrictions placed on those nutrients.

When you communicate with someone who has renal disease, with a member of the client's family, or with another person on the health care team, it may not be necessary for you to know that the client is allowed exactly 20 grams of protein a day. What is important is to know *why* protein must be restricted. Whatever your place on the team, you are most effective if you truly understand the disease and the necessity of the renal diet.

Dialysis and Kidney Transplants

The kidneys are virtually irreplaceable. No perfect substitute for one's own kidneys has been found. However, although they fall short of the real thing, dialysis and kidney transplants can be lifesaving for the person with ESRD. Dialysis works on the principles of simple diffusion and osmosis through a semipermeable membrane. When the membrane that covers the abdominal organs (the peritoneum) serves as the semipermeable membrane, then the procedure is called *peritoneal dialysis.* A synthetic semipermeable membrane also can be used. In this case, blood leaves the person's artery and passes through tubing made of semipermeable membranes. The tubes are continually bathed by solutions which selectively remove unwanted material. The blood returns to the body through the person's vein after being cleansed. This procedure is called *hemodialysis.*

The way dialysis works is actually simple. A solution similar in composition to normal blood plasma, called the *dialysate,* is placed on one side of the semipermeable membrane; the person's blood flows by on the other side. The blood has a higher concentration of urea and electrolytes than the dialysate, so these substances diffuse from the blood into the dialysate. The dialysate also contains glucose; the higher the concentration of glucose in the dialysate, the more fluid will move from the blood into the dialysate by osmosis.

In hemodialysis, the blood is returned to the person's body after it has passed through the machine that houses the semipermeable membrane and dialysate. Oftentimes, the person with chronic renal failure on hemodialysis gets four- to eight-hour treatments three times a week.

In peritoneal dialysis, the dialysate is infused directly through a tube into the person's abdomen. The fluid is kept in the abdomen for about 30 minutes, then drained from the peritoneal cavity by gravity. One complete exchange takes about an hour. The total treatment takes from 24 to 72 hours.

Dialysis takes over two important functions of the kidney: waste removal and fluid removal. In so doing, dialysis reduces the symptoms of uremia, hypertension, and edema, as well as the risk of congestive heart failure. But the hormonal functions of the kidney are not restored. Anemia is a problem. Hypertension may still persist, and hypotension can be a problem if too much fluid is removed during dialysis.

A preferred alternative to dialysis in ESRD is a kidney transplant. Kidney transplants can successfully restore kidney function and normal growth. For this reason, transplants are particularly desirable in children. People who generally are not considered as candidates for kidney transplants are the elderly, people with other life-threatening conditions, or people who prefer dialysis. Given a choice, many would prefer transplants; however, a suitable kidney donor can't always be found.

Finding a suitable kidney donor is of paramount importance. Once a kidney has been transplanted, it will be rejected and treated as a foreign protein unless the cells of the donor and recipient are properly matched. Without such a match, a transplant cannot take place. So many advances have been made in the area of renal transplants, particularly the availability

dialysis (dye-AL-ih-sis): removal of waste from the blood using the principles of simple diffusion and osmosis through a semipermeable membrane.

peritoneal (PERR-ee-toe-NEE-al) **dialysis:** removal of waste from the blood using the peritoneum as a semipermeable membrane.

hemodialysis (HE-mow-dye-AL-ih-sis): removal of wastes from the blood by passing it outside the body through tubes made of semipermeable membranes submerged in a water solution.

Diffusion is illustrated on p. 183; osmosis, on p. 377.

of drugs that help guard against rejection of the new organ, that such procedures have become much safer and far more common in recent years.

After the new kidney is in place, the person must take very large doses of corticosteroids to prevent rejection. Muscular weakness, GI bleeding, carbohydrate intolerance, sodium retention, hypertension, and a characteristic puffy-faced appearance commonly occur due to the medical therapy. Infections and increased susceptibility to malignant tumors are also common. The kidney may be rejected or fail to function, in which case dialysis must be reinstituted.

The actual diet is highly individualized. The one most often prescribed is a protein-restricted diet in which total kcalories, sodium, potassium, phosphorus, and fluids are carefully controlled.

Energy and Protein

Providing the right amount of protein to the person in renal failure is like walking a tightrope. Too little protein, and the person develops malnutrition. Too much protein, and blood urea levels (the toxic waste product of protein metabolism) rise. Studies of adults with chronic renal failure have shown that people who eat unrestricted-protein diets show a more rapid decline in renal function than people maintained on diets containing from 0.55 to 0.60 grams of protein per kilogram of body weight per day.[1] Other studies have shown that diets containing from 0.4 to 0.6 grams of protein per kilogram of body weight per day delay or halt the progression of chronic renal failure.[2] Even a moderate protein restriction (1 gram per kilogram of body weight per day) has shown value in improving renal function in people with chronic renal failure.[3]

Ideally, the diet should provide enough essential amino acids to support normal nitrogen balance without causing BUN levels to rise. Protein is adjusted to the kidneys' ability to excrete wastes, as measured by the GFR. Just as important as the amount of protein in the diet is the quality of the protein. Sources of protein with high biological value, such as eggs, milk, meat, poultry, and fish, are given the greatest emphasis.

Clinicians disagree about when a low-protein diet becomes too low to maintain nutrition status. Some investigators believe that once the GFR falls below 4 to 5 milliliters per minute, dialysis is needed so that protein intake can be adequate without precipitating uremia. However, others continue to give diets low in protein (about 20 grams) to avoid the need for dialysis. Virtually all of the protein in this type of diet must be of high quality.

The concept of supplying a low-protein diet high in essential amino acids to people with renal failure was first introduced by Giordano, Giovannetti, and Maggiore.[4] The rationale of the diet (often called the G-G, or Giordano-Giovannetti, diet) is that excess urea in the blood, together with essential amino acids in the diet, can be used by the body to synthesize nonessential amino acids. In theory, by using urea in this way, blood urea levels can be reduced and adequate protein can be supplied at the same time. Unfortunately, it appears that the use of endogenous urea for protein synthesis is limited. Furthermore, these diets are restrictive and unpalatable. It is often difficult to get people to

The diet must provide just enough protein to maintain nutrition status without precipitating uremia.

Urea is the waste product, normally excreted, into which many of the body's unused amino groups (NH_2) are collected:

Urea

$$\underset{H_2N}{}\;\overset{\overset{\displaystyle O}{\|}}{C}\;\underset{NH_2}{}\quad \text{Amino Groups}$$

When you replace the amino group (NH_2) of an amino acid with a hydroxy group (OH), you have made a keto-acid analogue. For example, pyruvic acid is the keto-acid analogue of alanine:

Pyruvic Acid (keto-acid)

$$\begin{array}{c} COOH \\ | \\ HC - OH \\ | \\ CH_3 \end{array}$$

Alanine (amino acid)

$$\begin{array}{c} COOH \\ | \\ HC - NH_2 \\ | \\ CH_3 \end{array}$$

In renal failure, it is hoped that the body will draw upon its unexcreted urea to put NH_2 back on the keto-acid analogues, making the amino acids it needs.

E. H., an adult with chronic renal failure, is on peritoneal dialysis (see Table 26–1). At 155 lb, she has the following protein needs:
1.2 g/kg × 70 kg = 84 g.
1.5 g/kg × 70 kg = 105 g.

E. H. has the following energy needs:
35 kcal/kg × 70 kg = 2,450 kcal.
50 kcal/kg × 70 kg = 3,500 kcal.
For comparison, a 12-year-old child who weighs only 34 kg (75 lb) would require more than 2,500 kcal/day for optimal growth.

When urine volume is minimal, **oliguria** exists; **anuria** means that no urine at all is being excreted.

consume adequate kcalories on a very-low-protein diet; without enough kcalories, protein will be used for energy.

However, researchers have been expanding on this concept, and new approaches to diet show promise. Very-low-protein diets supplemented with keto-acid analogues of essential amino acids have been effective in the maintenance of acceptable nitrogen balance while reducing the symptoms of uremia.[5] More recently, a study suggests that the addition of keto-acids to a low-protein diet delays the rate of renal deterioration.[6] However, another study suggests that while a low-protein diet supplemented with keto-acid analogues may slow the decline in renal function in some people, muscle mass may also be lost.[7] Additional research is needed to define the risks and benefits of these diets.

Once the decision has been made to use dialysis, protein intake is less restrictive. Table 26–1 illustrates how protein needs change during dialysis. Regardless of the protein allowance, all people with renal failure need adequate energy to maintain or achieve ideal body weight and to prevent protein catabolism. For adults, at least 35 kcalories per kilogram of body weight per day should be given.[8] For children, energy intake should at least meet the RDA.[9] One hundred or even more kcalories per kilogram per day is often desirable, and about 80 kcalories per kilogram of body weight per day is considered a realistic intake. Below 40 kcalories per kilogram of body weight per day, a child cannot grow at all.

Because the renal diet often is low in protein, kcalories from nonprotein sources are very important. Recommend the frequent use of fats (margarine, cream, and butter) and concentrated sweets (hard candy and jelly) to improve kcalorie intake.

To provide adequate kcalories from nonprotein sources may not sound like a difficult task. However, the person with renal disease frequently also has diabetes. Furthermore, renal disease and diabetes are both associated with abnormal serum lipids (see Chapter 25) and atherosclerosis. For the person with renal disease with diabetes, concentrated sweets must be avoided. The best treatment of lipid abnormalities in renal disease is not known.

Fluid and Electrolytes

Renal disease causes disturbances in the sea of fluid and electrolytes that bathes the cells. Early in renal failure, the kidneys lose the ability to reabsorb sodium as normal kidneys do. Therefore, even though renal volume may be reduced somewhat, the person can maintain sodium balance on a moderate sodium intake. However, as ESRD approaches, less urine is excreted, and the person cannot handle normal amounts of sodium. This increases the risk of developing hypertension, edema, and heart failure. At this point, sodium and water are restricted. A typical diet will contain from 1 to 3 grams of sodium and 1,500 to 3,000 milliliters of fluid daily.

A person on dialysis excretes little or no urine and may need to further restrict sodium and fluids. Fluid intake is controlled to allow a weight gain of about 2 to 2 1/2 pounds between dialysis treatments. Foods that are considered part of the fluid allowance are listed in Table 26–2. Sodium is a special concern for the person on peritoneal dialysis, because sodium is not effectively removed by this type of dialysis. Table 26–1 shows how requirements of fluid and minerals vary in renal disease.

TABLE 26–1

Typical Nutrient Needs in Chronic Renal Failure

	Predialysis	Hemodialysis	Peritoneal Dialysis
Energy (kcal/kg)	35–50	35–50	35–50
Protein (g/kg)	0.55–0.60	1.0–1.2	1.2–1.5
Fluid (ml)	1,500–3,000	750–1,500	750–1,500
Sodium (g)	1.0–3.0	1.0–1.5	1.0–1.5
Potassium (g)	1.5–2.8	1.5–2.8	3.0–3.5
Phosphorus (mg)	600–1,200	600–1,200	600–1,200
Supplements			
Calcium (mg)	1,200–1,600	1,000	1,200–1,600
Folacin (mg)	1	1	1
Vitamin B_6 (mg)	5	10	10
Vitamin C (mg)	70–100	100	100
Other water-soluble			
vitamins	RDA	RDA	RDA
Vitamin D	As appropriate	As appropriate	As appropriate

*The actual amounts of these nutrients in the diet must be highly individualized based on each person's responses.
Source: Adapted from J. D. Kopple, Nutritional therapy in kidney failure, *Nutrition Reviews* 39 (1981): 193–206; D. J. Rodriguez and V. M. Hunter, Nutritional intervention in chronic renal failure, *Nursing Clinics of North America* 16 (1981): 573–585.

Individual needs vary, and the way that needs are determined is by carefully monitoring weight, blood pressure, and urine output. Body weight and blood pressure increase when sodium and fluid are retained and decrease if sodium intake is too low. Urine output is also useful as a basis for the estimation of daily fluid needs. Simply add 500 milliliters—for insensible water loss—to the 24-hour urine output.

Potassium is another electrolyte that may be of concern for the person with renal failure. Most people with renal failure do not have problems handling typical intakes of potassium. However, hyperkalemia can occur, and if it does, it can be fatal. Therefore, potassium is moderately restricted to about 1.5 to

The little girl beams with pleasure when Charlie, the nurse, comes into the room. This is one of the high points of her day. "Do you have a lollipop for me?" she asks.

"Yep," says Charlie, reaching into his pocket. "Your favorite color, red. Eat it all up, and I'll bring you another one."

Why is this nurse feeding the child candy? Because the child has renal disease and has a hard time getting enough kcalories to protect the protein she eats, the staff has been instructed to keep giving her sugar in whatever form she will accept it. A lollipop is like a clear liquid, because it melts in the mouth; it contains no protein or electrolytes to burden the kidney; but it offers sugar to help spare protein. Nothing could be more appropriate for this growing child's health.

TABLE 26–2

Foods and Beverages Controlled on Fluid-restricted Diets

Beverages	
Alcoholic beverages	Milk
Carbonated beverages	Tea
Coffee	Water
Juices	Any other

Foods*	
Ice cream (melts to ½ initial volume)	Popsicles
Ice milk (melts to ½ initial volume)	Sherbet (melts to ⅔ initial volume)
Jello	Soup

Other	
Cream	Ice (melts to 9/10 initial volume)

*Although all foods contain some water, these are the foods considered part of the fluid allowance on a fluid-restricted diet.

2.8 grams per day. Table 25–5 in Chapter 25 lists foods high in potassium. Recommend that the person with renal failure avoid these foods. However, individual needs vary. If the person is also on potassium-wasting diuretics (see Chapter 25), then potassium intake may need to be increased.

Phosphorus, Calcium, and Vitamin D

Normally, the body maintains a balance of phosphorus and calcium in the blood. When phosphorus levels rise, calcium falls, and vice versa. The parathyroid hormone (PTH) and active vitamin D play essential roles in maintaining this balance, which, in turn, is extremely important in the maintenance of bone structure. Bone disease frequently occurs in the person with chronic renal failure, because this balance is upset. In recent years, the mechanisms involved in bone disease have been studied extensively but have not been clearly defined. Several factors seem to interact to cause bone disease.

First of all, phosphorus is normally excreted in the urine when serum levels are elevated. But in renal disease, phosphorus is retained. As serum phosphorus levels rise, serum calcium levels fall. The low serum calcium concentration triggers the release of PTH, which works to increase calcium levels by promoting the renal excretion of phosphorus.

For a while, this helps maintain lower serum phosphorus and higher serum calcium levels, but every time the GFR falls, more PTH is needed to maintain effectiveness. Hyperparathyroidism develops. Finally, as the GFR continues to drop, PTH becomes ineffective in reducing serum phosphorus levels.

These problems are compounded by the diseased kidney's making little or no active vitamin D. Under normal conditions, active vitamin D works with PTH to help mobilize calcium from bone and increase serum calcium levels. With less active vitamin D available, PTH has to work harder to maintain normal serum calcium levels. Calcium absorption in the GI tract is also impaired, further lowering serum calcium. Additionally, diets that are restricted in protein and phosphorus tend to be low in calcium as well.

Every day the renal team sees a group of adults and children. Many of the adults have had renal transplants, and their kidneys are now functioning well; before they received the transplants, however, they had already suffered irreversible growth failure. Many of the children are small for their age. They are suffering growth failure now, and the team must seize the chance to make up the deficit before the end of puberty.

The net result is that the normal bone matrix is disrupted. The bones become soft (demineralized) and fracture easily. Growth retardation is common. The person with renal bone disease may experience bone pain related to the hyperparathyroidism. The high levels of ineffective PTH can cause the total amount of phosphorus to stay high. When this happens, phosphorus and calcium may form a salt that is deposited in soft tissues and blood vessels. Figure 26–3 summarizes the events that lead to renal osteodystrophy, the defective bone development seen in renal disease.

The cycle of events leading to renal osteodystrophy is largely preventable through dietary control. Phosphorus levels are maintained in the low normal range (2 to 3 milligrams per 100 milliliters) by reduction of phosphorus intake. The amount of phosphorus given depends on the degree of renal function. (Generally, a low-protein diet is low in phosphorus anyway.) Table 26–3 lists foods high in phosphorus. Researchers have reported that the progression rate of advanced renal failure can be delayed if phosphorus is restricted along with protein.[10] If diet alone fails to keep phosphorus levels in check, the client may be asked to take phosphate binders, aluminum-containing antacids that work by binding phosphorus in the GI tract, thus making it unavailable for absorption.

renal osteodystrophies (OS-tee-oh-DIS-tro-fees): bone disorders resulting from calcium and phosphorus imbalances in renal disease.

One type of renal osteodystrophy that leads to a softening of the bones is called osteomalacia (see p. 355).

A type of renal osteodystrophy that results from hyperparathyroidism and is characterized by kidney stones, decalcification and softening of bones, and, sometimes, formation of cysts and tumors is called osteitis (os-tee-EYE-tis) fibrosis.

The deposition of phosphorus and calcium salts in soft tissue is called metastatic (MET-ah-STAT-ik) calcification.

FIGURE 26–3

Events leading to renal osteodystrophy.

TABLE 26-3

Foods High in Phosphorus

Chocolate	Milk and milk products
Cocoa	Nuts
Dried beans and peas	Organ meats
Dried fruit	Peanut butter
Fish, canned	Whole-grain breads
Game meats	Whole-grain cereals

Most people with renal disease receive 1,200 to 1,600 milligrams of calcium in supplement form each day to help prevent bone disease. Large doses of vitamin D (50,000 to 200,000 international units daily) can be given to improve the absorption and utilization of calcium. Recently, the active form of vitamin D has become available commercially, and its use is on the rise. Much smaller doses of active vitamin D or synthetic analogues can achieve the desired effect. The dosage must be carefully tailored to the individual to prevent hypercalcemia. (Active vitamin D is not given if serum phosphorus levels are high because further deterioration of renal function can occur under this circumstance.)

Other Nutrients

Vitamin deficiencies frequently develop in people with renal failure. The restrictive diet is partly responsible, since diets low in potassium also are low in water-soluble vitamins. Vitamins can also be lost during dialysis, and drug therapy can change nutrient needs. Uremia can affect the metabolism of nutrients. For these reasons, generous amounts of vitamin B_6 (5 milligrams), vitamin C (70 to 100 milligrams), and folacin (1 milligram) are given, along with the RDA of the remaining water-soluble vitamins. People on dialysis have higher needs for vitamin B_6 (10 milligrams) and vitamin C (100 milligrams). Other than vitamin D, supplementation of the fat-soluble vitamins is usually not necessary.

People with renal failure should never take antacids, laxatives, or enemas that are high in magnesium; serious hypermagnesemia can result.

Iron-deficiency anemia is frequently seen in people with chronic renal failure, and they often receive iron supplements. Many factors increase the risk of iron deficiency in renal failure. For one thing, the person may lose blood (and iron), because blood is drawn frequently for testing. Additionally, GI bleeding is fairly common. People on hemodialysis may lose some blood during dialysis. Finally, the intestinal absorption of iron may be impaired in people with uremia. Anemia unrelated to iron deficiency can also occur. The limited production of erythropoietin leads to reduced synthesis of red blood cells to carry oxygen. The toxins that accumulate in renal failure can shorten the life span of the existing red blood cells, thus compounding the problem.

Zinc may be deficient in people on dialysis. They frequently complain of anorexia and altered taste perceptions (dysgeusia); these features are typical of zinc deficiency. Studies of supplemental zinc as related to improved taste sensitivity and appetite have shown variable results and are inconclusive. However, for people with uremia, oral zinc supplements may help to restore cell-mediated immunity (see Highlight 19).[11]

Aluminum toxicity also may be a problem for people on dialysis. Contamination of the dialysate with aluminum has been linked to mental disturbances, bone fractures, and a severe anemia. The nutrient needs of people with renal disease are summarized in Table 26–1.

A deranged mental state seen in some people on dialysis and characterized by abnormal speech, muscle spasms, and convulsions—**dialysis encephalopathy**—has been associated with aluminum toxicity.

Nutrition and Kidney Transplants

The person with a kidney transplant is allowed a much freer choice of foods than the person on dialysis, provided that renal function is normal; however, the drugs that must be taken can cause some nutrition problems. Depending on the person's medical status, the following measures may be necessary:

- Restrict kcalories to avoid excessive weight gain. (Corticosteroids can stimulate the appetite.)
- Increase protein intake. (Corticosteroids can increase protein catabolism and lead to negative nitrogen balance.)
- Restrict sodium. (Hypertension and edema often accompany corticosteroid treatment.)
- Avoid concentrated sweets. (Glucose intolerance can develop in people taking corticosteroids.)
- Increase potassium. (Many people with renal transplants are on potassium-wasting diuretics.)

People with kidney transplants may develop temporary periods of kidney rejection, or they may permanently reject their new kidneys. During these times, they must go back on a renal failure diet. This may be difficult to accept, and clients should be prepared for this possibility before it occurs.

Helpful Hints

If you think a renal diet is difficult to plan, think of what it must be like to follow. The shock of finding out you have renal disease is quite enough. Being told about the restrictive diet makes matters worse. People who have just been told they have renal disease must cope with many changes. Don't expect them to understand instructions (including diet instructions) in one session. Explain the concept of the diet several times, and evaluate the person's compliance frequently.

Many people on a renal failure diet can comply with a sodium restriction by following a no-added-salt diet (see Table 25–4 in Chapter 25). However, caution the person not to use low-sodium products and salt substitutes, because they often contain potassium. Potassium can be kept in check if foods high in potassium are avoided (see Table 25–5 in Chapter 25). Similarly, phosphorus intake can be controlled (see Table 26–3). Encourage your clients to measure foods and to be sure kcaloric intake is adequate.

The severe thirst experienced by many people with renal failure makes compliance with fluid restriction extremely difficult. One method for helping people monitor their fluid intake is to have them fill a container with water in the amount of their total fluid allowance at the start of each day. For example, they can fill a jar with 1,500 milliliters of water if this is their fluid allowance. Every time they use a liquid food or drink, an equivalent amount of water is discarded from the container. They can look at the jar to see how much fluid they have

No doubt you have long since arrived at the conclusion that designing renal diets is a task for a specialist. The complexities pile up: the diet planner must raise/lower intakes of sodium, potassium, protein, kcalories, liquids, lipids, vitamins, and minerals. Then food combinations that will deliver the necessary amounts of these nutrients must be found. Not only that, these must be foods that *the individual on the diet will accept and enjoy.* The renal dietitian faces these challenges every day.

With all that hard work to do, the diet planner has still another task—communicating with, and especially listening to, the individual. Inside that tangled web of grossly altered metabolic processes, dialysis lines, and toxic waste products is a person—often, a frightened or discouraged one. One person will say he dreams of ice cream sodas, forbidden for their high sodium content; he needs at least to feel understood. Another says she feels guilty because her mother spends so much time preparing special foods for her; she, too, needs support. Another is fighting guilt and resentment because repeatedly, in spite of the rules he knows he should follow, he sneaks forbidden foods high in protein. If you have ever been on a diet, even though it wasn't a renal diet, you will appreciate some of the problems these people face.

The life the person with renal disease has to live involves many frustrations. Successful treatment often hinges on compliance with diet and drug orders. All the members of the health care team need to know what is involved, if they are to offer the most effective possible support.

left for the day. Remind the person to save some of the fluid allowance for taking medications. Some other suggestions to help control thirst:

- Chew gum or suck hard candy.
- Freeze fluids so that they take longer to consume.
- Add lemon juice to water to make it more refreshing.
- Gargle with refrigerated mouthwash.

Sample renal diet menu (60 grams of protein, sodium and potassium controlled). Increase the kcalories in this diet by preparing food with oil or unsalted margarine (regular margarine, if allowed) and using additional sugar or syrup whenever possible. For example, eating canned fruit packed in heavy syrup, rather than in juice, adds kcalories.

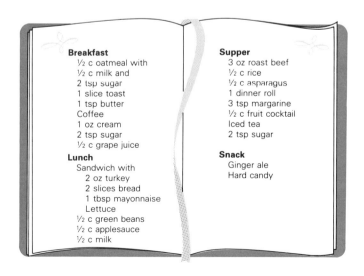

Breakfast
½ c oatmeal with
½ c milk and
2 tsp sugar
1 slice toast
1 tsp butter
Coffee
1 oz cream
2 tsp sugar
½ c grape juice

Lunch
Sandwich with
  2 oz turkey
  2 slices bread
  1 tbsp mayonnaise
  Lettuce
½ c green beans
½ c applesauce
½ c milk

Supper
3 oz roast beef
½ c rice
½ c asparagus
1 dinner roll
3 tsp margarine
½ c fruit cocktail
Iced tea
2 tsp sugar

Snack
Ginger ale
Hard candy

ickey is a nine-year-old child who developed chronic glomerulonephritis several months after suffering from a streptococcal infection (strep throat). Mickey's renal function has declined steadily over the last three years. Mickey's mother brought him in to see his physician because Mickey had been very tired, unable to eat, and complaining of stomach cramps and unpleasant taste sensations. Laboratory tests revealed the following information:

GFR : 4 ml/min (below normal).
BUN : 102 mg/dl (above normal).

Mickey was admitted to the hospital, and dialysis was begun. A search for a suitable kidney donor was also begun. Mickey is 3′8″ tall and weighs 40 lb. Before coming to the hospital, Mickey was following a 30-g-protein, no-

CASE STUDY

Chronic Renal Failure

added-salt, potassium- and fluid-restricted diet. His typical kcalorie intake is 1,100 kcal/day.

1. Describe chronic renal failure. How do the symptoms Mickey complained of relate to renal failure? Why does the GFR fall and why do the BUN levels rise in people with renal failure?
2. Look closely at Mickey's height and weight. How do they compare with the height and weight of a child his age without renal disease? (Use the growth charts in Appendix E or an estimate from the RDA table.) Discuss reasons why growth may be compromised in the child with renal failure.

3. Think about Mickey's diet before he came into the hospital. Describe the reasons why protein, sodium, and potassium were restricted. Calculate Mickey's kcalorie range, and compare this figure with Mickey's actual kcalorie intake. Consider the effect of Mickey's kcalorie intake on his growth.
4. Describe ways that Mickey's nutrient needs will change due to hemodialysis. How will his needs change if he receives a kidney transplant?
5. Discuss some diet strategies you can suggest to Mickey and his mother to help him comply with his diet.
6. Consider the impact of renal disease on Mickey and his family. How can all members of the health team help support Mickey and his family during this difficult crisis?

The renal failure diet can be extremely restrictive, unappealing, and monotonous. Try to provide exciting and appetizing changes. Special renal cookbooks can be a big help. Incorporate favorite foods whenever possible (this is especially important with children). Encourage people with renal disease and their families to eat together and to eat the same kinds of foods. Many times only the portion sizes will need to be adjusted. Spices and seasonings such as garlic and onion powder, chili powder, curry powder, oregano, pepper, and lemon juice can add zest to many foods. A sample renal diet is shown on the previous page.

Acute Renal Failure

Acute renal failure occurs suddenly and is the consequence of another medical condition. The typical victim of acute renal failure is hypercatabolic and has a major illness, such as an infection or a burn, or has suffered a cardiac arrest. Suddenly, the GFR drops, urine output decreases, blood pressure shoots up, and toxic waste products begin to build up in the blood. Acidosis is common. As the body's cells break down, potassium is released from the intracellular fluid, and the kidneys are unable to excrete it. Blood potassium levels rise sharply. Hiccups, anorexia, nausea, and vomiting are common clinical symptoms of acute renal failure. GI bleeding and diarrhea sometimes occur. Drowsiness, agitation, and confusion are frequently seen.

What went wrong? Many times acute renal failure is caused by problems that originate outside the kidney. For example, acute renal failure can develop when blood flow to the kidney is reduced. This can occur for many reasons, including heart failure, shock, or severe blood loss after trauma (surgery or accident). As less blood reaches the nephron, the pressure gradient between the glomerulus and the tubule is minimal. The body can't make normal amounts of urine.

Another cause of acute renal failure that originates outside the kidney is a urinary tract obstruction. In this case, the kidney can make urine, but the urine can't get out of the body.

Damage to the kidneys themselves can also cause acute renal failure; infections, toxins, some drugs, and environmental pollutants can damage kidney cells. Death of kidney cells from lack of blood flow to them, ischemia, can also lead to acute renal failure.

In the early stages of acute renal failure, urine volume often diminishes markedly. Later in the course of renal failure, the kidneys are unable to conserve water, and the person begins to excrete large amounts of urine and electrolytes. After this period, kidney function gradually improves over a 3- to 12-month period, provided that the person recovers.

In some cases, acute renal failure is reversible. In others, it progresses into chronic renal failure. About one-third of all people with acute renal failure die.[12] Death from acute renal failure occurs more often in people who develop the disorder after surgery, particularly GI surgery. In these people, the mortality rate is about 80 percent.

The primary concern in acute renal failure is to treat the underlying disorder to prevent permanent or further damage to the kidneys. For example, if severe blood loss is the problem, a blood transfusion is given to restore blood volume. Other measures must be taken to restore fluid and electrolyte balance and minimize levels of toxic waste products. In addition to the nutrition factors discussed below, diuretics are often used to mobilize fluids in the oliguric phase of acute renal failure. Dialysis (either peritoneal dialysis or hemodialysis) is necessary when blood urea, creatinine, or potassium is high.

Energy and Protein

As mentioned, the person in acute renal failure is often hypercatabolic and suffering from another major illness. Add to these conditions nausea, vomiting, and confusion, and you have a person who really needs kcalories but is unable to eat. It is particularly important for this person to receive enough kcalories to reverse the hypercatabolic state, because the breakdown of protein for energy contributes to the rising blood urea and potassium levels. The person's actual kcaloric needs depend on the rate of catabolism; usually 35 to 50 kcalories per kilogram of body weight are needed. Energy needs frequently increase to 50 to 100 percent above normal resting energy expenditure.

Protein needs also vary, depending on the catabolic rate. The protein requirement of people with acute renal failure is unknown. Generally, their diet is restricted to about 30 to 40 grams of protein per day. However, impaired wound healing, infection, muscular wasting, and negative nitrogen balance are commonly seen in these individuals. They often die. Some practitioners prefer to provide a higher protein intake, even though dialysis might be necessary. Once dialysis is instituted, a more liberal protein intake of 70 to 85 grams may be allowed.

Mrs. Calley is a 35-year-old homemaker admitted to the hospital's intensive care unit. She was first seen in the emergency room after she sustained many severe injuries in an auto accident. She had lost so much blood that she almost died before reaching the hospital. In addition to her injuries, which include a fractured leg, broken ribs, a collapsed lung, and internal bleeding, she has developed acute renal failure. Mrs. Calley is 5'3" tall and weighs 125 lb.

Mrs. Calley has a urine volume of less than 50 ml/day and has a BUN of 75 mg/dl. A test of GFR could not be

CASE STUDY

Acute Renal Failure

performed due to the low volume of urine excreted. She is receiving blood transfusions to maintain blood volume and will undergo surgery to uncover and correct the source of the internal bleeding.

1. Describe the most probable reason why Mrs. Calley developed acute renal failure. What other problems can cause acute renal failure?
2. Describe the phases of acute renal

failure. What are Mrs. Calley's dietary needs in the early phase? What waste products and electrolytes are of greatest concern? Why?
3. What factors do you have to keep in mind in determining Mrs. Calley's energy and protein needs during her episode of acute renal failure? How will these needs be changed if dialysis is begun?
4. How will her nutrient needs change as she progresses to the second stage of acute renal failure? Contrast Mrs. Calley's current nutrient needs with the nutrient needs of a person with chronic renal failure. Describe some of the differences between the two diets.

Fluid and Electrolytes

The total amount of fluid is carefully controlled to avoid overhydration or dehydration. You can determine fluid requirements by carefully measuring urine output. To the volume of urine, add about 400 to 500 milliliters for water lost through the skin, lungs, and perspiration. The person who is vomiting, has diarrhea, has a high fever, or otherwise loses fluids, needs extra water. In the oliguric stage, the person will need small volumes of fluids. But in the diuretic stage, up to 3 liters of urine may be lost daily, and large amounts of fluids will have to be provided.

Likewise, sodium may be restricted (500 to 1,000 milligrams) in the oliguric phase, but this may change as the person enters the diuretic phase. Pay special attention to potassium in the person with acute renal failure—hyperkalemia can be life threatening. In the oliguric phase, potassium may be restricted to less than 2 grams per day; however, potassium may have to be supplemented during the diuretic phase.

Drugs called *exchange resins* must sometimes be used to treat severe hyperkalemia. These drugs, which are placed rectally, cause sodium to be exchanged for potassium in the colon, and the potassium is then excreted in the stool. Another method that can temporarily reduce high potassium levels is to give IV dextrose and insulin. Potassium moves into the cells with glucose. However, this is only a temporary measure.

Enteral and Parenteral Nutrition in Renal Failure

When people with either acute or chronic renal failure are hypercatabolic or for other reasons are unable to eat adequately, then special nutrition support is in order. As discussed in Chapter 18, first you can try to supplement the diet or offer a liquid diet orally. Encourage the person to drink supplements between meals to increase the amount of energy received. Appendix L lists commercial formulas useful for this purpose. But remember, the person with renal failure who is only allowed a certain amount of fluid has to derive the maximum energy from a small volume: use products that provide more than 1 kcalorie per milliliter. Some products that are specially formulated for people with renal disease are available, and they can be taken orally or by tube. Other formulas also can be adapted for use by the person with renal disease. Remember to notice the amounts of vitamins and minerals delivered by these products, however; with some of them, added vitamin and mineral supplements are needed. The compositions of some vitamin and mineral supplements are given in Appendix J.

A growing interest in the use of TPN for people in renal failure has evolved. Early studies using essential amino acid solutions suggested that mortality rates could be reduced and dialysis deferred when this method was used.[13] The original study compared the essential amino acid solution with a glucose solution. Since then, other studies have suggested that using mixtures of both nonessential and essential amino acids (at lower concentrations than in standard TPN solutions) is comparable to using essential amino acids alone.[14] Animal studies have suggested that high doses of the amino acid lysine, present in high concentrations in standard TPN solutions, is capable of inducing renal failure.[15]

To prevent fluid overload during TPN, 70 percent, rather than 50 percent, glucose solutions are used. This way, more kcalories are provided in a smaller volume. Electrolytes are monitored closely and adjusted as necessary. Glucose intolerance and insulin resistance are common in both uremia and catabolic illnesses, so insulin must often be given with the TPN solution.

Nephrotic Syndrome

Nephrotic syndrome is not a disease, but rather a complex of symptoms caused by the loss of plasma protein into the urine. Many disorders can lead to nephrotic syndrome—glomerulonephritis, diabetes mellitus, infections, and renal vein thrombosis are some of these.

Normally, only small plasma proteins pass through the glomerulus into the filtrate. These proteins are then reabsorbed in the tubules and returned to the blood. But in nephrotic syndrome, the permeability of the glomerular capillaries is defective, and plasma proteins are lost in the urine. Since albumin is the major plasma protein, it is also the major protein lost in the urine.

The loss of protein in the urine is called **proteinuria**.

As plasma proteins are lost, blood levels of proteins fall sharply. Together with other factors, low blood protein levels cause fluid to move into the interstitial space, and edema develops. As protein loss continues, lean body mass breaks down. Losses of some plasma proteins, such as immunoglobulins, render the person with nephrotic syndrome prone to infections, which can compromise nutrition status further. The loss of transferrin, the iron-carrying protein, may lead to anemia (see Figure 26–4). Serum lipid levels rise markedly for unknown reasons.

FIGURE 26–4

Consequences of nephrotic syndrome.

Treatment of nephrotic syndrome depends largely on the underlying cause. Diet is always important in preventing protein malnutrition and alleviating edema. A diet high in kcalories (50 to 60 kcalories per kilogram of body weight) and high in protein (about 120 grams per day) is prescribed. Sodium restriction is important, because the body avidly retains sodium in nephrotic syndrome. In the early treatment, a diet low in sodium (250 milligrams) is used to help mobilize the fluid that has accumulated in the interstitial space. Diuretics also are used for this purpose. Once the person is free of edema and sodium balance has been achieved, the sodium restriction is liberalized to about 1,500 milligrams per day, which is still a fairly stringent sodium intake. Chapters 23 and 25 provide more information on low-sodium diets. If potassium-wasting diuretics are prescribed, foods high in potassium become important in the diet.

People with nephrotic syndrome often have hyperlipidemia—most commonly, type II or V (see Chapter 25). These people also are at high risk for atherosclerosis. Therefore, it is often recommended that they follow the diet appropriate for the type of hyperlipidemia they have.

Urinary Tract Infections

People with urinary tract infections should be encouraged to eat a well-balanced diet and to drink plenty of fluids. Fluids will help prevent stagnation and the growth of bacteria. Fluids also aid in delivering antibiotics to the urinary tract, where they are needed. Many antibiotics used for urinary tract infections work better in an acid urine; therefore, people with such infections may be encouraged to use acid-producing juices and foods. The effect of foods on acidity of the

See box entitled "A Note on Acid-formers and Base-formers" on p. 380.

The person with a urinary tract infection is typically told to drink plenty of cranberry juice. This suggestion stems from the widespread belief that cranberry juice can lower urinary pH more effectively than other foods and drinks. Furthermore, cranberry juice contains a precursor of an acid that has an antibacterial action in the urine.

Unfortunately, it is impractical to use cranberry juice for these purposes. Although cranberry juice has a high acidity, it is not dependable for consistently lowering urinary pH. The antibacterial potential of cranberry juice is never achieved, because the antibacterial product is not concentrated enough to be effective.[16]

urine is not clear (see Highlight 26). Drug therapy may be more effective for this purpose.

Nutrition Assessment

The person in renal failure is at high risk for malnutrition. It becomes essential that nutrition assessments be made frequently and that problems be prevented or promptly corrected, otherwise nutrient stores will be depleted. Some things you should consider carefully include:

- The diet history is extremely important. Try to determine the usual intake of kcalories, protein, sodium, potassium, phosphorus, calcium, and vitamin D. This will help you in adjusting the newly diagnosed person's current eating habits for better compliance in a restricted diet. For the person already following a renal diet, diet history helps to assess the understanding of, and compliance with, the diet.
- Anthropometric measurements taken on the person with renal failure will be significantly influenced by the state of hydration. Weights taken immediately after dialysis treatments will more accurately reflect true weight. This weight is sometimes called the "dry weight." When the person isn't on dialysis, weight may be deceptively normal or high because of water retention. Likewise, arm measurements are affected by edema. The person with nephrotic syndrome may be dehydrated; anthropometric measurements also are affected by dehydration.
- Weight changes are actually more useful in assessing the state of hydration than in determining body weight in people with renal failure. Weight gain and blood pressure elevations suggest fluid retention. Weight loss and low blood pressure suggest dehydration.
- Weight and height in children must be routinely assessed to ensure that their diets are adequate for growth. Remember that growth failure is common in children with renal failure. Weight loss often occurs in renal failure. Wasting is common in people with nephrotic syndrome who are not eating enough protein.

- Albumin and transferrin levels may be extremely low in people with nephrotic syndrome. Levels rise when protein intake is adequate. People with renal failure also have lower transferrin levels than healthy people do; these are even lower when malnutrition accompanies renal disease.
- Serum electrolytes, BUN, and creatinine must be carefully monitored in renal failure.
- Serum lipids are frequently elevated in both chronic renal failure and nephrotic syndrome.

People with chronic renal failure must be carefully monitored to prevent growth failure and renal osteodystrophy. Anemia also may be a problem that can be partially corrected by diet.

Study Questions

1. What functions do the kidneys perform? What is the role of the kidneys in maintaining chemical homeostasis?
2. What is renal failure? Why is it often difficult to detect renal failure in the early stages? What causes renal failure?
3. What happens in the end stage of renal failure? Describe some of the symptoms associated with the buildup of toxic metabolic products in the blood.
4. When is a special diet instituted in the course of renal failure? When is dialysis or a kidney transplant considered for the person with renal failure?
5. Describe some of the reasons why the metabolism of nutrients is affected by renal failure. What are the objectives of dietary treatment of chronic renal failure?
6. Why is the protein (nitrogen) intake of the person with chronic renal failure a particular concern? Describe the use of keto-acid analogues along with a low-protein diet for the treatment of chronic renal failure.
7. What are the energy needs of adults with chronic renal failure? Of children? What are the consequences of providing too little energy in the diet of the person with chronic renal failure?
8. What fluid and electrolyte modifications are made to the diet of the person with chronic renal failure? What modifications are made concerning phosphorus, calcium, and vitamin D? Why?
9. What other vitamins and minerals need special consideration in the diet of the person with chronic renal failure? Describe why each of the nutrients you list may be a problem.
10. Discuss the nutrient needs of the person with a kidney transplant.
11. What suggestions can you give people with chronic renal failure to help them comply with their restrictive diets?
12. Describe the differences between chronic renal failure and acute renal failure. List some causes of acute renal failure.
13. What are the nutrient needs of the person in the oliguric phase of acute renal failure? How do these needs change as the person progresses to the diuretic phase?
14. Can tube feedings and TPN be used safely in the person with renal failure? What special considerations must be made when selecting an enteral or parenteral formula for the person with kidney failure?
15. What is nephrotic syndrome? What are the consequences of nephrotic syndrome? What are the protein and energy needs of the person with nephrotic syndrome? What are the fluid and electrolyte needs of these individuals?
16. What dietary advice can benefit the person with a urinary tract infection?

Notes

1. L. Oldrizzi and coauthors, Progression of renal failure in patients with renal disease of diverse etiology on protein-restricted diets, *Kidney International* 27 (1985): 553–557; A. J. Williams and coauthors, Alteration of the course of chronic renal failure by dietary protein restriction, *Proceedings of the European Dialysis and Transplant Association* 21 (1985): 604–607; S. R. Acchiardo, L. W. Moore, and S. Cockrell, Does low protein diet halt the progression of renal insufficiency? *Clinical Nephrology* 25 (1986): 289–294.
2. J. B. Rosman and coauthors, Early protein restriction in chronic renal failure, *Proceedings of the European Dialysis and Transplant Association* 21 (1985): 567–573; C. Giordano, Early dietary protein restriction protects the failing kidney, *Kidney International* 28 (1985): 566–570.
3. G. Zakar, Effects of dietary protein restriction on the course of early renal failure, *Proceedings of the European Dialysis and Transplant Association* 21 (1985): 600–603.
4. C. Giordano, Use of exogenous and endogenous urea for protein synthesis in normal and uremic subjects, *Journal of Laboratory and Clinical Medicine* 62 (1963): 231–246; S. Giovannetti and Q. Maggiore, A low-nitrogen diet with proteins of high biological value for severe chronic uraemia, *Lancet* 1 (1964): 1000–1003.
5. P. Fürst and coauthors, Principles of essential amino acid therapy in uremia, *American Journal of Clinical Nutrition* 31 (1978): 1744–1755; M. Walser, Principles of keto acid

therapy in uremia, *American Journal of Clinical Nutrition* 31 (1978): 1756–1760.

6. P. T. Frohling and coauthors, Influence of phosphate restriction, keto acids and vitamin D on the progression of chronic renal failure, *Proceedings of the European Dialysis and Transplant Association* 21 (1985): 561–566.

7. P. A. Lucas and coauthors, The risks and benefits of a low-protein-essential amino acid-keto acid diet, *Kidney International* 29 (1986): 995-1003.

8. J. D. Kopple, F. J. Monteon, and J. K. Shaib, Effect of energy intake on nitrogen metabolism in nondialyzed patients with chronic renal failure, *Kidney International* 29 (1986): 734–742.

9. F. Santos, B. I. Friedman, and J. C. Chan, Management of chronic renal failure in children, *Current Problems in Pediatrics* 16 (1986): 237–301.

10. Frohling and coauthors, 1985; D. Lumlertgul and coauthors, Phosphate depletion arrests progression of chronic renal failure independent of protein intake, *Kidney International* 29 (1986): 658–666.

11. D. Grekas and coauthors, Effect of zinc treatment on cell mediated immunity of chronic renal failure patients, *Proceedings of the European Dialysis and Transplant Association* 21 (1985): 825–829.

12. J. S. Cameron, Acute renal failure in the intensive care unit today, *Intensive Care Medicine* 12 (1986): 64–70.

13. R. M. Abel and coauthors, Improved survival from acute renal failure after treatment with intravenous essential L-amino acids and glucose, *New England Journal of Medicine* 288 (1973): 695–699.

14. J. M. Mirtallo and coauthors, A comparison of essential and general amino acid infusions in the nutritional support of patients with compromised renal function, *Journal of Parenteral and Enteral Nutrition* 6 (1982): 109–113.

15. L. C. Racussen, A. Whelton, and K. Solez, Effects of lysine and other amino acids on kidney structure and function in the rat, *American Journal of Pathology* 120 (1985): 436–432.

16. Cranberries and urinary infections, *Nutrition and the MD*, August 1982, p. 3.

Nutrition in the Prevention and Treatment of Kidney Stones

Kidney stones are a common problem throughout the world. In the United States, about one in every 500 adults suffers from kidney stones, a painful and potentially dangerous condition. The person who has experienced a kidney stone may have a recurrence, but a large percentage of people with kidney stones report only a single episode. This suggests that with proper treatment, a recurrence of kidney stones may be preventable. The purpose of this highlight is to review some of the information that has been learned regarding the role of diet in the prevention and treatment of kidney stones. Much of the information is controversial, and research is still necessary to delineate the facts more fully.

What Are Kidney Stones?

Most kidney stones contain calcium oxalate (60 percent of all stones), calcium phosphate (9 percent), or a combination of both (11 percent). Less common stones are composed of uric acid, cystine, or magnesium ammonium phosphate. Calcium stones may form from a variety of underlying medical conditions that cause either elevated serum calcium levels, excessive urinary excretion of calcium, or deficiencies of substances in the urine that normally inhibit stone formation. Most frequently, calcium stones are associated with excessive urinary calcium excretion for which no cause can be identified (idiopathic hypercalciuria). Uric acid stones are associated with the excessive

urinary excretion of uric acid, an acid urine, and a low urine volume. Cystine stones occur as the result of a metabolic disorder that is characterized by the abnormal excretion of cystine in the urine (cystinuria). Table H26–1 summarizes some of the disorders that are associated with stone formation.

Stones that are small (less than 5 millimeters, or one-fifth of an inch in diameter) may pass through the ureters and be excreted in the urine. Larger stones cannot exit the body in this way. These may not cause problems if only a few are formed. However, if a larger stone enters a ureter (see Figure H26–1), a severe, stabbing pain, called *renal colic,* results. Pain can also occur when small pieces of the stone break off and travel down the ureters with urine. The pain normally starts in the back, just above the ribs, and follows the course of the stone. Once the stone reaches the bladder, the pain normally subsides. If a

TABLE H26–1

Disorders Associated with Kidney Stones

Bowel diseases causing malabsorption
Cystinuria
Glucocorticoid excess
Gout
Hyperparathyroidism
Hyperthyroidism
Immobilization
Malignancies (some types)
Osteoporosis
Paget's disease
Recurrent urinary tract infections
Renal tubular acidosis
Vitamin D intoxication

stone blocks the flow of urine or causes an infection, it must be removed either surgically or by newer techniques that use sound waves or shock waves to break up the stone so that it can be passed.

What Causes a Kidney Stone to Form?

The exact mechanisms by which kidney stones form are not clearly understood. Why is it, for example, that nearly all of us pass crystals in the urine, whereas only 10 percent of us actually develop kidney stones?[1] Three theories that help explain how kidney stones form are widely accepted by practitioners. They form the basis for the current treatment and prevention of kidney stones.

FIGURE H26–1

The urinary tract.

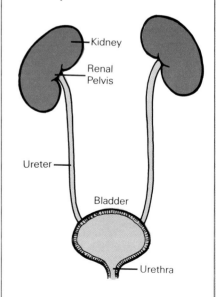

Kidney
Renal Pelvis
Ureter
Bladder
Urethra

One mechanism that is important in stone formation is called *supersaturation*. Stone constituents are relatively insoluble in urine. When their concentrations get high, they form crystals that eventually precipitate and get larger. The more concentrated a mineral is in the urine, the greater the likelihood that a stone will form.

Another mechanism that may be important in the formation of some stones is the formation of a small seed (sometimes called a *nucleus* or *nidus*) composed of a mineral different from that found in the remainder of the stone. The seed is formed from the crystallization of a mineral that is supersaturated in the urine. The crystalline structure then provides a matrix upon which a less saturated mineral can attach. In some cases, calcium oxalate stones have been found to form around a uric acid seed. The treatment of a stone of this type would involve the mineral found in the seed rather than the minerals that make up most of the stone.

Finally, it is widely believed that a deficiency of one or more naturally occurring stone inhibitors in the urine may contribute to stone formation. Citrate, a type of phosphate, and a type of polysaccharide are probable inhibitors.[2] Magnesium, zinc, and ribonucleic acid (RNA) might also have this effect. All of these substances have been identified as inhibitors of calcium oxalate stone formation.[3] What is not known is how important they are in the clinical situation. More research is needed to answer this question.

Diet and Kidney Stones

Can diet prevent the formation or recurrence of kidney stones? The answer to this question is complicated, because so many disorders can result in stone formation (see Table H26–1). Studies have shown differences between the diets of people with kidney stones and those without them.[4] In one study,

the diets of males with stones were significantly lower in thiamin than the diets of those in the control group. People with stones took vitamin C supplements more than twice as frequently as people in the control group. The same researchers then subdivided the group of stone formers further, based on the type of stone (calcium, oxalate, and uric acid).[5] They found that people with calcium oxalate stones without an identifiable underlying cause had lower intakes of dietary fiber, phytate, magnesium, phosphate, and thiamin than the control group. All the study group participants who excreted excessive urinary oxalate had a significantly higher intake of vitamin C than the control group. Although the significance of these findings is unclear at this time, the studies suggest that differences in diet may play a role in the development of kidney stones.

Universal agreement does exist on one aspect of diet in the prevention and treatment of kidney stone formation: a high fluid intake is encouraged. The person with a kidney stone is advised to drink enough fluid so that a urine volume of at least two liters per day is maintained. Furthermore, fluid intake should be spread out regularly throughout the day. Maintenance of a large urine volume ensures that the concentration of minerals in the urine will be diluted, and the risk of stone formation is thus reduced. Other aspects of diet in the treatment of kidney stones have been far more controversial and have changed dramatically in recent years. These aspects will be considered as we discuss the role of diet in different types of stones.

Diet and Calcium Stones

One of the most controversial topics in the treatment of stones concerns the role of calcium restriction for the person with a calcium-containing stone.

On the surface, it appears reasonable that the diet of a person who is excreting large amounts of calcium in the urine should be restricted in calcium. For years, people with calcium stones were routinely instructed to follow a low-calcium diet (400 to 600 milligrams of calcium). However, evidence suggests that a calcium restriction is indicated in only one type of kidney stone former—the person who regularly ingests high amounts of calcium. Even in this case, calcium intake is restricted to an average (not a low) calcium intake. The diet should meet, but not exceed, the RDA for calcium.

To restrict the calcium intake of other types of stone formers may actually be harmful. One ill effect is evident—a calcium deficiency could result and lead to bone disorders. Studies of people with excessive urinary calcium levels have suggested that these individuals lose more calcium from their bones than normal subjects, which raises urinary calcium, obviously making stone formation more, not less, likely. They also excrete more calcium than they ingest, which indicates that they are in negative calcium balance.[6]

Calcium restriction could cause other harmful effects for the person with a calcium oxalate stone. You may recall that calcium normally binds to oxalate in the intestine. It is possible that if dietary calcium is severely limited, oxalate absorption may increase resulting in enteric hyperoxaluria. This actually increases the likelihood that a calcium oxalate stone will form.[7] Rather than restrict calcium, people with calcium oxalate stones are advised to restrict their intakes of foods high in oxalate. Table H26–2 shows foods that contain considerable amounts of oxalate. Supplemental vitamin-mineral preparations and medicines containing calcium are discouraged. Vitamin D can increase calcium absorption from the GI tract, a problem for the person who forms calcium stones due to excessive

TABLE H26–2

Foods High in Oxalate

Vegetables

Baked beans canned in tomato sauce	Kale
Beans (green, wax, or dried)	Leeks
Beets	Mustard greens
Celery	Okra
Chard, Swiss	Parsley
Chives	Peppers, green
Collards	Potatoes, sweet
Dandelion greens	Rutabagas
Eggplant	Spinach
Escarole	Summer squash
	Watercress

Fruits

Blackberries	Lemon peel
Blueberries	Lime peel
Currants, red	Orange peel
Dewberries	Raspberries
Fruit cocktail	Rhubarb
Gooseberries	Strawberries
Grapes, Concord	Tangerines

Other

Chocolate	Pepper (more than 1 tsp/day)
Cocoa	Soybean crackers
Cola beverages	Soybean curd (tofu)
Draft beer	Tea
Fruit cake	Tomato soup
Grits	Vegetable soup
Peanut butter	Wheat germ

Source: Adapted from D. M. Ney, A. F. Hofmann, C. Fischer, and N. Stubblefield, *The Low Oxalate Diet Book* (San Diego: University of California, 1981).

absorption of calcium. Megadoses of vitamin C also have been reported to cause hyperoxaluria. Some people metabolize vitamin C to oxalate; therefore, people with hyperoxaluria should avoid vitamin C supplements. Calcium-containing antacids must also be avoided.

Thiazide diuretics are frequently prescribed for the person with calcium stones that are not associated with another medical condition. However, these diuretics can cause a deficiency of potassium, so they are sometimes given along with another type of diuretic that conserves potassium. People on thiazide diuretics are advised to follow a moderately restricted sodium diet, because a high sodium intake can offset the beneficial effects of the diuretic and can cause potassium to be excreted excessively.[8] Therefore, potassium levels are monitored closely, and potassium supplements are given, if necessary.

Sodium restriction may have another benefit: some evidence suggests that calcium excretion is linked to sodium excretion.[9] Therefore, a moderately restricted sodium diet might reduce excessive calcium levels in the urine, even for calcium stone formers not taking thiazide diuretics. Other studies have shown that a high protein intake increases the urinary excretion of calcium also. However, no studies have demonstrated a beneficial effect of protein restriction on calcium stone formation.

In summary, the calcium in the diet of a person with calcium stones who consumes excessive amounts of calcium is restricted to the RDA level. People with calcium oxalate stones are cautioned to limit their intakes of foods high in oxalate. Those on thiazide diuretics may benefit from a moderately restricted sodium intake, and possibly a potassium supplement, if potassium becomes deficient. Of course, fluid intake is encouraged.

Other Stones

Another common practice in the treatment of many types of kidney stones has been to prescribe diets that were meant to change the acidity of the urine. An acid ash diet, intended to make the urine more acid, centers on meat, cheese, eggs, whole grains, and some fruits. An alkaline ash diet, intended to reduce the acidity of the urine, emphasizes milk, vegetables, and most fruits. Diet can affect the acidity of the urine. However, current methods used to calculate the effect of different foods on the acidity of the urine are difficult to use, and they are inaccurate.[10] Until a better estimate of the effect of dietary components on urine acidity is available, drug therapy for this purpose will be more reliable; indeed, it is more frequently used today.

Uric acid stones can form when the urine is consistently acid and when excess uric acid is present in the urine. A metabolic disorder, gout, is frequently associated with uric acid stones. A generous fluid intake is encouraged. At one time, low-purine diets were commonly prescribed to

Miniglossary

cystinuria (SIS-te-NEW-ree-ah): a metabolic disorder in which large amounts of the amino acids cystine, lysine, arginine, and ornithine are excreted in the urine.

enteric hyperoxaluria: excessive urinary excretion of oxalate caused by excess oxalate absorption in the intestine; it occurs because calcium is unable to bind to oxalate in the intestine, thus allowing oxalate absorption.

gout: a metabolic disorder characterized by acute arthritis and inflammation of the joints that results in excess uric acid in the blood, and sometimes in the urine.

hyperparathyroidism (HIGH-per-para-THIGH-roy-dizm): a condition characterized by the excessive secretion of parathyroid hormone, which generally results in elevated serum calcium levels, low serum phosphorus levels, and abnormal bone metabolism.

hyperthyroidism: a condition characterized by the excessive secretion of thyroid hormones, which results in an accelerated metabolic rate.

idiopathic hypercalciuria (HIGH-per-kal-see-YOU-ree-ah): excessive urinary excretion of calcium not related to a known underlying medical condition.

nidus (NIGH-dus), **nucleus:** a small bit of a crystallized mineral that serves as a matrix for further crystallization.

Paget's (PAJ-ets) **disease:** a chronic inflammatory disease of the bones that may occur in elderly people, named for Sir James Paget, an English surgeon.

pH: see pp. 379-380.

renal colic: the severe pain that accompanies the movement of a kidney stone through the ureter.

renal tubular acidosis: a condition in which the nephron cannot maintain acid-base balance; it can lead to potassium depletion, rickets, or osteomalacia.

struvite: another name for magnesium ammonium phosphate.

supersaturation: a term that describes the concentration of a substance in a liquid at the point where it is too concentrated to stay in solution and instead precipitates.

---

reduce uric acid levels in the urine. A low-purine diet is restricted in red meats, particularly organ meats, anchovies, sardines, and meat extracts. The diet is restrictive, and benefits of such a diet have not been proven. Furthermore, drug therapy is now available that is effective in reducing uric acid levels. However, it may be useful to limit excessive protein, and a diet containing no more than 120 grams of protein per day is advisable.[11] Drug therapy may be prescribed to reduce the acidity of the urine.

Magnesium ammonium phosphate (struvite) stones can precipitate when the urine becomes alkaline. This most often occurs when the urinary tract becomes infected with microorganisms that release ammonia. No specific diet therapy other than a well-balanced diet is recommended for this type of kidney stone.

Cystine stones form as a result of a metabolic disorder called *cystinuria*. In cystinuria, large amounts of the amino acid cystine (in addition to other amino acids) are excreted in the urine. A diet low in the amino acid methionine is prescribed, because cystine, a nonessential amino acid, is produced from methionine. Drug therapy to reduce the acidity of the urine may also be beneficial.

As you can see, many connections between diet and kidney stones have been explored. Dramatic advances in the nonsurgical treatment of kidney stones have no doubt triggered a renewed interest in this area. A health care professional has an important responsibility to keep up with changes such as these so as to provide the best possible care for clients.

NOTES

1. B. Goldwasser, J. L. Weinerth, and C. C. Carson, Calcium stone disease: An overview, *Journal of Urology* 135 (1986): 1–9.

2. S. P. Kanig and R. L. Conn, Kidney stones: Medical management and newer options for stone removal, *Postgraduate Medicine* 78, no. 6 (1985): 38–51.

3. Goldwasser, Weinerth, and Carson, 1986.

4. H. M. Griffith and coauthors, A case-controlled study of dietary intake of renal stone patients: 1. Preliminary analysis, *Urology Research* 14 (1986): 67–74.

5. H. M. Griffith and coauthors, A case-controlled study of dietary intake of renal stone patients: 2. Urine biochemistry and stone analysis, *Urology Research* 14 (1986): 75–82.

6. F. L. Coe and J. H. Parks, Recurrent renal calculi: Causes and prevention, *Hospital Practice* 21, no. 3A (1986): 49–57.

7. P. Bataille and coauthors, Effect of calcium restriction on renal excretion of oxalate and the probability of stones in the various pathophysiological groups with calcium stones, *Journal of Urology* 130 (1983): 218–223.

8. Coe and Parks, 1986.

9. Kanig and Conn, 1985.

10. J. Dwyer and coauthors, Acid/alkaline ash diets: Time for assessment and change, *Journal of the American Dietetic Association* 85 (1985): 841–845.

11. Goldwasser, Weinerth, and Carson, 1986.

Nutrition for People with Cancer

27

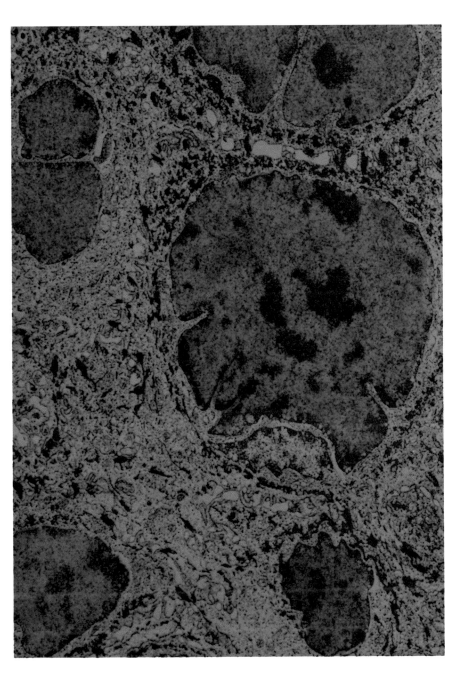

Cancer cells multiply within organs and spread to other organs, threatening their integrity and functions. Often, they rob the organs of needed nutrients, causing local starvation. Shown here is a cervical cancer cell.

FIGURE 27–1

Causes of the cancer cachexia syndrome. Anorexia and cachexia contribute to each other. Cancer itself and the available treatments for it make both problems worse.

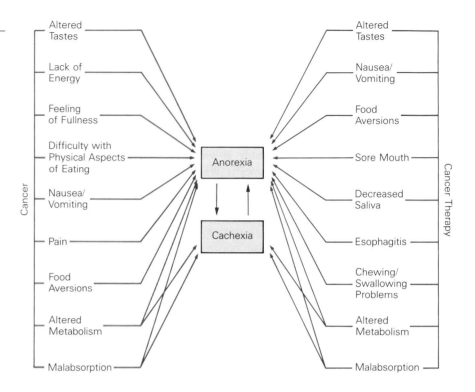

Loss of strength is called **asthenia** (as-THEE-nee-ah).

radiation therapy: the use of radiation to arrest or destroy cancer cells.

chemotherapy: the use of drugs to arrest or destroy cancer cells. Drugs used for chemotherapy are called **chemotherapeutic** or **antineoplastic agents.**
chemo = chemical

Another problem is a premature feeling of fullness: "I feel hungry, but I take a few bites and I'm full." Sometimes the person feels full for a good reason. For example, the tumor may be pressing against the stomach. But for the most part, the reason for this complaint is unknown.

The person with cancer often tires easily. This may interfere with meal preparation and consumption. Many hospitalized people with cancer have the most energy and feel the least full in the morning. As the day progresses, they become drained and feel full rapidly. The situation may be different for some people at home. One author reports that female homemakers with cancer eat breakfast poorly but eat more for dinner.[3]

Anorexia can be the result of pain associated with a tumor. A person in pain may have little interest in food, particularly if eating makes the pain worse.

Some types of cancer can result in anorexia because they cause an obstruction in the GI tract. For example, a tumor of the esophagus may cause a partial or complete obstruction; the person with such a tumor is unable to eat or has difficulty swallowing. A tumor obstructing the lower GI tract may cause nausea and vomiting.

Cancer itself is not the only factor that interferes with food intake. The treatment the person receives for cancer generally has many detrimental effects.

Anorexia Caused by Cancer Therapy

The treatment for cancer often involves radiation therapy, chemotherapy, surgery, or any combination of the three. Through their use, cancer can sometimes be arrested and nutrition problems corrected on a long-term basis. But ironically, any of these treatments can also cause major nutrition problems. In this section, we will discuss how these therapies cause anorexia. The ways they affect digestion, absorption, and metabolism are discussed later.

Radiation therapy works by disrupting the chemical bonds necessary to form DNA. This is why radiation works best on cells that are actively dividing and making new DNA, like tumor cells. It is also why radiation damages normal body cells that divide actively, such as the cells of the GI tract. The cancer cells divide fastest, so they are the most affected by radiation, but other actively dividing cells are also susceptible. The nutrition (and other) side effects of radiation depend on many factors, such as the type of radiation; the area of the body being irradiated; the size of the area; the dose; and the clinical status of the person in therapy.

Many chemotherapeutic drugs work the same way as radiation—they destroy dividing cells by interfering with DNA or RNA synthesis. Among the types of chemotherapeutic agents are antibiotics, alkaloids, alkylating agents, antimetabolites, steroids, and others. Like radiation, these drugs also affect normal cells, and those that divide rapidly are most likely to be affected. The current trend in chemotherapy is to use high doses of several chemotherapeutic agents together in cycles. This helps ensure that malignant cells will be killed. Although these treatments are effective in many cases, they also may intensify undesirable side effects.

Radiation and chemotherapy can cause anorexia, nausea, and vomiting. All of these symptoms, of course, tend to reduce food intake. Table 27–1 summarizes the possible effects of radiation and chemotherapy on nutrition status.

Cancer therapy can lead to anorexia by causing:
- Mouth blindness.
- Dry mouth.
- Esophagitis.
- Stomatitis.
- Mouth ulcers.
- Food aversions.

TABLE 27–1

Possible Effects of Radiation and Chemotherapy on Nutrition Status

Radiation	Chemotherapy
Reduced nutrient intake	
Anorexia	Abdominal pain
Damage to teeth and bone	Anorexia
Esophagitis	Intestinal ulcers
Nausea	Nausea
Reduced salivary secretions	Taste alterations
Taste alterations	Vomiting
Thick salivary secretions	
Vomiting	
Increased nutrient losses	
Chronic blood loss from intestine and bladder	Diarrhea
Diarrhea	Malabsorption
Fistula formation	
Intestinal obstructions	
Malabsorption	
Altered metabolism	
(Secondary to malnutrition)	Fluid and electrolyte imbalance
	Hyperglycemia
	Interference with vitamins or other metabolites
	Negative nitrogen and calcium balance

People receiving radiation therapy to the head and neck can develop other problems interfering with food intake. They frequently develop altered taste sensations and experience a diminished taste sensitivity. As a result of this "mouth blindness," foods they once liked may become unpleasant to them. An intolerance to meat, especially red meat, often develops. For some, food is just not sweet enough, and for others, many foods are too sweet.

Radiation to the head and neck area also can reduce the amount of saliva, and the saliva that remains is often thick. The person with this condition has trouble swallowing. The bones of the jaws and the teeth can also be damaged, further interfering with the ability to chew and swallow. Radiation can also cause mouth ulcers to form, another problem that makes eating quite painful.

Radiation to the esophagus can cause esophagitis (see Chapter 21). Many times this problem resolves itself when radiation therapy is stopped, but some people develop fibrosis and sometimes strictures, resulting in permanent swallowing problems. Fistulas can also develop, which may necessitate the use of a feeding tube or parenteral nutrition. When you consider that a person undergoing radiation therapy, particularly to the head and neck area, may suffer from several of these complications, you can see why nutrient intake is markedly affected.

Like radiation, chemotherapy can cause problems in addition to anorexia, nausea, and vomiting. It can inflame the lining of the mouth (stomatitis) and sometimes cause mouth ulcers, making chewing and swallowing painful. The person on chemotherapy may also experience abdominal pain or develop intestinal ulcers, which interfere with food intake. Finally, people on chemotherapy may develop a strong dislike for certain foods, tastes, and odors (see box entitled "Food Aversions").

Surgery can affect food intake in people with cancer, as it can in people having surgery for any other reason. It can cause anorexia, nausea, and vomiting. In addition, some types of surgery used almost exclusively in the treatment of cancer have special effects on food intake. Radical surgery of the head and neck falls into this category. Partial or total removal of the tongue, resection of the muscles of the mouth or esophagus and salivary glands, and removal of the lower jaw invariably create extensive problems with chewing and swallowing. People with these kinds of surgery may have to be maintained on tube feeding or TPN. Table 27–2 summarizes how some types of GI tract surgery for cancer can affect nutrition status.

Excess Nutrient Losses

The nutrition status of the person with cancer can be impaired not only because food intake is reduced, but also because nutrients may be excessively lost. These losses can be the result of the cancer itself or the treatment for it.

Depending on the location and type of cancer, maldigestion or malabsorption of nutrients can occur. For example, there may be a deficiency of pancreatic enzymes (cancer of the pancreas) or bile salts (cancer of the liver). In the Zollinger-Ellison syndrome, hypersecretion of gastric acid inactivates digestive

Zollinger-Ellison syndrome: a condition caused by pancreatic tumors secreting excess gastrin, which stimulates the stomach to release great amounts of HCl acid and pepsin.

Food Aversions

For many years, researchers have looked for physiologic causes to explain the anorexia that frequently accompanies cancer. Today, an interesting new insight shows promise of having a major impact on the understanding and prevention of anorexia.

People with cancer frequently develop strong dislikes to certain foods, tastes, and odors. These aversions seem to develop when certain foods, tastes, or odors are associated with unpleasant symptoms, such as nausea and vomiting.[4] For example, if a certain food is eaten before a treatment that results in nausea (such as chemotherapy), the person learns to dislike that food.

If you think about it, this would normally be an adaptive reaction. An animal "learns" to avoid foods that make it sick by developing just such an aversion. Unfortunately, however, the person with cancer may be led to avoid foods that could help the recovery as well. Learning to hate foods because of their association with unpleasant body sensations worsens the anorexia.

Experiments in both human beings and animals have shown that food aversions can develop in association with chemotherapy. In one experiment, children were served an unusually flavored ice cream before receiving chemotherapy.[5] After one to four weeks, they were offered a choice between eating the same flavor of ice cream and playing a game. These children were one-third as likely to choose the ice cream as control children who had received the ice cream without a simultaneous chemotherapy treatment. Another set of children received chemotherapy but not ice cream; they were not averse to eating the ice cream later. The experiment showed clearly that food aversions do develop in people undergoing chemotherapy.

Animal studies have shown that radiation therapy and unpleasant symptoms caused by tumor growth itself can also cause food aversions.[6] Research indicates that similar reactions occur in human beings.[7]

Learned food aversions raise several important questions. What is the best way to prevent them? What foods are most likely to become aversive? Are food aversions permanent? How much influence do food aversions have on anorexia? While research into this new area of investigation continues, it seems wise to let people know that they may develop food aversions. Suggest that they "save" their favorite foods for periods when they are feeling relatively good and not eat within an hour or two of (either before or after) scheduled radiation therapy or chemotherapy treatments.

enzymes. Tumors of the small bowel can lead to malabsorption, too. Malabsorption caused by blind loop syndrome (see Chapter 22) can occur when a tumor obstructs the upper small intestine.

Some cancers cause severe vomiting, diarrhea, or both. For example, a tumor that obstructs the small bowel may cause vomiting, and some tumors can produce severe diarrhea. Such conditions may result in electrolyte imbalances and dehydration.

Excess nutrient losses can occur due to:
• Malabsorption.
• Severe vomiting or diarrhea.
• Radiation enteritis.

In addition to the many effects of cancer and cancer therapy we have described here, there are many other effects that you may never realize until you work with a person who has a particular type of cancer. To show just how varied these effects can be, we would like to share an example from a personal experience with you. Kathy was a 36-year-old, vibrant, intelligent woman who developed a malignant brain tumor that progressively affected her speech center and the right side of her body. Because this type of tumor progresses rapidly, the prognosis was poor, with an expected length of survival of 6 months.

As the ability to communicate declined, it became progressively more difficult for Kathy to express her desires and needs regarding foods she would like to eat. Simultaneously, she was less able to prepare and physically eat foods herself because of loss of function to the right side of the body. Kathy was right-handed, and learning to use the left hand, particularly to handle feeding utensils, was a difficult task. One solution to this problem was to serve foods that could be finger fed. The type of food was important in preserving Kathy's dignity—she was an intelligent adult who did not want to be treated as a child. Breads, cheeses, fruit, and luncheon meats were easy to handle. Depression that resulted from the inability to communicate made it even more difficult to eat.

Another problem occurred if foods were too small. Kathy lost the ability to move her tongue back and forth, and if small foods lodged in the right side of the back of her mouth, she could not feel them, and could choke.

Kathy was taking a steroid medication to reduce swelling in the brain, as well as narcotics to deal with the severe headaches associated with the tumor. Both the tumor itself and the steroids caused nausea, although in Kathy's case, she ate more rather than less due to the nausea. She stated that she felt much more nauseated when she had an empty stomach. The tumor itself and the narcotics made Kathy sleepy, which compounded the difficulty she had with the physical aspects of eating.

As you can see, many factors affect nutrition in the person with cancer. In this case, prognosis was poor, so the effects on long-term nutrition status were not as critical as helping Kathy preserve feelings of self-esteem, dignity, and independence. These considerations are certainly important, particularly for the person whose disease is terminal. When time is short, you want the person to enjoy, rather than be burdened by, the routine experiences of everyday life.

Changes in the structure of the small bowel caused by radiation therapy are referred to as **radiation enteritis**.

Radiation to the small bowel often interferes with normal intestinal function, resulting in diarrhea and vomiting. Many times, intestinal function returns after radiation therapy ends, but for some people, changes may be permanent. After radiation therapy to the intestine, the structure of the intestine changes. The intestinal wall becomes thick and fibrotic, and the small intestinal arteries may become so inflamed that blood flow to some sections of the bowel is cut off. The intestine may narrow and become obstructed, or a fistula may form. Mal-

TABLE 27–2

Possible Effects of Some Types of GI Tract Surgery on Nutrition Status

Head and neck resection

Difficulty in chewing/swallowing
Inability to chew/swallow

Esophageal resection

Decreased gastric acid production	Fistula formation
Decreased stomach motility	Steatorrhea
Diarrhea	Stenosis

Stomach resection

Dumping syndrome	General malabsorption
Hypoglycemia	Vitamin B_{12} malabsorption
Lack of gastric acid	

Intestinal resection

Blind loop syndrome	General malabsorption
Diarrhea	Hyperoxaluria
Fluid and electrolyte imbalance	Steatorrhea

Pancreatic resection

General malabsorption
Diabetes mellitus

absorption and chronic blood loss from the intestine and bladder can result in malnutrition, as well as fluid and electrolyte imbalances.

The person on chemotherapy also may develop diarrhea and malabsorption. This is because the cells of the intestine cannot regenerate as they normally do, and nutrient absorption is impaired. As shown in Chapters 21 and 22, surgery to the GI tract also can have many ill effects on nutrition status. (These effects are summarized in Table 27–2.)

Thus, all these forms of treatment for cancer, as well as cancer itself, point in the same direction: malnutrition. In fact, it has been estimated that more than half of all the deaths attributed to cancer are actually caused by starvation.

Metabolic Consequences of Cancer

So far we have seen how a reduced intake of food and excessive losses of nutrients can contribute to cancer cachexia. Now let's look at how metabolic changes in cancer may further aggravate the cancer cachexia syndrome.

Although research has not revealed the underlying reasons, it appears that people with cancer have increased energy expenditure. In other words, they use more energy than healthy persons do. The tumor demands some energy, but the metabolic needs of the host are raised as well, sometimes even before the tumor is large enough to be detected. (This is one reason why, in preventive medicine, an important question in the dietary interview is: Have you experienced any recent changes in appetite or body weight?)

If reduced food intake were the only problem in people with cancer, then weight loss would largely occur at the expense of body fat. But in cancer, muscle wasting is extreme. This wasting is accounted for, in part, by metabolic changes that occur in cancer.

In normal cells, energy is derived through the cycle that uses oxygen (the TCA cycle; see Chapter 7 and Appendix C) rather than through the pathway that involves no oxygen (the glycolytic pathway). The TCA cycle is the more efficient of the two and can metabolize either glucose or fat for energy. But tumor cells use the glycolytic pathway to make energy. This pathway produces less energy and relies on glucose as an energy substrate. After the host's glycogen stores are depleted to provide this glucose, muscle catabolism begins to provide the amino acids necessary to make new glucose. Additionally, studies have shown that tumor tissues show a selective uptake of amino acids used for protein synthesis and making new glucose.[8] The host's muscle mass becomes progressively depleted, and negative nitrogen balance ensues.

As the tumor metabolizes glucose by way of glycolysis, lactic acid (lactate) is produced. This lactate is then returned to the liver, where it is reconverted to glucose in an energy-requiring process. Thus a demand is placed on the host to provide this energy. Accumulated lactate also may contribute to nausea.[9] (Sensations of nausea have even been experienced by healthy volunteers given an infusion of lactate.)

Another problem is that many people with cancer are hyperglycemic, probably for two reasons. For one thing, they tend to be insulin resistant; for another, they display reduced insulin release in response to a glucose load. Hunger generally corresponds to a return of blood glucose to fasting levels, and in the person with cancer, this return may be delayed—hence the person's lack of appetite.

One author postulates that people with cancer produce excessive body heat after a meal.[10] The excess heat produces an unpleasant sensation that they learn to avoid by eating less. This theory ties in well with the idea that cancer clients develop learned food aversions.

The energy needs of people with cancer may be high for other reasons—emotional or physiologic stress or surgery, for example. Both chemotherapy and radiation can interfere with the immune system, and infections can easily occur, again raising energy and nutrient needs further (see Chapter 20).

Chemotherapy using vitamin antagonists (see Chapter 19, Figure 19–1) can result in nutrient deficiencies and block normal metabolic pathways. This further interferes with nutrition status; anemias caused by a variety of vitamin deficiencies are frequently seen in people with cancer.

Some tumors produce hormones that can affect normal body functions. For example, as previously discussed, the Zollinger-Ellison syndrome is caused by tumors that secrete gastrin; the gastrin triggers the production of excess gastric acid, and digestive enzymes become inactivated.

Obviously, the person with cancer is at extremely great risk for poor nutrition status. Nutrition care is often crucial to recovery.

Nutrition Care

For many years, the deteriorating nutrition status that accompanies cancer was largely ignored. Many practitioners believed that emaciation and physical debilitation were an inevitable result of cancer. Others believed that if you fed the host, you also fed the tumor, and that you should therefore starve the host. Another problem was the state of the art of how people could be fed. Remember that the widespread use of tube feedings and TPN is a fairly recent advance.

Today, attitudes regarding the benefits of nutrition for the person with cancer have changed dramatically. Attention to the diet can prevent or reverse poor nutrition status, and the advantages of maintaining optimal nutrition status are recognized. The person in good nutrition status:

- Enjoys a better quality of life. The malnourished person is less active and becomes weak, eats less, becomes weaker, and goes into a downward spiral.
- Is less susceptible to infections (see Highlight 19 and Chapter 20).
- Probably tolerates cancer therapies better (surgery, chemotherapy, and radiation therapy).

In animal studies, it has been shown that improved nutrition can result in increased tumor growth. However, in human beings, tumor growth is generally not accelerated markedly by improved nutrition.[11] Furthermore, it has been suggested that accelerated tumor growth may be beneficial for people receiving chemotherapy or radiation, since these treatments are more effective in rapidly dividing cells. Do not allow your clients with cancer to starve themselves in the mistaken belief that they will be starving their cancer.

Finally, in considering the value of nutrition support in cancer, it is important to remember that progressive malnutrition in people with cancer is a major cause of death.[12] In a study of people with head and neck cancer, adequate nutrition status was associated with a highly significant increased survival rate (57.5 percent of adequately nourished people lived for 2 years), as opposed to poor nutrition status (only 7.5 percent of those in poor nutrition status lived for 2 years).[13] In cancer, extreme malnutrition is a sign of impending death.[14] Therefore, feeding the person with cancer before nutrient depletion is particularly important.

Oral Diets during Therapy

A diet supplying 40 to 45 kcalories per kilogram of body weight per day with 1.5 to 2.0 grams of protein is frequently recommended.[15] A few general measures can help the person with cancer to maintain nutrition status during radiation

People with cancer, particularly those who feel they cannot be helped by therapy, are easy targets for peddlers of nutrition "cures." They may take massive doses of vitamins and minerals, some of which may be toxic. Generally, people will not volunteer information about their use of vitamin supplements. Be sure to find out what supplements, and what amounts of them, your clients may be taking.

or chemotherapy. For one, encourage people to eat extra food between chemotherapy treatments, to compensate for weight loss during treatments. For another, minimize the likelihood of learned food aversions by suggesting that the person fast for several hours before radiation therapy or chemotherapy.

Tube Feedings and Parenteral Nutrition

Whenever possible, people with cancer should be encouraged to eat regular foods to meet nutrient needs. But often, this is difficult. Sometimes giving liquid supplements between or with meals can be helpful. However, when anorexia persists, particularly during and immediately after treatment, tube feedings or parenteral nutrition may be indicated (see Chapter 18). Begin these measures before severe malnutrition sets in.

Although the use of enteral and parenteral nutrition may be beneficial for many people, there are some additional considerations. These measures may cause some people to gain fat and water weight rather than lean body mass.

Improving Appetite

When working with cancer clients who are anorectic, try to provide them with a good reason to eat. Explain that they may be better able to tolerate their

Tips for improving the appetite:
- Understand the reasons you need to eat.
- Eat most during times when you feel best.
- Use foods that are easy to prepare and eat.
- Eat smaller meals.
- Don't drink liquids with meals.
- Use nutritious liquids between meals.
- Use time-saving appliances.

Some important questions (in addition to those mentioned above) should be considered before aggressive measures are taken to provide the cancer client with tube feedings and parenteral nutrition. Is the person a candidate for anticancer therapy? Providing such aggressive nutrition support to a person with terminal cancer who cannot be given other treatments is often contraindicated.

But sometimes another question comes up. If aggressive support will help maintain the quality of life, should it be encouraged? This question is harder to answer. On the one hand, the person who is dying should be as comfortable as possible. On the other hand, TPN is expensive, and it may prolong life unnecessarily. (Such dilemmas are discussed in Highlight 20.) The person may have false hopes about what TPN might accomplish. The person with terminal cancer who is a candidate for TPN should be given the facts on which to base the decision of whether to accept TPN or not. The person's decision must be respected.

treatments if they eat well, and that they will stay stronger and be more able to maintain their activity levels.

Counsel clients to take advantage of times when they feel best to eat more and to prepare foods that can be eaten when they don't have the energy to prepare a meal. For many people, morning is the best time of the day. For them, eating a high-kcalorie, high-protein breakfast will help. As the day wears on and they begin to tire easily, they can eat foods that were prepared earlier or that are easy to prepare and eat. Canned, frozen, or convenience foods are good alternatives. Foods that are easy to chew can help ease the task of eating. Encourage clients to let friends and family help with meals whenever possible.

People who complain of fullness can eat smaller meals more often. Chewing foods slowly and saving liquids for after meals can also help. Replace empty-kcalorie liquids with juices, milk, milk shakes, instant breakfast drinks, or liquid supplements that add nutrients to the diet. Recommend that greasy, high-fat foods be avoided, because they slow down gastric motility.

Find out what appliances clients have that can help reduce the time it takes to fix a meal. Blenders, electric frying pans, toaster ovens, microwave ovens, and dishwashers are useful. People who do not have these appliances may be able to purchase them.

You can also give your clients hints on how they can add kcalories and protein to their diets. Some suggestions are given in Table 27–3.

People with cancer frequently complain of a bitter or metallic taste in their mouths. Because of this taste alteration, they frequently dislike red meat, and they may prefer to use fish, poultry, eggs, or dairy products in its place. Meat casseroles or soups and sauces added to meat may be more appealing than meat served alone, and meats served at room temperature or cold meats may taste better than hot meats. Suggest marinating poultry and meats in sweet wines, Italian dressing, or sweet-sour sauces. Using

Try these suggestions if you experience a bitter or metallic taste when you eat:
- Use eggs, fish, poultry, and dairy products in place of meats.
- Add sauces and seasonings to meat.
- Serve meat cold or at room temperature.
- Use a mouthwash or brush teeth before eating.

TABLE 27–3

Suggestions for Adding kCalories and Protein to the Diet

- Add 2 tablespoons of milk powder to the milk that you drink, use in recipes, or add to soups, puddings, and cereals.
- Add ground meats, chicken, fish, or grated cheese to sauces, soups, casseroles, or vegetables.
- Use extra butter, margarine, or cream cheese on bread.
- Eat peanut butter on fruit, celery, or crackers.
- Use butter or margarine whenever possible (on bread, potatoes, vegetables, pasta, and rice).
- Use yogurt, sour cream, or a sour cream dip with vegetables.
- Use mayonnaise as a salad dressing and on sandwiches.
- Add whipping cream to desserts and hot chocolate or use it to lighten coffee.
- Have snacks available at all times.
- Add nuts and dried fruits such as raisins to desserts or cereals.
- Use cream instead of milk with cereal.
- Try commercially available liquid supplements or instant breakfast mixes for between meal snacks.

strong seasonings such as oregano, basil, mint, or tarragon can help. Suggest that clients use a mouthwash or brush their teeth before eating, to start with a fresh, pleasant feeling.

Relieving Nausea, Vomiting, and Other GI Discomforts

Nausea and vomiting are common complaints of people on chemotherapy. Some people get so sick they decide to discontinue the therapy. Standard drugs normally used to control nausea and vomiting are frequently ineffective in people with cancer.

Some diet guidelines may help. Advise the person to eat small meals and avoid high-fat foods. Save liquids for between meals. When the person is nauseated, slowly sipping clear beverages such as ginger ale or sucking Popsicles or ice cubes made from a favorite liquid may help. Encourage people to use liquids to prevent dehydration when vomiting is a problem. For nausea, suggest that the person lie down with head elevated after eating. Loosening the clothing and getting fresh air can also help relieve nausea.

If the smell of certain foods causes nausea, these foods should be avoided. It may be best to let someone else do the cooking or use foods that can be eaten without cooking.

Take a brief history to determine if the person becomes nauseated or vomits at about the same time each day. If so, have the person avoid favorite foods near that time to prevent the development of learned food aversions.

People with cancer may complain of diarrhea, constipation, heartburn, or gas. Others, particularly those who have had radiation therapy to the small bowel, develop lactose intolerance. The nutrition recommendations for these problems are discussed in Chapters 21 and 22.

Overcoming Chewing and Swallowing Problems

We have already discussed the general guidelines for handling problems with chewing and swallowing (see Chapter 21). These same principles apply to people with cancer who have mouth sores, reduced salivary secretions, or resections that interfere with chewing and swallowing.

Hints to control nausea and vomiting:
- Eat small meals.
- Avoid high-fat foods.
- Sip clear liquids or suck Popsicles to prevent dehydration.
- Lie down after eating.
- Loosen clothing after eating.
- Get fresh air.
- Avoid smells that cause nausea.
- If nausea occurs at the same time each day, avoid favorite foods during that time.

If you have trouble swallowing:
- Try modifying the consistency of the foods you eat; chopped or pureed foods may be easier to handle.
- Try tilting your head forward or backward to see if positioning your head differently can ease swallowing.
- Use a straw for drinking.
- Use liquid supplements to increase your kcaloric intake.

As you read about ways of handling nutrition-related problems in the cancer client, you may be deceived into thinking that it's not that hard to get the person to eat. For example, if you want someone to get more kcalories, you recommend adding fats to the diet. But think again. What if the person is nauseated and feels full after taking a few bites? For this person, a low-fat diet is recommended. That cuts out many ways for adding kcalories to the diet. A similar problem occurs in the lactose-intolerant person who needs to add more protein to the diet: milk shakes are the ideal way to add nourishment, but this person gets sick from drinking milk.

So, you see, getting a person with cancer to eat is a lot harder than it appears. The health professional has to work closely with the individual to find acceptable food choices that provide for a well-balanced diet.

Cancer

Mr. Wayne is a retired newsman who first visited his doctor when he noticed that he was losing weight rapidly and that he seemed to be drained of energy. He also had a lesion in his mouth that wouldn't heal. Mr. Wayne has a history of alcohol and cigarette abuse. After being admitted to the hospital, tests confirmed a diagnosis of cancer of the mouth. The doctor would like to prepare Mr. Wayne nutritionally before proceeding with radiation therapy. Radical surgery is a possibility. A thorough nutrition assessment revealed that Mr. Wayne was suffering from severe PCM that was classified as kwashiorkor-marasmus mix. His height and weight are 5'10" and 125 lb, respectively.

1. What is Mr. Wayne's ideal weight? His %IBW? What other anthropometric measurements would you expect to see affected? Will serum protein levels be low? What other lab test results would you expect to see affected?
2. How might Mr. Wayne's past history have affected his nutrition status before he developed cancer? In what ways can cancer affect his nutrition status? How can radiation therapy affect his nutrition status?

Discuss the possible impact of radical head and neck surgery on his nutrition status.
3. Describe cancer cachexia. What are some of its causes? What are the benefits of preventing or correcting it?
4. Discuss the possible feeding routes for replenishing Mr. Wayne's nutrient stores prior to treatment. How might radiation therapy or radical surgery narrow the choice of feeding routes?
5. If Mr. Wayne is able to take food by mouth, what suggestions will you give him for dealing with poor appetite, nausea and vomiting, dry and sore mouth, and chewing and swallowing problems? Is he likely to develop lactose intolerance or radiation enteritis? Why or why not?

People with chewing and swallowing difficulties may need softer foods to which sauces and gravies have been added. They may tolerate casseroles well. Spicy, acidic, or coarse foods, as well as foods with seeds, should be avoided by people with mouth sores. Suggest that the person who has trouble swallowing try tilting the head back or forward to see if this helps. Using a straw makes drinking easier. Smoking and alcoholic beverages can irritate the throat. Liquid supplements or tube feedings may sometimes be necessary.

People who have a reduced saliva flow may feel better if they rinse their mouths frequently. One author recommends swabbing the mouth with meat tenderizer to help relieve dry mouth.[16] The meat tenderizer contains an enzyme (papain) that helps break up thick mucous secretions. Artificial saliva is available to help reduce irritation and ease chewing and swallowing. In people with little saliva, special attention should be paid to oral hygiene, because they are more susceptible to dental caries. Therefore, concentrated sweets should also be avoided.

With mouth ulcers, avoid foods that are spicy, acidic, or coarse, or that contain small seeds that can be trapped in an ulcer.

If your mouth is dry due to a reduced flow of saliva, try rinsing your mouth frequently. Talk with your doctor about using artificial saliva, and avoid concentrated sweets.

Nutrition Assessment

The nutrition assessment of the person with cancer is particularly important in preventing severe malnutrition. Some areas that deserve special consideration include:

- Examine the person's diet history. Look for the adequacy of the diet and any foods that cause problems.
- Check to see what type of therapy the person has been receiving or will receive to determine how nutrition status may be affected.
- Check the person's weight history, noting any weight loss that has occurred unintentionally as a result of cancer or its treatment.
- Ask clients about special diets they may be following, and ask if they are taking any vitamin or mineral supplements.
- Record anthropometric measurements regularly. This will help determine if the person's energy and protein needs are being met. Step in to correct problems early, before they become severe.
- Edema may be present in certain types of cancer and can affect anthropometric measurements.
- People with severe vomiting or diarrhea may be dehydrated. Biochemical parameters in dehydrated people may falsely appear to be normal.

The person with cancer is frequently at high risk for malnutrition. The health care team should be alert to the possibility of malnutrition and should take corrective measures to avoid nutrition problems whenever possible.

Study Questions

1. What is cancer? What events are believed to lead to cancer?
2. What is cancer cachexia? What factors contribute to the development of cancer cachexia? Can nutrition intervention help prevent this problem?
3. Describe the anorexia that is associated with cancer. How does it differ from anorexia in other disease states? Discuss how cancer itself and the therapy for cancer contributes to anorexia.
4. How can cancer result in excess nutrient losses, and how do these losses contribute to the cancer cachexia syndrome?
5. What are food aversions, and how can they be dealt with?
6. Describe the metabolic changes that occur in the person with cancer, and discuss their role in the cancer cachexia syndrome.
7. What advantages does good nutrition status hold for the person with cancer? In what ways are people with cancer fed to prevent them from developing severe nutrient deficiencies?
8. What recommendations and other strategies can help the person with cancer who has anorexia? Bitter or metallic taste in the mouth? Nausea and vomiting? Problems with chewing and swallowing? Mouth ulcers? Reduced flow of saliva?

Notes

1. American Cancer Society, *1986 Cancer Facts and Figures* (New York: American Cancer Society, 1986), p. 3.
2. A. Theologides, Anorexia-producing intermediary metabolites, *American Journal of Clinical Nutrition* 29 (1976): 552–558.
3. M. E. Shils, How to nourish the cancer patient, *Nutrition Today*, May-June 1981, pp. 4–15.
4. I. L. Bernstein and R. A. Sigmundi, Tumor anorexia: A learned food aversion? *Science* 209 (1980): 416–418.
5. I. L. Bernstein, Physiological and psychological mechanisms of cancer anorexia, *Cancer Research* 42 (1982): 715s–720s.
6. Bernstein, 1982.
7. J. C. Smith and coauthors, Radiation-induced taste aversion as a factor in cancer therapy, *Cancer Treatment Reports* 68 (1984): 1219–1227.
8. J. A. Norlon, M. E. Burt, and M. F. Brennan, In vivo utilization of substrate by human sarcoma-bearing limbs, *Cancer* 45 (1980): 2934–2939.
9. W. D. DeWys, Pathophysiology of cancer cachexia: Current understanding and areas for future research, *Cancer Research* 42 (1982): 721s–726s.
10. DeWys, 1982.
11. Shils, 1981.
12. R. M. Faulk, Nutritional therapy in cancer, *Postgraduate Medicine* 78, no. 1 (1985): 83–87.
13. G. B. Brookes, Nutritional status—A prognostic indicator in head and neck cancer, *Otolaryngology Head and Neck Surgery* 93 (1985): 69–73.
14. J. van Eys, Effect of nutritional status on response to therapy, *Cancer Research* 42 (1982): 747s–753s.
15. Faulk, 1985.
16. G. L. Larsen, Rehabilitation for the patient with head and neck cancer, *American Journal of Nursing* 82 (1982): 119–121.

Therapeutic Diets in Perspective

Throughout the later part of this book, you have seen how modified diets can be used as a part of therapy in the treatment of a variety of disorders. You have been exposed to many facts about diets and disorders. You may have the impression that if a person has disorder A, then symptoms X, Y, and Z will appear. When given diet Q, the person recovers beautifully. In reality, nothing could be farther from the truth. The way a disorder manifests itself from one person to the next is as unique as individuals are. Two people do not respond to a set diet simply because they both have the same disorder.

Of all the highlights in this book, this one contains the most opinion and the fewest facts. Its purpose is to help you see how important it is to individualize therapeutic diets and learn how to develop a set of priorities to decide when a diet is of critical importance, when it is only slightly helpful, and when it may even be contraindicated.

Such a decision is first based on all the available facts. What are the proven benefits of the diet in question? What are its negative effects? What are the proven risks of *not* following the diet? Even after you have reflected on these questions, other considerations still arise. These are the intangible, human factors of real-life situations; that is, you must exercise clinical judgment in deciding how important a diet is to a client's health. From your evaluation, you can learn when a client's dietary indiscretions are real concerns that require further intervention, and when it may be best to leave well enough

alone. It is a matter of opinion, and opinions differ. Three examples follow.

Ted

Ted is a busy executive who leads a hectic life and is constantly on the go. Last year, Ted found out that he had a peptic ulcer. His doctor prescribed a traditional bland diet with six small meals a day and told Ted to drink plenty of milk and to take antacids between meals.

Ted is upset about the diet. You have gotten to know him pretty well during his hospital stay and can relate to some of his problems. He barely has time to eat three meals a day, let alone six. He hates milk. The only thing he likes about the diet is that he can still have his usual bedtime snack. Ted confided in you that he has no intention of following the diet. He was outraged when the nurses refused to bring him his morning coffee.

What should you say to Ted? First of all, review the facts. The traditional bland diet is of little proven value. Eating frequent meals and drinking

DO THE BENEFITS OUTWEIGH THE DISADVANTAGES?

milk may actually increase gastric acid secretion (see Chapter 21). Couple these facts with your knowledge that Ted won't follow the diet anyway, and you have identified several major factors weighing against Ted's proposed dietary regimen.

What about coffee? It is true that coffee, even if decaffeinated, stimulates gastric acid secretion. But will Ted's stomach secrete even more acid if he gets worked up about not having coffee? You can't know the answer to this question, but you do know Ted, so you must draw a conclusion from what you know. All in all, it seems to you that the minuses outweigh the pluses in the case of this diet.

You decide to discuss your concerns with the dietitian. The dietitian contacts Ted's physician and suggests an alternative approach. The dietitian then instructs Ted to follow a liberal bland diet with three meals a day. As for coffee, you reinforce what the dietitian told Ted—it's not recommended—and you then tell him why. But you add that if he does drink coffee, he should limit it to his one favorite cup in the

THIS DIET NEEDS WORK!

morning and not to drink it on an empty stomach.

The situation changes if the diagnosis is different. Suppose that Ted doesn't have an ulcer, but rather a hiatal hernia. This time the doctor prescribes a liberal bland diet with five small meals and no eating before bedtime. Ted still does not see how he can squeeze in two extra meals, and he does not want to give up his bedtime snack; however, now the ratio of benefits to disadvantages has changed. You decide to tell Ted why.

This time, the diet is more justifiable. Smaller feedings will help prevent stomach distension, which can aggravate the hiatal hernia. Furthermore, heartburn can result if the diet is not followed, and it can be quite painful. Lying down after eating increases the risk of reflux esophagitis and heartburn, so a bedtime snack is unwise. Coffee lowers the cardiac sphincter pressure, which also aggravates the problem.

The major drawback of the diet is that Ted will have to change his lifestyle slightly. He will have to find time to squeeze in extra feedings and to live without his morning cup of coffee and a bedtime snack. This time, the benefits of the diet outweigh the disadvantages. If Ted wishes to avoid the pain of heartburn and the possible

complications of hiatal hernia, he will have to find a way to make the necessary adjustments. Ask the dietitian to talk with Ted. The dietitian can suggest foods that are convenient for Ted to eat. You can reinforce the dietitian's suggestions.

Jennifer

Jennifer is a healthy young woman of 25. She was born with phenylketonuria (PKU), but it was diagnosed within three days' time; her parents instituted the PKU diet immediately to promote Jennifer's normal development (see Highlight 24). The diet was discontinued when Jennifer was six years old, and she has led quite a normal life since then. Now she is pregnant, and her doctor has told her she must go back on the PKU diet. She is expressing resentment to you at the necessity of following the diet's myriad rules and using its expensive special products. She remembers that the diet cramped her lifestyle and prevented her from participating fully in many social activities, even when she was only five.

What should you say to Jennifer? First, consult the facts. Obviously, to evade the doctor's orders would, in this case, pose considerable risks—not to

Jennifer herself, but to her unborn infant. The diet will not provide a perfect guarantee that Jennifer's baby will be mentally and physically normal, but severe disability is inevitable if she does not follow the diet. It is your responsibility to present her with the facts and to make sure that she receives meticulous instructions about the intricacies of the diet. Jennifer will make her own decision, but you can't in good conscience support her in a choice not to comply with the doctor's orders. Inform the other members of the health care team about Jennifer's feelings so that all of you can work together to help Jennifer through a difficult time.

Other diets that are of critical importance are those that bring about life-sustaining changes in metabolism. Among these diets are those for liver failure, renal failure, and IDDM. All of your efforts should be directed at ensuring compliance with these diets. A person's complaint that such a diet is restrictive is not a cue for you to tell the person, "Never mind, it's all right not to follow the diet." Rather, remember that no diet is so rigid that it cannot be planned to some extent around the individual's lifestyle and preferences. There are no foods that can't be worked into most diets on occasion with careful planning. The key is that "forbidden" foods should be used on occasion only, in limited amounts, and only when their inclusion in the diet is planned. An occasional lapse from the diet rules will not be fatal, but the better the compliance with a metabolism-normalizing diet, the better supported is the person's recovery and health.

Martha

Martha's case illustrates another set of considerations that enter into decision making about therapeutic diets. You have seen Martha in the hospital several times over the last few years. She is a

TED NEEDS TO ADJUST HIS LIFESTYLE FOR THIS DIET.

JENNIFER, THIS DIET IS VERY IMPORTANT!

sweet, elderly lady (70 years old) with several problems:

- Obesity.
- NIDDM.
- A hiatal hernia.
- Type IV hyperlipidemia.
- Chronic constipation.

For the first time, her doctor is recommending that she be put on a special diet. Considering her multiple problems, the diet that might be appropriate for Martha is:

- Low in kcalories.
- Low in cholesterol and total fat, with an even distribution of fat kcalories from saturated, monosaturated, and polyunsaturated fat.
- Low in concentrated sweets.
- Restricted in foods that cause gastric acid secretion.
- High in fiber.

These changes entail several problems, however. For one thing, these are quite a few changes to inflict on someone who has already lived seventy years. For another, Martha could get confused trying to obey all those rules at once. Let's analyze the pros and cons and establish priorities before deciding what kind of diet would be useful to Martha.

To make the diet low in kcalories would help with four of Martha's five problems, because a low-kcalorie diet would bring about weight loss, normalize blood glucose, bring down her high lipids, and reduce abdominal pressure to improve her hernia. Three of these four advantages would also be gained by making the diet low in concentrated sweets: weight loss; blood glucose control; and, possibly, lower triglyceride levels. It would seem advisable, then, to help Martha to work out a low-kcalorie, low-concentrated-sweets diet. This would be a fairly simple process and would not be too overwhelming to her at first.

To make Martha's diet high in fiber as well would help with her constipation problem, would facilitate weight loss by displacing kcalorie-rich foods, and might improve her blood glucose control—three of the five goals chosen for her. Martha could probably understand this diet and, with help, might incorporate these changes into her eating habits, especially if you gave her reason to hope that she would notice an improvement in her health.

What about all the proposed changes in the kinds and amounts of fat proposed for Martha's diet? A review of the facts on similar cases suggests that a fat-controlled diet for a woman Martha's age might not significantly reduce the risk of atherosclerosis. In this case, asking her to change menus she has used for years might not be worth the trouble. As for eliminating irritating foods to help with the hiatal hernia, perhaps you could discuss this with her. You and Martha might work out a low-kcalorie diet in which high-fiber foods are emphasized and concentrated sweets are discouraged. You might make Martha aware of the foods likely to irritate her hiatal hernia and leave the use of these foods to her discretion.

If you care enough to provide the best nutrition therapy for your clients, you will work hard to develop skill in giving diet advice. You won't simply give everyone who has the same "label" the same diet. Furthermore, because research in diet therapy is an active and fast-moving area, you will keep your eyes and ears open for new information on the benefits and risks of alternatives in diet. You will develop your clinical judgment as all good judges do: by allowing each new fact and each new case to find its proper place in your decision making.

Cells, Hormones, and Nerves

This appendix is offered as an optional chapter for readers who want to enhance their understanding of the body's ways of coordinating its activities. It presents a brief summary of the structure and function of the body's basic working unit—the cell, and of its two major regulatory systems—the hormonal system and the nervous system.

cell: the basic unit of life, of which all living things are composed. Every cell is surrounded by a membrane and contains cytoplasm, within which are organelles and a nucleus; the cell nucleus contains chromosomes.

The Cell

Every body organ is made up of millions of cells and of materials produced by them. Each organ's cells are specialized to perform that organ's functions, but all cells have basic things in common (see Figure A-1). Every cell is contained within a cell membrane. Inside the membrane lies the cytoplasm or cell "fluid," and another membrane-enclosed body, the nucleus. Inside the nucleus are the chromosomes, which contain the genetic material, DNA. The DNA encodes all the instructions for carrying out the cell's activities.

The cell membrane's functions in moving materials into and out of the cell, and some of its special proteins such as "pumps," were described in Chapter 5. Also described earlier were specializations of the cell membrane, such as microvilli (Chapter 6) and cilia (Chapter 10), which permit cells to interact with other cells and with their environments in highly specific ways.

The role of DNA in coding for cell proteins was summarized in Chapter 5, Figure 5-4. Chapter 5 also described the variety of proteins produced by cells and the ways they perform the body's work.

The cytoplasm contains much more than just fluid. It is a highly organized system of fibers, tubes, membranes, particles, and subcellular organelles as complex as a city. These parts intercommunicate, manufacture and exchange materials, package and prepare materials for export, and maintain and repair themselves.

Among the organelles are ribosomes, mitochondria, and lysosomes. Figure 5-4 briefly referred to the ribosomes; they assemble amino acids into proteins, following directions conveyed to them by RNA copies from the DNA in the chromosomes.

cell membrane: the membrane that surrounds the cell and encloses its contents; made primarily of lipid and protein.

cytoplasm (SIGH-toe-plazm): the cell contents, except for the nucleus.
cyto = cell
plasm = a form

nucleus: a major membrane-enclosed body within every cell, which contains the cell's genetic material, DNA, embedded in chromosomes.
nucleus = a kernel

chromosomes: a set of structures within the nucleus of every cell that contain the cell's genetic material, DNA, associated with other materials (primarily proteins).

organelles: subcellular structures such as ribosomes, mitochondria, and lysosomes.
organelle = little organ

ribosomes: protein-making organelles in cells; composed of RNA and protein.
ribo = containing the sugar ribose (in RNA)
some = body

A

FIGURE A-1.

The structure of a typical cell. The cell shown might be one in a gland (such as the pancreas) that produces secretory products (enzymes) for export (to the intestine). The rough endoplasmic reticulum with its ribosomes produces the enzymes; the smooth reticulum conducts them to the Golgi region; the Golgi membranes merge with the cell membrane; where the enzymes can be released into the extracellular fluid.

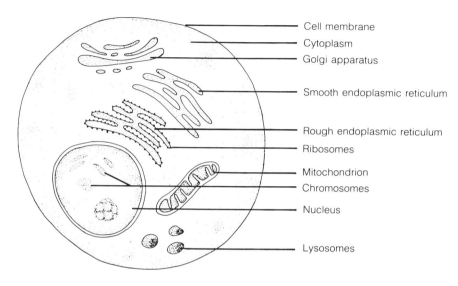

Cell membrane
Cytoplasm
Golgi apparatus

Smooth endoplasmic reticulum

Rough endoplasmic reticulum
Ribosomes

Mitochondrion
Chromosomes

Nucleus

Lysosomes

mitochondria (my-toe-KON-dree-uh); singular **mitochondrion**): the cellular organelles responsible for producing ATP aerobically; made of membranes (lipid and protein) with enzymes mounted on them.
mitos = thread (referring to their slender shape)
chondros = cartilage (referring to their external appearance)

lysosomes: cellular organelles, membrane-enclosed sacs of degradative enzymes.
lysis = dissolution

rough endoplasmic reticulum (en-doh-PLAZ-mic reh-TIC-you-lum): intracellular membranes on which ribosomes are mounted, where protein synthesis takes place.
endo = inside
plasm = the cytoplasm

The mitochondria are made of intricately folded membranes which bear thousands of highly organized sets of enzymes on their inner and outer surfaces. Although not often referred to in this book's chapters, their presence is implied whenever the enzymes of the TCA cycle and electron transport chain are mentioned, for the mitochondria house all these enzymes.* Mitochondria are therefore crucial to aerobic metabolism, described in Chapter 7, and muscles conditioned to work aerobically are packed with them. Several chapter-opening photographs depict mitochondria in different kinds of cells.

The lysosomes are membranes enclosing degradative enzymes. When a cell needs to self-destruct, or to digest materials in its surroundings, its lysosomes free their enzymes. Lysosomes are active when tissue repair or remodeling is taking place—for example, in cleaning up infections, healing wounds, shaping embryonic organs, and remodeling bones.

Besides these and other cellular organelles, the cell's cytoplasm contains a highly organized system of membranes, the endoplasmic reticulum. The ribosomes may either float free in the cytoplasm or may be seated on these membranes. A membranous surface dotted with ribosomes looks speckled under the microscope and is called "rough" endoplasmic reticulum; such a

*For the reactions of glycolysis, the TCA cycle, and the electron transport chain, see Chapter 7 and Appendix C. The reactions of glycolysis take place in the cytoplasm; the end product acetyl CoA moves into the mitochondrion; and the TCA and electron transport reactions take place there. The mitochondrion then releases carbon dioxide, water, and ATP as its end products.

surface without ribosomes is called "smooth." Some intracellular membranes are organized into tubules that collect cellular materials, merge with the cell membrane, and discharge their contents to the outside of the cell; these membrane systems are named the Golgi complex for the person who first described them. The rough and smooth endoplasmic reticulum and the Golgi complex are continuous with one another, so that secretions produced deep in the interior of the cell can be efficiently transported to the outside and released.

These and other cell structures enable cells to perform the multitudes of functions for which they are specialized. The illustrations at the start of each chapter depict further details of cell structure and function.

The actions of cells are coordinated by both hormones and nerves, as the next sections show. Among specializations of cellular organelles are receptors for hormones that deliver instructions originating elsewhere in the body. Some hormones penetrate the cell and nucleus, and attach to receptors on chromosomes, from which they activate certain genes to initiate, stop, speed up, or slow down synthesis of certain proteins as needed. Other hormones attach to receptors on the cell surface and transmit their messages from there. The hormones are described in the next section; the nerves in the one following.

smooth endoplasmic reticulum: smooth intracellular membranes bearing no ribosomes.

Golgi (GOAL-gee) **apparatus:** a set of membranes within the cell where secretory materials are packaged for export.

The Hormones

The hormones insulin and glucagon have already been introduced. Insulin lowers blood glucose by driving it into cells and promoting its conversion to glycogen and fat; glucagon raises it by enhancing the breakdown and release of stored glycogen and the conversion of amino acids to glucose. These hormones work rapidly and they work on cells all over the body as hormones typically do. They can do this because they are secreted directly into the blood by their producing organs—the endocrine glands—so they reach all cells without fail.

The hormones, the glands they originate in, and their target organs and effects are described in the next sections. All the hormones you might be interested in are included, but only a few are discussed in detail. Figure A-2 identifies the glands that produce the hormones discussed in these sections.

The whole picture is of a complex system in which many of the parts interact with each other. For example, several hormones are produced in the anterior pituitary gland in the brain. All of these are regulated by hormones produced in another part of the brain, the hypothalamus. Furthermore, each of the pituitary gland hormones has effects on the production of compounds elsewhere in the body. Some of these compounds are also hormones that will affect still other body parts. A hormone may travel far from its point of origin and ultimately have profound, even unexpected, effects.

insulin, glucagon: see pages 53-54

hormone: a chemical messenger. Hormones are secreted in response to altered conditions by a variety of endocrine glands in the body. Each affects one or more specific target tissues or organs and elicits specific responses to restore normal conditions.

endocrine: with reference to a gland, one that secretes its product directly into (endo) the blood, like the pancreas cells that produce insulin. An **exocrine** gland secretes its product(s) out (exo) of the blood through a duct into a cavity; the sweat glands of the skin and the enzyme-producing glands of the pancreas are both examples. The pancreas is therefore both an endocrine and an exocrine gland.

Endocrinology is the study of hormones and their effects, and the system of glands and hormones that regulates body processes is the **endocrine system.**

A

The endocrine system

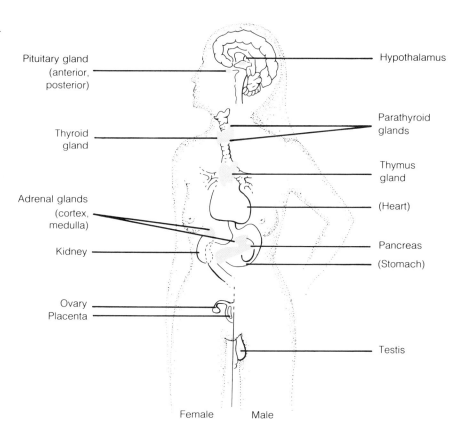

Pituitary gland
(anterior,
posterior)

Hypothalamus

Thyroid
gland

Parathyroid
glands

Thymus
gland

(Heart)

Adrenal glands
(cortex,
medulla)

Kidney

Pancreas

(Stomach)

Ovary
Placenta

Testis

Female   Male

The **pituitary** gland in the brain has two parts—the **anterior** (front) and the **posterior** (hind) part.

adrenocorticotropin: so named because it stimulates (*trope*) the adrenal cortex.

follicle: that part of the female reproductive system where the ovary lies and eggs are produced.

luteinizing: so called because the follicle turns orange as it matures.
lutein = an orange pigment

prolactin: so named because it promotes (*pro*) the production of milk (*lacto*).

melanocyte (MEL-an-oh-cite): a cell containing the pigment melanin.
cyte = cell

cortex: The adrenal gland, like the pituitary, has two parts, in this case an outer portion (*cortex*) and an inner core (*medulla*).

Hormones of the Pituitary Gland and Hypothalamus

The anterior pituitary gland produces the hormones:

- Adrenocorticotropin (ACTH).
- Thyroid-stimulating hormone (TSH).
- Growth hormone (GH).
- Follicle-stimulating hormone (FSH).
- Luteinizing hormone (LH).
- Prolactin.
- Melanocyte-stimulating hormone (MSH).

Each of these hormones acts on one or more target organs and elicits a characteristic response. ACTH acts on the adrenal cortex, promoting the making and release of its hormones. TSH acts on the thyroid gland, promoting the making and release of thyroid hormone. GH works on all tissues, promoting growth, fat breakdown, and the formation of antibodies. FSH works on the ovaries in the female, promoting their maturation, and on the testicles in the male, promoting sperm formation. LH also acts on the ovaries, forwarding their maturation, the making of progesterone and estrogens, and ovulation; and on the testicles, promoting the making and release of androgens (male hormones). Prolactin, secreted in the female after she has borne a baby, acts on the mammary glands to stimulate their growth and the making of milk. Finally, MSH acts on the pigment cells, promoting the making and dispersal of pigment.

A

The controls over this array of actions are sensitive and specific. Each of the seven hormones itemized above has one or more signals that turn it on and another (or others) that turn it off.

Among the controlling signals are several hormones from the hypothalamus:

- Corticotropin-releasing hormone (CRH), which promotes release of ACTH. This is itself turned on by stress, and off by ACTH when enough has been released.
- TSH-releasing hormone (TRH), which promotes release of TSH. This is turned on by large meals or low body temperature.
- GH-releasing hormone (GRH), which is turned on by insulin.
- FSH/LH-releasing hormone (FSH/LH-RH), which is turned on in the female by nerve messages or low estrogen and in the male by low testosterone.
- GH-inhibiting hormone (GIH or somatostatin), which inhibits the release of GSH and interferes with the release of TSH. This is turned on by hypoglycemia and/or exercise, and is rapidly destroyed by body tissues so that it does not accumulate.
- Prolactin-release-inhibiting hormone (PIH), which is turned on by high prolactin levels and off by estrogen, testosterone, and suckling (by way of nerve messages).
- MSH-release-inhibiting hormone (MIH), which is turned on by melatonin.

Let's examine some of these controls. PIH, for example, responds to high prolactin levels (remember, prolactin promotes the making of milk). High prolactin levels will ensure that milk is made and—by calling forth PIH—will ensure that they don't get too high. But when the infant is suckling—and creating a demand for milk—then PIH is not allowed to work (suckling turns off PIH). The consequence: prolactin remains high and milk manufacture continues. Demand from the infant thus directly adjusts the infant's supply of milk. This example shows not only how the need is met but also illustrates the cooperation between nerves and hormones that achieves this effect.

As another example, take CRH. Stress, perceived in the brain and relayed to the hypothalamus, switches on CRH. CRH, on arriving at the pituitary, switches on ACTH. Then ACTH acts on its target organ, the adrenal cortex, which responds by producing and releasing stress hormones, and the stress response is under way. Events cascading from there involve every body cell and many other hormones (see Chapter 6).

You may wonder why so many steps are required to set the stress response in motion. Having many steps makes it possible for the body to fine-tune the stress response, because control can be exerted at each step. These are just two examples of what the body can do in response to two different stimuli—producing milk in response to an infant's need, and gearing up for action in an emergency.

Two hormones produced by the posterior pituitary gland are:

- Antidiuretic hormone (ADH), or vasopressin.
- Oxytocin.

hypothalamus: a brain region (see Figure 2) that is connected by a channel to the pituitary and can produce many hormones in response to signals from it or from other body conditions.
hypo = below
thalamus = another brain region

Hormones that are turned off by their own effects are said to be regulated by **negative feedback.** For example, when a pituitary gland hormone has caused the release of a substance from a target organ, that substance itself switches off the original hormone signal (that is, it feeds back, negatively).

somatostatin (GIH): the opposite of **somatotropin.**
somato = body
stat = keep the same
tropin = make more

antidiuretic hormone (ADH): the hormone that prevents water loss in urine (also **vasopressin**).
anti = against
di = through
ure = urine
vaso = blood vessels
pressin = pressure

A

oxytocin: the hormone of childbirth.
oxy = quick
tocin = childbirth

progesterone: the hormone of gestation (pregnancy).
pro = promoting
gest = gestation (pregnancy)
sterone = a steroid hormone

cervix: the circular muscle that guards the opening of the uterus. When a baby is about to be born, the cervix begins to stretch.
cervic = neck

Norepinephrine and epinephrine were formerly called noradrenalin and adrenalin.

glucocorticoid: hormone from the adrenal cortex affecting the body's management of glucose.
gluco = glucose
corticoid = from the cortex

calcitonin: so called because it regulates (tones) calcium level.

parathyroid: named for their location, the four parathyroid glands nestle in the surface layers of the two thyroid lobes in the neck.
para = beside, next to

ADH promotes contraction of arteries and acts on the kidney to prevent water from being excreted. It is turned on whenever the blood volume is depleted, or the blood pressure is low, or the salt concentration of the blood is too high. It is turned off by correction of these deviations from normal. Oxytocin is produced in response to reduced progesterone levels, suckling, or the stretching of the cervix, and acts on two target organs. One, the uterus, contracts in response; the other, the mammary glands, eject milk. Oxytocin is turned off by raised progesterone.

Hormones That Regulate Energy Metabolism

Hormones produced by a number of different glands have effects on energy metabolism:

- Insulin, from the pancreas beta cells.
- Glucagon, from the pancreas alpha cells.
- Thyroxine, from the thyroid gland.
- Norepinephrine and epinephrine, from the adrenal medulla.
- Growth hormone (GH), from the anterior pituitary (already mentioned).
- Glucocorticoids, from the adrenal cortex.

Insulin is turned on by many stimuli including raised blood glucose, high levels of its opposing hormone glucagon, and several other hormones; and acts on all cells to increase glucose and amino acid uptake into cells and to promote the secretion of GRH. Glucagon responds to low blood glucose and to its opposing hormone insulin and acts on the liver to promote the breakdown of glycogen to glucose, the conversion of amino acids to glucose, and the release of glucose. Thyroxine responds to TSH and acts on many cells to increase their metabolic rate, growth, and heat production. The hormones norepinephrine and epinephrine respond to stimulation by sympathetic nerves and produce reactions in many cells that facilitate the body's readiness for fight or flight: increased heart activity, blood vessel constriction, breakdown of glycogen and glucose, raised blood glucose levels, and fat breakdown; they also influence the secretion of the many hormones from the hypothalamus that exert control on the body's other systems.

Every body part is affected by these hormones. Different hormones each have unique effects, and hormones that oppose each other can be produced in carefully regulated amounts, so each part can respond to the exact degree that is appropriate to the occasion.

Hormones That Adjust Other Body Balances

Three hormones are involved in moving calcium in and out of the body's storage deposits in the bones:

- Calcitonin (CT), from the thyroid gland.
- Parathyroid hormone (PTH), from the parathyroid gland.
- Vitamin D, from the kidney.

One of calcitonin's target tissues is the bones, which respond by storing calcium from the bloodstream whenever blood calcium rises above the normal range. Calcitonin also acts on the kidney to increase excretion of both calcium and phosphorus in the urine. Parathyroid hormone responds to the opposite condition—lowered blood calcium—and acts on three targets: the bones, which release stored calcium into the blood; the kidney, which slows its excretion of calcium; and the intestine, which increases its calcium absorption. Vitamin D acts with parathyroid hormone and is essential for the absorption of calcium in the intestine.

Another hormone has effects on blood-making activity:

- Erythropoietin, from the kidney.

Erythropoietin is responsive to oxygen depletion of the blood and to anemia, and acts on the bone marrow to stimulate its making of red blood cells.

Another hormone, special for pregnancy, is:

- Relaxin, from the ovary.

This hormone is secreted in response to the raised progesterone and estrogen levels of late pregnancy, and acts on the cervix and pelvic ligaments to allow them to stretch so that they can accommodate the birth process without strain.

Other agents also help regulate blood pressure:

- Renin (enzyme), from the kidney in cooperation with angiotensin in the blood.
- Aldosterone, a hormone from the adrenal cortex.

Renin responds to a reduced blood supply experienced by the kidney, and acts in several ways. Encountering the inactive form of angiotensin in the blood stream, it converts this molecule to active angiotensin I and then to the very active angiotensin II. The angiotensins constrict the blood vessels, thus raising the blood pressure. They also stimulate thirst, leading to increased water intake, another way of raising the blood pressure. The angiotensins also cause the kidneys to retain water and salt. Thus the angiotensins increase blood pressure by several means at once.

Renin and angiotensin also stimulate the adrenal cortex to secrete the hormone aldosterone. This hormone's target is also the kidney which responds by excreting less sodium, and with it, less water. The effect is to retain more water in the bloodstream—thus, again, raising the blood pressure.

The Gastrointestinal Hormones

Three hormones are known to be produced in the stomach and intestines in response to the presence of food or the components of food:

- Gastrin, from the stomach and duodenum.
- Cholecystokinin, from the duodenum.
- Secretin (enterogastrone), from the duodenum.

Gastrin stimulates the stomach to make and release its acid and digestive juices and to move and churn its contents actively. Cholecystokinin signals the gall bladder and pancreas to release their contents into the intestine to

---

Vitamin D, once thought to be a nutrient, is now viewed as a hormone, because it is produced in one body organ and regulates others. For details, see Chapter 11.

erythropoietin (eh-REE-throw-POY-eh-tin): named for its red-blood-cell-making function.
erythro = red (blood cell)
poiesis = creating (like poetry)

relaxin: the hormone of late pregnancy.

renin (REEN-in): an enzyme from the kidney, which works by activating angiotensin.
ren = kidney

angiotensin: a hormone involved in blood pressure regulation.
angio = blood vessels
tensin = pressure

aldosterone: a hormone from the adrenal gland, involved in blood pressure regulation.
aldo = aldehyde

A

aid in digestion. Secretin calls forth acid-neutralizing bicarbonate from the pancreas into the intestine, and slows the action of the stomach and its secretion of acid and digestive juices. These hormones are dealt with in more detail in Chapter 6.

The Sex Hormones

The three major sex hormones are:

- Testosterone, from the testes.
- Estrogen, from the ovary.
- Progesterone, from the ovary's corpus luteum in preparation for, and during, pregnancy.

Testosterone, in the male, in response to LH (described earlier) acts on all the tissues that are involved in male sexuality and promotes their sexual development and maintenance. Estrogens, in response to both FSH and LH, do the same thing in the female. Progesterone, in response to raised LH and prolactin, acts on the uterus and mammary glands, stimulating them to grow and develop.

testosterone: a steroid hormone from the testes. The steroids, as explained in Chapter 4, are chemically related to, and some are derived from, the lipid cholesterol.
sterone = a steroid hormone

estrogens: hormones responsible for the menstrual cycle and other female characteristics.
oestrus = the egg-making cycle
gen = gives rise to

progesterone: see page A-6.

The Prostaglandins

The prostaglandins are a group of hormones produced by many different body organs with a multitude of diverse effects. More recently discovered than the other hormones, they don't have descriptive names but are designated by letters and numbers: E_1, E_2, and so forth. One, produced in the kidney in response to angiotensin and increased epinephrine, dilates and/or constricts blood vessels, working especially on those of the kidney itself. The lung and liver rapidly inactivate this hormone so that it will not work in these organs. Another prostaglandin, produced in the neural tissue in response to certain nerve activity, alters transmission of nerve impulses. Still another, produced by many of the body's cells, alters their response to hormones. The prostaglandins are all derived from the polyunsaturated fatty acids, and account in part for the essentiality of these fatty acids in the diet.

prostaglandin: see p. 98.

The description of the hormones just given names the major ones and lists a function or two for each. This should suffice to provide an awareness of the enormous impact these compounds have on body processes. The other overall regualting agency is the nervous system.

The Nervous System

The nervous system has a central control system—a sort of computer—that can evaluate information about conditions within and outside the body, and a vast system of wiring by means of which it receives information and sends

central nervous system: the central part of the nervous system, the brain and spinal cord.

A

instructions. The control unit is the brain and spinal cord, called the central nervous system; and the vast complex of wiring between the center and the parts is the peripheral nervous system.

The nervous system has several functions; it controls voluntary muscles in response to sensory stimuli from them, and it controls involuntary, internal muscles and glands in response to nerve-borne and chemical signals about their status. In fact, it is best understood as two systems that use the same or similar pathways to receive and transmit their messages. The somatic nervous system controls the voluntary muscles; the autonomic nervous system controls the internal organs.

When scientists were first studying the autonomic nervous system, they noticed that when something hurt one organ of the body, some of the other organs reacted as if in sympathy for the afflicted one. They therefore named the nerve network they were studying the sympathetic nervous system. The term is still used today to refer to that branch of the autonomic nervous system that responds to pain and stress. The other branch is called parasympathetic nervous system. (Both transmit their messages through the brain and spinal cord.) Nerves of the two branches travel side by side along the same pathways to transmit their messages, but they oppose each other's actions (see Figure A-3).

peripheral (puh-RIFF-er-ul) **nervous system:** the peripheral (outermost) part of the nervous system, the vast complex of wiring that extends from the central nervous system to the body's outermost areas. It contains both somatic and autonomic components (defined next).

somatic (so-MAT-ick) **nervous system:** the division of the nervous system that controls the voluntary muscles, as distinguished from the autonomic nervous system, which controls involuntary functions.
soma = body

autonomic nervous system: the division of the nervous system that controls the body's automatic responses. Its two branches are the **sympathetic** branch, which helps the body respond to stressors from the outside environment, and the **parasympathetic** branch, which regulates normal body activities between stressful times.
autonomos = self-governing

FIGURE A-3.

The organization of the nervous system.

Brain

Spinal cord

Peripheral nerves

Physical structures, such as brain and nerves, make up all the nervous system divisions. They can be separated by function.

Somatic nervous system (conscious control)

Autonomic nervous system (automatic control)

Sympathetic nervous system

Parasympathetic nervous system

A

An example will show how the two branches of the nervous system's autonomic division work in balance to maintain homeostasis. When you go outside in cold weather, your skin's temperature receptors send "cold" messages to the spinal cord and brain. Your conscious mind may intervene at this point to tell you to wrap your sweater more closely around you, but let's say you have no sweater. You're cold, and the maintenance of your body temperature is essential to life, so your sympathetic nervous system reacts to this external stressor, the cold. To conserve heat, it signals your skin-surface capillaries to shut down so your blood will circulate deeper in your tissues, where it won't lose heat. It also signals involuntary contractions of the small muscles just under the skin surface. The product of these muscle contractions is heat, and the visible result is goose bumps. If these measures don't raise your body temperature enough, then the sympathetic nerves signal your large muscle groups to shiver; the contractions of these large muscles produce still more heat. All of this activity adds up to a set of adjustments that maintain your homeostasis (with respect to temperature) under conditions of external extremes that would throw it off balance (cold). The cold was a stressor; the body's response was resistance.

Now let's say you come in and sit by a fire and drink hot cocoa. Homeostasis would no longer be promoted by sympathetic activity. At this point, your parasympathetic nerves take over; they signal your skin surface capillaries to dilate again, your goosebumps to subside, and your muscles to relax. Your body has returned to normal. This is recovery.

Basic Chemistry Concepts

This appendix is intended to provide the background in basic chemistry that you need to understand the nutrition concepts presented in this book.

Chemistry is the branch of natural science that is concerned with the description and classification of matter, with the changes that matter undergoes, and with the energy associated with these changes. **Matter** is anything that takes up space and has mass. **Energy** is the ability to do work.

Matter: The Properties of Atoms

Every substance has characteristics or properties that distinguish it from all other substances and thus give it a unique identity. These properties are both physical and chemical. The physical properties include such characteristics as color, taste, texture, and odor, as well as the temperatures at which a substance changes its state (changes from a solid to a liquid or from a liquid to a gas) and the weight of a unit volume (its density). The chemical properties of a substance have to do with how it reacts with other substances or responds to a change in its environment so that new substances with different sets of properties are produced.

A physical change is one that does not change a substance's chemical composition. For example, when ice changes to liquid water and to steam, two hydrogen atoms and one oxygen atom remain bound together in all three states. However, a chemical change does occur if an electric current is passed through water. The water disappears, and two different substances are formed: hydrogen gas, which is flammable, and oxygen gas, which supports life. Chemical changes are also referred to as **chemical reactions**.

Substances: Elements and Compounds

Molecules are one or more atoms constituting the smallest part of an element or compound that can exist separately without losing its chemical properties. If the molecules of a substance are composed of atoms that are all alike, the sub-

Contents

stance is an **element**. If the molecules are composed of two or more different kinds of atoms, the substance is a **compound**.

Just over 100 elements are known, and these are listed in Table B–1. A familiar example is hydrogen, whose molecules are composed only of hydrogen atoms linked together in pairs (H_2). On the other hand, over a million compounds are known. An example is the sugar glucose. Each of its molecules is composed of 6 carbon, 6 oxygen, and 12 hydrogen atoms linked together in a specific arrangement (as described in Chapter 3).

The Nature of Atoms

Atoms themselves are made of smaller particles. The atomic nucleus contains **protons** (positively charged particles); and **electrons** (negatively charged particles) surround the nucleus. Because opposite charges attract, the number of protons ($+$) in the nucleus of an atom determines the number of electrons ($-$) around it. The positive charge on a proton is equal to the negative charge on an electron, so that the charges cancel each other out and leave the atom neutral.

The nucleus may also include **neutrons**, subatomic parti-

TABLE B–1

Chemical Symbols for the Elements

Number of Protons (Atomic Number)	Element	Number of Electrons In Outer Shell	Number of Protons (atomic Number)	Element	Number of Electrons In Outer Shell
1	Hydrogen (H)	1	49	Indium (In)	3
2	Helium (He)	2	50	Tin (Sn)	4
3	Lithium (Li)	1	51	Antimony (Sb)	5
4	Beryllium (Be)	2	52	Tellurium (Te)	6
5	Boron (B)	3	53	Iodine (I)	7
6	Carbon (C)	4	54	Xenon (Xe)	8
7	Nitrogen (N)	5	55	Cesium (Cs)	1
8	Oxygen (O)	6	56	Barium (Ba)	2
9	Fluorine (F)	7	57	Lanthanum (La)	2
10	Neon (Ne)	8	58	Cerium (Ce)	2
11	Sodium (Na)	1	59	Praseodymium (Pr)	2
12	Magnesium (Mg)	2	60	Neodymium (Nd)	2
13	Aluminum (Al)	3	61	Promethium (Pm)	2
14	Silicon (Si)	4	62	Samarium (Sm)	2
15	Phosphorus (P)	5	63	Europium (Eu)	2
16	Sulfur (S)	6	64	Gadolinium (Gd)	2
17	Chlorine (Cl)	7	65	Terbium (Tb)	2
18	Argon (Ar)	8	66	Dysprosium (Dy)	2
19	Potassium (K)	1	67	Holmium (Ho)	2
20	Calcium (Ca)	2	68	Erbium (Er)	2
21	Scandium (Sc)	2	69	Thulium (Tm)	2
22	Titanium (Ti)	2	70	Ytterbium (Yb)	2
23	Vanadium (V)	2	71	Lutetium (Lu)	2
24	Chromium (Cr)	1	72	Hafnium (Hf)	2
25	Manganese (Mn)	2	73	Tantalum (Ta)	2
26	Iron (Fe)	2	74	Tungsten (W)	2
27	Cobalt (Co)	2	75	Rhenium (Re)	2
28	Nickel (Ni)	2	76	Osmium (Os)	2
29	Copper (Cu)	1	77	Iridium (Ir)	2
30	Zinc (Zn)	2	78	Platinum (Pt)	1
31	Gallium (Ga)	3	79	Gold (Au)	1
32	Germanium (Ge)	4	80	Mercury (Hg)	2
33	Arsenic (As)	5	81	Thallium (Tl)	3
34	Selenium (Se)	6	82	Lead (Pb)	4
35	Bromine (Br)	7	83	Bismuth (Bi)	5
36	Krypton (Kr)	8	84	Polonium (Po)	6
37	Rubidium (Rb)	1	85	Astatine (At)	7
38	Strontium (Sr)	2	86	Radon (Rn)	8
39	Yttrium (Y)	2	87	Francium (Fr)	1
40	Zirconium (Zr)	2	88	Radium (Ra)	2
41	Niobium (Nb)	1	89	Actinium (Ac)	2
42	Molybdenum (Mo)	1	90	Thorium (Th)	2
43	Technetium (Tc)	1	91	Protactinium (Pa)	2
44	Ruthenium (Ru)	1	92	Uranium (U)	2
45	Rhodium (Rh)	1	93	Neptunium (Np)	2
46	Palladium (Pd)	—	94	Plutonium (Pu)	2
47	Silver (Ag)	1	95	Americium (Am)	2
48	Cadmium (Cd)	2	96	Curium (Cm)	2

TABLE B–1

(continued)

Number of Protons (Atomic Number)	Element	Number of Electrons In Outer Shell	Number of Protons (atomic Number)	Element	Number of Electrons In Outer Shell
97	Berkelium (Bk)	2	100	Fermium (Fm)	2
98	Californium (Cf)	2	101	Mendelevium (Md)	2
99	Einsteinium (Es)	2	102	Nobelium (No)	2

cles that have no charge. Protons and neutrons are of equal mass, and together they give an atom its weight. Electrons bond atoms together to make molecules and they are involved in chemical reactions.

Each type of atom has a characteristic number of protons in its nucleus. The hydrogen atom (symbol H) is the simplest of all. It possesses a single proton, with a single electron associated with it:

Hydrogen atom (H), atomic number 1.

Just as hydrogen always has one proton, helium always has two, lithium three, and so on. The **atomic number** of each type of atom represents the number of protons it contains. The atomic number never changes; it gives the atom its identity. The atomic numbers for the known elements are listed in Table B–1.

All atoms except hydrogen also have neutrons in their nuclei, and these contribute to their atomic weight. Helium, for example, has two neutrons in its nucleus in addition to its two protons, for a total of four nuclear particles and an atomic weight of 4. However, only the two protons are charged, and these determine the number of electrons the atom has. The number of electrons determines how the atom will chemically react with other atoms. Hence the atomic number, not the weight, is what gives an atom its chemical nature.

Besides hydrogen, the atoms most common in living things are carbon (C), nitrogen (N), and oxygen (O), whose atomic numbers are 6, 7, and 8 respectively. Their structures are more complicated than that of hydrogen. Each possesses a number of electrons equal to the number of protons in its nucleus. These electrons have two energy levels, symbolized in the following diagrams as two orbits, or shells:

Carbon atom (C), atomic number 6.

Nitrogen atom (N), atomic number 7.

Oxygen atom (O), atomic number 8.

In these and all diagrams of atoms that follow, only the protons and electrons are shown. The neutrons, which contribute only to atomic weight, not to charge, are omitted.

The shells closest to the nucleus are occupied by electrons of lesser energy. Thus the two electrons in the first shells of carbon, nitrogen, and oxygen have less energy than the electrons in their second, or outer, shells. Also, the first shell can hold only two electrons; when it is full, it is in a very stable energy state, or a state of lowest energy.

B

The most important structural feature of an atom for determining its chemical behavior is the number of electrons in its outer shell. The first shell is full when it is occupied by two electrons; so an atom with three protons has a filled first shell. Its third electron possesses greater energy and has a greater probability of being farther from the nucleus. In other words, the third electron is not so tightly bound as the first two and has a high probability of flying off to join other substances in chemical reactions. As a matter of fact, lithium, atomic number 3, is just such a highly reactive element.

The second shell is completely full when it has eight electrons. A substance that has a full outer shell tends to enter into no chemical reactions. Atomic number 10, neon, is a chemically inert substance, because its outer shell is complete. Fluorine, atomic number 9, has a great tendency to draw an electron from other substances to complete its outer shell and thus is highly reactive. Carbon has a half-full outer shell, which helps explain its great versatility; it can combine with other elements in a great variety of ways to form a large number of compounds.

Atoms seek to reach a state of maximum stability or of lowest energy in the same way that a ball will roll down a hill until it reaches the lowest place. An atom achieves a state of maximum stability:

- By having a filled outer shell (occupied by the maximum number of electrons it can hold).
- By having an entirely empty outer shell (by completely donating or transferring its outer shell electrons to other atoms).
- By sharing its electrons through bonding together with other atoms.

Methane molecule. The **chemical formula** for methane is CH_4. (Note that with the sharing of electrons, every atom has a filled outer shell.)

Chemical Bonding

Atoms often complete their outer shells by sharing electrons with other atoms. In order to complete its outer shell, a carbon atom requires four electrons. A hydrogen atom requires one. Thus when a carbon atom shares electrons with four hydrogen atoms, each completes its outer shell:

This electron sharing binds the atoms together and satisfies the conditions of maximum stability for the molecule. The outer shell of each atom is complete, since hydrogen effectively has the required two electrons in its first and outer shell and carbon has eight electrons in its second and outer shell; and the molecule is electrically neutral, with a total of ten protons and ten electrons.

B

Bonds that involve the sharing of electrons, like the bond between carbon and hydrogen, are the most stable kind of association that atoms can form with one another. They are sometimes called **covalent bonds**, and the resulting combinations of atoms are called molecules. A single pair of shared electrons forms a **single bond**. A simplified way to represent a single bond is with a single line. Thus the structure of methane could be represented like this (ignoring the inner-shell electrons, which do not participate in bonding):

```
        H
        |
   H —  C — H
        |
        H
```

Methane (**chemical structure**).

Similarly, one nitrogen atom and three hydrogen atoms can share electrons to form one molecule of ammonia:

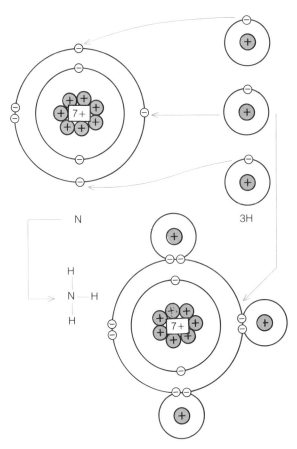

Ammonia molecule (NH_3). Count the electrons in each atom's outer shell.

One oxygen atom may be bonded to two hydrogen atoms to form one molecule of water:

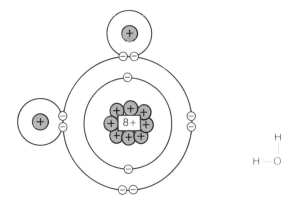

Water molecule (H_2O).

When two oxygen atoms form a molecule of oxygen, they must share two pairs of electrons. This **double bond** may be represented as two single lines:

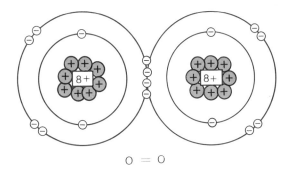

```
O = O
```

Oxygen molecule (O_2).

Small atoms form the tightest, most stable bonds. H, O, N, and C are the smallest atoms capable of forming one, two, three, and four electron-pair bonds (respectively). This fact is the basis for the simple statement in Chapter 3 that when you draw compounds containing these atoms, hydrogen must always have one, oxygen two, nitrogen three, and carbon four lines radiating to other atoms.

```
                   |         |
H —    — O —    N —      — C —
                   |         |
```

The stability of the associations between these small atoms and the versatility with which they can combine make them very common in living things. Interestingly, all cells, whether they come from animals, plants, or bacteria, contain the same

B

elements in very nearly the same proportions.[1] The atomic elements found in living things are shown in Table B–2.

Formation of Ions

An atom such as sodium (Na, atomic number 11) is more likely to lose an electron than to share electrons. Sodium possesses a filled inner shell of two electrons and a filled second shell of eight; there is only one electron in its outermost shell:

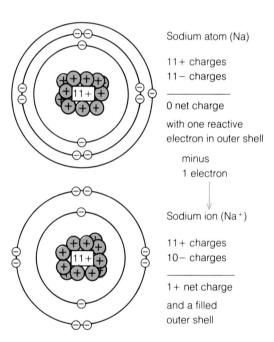

Sodium atom (Na)

11+ charges
11− charges
_____
0 net charge

with one reactive electron in outer shell

minus
1 electron

Sodium ion (Na$^+$)

11+ charges
10− charges
_____
1+ net charge

and a filled outer shell

If sodium loses this electron, it satisfies one condition for stability: a filled outer shell (now its second shell counts as the outer shell). However, it is not electrically neutral. It has 11 protons (positive) and only 10 electrons (negative). It therefore is positively charged. Such a structure is called an **ion**— an atom or molecule that has lost or gained one or more electrons and so is electrically charged.

An atom such as chlorine (Cl, atomic number 17) is likely to gain an electron for a similar reason. It possesses filled inner shells of two and eight electrons and has seven electrons in its outermost shell. Gaining one electron makes its outer

shell complete and thus makes it a negatively charged ion:

Chlorine atom (Cl)

17+ charges
17− charges
_____
0 net charges

but lacks one electron to fill outer shell

plus 1
electron

Chloride ion (Cl$^-$)

17+ charges
18− charges
_____
1− net charge

and a filled outer shell

A positively charged ion such as a sodium ion (Na$^+$) is a **cation**; a negatively charged ion such as a chloride ion (Cl$^-$) is an **anion**. Cations and anions attract one another to form **salts**:

Na$^+$

Sodium chloride (Na$^+$Cl$^-$)

28+ charges
28− charges
_____
0 net charge

and filled outer shells

Cl$^-$

[1]V. Rodwell, Appendix: Organic chemistry (a brief review), in *Review of Physiological Chemistry*, ed. H. Harper (Los Altos, Calif.: Lange Medical Publications, 1971), p. 499.

With all its electrons, sodium is a shiny, highly reactive metal; chlorine is the poisonous greenish-yellow gas that was used in World War I. But after they have transferred electrons, they form the harmless white salt familiar to you as table salt, or sodium chloride (Na^+Cl^-). The dramatic difference illustrates how profoundly the electron arrangement can influence the nature of a substance. The wide distribution of salt in nature attests to the stability of the union between the ions. Each meets the other's needs (a good marriage).

When dry, salt exists as crystals; its ions are stacked very regularly into a lattice, with positive and negative ions alternating in a sort of three-dimensional checkerboard structure. In water, however, the salt quickly dissolves, and its ions separate from each other, forming an electrolyte solution in which they move about freely. Covalently bonded molecules rarely dissociate like this in water solution. The most common exception is when they behave as acids and release H ions, as discussed in the next section. Molecules and ion pairs (salts) behave very differently in many ways.

An ion can also be a group of atoms bound together in such a way that the group has a charge and enters into reactions as a single unit. Many such groups are active in the fluids of the body. The bicarbonate ion is composed of five atoms—one H, one C, and three Os—and has a net charge of -1 (HCO_3^-). Another important ion of this type is a phosphate ion with one H, one P, and four Os, and a net charge of -2 (HPO_4^{-2}).

TABLE B–2

Elemental Composition of Living Cells

Element	Chemical Symbol	Composition by Weight (%)
Oxygen	O	65
Carbon	C	18
Hydrogen	H	10
Nitrogen	N	3
Calcium	Ca	1.5
Phosphorus	P	1.0
Sulfur	S	0.25
Sodium	Na	0.15
Magnesium	Mg	0.05
TOTAL		99.30[a]

[a]The remaining 0.70% by weight is contributed by the trace elements: copper (Cu), zinc (Zn), selenium (Se), molybdenum (Mo), fluorine (F), chlorine (Cl), iodine (I), manganese (Mn), cobalt (Co), iron (Fe). There are also variable traces of some of the following in cells: lithium (Li), strontium (Sr), aluminum (Al), silicon (Si), lead (Pb), vanadium (V), arsenic (As), bromium (Br), and others.

Whereas many elements have only one configuration in the outer shell and thus only one way to bond with other elements, some elements have the possibility of varied configurations. Iron is such an element. Under some conditions iron loses two electrons, and under other circumstances it loses three. If iron loses two electrons, it then has a net charge of $+2$, and we call it ferrous iron. If it donates three electrons to another atom, it becomes the $+3$ ion, or ferric iron.

(Note: It is important to remember that a positive charge on an ion means that negative charges—electrons—have been lost and not that positive charges have been added. If you could add two protons to an iron atom, they would go to the nucleus, adding 2 to its atomic number. Then it would no longer be iron, atomic number 26, but nickel, atomic number 28—and it would gain two more electrons to balance its positive charges.)

$$Fe^{++} \qquad\qquad Fe^{+++}$$

Ferrous iron (Fe^{++}) (had 2 outer-shell electrons but has lost them)	Ferric iron (Fe^{+++}) (had 3 outer-shell electrons but has lost them)
26+ charges 24− charges	26+ charges 23− charges
2+ net charge	3+ net charge

Water, Acids, and Bases

The water molecule is electrically neutral, having equal numbers of protons and electrons. However, if the hydrogen atom shares its one electron with oxygen, that electron will spend most of its time near the large positively charged oxygen nucleus on the oxygen side of the hydrogen atom. This leaves the positive proton (nucleus of the hydrogen atom) exposed on the outer part of the water molecule. We know, too, that the two hydrogens both bond toward the same side of the oxygen. These two ideas explain the fact that water molecules are **polar**: they have regions of more positive and more negative charge.

Polar molecules like water are drawn to one another by the attractive forces between the positive polar areas of one and the negative poles of another. These attractive forces, sometimes known as polar or **hydrogen bonds**, occur among many molecules and also within the different parts of single large molecules. Although very weak in comparison with covalent bonds, polar bonds may occur in such abundance that they become exceedingly important in determining the structure of such large molecules as proteins and DNA.

B

H (Slight net + charge)

↓

H ———————→ O (Slight net − charge)

(Slight net + charge)

Water (H_2O).

The arrows on the diagram of the polar molecule show displacement of electrons toward the O nucleus; so the negative region is near the O, the positive region near the Hs.

Water molecules have a slight tendency to ionize, separating into positive and negative ions. In any given amount of pure water, a small but constant number of these ions is present, and the number of positive ions exactly equals the number of negative ions.

An **acid** is a substance that releases H^+ ions (protons) in water solution. Hydrochloric acid (HCl) is such a substance, because it dissociates in water solution into H^+ and Cl^- ions. Acetic acid is also an acid, because it ionizes in water to acetate ions and free H^+:

H   O   H   O
| ‖ | ‖
H—C—C—O—H ⟶ H—C—C—O⁻ + H^+
| |
H   H

Acetic acid dissociates into an acetate ion and a hydrogen ion.

The more H^+ ions free in a water solution, the stronger the acid.

Chemists define degrees of acidity by means of the **pH scale**. The pH scale runs from 0 to 14. A pH of 1 is extremely acidic, 7 is neutral, and 13 is very basic. There is a tenfold difference between points on this scale. A solution with pH 3, for example, has *ten times* as many H^+ ions as a solution with pH 4. At pH 7, the concentrations of free H^+ and OH^- are exactly the same—1/10,000,000 moles per liter (10^{-7} moles per liter).[2] At pH 4, the concentration of free H^+ ions is 1/10,000 (10^{-4}) moles per liter. This is a higher concentration of H^+ ions, and the solution is therefore acidic.

A **base** is a substance that can soak up or combine with H^+

[2]A mole is a certain number (about 6×10^{23}) of molecules. The pH of a solution is defined as the negative logarithm of the hydrogen ion concentration of the solution. Thus if the concentration is 10^{-2} (moles per liter), the pH is 2; if 10^{-8}, the pH is 8; and so on.

ions, thus reducing the acidity of a solution. The compound ammonia is such a substance. The ammonia molecule has two electrons that are not shared with any other atom; a hydrogen ion (H^+) is just a naked proton with no shell of electrons at

H   H
| |
: N—H   +   H·   ⟶   H—N·—H
| |
H   H

Ammonia captures a hydrogen ion from water.

The two dots here represent the two electrons not shared with another atom. These are ordinarily not shown in chemical structure drawings. Compare this with the earlier diagram of an ammonia molecule.

all. Thus the proton readily combines with the ammonia molecule to form an ammonium ion and so is withdrawn from the solution as a free proton and no longer contributes to its acidity. Many compounds containing nitrogen are important bases in living systems. Acids and bases neutralize each other to produce substances that are neither acid nor base.

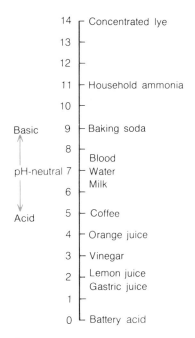

The pH scale.

Note: Each step is ten times as concentrated in base (1/10 as much acid, H^+) as the one below it.

B

Chemical Reactions

Structures:

Formulas: $2 H_2 + O_2 \longrightarrow 2 H_2O$

A chemical reaction, or chemical change, results in the disappearance of substances and the formation of new ones. Almost all such reactions involve a change in the bonding of atoms. Old bonds are broken, and new ones are formed. The nuclei of atoms are never involved in chemical reactions—only their outer-shell electrons. At the end of a reaction there is always the same number of atoms of each type as there was at the beginning. For example, two hydrogen molecules can react with one oxygen molecule to form two water molecules. In this reaction two substances (hydrogen and oxygen) disappear, and a new one (water) is formed, but at the end of the reaction there are still four H atoms and two O atoms, just as there were at the beginning. The only difference is in how they are linked.

In many instances chemical reactions involve not the relinking of molecules but the exchanging of electrons or protons among them. In such reactions, the molecule that gains one or more electrons (or loses one or more hydrogen ions) is said to be reduced; the molecule that loses electrons (or gains

protons) is oxidized. (A hydrogen ion is equivalent to a proton.) Oxidation and reduction take place simultaneously, because an electron or proton that is lost by one molecule is accepted by another. The addition of an atom of oxygen is also oxidation, because oxygen (with six electrons in the outer shell) accepts two electrons in becoming bonded. **Oxidation**, then, is loss of electrons, gain of protons, or addition of oxygen (with six electrons); **reduction** is the opposite—gain of electrons, loss of protons, or loss of oxygen. The addition of hydrogen atoms to oxygen to form water can thus be described as the reduction of oxygen—or the oxidation of hydrogen.

If a reaction results in a net increase in the energy of a compound, it is called an **endergonic**, or "uphill," reaction (energy, *erg*, is added into, *endo*, the compound). An example is the chief result of photosynthesis, the making of sugar in a plant from carbon dioxide and water using the energy of sunlight. Conversely, the oxidation of sugar to carbon dioxide and water is an **exergonic**, or "downhill," reaction, because the end products have less energy than the starting products. Oftentimes, but not always, reduction reactions are endergonic, resulting in an increase in the energy of the products. Oxidation reactions often, but not always, are exergonic.

Chemical reactions tend to occur spontaneously if the end products are in a lower energy state (are more stable) than the reacting compounds were. These reactions often give off energy in the form of heat as they occur. The generation of heat by wood burning in a fireplace and the maintenance of human body warmth both depend on energy-yielding chemical reactions. These downhill reactions occur easily, although they may require some activation energy to get them started, just as a ball requires a push to get started rolling downhill.

Uphill reactions, in which the products contain more energy than the reacting compounds started with, do not occur until an energy source is provided. An example of such an energy source is the sunlight used in photosynthesis, where carbon dioxide and water (low-energy compounds) are combined to form the sugar glucose (a higher-energy compound). Another example is the use of the energy in glucose to combine two low-energy compounds in the body into the high-energy compound ATP. The energy in ATP may be used to power many other energy-requiring, uphill reactions. Clearly, any of many different molecules can be used as a temporary storage place for energy.

Hydrogen and oxygen react to form water.

B

Energy Change as Reaction Occurs

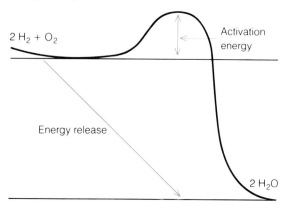

Activation energy

$2 H_2 + O_2$

Energy release

$2 H_2O$

Start of reaction → End of reaction

Reactants → Products

$2 H_2 + O_2 \rightarrow 2 H_2O$

Neither downhill nor uphill reactions occur until something sets them off (activation) or until a path is provided for them to follow. The body uses enzymes as a means of providing paths and controlling chemical reactions (see Chapter 5). By controlling the availability and the action of its enzymes, the body can "decide" which chemical reactions to prevent and which to promote.

Formation of Free Radicals

Normally, when a chemical reaction takes place, bonds break and reform with some redistribution of atoms and rearrangement of bonds to form new, stable compounds. Normally, bonds don't split in such a way as to leave a molecule with an

$$H-O-O-H \xrightarrow{\text{Heat or light}} H-O\bullet \; + \; \bullet O-H$$
or   or
$$R-O-O-H \longrightarrow R-O\bullet \; + \; \bullet O-H$$

Hydrogen peroxide or any hydroperoxide (R is any carbon chain with appropriate numbers of Hs.)

Two free radicals

Free radicals are formed. The dots represent single electrons that are available for sharing (the atom also needs another electron to fill its outer shell).

odd, unpaired electron. However, weak bonds can split this way, and when they do, **free radicals** are formed. Free radicals are highly unstable and quickly react with other compounds, forming more free radicals in a chain reaction.

A physical event such as the arrival of an energy-carrying particle of light or other radiation starts the process by breaking a weak bond so that free radicals are formed. A cascade may ensue in which many highly reactive radicals are generated, resulting finally in the disruption of a living structure such as a cell membrane.

$$H-O\bullet \; + \; H-\overset{\displaystyle H}{\underset{\displaystyle H}{C}}-H \longrightarrow H-O-H \; + \; H-\overset{\displaystyle H}{\underset{\displaystyle H}{C}}\bullet$$

or   or

$$R-H \hspace{6cm} R\bullet$$

| Free radical | Compound with weak bond (perhaps an unsaturated fatty acid) | New stable compound (water or an alcohol) | Free radical |

Destruction of biological compounds by free radicals. The free radical attacks a weak bond in a biological compound, disrupting it and forming a new stable molecule and another free radical. This can attack another biological compound, and so on.

Oxidation of some compounds can be induced by air at room temperature in the presence of light. Such reactions are thought to take place through the formation of compounds called peroxides:

Peroxides:

$H-O-O-H$ — Hydrogen peroxide

$R-O-O-H$ — Hydroperoxides (R is any carbon chain with appropriate numbers of Hs.)

$R-O-O-R$ — Peroxide

Some peroxides readily disintegrate into free radicals, initiating chain reactions like those just described.

Free radicals are of special interest in nutrition because the antioxidant properties of vitamin E are thought to protect against their destructive effects. Vitamin E on the surface of the lungs reacts with (and is destroyed by) free radicals, thus preventing them from reaching underlying cells and oxidizing the lipids in their membranes.

Biochemical Structures and Pathways

The diagrams of nutrients presented here are meant to enhance your understanding of the most important organic molecules in the human diet. The names used are those agreed on by the American Institute of Nutrition and other scientific organizations in 1976.[1] Following the diagrams of nutrients are sections on the major metabolic pathways mentioned in Chapter 7—glycolysis, the TCA cycle, and the electron transport chain.

Contents

Carbohydrates

Monosaccharides

Glucose (alpha form). The ring would be at right angles to the plane of the paper. The bonds directed upward are above the plane; those directed downward are below the plane. This molecule is considered an alpha form because the OH carbon 1 points downward.

Glucose (beta form). The OH on carbon 1 points upward.

Fructose, galactose: see Chapter 2.

[1]Nomenclature policy: Generic descriptors and trivial names for vitamins and related compounds, *Journal of Nutrition* 112 (1982): 7–14; Nomenclature policy: Abbreviated designations of amino acids, in the same journal, p. 15.

C

Disaccharides

Maltose.

Lactose (alpha form).

Sucrose.

Polysaccharides

As described in Chapter 3, starch, glycogen, and cellulose are all long chains of glucose molecules covalently linked together.

Amylose

Amylopectin

Starch. Two kinds of covalent linkages occur between glucose molecules in starch, giving rise to two kinds of chains. Amylose is composed of straight chains, with carbon 1 of one glucose linked to carbon 4 of the next. Amylopectin is made up of straight chains like amylose but has occasional branches arising where the carbon 6 of a glucose is also linked to the carbon 1 of another glucose. On amylopectin, some of the H have been left off, for simplicity's sake. (See the rules for simplified chemical structures on p. 58).

Glycogen: like amylopectin but with longer chains and many more branches.

C

C

Cellulose.

Mucopolysaccharides

Hyaluronic acid

Repeating units of hyaluronic acid. Such structures are typical of mucopolysaccharides.

Lipids

TABLE C-1

Saturated Fatty Acids Found in Natural Fats

Saturated Fatty Acid	Chemical Formula	Source
Butyric	C_3H_7COOH	Butter fat
Caproic	$C_5H_{11}COOH$	Butter fat
Caprylic	$C_7H_{15}COOH$	Coconut oil
Capric	$C_9H_{19}COOH$	Palm oil
Lauric	$C_{11}H_{23}COOH$	Coconut oil
Myristic[a]	$C_{13}H_{27}COOH$	Nutmeg oil, animal fat (butter)
Palmitic[a]	$C_{15}H_{31}COOH$	Animal and vegetable fat
Stearic[a]	$C_{17}H_{35}COOH$	Animal and vegetable fat
Arachidic	$C_{19}H_{39}COOH$	Peanut oil

[a]Most common saturated fatty acids.

TABLE C-2

Unsaturated Fatty Acids Found in Natural Fats

Unsaturated Fatty Acid	Chemical Formula	Position Of Double Bonds	Source
Palmitoleic	$C_{15}H_{29}COOH$	C_9-C_{10}	Butter fat
Oleic	$C_{17}H_{33}COOH$	C_9-C_{10}	Olive oil
Linoleic	$C_{17}H_{31}COOH$	C_9-C_{10} C_{12}-C_{13}	Linseed oil
Linolenic	$C_{17}H_{29}COOH$	C_9-C_{10} C_{12}-C_{13} C_{15}-C_{16}	Linseed oil
Arachidonic	$C_{19}H_{31}COOH$	C_5-C_6 C_8-C_9 C_{11}-C_{12} C_{14}-C_{15}	Lecithin
Eicosapentanoic	$C_{19}H_{29}COOH$	C_3-C_4 C_5-C_6 C_8-C_9 C_{11}-C_{12} C_{14}-C_{15}	Fish oils (fatty fish)

Acids are numbered from the methyl end.

Proteins: Amino Acids

The common amino acids may be classified into the seven groups listed below.[2] Amino acids marked with an asterisk (*) are essential, because human beings cannot synthesize them.

1. With aliphatic side chains, which consist of hydrogen and carbon atoms (hydrocarbons).

Glycine (Gly).

Alanine (Ala).

Valine* (Val).

Leucine* (Leu).

Isoleucine* (Ile).

2. With hydroxylic (OH) side chains.

Serine (Ser).

Threonine* (Thr).

[2]A discussion of the designated abbreviations for the common amino acids presented here is found in: Nomenclature policy: Abbreviated designations of amino acids, 1982.

C

3. With side chains containing acidic groups or their amides, which contain the group NH_2.

$$HO-\overset{\overset{O}{\|}}{C}-CH_2-\overset{\overset{H}{|}}{\underset{\underset{NH_2}{|}}{C}}-\overset{\overset{O}{\|}}{C}-OH$$

Aspartic acid (Asp).

$$HO-\overset{\overset{O}{\|}}{C}-CH_2-CH_2-\overset{\overset{H}{|}}{\underset{\underset{NH_2}{|}}{C}}-\overset{\overset{O}{\|}}{C}-OH$$

Glutamic acid (Glu).

$$NH_2-\underset{\underset{O}{\|}}{C}-CH_2-\overset{\overset{H}{|}}{\underset{\underset{NH_2}{|}}{C}}-\overset{\overset{O}{\|}}{C}-OH$$

Asparagine (Asn).

$$NH_2-\underset{\underset{O}{\|}}{C}-CH_2-CH_2-\overset{\overset{H}{|}}{\underset{\underset{NH_2}{|}}{C}}-\overset{\overset{O}{\|}}{C}-OH$$

Glutamine (Gln).

4. With basic side chains.

$$NH_2-CH_2-CH_2-CH_2-CH_2-\overset{\overset{H}{|}}{\underset{\underset{NH_2}{|}}{C}}-\overset{\overset{O}{\|}}{C}-OH$$

Lysine* (Lys).

$$NH_2-\underset{\underset{NH}{\|}}{C}-NH-CH_2-CH_2-\overset{\overset{H}{|}}{\underset{\underset{NH_2}{|}}{C}}-\overset{\overset{O}{\|}}{C}-OH$$

Arginine (Arg).

$$H-C=C-CH_2-\overset{\overset{H}{|}}{\underset{\underset{NH_2}{|}}{C}}-\overset{\overset{O}{\|}}{C}-OH$$

Histidine* (His).

$$NH_2-CH_2-CH_2-CH_2-\overset{\overset{H}{|}}{\underset{\underset{NH_2}{|}}{C}}-\overset{\overset{O}{\|}}{C}-OH$$

Ornithine (Orn).

5. With aromatic side chains, which are characterized by the presence of at least one cyclical (ring) structure.

Phenylalanine* (Phe).

Tyrosine (Tyr).

Tryptophan* (Trp).

6. With side chains containing sulfur atoms.

$$HS-CH_2-\overset{\overset{H}{|}}{\underset{\underset{NH_2}{|}}{C}}-\overset{\overset{O}{\|}}{C}-OH$$

Cysteine (Cys).

$$\begin{array}{l}CH_2-\overset{\overset{O}{\|}}{\underset{\underset{NH_2}{|}}{C}}-C-OH\\ |\\ S\\ |\\ S\\ |\\ CH_2-\overset{\overset{O}{\|}}{\underset{\underset{NH_2}{|}}{C}}-C-OH\end{array}$$

Cystine (Cys-Cys).

$$CH_3-S-CH_2-CH_2-\overset{\overset{H}{|}}{\underset{\underset{NH_2}{|}}{C}}-\overset{\overset{O}{\|}}{C}-OH$$

Methionine* (Met).

7. Imino acids.

Proline (Pro).[3]

C

Vitamins and Coenzymes

Vitamin A: retinol.

Vitamin A: retinal.

[3]Proline has the same H_2N-C-COOH structure as the other amino acids, but its amino group has given up a hydrogen to form a ring, as shown.

C

CH₃   CH₃   CH₃   CH₃
  C   C   C   CH
H   CH   CH   CH   CH
H—C   C   CH   CH   CH   CH
              ‖
H—C   C—CH₃
  H   C
      H   H

CH₃   CH₃   CH₃   CH₃
  C   C   C   CH
H   CH   CH   CH   CH
H—C   C   CH   CH   CH   CH
              ‖
H—C   C—CH₃
  H   C
      H   H

Vitamin A: beta-carotene.

Thiamin hydrochloride. Chloride ions (Cl⁻) are shown nearby because two of the nitrogens in this compound have donated their spare outer-shell electrons to bond with positively charged ions (see Appendix B). Thus the whole molecule is positively charged (+2) and will attract two negatively charged ions (Cl⁻) into its vicinity. When crystallized out of water solution, this complex precipitates as the salt thiamin hydrochloride. This chemical name usually appears on vitamin bottles containing thiamin.

Thiamin pyrophosphate (TPP). TPP is a coenzyme that includes the thiamin molecule as part of its structure.

C

Riboflavin. This molecule is a part of two coenzymes—flavin mononucleotide (FMN) and flavin adenine dinucleotide (FAD).

Flavin mononucleotide (FMN).

Flavin adenine dinucleotide (FAD).

becomes

in FADH$_2$

C

Nicotinic acid

Nicotinamide

Niacin (nicotinic acid and nicotinamide). These molecules are a part of two coenzymes—nicotinamide adenine dinucleotide (NAD^+) and nicotinamide adenine dinucleotide phosphate ($NADP^+$).

Nicotinamide

Adenine

D-ribose

D-ribose

Pyrophosphate

Nicotinamide adenine dinucleotide (NAD^+) and nicotinamide adenine dinucleotide phosphate ($NADP^+$). NAD has also been called coenzyme I and DPN; NADP has been called coenzyme II and TPN. NADP has the same structure as NAD but with a phosphate group attached at the dagger (†).

NAD^+

NADH

Reduced NAD^+ (NADH). When NAD^+ is reduced, by the addition of H^+ and two electrons, it becomes the coenzyme NADH. (The dots on the Hs entering this reaction represent electrons—see Appendix B.)

C

Pyridoxine

CH_2-OH

$HO-C$ $C-CH_2-OH$

CH_3-C $C-H$

N

Pyridoxine

Pyridoxal

H

$C=O$

$HO-C$ $C-CH_2-OH$

CH_3-C $C-H$

N

Pyridoxal

Pyridoxamine

CH_2-NH_2

$HO-C$ $C-CH_2-OH$

CH_3-C $C-H$

N

Pyridoxamine

Vitamin B_6 (a general name for three compounds—pyridoxine, pyridoxal, and pyridoxamine).

Pyridoxal phosphate

H

$C=O$

$HO-C$ $C-CH_2-O-P-OH$

CH_3-C $C-H$ OH

N

Pyridoxal phosphate

NH_3

O

NH_3

O

Pyridoxamine phosphate

CH_2-NH_2

$HO-C$ $C-CH_2-O-P-OH$

CH_3-C $C-H$ OH

N

Pyridoxamine phosphate

Pyridoxal phosphate and pyridoxamine phosphate are the coenzymes necessary for transamination and other important processes.

C

Vitamin B₁₂ (cyanocobalamin). The arrows in this diagram indicate that the spare electron pairs on the nitrogens attract them to the cobalt.

Folacin (folic acid).[4]

C

Tetrahydrofolic acid, the active coenzyme form of folacin. (The four hydrogens added to folacin are circled. An intermediate form, dihydrofolate, has two of these hydrogens added.)

Pantothenic acid

Coenzyme A (CoA). This molecule is made up in part of pantothenic acid.

[4]The term *folacin* is to be used as the generic descriptor for folic acid and related compounds. For further discussion, see: Nomenclature policy: Generic descriptors and trivial names for vitamins and related compounds, 1982.

C

Biotin.

Vitamin C   Dehydroascorbic acid

Vitamin C (ascorbic acid).[5] The oxidized form of vitamin C is dehydroascorbic acid. (The dots on the Hs indicate that two hydrogen atoms, complete with their electrons, are lost when ascorbic acid is oxidized and gained when it is reduced again.)

[5]The term *vitamin C* should be used for all compounds with the biological activity of ascorbic acid. See: Nomenclature policy: Generic descriptors and trivial names for vitamins and related compounds, 1982.

C

Active vitamin D and its precursors, beginning with 7-dehydrocholesterol. (The carbon atoms at which changes occur are numbered.) Compare the structure of 7-dehydrocholesterol with that of cholesterol, p. 103.

Vitamin E (alpha-tocopherol).

C

Vitamin K, a naturally occurring compound.

Menadione, a synthetic compound that exhibits vitamin K activity.

Adenosine triphosphate (ATP), the energy carrier. The cleavage point marks the bond that is broken when ATP splits to become ADP + P.

C

OH
|
HO – P =O
|
O
|
HO – P = O
|
O

cleavage

+ H – O – H
   (Water)

OH
|
HO – P =O
|
O⁻   H⁺

Phosphate
+
OH
|
HO – P =O

ADP

Adenosine diphosphate (ADP).

Glycolysis

Energy of falling water dissipated without doing work.

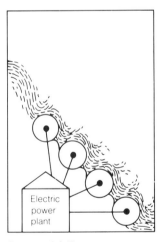

Energy of falling water coupled to the turning of a series of water wheels.

Analogy for a coupled reaction. Breakdown of glucose is coupled to making of ATP—or—breakdown of ATP is coupled to activation of glucose (making glucose-P).

Figure C–1 depicts the events of glycolysis. First, glucose must be given some activation energy before it can proceed toward the release of its own energy, just as a log must be given some heat from twigs and paper before it will burn spontaneously. This activation of glucose is accomplished in a coupled reaction with ATP. (A **coupled reaction** is a chemical event in which an enzyme complex catalyzes two reactions simultaneously. It often involves the breakdown of one compound to two and the synthesis of another from two.)

In the process of activation, a phosphate is attached to the carbon that chemists call number 6. The product is called, logically enough, glucose-6-phosphate. In the next step, glucose-6-phosphate is rearranged by an enzyme, and a phosphate is added in another coupled reaction with ATP. The product this time is fructose-1,6-diphosphate. At this point the six-carbon sugar has been activated. It has a phosphate group on its first and sixth carbons and enough energy to break apart. Two ATPs have been used to accomplish this.

This is the way chemists number the carbons in a glucose molecule

(From this point to the production of pyruvate we will use letters in place of compound names. The names are in Figure C–1, for those who wish to know them.)

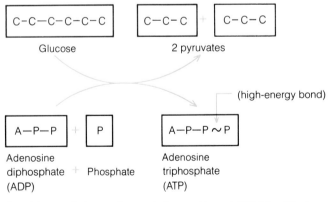

Breakdown of glucose is coupled to making of ATP (simplified). Actually 2 ATP are used to activate glucose, and 4 ATP are gained in catabolism to 2 pyruvate.

C

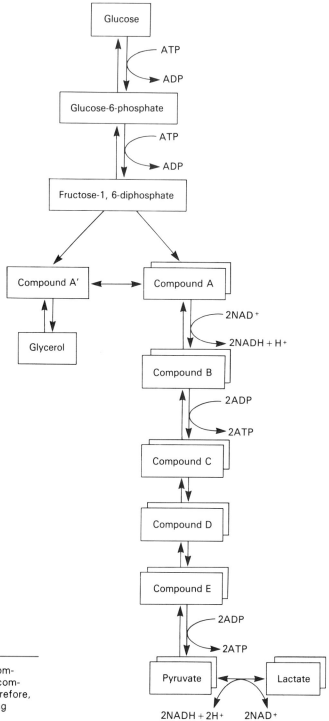

FIGURE C–1

Glycolysis. Two molecules of compound A are produced (because compound A′ converts to A), and therefore, two molecules of each succeeding compound.

A = glyceraldehyde-3-phosphate.
A′ = dihydroxyacetone phosphate.
B = 1,3-diphosphoglyceric acid.
C = 3-phosphoglyceric acid.
D = 2-phosphoglyceric acid.
E = phosphoenol pyruvic acid.

When fructose-1,6-diphosphate breaks in half, the two three-carbon compounds (A and A′) are not identical. Each has a phosphate group attached, but only one converts directly to pyruvate. The other compound converts easily to the first. (Compound A′ is usually ignored, except for its role as the point of entry for glycerol; we say that two molecules of compound A are derived from one glucose.)

In the step from compound A to compound B, enough energy is released to convert NAD^+ to $NADH + H^+$. Also, in the steps from B to C and from E to pyruvate, ATP is regenerated. Remember that there are effectively two molecules of compound A coming from glucose; therefore, four ATP molecules are generated. Two ATPs were needed to get the sequence started, so the net gain at this point is two ATPs and two molecules of $NADH + H^+$.

So far, no oxygen has been used; the process has been anaerobic. But at this point, oxygen is needed. If oxygen is not immediately available, pyruvate converts to lactic acid, to soak up the hydrogens from the $NADH + H^+$ that was generated. Lactic acid accumulates until oxygen becomes available. However, in the energy path from glucose to carbon dioxide, this side step usually is not necessary. As you will see later, each $NADH + H^+$ moves to the electron transport chain to unload its hydrogens onto oxygen. The associated energy produces two ATPs, making the total yield eight ATPs for the process from glucose to pyruvate.

The TCA Cycle

The step from pyruvate to acetyl CoA is exceedingly complex. We have included only those substances that will help you understand the transfer of energy from the nutrients. When pyruvate is in the presence of oxygen, it loses a carbon in the form of carbon dioxide, and CoA is attached. In the process, NAD^+ picks up two hydrogens with their associated energy, becoming $NADH + H^+$.

As the acetyl CoA breaks down to carbon dioxide and water, its energy is captured in ATP. Let's follow the steps by which this occurs (see Figure C–2).

The tricarboxylic acid, or TCA, cycle (Figure C–2) is the name given to the set of reactions involving oxygen and leading from acetyl CoA to carbon dioxide (and water). To link glycolysis to the TCA cycle, pyruvate is converted to acetyl CoA. This set of aerobic reactions is not restricted to the metabolism of carbohydrate. It also includes fat and protein. Any substance that can be converted to acetyl CoA directly, or indirectly through pyruvate, may enter the cycle.

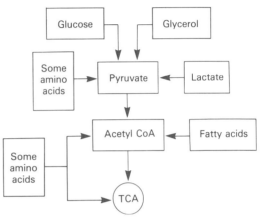

Any substance that can be converted to acetyl CoA either directly, or indirectly through pyruvate, may enter the TCA cycle.

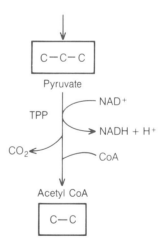

The step from pyruvate to acetyl CoA.

(TPP is a helper compound containing the B vitamin thiamin.)

C

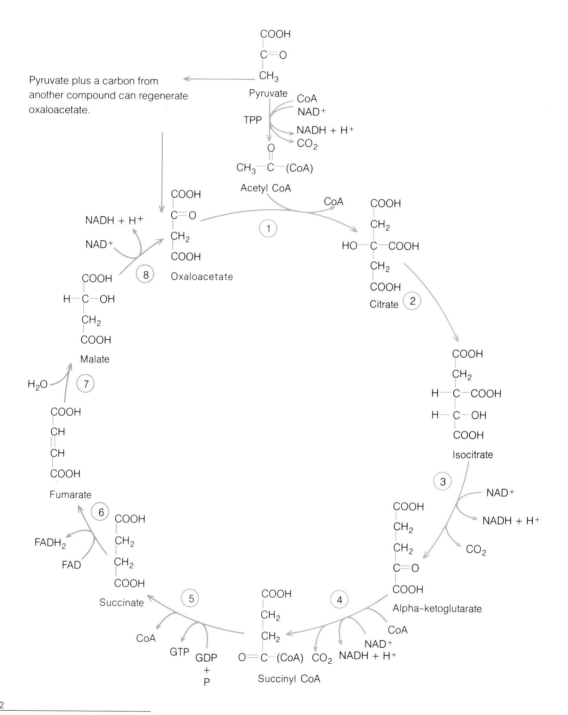

FIGURE C–2

The TCA cycle.

C

1. Acetyl CoA combines with a four-carbon compound, oxaloacetate. The CoA comes off, and the product is a six-carbon compound, citrate.

2. The atoms of citrate are rearranged to form isocitrate.

3. Now NAD^+ reacts with isocitrate. Two Hs and two electrons are removed from the isocitrate. One H becomes attached to the NAD^+ with the two electrons; the other H is released as a free proton. Thus NAD^+ becomes $NADH + H^+$. *(Remember this $NADH + H^+$. It is carrying the Hs and the energy from the last reaction. But let's follow the carbons first.)* A carbon is removed and combined with oxygen, forming carbon dioxide (which diffuses away in the blood and is exhaled). What is left is the five-carbon compound alpha-ketoglutarate.

4. Now two compounds interact with alpha-ketoglutarate —a molecule of CoA and a molecule of NAD^+. In this complex reaction, a carbon is removed and combined with oxygen (forming carbon dioxide); two Hs are removed and go to NAD^+ (forming $NADH + H^+$); and the CoA is attached to the remaining four-carbon compound, forming succinyl CoA. *(Remember this $NADH + H^+$ also. You will see later what happens to it.)*

5. Now two molecules react with succinyl CoA—a molecule called GDP and one of phosphate (P). The CoA comes off, the GDP and P combine to form the high-energy compound GTP, and succinate remains. *(Remember this GTP.)*

6. In the next reaction, two Hs with their energy are removed from succinate and are transferred to a molecule called FAD (an electron-hydrogen receiver like NAD^+) to form $FADH_2$. The product that remains is fumarate. *(Remember this $FADH_2$.)*

7. Next a molecule of water is added to fumarate, forming malate.

8. A molecule of NAD^+ reacts with the malate; two Hs with their associated energy are removed from the malate and form $NADH + H^+$. The product that remains is the four-carbon compound oxaloacetate. *(Remember this $NADH + H^+$.)*

We are back where we started. The oxaloacetate formed in this process can combine with another molecule of acetyl CoA (step 1), and the cycle can begin again. (The whole scheme is shown in Figure C–2.)

So far, what you have seen is that two carbons are brought in with acetyl CoA and that two carbons end up in carbon dioxide. But where is the energy and the ATP we promised you?

Each time a pair of hydrogen atoms is removed from one of the compounds in the cycle, it carries a pair of electrons with it. This chemical bond energy is thus captured into the compound to which the Hs become attached. A review of the eight steps of the cycle shows that energy is thus transferred into other compounds in steps 3, 4, 6, and 8. In step 5, energy is harnessed to bind GDP and P together to form GTP. Thus the compounds $NADH + H^+$ (three molecules) $FADH_2$, and GTP are built with energy originally found in acetyl CoA. To see how this energy ends up in ATP, we must follow the electrons further. Let us take those attached to NAD^+ as an example.

The Electron Transport Chain

The six reactions described here are those of the **electron transport chain**. Since oxygen is required for these reactions and ADP and P are combined to form ATP in several of them (ADP is phosphorylated), they are also called **oxidative phosphorylation**.

An important concept to remember at this point is that an electron is not a fixed amount of energy. The electrons that bond the H to NAD^+ in NADH have a relatively large amount of energy. In the series of reactions that follow, they lose this energy in small amounts, until at the end they are attached (with Hs) to oxygen (O) to make water (H_2O). In some of the steps, the energy they lose is captured into ATP in coupled reactions.

In the first step of the electron transport chain, NADH reacts with a molecule called a flavoprotein, losing its electrons (and their Hs). The products are NAD^+ and reduced flavoprotein. A little energy is lost as heat in this reaction.

The flavoprotein passes on the electrons to a molecule called coenzyme Q. Again they lose some energy as heat, but ADP and P participate in this reaction and gain much of the energy to bond together and form ATP. This is a coupled reaction: $ADP + P \rightarrow ATP$.

Coenzyme Q passes the electrons to cytochrome *b*. Again the electrons lose energy.

Cytochrome *b* passes the electrons to cytochrome *c* in a coupled reaction in which ATP is formed: $ADP + P \rightarrow ATP$.

Cytochrome *c* passes the electrons to cytochrome *a*.

Cytochrome *a* passes them (with their Hs) to an atom of oxygen (O), forming water (H_2O). This is a coupled reaction in which ATP is formed: $ADP + P \rightarrow ATP$.

FIGURE C–3

The electron transport chain.

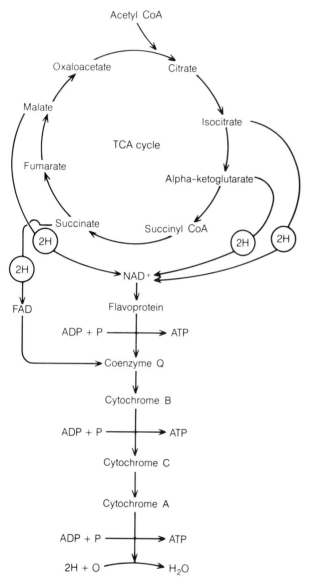

Cytochrome c passes the electrons to cytochrome a.

Cytochrome a passes them (with their Hs) to an atom of oxygen (O), forming water (H_2O). This is a coupled reaction in which ATP is formed: ADP + P → ATP.

The entire electron transport chain is diagramed in Figure C–3. As you can see, each time NADH is oxidized (loses its electrons) by this means, the energy it loses is parceled out

into three ATP molecules. When the electrons are passed on to water at the end, they have much less energy than they had to begin with. This completes the story of the electrons from NADH.

As for $FADH_2$, its electrons enter the electron transport chain at coenzyme Q. From coenzyme Q to water there are only two steps in which ATP is generated. Therefore, $FADH_2$ coming out of the TCA cycle yields just two ATP molecules.

One energy-receiving compound of the TCA cycle (GTP) does not enter the electron transport chain but gives its energy directly to ADP in a simple phosphorylation reaction, yielding one ATP.

It is now possible to draw up a balance sheet of glucose metabolism (see Table C–3). Glycolysis has yielded 4 NADH + H^+ and 4 ATP molecules and has spent 2 ATPs. The 2 acetyl CoAs going through the TCA cycle have yielded 6 NADH + H^+, 2 $FADH_2$, and 2 GTP molecules. After the NADH + H^+ and $FADH_2$ have gone through the electron transport chain, there are 34 ATPs. Added to these are the 4 ATPs from glycolysis and the 2 ATPs from GTP, making the

TABLE C–3

Balance Sheet for Glucose Metabolism

	Expend-itures	In-come
Glycolysis:		
1 glucose	2 ATP	4 ATP
1 fructose-1,6-diphosphate		2 NADH + H^+
2 pyruvate		2 NADH + H^+
TCA cycle:		
2 isocitrate		2 NADH + H^+
2 alpha-ketoglutarate		2 NADH + H^+
2 succinyl CoA		2 GTP
2 succinate		2 $FADH_2$
2 malate		2 NADH + H^+
Total ATP collected:		
From glycolysis	2 ATP	4 ATP
From 2 NADH + H^+		4–6 ATP[a]
From 8 NADH + H^+		24 ATP
From 2 GTP		2 ATP
From 2 $FADH_2$		4 ATP
Totals:	2 ATP	38–40 ATP
Balance on hand from 1 molecule glucose:	36–38 ATP	

[a]Each NADH + H^+ from glycolysis can yield 2 or 3 ATP. See accompanying text.

total 40 ATPs generated from one molecule of glucose. After the expense of 2 ATPs is subtracted, there is a net gain of 38 ATPs.*

The TCA cycle and the electron transport chain are the body's major means of capturing the energy from nutrients in ATP molecules. Other means, such as anaerobic glycolysis, contribute, but the aerobic processes are the most efficient. Biologists and chemists understand much more about these processes than has been presented here.

The Urea Cycle

Chapter 7 summed up how waste nitrogen is eliminated from the body by stating that ammonia molecules combine with carbon dioxide to produce urea. This is true, but it is not the whole story. Urea is produced in a multistep process within the cells of the kidney.

Ammonia, freed from an amino acid or other compound during metabolism anywhere in the body, arrives at the kidney by way of the bloodstream and is taken into a kidney cell. There, it is first combined with carbon dioxide and a phosphate group from ATP to form carbamyl phosphate:

Figure C–4 shows the cycle of four reactions that follow. In the first step, carbamyl phosphate combines with the amino acid ornithine, losing its phosphate group. The compound formed is citrulline.

In the second step, citrulline combines with the amino acid aspartic acid, to form argininosuccinate. The reaction

---

*The total may sometimes be 36 or 37, rather than 38, ATPs. The NADH + H$^+$ generated in the cytoplasm during glycolysis pass their electrons on to shuttle molecules, which move them into the mitochondria. One shuttle, malate, contributes its electrons to the electron transport chain before the first site of ATP synthesis. Another, glycerol phosphate, adds them into the chain beyond that first site. Thus sometimes 3, and sometimes only 2, ATP result from the NADH + H$^+$ that arises from glycolysis.

C

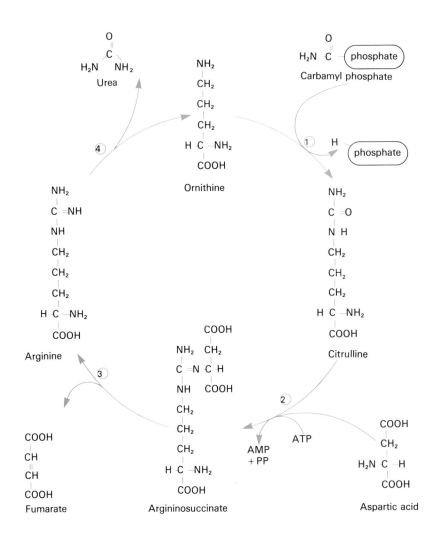

FIGURE C–4

The urea cycle.

requires energy from ATP. (ATP has been shown, before, to lose one phosphorus atom in a phosphate group, P, becoming ADP. In this reaction, it loses two phosphorus atoms joined together, PP, and becomes adenosine monophosphate, AMP.)

In the third step, argininosuccinate is split, forming another acid, fumaric acid, and the amino acid arginine.

In the fourth step, arginine loses its terminal carbon with two attached amino groups. This is urea, which the kidney excretes in the urine. The compound that remains is ornithine, identical to the ornithine with which this series of reactions began, ready to react with another molecule of carbamyl phosphate and turn the cycle again.

CoA condenses with another acetyl CoA to form a 6-carbon intermediate, beta-hydroxy-beta-methyl glutaryl CoA. In step 2, this intermediate is cleaved to acetyl CoA and acetoacetic acid. This product can be metabolized either to beta-hydroxybutyric acid (step 3a) or to acetone (3b).

The three last-named compounds are the three so-called ketone bodies of ketosis. Two are real ketones (they have a C=O group between two carbons); the other is a ketone-like compound (actually, an alcohol); hence the term ketone bodies to describe the three of them, rather than ketones. There are many other ketones in nature; these three are the ones characteristic of ketosis in the body.

C

Formation of Ketone Bodies

Normally, fatty acid oxidation proceeds all the way to carbon dioxide and water. However, in ketosis, an intermediate is formed from the condensation of two molecules of acetyl CoA: acetoacetyl CoA. Figure C–5 shows the formation of ketone bodies from that intermediate. In step 1, acetoacetyl

FIGURE C–5

Formation of ketone bodies.

Aids to
Calculation

Many mathematical problems have been worked out for you as examples at appropriate places in the text. This appendix aims to help with the use of the metric system and with those problems not fully explained elsewhere.

Contents

Conversion Factors

Conversion factors are useful mathematical tools in everyday calculations, like the ones encountered in the study of nutrition. Skill in the use of conversion factors is especially desirable as the United States and Canada "go metric."

A conversion factor is a fraction in which the numerator (top) and the denominator (bottom) express the same quantity in different units. For example, 2.2 pounds (lb) and 1 kilogram (kg) are equivalent; they express the same weight. The conversion factor used to change pounds to kilograms or vice versa is:

$$\frac{2.2 \text{ lb}}{1 \text{ kg}} \text{ or } \frac{1 \text{ kg}}{2.2 \text{ lb}}$$

Because both factors equal 1, measurements can be multiplied by the factor without changing the value of the measurement. Thus the units can be changed.

The correct factor to use in a problem is the one with the unit you are seeking in the numerator (top) of the fraction.

Following are two examples of problems commonly encountered in nutrition study; they illustrate the usefulness of conversion factors.

Example 1 Convert weight of 130 pounds to kilograms.

1. Choose the conversion factor in which the unit you are seeking is on top:

$$\frac{1 \text{ kg}}{2.2 \text{ lb}}$$

2. Multiply 130 pounds by the factor:

$$130 \text{ lb} \times \frac{1 \text{ kg}}{2.2 \text{ lb}} = \frac{130}{2.2} = \begin{array}{l} 59 \text{ kg (rounded off to} \\ \text{nearest whole number).} \end{array}$$

Example 2 How many grams (g) of saturated fat are contained in a 3-ounce (oz) hamburger?

1. Appendix H shows that a 4-ounce hamburger contains 7 grams of saturated fat. You are seeking grams of saturated fat; therefore, the conversion factor is:

$$\frac{7 \text{ g saturated fat}}{4 \text{ oz hamburger}}$$

2. Multiply 3 ounces of hamburger by the conversion factor:

$$3 \text{ oz hamburger} \times \frac{7 \text{ g saturated fat}}{4 \text{ oz hamburger}} = \frac{3 \times 7}{4}$$

$$= \begin{array}{l} 5 \text{ g saturated fat} \\ \text{(rounded off to} \\ \text{nearest whole} \\ \text{number).} \end{array}$$

Percentages

A percentage is a comparison between a number of items (perhaps your intake of energy) and a standard number (perhaps

D

the number of kcalories recommended for your age and sex—your energy RDA). The standard number is the number you divide by. The answer you get after the division must be multiplied by 100 to be stated as a percentage (*percent* means "per 100"):

Example 3 What percentage of the RDA for energy is your energy intake?

1. Find your energy RDA (Appendix I). We'll use 2,100 kcalories to demonstrate.
2. Total your energy intake for a day—for example, 1,200 kcalories.
3. Divide your kcalorie intake by the RDA kcalories:

   1,200 kcal (your intake) ÷ 2,100 kcal (RDA) = 0.573.

4. Multiply your answer by 100 to state it as a percentage:

   $0.573 \times 100 = 57.3 = $ 57% (rounded off to the nearest whole number).

In some problems in nutrition, the percentage may be more than 100. For example, suppose your daily intake of vitamin A is 3,200 RE and your RDA (male) is 1,000 RE. Your intake as a percentage of the RDA is more than 100 percent (that is, you consume more than 100 percent of your vitamin A RDA). The following calculations show your vitamin A intake as a percentage of the RDA:

3,200 ÷ 1,000 = 3.2.

$3.2 \times 100 = $ 320% of RDA.

Sometimes the comparison is between a part of a whole (for example, your kcalories from protein) and the total amount (your total kcalories). In this case, the total number is the one you divide by.

Example 4 What percentages of your total kcalories for the day come from protein, fat, and carbohydrate?

1. Using Appendix H and your diet record, find the total grams of protein, fat, and carbohydrate you consumed —for example, 60 grams protein, 80 grams fat, and 285 grams carbohydrate.
2. Multiply the number of grams by the number of kcalories from 1 gram of each energy nutrient (conversion factors):

   $60 \text{ g protein} \times \dfrac{4 \text{ kcal}}{1 \text{ g protein}} = 240 \text{ kcal.}$

   $80 \text{ g fat} \times \dfrac{9 \text{ kcal}}{1 \text{ g fat}} = 720 \text{ kcal.}$

$285 \text{ g carbohydrate} \times \dfrac{4 \text{ kcal}}{1 \text{ g carbohydrate}} = 1,140 \text{ kcal.}$

240 + 720 + 1140 = 2,100 kcal.

3. Find the percentage of total kcalories from each energy nutrient (see example 3).

   Protein: $240 \div 2,100 = 0.114 \times 100 = 11.4 = $ 11% of kcal.

   Fat: $720 \div 2,100 = 0.342 \times 100 = 34.2 = $ 34% of kcal.

   Carbohydrate: $1,140 \div 2,100 = 0.542 \times 100 = 54.2$

   = 54% of kcal.

   11% + 34% + 54% = 99% of kcal (total).

The percentages total 99 percent rather than 100 percent because a little was lost from each number in rounding off. This is a reasonable error.

Ratios

A ratio is a comparison of two or three values in which one of the values is reduced to 1. A ratio compares identical units and so is expressed without units. For example, the P:S ratio is a comparison of the grams of polyunsaturated fat to grams of saturated fat in the diet:

Example 5 Find the P:S ratio of your diet.

1. Using Appendix H and your diet record, find the grams polyunsaturated fat and grams saturated fat. Say they are 32 grams polyunsaturated fat and 25 grams saturated fat.
2. Divide the larger of the amounts above by the smaller —divide polyunsaturated fat grams by saturated fat grams:

   Polyunsaturated fat (g) ÷ saturated fat (g).

   32 g ÷ 25 g = 1.28.

3. The P:S ratio is usually expressed as correct to one decimal place: 1.28 = 1.3.
   The P:S ratio of your diet is 1.3:1 (read as "one point three to one" or simply "one point three").

Nutrition Assessment

Competent medical care includes attention to nutrition. A client's nutrition status can be evaluated by a dietitian or other qualified health care professional using the information gathered from several nutrition assessment sources. The accurate gathering of this information and its careful interpretation are the basis for a meaningful evaluation. This appendix provides a sample of the procedures, standards, charts, and other forms commonly used in nutrition assessment, and concludes with some cautions relating to their use by unqualified people.

Nutrition assessment involves four techniques:

- History taking.
- Anthropometric measures.
- Physical examination.
- Biochemical analysis (clinical or lab tests).

Each of these involves collecting data in a variety of ways and interpreting the findings in relation to the total picture.

Historical Data

Many clues about a person's present nutrition status are revealed in the historical data. A client's history is explored from several angles: medical, social, and drug, as well as diet. Table E–1 lists risk factors associated with poor nutrition status that might be identified in a history and Form E–1 shows how such information might be collected. As you can see, many circumstances in a person's life have an impact on nutrition status and provide the assessor with clues to possible problems.

TABLE E-1

Risk Factors for Poor Nutrition Status

Medical History	Diet History	Social/Economic History	Drug History
Recent major illness	Chewing or swallowing difficulties (including poorly fitted dentures, dental caries, and missing teeth)	Inadequate food budget	Antibiotics
Recent major surgery		Inadequate food preparation facilities	Anticancer agents
Surgery of the GI tract		Inadequate food storage facilities	Anticonvulsants
Overweight	Inadequate food intake		Antihypertensive agents
Underweight	Restricted or fad diets	Elderly	Catabolic steroids
Recent weight loss or gain	Frequently eating out	Living (eating) alone	Oral contraceptives
Anorexia	No intake for 10 or more days	Poor education	Vitamin and other nutrient preparations
Nausea	Intravenous fluids (other than total parenteral nutrition) for 10 or more days		
Vomiting			
Diarrhea			
Alcoholism			
Cancer			
Circulatory problems			
Liver disease			
Lung disease			
Kidney disease			
Diabetes			
Heart disease			
Heavy smoking			
Hormonal imbalance			
Hyperlipidemia			
Hypertension			
Mental retardation			
Multiple pregnancies[a]			
Neurologic disorders			
Pancreatic insufficiency			
Paralysis			
Physical disability			
Radiation therapy			
Teenage pregnancies[a]			

[a]See also Risk Factors for Poor Nutrition Status in Pregnancy, Chapter 14, p. 500.

FORM E-1

History

Name _____ Today's date _____

Address _____ Age _____

_____ Sex _____

_____ Phone _____

Date of last medical checkup _____ Height _____

Reason for coming in _____ Weight _____

_____ Usual Weight _____

PERSONAL DATA

1. Last grade of school completed _____ Still in school? _____

2. Are you employed? _____ Occupation _____

3. Does someone else live at your home? _____ Who? _____

4. Do you smoke in any way? _____ How much? _____

5. Have you recently lost or gained more than 10 lbs? _____ If yes, please explain how _____

6. Are you pregnant? _____ How many months? _____

7. How many pregnancies have you carried to term? _____

8. Are your menstrual periods normal? _____ If not, please explain _____

_____

9. Have you been told that you have (check any that apply):

   Diabetes _____ High blood pressure _____ Hardening of the arteries _____

   Lung disease _____ Kidney disease _____ Liver disease _____ Ulcers _____

   Cancer _____ Other _____

10. Do you eat at regular times each day? _____ How many times per day? _____

11. Do you usually eat snacks? _____ When? _____

12. Where do you usually eat your meal?

   Morning _____ Noon _____ Night _____
   With whom?
   Morning _____ Noon _____ Night _____

13. Would you say your appetite is good? _____ Fair? _____ Poor? _____

   If poor, please explain _____

14. What foods do you particularly dislike? _____

15. Are there foods you don't eat for other reasons? _____

16. Do you have any difficulty eating? _____

17. How would you describe your feelings about food? _____

_____

_____

E

FORM E–1

(continued)

18. Who prepares your meals? _____

19. Are you, or is any member of your family, on a special diet? _____

    If yes, who and what kind? _____

20. Do you drink alcohol? _____ How many drinks per day? _____

    Do you ever drink alcohol excessively? _____ How often? _____

21. Do you take any kind of medication, either prescribed by a doctor or over the counter, for any condition? _____

22. How would you describe your exercise habits?

    Kind of exercise _____ How intense? _____

    How long at a time? _____ How often? _____

23. Are there any other facts about your lifestyle that you think might be related to you nutritional health? _____ Explain _____

Medical and social histories can often be obtained from records completed by the attending physician, nurse, or other health care workers. Additional information can be gathered through an interview.

The drug history requires special attention. Hundreds of drugs interact with nutrients, creating the possibility of imbalances or deficiencies. They must not be overlooked in assessing a person's nutrition status. Form E–2 elicits the necessary information regarding drugs and Table E–2 identifies commonly used drugs and their effects on nutrition.

Drug History

1a. Do you have any health problems for which you are taking prescription medications at the present time? Yes _____ No _____
If yes:

Health problem	Proprietary name of drug	Generic name of drug	Dose Frequency	Duration of intake

1b. Are you taking any other medication a doctor has prescribed (name of drug unknown, reason for taking unknown)? Yes _____ No _____
If yes:

Description of drug	Dose	Frequency	Duration of intake

2a. Have you taken prescription medication for any of the health problems listed below within the past three months? Yes _____ No _____
If yes:

Health problem	Drug name	Duration of intake	When discontinued	Reason for stopping	Still taking[a]
Asthma					
Arthritis					
High blood pressure					
Fluid retention					
Infection (specify)					
Tuberculosis					
Malaria					
Psoriasis					
Colitis					
High cholesterol					
Parkinson's disease					
Liver disease					
Kidney disease					
Blood disease					
Bone disease					
Gout					
Blood clots					
Diabetes					
Other (specify)					

[a]Check (✔) if still taking.

2b. Have you taken any other medication within the past three months that a doctor has prescribed (name of drug unknown, reason for taking unknown)? Yes _____ No _____

Description	Dose	Frequency	Duration of intake

3a. Do you take medications, self-prescribed, for any reason? Yes _____ No _____

If yes:

Complaint	Constantly	Frequently	Occasionally
Constipation			
Indigestion			
Headache			
Nervousness			
Insomnia			
Pain			
Menstrual cramps			
Colds and sinus trouble			
Other (state)			

E

(continued)

3b. If response to 3a is positive in one or more categories, what medication do you take to relieve these complaints, and how much do you need to gain relief?

Complaint	Drug	Dose	Frequency	Duration
Constipation				
Indigestion				
Headache				
Nervousness				
Insomnia				
Pain				
Menstrual cramps				
Colds and sinus trouble				
Other (state)				

4. Are you taking birth control pills now? Yes _____ No _____

If yes:
  Name:
  Duration of intake:

Have you taken birth control pills within the past six months? Yes _____ No _____

If yes:
  Name:
  Duration of intake:
  Date discontinued:
  Reason for stopping:

Source: Adapted from D. Roe, *Drug-Induced Nutritional Deficiencies* (Westport, Conn.: AVI Publishing Company, 1976), Table 4.2, pp. 106—108.

TABLE E–2

Selected Drug-Nutrient Interactions

Drug		Effect on nutrition
Alcohol	Energy	↓intake
	Protein	↓intake
	Fat	↑buildup in liver
		↓absorption
	Thiamin	↓absorption ↓storage
	Vitamin B$_6$	↓activation
	Folacin	↓absorption, utilization
	Vitamin B$_{12}$	↓absorption
	Magnesium	↑urinary excretion
	Zinc	↑urinary excretion
Analgesics		
Aspirin	Folacin	↓serum levels; altered transport
	Vitamin C	↑urinary excretion
	Thiamin	↑urinary excretion
	Vitamin K	↑urinary excretion
	Iron	may cause blood loss
Amphetamines	↓Intake	causes anorexia, dry mouth, metallic taste, nausea, vomiting
Antacids		
Aluminum hydroxide	Phosphorus	↓absorption
Other types	Thiamin	↑destruction
Anticoagulants	Vitamin K	↓conversion to active form
Anticonvulsants	Folacin	↓serum levels
	Vitamin B$_6$	↓serum levels
	Vitamin B$_{12}$	↓serum levels
	Vitamin D	↓conversion to active forms
	Vitamin K	↑requirement
Antimicrobials		
Chloramphenicol	Riboflavin	↑requirement (?)
	Vitamin B$_6$	↑requirement (?)
	Vitamin B$_{12}$	↑requirement (?)
Penicillin	Potassium	↑urinary excretion
Neomycin	Fats	↓absorption
	Nitrogen	↓absorption
	Carbohydrates	↓absorption
	Folacin	↓absorption
	Vitamin B$_{12}$	↓absorption
	Fat-soluble vitamins	↓absorption
	Calcium	↓absorption
	Iron	↓absorption
	Potassium	↓absorption
	Vitamin K	↓intestinal synthesis
Tetracycline	Fat	↓absorption
	Amino acids	↓absorption
	Calcium	↓absorption
	Iron	↓absorption
	Magnesium	↓absorption
	Zinc	↓absorption
	Niacin	↑urinary excretion
	Riboflavin	↑urinary excretion
	Folacin	↑urinary excretion
	Vitamin C	↑urinary excretion

E

E

TABLE E–2

(continued)

Drug		Effect on nutrition
Antineoplastic agents		
Methotrexate and pyrimethamine	Folacin	folacin antagonist
	Vitamin B$_{12}$	↓absorption
	Fat	↓absorption
	↓Intake and general malabsorption	anorexia, nausea, vomiting, mouth sores
S-Fluorouracil	Protein	↓absorption and synthesis
Antitubercular drugs		
Cycloserine	Vitamin B$_6$	vitamin B$_6$ antagonist
	Protein	↓synthesis
	Calcium	↓absorption (?)
	Magnesium	↓absorption (?)
	Vitamin B$_6$	↓serum levels (?)
	Folacin	↓serum levels (?)
	Vitamin B$_{12}$	↓serum levels (?)
Isonicotinic acid hydrazide (INH)	Vitamin B$_6$	Vitamin B$_6$ antagonist
		↑urinary excretion
		causes deficiency
	Niacin	causes deficiency
	Vitamin B$_{12}$	↓absorption
		↓serum levels
Para-aminosalicylic acid	Folacin	↓absorption
	Vitamin B$_{12}$	↓absorption
	Fat	↓absorption
	Iron	↓absorption
Chelating agents		
Penicillamine	Vitamin B$_6$	↑requirement
		↑urinary excretion
	Zinc	↑urinary excretion
	Iron	↑urinary excretion
	Copper	↑urinary excretion
	↓Intake	alters taste; causes anorexia, nausea, vomiting
Cholesterol-lowering agents		
Cholestyramine	Fat and cholesterol	↓absorption
	Fat-soluble vitamins	↓absorption
	Folacin	↓absorption
	Iron	↓absorption
	Vitamin B$_{12}$	↓absorption
		↓blood levels
	Calcium	↑urinary excretion
		↓blood levels
Clofibrate	Vitamin B$_{12}$	↓absorption
	Iron	↓absorption
	↓Intake	alters taste; causes nausea and GI irritation
Colchicine	Fat	↓absorption
	Nitrogen	↓absorption
	Folacin	↓absorption
	Vitamin B$_{12}$	↓absorption
	Sodium	↓absorption
	Potassium	↓absorption

TABLE E–2

(continued)

Drug		Effect on nutrition
Corticosteirods	Vitamin D	↑metabolism
		↑requirement
	Vitamin B$_6$	↑requirement
	Vitamin C	↑requirement
		↑urinary excretion
	Calcium	↓absorption
		↑urinary excretion
	Phosphorus	↓absorption
	Zinc	↑urinary excretion
		↓serum levels
	Glucose	↑serum levels
	Triglycerides	↑serum levels
	Cholesterol	↑serum levels
	Potassium	↑urinary excretion
	Nitrogen	↑urinary excretion
Diuretics		
Furosemide	Calcium	↑urinary excretion
	Sodium	↑urinary excretion
	Potassium	↓serum levels
	Chloride	↓serum levels
	Magnesium	↓serum levels
	Zinc	↑serum levels
		↓storage in liver
Mercurials	Thiamin	↑urinary excretion
	Calcium	↑urinary excretion
	Sodium	↑urinary excretion
	Potassium	↑urinary excretion
	Chloride	↑urinary excretion
	Magnesium	↑urinary excretion
Thiazides	Sodium	↑urinary excretion
	Potassium	↓blood levels
	Chloride	↓blood levels
	Calcium	↑urinary excretion
		↑blood levels
	Magnesium	↑urinary excretion
	Phosphorus	↓blood levels
	Glucose	↑blood levels(?)
Triamterene	Sodium	↑urinary excretion
	Folacin	↓serum levels
	Vitamin B$_{12}$	↓serum levels
Glutethimide	Vitamin D	↑metabolsim
Hypoglycemics		
Phenformin and		
metformin	Vitamin B$_{12}$	↓absorption
Hydralazine	Vitamin B$_6$	↑urinary excretion

E

TABLE E-2

(continued)

Drug		Effect on nutrition
Laxatives		
Cathartics	Fat	↓absorption
	Glucose	↓absorption
	Vitamin D	↓absorption
	Calcium	↓absorption
	Potassium	↓absorption
Mineral oil	Fat-soluble vitamins	↓absorption
	Calcium	↓absorption
	Phosphates	↓absorption
Levodopa	Amino acids	↑requirement
	Vitamin B$_6$	↑requirement
	Vitamin C	↑requirement
	Sodium	↓urinary excretion
	Potassium	↓urinary excretion
Oral contraceptives	Vitamin B$_6$	↑requirement
		↓blood levels
	Riboflavin	↑requirement
		↓blood levels
	Folacin	↓absorption
		↓blood levels
	Vitamin B$_{12}$	↓blood levels
	Vitamin C	↓blood levels
	Vitamin A	↑blood levels
	Calcium	↑absorption
	Iron	↑serum levels
	Copper	↑serum levels
	Magnesium	↓blood levels(?)
	Zinc	↓blood levels(?)
Potassium salts	Vitamin B$_{12}$	↓absorption
Sulfonamides		
Salicylazosulfapyridine	Folacin	↓absorption
		↓blood levels
	Iron	↓blood levels
Others	Folacin	↓intestinal synthesis
	Vitamin K	↓intestinal synthesis
	B vitamins	↓intestinal synthesis

↑ increases
↓ decreases
(?) possible effect

Sources: Data from R. E. Hodges, Drug-nutrient interactions, in *Nutrition in Medical Practice* (Philadelphia: Saunders, 1980), pp. 323-331; R. C. Theuer and J. J. Vitale, Drug and nutrient interactions, in *Nutritional Support of Medical Practice,* eds. H. A. Schneider, C. E. Anderson, and D. B. Coursin (Hagerstown, Md.: Harper & Row, 1977), pp. 297–305; A. O. Moore and D. E. Powers, *Food-Medication Interactions,* ed. C. H. Smith (Tempe, Ariz.: A. O. Moore and D. E. Powers, 1981); A. Grant, *Nutritional Assessment Guidelines* (Seattle: A. Grant, 1979), pp. 63–96; D. C. March, *Handbook: Interactions of Selected Drugs with Nutritional Status in Man* (Chicago: American Dietetic Association, 1978).

As for the diet history, there are several means of obtaining food intake data, including the 24-hour recall, the usual intake record, the food frequency checklist, and the food diary. Great skill is required to obtain accurate food intake data. The dietitian trained in these techniques often uses food models or photos and measuring devices to help clients identify serving sizes of food consumed.

The most commonly used method of obtaining food intake data is the 24-hour recall. To use this method the assessor asks the client to recount everything eaten or drunk in the past 24 hours or for the previous day. (Form E-3 shows a typical 24-hour recall form.) This method does not provide enough accurate information to allow generalizations about an individual's usual food intake, however. It is more often used in nutrition surveys to obtain estimates of the typical food intakes of large numbers of people in given populations.

Food Intake for a 24-Hour Recall or Usual Intake Pattern

Name and address _____   Date _____

_____

_____

Did you take a vitamin/mineral supplement? _____

If yes, what kind? _____   Dose _____

Please record the amount and type of foods and beverages consumed today. [Or: Please record the amount and type of foods and beverages you typically consume each day.]

FOOD	AMOUNT (c, tbsp, or piece)	DESCRIPTION (how cooked, how served)

(etc.)

An advantage of the 24-hour recall is that it is easy to obtain. It is also less frustrating to elicit information from the past 24 hours than to require a person to estimate his intake over a long period of time. However, the previous day's intake may not be the usual intake; the subject may be unable to accurately estimate the amounts of food eaten; or the subject may conceal facts about what was consumed. As a result, sometimes the information gathered in a 24-hour recall does not truly reflect a person's usual intake.

Another method is to obtain a "usual intake pattern." An inquiry on usual intake might begin with "What is the first thing you usually eat or drink during the day?" Similar questions follow until a typical daily intake pattern is obtained. This method is similar to the 24-hour recall and can be recorded on the same form (Form E–3). A skilled and patient interviewer can obtain much useful information from it. For a person whose intake varies widely from day to day,

however, it may be hard to answer the questions, and in such a case the data obtained may be useless in estimating nutrient intake. However, the usual intake method is useful in verifying food intake when the past 24 hours have been atypical.

Another approach is to use a food frequency checklist. The purpose of this record is to ascertain how often an individual eats a specific type of food per day, week, month, or year. Subjects are asked to state how often they eat a certain food or food type, and a long list of foods is used to cover all possibilities. This information can help pinpoint nutrients that may be excessive or deficient in the diet. If used in conjunction with the usual intake or 24-hour recall, the food frequency record permits double-checking the accuracy of the information obtained. Form E–4 is a food frequency checklist.

FORM E–4

Food Frequency Checklist

The following information will help us to understand your regular eating habits so that we may offer you the best service possible. If you have any doubt about some items, be sure to underestimate the "goodness" of your habits rather than to overestimate.

1. How many times *per week* do you eat the following foods? Circle the appropriate number:

PER WEEK

Poultry	0	<1	1	2	3	4	5	6	7	8	9	>9	_____
Fish	0	<1	1	2	3	4	5	6	7	8	9	>9	_____
Hot dogs	0	<1	1	2	3	4	5	6	7	8	9	>9	_____
Bacon	0	<1	1	2	3	4	5	6	7	8	9	>9	_____
Lunch meat	0	<1	1	2	3	4	5	6	7	8	9	>9	_____
Sausage	0	<1	1	2	3	4	5	6	7	8	9	>9	_____
Pork or ham	0	<1	1	2	3	4	5	6	7	8	9	>9	_____
Salt pork	0	<1	1	2	3	4	5	6	7	8	9	>9	_____
Liver	0	<1	1	2	3	4	5	6	7	8	9	>9	_____
Beef or veal	0	<1	1	2	3	4	5	6	7	8	9	>9	_____
Other meats (which?) _____	0	<1	1	2	3	4	5	6	7	8	9	>9	_____
Eggs	0	<1	1	2	3	4	5	6	7	8	9	>9	_____
Fast foods?	0	<1	1	2	3	4	5	6	7	8	9	>9	_____

2. How many times *per day* do you eat the following foods? Circle the appropriate number:

PER WEEK

Bread, toast, rolls, muffins	0	<1	1	2	3	4	5	6	7	8	9	>9	_____
Milk (including on cereal)	0	<1	1	2	3	4	5	6	7	8	9	>9	_____
Yogurt or tofu	0	<1	1	2	3	4	5	6	7	8	9	>9	_____
Cheese or cheese dishes	0	<1	1	2	3	4	5	6	7	8	9	>9	_____
Sugar, jam, jelly, syrup, honey	0	<1	1	2	3	4	5	6	7	8	9	>9	_____
Butter or margarine	0	<1	1	2	3	4	5	6	7	8	9	>9	_____

3. How many times *per week* do you eat the following foods? Circle the appropriate number:

PER WEEK

Fruit or fruit juice	0	<1	1	2	3	4	5	6	7	8	9	>9	_____
Vegetables other than potato	0	<1	1	2	3	4	5	6	7	8	9	>9	_____
Potatoes and other starchy vegetables	0	<1	1	2	3	4	5	6	7	8	9	>9	_____
Salads or raw vegetables	0	<1	1	2	3	4	5	6	7	8	9	>9	_____
Cereal (which kind?)_____	0	<1	1	2	3	4	5	6	7	8	9	>9	_____
Pancakes or waffles	0	<1	1	2	3	4	5	6	7	8	9	>9	_____

(continued)

Rice or other cooked grains . . . . 0 <1 1 2 3 4 5 6 7 8 9 >9 _____

Noodles (macaroni, spaghetti) . . . . 0 <1 1 2 3 4 5 6 7 8 9 >9 _____

Crackers or pretzels . . . . 0 <1 1 2 3 4 5 6 7 8 9 >9 _____

Sweet rolls or doughnuts . . . . 0 <1 1 2 3 4 5 6 7 8 9 >9 _____

Cooked dry beans or peas . . . . 0 <1 1 2 3 4 5 6 7 8 9 >9 _____

Peanut butter or nuts . . . . 0 <1 1 2 3 4 5 6 7 8 9 >9 _____

Milk or milk products . . . . 0 <1 1 2 3 4 5 6 7 8 9 >9 _____

TV dinners, pot pies, other prepared meals . . . . 0 <1 1 2 3 4 5 6 7 8 9 >9 _____

Sweet bakery goods (cake, cookies) . . . . 0 <1 1 2 3 4 5 6 7 8 9 >9 _____

Snack foods (potato or corn chips) . . . . 0 <1 1 2 3 4 5 6 7 8 9 >9 _____

Candy . . . . 0 <1 1 2 3 4 5 6 7 8 9 >9 _____

Soft drinks (which?) _____ . . . . 0 <1 1 2 3 4 5 6 7 8 9 >9 _____

Coffee or tea . . . . 0 <1 1 2 3 4 5 6 7 8 9 >9 _____

Frozen sweets (which?) _____ . . . . 0 <1 1 2 3 4 5 6 7 8 9 >9 _____

Instant meals such as breakfast bars or diet meal beverages
(which?)_____ . . . . 0 <1 1 2 3 4 5 6 7 8 9 >9 _____

Wine . . . . 0 <1 1 2 3 4 5 6 7 8 9 >9 _____

Beer . . . . 0 <1 1 2 3 4 5 6 7 8 9 >9 _____

Whiskey, vodka, rum, etc. . . . . 0 <1 1 2 3 4 5 6 7 8 9 >9 _____

4. What specific kinds of the following foods do you eat most often? Include the name of the food; whether it is fresh, canned, or frozen; and how it is prepared.

　　Fruits and fruit juices _____

　　Vegetables _____

　　Milk and Milk products _____

　　Meats _____

　　Breads and cereals _____

　　Desserts _____

　　Snack foods _____

5. Please list the names of any liquid, powder, or pill form of vitamin or mineral product you take, and state how often you take it. Please list also any diet supplement you use (such as protein milk shakes or brewer's yeast), how much you use, and how often you use it. _____

6. Is there anything else we should know about your food/nutrient intake? _____

Still another alternative is the food diary. (An example is provided in Form E–5.) Completion of a diary often helps to determine factors associated with food intake (time of day, place eaten, mood, others present). The person keeping the diary is instructed to write down the required information immediately after eating. A food diary works well with cooperative people but requires considerable time and effort on their part.

The advantages of the food diary are that the diary keeper assumes an active role; the person may for the first time begin to see and understand personal food habits; and that the assessor obtains an accurate picture of the diary keeper's lifestyle and factors that affect food intake. For these reasons, food diaries are particularly useful in outpatient counseling for such nutrition problems as overweight, underweight, or food allergy. The major disadvantages stem from poor compliance in recording the data and conscious or unconscious changes in eating habits that may occur while the diary is being kept.

After food intake data have been collected, they are used to determine nutrient intake, if appropriate. Comparison of the nutrients in the foods eaten (Appendix H) with standards such as the RDA (inside front cover) or the Canadian RNI (Appendix I) is the next step. The comparison is made either by a skilled dietitian estimating or manually calculating the amount of each nutrient obtained from each food or through the use of a nutrient analysis computer program.

Such a dietary analysis tends to imply an accuracy greater than can actually be obtained from data as uncertain as those that provide the starting information. Nutrient contents of foods listed in tables of food composition are averages. Foods vary. Furthermore, the person who reports eating "a serving" of greens may not know the difference between a quarter-cup and two whole cups; only trained individuals can accurately estimate serving sizes. Thus there are many sources of error in comparing nutrient intakes with nutrient needs in this way.

FORM E–5

Food Diary

Name _____

Date _____

TIME	PLACE	WITH WHOM	EMOTIONAL STATE	HUNGRY OR NOT HUNGRY	FOOD EATEN (AMOUNT)

(etc.)

E

Most history-takers learn to use shortcut systems to obtain rough estimates of nutrient intakes and then use the calculation method to pin down any suspected nutrient deficiencies or imbalances.

Once an estimate of nutrient intakes has been obtained by means of a diet history, it has to be combined with other sources of information to confirm or eliminate the possibility of suspected nutrition problems. The assessor must constantly remember that a sufficient intake of a nutrient does not guarantee adequate nutrient status for an individual. Each person digests, absorbs, metabolizes, and excretes nutrients in a unique way; individual needs vary.

Anthropometric Measures

One use of anthropometric measures is to assess growth in children. Although special equipment is available to measure an infant's length (see Figure E–1), in many settings a less accurate method is used: with the infant lying on a flat surface, a measuring tape is run along the side of the baby from the top of the head to the heel of the foot. Care is taken to ensure that the infant's legs and body are straight. Since this is difficult to accomplish, it requires two people to obtain an accurate measurement.

FIGURE E–1

Measurement of an infant. An infant is measured lying down by use of a length measuring device with a fixed headboard and movable footboard. Note that two people are needed to measure the infant's length.

Illustration courtesy of Ross Laboratories.

A child that can stand erect and cooperate can be measured in the same manner as an adult. The best way to measure height standing, is to have the person being measured stand against a flat wall to which a measuring tape or stick has been affixed (see Figure E–2). The person should not be wearing shoes and should stand erect with heels

FIGURE E–2

Measurement of an adult. Height is measured most accurately when the person stands against a flat wall to which a measuring tape has been affixed. When the person is taller than the measurer, the measurer can stand on a stool to help insure that the proper height measurement is obtained.

together. The person's line of sight should be horizontal, and the heels, buttocks, shoulders, and head should be touching the wall. After carefully checking the height measurement, the assessor should record the result immediately to avoid misplacing or forgetting the measurement. Height is recorded in either inches or centimeters, depending on the policy of the institution.

Although less desirable, the measuring rod of a scale can be used to measure height by using the same general procedure. The person should be facing away from the scale and extra care should be taken to ensure that the person is standing as straight as possible.

Unfortunately, it is a common and inexcusable practice in many health care institutions to ask clients how tall they are, rather than measuring their height. Self-reported height should be used only as a last resort when measurement is not practical (in the case of an uncooperative patient, an emergency admission, or the like).

In adults, weight measurements should be taken on a beam balance that frequently is checked for accuracy (see Figure E–3). Standardized conditions under which people are

E

weighed increase the usability of repeated weight measurements. Whenever possible, a person should be weighed at the same time of day (preferably before breakfast), in the same amount of clothing (hospital gown, without shoes), after having voided, and on the same scale. Bedridden patients can be measured with metabolic scales (see Figure E–4). Bathroom scales are not accurate and should not be used. Like all measurements, observed weight should be recorded immediately. Weight is recorded in either pounds or kilograms, depending on the policy of the institution.

FIGURE E–4

Weighing an adult using metabolic scales. Metabolic bed scales are used to measure patients who cannot get out of bed.

To assess growth in infants and children use Figures E–5 (A and B), E–6 (A and B), E–7 (A and B) and E–8 (A and B). Follow these steps:

- Select the appropriate figure based on age and sex. For example, for a 3-month-old female infant weighing 12 pounds with a length of 23 inches, you would use the chart for girls, birth to 36 months (Figure E–5A).
- Locate the child's age on the bottom or top of the chart (in our example, 3 months).
- Locate the child's weight in pounds or kilograms on the lower left or right side of the chart (in our example, 12 pounds).
- Mark the chart where the age and weight lines intersect. (In our example, this is just above the 50th percentile. Note where the chart is marked.)
- To find the child's percentile for length or height and age, start by locating the child's age on the top of the chart and the length on the upper right or left side. Proceed as you did when you were comparing age and weight. (Note the mark on the chart for the baby in the example.)

FIGURE E–3

Weighing an adult. Whenever possible, subjects are measured on beam balance scales to insure accuracy.

E

GIRLS: BIRTH TO 36 MONTHS
PHYSICAL GROWTH
NCHS PERCENTILES*

NAME _____ RECORD # _____

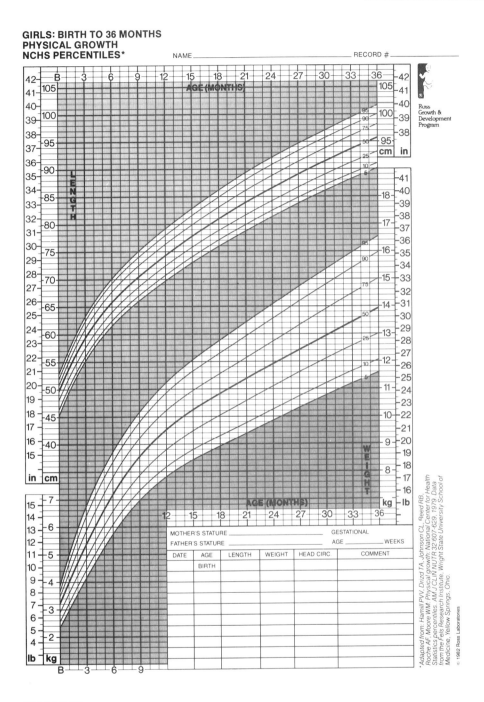

FIGURE E–5A

Girls: Birth to 36 Months Physical Growth NCHS Percentiles—Length and Weight for Age.

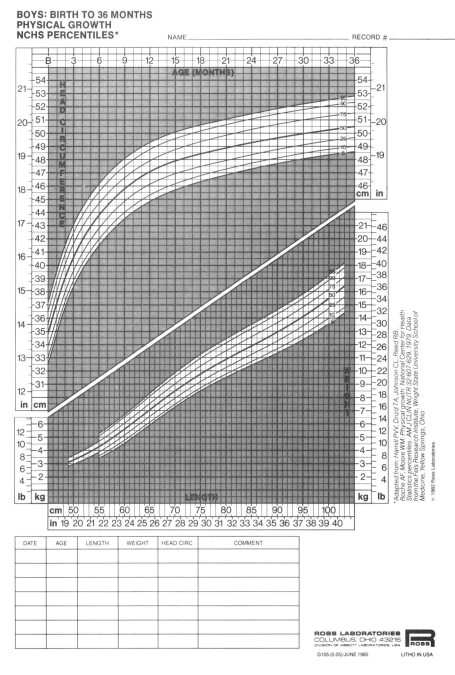

BOYS: BIRTH TO 36 MONTHS
PHYSICAL GROWTH
NCHS PERCENTILES*

NAME _____   RECORD # _____

*Adapted from: Hamill PVV, Drizd TA, Johnson CL, Reed RB, Roche AF, Moore WM. Physical growth: National Center for Health Statistics percentiles. AM J CLIN NUTR 32:607-629, 1979. Data from the Fels Research Institute, Wright State University School of Medicine, Yellow Springs, Ohio.

© 1982 Ross Laboratories

DATE	AGE	LENGTH	WEIGHT	HEAD CIRC	COMMENT

ROSS LABORATORIES
COLUMBUS, OHIO 43216
DIVISION OF ABBOTT LABORATORIES, USA

G105 (0.05)/JUNE 1985   LITHO IN USA

FIGURE E–6B

Boys: Birth to 36 Months Physical Growth NCHS Percentiles—Head Circumference for Age and Weight for Length.

**GIRLS: 2 TO 18 YEARS
PHYSICAL GROWTH
NCHS PERCENTILES***

NAME _____ RECORD # _____

FIGURE E–7A

Girls: 2 to 18 Years Physical Growth NCHS Percentiles—Height and Weight for Age.

E

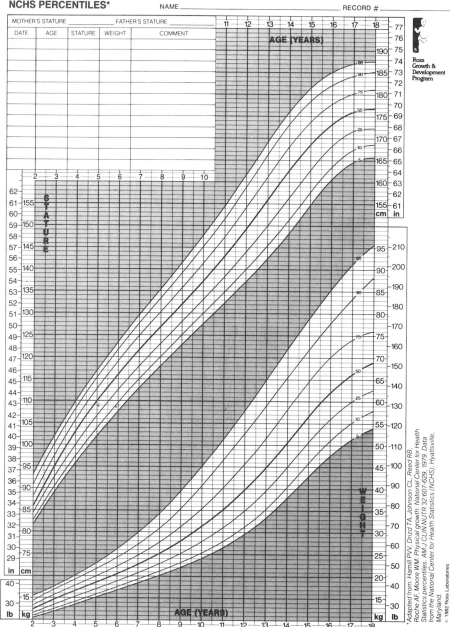

**BOYS: 2 TO 18 YEARS
PHYSICAL GROWTH
NCHS PERCENTILES***

FIGURE E–7B

Boys: 2 to 18 Years Physical Growth NCHS Percentiles—Height and Weight for Age.

E

**GIRLS: PREPUBESCENT
PHYSICAL GROWTH
NCHS PERCENTILES***

NAME _____ RECORD # _____

*Adapted from: Hamill PVV, Drizd TA, Johnson CL, Reed RB,
Roche AF, Moore WM. Physical growth: National Center for Health
Statistics percentiles. AM J CLIN NUTR 32:607-629, 1979. Data
from the National Center for Health Statistics (NCHS), Hyattsville,
Maryland*

© 1982 Ross Laboratories

ROSS LABORATORIES
COLUMBUS, OHIO 43216
DIVISION OF ABBOTT LABORATORIES USA

G108 (0.05)/JUNE 1985   LITHO IN USA

FIGURE E-8A

Girls: Prepubescent Physical Growth NCHS Percentiles—Weight for Height.

E

**BOYS: PREPUBESCENT
PHYSICAL GROWTH
NCHS PERCENTILES***

NAME _____ RECORD # _____

*Adapted from: Hamill PVV, Drizd TA, Johnson CL, Reed RB Roche AF, Moore WM. Physical growth: National Center for Health Statistics percentiles. AM J CLIN NUTR 32:607-629, 1979. Data from the National Center for Health Statistics (NCHS), Hyattsville, Maryland.

© 1982 Ross Laboratories

ROSS LABORATORIES
COLUMBUS, OHIO 43216
DIVISION OF ABBOTT LABORATORIES USA

G107 (0.05)/JUNE 1985   LITHO IN USA

FIGURE E–8B

Boys: Prepubescent Physical Growth NCHS Percentiles—Weight for Height.

In pregnancy, satisfactory growth of the fetus is normally assumed if the pregnant woman's weight gain is normal. Figure E–9 is a weight-gain grid used for assessment purposes.

Among the standards used for anthropometric measures are several already presented. A table of average weights for height (inside back cover) is often used as a standard for individual people's weight. To use the height-weight table, the assessor refers to a table of frame sizes such as the one based

E

FIGURE E–9

Prenatal weight gain grid.

on elbow breadth (Table 8–2) or the one that compares wrist circumference to height (see Figure E–10 and Table E–3).

place tape here

Styloid process ("wristbone")

FIGURE E–10

Wrist circumference. The wrist circumference is measured as shown above.

TABLE E–3

Frame Size from Height-Wrist Circumference Ratios (r)

	MALE r VALUES[a]	FEMALE r VALUES[a]
Small	>10.4	>11.0
Medium	9.6–10.4	10.1–11.0
Large	<9.6	<10.1

[a] $r = \dfrac{\text{Height (cm)}}{\text{Wrist circumference (cm)}^b}$

[b]The wrist is measured where it bends (distal to the styloid process), on the right arm.
Source: Adapted from J. P. Grant, Patient selection, *Handbook of Total Parenteral Nutrition* (Philadelphia: Saunders, 1980), p. 15.

The table of average weights for height may not be useful in cases where a person has weighed much more or much less than the average throughout life. To assess such a person's weight, it may be more informative to compare the present weight, not with an "ideal" body weight, but with the usual body weight. The percentages of a person's actual weight compared with ideal or usual body weight are useful indicators of malnutrition (Table E–4).

TABLE E–4

Weight as an Indicator of Malnutrition

%IBW[a]	%UBW[b]	DEGREE OF UNDERNUTRITION
80–90%	85–95%	Mildly depleted
70–79%	75–84%	Moderately depleted
<70%	<75%	Severely depleted

[a]Percent ideal body weight.
[b]Percent usual body weight.
Source: Adapted from J. P. Grant, Patient selection, *Handbook of Total Parenteral Nutrition* (Philadelphia: Saunders, 1980), p. 11.

The height-weight tables just mentioned are useful for identifying both under- and overnutrition. A standard derived from height and weight, which is especially useful for estimating the risk to health associated with overnutrition, is the body mass index (BMI), presented in Chapter 8. Nomograms for determining the BMI are presented in Figure 8–3.

The triceps fatfold measurement provides an estimate of body fat (see Figure E–11). Triceps fatfold percentiles are given in Table 8–3. The midarm circumference (MAC) provides an index of the arm's total area (see Figure E–12 and Table E–5); and an arithmetical calculation subtracts the fat from the total area, leaving an estimate of the lean tissue in the arm—the mid-arm muscle circumference (MAMC). The MAMC (see Figures E–13 and E–14 and Table E–6) reflects the body's total skeletal muscle mass.

To assess protein-kcalorie malnutrition, several lab tests are used in conjunction with these anthropometric measures. Table E–7 shows that different compartments are depleted, depending on whether the person has kwashiorkor (from protein deficiency as reflected in skeletal muscle and visceral protein), marasmus (from kcalorie deficiency as reflected in body fat), or a mixture of the two. A form such as Form E–6 summarizes the anthropometric and biochemical data used to classify protein-kcalorie malnutrition.

FIGURE E-11

How to measure the triceps fatfold.
A. Find the midpoint of the arm:
1. Ask the subject to bend his arm at the elbow and lay his hand across his stomach. (If he is right-handed, measure the left arm, and vice versa.)
2. Feel the shoulder to locate the acromial process. It helps to slide your fingers along the clavicle to find the acromial process. The olecranon process is the tip of the elbow.
3. Place a measuring tape from the acromial process to the tip of the elbow. Divide this measurement by 2 and mark the midpoint of the arm with a pen.

B. Measure the fat fold:
1. Ask the subject to let his arm hang loosely at his side.
2. Grasp a fold of skin and subcutaneous fat between the thumb and forefinger slightly above the midpoint mark. Gently pull the skin away from the underlying muscle. (This step takes a lot of practice. If you want to be sure you don't have muscle as well as fat, ask the subject to contract and relax his muscle. You should be able to feel if you are pinching muscle.)
3. Place the calipers over the fatfold at the midpoint mark and read the measurement to the nearest 1.0 mm in two to three seconds. (If using plastic calipers, align pressure lines and read measurement to the nearest 1.0 mm in two to three seconds.)
4. Repeat steps 2 to 4 twice more. Add the three readings and then divide by 3 to find the average.

FIGURE E-12

How to measure the midarm circumference. Ask the subject to let his arm hang loosely at his side. Place the measuring tape horizontally around the arm at the midpoint mark. This measurement is the midarm circumference.

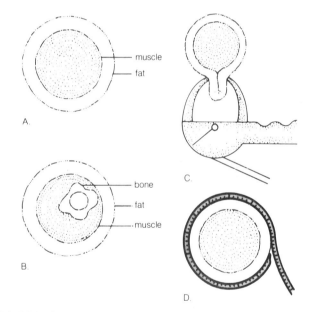

FIGURE E-13

How the midarm muscle circumference is derived.
A. The arm is visualized as an inner circle of muscle surrounded by an outer circle of fat.
B. In reality, the arm is not circular, and there is some bone, but the simplified picture is approximately correct.
C. This measurement (the fatfold) gives you two times the thickness of the fat.
D. This measurement (the tape-measured outer circumference of the arm) gives you the outer circumference (muscle plus fat).
E. An equation then derives the *circumference of the muscle*, an index of the body's total skeletal muscle mass. The equation is:

midarm muscle circumference(cm) =
midarm circumference(cm) − [0.314* × triceps fatfold(mm)]

*This factor converts the fatfold measurement and also converts millimeters to centimeters.

FORM E-6

Nutrition Assessment Summary

Date _____ Admitting date _____

Client _____ Room _____

Height _____ Admitting weight _____

Current weight _____ Usual body weight _____

Admitting diagnosis _____

Somatic protein and fat	Client value	Degree of depletion			
		None	Mild	Moderate	Severe
Weight as % IBW					
Weight as % UBW					
Midarm circumference					
Triceps fatfold					
Midarm muscle circumference					
Urinary creatinine					
Creatinine-height index					

Visceral protein					
Serum albumin					
Total iron binding capacity					
Transferrin (serum or calculated)					
Total lymphocyte count					
Cell mediated immunity					

Nitrogen balance: _____

Protein-kcalorie nutrition status

☐ Adequate

☐ Marasmus
  Somatic protein and fat depleted; visceral protein adequate

☐ Kwashiorkor
  Somatic protein and fat adequate; visceral proteins depleted

☐ Kwashiorkor-marasmus mix
  Somatic and visceral protein depleted

Other findings and comments

(Include pertinent food intake data, other laboratory tests, and physical findings.)

_____

_____
Signature of Assessor

TABLE E–5

Midarm Circumference (MAC) (centimeters)

	MALE					FEMALE				
Age	5th	25th	50th	75th	95th	5th	25th	50th	75th	95th
1–1.9	14.2	15.0	15.9	17.0	18.3	13.8	14.8	15.6	16.4	17.7
2–2.9	14.1	15.3	16.2	17.0	18.5	14.2	15.2	16.0	16.7	18.4
3–3.9	15.0	16.0	16.7	17.5	19.0	14.3	15.8	16.7	17.5	18.9
4–4.9	14.9	16.2	17.1	18.0	19.2	14.9	16.0	16.9	17.7	19.1
5–5.9	15.3	16.7	17.5	18.5	20.4	15.3	16.5	17.5	18.5	21.1
6–6.9	15.5	16.7	17.9	18.8	22.8	15.6	17.0	17.6	18.7	21.1
7–7.9	16.2	17.7	18.7	20.1	23.0	16.4	17.4	18.3	19.9	23.1
8–8.9	16.2	17.7	19.0	20.2	24.5	16.8	18.3	19.5	21.4	26.1
9–9.9	17.5	18.7	20.0	21.7	25.7	17.8	19.4	21.1	22.4	26.0
10–10.9	18.1	19.6	21.0	23.1	27.4	17.4	19.3	21.0	22.8	26.5
11–11.9	18.6	20.2	22.3	24.4	28.0	18.5	20.8	22.4	24.8	30.3
12–12.9	19.3	21.4	23.2	25.4	30.3	19.4	21.6	23.7	25.6	29.4
13–13.9	19.4	22.8	24.7	26.3	30.1	20.2	22.3	24.3	27.1	33.8
14–14.9	22.0	23.7	25.3	28.3	32.3	21.4	23.7	25.2	27.2	32.2
15–15.9	22.2	24.4	26.4	28.4	32.0	20.8	23.9	25.4	27.9	32.2
16–16.9	24.4	26.2	27.8	30.3	34.3	21.8	24.1	25.8	28.3	33.4
17–17.9	24.6	26.7	28.5	30.8	34.7	22.0	24.1	26.4	29.5	35.0
18–18.9	24.5	27.6	29.7	32.1	37.9	22.2	24.1	25.8	28.1	32.5
19–24.9	26.2	28.8	30.8	33.1	37.2	21.1	24.7	26.5	29.0	34.5
25–34.9	27.1	30.0	31.9	34.2	37.5	23.3	25.6	27.7	30.4	36.8
35–44.9	27.8	30.5	32.6	34.5	37.4	24.1	26.7	29.0	31.7	37.8
45–54.9	26.7	30.1	32.2	34.2	37.6	24.2	27.4	29.9	32.8	38.4
55–64.9	25.8	29.6	31.7	33.6	36.9	24.3	28.0	30.3	33.5	38.5
65–74.9	24.8	28.5	30.7	32.5	35.5	24.0	27.4	29.9	32.6	37.3

Source: Adapted from A. R. Frisancho, New norms of upper limb fat and muscle areas for assessment of nutritional status, *American Journal of Clinical Nutrition* 34 (1981): 2540–2545.

E

FIGURE E–14

Nomograms for determination of midarm muscle circumference (MAMC) To obtain muscle circumference using either nomogram, lay ruler between values of arm circumference and fatfold and read off muscle circumference.

Source: Reproduced with permission from J. Gurney and D. Jelliffe, Arm anthropometry in nutritional asessment; nomogram for rapid calculation of muscle circumference and cross-sectional muscle and fat areas, *American Journal of Clinical Nutrition* 26 (1973): 912, as adapted by A. Grant, *Nutritional Assessment Guidelines*, 2nd ed., 1979 (available from P.O. Box 25057, Northgate Station, Seattle, WA 98125).

TABLE E-6

Midarm Muscle Circumference (MAMC) (centimeters)

Age	\multicolumn{5}{c}{MALE}					\multicolumn{5}{c}{FEMALE}				
	5th	25th	50th	75th	95th	5th	25th	50th	75th	95th
1–1.9	11.0	11.9	12.7	13.5	14.7	10.5	11.7	12.4	13.9	14.3
2–2.9	11.1	12.2	13.0	14.0	15.0	11.1	11.9	12.6	13.3	14.7
3–3.9	11.7	13.1	13.7	14.3	15.3	11.3	12.4	13.2	14.0	15.2
4–4.9	12.3	13.3	14.1	14.8	15.9	11.5	12.8	13.6	14.4	15.7
5–5.9	12.8	14.0	14.7	15.4	16.9	12.5	13.4	14.2	15.1	16.5
6–6.9	13.1	14.2	15.1	16.1	17.7	13.0	13.8	14.5	15.4	17.1
7–7.9	13.7	15.1	16.0	16.8	19.0	12.9	14.2	15.1	16.0	17.6
8–8.9	14.0	15.4	16.2	17.0	18.7	13.8	15.1	16.0	17.1	19.4
9–9.9	15.1	16.1	17.0	18.3	20.2	14.7	15.8	16.7	18.0	19.8
10–10.9	15.6	16.6	18.0	19.1	22.1	14.8	15.9	17.0	18.0	19.7
11–11.9	15.9	17.3	18.3	19.5	23.0	15.0	17.1	18.1	19.6	22.3
12–12.9	16.7	18.2	19.5	21.0	24.1	16.2	18.0	19.1	20.1	22.0
13–13.9	17.2	19.6	21.1	22.6	24.5	16.9	18.3	19.8	21.1	24.0
14–14.9	18.9	21.2	22.3	24.0	26.4	17.4	19.0	20.1	21.6	24.7
15–15.9	19.9	21.8	23.7	25.4	27.2	17.5	18.9	20.2	21.5	24.4
16–16.9	21.3	23.4	24.9	26.9	29.6	17.0	19.0	20.2	21.6	24.9
17–17.9	22.4	24.5	25.8	27.3	31.2	17.5	19.4	20.5	22.1	25.7
18–18.9	22.6	25.2	26.4	28.3	32.4	17.4	19.1	20.2	21.5	24.5
19–24.9	23.8	25.7	27.3	28.9	32.1	17.9	19.5	20.7	22.1	24.9
25–34.9	24.3	26.4	27.9	29.8	32.6	18.3	19.9	21.2	22.8	26.4
35–44.9	24.7	26.9	28.6	30.2	32.7	18.6	20.5	21.8	23.6	27.2
45–54.9	23.9	26.5	28.1	30.0	32.6	18.7	20.6	22.0	23.8	27.4
55–64.9	23.6	26.0	27.8	29.5	32.0	18.7	20.9	22.5	24.4	28.0
65–74.9	22.3	25.1	26.8	28.4	30.6	18.5	20.8	22.5	24.4	27.9

Source: Adapted from A. R. Frisancho, New norms of upper limb fat and muscle areas for assessment of nutritional status, *American Journal of Clinical Nutrition* 34 (1981): 2540–2545.

TABLE E-7

Anthropometric and Biochemical Measures Used to Assess Protein-kCalorie Malnutrition (PCM)

Measure	\multicolumn{3}{c}{Body Compartment Measured}		
	Body Fat	Skeletal Muscle	Visceral Protein
Anthropometrics			
Weight[a]	x	x	
Triceps skinfold	x		
Midarm circumference	x	x	
Midarm muscle circumference		x	
Lab tests			
Serum albumin			x
Serum transferrin			x
Total lymphocyte count			x
Creatinine-height index[b]		x	

[a]A standard table of weight for height appears on the inside back cover.
[b]The amount of creatinine excreted is thought to reflect total skeletal mass. It therefore should be proportional to height. If creatinine excreted (for a person of a given height) is low, this reflects depleted skeletal muscle. Table E–11 presents standards.

Physical Examination

Chapters 9 to 12 discussed some symptoms of vitamin and mineral deficiencies and toxicities, revealing that many tissues and organs reflect signs of malnutrition. Table E–8 presents some of the signs of vitamin/mineral malnutrition, body system by body system.

TABLE E–8

Physical Findings Associated with Various Nutrient Imbalances

PHYSICAL FINDINGS	PROTEIN-kCALORIE	VITAMIN A	B VITAMINS	VITAMIN C	VITAMIN D	IRON	OTHER
Hair							
Dull, dry, sparse, readily plucked, lighter and darker bands (flag sign), depigmented	X						
Face							
Swollen	X						
Dark areas of skin over eyes and under cheeks, flaky skin around nose		X					
Pale		X				X	
Eyes							
Night blindness		X					Zinc
Triangular, shiny gray spots on exposed portion of conjunctiva (mucous membrane lining eyelid)		X					
Dull, opaque, or dry cornea		X					
Softening of cornea, inner eyelids		X					
Inner eyelids and whites dry and pigmented		X					
Cracked and red at corners			X				
Pale conjunctiva		X				X	
White ring around iris							Elevated blood lipids
Raised yellow spots on eye							Elevated blood lipids
Lips							
Bilateral redness, cracking, scaling, or scarring at corners of mouth			X				
Swollen, red lips with vertical cracks			X				
Tongue							
Swollen, magenta colored			X				
Smooth surface			X				
Atrophy of the surface structures			X				
Bright red, painful			X				

TABLE E–8

(continued)

PHYSICAL FINDINGS	PROTEIN-kCALORIE	VITAMIN A	B VITAMINS	VITAMIN C	VITAMIN D	IRON	OTHER
Teeth							
Caries							Excess sugar
Mottled enamel							Excess fluoride
Gums							
Bleeding, spongy, receding				X			
Glands							
Enlarged thyroid gland (located at front of neck)							Iodine
Enlarged parotid gland (located just below earlobes)	X						General undernutrition
Skin							
Depigmentation, patches of hyperpigmented skin that peels off (flaky-paint dermatosis)	X						
Dry, scaling, rough (skin may appear to have permanent goosebumps)		X					Essential fatty acids
Bilateral hyperpigmentation with redness and swelling on body areas exposed to sunlight; scrotal or vulval dermatosis			X				
Small red or purple skin hemorrhages				X			
Nails							
Spoon-shaped, brittle, ridged						X	
Pale nail bed						X	
Subcutaneous tissue							
Edematous (swollen)	X						
Decreased fat stores	X						
Excessive fat stores							Obesity

Biochemical (Lab) Tests

Biochemical or clinical lab tests help to determine what is really happening inside the body. Blood and urine samples are most often used to directly measure nutrients or metabolites that are affected by poor nutrition. Table E–9 summarizes the biochemical tests used to assess vitamin-mineral status.

Standards for determining the severity of depletion of serum albumin and transferrin are given in Table E–10. Creatinine-height index standards are given in Table E–11A and Table E–11B.

TABLE E–9

Laboratory Tests Useful for Assessing Some Vitamin and Mineral Deficiencies

Vitamins	Tests
Vitamin A	Serum vitamin A, serum carotene, retinol binding protein
Thiamin	Erythrocyte transketolase
Riboflavin	Erythrocyte glutathione reductase
Niacin	Urinary N-methylnicotinamide, urinary 2-pyridone
Vitamin B_6	Tryptophan load test, serum vitamin B_6
Folacin	Erythrocyte folate, vitamin B_{12} status, serum free folate
Vitamin B_{12}	Deoxyuridine suppression test
Vitamin C	Leukocyte vitamin C, serum vitamin C
Vitamin D	Serum alkaline phosphatase
Vitamin E	Erythrocyte hemolysis test, plasma or serum tocopherol
Vitamin K	Prothrombin time

Minerals	Tests
Calcium	Serum calcium; bone tests under development
Potassium	Serum potassium
Magnesium	Serum magnesium
Iron	Hemoglobin, hematocrit, total iron-binding capacity (TIBC), transferrin saturation, erythrocyte protoporphyrin, leukocyte ferritin
Iodine	Serum protein-bound iodine, radioiodine uptake
Zinc	Serum or plasma zinc, hair zinc

TABLE E–10

Relationship between Degree of Undernutrition and Serum Proteins

DEGREE OF DEPLETION	INDICATOR	
	Albumin (g/100 ml)	Transferrin (mg/100 ml)
Mild	2.8–3.4	150–200
Moderate	2.1–2.7	100–149
Severe	<2.1	<100

TABLE E–11A

Creatinine-Height Index Standards for Men

HEIGHT		SMALL FRAME		MEDIUM FRAME		LARGE FRAME	
in	cm	Ideal weight (kg)	Creatinine (mg per 24 hr)	Ideal weight (kg)	Creatinine (mg per 24 hr)	Ideal weight (kg)	Creatinine (mg per 24 hr)
61	154.9	52.7	1,212	56.1	1,290	60.7	1,396
62	157.5	54.1	1,244	57.7	1,327	62.0	1,426
63	160.0	55.4	1,274	59.1	1,359	63.6	1,463
64	162.5	56.8	1,306	60.4	1,389	65.2	1,500
65	165.1	58.4	1,343	62.0	1,426	66.8	1,536
66	167.6	60.2	1,385	63.9	1,470	68.9	1,585
67	170.2	62.0	1,426	65.9	1,516	71.1	1,635
68	172.7	63.9	1,470	67.7	1,557	72.9	1,677
69	175.3	65.9	1,516	69.5	1,598	74.8	1,720
70	177.8	67.7	1,557	71.6	1,647	76.8	1,766
71	180.3	69.5	1,599	73.6	1,693	79.1	1,819
72	182.9	71.4	1,642	75.7	1,741	81.1	1,865
73	185.4	73.4	1,688	77.7	1,787	83.4	1,918
74	187.9	75.2	1,730	80.0	1,846	85.7	1,971
75	190.5	77.0	1,771	82.3	1,893	87.7	2,017

TABLE E–11B

Creatinine-Height Index Standards for Women

HEIGHT		SMALL FRAME		MEDIUM FRAME		LARGE FRAME	
in	cm	Ideal weight (kg)	Creatinine (mg per 24 hr)	Ideal weight (kg)	Creatinine (mg per 24 hr)	Ideal weight (kg)	Creatinine (mg per 24 hr)
56	142.2	43.2	778	46.1	830	50.7	913
57	144.8	44.3	797	47.3	851	51.8	932
58	147.3	45.4	817	48.6	875	53.2	958
59	149.8	46.8	842	50.0	900	54.5	981
60	152.4	48.2	868	51.4	925	55.9	1,006
61	154.9	49.5	891	52.7	949	57.3	1,031
62	157.5	50.9	916	54.3	977	58.9	1,060
63	160.0	52.3	941	55.9	1,006	60.6	1,091
64	162.5	53.9	970	57.9	1,042	62.5	1,125
65	165.1	55.7	1,003	59.8	1,076	64.3	1,157
66	167.6	57.5	1,035	61.6	1,109	66.1	1,190
67	170.2	59.3	1,067	63.4	1,141	67.9	1,222
68	172.7	61.4	1,105	65.2	1,174	70.0	1,260
69	175.2	63.2	1,138	67.0	1,206	72.0	1,296
70	177.8	65.0	1,170	68.9	1,240	74.1	1,334

Source: A. Grant, *Nutritional Assessment Guidelines*, 2nd ed., 1979 (available from P.O. Box 25057, Northgate Station, Seattle, WA 98125).

Cautions about Nutrition Assessment

To give all the details of nutrition assessment procedures would entail writing another textbook. Whole graduate courses are taught in the subject, and hundreds of pages of reading are required. However, any student of nutrition should know the basics of a proper nutrition assessment procedure, for two reasons.

For one thing, competent medical care includes attention to nutrition. The physician should employ a person skilled in nutrition assessment techniques or refer all patients to such a person, to make sure their nutritional health is sound, while the health care organization (hospital or other) should make nutrition assessment a routine part of its workup on every client, so that nutrition handicaps will not hinder the response to medical treatment and the recovery from illness.

Second, because nutrition is such a popular subject today ("everybody's doing it"), fraudulent practices are even more abundant in this area than they have been in the past (and they have always been rampant). The knowledgeable consumer needs to know what procedures he or she can expect in a nutrition assessment, and what kinds of information they can yield. This appendix has presented the basics of nutrition assessment techniques for these reasons.

The caution should be added, that the tests outlined here yield, in all cases, information that only becomes meaningful when integrated into a whole picture by a skilled, experienced, and educated interpreter. Sources of error are many, from the taking of the initial data to its reporting and analysis. For example, the calculation of nutrients consumed from a diet history has to be combined with other sources of information to confirm or eliminate the possibility of suspected nutrition problems. The assessor must constantly remember that a sufficient intake of a nutrient does not guarantee adequate nutrient status for an individual. Conversely, the apparent inadequate intake of a nutrient does not, by itself, establish that a deficiency exists.

Similarly, the accuracy and value of anthropometric measures are limited by many uncertainties, by the skills of the measurer, and by the perspective of the interpreter. This is even more true of the results of the physical examination. Physical symptoms suggestive of malnutrition are nonspecific: they can be associated with nutrient deficiencies but may be totally unrelated to nutrition. Physical findings can only be interpreted in light of other assessment findings. Finally, the usefulness of clinical tests is also limited. For example, many factors other than nutrition can interfere with the immune response, and the value of skin testing as an index of nutrition status has been questioned. No studies to date have considered all the factors that might affect skin test results. Among known factors are age, certain allergies, and certain drug regimens. For biochemical tests of vitamin and mineral status, too, the assessor must use caution in interpreting results.

Vitamin and mineral levels present in the blood may reflect disease processes, abnormal hormone levels, or other aberrations rather than dietary intake. Even if they reflect dietary intake, they may be affected by what the person has been eating recently, and may not give a true picture of the state of the person's nutrient stores; this sometimes makes it difficult to detect a subclinical deficiency. Furthermore, many nutrients interact. The assessor has to keep in mind that an abnormal lab value for one nutrient may reflect abnormal status with respect to other nutrients. The ultimate diagnosis obtained is therefore appropriately tentative and is confirmed only after careful remedial steps have been taken and have been shown to successfully alleviate the observed problems.

The responsible use of nutrition assessment procedures is a far cry from the kind of experience the man on the street may encounter when he walks into a "nutrition clinic" and is offered a "nutrition assessment" by a "nutritionist." People today are easily led to believe that computers or "hair analysis" will accurately determine their nutrition status. They do not understand all the processes involved in doing such tests but they see that the "experts" seem to know a lot and that the systems being used are very complicated, and so they think there must be some validity to the "results."

A single example of a fraudulent nutrition assessment technique is hair analysis--except in strictly limited applications. Hair analyses are still in the experimental stage. They are being studied to determine what their validity and usefulness may be. One way in which nutrition researchers can use hairs for nutrition assessment is to pull them out and measure the size or protein content of the roots. This provides a clue to protein nutrition status, because hair roots diminish in size and protein content early in a developing protein deficiency. However, the minerals in the shaft of the hair do not reflect accurately the body's total content of minerals, except in the case of some toxic metal contaminants and possibly zinc—and then only for populations, not individuals. Hair analysis is a valuable method in research and shows promise as an assessment tool if the problems can be worked out, but at present it is not suitable for use in individual nutrition assessments. In several instances, hair contents of minerals have been demonstrated *not* to reflect body content in any consistent way.[1] Too many confounding variables interfere: air and water pollution, shampoos and dyes, water hardness, and many others.

Hair analysis is only one practice that is being used by unscrupulous practitioners to elicit belief and extract money from an unsuspecting public. There are many other examples. The rule for the cautious consumer should be to stay skeptical. The fact that you do not understand, or haven't heard of, the method a "nutritionist" is using to test nutrition status may not be a reflection on your limited knowledge. The test may simply be a fraud.

---

[1]R. S. Gibson, B. M. Anderson, and C. A. Scythes, Regional differences in hair zinc concentrations: A possible effect of water hardness, *American Journal of Clinical Nutrition* 37 (1983): 37–42; K. M. Hambidge, Hair analyses: Worthless for vitamins, limited for minerals, *American Journal of Clinical Nutrition* 36 (1982): 943–949.

Nutrition Resources

Appendix *F*

F

Contents

Books

Journals

Addresses

People interested in nutrition often want to know where, in their own town or county, they can find reliable nutrition information. One place you are not likely to find it is the local library, where fad diet books sit side by side on the shelf with books of facts. However, wherever you live, there are several sources you can turn to:

- The Department of Health may have a nutrition expert.
- The local extension agent is often an expert.
- The food editor of your local paper may be well informed.
- The dietitian at the local hospital had to fulfill a set of qualifications before he or she became an R.D. (Registered Dietitian).
- There may be knowledgeable professors of nutrition or biochemistry at a nearby college or university.

The syndicated column on nutrition by J. Mayer and J. Dwyer, which appears in many newspapers, presents well-researched, reliable answers to current questions. The column by R. Alfin-Slater and Jelliffe is also accurate and trustworthy. In addition, you may be interested in building a nutrition library of your own. Books you can buy, journals you can subscribe to, and addresses you can write to for general information are given below.

Books

A 54-page list of references with critiques of each, *Nutrition References and Book Reviews*, is available for purchase from the Chicago Nutrition Association. (See "Addresses," below.)

This 900-page paperback has a chapter on each of 58 topics, including energy, obesity, 32 nutrients, several diseases, malnutrition, growth and its assessment, immunity, alcohol, fiber, dental health, drugs, and toxins. The only major omis-

sions seem to be nutrition and food intake and national nutrition status surveys. Watch for an update; these come out every several years:

- *Nutrition Reviews' Present Knowledge in Nutrition*, 5th ed. Washington, D.C.: Nutrition Foundation, 1984.

A scholarly volume from the *Journal of Nutrition*, five times larger than *Present Knowledge*, is:

- *Nutritional Requirements of Man, a Conspectus of Research*. New York and Washington, D.C.: Nutrition Foundation, 1980.

The *Conspectus* has major review articles on human requirements for protein, amino acids, vitamin A, calcium, zinc, vitamin C, iron, folacin, and copper.

This 1153-page volume (about $50) is a major technical reference book on nutrition topics, containing 40 encyclopedic articles on the nutrients, foods, the diet, metabolism, malnutrition, age-related needs, and nutrition in disease, with 28 appendixes:

- Goodhart, R. S., and Shils, M. E., eds. *Modern Nutrition in Health and Disease*, 6th ed. Philadelphia: Lea and Febiger, 1980.

F

We also recommend:

■ Davidson, S., Passmore, R., Brock, J. F., and Truswell, A. S. *Human Nutrition and Dietetics*, 7th ed. New York: Churchill Livingstone, 1979.

This entertaining paperback would make an excellent discussion-topic source for a nutrition course; it includes articles by recognized authorities on the RDA, fast foods, additives, infant nutrition, fad diets, sugar, alcohol, and most of the other topics treated in this book's Highlights:

■ Hofmann, L., ed. *The Great American Nutrition Hassle*. Palo Alto, Calif.: Mayfield, 1978.

Another book that readers may wish to add to their libraries is the latest edition of *Recommended Dietary Allowances*, available from the National Academy of Sciences (see "Addresses," below).

We also recommend our own book, which explores current nutrition topics other than those treated here. The 4th edition is slated for publication in 1987:

■ Hamilton, E. M. N., Whitney, E. N., and Sizer, F. S. *Nutrition: Concepts and Controversies*, 3rd ed. St. Paul, Minn.: West, 1985.

An excellent cookbook for families wishing to prepare truly healthful meals is:

■ White, A., and the Society for Nutrition Education. *The Family Health Cookbook*. New York: David McKay Company, 1980.

Journals

Nutrition Today, the publication of the Nutrition Today Society, is an excellent magazine for the interested layperson. It makes a point of raising controversial issues and providing a forum for conflicting opinions. References are seldom printed in the magazine but are available on request. Six issues per year, from Director of Membership Services, Nutrition Today Society. (See "Addresses," below.)

The *Journal of the American Dietetic Association*, the official publication of the ADA, contains articles of interest to dietitians and nutritionists, news of legislative action on food and nutrition, and a very useful section of abstracts of articles from many other journals of nutrition and related areas. Twelve issues per year, from the American Dietetic Association. (See "Addresses," below.)

Nutrition Reviews, a publication of The Nutrition Foundation, Inc., does much of the work for the library researcher, compiling recent evidence on current topics and presenting extensive bibliographies. Twelve issues per year, from the Nutrition Foundation. (See "Addresses," below.)

Nutrition and the MD is a monthly newsletter that provides up-to-date, easy to read, and practical information on nutrition for health care providers. It is available from PM, Inc. (See "Addresses," below.)

Other journals that deserve mention here are the *Journal of Nutrition*, *Food Technology*, the *American Journal of Clinical Nutrition*, and the *Journal of Nutrition Education*. *FDA Consumer*, a government publication with many articles of interest to the consumer, is available from the Food and Drug Administration (see "Addresses," below). Many other journals of value are referred to throughout this book.

Some of this book's Highlights as well as other articles of interest to consumers, are available as individual booklets called *Nutrition Clinics*. You can write for a free publication list from The George F. Stickley Company (address below). Many of the other organizations listed below will also provide publication lists free on request.

Addresses

U.S. Government

The U.S. Department of Agriculture (USDA) has several divisions. USDA's Food Safety and Inspection Service (FSIS) inspects and analyzes domestic and imported meat, poultry, and meat and poultry food products; establishes standards and approves recipes and labels of processed meat and poultry products; and monitors the meat and poultry industries for violations of inspection laws. To obtain publications or ask questions, write or call:

■ FSIS Consumer Inquiries
USDA
Washington, DC 20250
(202) 472–4485

USDA's Agricultural Research Service (ARS) conducts research to fulfill the diverse needs of agricultural users—from farmers to consumers—in the areas of crop and animal production, protection, processing, and distribution; food safety and quality; and natural resources conservation. Write to the Information Division, ARS, USDA (same address).

USDA's Human Nutrition Information Service (HNIS) maintains USDA's Nutrient Data Bank; conducts the Nationwide Food Consumption Survey; monitors nutrient content of the U.S. food supply; provides nutrition guidelines for education and action programs; collects and disseminates food and nutrition materials; and conducts nutrition education research. Write to:

- HNIS, USDA
  Federal Center Building
  Hyattsville, MD 20782

USDA's Food and Nutrition Service (FNS) administers the food stamp program; the national school lunch and school breakfast programs; the special supplemental food program for women, infants, and children (WIC); and the food distribution, child care food, summer food service, and special milk programs. Write to:

- FNS, USDA
  500 12th Street SW
  Washington, DC 20250

USDA's Agricultural Marketing Service (AMS) operates a variety of marketing programs and services—several of interest to consumers—that include developing grades and standards for the trading of food and other farm products and carrying out grading services on request from packers and processors; inspecting egg products for wholesomeness; administering marketing orders that aid in the marketing of milk, fruits, vegetables, and related specialty crops like nuts; and administering truth-in-seed labeling and other regulatory programs. Write to:

- Information Division, AMS, USDA
  Washington, DC 20250

USDA's *Food News for Consumers*, a quarterly newsletter, is available from the Government Printing Office.

Other government addresses are:

- Food and Drug Administration (FDA)
  5600 Fishers Lane
  Rockville, MD 20852
- The Food and Nutrition Information Education Resources Center (FNIERC)
  National Agriculture Library
  10301 Baltimore Boulevard, Room 304
  Beltsville, MD 20705
  Tel: (301) 344-3719
- National Academy of Sciences/National Research Council (NAS/NRC)
  2101 Constitution Avenue NW
  Washington, DC 20418
- National Center for Health Statistics (NCHS)
  U.S. Department of Health and Human Services (USDHHS)

- Public Health Service
  3700 East–West Highway
  Hyattsville, MD 20782
- U.S. Government Printing Office
  The Superintendent of Documents
  Washington, DC 20402

Canadian Government

- Nutrition Programs
  446 Jeanne Mance Building
  Tunney's Pasture
  OTTAWA, Ontario K1A 1B4
- Nutrition Services
  Box 488
  HALIFAX, Nova Scotia
  B3J 3R8
- Nutrition Services
  P.O. Box 6000
  FREDERICTON, New Brunswick
  E3B 5H1
- Department of Community Health
  1075 Ste-Foy Road, 7th floor
  QUEBEC, Quebec
  G1S 2M1
- Public Health Resource Service
  5th floor, 15 Overlea Blvd.
  TORONTO, Ontario
  M4H 1A9
- Home Economics Directorate
  2nd floor, 880 Portage Avenue
  WINNIPEG, Manitoba
  R3G 0P1

Consumer and Advocacy Groups

- Action for Children's Television (ACT)
  46 Austin Street
  Newtonville, MA 02160
- California Council against Health Fraud, Inc.
  PO Box 1276
  Loma Linda, CA 92354
- Center for Science in the Public Interest (CSPI)
  1755 S Street NW
  Washington, DC 20009
- Children's Foundation
  1420 New York Avenue NW
  Suite 800
  Washington, DC 20005
- Community Nutrition Institute
  1146 19th Street NW
  Washington, DC 20036

F

F

- The Consumer Information Center
  Department 609K
  Pueblo, Colorado 81009
- Food Research and Action Center (FRAC)
  2011 I Street NW
  Washington, DC 20006
- National Self-Help Clearinghouse
  33 West 42nd St., Room 1227
  New York, NY 10036

Professional and Service Organizations

- Alcoholics Anonymous World Services
  P.O. Box 459
  Grand Central Station
  New York, NY 10017
- Al-Anon Family Group Headquarters
  P.O. Box 182
  Madison Square Station
  New York, NY 10010
- American Academy of Pediatrics
  PO Box 1034
  Evanston, IL 60204
- American College of Nutrition
  100 Manhattan Avenue #1606
  Union City, NJ 07087
- American Dental Association
  211 East Chicago Avenue
  Chicago, IL 60611
- American Diabetes Association
  2 Park Avenue
  New York, NY 10016
- American Dietetic Association
  430 North Michigan Avenue
  Chicago, IL 60611
- American Heart Association
  7320 Greenville Avenue
  Dallas, TX 75231
- American Home Economics Association
  2010 Massachusetts Avenue NW
  Washington, DC 20036
- American Institute for Cancer Research
  803 W. Broad St.
  Falls Church, VA 22046
- American Institute of Nutrition
  9650 Rockville Pike
  Bethesda, MD 20014
- American Medical Association
  Nutrition Information Section
  535 North Dearborn Street
  Chicago, IL 60610

- The American National Red Cross
  Food and Nutrition Consultant
  National Headquarters
  Washington, DC 20006
- American Public Health Association
  1015 Fifteenth Street NW
  Washington, DC 20005
- American Society for Clinical Nutrition
  9650 Rockville Pike
  Bethesda, MD 20014
- The Canadian Diabetes Association
  123 Edward Street, Suite 601
  Toronto, Ontario M5G 1E2 Canada
- The Canadian Dietetic Association
  385 Yonge Street
  Toronto, Ontario M4T 1Z5 Canada
- The Chicago Nutrition Association
  8158 Kedzie Avenue
  Chicago, IL 60652
- Institute of Food Technologists
  221 North La Salle Street
  Chicago, IL 60601
- George F. Stickley Company
  210 West Washington Square
  Philadelphia, PA 19106
- La Leche League International, Inc.
  9616 Minneapolis Avenue
  Franklin Park, IL 60131
- March of Dimes Birth Defects Foundation (National Headquarters)
  1275 Mamaroneck Avenue
  White Plains, NY 10605
- National Clearinghouse for Alcohol Information
  Box 2345
  Rockville, MD 20850
- National Council on Alcoholism
  733 Third Avenue
  New York, NY 10017
- National Nutrition Consortium
  1635 P Street NW, Suite 1
  Washington, DC 20036
- Nutrition Foundation, Inc.
  1126 Sixteenth St., NW, Suite 111
  Washington, DC 20036
- Nutrition Today Society
  428 E. Preston St.
  Baltimore, MD 21202
- Overeaters Anonymous (OA)
  2190 190th Street
  Torrance, CA 90504
  (213) 320-7941
- PM, Inc. (Publisher of *Nutrition and the MD*)
  14545 Friar, #106
  Van Nuys, CA 91411

- Society for Nutrition Education
  1736 Franklin Street
  Oakland, CA 94612
- Technical Information Center
  Office on Smoking and Health
  5600 Fishers Lane, Room 1–16
  Rockville, MD 20857

Trade Organizations

Trade organizations produce many excellent free materials on nutrition. Naturally, they also promote their own products. The student must learn to differentiate between slanted and valid information. We find the brief reviews in *Contemporary Nutrition* (General Mills), the *Dairy Council Digest*, Ross Laboratories' *Dietetic Currents*, and R. A. Seelig's reviews from the United Fresh Fruit and Vegetable Association to be generally reliable and very useful.

- ABC Corporation
  1330 Avenue of the Americas
  New York, NY 10019
- American Egg Board
  1460 Renaissance St.
  Park Ridge, IL 60068
- American Meat Institute
  P.O. Box 3556
  Washington, DC 20007
- Best Foods
  Consumer Service Department
  Division of CPC International
  Internation Plaza
  Englewood Cliffs, NJ 07623
- Borden Farm Products
  Borden Company, Consumer Affairs
  180 E. Broad Street
  Columbus, OH 43215
- Campbell Soup Company
  Food Service Products Division
  375 Memorial Avenue
  Camden, NJ 08101
- Del Monte Teaching Aids
  PO Box 9075
  Clinton, IA 52736
- Fleischmann's Margarines
  Standard Brands, Inc.
  625 Madison Avenue
  New York, NY 10022
- General Foods Consumer Center
  250 North Street
  White Plains, NY 10625
- General Mills
  PO Box 113
  Minneapolis, MN 55440

- Gerber Products Company
  445 State Street
  Fremont, MI 49412
- H. J. Heinz
  Consumer Relations
  PO Box 57
  Pittsburgh, PA 15230
- Hunt–Wesson Foods
  Educational Services
  1645 West Valencia Drive
  Fullerton, CA 92634
- Kellogg Company
  Department of Home Economics Services
  Battle Creek, MI 49016
- McGraw–Hill Films
  Care of Association Films, Inc.
  600 Grand Avenue
  Ridgefield, NJ 07657
- Mead Johnson Nutritionals
  2404 Pennsylvania Avenue
  Evansville, IN 47721
- National Commission on Egg Nutrition
  205 Touvy Avenue
  Park Ridge, IL 60668
- National Dairy Council
  6300 North River Road
  Rosemont, IL 60018–4233
- Nestle Company
  Home Economics Division
  100 Bloomingdale Road
  White Plains, NY 10605
- Oscar Mayer Company
  Consumer Service
  PO Box 1409
  Madison, WI 53701
- Pillsbury Company
  1177 Pillsbury Building
  608 Second Avenue South
  Minneapolis, MN 55402
- The Potato Board
  1385 South Colorado Boulevard
  Suite 512
  Denver, CO 80222
- Rice Council
  PO Box 22802
  Houston, TX 77027
- Ross Laboratories
  Director of Professional Services
  625 Cleveland Avenue
  Columbus, OH 43216
- Sister Kenny Institute
  Chicago Avenue at 27th Street
  Minneapolis, MN 55407

F

F

- Soy Protein Council
  1800 M Street NW
  Washington, DC 20036
- Sunkist Growers
  Consumer Service, Division BB
  Box 7888
  Valley Annex
  Van Nuys, CA 91409
- VNIS (Vitamin Nutrition Information Service)
  Hoffmann–LaRoche
  340 Kingsland Avenue
  Nutley, NJ 07110
- United Fresh Fruit and Vegetable Association
  727 N. Washington Street
  Alexandria, VA 22314
- Vitamin Information Bureau
  383 Madison Avenue
  New York, NY 10017
- Wheat Flour Institute
  600 Maryland Avenue
  Washington, DC 20024

Organizations Concerned with World Hunger

- Bread for the World
  802 Rhode Island Avenue NE
  Washington, DC 20018
- Institute for Food and Development Policy
  1885 Mission Street
  San Francisco, CA 94103

- Interreligious Taskforce on U.S. Food Policy
  110 Maryland Avenue NE
  Washington, DC 20002
- Meals for Millions/Freedom from Hunger Foundation
  1800 Olympic Boulevard
  PO Drawer 680
  Santa Monica, CA 90406
- Oxfam America
  115 Broadway
  Boston, MA 02116
- The Hunger Project
  2015 Steiner Street
  San Francisco, CA 94115
- Worldwatch Institute
  1776 Massachusetts Avenue NW
  Washington, DC 20036

United Nations

- Food and Agriculture Organization (FAO)
  North American Regional Office
  1325 C Street SW
  Washington, DC 20025
- World Health Organization (WHO)
  1211 Geneva 27
  Switzerland

Food Exchange Systems

For an introduction to the use of exchange systems, see Chapter 2. The U.S. Exchange System and the Canadian Food Group System are presented here. For a complete description of the U.S. Four Food Group Plan, see Chapter 2.

The U.S. Exchange System

The United States system divides the foods suitable for use in planning a healthy diet into six lists—the starch/bread, meat, vegetable, fruit, milk, and fat lists.[1] These lists are shown in Tables G-1 through G-6. Following these lists are three other sets of foods: free foods, combination foods, and foods for occasional use.

TABLE G–1

Starch/Bread List (15 g carbohydrate, 3 g protein, 80 kcal)

Amount	Food
Cereals/Grains/Pasta	
⅓ c	Bran cereals, concentrated[w]
½ c	Bran cereals, flaked[w]
½ c	Bulgur (cooked)
½ c	Cooked cereals
2½ tbsp	Cornmeal (dry)
3 tbsp	Grapenuts
½ c	Grits (cooked)
¾ c	Other ready-to-eat unsweetened cereals
½ c	Pasta (cooked)
1½ c	Puffed cereal
⅓ c	Rice, white or brown (cooked)
½ c	Shredded wheat
3 tbsp	Wheat germ[w]

[1]The exchange lists are the basis of a meal planning system designed by a committee of the American Diabetes Association and the American Dietetic Association. While designed primarily for people with diabetes and others who must follow special diets, the exchange lists are based on principles of good nutrition that apply to everyone. © 1986 American Diabetes Association, American Dietetic Association.

Amount	Food
Dried Beans/Peas/Lentils	
⅓ c	Beans and peas (cooked) (such as kidney, white, split, blackeye)[w]
⅓ c	Lentils (cooked)[w]
¼ c	Baked beans[w]
Starchy Vegetables	
½ c	Corn[w]
1 cob	Corn on cob, 6 in. long[w]
½ c	Lima beans[w]
½ c	Peas, green (canned or frozen)[w]
½ c	Plantain[w]
1 small (3 oz)	Potato, baked
½ c	Potato, mashed
¾ c	Squash, winter (acorn, butternut)
⅓ c	Yam, sweet potato, plain
Bread	
½ (1 oz)	Bagel
2 (⅔ oz)	Bread sticks, crisp, 4 in. long × ½ in.
1 c	Croutons, low fat
½ muffin	English muffin
½ (1 oz)	Frankfurter or hamburger bun
½ loaf	Pita, 6 in. across
1 (1 oz)	Plain roll, small
1 slice (1 oz)	Raisin, unfrosted
1 slice (1 oz)	Rye, pumpernickel[w]
1 tortilla	Tortilla, 6 in. across
1 slice (1 oz)	White (including French, Italian)
1 slice (1 oz)	Whole wheat
Crackers/Snacks	
8 crackers	Animal crackers
3 crackers	Graham crackers, 2½ in. square
¾ oz	Matzoth
5 slices	Melba toast
24 crackers	Oyster crackers
3 c	Popcorn (popped, no fat added)
¾ oz	Pretzels
4 crackers	Rye crisp, 2 in. × 3½ in.
6 crackers	Saltine-type crackers
2-4 slices (¾ oz)	Whole wheat crackers, no fat added (crisp breads)

TABLE G–1

(continued)

Amount	Food
Starch Foods Prepared With Fat	
(Count as 1 starch/bread serving, plus 1 fat serving.)	
1 biscuit	Biscuit, 2½ in. across
½ c	Chow mein noodles
1 (2 oz)	Corn bread, 2 in. cube
6 crackers	Cracker, round butter type
10 (1½ oz)	French fried potatoes, 2 in. to 3½ in. long
1 muffin	Muffin, plain, small
2 pancakes	Pancake, 4 in. across
¼ c	Stuffing, bread (prepared)
2 tacos	Taco shell, 6 in. across
1 waffle	Waffle, 4½ in. square
4-6 crackers (1 oz)	Whole wheat crackers, fat added

w3 grams or more of dietary fiber per serving. Average fiber contents of whole grain products is 2 grams per serving. For starch foods not on this list, the general rule is that ½ cup of cereal grain, or pasta is one serving; 1 ounce of a bread product is one serving.

TABLE G–2.

Meat/Meat Alternate Lists (Lean meat = 7 g protein, 3 g fat, 55 kcal. Medium-fat meat = 7 g protein, 5 g fat, 75 kcal. High-fat meat = 7 g protein, 8 g fat, 100 kcal.)

Lean Meat and Alternates

Beef:	1 oz	USDA Good or Choice grades of lean beef, such as round, sirloin, and flank steak; tenderloin; and chipped beef[s].
Pork:	1 oz	Lean pork, such as fresh ham; canned, cured or boiled ham[s]; Canadian bacon[s], tenderloin.
Veal:	1 oz	All cuts are lean except for veal cutlets (ground or cubed). Examples of lean veal are chops and roasts.
Poultry:	1 oz	Chicken, turkey, Cornish hen (without skin)
Fish:	1 oz	All fresh and frozen fish
	2 oz	Crab, lobster, scallops, shrimp, clams (fresh or canned in water[s])
	6 medium	Oysters
	¼ c	Tuna[s] (canned in water)
	1 oz	Herring (uncreamed or smoked)
	2 medium	Sardines (canned)
Wild Game:	1 oz	Venison, rabbit, squirrel
	1 oz	Pheasant, duck, goose (without skin)
Cheese:	¼ c	Any cottage cheese
	2 tbsp	Grated parmesan
	1 oz	Diet cheeses[s] (with less than 55 calories per ounce)
Other:	1 oz	95% fat-free luncheon meat
	3 whites	Egg whites
	¼ c	Egg substitutes with less than 55 calories per ¼ cup

Medium-Fat Meat and Alternates

Beef:	1 oz	Most beef products fall into this category. Examples are: all ground beef, roast (rib, chuck, rump), steak (cubed, Porterhouse, T-bone), and meatloaf.
Pork:	1 oz	Most pork products fall into this category. Examples are: chops, loin roast, Boston butt, cutlets
Lamb:	1 oz	Most lamb products fall into this category. Examples are: chops, leg, and roast.
Veal:	1 oz	Cutlet (ground or cubed, unbreaded)
Poultry:	1 oz	Chicken (with skin), domestic duck or goose (well-drained of fat), ground turkey
Fish:	¼ c	Tuna[s] (canned in oil and drained)
	¼ c	Salmon[s] (canned)
Cheese:		Skim or part-skim milk cheeses, such as:
	¼ c	Ricotta
	1 oz	Mozzarella
	1 oz	Diet cheeses[s] (with 56-80 calories per ounce)
Other:	1 oz	86% fat-free luncheon meat[s]
	1	Egg (high in cholesterol, limit to 3 per week)
	¼ c	Egg substitutes with 56-80 calories per ¼ cup
	4 oz	Tofu (2½ in. × 2¾ in. × 1 in.)
	1 oz	Liver, heart, kidney, sweetbreads (high in cholesterol)

High-Fat Meat and Alternates

Beef:	1 oz	Most USDA Prime cuts of beef, such as ribs, corned beef[s]
Pork:	1 oz	Spareribs, ground pork, pork sausage[s] (patty or link)
Lamb:	1 oz	Patties (ground lamb)
Fish:	1 oz	Any fried fish product
Cheese:	1 oz	All regular cheeses[s], such as American, Blue, Cheddar, Monterey, Swiss
Other:	1 oz	Luncheon meat[s], such as bologna, salami, pimento loaf
	1 oz	Sausage[s], such as Polish, Italian
	1 oz	Knockwurst, smoked
	1 oz	Bratwurst[s]
	1 frank (10/lb)	Frankfurter[s] (turkey or chicken)
	1 tbsp	Peanut butter (contains unsaturated fat)

Count as one high-fat meat plus one fat exchange:

1 frank	(10/lb)	Frankfurter[s] (beef, pork, or combination)

s400 mg or more of sodium per exchange. Meats contribute no fiber to the diet.

TABLE G–3.

Vegetable List (5 g carbohydrate, 2 g protein, 25 kcal)
All portion sizes, except as otherwise noted, are: ½ c of any cooked
vegetable or vegetable juice, 1 c of any raw vegetable.

Artichoke (½ medium)	Mushrooms, cooked
Asparagus	Okra
Beans (green, wax, Italian)	Onions
Bean sprouts	Pea pods
Beets	Peppers (green)
Broccoli	Rutabaga
Brussels sprouts	Sauerkraut^s
Cabbage, cooked	Spinach, cooked
Carrots	Summer squash (crookneck)
Cauliflower	Tomato (one large)
Eggplant	Tomato/vegetable juice^s
Greens (collard, mustard, turnip)	Turnips
Kohlrabi	Water chestnuts
Leeks	Zucchini, cooked

Starchy vegetables such as corn, peas, and potatoes are found on the
    Starch/Bread List.
For free vegetables, see Free Food List.

^{s}400 mg or more of sodium per serving. Most vegetable servings
contain 2 to 3 g of dietary fiber.

TABLE G–4.

Fruit List (15 g carbohydrate, 60 kcal)
All portion sizes, unless otherwise noted, are: ½ c of fresh fruit or
fruit juice, ¼ c of dried fruit.

Amount	Food
Fresh, Frozen and Unsweetened Canned Fruit	
1 apple	Apple (raw, 2 in. across)
½ c	Applesauce (unsweetened)
4 apricots	Apricots (medium, raw) or
½ c, or 4 halves	Apricots (canned)
½ banana	Banana (9 in. long)
¾ c	Blackberries (raw)^w
¾ c	Blueberries (raw)^w
⅓ melon	Cantaloupe (5 in. across)
1 c	(cubes)
12 cherries	Cherries (large, raw)
½ c	Cherries (canned)
2 figs	Figs (raw, 2 in. across)
½ c	Fruit cocktail (canned)
½ grapefruit	Grapefruit (medium)
¾ c	Grapefruit (segments)
15 grapes	Grapes (small)
⅛ melon	Honeydew melon (medium)
1 cup	(cubes)
1 kiwi	Kiwi (large)
¾ c	Mandarin oranges
½ mango	Mango (small)

1 nectarine	Nectarine (1½ in. across)^w
1 orange	Orange (2½ in. across)
1 c	Papaya
1 peach, or ¾ c	Peach (2¾ in. across)
½ c, or 2 halves	Peaches (canned)
½ large, or 1 small	Pear
½ c or 2 halves	Pears (canned)
2 persimmons	Persimmon (medium, native)
¾ c	Pineapple (raw)
⅓ c	Pineapple (canned)
2 plums	Plum (raw, 2 in. across)
½ pomegranate	Pomegranate^w
1 c	Raspberries (raw)^w
1¼ c	Strawberries (raw, whole)^w
2 tangerines	Tangerine (2½ in. across)
1¼ c	Watermelon (cubes)

Dried Fruit

4 rings	Apples^w
7 halves	Apricots^w
2½ medium	Dates
1½ figs	Figs^w
3 medium	Prunes^w
2 tbsp	Raisins

Fruit Juice

½ c	Apple juice/cider
⅓ c	Cranberry juice cocktail
½ c	Grapefruit juice
⅓ c	Grape juice
½ c	Orange juice
½ c	Pineapple juice
⅓ c	Prune juice

^{w}3 or more grams of dietary fiber per serving. Average fiber contents
of fresh, frozen, and dry fruits: 2 g per serving.

G

TABLE G–5.

Milk List Nonfat and very lowfat milk = 12 g carbohydrate, 8 g protein, trace fat, 90 kcal. Lowfat milk = 12 g carbohydrate, 8 g protein, 5 g fat, 120 kcal. Whole milk = 12 g carbohydrate, 8 g protein, 8 g fat, 150 kcal.

Amount	Food
Nonfat and Very Lowfat Milk	
1 c	Nonfat milk
1 c	½% milk
1 c	1% milk
1 c	Lowfat buttermilk
½ c	Evaporated nonfat milk
⅓ c	Dry nonfat milk
8 oz	Plain nonfat yogurt
Lowfat Milk	
1 c fluid	2% milk
8 oz	Plain lowfat yogurt (with added nonfat milk solids)
Whole Milk	
1 c	Whole milk
½ c	Evaporated whole milk
8 oz	Whole plain yogurt

TABLE G–6.

Fat List (5 g fat, 45 kcal)

Amount	Food
Unsaturated Fats	
⅛ medium	Avocado
1 tsp	Margarine
1 tbsp	Margarine, diet*
1 tsp	Mayonnaise
1 tbsp	Mayonnaise, reduced-kcalorie*
	Nuts and Seeds:
6 whole	Almonds, dry roasted
1 tbsp	Cashews, dry roasted
2 whole	Pecans
20 small or 10 large	Peanuts
2 whole	Walnuts
1 tbsp	Other nuts
1 tbsp	Seeds, pine nuts, sunflower (without shells)
2 tsp	Pumpkin seeds
1 tsp	Oil (corn, cottonseed, safflower, soybean, sunflower, olive, peanut)
10 small or 5 large	Olives*
2 tsp	Salad dressing, mayonnaise-type
1 tbsp	Salad dressing, mayonnaise-type, reduced-calorie
1 tbsp	Salad dressing (all varieties)*
2 tbsp	Salad dressing, reduced-kcalorie$

Amount	Food
Saturated Fats	
1 tsp	Butter
1 slice	Bacon*
½ oz	Chitterlings
2 tbsp	Coconut, shredded
2 tbsp	Coffee whitener, liquid
4 tsp	Coffee whitener, powder
2 tbsp	Cream (light, coffee, table)
2 tbsp	Cream, sour
1 tbsp	Cream (heavy, whipping)
1 tbsp	Cream cheese
¼ oz	Salt pork*

(Two tablespoons of low-kcalorie salad dressing is a free food.)
*If more than one or two servings are eaten, these foods have 400 mg or more of sodium.
$400 mg or more of sodium per serving.

Free Foods

A free food is any food or drink that contains less than 20 kcalories per serving. People with diabetes are advised to eat as much as they want of those items that have no serving size specified. They may eat two or three servings per day of those items that have a specific serving size. It is suggested that they spread them out through the day.

Drinks:
	Bouillon$ or broth without fat
	Bouillon, low-sodium
	Carbonated drinks, sugar-free
	Carbonated water
	Club soda
1 tbsp	Cocoa powder, unsweetened
	Coffee/Tea
	Drink mixes, sugar-free
	Tonic water, sugar-free

Nonstick pan spray
Fruit:
½ c	Cranberries, unsweetened
½ c	Rhubarb, unsweetened

Vegetables:
(raw, 1 c)
	Cabbage
	Celery
	Chinese cabbage^w
	Cucumber
	Green onion
	Hot peppers
	Mushrooms
	Radishes
	Zucchini^w

Salad greens:
	Endive
	Escarole
	Lettuce

Romaine
Spinach

Sweet Substitutes:

Candy, hard, sugar-free
Gelatin, sugar-free
Gum, sugar free
2 tsp   Jam/Jelly, sugar-free
1-2 tbsp   Pancake syrup, sugar-free
Sugar substitutes (saccharin, aspartame)
2 tbsp   Whipped topping

Condiments:

1 tbsp   Catsup
Horseradish
Mustard
Pickles⁵, dill, unsweetened
2 tbsp   Salad dressing, low-kcalorie
1 tbsp   Taco sauce
Vinegar

Seasonings:

Basil (fresh)
Celery seeds
Cinnamon
Chili powder
Chives
Curry
Dill
Flavoring extracts (vanilla, almond, walnut, pepper-mint, butter, lemon, etc.)
Garlic
Garlic powder
Herbs
Hot pepper sauce
Lemon
Lemon juice
Lemon pepper
Lime
Lime juice
Mint
Onion powder
Oregano
Paprika
Pepper
Pimento
Spices
Soy sauce⁵
Soy sauce, low sodium ("lite")
¼ c   Wine, used in cooking
Worcestershire sauce

ᵂ3 grams or more of fiber per serving
⁵400 mg or more of sodium per serving

Combination Foods

Much of the food we eat is mixed together in various combinations. These combination foods do not fit into only one exchange list. It can be quite hard to tell what is in a certain casserole dish or baked food item. This is a list of average values for some typical combination foods. This list will help you fit these foods into your meal plan. Ask your dietitian for information about any other foods you'd like to eat. The *American Diabetes Association/American Dietetic Association Family Cookbooks* and the *American Diabetes Association Holiday Cookbook* have many recipes and further information about many foods, including combination foods. Check your library or local bookstore.

Food	Amount	Exchanges
Casseroles	1 c (8 oz)	2 starch, 2 medium-fat meat, 1 fat
Cheese pizza⁵, thin crust	¼ of 15 oz, or ¼ of 10″	2 starch, 1 medium-fat meat, 1 fat
Chili with beansᵂˢ (commercial)	1 c (8 oz)	2 starch, 2 medium-fat meat, 2 fat
Chow meinᵂˢ (without noodles or rice)	2 c (16 oz)	1 starch, 2 vegetable, 2 lean meat
Macaroni and cheese⁵	1 c (8 oz)	2 starch, 1 medium-fat meat, 2 fat
Soup:		
Beanᵂˢ	1 c (8 oz)	1 starch, 1 vegetable, 1 lean meat
Chunky, all varieties⁵	10¾ oz can	1 starch, 1 vegetable, 1 medium-fat meat
Cream⁵ (made with water)	1 c (8 oz)	1 starch, 1 fat
Vegetable⁵ or broth⁵	1 c (8 oz)	1 starch
Spaghetti and meatballs⁵ (canned)	1 c (8 oz)	2 starch, 1 medium-fat meat, 1 fat
Sugar-free pudding (made with nonfat milk)	½ c	1 starch
If beans are used as a meat substitute:		
Dried beansᵂ, peasᵂ, lentilsᵂ	1 c (cooked)	2 starch, 1 lean meat

ᵂ3 grams or more of fiber per serving
⁵400 mg or more of sodium per serving

G

Foods for Occasional Use

Food	Amount	Exchanges
Angel food cake	1/12 cake	2 starch
Cake, no icing	1/12 cake, or a 3″ square	2 starch, 2 fat
Cookies	2 small (1¾″ across)	1 starch, 1 fat
Frozen fruit yogurt	⅓ c	1 starch
Gingersnaps	3 cookies	1 starch
Granola	¼ c	1 starch, 1 fat
Granola bars	1 small	1 starch, 1 fat
Ice cream, any flavor	½ c	1 starch, 2 fat
Ice milk, any flavor	½ c	1 starch, 1 fat
Sherbet, any flavor	¼ c	1 starch
Snack chips[s], all varieties	1 oz	1 starch, 2 fat
Vanilla wafers	6 small	1 starch, 1 fat

[s]If more than one serving is eaten, these foods have 400 mg. or more of sodium.

G

The Canadian Food Group System

The Canadian food group system is similar to the U.S. exchange system, but the serving sizes and some of the foods listed are different. This food group system, as explained in the handbook *Good Health Eating Guide*, is a revision of the Canadian exchange system of meal planning.[1] Features of the new system similar to those of the exchange system include the following:

- Foods are divided into six groups according to carbohydrate, protein, and fat content.
- Foods are interchangeable within a group.
- Most foods are eaten in measured amounts.

New features of the food group system include the following:

- An energy value is given for each food group.
- Protein foods low in fat are emphasized in the protein foods group. Protein foods containing extra fat are identified.
- The user is able to distinguish between complex and simple carbohydrates (starches and sugars).

[1]The tables for the Canadian Food Group System are taken from *Good Health Eating Guide* (Toronto, Ontario: Canadian Diabetes Association, 1981), and are used with the association's permission.

TABLE G–7

Protein Foods Group (7 g protein, 3 g fat, 55 kcal)

Food	Measure	Mass (Weight)
Cheese		
All types, made from partly skim milk, e.g. mozzarella, part-skim	1 piece, 5 cm × 2 cm × 2 cm (2″ × ¾″ × ¾″)	25 g
Cottage cheese, all types	50 mL (¼ cup)	55 g
Fish		
Anchovy (see extras)		
Canned, drained, e.g. chicken haddie, mackerel, salmon, tuna	50 mL (¼ cup)	30 g
Cod tongues/cheeks	75 mL (⅓ cup)	50 g
Fillet or Steak, e.g. Boston blue, cod, flounder, haddock, halibut, perch, pickerel, pike, salmon, shad, sole, trout, whitefish	1 piece, 6 cm × 2 cm × 2 cm (2½″ × ¾″ × ¾″)	30 g
Herring	⅓ fish	30 g
Octopus	50 mL (¼ cup)	40 g
Sardines	2 medium or 3 small	30 g
Seal, walrus	1 slice, 6 cm × 4 cm × 1 cm (2½″ × 1½″ × ½″)	25 g
Smelts	2 medium	30 g
Squid	50 mL (¼ cup)	40 g
Shellfish		
Clams, mussels, oysters, scallops, snails	3 medium	30 g
Crab, lobster, flaked	50 mL (¼ cup)	30 g
Shrimp, fresh	5 large	30 g
frozen	10 medium	30 g
canned	18 small	30 g
dry pack	50 mL (¼ cup)	30 g
Meat and poultry, e.g. beef, chicken, ham, lamb, pork, turkey, veal, wild game		
Back bacon	3 slices, thin	25 g
Chop	½ chop, with bone	35 g
Minced or ground, lean	30 mL (2 tbsps.)	25 g
Sliced, lean	1 slice, 10 cm × 5 cm × 5 mm (4″ × 2″ × ¼″)	25 g
Steak, lean	1 piece, 4 cm × 3 cm × 2 cm (1½″ × 1¼″ × ¾″)	25 g
Organ Meats		
Heart, liver	1 slice, 5 cm × 5 cm × 1 cm (2″ × 2″ × ½″)	25 g
Kidney, sweet breads, chopped	50 mL (¼ cup)	25 g
Tongue	1 slice, 8 cm × 6 cm × 5 mm (3¼″ × 2½″ × ¼″)	25 g
Tripe, 1 piece = 4 cm × 4 cm × 8 mm (1½″ × 1½″ × ⅜″)	5 pieces	50 g
Soyabean		
Bean curd or tofu, 1 block = 6 cm × 6 cm × 4 cm (2½″ × 2½″ × 1½″)	½ block	70 g

TABLE G–7

(continued)

Food	Measure	Mass (Weight)
The following choices contain extra fat, so use them less often.		
Cheese		
Cheese, all types made from whole milk, e.g. brick, brie, camembert, cheddar, edam, tilsit	1 piece 5 cm × 2 cm × 2 cm (2″ × ¾″ × ¾″)	25 g
Cheese, coarsely grated, e.g. cheddar	75 mL (⅓ cup)	25 g
Cheese, dry, finely grated, e.g. parmesan	45 mL (3 tbsps.)	15 g
Cheese, ricotta	50 mL (¼ cup)	55 g
Egg		
Egg, in shell, raw or cooked	1 medium	50 g
Egg, without shell, cooked or poached in water	1 medium	45 g
Egg, scrambled	50 mL (¼ cup)	55 g
Fish		
Eel	5 cm, 4 cm diameter (2″, 1½″ diameter)	50 g
Meat		
Bologna	1 slice, 5 mm, 10 cm diameter (¼″, 4″ diameter)	40 g
Canned luncheon meat	1 slice, 85 mm × 45 mm × 10 mm (3½″ × 1¾″ × ½″)	40 g
Corned beef, fresh	1 slice, 10 cm × 5 cm × 5 mm (4″ × 2″ × ¼″)	25 g
Corned beef, canned	1 slice, 75 mm × 55 mm × 5 mm (3″ × 2¼″ × ¼″)	25 g
Ground beef, medium fat	30 mL (2 tbsps.)	25 g
Meat spreads, canned	45 mL (3 tbsps.)	35 g
Pate (see fats and oils group)		
Sausage, pork, link	1 link	25 g
Sausage, garlic, Polish or knockwurst	1 slice, 1 cm, 5 cm diameter (½″, 2″ diameter)	50 g
Summer sausage or salami	1 slice, 5 mm, 10 cm diameter (¼″, 4″ diameter)	40 g
Spareribs or shortribs, with bone	10 cm × 6 cm (4″ × 2½″)	65 g
Stewing beef	1 cube, 25 mm (1″)	25 g
Wiener	½ medium	25 g
Miscellaneous		
Blood pudding	1 slice, 5 cm × 1 cm (2″ × ½″)	25 g
Peanut butter, all kinds	15 mL (1 tbsp.)	15 g

G

TABLE G–8

Starchy Foods Group 15 g carbohydrate (starch), 2 g protein, 68 kcal

Food	Measure	Mass (Weight)
Breads		
Bagel	½	25 g
Bread crumbs	50 mL (¼ cup)	25 g
Bread cubes	250 mL (1 cup)	25 g
Bread sticks, 11 cm × 1 cm (4½″ × ½″)	2	20 g
Brewis, cooked	50 mL (¼ cup)	45 g
English muffin, crumpet	½	25 g
Flour	40 mL (2½ tbsps.)	20 g
Hamburger bun	½	30 g
Hot dog bun	½	30 g
Kaiser roll	½	25 g
Matzoh, 15 cm (6″ square)	1	20 g
Melba toast, rectangular	4	15 g
Pita, 20 cm diameter (8″ diameter)	¼	25 g
Plain roll	1 small	25 g
Raisin bread	1 slice	25 g
Rusks	2	20 g
Rye, coarse or pumpernickel, 10 cm × 10 cm × 8 mm (4″ × 4″ × ⅜″)	½ slice	25 g
Tortilla, 15 cm (6″)	1	20 g
White (French and Italian)	1 slice	25 g
Whole wheat, cracked wheat, rye, white enriched	1 slice	25 g
Cereals		
Bran flakes, 40% bran	125 mL (½ cup)	20 g
Cooked cereals, cooked	125 mL (½ cup)	125 g
dry	30 mL (2 tbsps.)	20 g
Cornmeal, cooked	125 mL (½ cup)	125 g
dry	30 mL (2 tbsps.)	20 g
Ready-to-eat unsweetened cereal	250 mL (1 cup)	20 g
Shredded wheat biscuit, rectangular or round	1	20 g
Shredded wheat bite size	125 mL (½ cup)	20 g
Wheat germ	75 mL (⅓ cup)	30 g
Cookies and biscuits		
See "Prepared Foods" [below].		
Grains		
Barley, cooked	125 mL (½ cup)	120 g
dry	30 mL (2 tbsps.)	20 g
Bulgar, kasha, cooked, moist	125 mL (½ cup)	70 g
cooked, crumbly	75 mL (⅓ cup)	40 g
dry	30 mL (2 tbsps.)	20 g
Rice, cooked, loosely packed	125 mL (½ cup)	105 g
cooked, tightly packed	75 mL (⅓ cup)	70 g
Tapioca, pearl and granulated, quick cooking, dry	30 mL (2 tbsps.)	15 g
Pastas		
Macaroni, cooked	125 mL (½ cup)	70 g
Noodles, cooked	125 mL (½ cup)	80 g
Spaghetti, cooked	125 mL (½ cup)	70 g

G

TABLE G–8

(continued)

Food	Measure	Mass (Weight)
Starchy Vegetables		
Beans and peas (dried), cooked	125 mL (½ cup)	80 g
Breadfruit	1 slice	75 g
Corn, canned, whole kernel	125 mL (½ cup)	85 g
canned, creamed	75 mL (¼ cup)	60 g
Corn, on the cob, 13 cm, 4 cm diameter (5″, 1½″ diameter)	1 small cob	140 g
Cornstarch	30 mL (2 tbsps.)	15 g
Plantain	⅓ small	50 g
Popcorn, unbuttered, large kernel	750 mL (3 cups)	20 g
Potatoes, whipped	125 mL (½ cup)	105 g
Potatoes, whole, 13 cm, 5 cm diameter (5″, 2″ diameter)	½	95 g
Yam, sweet potatoes 13 cm, 5 cm diameter (5″, 2″ diameter)	½	75 g

Starchy Foods Group (add 1 fats and oils choice)

Food	Measure	Mass (Weight)
Prepared foods		
Baking powder biscuit, 5 cm diameter (2″ diameter)	1	30 g
Cookies, plain, (e.g., digestive, oatmeal)	2	20 g
Cup cake, un-iced, 5 cm diameter (2″ diameter)	1 small	35 g
Donut, cake type, plain, 7 cm diameter (2¾″ diameter)	1	30 g
Muffin, plain, 6 cm diameter (2½″ diameter)	1 small	40 g
Pancake, homemade using 50 mL (¼ cup) batter	1 small	50 g
Potatoes, french fried, 5 cm × 9 cm (2″ × 3½″)	10	65 g
Soup, canned (prepared with equal volume of water)	250 mL (1 cup)	260 g
Waffle, homemade, using 50 mL (¼ cup) batter	1 small	35 g

TABLE G–9

Milk Group

Type of Milk	Carbohydrate	Protein	Fat	Energy
Nonfat	6 g	4 g	0 g	40 kcalories
2%	6 g	4 g	2 g	58 kcalories
Whole	6 g	4 g	4 g	76 kcalories

Food	Measure	Mass (Weight)
Milk	125 mL (½ cup)	125 g
Buttermilk	125 mL (½ cup)	125 g
Evaporated milk	50 mL (¼ cup)	50 g
Powdered milk, regular	30 mL (2 tbsps.)	15 g
instant	50 mL (¼ cup)	15 g
Unflavoured yogurt	125 mL (½ cup)	125 g

TABLE G-10

Fruits and Vegetables Group 10 g carbohydrate (simple sugar), 1 g protein, 44 kcal

Food	Measure	Mass (Weight)
Fruits (fresh, frozen without sugar, canned in water)		
Apple, raw	½ medium	75 g
raw, without skin and core	½ medium	65 g
sauce	125 mL (½ cup)	120 g
Apricot, raw	2 medium	115 g
canned, in water	4 halves, plus 30 mL (2 tbsps.) liquid	110 g
Bake-apple (cloudberries), raw	125 mL (½ cup)	120 g
Banana, 15 cm (6″), with peel	½ small	75 g
peeled	½ small	50 g
Blackberries, raw	125 mL (½ cup)	70 g
canned, in water	125 mL (½ cup), includes 30 mL (2 tbsps.) liquid	100 g
Blueberries, raw	125 mL (½ cup)	120 g
Boysenberries, raw	125 mL (½ cup)	70 g
canned, in water	125 mL (½ cup), includes 30 mL (2 tbsps.) liquid	100 g
Cantaloupe, wedge with rind, 13 cm diameter (5″ diameter)	¼	240 g
cubed or diced	250 mL (1 cup)	160 g
Cherries, raw, with pits	10	75 g
raw, without pits	10	70 g
canned, in water, with pits	75 mL (⅓ cup) includes 30 mL (2 tbsps.) liquid	90 g
canned, in water, without pits	75 mL (⅓ cup), includes 30 mL (2 tbsps.) liquid	85 g
Crabapple, raw	1 small	55 g
Cranberries, raw	250 mL (1 cup)	100 g
Figs, raw	1 medium	50 g
canned, in water	3 medium, plus 30 mL (2 tbsps.) liquid	100 g
Foxberries, raw	250 mL (1 cup)	100 g
Fruit cocktail, canned, in water	125 mL (½ cup), includes 30 mL (2 tbsps.) liquid	120 g
Fruit, mixed, cut-up	125 mL (½ cup)	120 g
Gooseberries, raw	250 mL (1 cup)	150 g
canned, in water	250 mL (1 cup), includes 30 mL (2 tbsps.) liquid	230 g
Grapefruit, raw, with rind	½ small	185 g
raw, sectioned	125 mL (½ cup)	100 g
canned, in water	125 mL (½ cup), includes 30 mL (2 tbsps.) liquid	120 g
Grapes, raw, slip skin	125 mL (½ cup)	75 g
raw, seedless	125 mL (½ cup)	75 g
canned, in water	75 mL (⅓ cup), includes 30 mL (2 tbsps.) liquid	115 g
Honeydew melon, raw, with rind	1/10	225 g
cubed or diced	250 mL (1 cup)	170 g
Guava, raw	½	50 g
Kiwi, raw, with skin	2	155 g
Kumquats, raw	3	60 g
Huckleberries, raw	125 mL (½ cup)	70 g
Loganberries, raw	125 mL (½ cup)	70 g
Loquats, raw	8	130 g
Lychee fruit, raw	8	120 g
Mandarin oranges, raw, with rind	1	135 g
raw, sectioned	125 mL (½ cup)	100 g
canned, in water	125 mL (½ cup), includes 30 mL (2 tbsps.) liquid	100 g
Mango, raw, without skin and seed	⅓	65 g
diced	75 mL (⅓ cup)	65 g
Nectarine	½ medium	75 g
Orange, raw, with rind	1 small	90 g
raw, sectioned	125 mL (½ cup)	90 g

G

TABLE G-10

(continued)

Food	Measure	Mass (Weight)
Papaya, raw, with skin and seeds	¼ medium	150 g
raw, without skin and seeds	¼ medium	100 g
cubed or diced	125 mL (½ cup)	100 g
Peaches, raw with seed and skin, 6 cm (2½″) diameter	1 large	130 g
raw, sliced, diced	125 mL (½ cup)	100 g
canned, in water, halves or slices	125 mL (½ cup), includes 30 mL (2 tbsps.) liquid	120 g
Pear, raw with skin and core	½	90 g
raw, without skin and core	½	85 g
canned, in water, halves	2 halves, plus 30 mL (2 tbsps.) liquid	90 g
Persimmons, raw, native	1	30 g
raw, Japanese	¼	50 g
Pineapple, raw	1 slice, 8 cm diameter, 2 cm thick (3⅓″ diameter, ¾″ thick)	75 g
raw, diced	125 mL (½ cup)	75 g
canned, in water, sliced	2 slices, plus 15 mL (1 tbsp.) liquid	100 g
canned, in water, diced	125 mL (½ cup), includes 30 mL (2 tbsps.) liquid	100 g
canned, in juice, sliced	1 slice, plus 15 mL (1 tbsp.) liquid	55 g
canned, in juice, diced	75 mL (⅓ cup), includes 15 mL (1 tbsp.) liquid	55 g
Plums, raw, prune type	2	60 g
damson	6	65 g
Japanese	1	70 g
canned, in water	3, plus 30 mL (2 tbsps.) liquid	100 g
canned, in apple juice	2, plus 30 mL (2 tbsps.) liquid	70 g
Pomegranate, raw	½	140 g
Raspberries, raw, black or red	125 mL (½ cup)	65 g
canned, in water	125 mL (½ cup), includes 30 mL (2 tbsps.) liquid	100 g
Saskatoons (see blueberries)		
Strawberries, raw	250 mL (1 cup)	150 g
canned, in water	250 mL (1 cup), includes 30 mL (2 tbsps.) liquid	240 g
Tangelo, raw	1	205 g
Tangerine, raw	1	115 g
raw, sectioned	125 mL (½ cup)	100 g
Watermelon, raw with rind	1 wedge, 125 mm triangle, 22 mm thick (5″ triangle, 1″ thick)	310 g
cubed or diced	250 mL (1 cup)	160 g
Dried Fruit		
Apple	5 pieces	15 g
Apricot	4 halves	15 g
Banana flakes	30 mL (2 tbsps.)	15 g
Currants	30 mL (2 tbsps.)	15 g
Dates, without pits	2	15 g
Peach	1 half	15 g
Pear	1 half	15 g
Prunes, raw, with pits	2	15 g
raw, without pits	2	10 g
stewed, no liquid	2	20 g
stewed, with liquid	2, plus 15 mL (1 tbsp.) liquid	35 g
Raisins	30 mL (2 tbsps.)	15 g

G

TABLE G–10

(continued)

Food	Measure	Mass (Weight)
Juices (no sugar added or unsweetened)		
Apricot, grape, guava, mango, prune	50 mL (¼ cup)	55 g
Apple, carrot, papaya, pear, pineapple, pomegranate	75 mL (⅓ cup)	80 g
Grapefruit, loganberry, orange, raspberry, tangelo, tangerine	125 mL (½ cup)	130 g
Tomato, tomato based mixed vegetables	250 mL (1 cup)	255 g
Vegetables (fresh, frozen, or canned)		
Artichokes, Jerusalem, mature or late season[a]	2 small	50 g
Beets, diced or sliced	125 mL (½ cup)	85 g
Carrots, diced	125 mL (½ cup)	75 g
Parsnips, mashed	125 mL (½ cup)	80 g
Peas, fresh or frozen	125 mL (½ cup)	80 g
canned	75 mL (⅓ cup)	55 g
Pumpkin, mashed	125 mL (½ cup)	45 g
Rutabagas, mashed	125 mL (½ cup)	85 g
Sauerkraut	250 mL (1 cup)	235 g
Snowpeas	10 pods	100 g
Squash, yellow or winter, mashed	125 mL (½ cup)	115 g
Succotash	75 mL (⅓ cup)	55 g
Tomatoes, canned	250 mL (1 cup)	240 g
Turnip, mashed	125 mL (½ cup)	115 g
Vegetables, mixed	125 mL (½ cup)	90 g
Water chestnuts	8 medium	50 g

[a]Jerusalem artichokes contain inulin which converts to carbohydrate during storage, in or out of ground. Jerusalem artichokes in early season (autumn) are low in carbohydrate but in late season (winter/spring) they become a Fruits and Vegetables Choice.

TABLE G–11

Extra Vegetables Group (½ cup, 3.5 g carbohydrate, 14 kcal)

Artichokes, globe or french
Artichokes, Jerusalem, early season[a]
Asparagus
Bamboo shoots
Beans, string, green or yellow
Bean sprouts, mung or soya
Bitter melon (balsam pear)
Bok Choy
Broccoli
Brussels sprouts
Cabbage
Cauliflower
Celery
Chard
Cucumber
Eggplant
Endive
Fiddleheads
Greens: beet, collard, dandelion, mustard, turnip, etc.
Kale
Kohlrabi
Leeks
Lettuce
Mushrooms
Okra
Onions, green or mature
Parsley
Pepper, green or red
Radish
Rhubarb
Shallots
Spinach
Sprouts: alfalfa, radish, etc.
Tomato, raw
Vegetable marrow
Watercress
Zucchini

If eaten in large amounts, the following foods must be counted as 1 fruits and vegetables choice.

Brussels sprouts, cooked, 250 mL (1 cup)	155 g
Eggplant, cooked, diced, 250 mL (1 cup)	200 g
Kohlrabi, cooked, diced, 250 mL (1 cup)	140 g
Leeks, cooked, edible parts of 4 leeks	100 g
Okra, cooked, sliced, 250 mL (1 cup)	160 g
Onion, mature, cooked, 250 mL (1 cup)	210 g
Rhubarb, cooked, no sugar added, 250 mL (1 cup)	244 g
Tomato, raw, 2 medium (6 cm or 2½″ diameter) or 1 large (13 cm or 5″ diameter)	270 g

[a]Jerusalem artichokes contain inulin which converts to carbohydrate during storage, in or out of ground. Jerusalem artichokes in early season (autumn) are low in carbohydrate but in late season (winter/spring) they become a Fruits and Vegetables Choice.

TABLE G-12

Fats and Oils Group (5 g fat, 45 kcal)

Food	Measure	Mass (Weight)
Avocado pear	⅛	30 g
Bacon, side, crisp	1 slice	5 g
Butter	5 mL (1 tsp.)	5 g
Cheese spread	15 mL (1 tbsp.)	15 g
Coconut, fresh	45 mL (3 tbsps.)	15 g
dried	15 mL (1 tbsp.)	10 g
Cream, half and half (cereal) 10%	30 mL (2 tbsps.)	30 g
light (coffee) 20%	15 mL (1 tbsp.)	15 g
whipping 32-37%	15 mL (1 tbsp.)	15 g
sour 12-14%	45 mL (3 tbsps.)	35 g
Cream cheese	15 mL (1 tbsp.)	15 g
Gravy	30 mL (2 tbsps.)	30 g
Lard	5 mL (1 tsp.)	5 g
Margarine	5 mL (1 tsp.)	5 g
Nuts, shelled:		
almonds	8 nuts	20 g
Brazil nuts	2 nuts	5 g
cashews	5 nuts	10 g
filberts, hazelnuts	5 nuts	10 g
macadamia	3 nuts	5 g
peanuts	10 nuts	10 g
pecans	5 halves	5 g
pignolias, pine nuts	25 mL (5 tsps.)	10 g
pistachios, shelled	20 nuts	10 g
in shell	20 nuts	20 g
pumpkin and squash seeds	20 mL (4 tsps.)	10 g
sesame seeds	15 mL (1 tbsp.)	10 g
sunflower seeds, shelled	15 mL (1 tbsp.)	10 g
in shell	45 mL (3 tbsps.)	15 g
walnuts	4 halves	10 g
Oil, cooking and salad	5 mL	5 g
Olives, green	10	45 g
ripe	7	40 g
Pate, liverwurst, meat spreads	15 mL (1 tbsp.)	15 g
Salad dressing: blue, French, Italian, mayonnaise, thousand island	5 mL (1 tsp.)	5 g
Salt pork, raw or cooked	5 mL	5 g
Sesame oil	5 mL	5 g

TABLE G-13

Extras (may be used without measuring)

Beverages
Bouillon or clear broth
Bouillon from cube, powder or liquid
Coffee, clear
Consomme
Herbal teas, unsweetened
Mineral water
Soda water, club soda
Sugar-free soft drink
Tea, clear
Water

Condiments
Chow chow, unsweetened tomato pickles
Garlic
Gelatin, unsweetened
Ginger root
Horseradish, uncreamed
Lemon juice or lemon wedge
Lime juice or lime wedge
Mustard
Parsley
Pickles, unsweetened dill pickles or sour cucumber pickles
Pimentos
Soya sauce
Vinegar
Worcestershire sauce

Herbs and spices
Salt, pepper, thyme, marjoram, cinammon, etc.

Miscellaneous
Artificial sweetener, such as cyclamate or saccharin
Baking powder, baking soda
Dulse
Flavourings and extracts, e.g. vanilla
Rennet

TABLE G–14

Extras (2.5 g carbohydrate, 15 kcal, limited to amount indicated)

Anchovy	2 fillets
Barbecue sauce	15 mL (1 tbsp.)
Bran, natural	30 mL (2 tbsps.)
Brewers yeast	5 mL (1 tsp.)
Carob powder	5 ml (1 tsp.)
Chili sauce	5 mL (1 tsp.)
Cocoa powder	5 mL (1 tsp.)
Cranberry sauce, unsweetened	15 mL (1 tbsp.)
Dietetic fruit spreads	5 mL (1 tsp.)
Ketchup	5 mL (1 tsp.)
Maraschino cherry	1 cherry
Nuts, chopped pieces	5 mL (1 tsp.)
Non-dairy coffee whitener	5 mL (1 tsp.)
Relish	5 mL (1 tsp.)
Sugar substitutes, granular	5 mL (1 tsp.) (3 to 4 packages)
Whipped topping	15 mL (1 tbsp.)
Yogurt, plain	30 mL (2 tbsps.)

G

Table of Food Composition

This table of food composition is not the standard table found in most nutrition textbooks. The list of foods chosen is an expanded version of that presented in the 1985 edition of the USDA *Home and Garden Bulletin Number 72, Nutritive Value of Foods*. The *Bulletin,* however, does not contain all the foods listed here nor the values for dietary fiber, vitamin B₆, folacin, magnesium or zinc.

To achieve a complete and reliable listing of nutrients for all the foods, many sources of information had to be researched. Government sources of information are the primary base for all the data: USDA *Handbooks 8-1* through *8-11, Handbook 8-14* (it was released before 8-12 and 8-13), and the 1986 release of USDA's *Home and Garden Bulletin Number 72, Nutritive Value of Foods*. In addition, provisional USDA information of nutrient values—both published and unpublished—and many conversations with the staff members at USDA, Human Nutrition Information Service in Hyattsville, Maryland, have provided professional assistance to refine the data.

Even with all the government sources available, there are still many missing nutrient values, and as the various government data are updated, conflicting values are reported from the USDA for the same items. To fill in the missing values and resolve discrepancies, other sources of information were used. These reliable sources include refereed journal articles, food composition tables from Canada and England, information from other nutrient data banks and publications, unpublished scientific data, and manufacturers' data.

Estimates of nutrient amounts for foods and nutrients include all possible adjustments in the interest of accuracy. When multiple values were reported for a nutrient, the numbers were averaged and weighted with consideration of the original number of samples in the separate sources. Whenever water percentages were available, estimates of nutrient amounts were adjusted for water content. When no water was given, water percentage was assumed to be that shown in the table. Whenever a reported weight appeared inconsistent (cooked eggplant and collards) many kitchen tests were made and the average weight of the typical product was given as tested.

When estimates of nutrient amounts in cooked foods were derived from reported amounts in raw foods, published retention factors were applied. Some reported data for combination foods were modified in this table to include newer data available for major ingredients. For example, since the "pies" were analyzed and reported, newer data on fruits have been published. Older reported data on certain bakery items were updated for the new enrichment levels for certain nutrients.

Considerable effort has been made to report the most accurate data available and to eliminate missing values. There will always be changes in the future and the authors* welcome any suggestions or comments for the future.

It is important to know

that there can be many different nutrient values reported for foods. Many factors influence the amounts of nutrients in foods, including: the mineral content of the soil, the method of processing, genetics, diet of the animal or fertilizer of the plant, season of the year, methods of analysis, difference in moisture content of the samples analyzed, length and method of storage, and methods of cooking the food.

As a result, different nutrient values for the same food item are reported, even by reliable sources. Although each nutrient from USDA government data is presented as a single number in some of their publications, it is actually an average of a range of data. In the more detailed reports (Handbook 8 series), the number of samples is identified and the standard deviation of the data is also noted. USDA data will have different reported values for foods as well, as older information is replaced with newer data in the more recent publications.

---

*This table has been prepared for The West Publishing Company and is copyrighted by ESHA Research in Salem, Oregon—the developer and publisher of "The Food Processor®" computerized nutrition systems. The major sources for the data from the U.S. Department of Agriculture are supplemented by over 300 additional sources of information. Because the list of references is so extensive, it is not provided here, but it is available from the publisher.

Therefore, nutrient data should be viewed and used only as a guide, a close approximation of nutrient content.

Dietary fiber deserves a special word. Estimates of dietary fiber are included for all the foods in this table. The sources of this information are primarily from Southgate (England), many journal articles, some of the latest published data from the USDA, and extensive unpublished information from the USDA Human Nutrition Information Service in Hyattsville, Maryland.

It is important to know that this is emerging data, and to expect additional research and refinement of analytical techniques to modify the data in the future. Dietary fiber is composed of cellulose, hemicellulose, lignin, pectin, gums, and mucilages. Very little data is yet available on the gum and mucilage components in foods, but there is considerable data on the other components.

Many different analytical techniques are used to measure various components of fiber, and these methods are undergoing their own review of accuracy in the scientific community. In this table, either an estimate of the total dietary fiber (a specific analytical technique) or a combination of measures for the insoluble components and pectin, when available, is used.

Vitamin A is reported in Retinol Equivalents. The amount of this vitamin can vary by the season of the year. Reported values in both dairy products and plants are higher in summer and early fall than in winter. The values reported here represent year-round averages. In the organ meats of all animal products (liver especially) there is a large amount of vitamin A and these amounts vary widely depending on the background of the animal. The vitamin is present in very small amounts in regular meat and is often reported as a trace.

Newer reported vitamin A values for some plant foods have increased significantly due to additional information and sometimes to newer plant genetics. New vitamin A values for canned pumpkin are 3.5 times greater than the previously reported values. This information was used to modify the vitamin A value of pumpkin pie, which was not yet updated.

The energy and nutrients in recipes and combination foods vary widely depending on the ingredients. The various fatty acids and cholesterol are influenced by the type of fat used (the specific type of oil, vegetable shortening, butter, margarine, etc.).

Total fats, as well as the breakdown of total fats to saturated, mono-unsaturated, and poly-unsaturated fats, are listed in the table. The fatty acids seldom add up exactly to the total. This is due to rounding and to the existence of small amounts of other fatty acid components that are not included in the basic three categories.

Niacin values are for preformed niacin and do not include additional niacin that may form in the body from the conversion of tryptophan.

TABLE H–1

Food Composition

Grp	Ref	Name	Measure	Wt (g)	H₂O (%)	Ener (kcal)	Prot (g)	Carb (g)	Fiber (g)	Fat (g)	Fat Breakdown (g) Sat	Mono	Poly
		BEVERAGES											
		Alcoholic:											
		Beer:											
1	1	Regular (12 fl oz)	1½ cups	356	92	146	.9	13.2	.71	0	0	0	0
1	2	Light (12 fl oz)	1½ cups	354	95	100[1]	.7	4.6	.25	0	0	0	0
		Gin, rum, vodka, whiskey:											
1	3	80 proof	1½ fl oz	42	67	97	0	<.1	0	0	0	0	0
1	4	86 proof	1½ fl oz	42	64	105	0	<.1	0	0	0	0	0
1	5	90 proof	1½ fl oz	42	62	110	0	<.1	0	0	0	0	0
		Wine:											
1	6	Dessert (4 fl oz)	½ cup	118	72	181[2]	.2	13.9[2]	0	0	0	0	0
1	7	Red	3½ fl oz	103	88	74	.2	1.8	0	0	0	0	0
1	8	Rosé	3½ fl oz	103	89	73	.2	1.5	0	0	0	0	0
1	9	White medium	3½ fl oz	103	90	70	.1	.8	0	0	0	0	0
		Carbonated[3]:											
1	10	Club soda (12 fl oz)	1½ cups	355	100	0	0	0	0	0	0	0	0
1	11	Cola beverage (12 fl oz)	1½ cups	370	89	151	.1	38.5	0	0	0	0	0
1	12	Diet cola (12 fl oz)	1½ cups	355	100	2	.2	.3	0	0	0	0	0
1	13	Diet soda pop-average (12 fl oz)	1½ cups	355	100	2	.1	.3	0	0	0	0	0
1	14	Ginger ale (12 fl oz)	1½ cups	366	91	124	.1	31.9	0	0	0	0	0
1	15	Grape soda (12 fl oz)	1½ cups	372	89	161	0	41.7	0	0	0	0	0
1	16	Lemon-lime (12 fl oz)	1½ cups	368	90	149	0	38.4	0	0	0	0	0
1	17	Orange (12 fl oz)	1½ cups	372	88	177	0	45.8	0	0	0	0	0
1	18	Pepper type soda (12 fl oz)	1½ cups	368	89	151	0	38.2	0	0	0	0	0
1	19	Root beer (12 fl oz)	1½ cups	370	89	152	.1	39.2	0	0	0	0	0
		Coffee:[3]											
1	20	Brewed	1 cup	240	99	2[5]	.1	1.1	.02	.01	<.01	0	<.01
1	21	Prepared from instant	1 cup	240	99	2[5]	.3	.9	0	.01	<.01	0	<.01
		Fruit drinks,[6] noncarbonated:											
1	22	Fruit punch drink, canned	1 cup	253	88	118	.1	30.1	0	.06	<.01	<.01	<.01
1	23	Grape drink, canned	1 cup	250	88	112	0	34.7	.25	.04	<.01	<.01	<.01
1	24	Pineapple grapefruit, canned	1 cup	250	88	117	.6	29	0	.20	.01	.03	.07
1	25	Pineapple orange, canned	1 cup	250	87	125	3.1	29.4	0	.24	.03	.04	.05
		Lemonade, frozen:											
1	26	Concentrate (6 oz can)	¾ cup	219	52	397	.6	103	.88	.40	.06	.02	.13
1	27	Lemonade, prepared from frozen concentrate	1 cup	248	89	100	.1	26	.29	.10	.01	<.01	.03
		Limeade, frozen:											
1	28	Concentrate (6 oz can)	¾ cup	218	50	408	.4	108	.88[8]	.20	.02	.02	.06
1	29	Limeade prepared from frozen concentrate	1 cup	247	89	102	.1	27.1	.29[8]	.10	<.01	<.01	.01
		Fruit and vegetable juices; see Fruit and Vegetable sections.											
		Tea:[3]											
1	30	Brewed	1 cup	240	100[3]	2[5]	t	.5	0	0	<.01	<.01	<.01
1	31	From instant, unsweetened	1 cup	237	100[3]	2[5]	.1	.4	0	t	t	t	t
1	32	From instant, sweetened	1 cup	262	91	86	t	22.1	0	.07	t	t	t

[1] kCalories can vary from 78 to 131 for 12 fluid ounces.
[2] Values for sweet dessert wine. Dry dessert wines contain 149 kcalories, 4.8 g of carbohydrate.
[3] Mineral content varies depending on water source.
[5] kCalorie values are not available: these are USDA estimates.
[6] Usually less than 10% fruit juice.
[8] Dietary fiber values are estimated from values for lemonade.

(For purposes of calculations, use "0" for t, <1, <.1, <.01, etc.)

KEY: 1 = BEV 2 = DAIRY 3 = EGGS 4 = FAT/OIL 5 = FRUIT 6 = BAKERY 7 = GRAIN 8 = FISH 9 = BEEF 10 = POULTRY
11 = SAUSAGE 12 = MIXED 13 = NUTS/SEEDS 14 = SWEETS 15 = VEG/LEG 16 = MISC 22 = SOUP/SAUCE

Chol (mg)	Calc (mg)	Iron (mg)	Magn (mg)	Phos (mg)	Pota (mg)	Sodi (mg)	Zinc (mg)	VT-A (RE)	Thia (mg)	Ribo (mg)	Niac (mg)	V-B6 (mg)	Fola (µg)	VT-C (mg)
0	18	.11	23	44	89	19	.07	0	.02	.09	1.61	.18	21	0
0	18	.14	18	43	64	10	.11	0	.03	.11	1.39	.12	15	0
0	0	.02	0	2	1	.4	.02	0	<.01	<.01	<.01	t	0	0
0	0	.02	0	2	1	.4	.02	0	<.01	<.01	<.01	0	0	0
0	0	.02	0	2	1	.4	.02	0	<.01	<.01	<.01	0	0	0
0	9	.28	11	11	109	11	.08	0	.02	.02	.25	0	<1	0
0	8	.44	13	14	115	6	.09	0	<.01	.03	.08	.04	2	0
0	9	.39	10	15	102	5	.06	0	<.01	.02	.08	.03	1	0
0	9	.33	11	14	82	5	.07	0	<.01	<.01	.07	.01	<1	0
0	17	.15	4	0	6	75	.36	0	0	0	0	0	0	0
0	9	.13	3	46	4	14	.05	0	0	0	0	0	0	0
0	12	.11	4	30	0	214[4]	.28	0	.02	.08	0	0	0	0
0	14	.14	3	38	7	214[4]	.18	0	0	0	0	0	0	0
0	12	.66	3	1	5	25	.18	0	0	0	0	0	0	0
0	12	.31	4	0	3	57	.26	0	0	0	0	0	0	0
0	9	.25	2	1	4	41	.18	0	0	0	.06	0	0	0
0	19	.23	4	4	9	46	.38	0	0	0	0	0	0	0
0	12	.14	1	41	2	38	.15	0	0	0	0	0	0	0
0	19	.18	4	2	3	49	.26	0	0	0	0	0	0	0
0	4	.98	14	2	130	5	.04	0	0	0	.53	0	<1	0
0	8	.12	11	8	87	8	.07	0	0	<.01	.69	0	0	0
0	19	.52	5	2	64	56	.31	4	.06	.06	.05	0	3	75
0	3	.41	5	3	13	16	.28	t	.08	.01	.07	.01	<1	85
0	18	.77	15	14	154	34	.15	9	.07	.04	.67	.10	26	115
0	13	.67	14	10	116	9	.14	133	.07	.05	.52	.12	27	56
0	15	1.58	11	19	148	8	.17	21	.06	.21	.16	.06	22	397
0	8	.41	5	5	38	8	.09	5	.01	.05	.04	.01	6	107
0	11	.22	60	13	129	.003	.11	t	.02	.02	.22	.11	24	26
0	7	.06	2	3	33	6	.05	t	<.01	<.01	.05	.03	7	7
0	0	.05	7	1	89	6.7	.05	0	0	.03	.1	0	12	0
0	5	.05	5	3	47	8	.07	0	0	<.01	<.01	<.09	<1	0
0	1	.04	3	3	49	t	.02	0	0	.04	.09	0	5	0

[4]Value for product sweetened with aspartame only; sodium is 32 mg if a blend of aspartame and sodium saccharin is used; 75 mg if just sodium saccharin is used.

[7]Vitamin C can range from 5 to 72 mg in a small can of frozen concentrate; and from 1 to 18 mg in 1 cup lemonade.

H

(For purposes of calculations, use "0" for t, <1, <.1, <.01, etc.)

TABLE H–1

Food Composition

Grp	Ref	Name	Measure	Wt (g)	H₂O (%)	Ener (kcal)	Prot (g)	Carb (g)	Fiber (g)	Fat (g)	Fat Breakdown (g)		
											Sat	Mono	Poly
DAIRY													
		Butter: see Fats and Oils, # 158, 159, 160:											
		Cheese, natural:											
2	33	Blue	1 oz	28	42	100	6.1	.7	0	8.15	5.30	2.21	.23
2	34	Brick	1 oz	28	41	105	6.4	.8	0	8.41	5.32	2.44	.22
2	35	Brie	1 oz	28	48	95	5.9	.1	0	7.85	4.95	2.29	.25
2	36	Camembert	1 oz	28	52	85	5.6	.1	0	6.87	4.33	2	.20
		Cheddar:											
2	37	Cut pieces	1 oz	28	37	114	7.1	.4	0	9.40	5.98	2.66	.27
2	38	1″ cube	1 ea	17	37	69	4.3	.2	0	5.70	3.63	1.62	.16
2	39	Shredded	1 cup	113	37	455	28.1	1.4	0	37.5	23.8	10.6	1.06
		Cottage:											
2	40	Creamed, large curd	1 cup	225	79	235	28	6.0	0	9.60	6.42	2.9	.31
2	41	Creamed, small curd	1 cup	210	79	215	26.2	5.6	0	8.93	5.99	2.7	.29
2	42	With fruit	1 cup	226	72	279	22.4	30.1	0	7.68	4.86	2.19	.24
2	43	Lowfat 2%	1 cup	226	79	205	31.1	8.2	0	4.36	2.76	1.24	.13
2	44	Lowfat 1%	1 cup	226	82	164	28	6.2	0	2.30	1.46	.66	.07
2	45	Dry curd	1 cup	145	80	123	25	2.7	0	.61	.40	.16	.02
2	46	Cream	1 oz	28	54	99	2.1	.8	0	9.89	6.23	2.79	.36
2	47	Edam	1 oz	28	42	101	7.1	.4	0	7.80	4.98	2.3	.19
2	48	Feta	1 oz	28	55	75	4.5	1.2	0	6.20	4.24	1.31	.17
2	49	Gouda	1 oz	28	42	101	7.1	.6	0	7.73	4.99	2.2	.19
2	50	Gruyere	1 oz	28	33	117	8.4	.1	0	9.07	5.36	2.85	.49
2	51	Gorgonzola	1 oz	28	39	111	7	0	0	9	5.50	2.4	.50
2	52	Liederkranz	1 oz	28	53	87	5	0	0	8	5.30	2.2	.23
2	53	Monterey jack	1 oz	28	41	106	6.9	.2	0	8.58	5.43	2.35	.24
		Mozzarella, made with:											
2	54	Whole milk	1 oz	28	54	80	5.5	.6	0	5.76	3.73	1.86	.22
2	55	Part skim milk, low moisture	1 oz	28	49	80	7.6	.9	0	4.68	3.08	1.38	.14
2	56	Muenster	1 oz	28	42	104	6.4	.3	0	8.43	5.42	2.47	.19
		Parmesan, grated:											
2	57	Cup, not pressed down	1 cup	100	18	455	41.6	3.7	0	30.0	19.1	8.73	.70
2	58	Tablespoon	1 tbsp	5	18	23	2.1	.2	0	1.50	1	.44	.04
2	59	Ounce	1 oz	28	18	129	11.8	1.1	0	8.51	5.40	2.5	.20
2	60	Provolone	1 oz	28	41	100	7.1	.6	0	7.55	4.84	2.1	.22
		Ricotta, made with:											
2	61	Whole milk	1 cup	246	72	428	27.7	7.5	0	31.9	20.4	8.92	.95
2	62	Part skim milk	1 cup	246	74	340	28	12.6	0	19.5	12.1	5.69	.64
2	63	Romano	1 oz	28	31	110	9	1	0	7.64	4.85	2.22	.17
2	64	Swiss	1 oz	28	37	107	8	1	0	7.80	5.04	2.06	.28
		Pasteurized processed cheese products:											
2	65	American	1 oz	28	39	106	6.3	.5	0	8.86	5.58	2.54	.28
2	66	Swiss	1 oz	28	42	95	7	.6	0	6.98	4.55	2	.18
2	67	American cheese food	1 oz	28	44	93	5.6	2.1	0	6.97	4.38	2.04	.20
2	68	American cheese spread	1 oz	28	48	82	5.2	2.5	0	6.02	3.78	1.76	.18
		Cream, sweet:											
		Half and half (cream and milk):											
2	69	Cup	1 cup	242	81	315	7.2	10.4	0	27.8	17.3	8.04	1.03
2	70	Tablespoon	1 tbsp	15	81	20	.4	.7	0	1.74	1.10	.50	.10
		Light, coffee or table:											
2	71	Cup	1 cup	240	74	469	6.5	8.8	0	46.3	28.9	13.4	1.72
2	72	Tablespoon	1 tbsp	15	74	30	.4	.6	0	2.89	1.81	.84	.11
		Light whipping cream, liquid:											
2	73	Cup	1 cup	239	64	699	5.2	7.1	0	73.9	46.2	21.7	2.11
2	74	Tablespoon	1 tbsp	15	64	44	.3	.4	0	4.62	2.9	1.36	.13

(For purposes of calculations, use "0" for t, <1, <.1, <.01, etc.)

KEY: 1 = BEV 2 = DAIRY 3 = EGGS 4 = FAT/OIL 5 = FRUIT 6 = BAKERY 7 = GRAIN 8 = FISH 9 = BEEF 10 = POULTRY 11 = SAUSAGE 12 = MIXED 13 = NUTS/SEEDS 14 = SWEETS 15 = VEG/LEG 16 = MISC 22 = SOUP/SAUCE

Chol (mg)	Calc (mg)	Iron (mg)	Magn (mg)	Phos (mg)	Pota (mg)	Sodi (mg)	Zinc (mg)	VT-A (RE)	Thia (mg)	Ribo (mg)	Niac (mg)	V-B6 (mg)	Fola (µg)	VT-C (mg)
21	150	.09	7	110	73	396	.75	65	<.01	.11	.29	.05	10	0
27	191	.13	7	128	38	159	.73	86	<.01	.1	.03	.02	6	0
28	52	.14	6	53	43	178	.7	57	.02	.15	.11	.07	18	0
20	110	.09	6	98	53	236	.68	71	<.01	.14	.18	.06	18	0
30	204	.20	8	146	28	176	.92	86	<.01	.11	.02	.02	5	0
18	124	.12	5	88	17	107	.54	52	<.01	.07	.01	.01	3	0
119	815	.77	31	579	111	701	3.51	342	.03	.42	.09	.08	21	0
34	135	.26	11	297	190	911	.8	108	.05	.37	.30	.14	27	t
31	126	.29	11	277	177	850	.8	101	.04	.34	.27	.14	26	t
25	108	.25	9	236	151	915	.66	81	.04	.29	.23	.12	22	t
19	155	.36	14	340	217	918	.95	45	.05	.42	.33	.17	30	0
10	138	.32	12	302	193	918	.86	25	.05	.37	.29	.15	28	t
10	46	.33	6	151	47	19	.68	12	.04	.21	.23	.12	21	0
31	23	.34	2	30	34	84	.33	124	<.01	.06	.03	.01	4	0
25	207	.12	8	152	53	274	1.06	72	.01	.11	.02	.02	5	0
25	140	.18	5	96	18	316	.81	36	.04	.23	.29	.02	3	0
32	198	.07	8	155	34	232	1.1	49	<.01	.10	.02	.02	6	0
31	287	.06	4	172	23	95	1	98	.02	.08	.03	.02	3	0
25	149	.12	8	121	26	513	.57	103	.01	.09	.2	.04	9	0
21	110	.12	7	100	68	390	.7	91	.01	.18	.1	.04	34	0
26	212	.2	8	126	23	152	.85	81	<.01	.11	.02	.02	3	0
22	147	.05	5	105	19	106	.7	68	<.01	.07	.02	.02	2	0
15	207	.08	8	149	27	150	.82	54	<.01	.1	.03	.02	3	0
27	203	.12	8	133	38	178	.84	90	<.01	.09	.03	.02	3	0
79	1376	.95	51	807	107	1862	3.19	173	.04	.39	.32	.1	8	0
4	69	.05	3	40	5	93	.16	9	<.01	.02	.02	<.01	<1	0
22	390	.27	14	229	30	528	1	49	.01	.11	.09	.03	2	0
20	214	.15	8	141	39	248	.89	75	<.01	.09	.04	.02	3	0
124	509	.94	28	389	257	207	2.85	330	.03	.48	.26	.11	14	0
76	669	1.09	4	449	307	307	3.29	278	.05	.46	.19	.05	14	0
29	302	.23	12	215	26	340	1	40	.01	.1	.02	.03	2	0
26	272	.05	10	171	31	74	1.1	72	<.01	.1	.03	.02	2	0
27	174	.11	6	211	46	406	.93	82	<.01	.1	.02	.02	2	0
24	219	.17	8	216	61	388	1.02	65	<.01	.08	.01	.01	2	0
18	163	.24	9	130	79	337	.85	62	<.01	.12	.04	.02	2	0
16	159	.09	8	201	69	381	.78	54	.01	.12	.04	.03	2	0
89	254	.17	25	230	314	98	1.23	259	.09	.36	.19	.09	6	2
6	16	.01	2	14	20	6	.08	16	<.01	.02	.01	<.01	<1	t
159	231	.1	21	192	292	95	.65	437	.08	.35	.14	.08	6	2
10	14	<.01	1	12	18	6	.04	27	<.01	.02	<.01	<.01	<1	t
265	166	.07	17	146	231	82	.60	705	.06	.30	.1	.07	9	1
17	10	<.01	1	9	15	5	.04	44	<.01	.02	<.01	<.01	<1	t

H

(For purposes of calculations, use "0" for t, <1, <.1, <.01, etc.)

TABLE H-1

Food Composition

Grp	Ref	Name	Measure	Wt (g)	H₂O (%)	Ener (kcal)	Prot (g)	Carb (g)	Fiber (g)	Fat (g)	Fat Breakdown (g) Sat	Mono	Poly
DAIRY—Con.													
		Heavy whipping cream, liquid:											
2	75	Cup	1 cup	238	58	821	4.9	6.6	0	88	54.8	25.4	3.27
2	76	Tablespoon	1 tbsp	15	58	51	.3	.4	0	5.5	3.5	1.60	.2
		Whipped cream, pressurized:											
2	77	Cup	1 cup	60	61	154	1.9	7.5	0	13.3	8.3	3.85	.5
2	78	Tablespoon	1 tbsp	4	61	10	.1	.5	0	.83	.52	.24	.03
		Cream, sour, cultured:											
2	79	Cup	1 cup	230	71	493	7.3	9.8	0	48.2	30	13.9	1.8
2	80	Tablespoon	1 tbsp	14	71	30	.4	.6	0	2.93	1.83	.85	.11
		Cream products-imitation and part dairy:											
		Coffee whitener:											
2	81	Frozen or liquid	1 tbsp	15	77	20	.1	1.7	0	1.5	1.4	.02	t
2	82	Powdered	1 tsp	2	2	11	<.1	1	0	.7	.64	.02	t
		Dessert topping, frozen:											
2	83	Cup	1 cup	75	50	239	.9	17.3	0	19	16.3	1.21	.39
2	84	Tablespoon	1 tbsp	4.7	50	15	<.1	1.1	0	1.19	1.02	.08	.02
		Dessert topping from mix:											
2	85	Cup	1 cup	80	67	151	2.9	13.2	0	9.93	8.55	.68	.16
2	86	Tablespoon	1 tbsp	5	67	9	.2	.8	0	.62	.53	.04	.01
		Dessert topping, pressurized:											
2	87	Cup	1 cup	70	60	185	.7	11.2	0	15.6	13.2	1.35	.17
2	88	Tablespoon	1 tbsp	4	60	11	<.1	.7	0	.98	.83	.08	.01
		Sour dressing, part dairy:											
2	89	Cup	1 cup	235	75	416	7.6	11	0	39	31.2	4.60	1.1
2	90	Tablespoon	1 tbsp	15	75	25	.5	.7	0	2.44	1.95	.29	.07
		Imitation sour cream:											
2	91	Cup	1 cup	230	71	479	5.5	15.3	0	44.9	40.9	1.35	.13
2	92	Tablespoon	1 tbsp	14	71	29	.3	.9	0	2.73	2.49	.08	<.01
		Milk, fluid:											
2	93	Whole milk	1 cup	244	88	150	8	11.4	0	8.15	5.07	2.35	.30
2	94	2% Lowfat milk	1 cup	244	89	121	8.1	11.7	0	4.78	2.92	1.35	.17
2	95	2% Milk-solids added[9a]	1 cup	245	89	125	8.5	12.2	0	4.7	2.94	1.37	.18
2	96	1% Lowfat milk	1 cup	244	90	102	8	11.7	0	2.54	1.61	.75	.1
2	97	1% Milk-solids added[9a]	1 cup	245	90	105	8.5	12.2	0	2.3	1.48	.69	.1
2	98	Skim milk	1 cup	245	91	86	8.3	11.9	0	.44	.29	.12	.02
2	99	Skim milk-solids added[9a]	1 cup	245	90	91	8.8	12.3	0	.61	.4	.16	.02
2	100	Buttermilk	1 cup	245	90	99	8.1	11.7	0	2.16	1.34	.62	.08
		Milk, canned:											
2	101	Sweetened condensed	1 cup	306	27	982	24.2	166	0	26.6	16.8	7.43	1.03
2	102	Evaporated, whole	1 cup	252	74	340	17	25	0	19.6	11.6	5.88	.62
2	103	Evaporated, skim	1 cup	255	79	200	19	29	0	.52	.31	.16	.02
		Milk, dried:											
2	104	Buttermilk	1 cup	120	3	464	41.2	58.8	0	6.65	432	2.01	.26
		Instant, nonfat:											
2	105	Envelope[10]	1 ea	91	4	326	31.9	47.5	0	.66	.43	.17	.03
2	106	Cup	1 cup	68	4	244	23.9	35.5	0	.51	.32	.17	.02
2	107	Goat milk	1 cup	244	87	168	8.7	10.9	0	10.1	6.51	2.71	.36
2	108	Kefir[12]	1 cup	233	82	160	9.3	8.8	0	4.5	2.91	1.23	.12

[9a] Milk solids added, label claim less than 10 grams of protein per cup.
[10] Yields 1 qt of fluid milk when reconstituted according to package directions.
[12] Most values provided by product labeling.

(For purposes of calculations, use "0" for t, <1, <.1, <.01, etc.)

KEY: 1 = BEV 2 = DAIRY 3 = EGGS 4 = FAT/OIL 5 = FRUIT 6 = BAKERY 7 = GRAIN 8 = FISH 9 = BEEF 10 = POULTRY
11 = SAUSAGE 12 = MIXED 13 = NUTS/SEEDS 14 = SWEETS 15 = VEG/LEG 16 = MISC 22 = SOUP/SAUCE

Chol (mg)	Calc (mg)	Iron (mg)	Magn (mg)	Phos (mg)	Pota (mg)	Sodi (mg)	Zinc (mg)	VT-A (RE)	Thia (mg)	Ribo (mg)	Niac (mg)	V-B6 (mg)	Fola (µg)	VT-C (mg)
326	154	.07	17	149	179	89	.55	1002	.05	.26	.09	.06	10	1
20	10	<.01	1	9	11	6	.03	63	<.01	.02	<.01	<.01	<1	t
46	61	.03	6	54	88	78	.22	124	.02	.04	.04	.03	1	0
3	4	<.01	<1	3	5	5	.01	8	<.01	<.01	<.01	<.01	<1	0
102	268	.14	26	195	331	123	.69	448	.08	.34	.15	.04	25	2
6	16	<.01	2	12	20	7	.04	27	<.01	.02	<.01	<.01	2	t
0	1.4	<.01	<1	10	29	12	<.01	1[9]	0	0	0	0	0	0
0	.4	.02	<1	8	16	4	.01	.4[9]	0	<.01	0	0	0	0
0	5	.09	1	6	14	19	.03	65[9]	0	0	0	0	0	0
0	.3	<.01	<1	.4	.9	1	<.01	4[9]	0	0	0	0	0	0
8	72	.03	8	69	121	53	.22	39[9]	.02	.09	.05	.02	3	.5
.5	4.5	<.01	<1	4	8	3	.14	2[9]	<.01	<.01	<.01	<.01	<1	t
0	4	.01	1	13	13	43	.01	33[9]	0	0	0	0	0	0
0	.2	<.01	<1	1	1	2.7	<.01	2[9]	0	0	0	0	0	0
13	266	.07	23	205	381	113	.87	5[9]	.09	.38	.17	.04	28	2
.8	17	<.01	2	13	24	7	.05	t[9]	<.01	.02	.01	<.01	2	t
0	6	.01	—	102	369	235	0	0	0	0	0	0	0	0
0	.4	<.01	—	6	22	14	0	0	0	0	0	0	0	0
33	291	.12	33	228	370	120	.94	76	.09	.4	.2	.1	12	2
22	297	.12	33	232	377	122	.96	140	.1	.4	.21	.1	12	2
18	314	.12	35	245	397	128	.98	140	.1	.42	.22	.11	12	2
10	300	.12	34	235	381	123	.96	145	.1	.41	.21	.1	12	2
10	314	.12	35	245	397	128	.98	145	.1	.42	.22	.11	12	2
4	302	.1	28	247	406	126	.92	149	.09	.34	.22	.1	14	2
5	316	.12	37	255	419	130	1	149	.1	.43	.22	.11	12	2
9	285	.12	26	219	371	257	1.03	20	.08	.38	.14	.08	12	2
104	868	.58	78	775	1136	389	2.88	248	.28	1.27	.64	.16	34	8
74	657	.48	60	510	764	267	1.94	136	.12	.8	.49	.13	18	5
10	738	.7	68	497	845	293	2.18	300	.11	.8	.4	.14	22	3
83	1421	.36	131	1119	1910	621	4.82	65	.47	1.9	1.05	.41	57	7
16	1120	.28	107	896	1552	500	4.01	646[11]	.38	1.59	.81	.31	45	5
12	837	.21	80	670	1160	373	3.06	483[11]	.28	1.19	.61	.23	34	4
28	326	.12	34	270	499	122	.73	137	.12	.34	.68	.11	2	3
10	350	.5	28	319	205	50	.9	155	.45	.44	.3	.09	20	6

H

[9]Vitamin A value is largely from beta-carotene used for coloring.
[11]With added vitamin A.

(For purposes of calculations, use "0" for t, <1, <.1, <.01, etc.)

TABLE H–1

Food Composition

Grp	Ref	Name	Measure	Wt (g)	H₂O (%)	Ener (kcal)	Prot (g)	Carb (g)	Fiber (g)	Fat (g)	Fat Breakdown (g)		
											Sat	Mono	Poly
DAIRY—Con.													
		Milk beverages and powdered mixes:											
		Chocolate:											
2	109	Whole	1 cup	250	82	210	7.9	25.9	.15	8.48	5.26	2.48	.31
2	110	2% Fat	1 cup	250	84	180	8	26	.15	5	3.1	1.47	.18
2	111	1% Fat	1 cup	250	84	160	8.1	26.1	.15	2.5	1.54	.75	.09
		Chocolate flavored beverages:											
2	112	Powder containing nonfat dry milk	1 oz	28.4	1	100	3.6	22.7	.14	1.1	.68	.38	.03
2	113	Choc drink prepared with water	¾ cup	206	86	100	3.6	22.7	.14	1.1	.68	.38	t
2	114	Powder without nonfat dry milk	¾ oz	21.6	<1	75	.7	19.5	.08	.7	.4	.22	.02
2	115	Choc drink prepared with whole milk	1 cup	266	81	226	8.8	30.9	.08	8.8	5.48	2.58	.32
2	116	Egg nog, commercial	1 cup	254	74	342	9.7	34.4	0	19	11.3	5.67	.86
		Malted milk, chocolate flavor:											
2	117	Powder[12a]	¾ oz or 3 heaping tsp	21	1	79	1.1	18.4	.10	.8	.45	.22	.07
2	118	Malted milk prepared with whole milk	1 cup	265	81	229	9.3	29.8	.10	8.9	5.23	2.57	.38
		Malted milk, natural flavor:											
2	119	Powder[12a]	¾ oz or 3 heaping tsp	21	2	87	2.3	15.9	0	1.7	.88	.43	.25
2	120	Malted milk prepared with whole milk	1 cup	265	81	237	10.4	27.3	0	9.8	5.96	2.78	.56
		Milk shakes:											
2	121	Chocolate (10 fl oz)	1¼ cups	283	72	360	9.6	57.9	.29	10.5	6.55	3.04	.4
2	122	Vanilla (10 fl oz)	1¼ cups	283	75	314	9.8	50.8	.19	8.4	5.26	2.44	.31
		Milk desserts, frozen:											
		Ice cream, regular (about 11% fat) vanilla:											
		Hardened:											
2	123	½ Gallon	½ gal	1064	61	2153	38.4	254	0	115	71.3	33.1	4.3
2	124	Cup	1 cup	133	61	269	4.8	31.7	0	14.3	8.29	4.14	.53
2	125	Fluid ounces	3 oz	50	61	101	1.8	11.9	0	5.4	3.35	1.56	.2
2	126	Soft Serve	1 cup	173	60	377	7	38.3	0	22.5	13.5	6.68	.98
		Ice cream, rich vanilla (about 16% fat): hardened:											
2	127	½ Gallon	½ gallon	1188	59	2805	33.1	256	0	190	118	54.9	7.1
2	128	Cup	1 cup	148	59	349	4.1	32	0	23.7	14.7	6.84	.88
		Ice milk, vanilla (about 4% fat):											
		Hardened:											
2	129	½ Gallon	½ gallon	1048	69	1467	41.3	232	0	45.1	28.1	13	1.67
2	130	Cup	1 cup	131	69	184	5.2	29	0	5.6	3.51	1.63	.21
2	131	Soft serve (about 3% fat)	1 cup	175	70	223	8	38.4	0	4.6	2.88	1.33	.17
		Sherbet (2% fat):											
2	132	½ Gallon	½ gallon	1542	66	2158	17.3	469	0	30.5	19	8.82	1.13
2	133	Cup	1 cup	193	66	270	2.2	58.7	0	3.8	2.38	1.1	.14

[12a]The latest USDA data from Handbook 8-14 on beverages updates previous USDA data.

(For purposes of calculations, use "0" for t, <1, <.1, <.01, etc.)

KEY: 1 = BEV 2 = DAIRY 3 = EGGS 4 = FAT/OIL 5 = FRUIT 6 = BAKERY 7 = GRAIN 8 = FISH 9 = BEEF 10 = POULTRY
11 = SAUSAGE 12 = MIXED 13 = NUTS/SEEDS 14 = SWEETS 15 = VEG/LEG 16 = MISC 22 = SOUP/SAUCE

Chol (mg)	Calc (mg)	Iron (mg)	Magn (mg)	Phos (mg)	Pota (mg)	Sodi (mg)	Zinc (mg)	VT-A (RE)	Thia (mg)	Ribo (mg)	Niac (mg)	V-B6 (mg)	Fola (µg)	VT-C (mg)
31	280	.6	33	251	417	149	1.02	73	.09	.41	.31	.1	12	2
17	284	.6	33	254	422	151	.91	143	.09	.41	.32	.1	12	2
7	287	.6	33	256	425	152	1.02	148	.1	.41	.32	.1	12	2
1	89	.29	23	88	223	139	.46	.3	.03	.17	.18	.04	3	.6
1	89	.29	23	88	223	139	.46	.3	.03	.17	.18	.04	3	.6
0	8	.68	21	28	128	45	.33	.4	<.01	.03	.11	<.01	4	t
33	300	.8	54	256	498	165	1.26	76	.1	.43	.32	.1	12	3
149	330	.51	47	278	420	138	1.17	203	.09	.48	.27	.13	2	4
1	13	.48	15	37	130	53	.17	4	.04	.04	.42	.04	4	t
34	304	.6	47	265	499	172	1.09	80	.13	.44	.62	.14	16	3
4	63	.15	20	75	159	103	.21	19	.11	.19	1.1	.08	10	.6
37	354	.27	52	303	529	223	1.14	94	.2	.59	1.31	.19	22	3
37	319	.88	47	288	567	273	1.15	64	.16	.69	.46	.14	10	1
32	344	.26	35	289	492	232	1.01	90	.13	.52	.52	.15	9	2
478	1405	.96	149	1075	2053	926	11.3	1064	.41	2.63	1.08	.49	22	6
59	176	.12	18	134	257	116	1.41	133	.05	.33	.13	.06	3	1
22	66	.04	7	50	97	44	.53	50	.02	.12	.05	.02	1	t
153	236	.43	25	199	338	153	1.99	199	.08	.45	.18	.1	9	1
701	1212	.83	131	927	1770	867	9.74	1758	.36	2.27	.93	.43	23	5
88	151	.1	16	115	221	108	1.21	219	.04	.28	.12	.05	2	1
146	1404	1.47	147	1035	2117	838	4.40	419	.61	2.78	.94	.68	21	6
18	176	.18	19	129	265	105	.55	52	.08	.35	.12	.09	3	1
13	274	.28	29	202	412	163	.86	44	.12	.54	.18	.13	5	1
113	827	2.47	124	594	1588	709	10.6	308	.26	.71	1.05	.2	108	31
14	103	.31	15	74	198	88	1.33	39	.03	.09	.13	.03	14	4

H

(For purposes of calculations, use "0" for t, <1, <.1, <.01, etc.)

TABLE H-1

Food Composition

Grp	Ref	Name	Measure	Wt (g)	H$_2$O (%)	Ener (kcal)	Prot (g)	Carb (g)	Fiber (g)	Fat (g)	Fat Breakdown (g)		
											Sat	Mono	Poly
DAIRY—Con.													
		Milk desserts, other:											
2	134	Custard, baked	1 cup	265	77	305	14	29	0	15	6.8	5.4	.7
		Pudding, canned:											
2	135	Chocolate	5 oz	142	68	205	3	30	.07	11	9.5	.5	.1
2	136	Tapioca	5 oz	142	74	160	3	28	0	5	4.8	.01	.01
2	137	Vanilla	5 oz	142	69	220	2	33	0	10	9.5	.25	.1
		Puddings, prepared from dry mix with whole milk:											
2	138	Chocolate, instant	1 cup	260	71	310	7.8	54	.26	7.5	4.6	2.2	.4
2	139	Chocolate, regular, cooked	½ cup	130	73	150	4	25	.14	4	2.4	1.1	.1
2	140	Rice	½ cup	132	73	155	4	27	.10	4	2.3	1.1	.1
2	141	Tapioca	½ cup	130	75	145	4	25	0	4	2.3	1.1	.1
2	142	Vanilla, instant	½ cup	130	73	150	4	27	0	4	2.2	1.1	.2
2	143	Vanilla, regular, cooked	½ cup	130	74	145	4	25	0	4	2.3	1	.1
2	144	Soybean milk	1 cup	263	92	87	8.9	5.8	0	4	.51	.74	2.08
		Yogurt, lowfat:											
2	145	Fruit added[13]	1 cup	227	74	231	9.9	43	.27	2.5	1.58	.67	.07
2	146	Plain	1 cup	227	85	144	11.9	16	0	3.5	2.27	.97	.1
2	147	Vanilla or coffee flavor	1 cup	227	79	193	11.2	31.3	0	2.8	1.84	.77	.09
2	148	Yogurt, made with nonfat milk	1 cup	227	85	127	13	17.4	0	.41	.26	.11	.01
2	149	Yogurt, made with whole milk	1 cup	227	88	138	7.9	10.6	0	7.4	4.76	2.02	.2
EGGS													
		Raw, large:											
3	150	Whole, without shell	1 ea	50	75	79	6.1	.6	0	5.6	1.67	2.23	.72
3	151	White	1 ea	33	88	16	3.4	.4	0	<.1	0	0	0
3	152	Yolk	1 ea	17	49	63	2.8	<.1	0	5.6	1.68	2.24	.73
		Cooked:											
3	153	Fried in butter	1 ea	46	72	95	5.4	.5	0	6.4	2.41	2.4	.7
3	154	Hard-cooked, shell removed	1 ea	50	75	79	6.1	.6	0	5.6	1.67	2.23	.72
3	155	Hard-cooked, chopped	1 cup	136	75	215	16.5	1.6	0	15.2	4.55	6.06	1.97
3	156	Poached	1 ea	50	74	79	6	.6	0	5.5	1.67	2.22	.72
3	157	Scrambled with milk and butter (also omelet)	1 ea	64	73	95	6	1.4	0	7.1	3.01	2.75	.76
FATS and OILS													
		Butter:											
4	158	Stick	½ cup	113	16	813	1	<.1	0	92	57.3	26.6	3.42
4	159	Tablespoon	1 tbsp	14.2	16	100	.1	<.1	0	11.5	7.18	3.33	.41
4	160	Pat (about 1 tsp)[15a]	1 ea	5	16	34	<.1	<.1	0	3.8	2.53	1.18	.15
		Fats, cooking (vegetable shortening):											
4	161	Cup	1 cup	205	0	1812	0	0	0	205	51.3	91.3	53.8
4	162	Tablespoon	1 tbsp	13	0	115	0	0	0	13	3.3	5.8	3.4
		Lard:											
4	163	Cup	1 cup	205	0	1849	0	0	0	205	80.4	92.5	23
4	164	Tablespoon	1 tbsp	13	0	115	0	0	0	13	5.1	5.9	1.5
		Margarine:											
		Imitation (about 40% fat) soft:											
4	165	8 ounce container	8 oz	227	58	785	1.1	.9	0	88	17.5	35.6	31.3
4	166	Tablespoon	1 tbsp	14.2	58	50	<.1	<.1	0	5.5	1.09	2.23	1.96
		Regular, hard (about 80% fat):											
4	167	Cup	½ cup	113	16	812	1	1	0	91	17.9	40.6	28.8
4	168	Tablespoon	1 tbsp	14	16	100	.1	.1	0	11.4	2.25	5.09	3.61
4	169	Pat[15a]	1 ea	5	16	36	<.1	<.1	0	4	.79	1.79	1.27

[13]Carbohydrate and kcalories vary widely—consult label if more precise values are needed.
[15a]Pat is 1 in square, ⅓ in high; 90 per lb.

(For purposes of calculations, use "0" for t, <1, <.1, <.01, etc.)

KEY: 1 = BEV 2 = DAIRY 3 = EGGS 4 = FAT/OIL 5 = FRUIT 6 = BAKERY 7 = GRAIN 8 = FISH 9 = BEEF 10 = POULTRY 11 = SAUSAGE 12 = MIXED 13 = NUTS/SEEDS 14 = SWEETS 15 = VEG/LEG 16 = MISC 22 = SOUP/SAUCE

Chol (mg)	Calc (mg)	Iron (mg)	Magn (mg)	Phos (mg)	Pota (mg)	Sodi (mg)	Zinc (mg)	VT-A (RE)	Thia (mg)	Ribo (mg)	Niac (mg)	V-B6 (mg)	Fola (µg)	VT-C (mg)
278	297	1.1	37	310	387	209	1.53	146	.11	.5	.3	.13	24	1
1	74	1.2	24	117	254	285	.70	31	.04	.17	.6	.03	3	t
1	119	.3	24	113	212	252	.70	t	.03	.14	.4	.03	3	t
1	79	.2	24	94	155	305	.70	t	.03	.12	.6	.03	3	t
28	260	.6	48	658	352	880	1.18	66	.08	.36	.22	.13	10	2
15	146	.4	24	120	190	167	.59	34	.05	.2	.1	.06	5	1
15	133	.5	16	110	165	140	.60	33	.10	.18	.6	.05	6	1
15	131	.1	16	103	167	152	.50	34	.04	.18	.1	.05	6	1
15	129	.1	16	273	164	375	.50	33	.04	.17	.1	.05	6	1
15	132	.1	16	102	166	178	.50	34	.04	.18	.1	.05	6	1
0	55	.8	57	126	340	55	.40	10	.02	.08	.5	.28	28	0
10	345	.16	33	271	442	133	1.68	25	.08	.4	.22	.09	21	2
14	415	.18	40	326	531	159	2.02	36	.10	.49	.26	.11	25	2
11	388	.16	36	306	497	150	1.88	30	.10	.46	.24	.1	23	2
4	452	.2	43	354	579	173	2.20	5	.11	.53	.28	.12	28	2
29	275	.11	27	216	352	104	1.34	68	.07	.32	.17	.07	16	1
274	28	1.04	6	90	65	69	.61	78	.04	.15	.03	.06	32	0
0	4	.01	3	4	45	50	.06	0	<.01	.09	.03	<.01	5	0
272	26	.95	3	86	15	8	.55	94	.04	.07	.01	.05	26	0
278	28	.92	5	90	58	162	.64	94	.04	.13	.03	.05	22	0
274	28	1.04	6	90	65	69	.72	78	.04	.14	.03	.06	24	0
745	76	2.84	17	245	177	188	1.96	212	.10	.39	.08	.15	67	0
273	28	1.04	6	90	65	146	.72	78	.04	.13	.03	.05	24	0
282	54	.93	109	109	97	176	.7	102	.04	.18	.04	.06	22	t
247	27	.18	2	26	29	933[14]	.06	852[15]	<.01	.04	.05	<.01	3	0
31	3	.02	<1	3	4	116[14]	<.01	106[15]	<.01	<.01	<.01	t	<1	0
11	1	<.01	<1	1	1	41[14]	<.01	38[15]	t	<.01	<.01	t	<1	0
0	0	0	0	0	0	0	.1	0	0	0	0	0	0	0
0	0	0	0	0	0	0	0	0	0	0	0	0	0	0
195	t	0	<1	6	t	t	.23	0	0	0	0	0	0	0
12	t	0	<1	<1	t	t	.01	0	0	0	0	0	0	0
0	40	0	2	31	57	2178[16]	.23	2254[17]	.01	.05	.03	.01	2	t
0	2.5	0	<1	2	4	136[16]	.03	141[17]	<.01	<.01	<.01	<.01	<1	t
0	34	.07	3	26	48	1066[16]	.23	1122[17]	.01	.04	.03	.01	1	t
0	4.2	<.01	<1	3	6	133[16]	.03	139[17]	<.01	<.01	<.01	<.01	<1	t
0	1.5	<.01	<1	1	2	47[16]	.01	50[17]	t	<.01	<.01	t	<1	t

H

(14)For salted butter; unsalted butter contains 12 mg sodium per stick or ½ cup, 1.5 mg per tablespoon, or .5 mg per pat.
(15)Values for vitamin A are a year-round average.
(16)For salted margarine.
(17)Based on average vitamin A content of fortified margarine. Federal specifications require a minimum of 15,000 IU per pound.

(For purposes of calculations, use "0" for t, <1, <.1, <.01, etc.)

TABLE H–1

Food Composition

Grp	Ref	Name	Measure	Wt (g)	H₂O (%)	Ener (kcal)	Prot (g)	Carb (g)	Fiber (g)	Fat (g)	Fat Breakdown (g)		
											Sat	Mono	Poly
FATS and OILS—Con.													
		Margarine:—continued											
		Regular, soft (about 80% fat):											
4	170	8 ounce container	8 oz	227	16	1626	1.8	1.1	0	183	31.3	64.7	78.5
4	171	Tablespoon	1 tbsp	14	16	100	1.1	<.1	0	11.4	1.96	4.04	4.91
		Spread (about 60% fat), hard:											
4	172	Cup	½ cup	113	37	610	.7	0	0	68.7	15.9	29.3	20.4
4	173	Tablespoon	1 tbsp	14	37	75	<.1	0	0	8.5	1.97	3.6	2.52
4	174	Pat[15a]	1 ea	5	37	25	<.1	0	0	3	.71	1.31	.91
		Spread (about 60% fat) soft:											
4	175	8 ounce container	8 oz	227	37	1225	1.4	0	0	138	29.1	71.5	31.3
4	176	Tablespoon	1 tbsp	14	37	75	<.1	0	0	8.5	1.79	4.41	1.93
		Oils:											
		Corn:											
4	177	Cup	1 cup	218	0	1927	0	0	0	218	27.7	52.7	128
4	178	Tablespoon	1 tbsp	14	0	125	0	0	0	14	1.8	3.4	8.2
		Olive:											
4	179	Cup	1 cup	216	0	1909	0	0	0	216	29.2	159	18.1
4	180	Tablespoon	1 tbsp	14	0	125	0	0	0	14	1.9	10.3	1.2
		Peanut:											
4	181	Cup	1 cup	216	0	1909	0	0	0	216	36.4	99.9	69.2
4	182	Tablespoon	1 tbsp	14	0	125	0	0	0	14	2.4	6.5	4.5
		Safflower:											
4	183	Cup	1 cup	218	0	1927	0	0	0	218	19.8	26.4	162
4	184	Tablespoon	1 tbsp	14	0	125	0	0	0	14	1.3	1.7	10.4
		Soybean:											
4	185	Cup	1 cup	218	0	1927	0	0	0	218	32.5	93.8	82
4	186	Tablespoon	1 tbsp	14	0	125	0	0	0	14	2.1	6	5.3
		Soybean/cottonseed:											
4	187	Cup	1 cup	218	0	1927	0	0	0	218	39.2	64.4	105
4	188	Tablespoon	1 tbsp	14	0	125	0	0	0	14	2.5	4.1	6.7
		Sunflower:											
4	189	Cup	1 cup	218	0	1927	0	0	0	218	22.5	42.6	143
4	190	Tablespoon	1 tbsp	14	0	125	0	0	0	14	1.4	2.7	9.2
		Salad dressings/sandwich spreads:											
4	191	Blue cheese:	1 tbsp	15	32	75	.7	1.1	.01	8	1.5	1.9	4.3
		French:											
4	192	Regular	1 tbsp	16	35	85	<.1	1	.13	9	1.4	4	3.5
4	193	Low calorie	1 tbsp	16	75	24	<.1	2.5	.05	2	.2	.3	1
		Italian:											
4	194	Regular	1 tbsp	14	34	80	.1	1	.03	9.	1.3	3.7	3.2
4	195	Low calorie	1 tbsp	15	86	5	<.1	.7	.04	.9	.12	.18	.54
		Mayonnaise:											
4	196	Regular	1 tbsp	13.8	15	100	.2	.4	0	11	1.7	3.2	5.8
4	197	Imitation	1 tbsp	15	63	35	0	2	0	3	.5	.7	1.6
4	198	Ranch style	½ cup	119	35	435	3.6	5.5	0	45.1	6.72	19.4	17
4	199	Salad dressing-mayo type	1 tbsp	15	40	58	.1	3.5	0	4.9	.7	1.4	2.7
4	200	Tartar sauce	1 tbsp	14	34	74	.2	.6	.04	8.1	1.2	2.6	3.9
		Thousand Island:											
4	201	Regular	1 tbsp	16	46	60	.1	2.4	.03	5.7	.97	1.32	3.17
4	202	Low calorie	1 tbsp	15	69	25	.1	2.5	.18	1.6	.24	.4	.9
		Salad dressings, prepared from home recipe:											
4	203	Cooked type[18]	1 tbsp	16	69	25	.7	2.4	0	1.5	.5	.6	.3
4	204	Vinegar & oil	1 tbsp	16	47	70	0	0	0	8	1.5	2.4	3.9

[18]Fatty acid values apply to product made with regular margarine.

(For purposes of calculations, use "0" for t, <1, <.1, <.01, etc.)

KEY: 1 = BEV 2 = DAIRY 3 = EGGS 4 = FAT/OIL 5 = FRUIT 6 = BAKERY 7 = GRAIN 8 = FISH 9 = BEEF 10 = POULTRY 11 = SAUSAGE 12 = MIXED 13 = NUTS/SEEDS 14 = SWEETS 15 = VEG/LEG 16 = MISC 22 = SOUP/SAUCE

Chol (mg)	Calc (mg)	Iron (mg)	Magn (mg)	Phos (mg)	Pota (mg)	Sodi (mg)	Zinc (mg)	VT-A (RE)	Thia (mg)	Ribo (mg)	Niac (mg)	V-B6 (mg)	Fola (µg)	VT-C (mg)
0	60	0	5	46	86	2448[16]	.46	2254[17]	.02	.07	.04	.02	2	t
0	4	0	<1	3	5	153[16]	.03	140[17]	<.01	<.01	<.01	<.01	<1	t
0	24	0	2	18	34	1123[16]	.17	1122[17]	<.01	.03	.02	<.01	<1	t
0	3	0	<1	2	4	139[16]	.02	139[17]	<.01	<.01	<.01	<.01	<1	t
0	1	0	<1	1	1	50[16]	<.01	50[17]	t	<.01	<.01	t	<1	t
0	47	0	4	37	68	2256[16]	.34	2254[17]	.16	.06	.04	.01	2	t
0	3	0	<1	2	4	139[16]	.02	139[17]	.01	<.01	<.01	<.01	<1	t
0	0	0	—	0	0	0	.4	0	0	0	0	0	<1	0
0	0	0	—	0	0	0	.03	0	0	0	0	0	0	0
0	.4	.83	<1	3	0	0	.13	0	0	0	0	0	<1	0
0	t	.05	<1	t	0	0	<.01	0	0	0	0	0	0	0
0	t	.06	<1	0	0	0	.02	t	0	0	0	0	<1	0
0	t	<.01	<1	0	0	0	<.01	t	0	0	0	0	0	0
0	0	0	—	0	0	0	.41	0	0	0	0	0	0	0
0	0	0	—	0	0	0	.03	0	0	0	0	0	0	0
0	.1	.05	<1	1	0	0	.4	0	0	0	0	0	<1	0
0	t	0	<1	t	0	0	.03	0	0	0	0	0	t	0
0	0	0	—	0	0	0	.4	0	0	0	0	0	<1	0
0	0	0	—	0	0	0	.03	0	0	0	0	0	0	0
0	0	0	0	0	0	0	—	0	0	0	0	0	0	0
0	0	0	0	0	0	0	—	0	0	0	0	0	0	0
3	12	.03	<1	11	6	.3	.28	10	<.01	.02	.01	<.01	8	t
0	2	.06	<1	1	2	188	.01	t	t	t	t	<.01	0	t
0	6	.07	—	5	3	306	.03	t	t	t	t	0	t	t
0	1	.03	<1	1	5	162	.02	3	t	t	t	.03	0	t
0	1	.03	<1	1	4	136	0	t	t	t	t	0	t	t
8	2	.07	<1	4	5	80	.02	12	<.01	<.01	<.01	<.01	<1	0
4	0	0	—	0	2	75	—	0	0	0	0	0	t	0
47	119	.31	12	100	158	522	.43	86	.04	.17	.08	.05	6	1
4	2	.03	<1	4	1	105	0	13	<.01	<.01	t	<.01	t	0
4	3	.1	<1	4	11	182	.02	9	<.01	<.01	<.01	<.01	<1	t
4	2	.09	<1	3	18	110	.03	15	<.01	<.01	.03	<.01	6	t
2	2	.09	<1	3	17	153	0	14	<.01	<.01	.03	<.01	<1	t
9	13	.08	—	14	19	117	0	20	.01	.02	.04	0	<1	t
0	0	0	—	0	1	0	—	0	0	0	0	0	—	0

[16] For salted margarine.
[17] Based on average vitamin A content of fortified margarine. Federal specifications require a minimum of 15,000 IU per pound.

(For purposes of calculations, use "0" for t, <1, <.1, <.01, etc.)

H

TABLE H–1

Food Composition

Grp	Ref	Name	Measure	Wt (g)	H₂O (%)	Ener (kcal)	Prot (g)	Carb (g)	Fiber (g)	Fat (g)	Fat Breakdown (g) Sat	Mono	Poly
		FRUITS and FRUIT JUICES											
		Apples:											
		Raw, with peel:											
5	205	2¾″ diam (about 3 per lb with cores)	1 ea	138	84	80	.3	21	4.28	.5	.1	.02	.14
5	206	3¼″ diam (about 2 per lb with cores)	1 ea	212	84	125	.4	32	6.58	.8	.12	.03	.22
5	207	Raw, peeled slices	1 cup	110	84	65	.2	16	2.92	.3	.06	.01	.1
5	208	Dried, sulfured	10 ea	64	32	155	.6	42.2	9.01	.2	.03	<.01	.06
5	209	Apple juice, bottled or canned[21]	1 cup	248	88	116	.1	29	.52	.3	.05	.01	.08
		Applesauce:											
5	210	Sweetened	1 cup	255	80	195	.5	51	3.6	.5	.08	.02	.14
5	211	Unsweetened	1 cup	244	88	106	.4	27.5	5.12	.1	.02	<.01	.03
		Apricots:											
5	212	Raw, without pits (about 12 per lb with pits)	3 ea	106	86	51	1.5	11.8	2.23	.4	.03	.18	.08
		Canned (fruit and liquid):											
5	213	Heavy syrup	1 cup	258	78	214	1.4	55.4	4.3	.2	.01	.09	.04
5	214	Halves	3 ea	85	78	70	.5	18.3	1.42	<.1	<.01	.03	.01
5	215	Juice pack	1 cup	248	87	119	1.6	30.6	4.38	<.1	<.01	.04	.02
5	216	Halves	3 ea	84	87	40	.5	10.4	1.45	<.1	<.01	.01	<.01
		Dried:											
5	217	Dried halves	10 ea	35	31	83	1.3	21.6	3.5	.2	.01	.07	.03
5	218	Cooked, unsweetened, with liquid	1 cup	250	75	210	3.2	54.8	7.5	.4	.03	.18	.08
5	219	Apricot nectar, canned	1 cup	251	85	141	.9	36.1	1.51	.2	.01	.10	.04
		Avocado, raw, edible part only:											
5	220	California (½ lb with refuse)	1 ea	173	73	305	4	12	4.84	30	4.48	19.4	3.53
5	221	Florida (1 lb with refuse)	1 ea	304	80	340	5	27	8.51	27	5.34	14.8	4.5
5	222	Mashed, fresh, average	1 cup	230	74	370	4.6	17	6.43	35.2	5.61	22.1	4.5
		Bananas, raw, without peel:											
5	223	Whole, 8¾″ long (weighs 175g with peel)	1 ea	114	74	105	1.2	26.7	3.26	.5	.21	.05	.1
5	224	Slices	1 cup	150	74	138	1.6	35.1	4.29	.7	.28	.06	.13
5	225	Blackberries, raw	1 cup	144	86	74	1	18.4	9.72	.6	.25	.12	.14
		Blueberries:											
5	226	Raw	1 cup	145	85	82	1	20.5	4.93	.6	.04	.17	.34
		Frozen, sweetened:											
5	227	10 oz container	10 oz	284	77	230	1.2	62.4	8.52	.4	.07	.1	.2
5	228	Cup	1 cup	230	77	185	.9	50.5	6.9	.3	.06	.08	.17
		Cherries:											
5	229	Sour, red pitted, canned water pack	1 cup	244	90	90	1.9	21.8	2.68	.2	.06	.07	.07
5	230	Sweet, raw, without pits	10 ea	68	81	49	.8	11.3	1.25	.7	.1	.2	.2
		Cranberry juices:											
5	231	Cranberry juice cocktail[26]	1 cup	253	85	145	<.1[24]	36.6	.76	.1	.01	.03	.07
5	232	Cranberry-apple juice	1 cup	253	86	169	.1	43	.63	1.3[25]	.23	.06	.4
5	233	Cranberry sauce, canned, strained	1 cup	277	61	419	.6	108	2	.4	.05	.11	.24
		Dates:											
5	234	Whole, without pits	10 ea	83	22	228	1.6	61	7.23	.4	.16	.11	.02
5	235	Chopped	1 cup	178	22	489	3.5	131	15.5	.8	.35	.24	.05

[21]Also applies to pasteurized apple cider.
[24]The newest USDA Handbook 8-14 data on beverages indicates "0" for protein.
[25]The newest USDA Handbook 8-14 data on beverages indicates "0" for fat.
[26]Data here is from the newest USDA Handbook 8-14 on beverages. This data is somewhat different from that presented in Handbook 8-9 on fruits and fruit juices.

H

(For purposes of calculations, use "0" for t, <1, <.1, <.01, etc.)

KEY: 1 = BEV 2 = DAIRY 3 = EGGS 4 = FAT/OIL 5 = FRUIT 6 = BAKERY 7 = GRAIN 8 = FISH 9 = BEEF 10 = POULTRY
11 = SAUSAGE 12 = MIXED 13 = NUTS/SEEDS 14 = SWEETS 15 = VEG/LEG 16 = MISC 22 = SOUP/SAUCE

Chol (mg)	Calc (mg)	Iron (mg)	Magn (mg)	Phos (mg)	Pota (mg)	Sodi (mg)	Zinc (mg)	VT-A (RE)	Thia (mg)	Ribo (mg)	Niac (mg)	V-B6 (mg)	Fola (μg)	VT-C (mg)
0	10	.25	6	10	159	1	.05	7	.02	.02	.11	.07	4	8
0	15	.38	9	23	244	1.5	.08	11	.04	.03	.16	.1	6	12
0	4	.1	3	8	124	.8	.04	5	.02	.01	.1	.05	<1	4
0	9	.9	10	24	288	56[20]	.13	0	0	.1	.59	.08	<1	3
0	17	.92	8	17	295	7	.07	t	.05	.04	.25	.07	<1	2[19]
0	10	1	7	18	156	8	.1	3	.03	.07	.50	.07	2	4[19]
0	7	.29	7	18	183	5	.06	7	.03	.06	.46	.06	2	3[19]
0	15	.58	8	21	313	1	.28	277	.03	.04	.64	.06	9	10.6
0	23	.77	18	33	361	10	.27	317	.05	.06	.97	.14	4	8
0	7	.26	6	10	119	3	.09	105	.02	.02	.32	.05	1	3
0	30	.74	24	50	409	9	.27	419	.04	.05	.85	.18	5	12
0	10	.25	8	17	139	3	.1	142	.01	.02	.29	.06	2	4
0	16	1.65	16	41	482	3	.26	253	<.01	.05	1.05	.06	4	1
0	40	4.2	42	103	1222	8	.66	591	.01	.07	2.36	.28	0	4
0	18	.96	13	23	286	8	.23	330	.02	.04	.65	.16	3	2[22]
0	19	2.04	70	73	1097	21	.73	106	.19	.21	3.32	.48	113	14
0	33	1.6	104	119	1484	14	1.28	186	.33	.37	5.84	.85	162	24
0	25	2.3	90	95	1378	24	.97	141	.25	.28	4.42	.64	142	18
0	7	.35	32	22	451	1	.19	9	.05	.11	.62	.66	24	10
0	9	.46	43	29	593	1	.25	12	.07	.15	.81	.87	31	13
0	46	.8	29	30	282	0	.39	24	.04	.06	.58	.08	49	30
0	9	.24	7	15	129	9	.16	15	.07	.07	.7	.05	9	20
0	16	1.11	7	20	169	4	.14	12	.06	.15	.72	.17	19	3
0	13	.9	6	16	138	3	.14	10	.05	.12	.58	.14	16	2
0	27	3.34	15	25	240	17	.17	184	.04	.1	.43	.11	20	5
0	10	.3	8	13	152	0	.04	15	.03	.04	.3	.02	3	5
0	8	.38	5	5	45	5	.177	1	.02	.02	.09	.05	.5	90[23]
0	18	.15	5	7	68	5	.1	t	.01	.05	.15	.06	<1	81[23]
0	11	.61	8	17	72	80	.09	6	.04	.06	.28	.05	2	6
0	27	1	29	33	541	2	.24	4	.07	.08	1.83	.16	14	0
0	58	2.14	63	70	1161	5	.52	9	.16	.18	3.92	.34	29	0

[19]Value based on products without added ascorbic acid. Bottled apple juice with added ascorbic acid usually contains 41.6 mg/100 g or 103 mg vitamin C per cup. Check label for specific vitamin C values.
[20]Sodium bisulfite used to preserve color; unsulfured product would contain lower levels of sodium.
[22]Without added ascorbic acid. Products with added ascorbic acid contain 136 mg per cup. Check label.
[23]Source added.

(For purposes of calculations, use "0" for t, <1, <.1, <.01, etc.)

TABLE H-1

Food Composition

Grp	Ref	Name	Measure	Wt (g)	H₂O (%)	Ener (kcal)	Prot (g)	Carb (g)	Fiber (g)	Fat (g)	Fat Breakdown (g)		
											Sat	Mono	Poly
		FRUITS and FRUIT JUICES—Con.											
5	236	Figs, dried	10 ea	187	28	477	5.7	122	24	2.2	.44	.48	1.05
		Fruit cocktail, canned, fruit and liquid:											
5	237	Heavy syrup pack	1 cup	255	80	185	1	48.2	2.52	.2	.03	.03	.08
5	238	Juice pack	1 cup	248	87	115	1.1	29.4	2.52	<.1	<.01	<.01	.01
		Grapefruit:											
		Raw 3¾ in diam, whole fruit weighs 1 lb 1 oz with refuse (peel, membrane, seeds):											
5	239	Pink/red, half fruit[27], edible part	1 half	123	91	37	.7	9.4	1.53	.1	.02	.02	.03
5	240	White, half fruit[27], edible part	1 half	118	90	39	.8	9.9	1.46	.1	.02	.01	.03
5	241	Canned sections with liquid	1 cup	254	84	152	1.4	39.2	2.24	.2	.04	.03	.06
		Grapefruit juice:											
5	242	Raw	1 cup	247	90	96	1.2	22.7	.37	.2	.04	.03	.06
		Canned:											
5	243	Unsweetened	1 cup	247	90	93	1.3	22.1	.25	.2	.03	.03	.06
5	244	Sweetened	1 cup	250	87	115	1.4	27.8	.25	.2	.03	.03	.05
		Frozen concentrate, unsweetened:											
5	245	Undiluted, 6 fl oz can	¾ cup	207	62	300	4	72	.83	1	.13	.13	.23
5	246	Diluted with 3 cans water	1 cup	247	89	102	1.4	24	.25	.3	.05	.04	.08
		Grapes, raw, European type (adherent skin):											
5	247	Thompson seedless	10 ea	50	81	35	.3	8.9	1	.3	.1	.01	.09
5	248	Tokay/Emperor, seeded types	10 ea	57	81	40	.4	10.1	1.14	.3	.11	.01	.1
		Grape juice:											
5	249	Bottled or canned	1 cup	253	84	155	1.4	37.9	1.26	.2	.06	<.01	.06
		Frozen concentrate, sweetened:											
5	250	Undiluted, 6 fl oz can	¾ cup	216	54	385	1.4	95.8	3.75	.7	.22	.03	.2
5	251	Diluted with 3 cans water	1 cup	250	87	128	.5	31.9	1.25	.2	.07	.01	.07
5	252	Kiwi fruit, raw, peeled (about 5 per lb with skin):	1 ea	76	83	46	.8	11.3	1.16	.3	<.01	.14	.14
5	253	Lemons, raw, without peel and seeds (about 4 per lb whole)	1 ea	58	89	17	.6	5.4	1.19	.2	.02	<.01	.05
		Lemon juice:											
		Fresh:											
5	254	Cup	1 cup	244	91	60	.9	21.1	.85	0	0	0	0
5	255	Tablespoon	1 tbsp	15.2	91	4	<.1	1.3	.05	0	0	0	0
		Canned or bottled, unsweetened:											
5	256	Cup	1 cup	244	92	52	1	15.8	.73	.7	.09	.03	.21
5	257	Tablespoon	1 tbsp	15	92	5	<.1	1	.05	<.1	<.01	<.01	.13
		Frozen, single strength, unsweetened:											
5	258	Cup	1 cup	244	92	54	1.1	15.9	.79	.8	.1	.03	.24
5	259	Tablespoon	1 tbsp	15	92	3	<.1	1	.05	<.1	<.01	<.01	.01
		Lime juice:											
		Fresh:											
5	260	Cup	1 cup	246	90	65	1.1	22.2	.98	.2	.03	.03	.07
5	261	Tablespoon	1 tbsp	15	90	4	<.1	1.4	.06	<.1	<.01	<.01	<.01
5	262	Canned or bottled, unsweetened	1 cup	246	92	50	1	16	.86	1	.06	.05	.16

[27]Weight is for edible portion. Weight with rind is 241 grams for one half.

(For purposes of calculations, use "0" for t, <1, <.1, <.01, etc.)

KEY: 1 = BEV 2 = DAIRY 3 = EGGS 4 = FAT/OIL 5 = FRUIT 6 = BAKERY 7 = GRAIN 8 = FISH 9 = BEEF 10 = POULTRY
11 = SAUSAGE 12 = MIXED 13 = NUTS/SEEDS 14 = SWEETS 15 = VEG/LEG 16 = MISC 22 = SOUP/SAUCE

Chol (mg)	Calc (mg)	Iron (mg)	Magn (mg)	Phos (mg)	Pota (mg)	Sodi (mg)	Zinc (mg)	VT-A (RE)	Thia (mg)	Ribo (mg)	Niac (mg)	V-B6 (mg)	Fola (µg)	VT-C (mg)
0	269	4.18	111	128	1331	21	.94	25	.13	.17	1.3	.42	16	1
0	16	.73	14	28	224	15	.21	52	.05	.05	.95	.11	1	5
0	20	.53	17	34	235	10	.21	76	.03	.04	1	.13	2	7
0	13	.15	10	11	158	0	.09	32[28]	.04	.03	.23	.05	15	47
0	14	.07	11	9	175	0	.08	1	.04	.02	.32	.05	12	39
0	36	1.02	25	25	328	4	.21	0	.1	.05	.62	.05	22	54
0	22	.49	30	37	400	2	.13	2[29]	.1	.05	.49	.11	52	94
0	17	.49	24	27	378	2	.22	2	.1	.05	.57	.05	26	72
0	20	.9	24	28	405	5	.15	2	.1	.06	.8	.05	26	67
0	56	1.02	78	101	1002	6	.38	6	.3	.16	1.6	.32	26	248
0	20	.34	26	34	337	2	.12	2	.1	.05	.54	.11	52	83
0	5	.13	3	7	92	1	.03	4	.05	.03	.15	.06	4	5.4
0	6	.15	4	8	105	1	.03	4	.05	.03	.17	.06	4	6.2
0	22	.61	24	27	334	8	.13	2	.07	.09	.66	.16	6	t[30]
0	28	.78	32	32	160	15	.28	6	.11	.2	.93	.32	9	179[31]
0	10	.26	11	11	53	5	.10	2	.04	.07	.31	.1	4	60[31]
0	20	.3	23	30	252	4	.08[32]	13	.02	.04	.4	.04[32]	17[32]	74.5
0	15	.35	2	9	80	1	.06	2	.02	.01	.06	.05	7	31
0	18	.08	16	14	303	2	.12	5	.07	.02	.24	.12	32	112
0	1	<.01	1	1	19	.1	<.01	t	<.01	<.01	.01	<.01	2	7
0	26	.31	22	21	248	50[33]	.15	4	.10	.02	.48	.1	25	61
0	2	.02	1	1	15	3[33]	.01	t	<.01	<.01	.03	<.01	2	4
0	19	.30	20	20	218	4	.12	3	.14	.03	.33	.15	23	77
0	1	.02	1	1	14	.2	<.01	t	<.01	<.01	.02	<.01	1	5
0	22	.08	14	18	268	2	.15	3	.05	.03	.25	.11	21	72
0	1	<.01	1	1	17	.1	.01	t	<.01	<.01	.01	.08	1	4.5
0	30	.6	16	25	185	39[33]	.15	4	.08	.01	.4	.07	20	16

(28)Vitamin A in texas red grapefruit would be 74 RE.
(29)Vitamin A for white grapefruit juice; pink or red grapefruit juice = 109 RE per cup.
(30)Without added ascorbic acid.
(31)With added ascorbic acid.
(32)Data is estimated from other fruit data.
(33)Sodium benzoate and sodium bisulfite added as preservatives.

(For purposes of calculations, use "0" for t, <1, <.1, <.01, etc.)

TABLE H–1

Food Composition

Grp	Ref	Name	Measure	Wt (g)	H$_2$O (%)	Ener (kcal)	Prot (g)	Carb (g)	Fiber (g)	Fat (g)	Sat	Mono	Poly
											Fat Breakdown (g)		
		FRUITS and FRUIT JUICES—Con.											
5	263	Mango, raw, edible part (weighs 300g with skin and seed)	1 ea	207	82	135	1.1	35.2	2.86	.6	.14	.21	.11
		Melons, raw, without rind and cavity contents:												
5	264	Cantaloupe, 5 in diam (2⅛ lb whole, (with refuse) orange flesh:	½ ea	267	90	94	2.4	22.3	2.67	.7	.12	.14	.24
5	265	Honeydew, 6½ in diam (5¼ lb whole with refuse) slice = ¹⁄₁₀ melon	1 pce	129	90	45	.6	11.8	1.40	.1	.02	.02	.04
5	266	Nectarines, raw, without pits, 2½ in diam	1 ea	136	86	67	1.3	16	3.13	.6	.1	.2	.3
		Oranges, raw:												
5	267	Whole without peel and seeds 2⅝ in diam (weighs about 180g with peel and seeds)	1 ea	131	87	60	1.2	15.4	2.97	.2	.02	.03	.03
5	268	Sections, without membranes	1 cup	180	87	85	1.7	21.2	4.09	.2	.03	.04	.04
		Orange juice:												
5	269	Fresh, all varieties:	1 cup	248	88	111	1.7	25.8	.5	.5	.06	.09	.1
5	270	Canned, unsweetened	1 cup	249	89	105	1.5	24.5	.25	.4	.04	.06	.09
5	271	Chilled	1 cup	249	88	110	2	25	1	.7	.07	.12	.16
		Frozen concentrate:												
5	272	Undiluted (6 oz can)	¾ cup	213	58	339	5.1	81.3	2.99	.4	.05	.08	.09
5	273	Diluted with 3 parts water by volume	1 cup	249	88	110	1.7	26.8	1	.1	.02	.03	.03
5	274	Orange and grapefruit juice, canned	1 cup	247	89	105	1.5	25.4	.49	.2	.03	.04	.05
		Papaya, raw:												
5	275	½ in	1 cup	140	89	60	.9	13.7	2.38	.2	.06	.05	.04
5	276	Whole fruit, cubes, 3½ in diam by 5⅛ in, without seeds and skin, (1 lb with refuse)	1 ea	304	89	117	1.9	29.8	5.17	.4	.13	.12	.09
		Peaches:												
		Raw:												
5	277	Whole, 2½ in diam, peeled, pitted (about 4 per lb with peels and pits)	1 ea	87	88	37	.6	9.6	2	<.1	<.01	.03	.04
5	278	Sliced	1 cup	170	88	73	1.2	18.9	3.91	.2	.02	.06	.08
		Canned, fruit and liquid:												
		Heavy syrup pack												
5	279	Cup	1 cup	256	79	190	1.2	51	4.2	.2	.03	.09	.12
5	280	Half	1 ea	81	79	60	.4	16.2	1.33	<.1	<.01	.03	.04
		Juice pack												
5	281	Cup	1 cup	248	88	109	1.6	28.7	4.10	<.1	.01	.03	.04
5	282	Half	1 ea	77	88	34	.5	8.9	1.27	<.1	<.01	<.01	.01
		Dried:												
5	283	Uncooked	10 ea	130	32	311	4.7	79.7	10.3	1.0	.11	.36	.48
5	284	Cooked, fruit and liquid	1 cup	258	78	200	3	50.8	4.62	.6	.07	.23	.3
		Frozen, sliced, sweetened:												
5	285	10 oz package	1 ea	284	75	267	1.8	68	6.25	.4	.04	.14	.18
5	286	Cup, thawed measure	1 cup	250	75	235	1.6	60	5.50	.3	.04	.12	.16
		Pears:												
		Raw, with skin, cored:												
5	287	Bartlett, 2½ in diam (about 2½ per lb, whole)	1 ea	166	84	98	.7	25.1	4.98[36]	.7	.04	.14	.16

[36] Dietary fiber data varies 2.4-3.4 grams per 100 grams for fresh pears; 1.6-2.6 grams per 100 grams for canned pears.

(For purposes of calculations, use "0" for t, <1, <.1, <.01, etc.)

KEY: 1 = BEV 2 = DAIRY 3 = EGGS 4 = FAT/OIL 5 = FRUIT 6 = BAKERY 7 = GRAIN 8 = FISH 9 = BEEF 10 = POULTRY
11 = SAUSAGE 12 = MIXED 13 = NUTS/SEEDS 14 = SWEETS 15 = VEG/LEG 16 = MISC 22 = SOUP/SAUCE

Chol (mg)	Calc (mg)	Iron (mg)	Magn (mg)	Phos (mg)	Pota (mg)	Sodi (mg)	Zinc (mg)	VT-A (RE)	Thia (mg)	Ribo (mg)	Niac (mg)	V-B6 (mg)	Fola (µg)	VT-C (mg)
0	21	.26	18	22	323	4	.07	806	.12	.12	1.21	.28	39	57
0	29	.56	19	45	825	24	.43	861	.1	.06	1.53	.31	80	113
0	8	.09	9	13	350	13	.11	5	.1	.02	.77	.08	39	32
0	6	.21	11	22	288	0	.12	100	.02	.06	1.35	.03	5	7
0	52	.14	13	18	237	t	.09	27	.11	.05	.37	.08	40	70
0	72	.19	18	25	326	t	.4	37	.16	.07	.51	.11	83	96
0	27	.50	27	42	496	2	.12	50	.22	.07	.99	.1	109	124
0	20	1.1	27	35	436	5	.17	44	.15	.07	.78	.22	15	86
0	25	.42	28	27	473	2	.11	19[34]	.28	.05	.7	.13	45[34]	82[34]
0	68	.75	73	121	1436	6	.38	59	.6	.14	1.53	.33	331	294
0	22	.27	24	40	474	2	.13	19	.2	.04	.5	.11	109	97
0	20	1.1	24	35	390	7	.18	29	.14	.07	.83	.06	20	72
0	33	.3	14	12	247	9	.10	282	.04	.04	.47	.03	26	92
0	72	.3	31	16	780	8	.22	612	.08	.10	1.03	.06	48	188
0	4	.1	6	10	171	0	.12	47	.01	.04	.86	.02	3	6
0	9	.19	11	20	335	1	.18	91	.03	.07	1.68	.03	6	11
0	8	.69	13	29	235	16	.22	85	.03	.06	1.57	.05	8	7
0	2	.22	4	9	75	5	.07	27	<.01	.02	.5	.01	3	2
0	15	.72	18	43	317	11	.26	94	.02	.04	1.44	.05	8	9
0	5	.21	6	13	98	3	.09	29	<.01	.01	.45	.01	3	3
0	37	5.28	54	155	1295	9	.74	281	<.01	.28	5.69	.09	6	6
0	23	3.37	35	99	825	6	.46	51	.01	.05	3.92	.1	<1	10
0	9	1.05	14	31	369	17	.14	81	.04	.10	1.9	.05	9	268[35]
0	8	.93	12	28	325	16	.13	71	.03	.09	1.63	.04	8	236[35]
0	19	.41	9	18	208	1	.20	3	.03	.07	.17	.03	12	7

H

[34]Values for juice from California oranges indicates the following values for 1 cup: 36 RE of vitamin A, 72 µg of folacin and 106 mg of vitamin C.
[35]With added ascorbic acid.

(For purposes of calculations, use "0" for t, <1, <.1, <.01, etc.)

TABLE H–1

Food Composition

Grp	Ref	Name	Measure	Wt (g)	H$_2$O (%)	Ener (kcal)	Prot (g)	Carb (g)	Fiber (g)	Fat (g)	Sat	Mono	Poly
		FRUITS and FRUIT JUICES—Con.											
		Pears, raw, with skin, cored:— continued											
5	288	Bosc, 2½ in diam (about 3 per lb, whole)	1 ea	141	84	85	.6	21	4.23[36]	.5	.05	.1	.1
5	289	D'Anjou, 3 in diam (about ½ lb, whole)	1 ea	200	84	120	.8	30	6[36]	.7	.05	.2	.2
		Canned, fruit and liquid:											
		Heavy syrup pack:											
5	290	Cup	1 cup	255	80	188	.5	48.9	5[36]	.3	.02	.07	.08
5	291	Half	1 ea	79	80	59	.2	15.1	1.55[36]	.1	<.01	.02	.02
		Juice pack:											
5	292	Cup	1 cup	248	86	123	.8	32.1	5[36]	.2	.01	.04	.04
5	293	Half	1 ea	77	86	38	.3	10	1.55[36]	<.1	<.01	<.01	<.01
5	294	Dried halves	10 ca	175	27	459	3.3	122	19.1	1.1	.06	.23	.26
		Pineapple:											
5	295	Raw chunks, dices	1 cup	155	86	76	.6	19.2	2.95	.7	.05	.07	.23
		Canned, fruit and liquid:											
		Heavy syrup pack:											
5	296	Crushed, chunks, tidbits	1 cup	255	79	199	.9	51.5	2.43	.3	.02	.03	.10
5	297	Slices	1 ea	58	79	45	.2	11.7	.55	<.1	<.01	<.01	.02
		Juice pack:											
5	298	Crushed, chunks, tidbits	1 cup	250	84	150	1	39.2	2.48	.2	.01	.03	.07
5	299	Slices	1 ea	58	84	35	.2	9.1	.57	<.1	<.01	<.01	.02
5	300	Pineapple juice, canned, unsweetened	1 cup	250	86	140	.8	34.4	.75	.2	.01	.02	.07
		Plantains, without peel:											
5	301	Raw slices (one whole plantain weighs 179 g without peel)	1 cup	148	65	181	1.9	47.2	4.22[38]	.6	.25	.08	.08
5	302	Cooked, boiled, sliced	1 cup	154	67	179	1.2	48	4.29	.3	.13	.04	.05
		Plums, without pits:											
		Raw:											
5	303	Medium 2-⅛ in diam	1 ea	66	85	36	.5	8.6	1.45	.4	.03	.27	.09
5	304	Small 1-½ inch diam	1 ea	28	85	15	.2	3.6	.62	.2	.01	.11	.04
		Canned, purple, with liquid:											
		Heavy syrup pack:											
5	305	Cup	1 cup	258	76	230	.9	60	4.44	.3	.02	.17	.06
5	306	Plums	3 ea	110	76	98	.4	25	1.89	.1	<.01	.07	.02
		Juice pack:											
5	307	Cup	1 cup	252	84	146	1.3	38.2	5.54	<.1	<.01	.04	.01
5	308	Plums	3 ea	95	84	55	.5	14.4	2.09	<.1	<.01	.01	<.01
		Prunes, dried, pitted:											
5	309	Uncooked (10 prunes with pits weigh 97 g):	10 ea	84	32	201	2.2	52.7	13.5[40]	.4	.03	.29	.09
5	310	Cooked, unsweetened, fruit and liquid (250 g with pits)	1 cup	212	70	227	2.5	59.5	17.2	.5	.04	.32	.11
5	311	Prune juice-bottled or canned	1 cup	256	81	181	1.6	44.7	3	<.1	<.01	.05	.02
		Raisins, seedless:											
5	312	Cup, not pressed down	1 cup	145	15	435	4.7	115	9.6	.7	.22	.03	.20
5	313	One packet, ½ oz	½ oz	14	15	41	.5	11.1	.95	<.1	.02	<.01	.02
		Raspberries:											
5	314	Raw	1 cup	123	87	60	1.1	14.2	9.1	.7	.02	.07	.39
		Frozen, sweetened											
5	315	10 oz container	10 oz	284	73	293	2	74	14.8	.5	.01	.04	.3
5	316	Cup, thawed measure	1 cup	250	73	255	1.7	65.4	13.6	.4	.01	.04	.22
5	317	Rhubarb, cooked, added sugar	1 cup	240	68	279	.9	74.9	5.28	.1	<.01	<.01	.1

[36]Dietary fiber data varies 2.4-3.4 grams per 100 grams for fresh pears; 1.6-2.6 grams per 100 grams for canned pears.
[38]Dietary fiber data partially derived from bananas.
[40]Dietary fiber data can vary to a lower value of approx 8.1 grams for 10 prunes.

(For purposes of calculations, use "0" for t, <1, <.1, <.01, etc.)

KEY: 1 = BEV 2 = DAIRY 3 = EGGS 4 = FAT/OIL 5 = FRUIT 6 = BAKERY 7 = GRAIN 8 = FISH 9 = BEEF 10 = POULTRY
11 = SAUSAGE 12 = MIXED 13 = NUTS/SEEDS 14 = SWEETS 15 = VEG/LEG 16 = MISC 22 = SOUP/SAUCE

Chol (mg)	Calc (mg)	Iron (mg)	Magn (mg)	Phos (mg)	Pota (mg)	Sodi (mg)	Zinc (mg)	VT-A (RE)	Thia (mg)	Ribo (mg)	Niac (mg)	V-B6 (mg)	Fola (μg)	VT-C (mg)
0	16	.40	8	16	176	t	.17	3	.03	.06	.1	.03	10	6
0	22	.50	11	22	250	t	.24	4	.04	.08	.2	.04	14	8
0	13	.56	11	18	166	13	.21	1	.03	.06	.62	.04	3	3
0	4	.17	3	5	51	4	.06	t	.01	.02	.19	.01	<1	.9
0	22	.71	17	29	238	10	.22	1	.03	.03	.5	.04	5	4
0	7	.22	5	9	74	3	.07	t	<.01	<.01	.15	.01	2	1
0	59	3.68	58	103	932	10	.68	t	.01	.25	2.4	.01	21	12
0	11	.57	21	11	175	2	.12	4	.14	.06	.65	.14	16	24
0	36	.97	40	18	265	3	.31	4	.23	.06	.73	.19	12	19
0	8	.22	9	4	60	1	.70	1	.05	.01	.17	.04	3	4
0	35	.70	35	15	305	3	.25	10	.24	.05	.71	.19	12	24
0	8	.16	8	4	71	1	.06	2	.06	.01	.17	.04	3	6
0	43	.65	34	20	335	3	.28	1	.14	.06	.64	.24	58	27[37]
0	4	.89	55	50	739	6	.21	167[39]	.08	.08	1.02	.44	33	27
0	3	.89	49	43	716	8	.2	140	.07	.08	1.16	.37	40	17
0	3	.07	4	7	114	.4	.07	21	.03	.06	.33	.05	3	6
0	1	.03	2	3	48	.2	.03	9	.01	.03	.14	.02	<1	3
0	23	2.17	13	34	235	49	.18	67	.04	.1	.75	.07	6	1
0	10	.92	6	14	100	21	.08	29	.02	.04	.32	.03	3	.5
0	25	.86	20	38	388	3	.28	254	.06	.15	1.19	.1	8	7
0	10	.32	8	15	147	1	.1	96	.02	.06	.45	.04	3	3
0	43	2.08	38	66	626	3	.45	167	.07	.14	1.65	.22	3	3
0	49	2.35	43	74	708	4	.51	65	.05	.21	1.53	.46	<1	6
0	31	3.02	36	64	707	10	.54	t	.04	.18	2.01	.56	1	11
0	71	3.02	48	140	1089	17	.46	1	.23	.13	1.19	.36	5	5
0	7	.29	5	14	105	2	.04	t	.02	.01	.12	.04	<1	.5
0	27	.7	22	15	187	0	.57	16	.04	.11	1.11	.07	32	31
0	43	1.85	37	48	324	3	.51	17	.05	.13	.65	.1	74	47
0	38	1.62	32	43	285	3	.45	15	.05	.11	1.5	.09	65	41
0	348	.5	30	19	230	2	.19	17	.04	.06	.48	.05	13	8

[37]Without added ascorbic acid. If added, contains 96 mg per cup.
[39]Vitamin A values range from 1.5 RE for white fleshed varieties to 178 RE for yellow fleshed varieties.

(For purposes of calculations, use "0" for t, <1, <.1, <.01, etc.)

TABLE H–1

Food Composition

Grp	Ref	Name	Measure	Wt (g)	H$_2$O (%)	Ener (kcal)	Prot (g)	Carb (g)	Fiber (g)	Fat (g)	Fat Breakdown (g) Sat	Mono	Poly
		FRUITS and FRUIT JUICES—Con.											
		Strawberries:											
5	318	Raw, whole, capped	1 cup	149	92	45	.9	10.5	3.28	.6	.03	.08	.28
		Frozen, sliced, sweetened:											
5	319	10 oz container	10 oz	284	73	273	2	74	6.16	.3	.02	.1	.2
5	320	Cup, thawed measure	1 cup	255	73	245	1.4	66.1	5.53	.3	.02	.05	.16
		Tangerines, without peel and seeds:											
5	321	Raw (2⅜ in whole)	1 ea	84	88	37	.5	9.4	1.6	.2	.02	.03	.03
5	322	Canned, light syrup, fruit and liquid	1 cup	252	83	154	1.1	41	4.03	.2	.03	.04	.1
5	323	Tangerine juice, canned, sweetened	1 cup	249	87	125	1.2	29.9	.75	.5	.03	.04	.06
		Watermelon, raw, without rind and seeds											
5	324	Piece, 1″ thick by 10″ diam (weighs 2 lb with refuse)	1 pce	482[41]	92	152	3	34.6	2.41	2.1	.3	.2	1
5	325	Diced	1 cup	160	92	50	1	11.5	.80	.7	.1	.12	.35
		BAKED GOODS-BREADS, CAKES, COOKIES, CRACKERS, PIES, PANCAKES, TORTILLAS											
6	326	Bagel, plain, enriched, 3½ in diam	1 ea	68	29	200	7.5	38.2	.74	1.75	.3	.5	.7
		Biscuits:											
6	327	From home recipe-homemade	1 ea	28	28	100	2	13	.7	5	1.2	2	1.3
6	328	From mix	1 ea	28	29	94	2.1	13.7	.6	3.1	.8	1.4	.9
6	329	From refrigerated dough	1 ea	20	30	65	1.4	9.7	.54	2.1	.6	.9	.6
6	330	Bread crumbs, dry grated (see 364,365 for soft crumbs)	1 cup	100	7	390	13	73	4.04	5	1.5	1.6	1
		Breads:											
6	331	Boston brown bread, canned, 3¼ in by ½ in slice	1 pce	45	45	95	2	21	1.7	.62	.26	.13	.14
		Cracked wheat bread (¼ cracked wheat flour, ¾ enr wheat flour):											
6	332	1 lb loaf	1 ea	454	35	1190	42	227	22.7	15.8	3.1	4.3	5.7
6	333	Slice (18 per loaf)	1 pce	25	35	65	2.3	12.5	1.25	.87	.17	.24	.31
6	334	Slice, toasted	1 pce	21	26	65	2.2	12.5	1.25	.87	.17	.24	.31
		French/Vienna bread, enriched:											
6	335	1 lb loaf	1 ea	454	34	1270	43	230	7.54	17.6	3.8	5.7	5.9
6	336	French, slice, 5x2½x1 in	1 pce	35	34	100	3.3	17.7	.58	1.36	.29	.44	.46
6	337	Vienna, slice 4¾x4x½ in	1 pce	25	34	70	2.4	12.7	.41	.97	.21	.31	.33
		French toast: see Mixed dishes item 691											
		Italian bread, enriched:											
6	338	1 lb loaf	1 ea	454	32	1255	41	256	4.95	4	.6	.3	1.6
6	339	Slice 4½x3¼x¾ in	1 pce	30	32	83	2.7	16.9	.33	.26	.04	.02	.11
		Mixed grain bread, enriched:											
6	340	1 lb loaf	1 ea	454	37	1165	45	212	18.2	16.9	3.2	4.1	6.5
6	341	Slice (18 per loaf)	1 pce	25	37	65	2	12	1	.93	.18	.23	.36
6	342	Slice, toasted	1 pce	23	27	65	2	12	1	.93	.18	.23	.36
		Oatmeal bread, enriched:											
6	343	1 lb loaf	1 ea	454	37	1145	38	212	15.6	20	3.7	7.1	8.2
6	344	Slice (18 per loaf)	1 pce	25	37	65	2.1	12	.86	1.1	.2	.39	.45
6	345	Slice, toasted	1 pce	23	30	65	2	12	.86	1.1	.2	.39	.45
6	346	Pita pocket bread, enr, 6½ in round	1 ea	60	31	165	6.2	33	.69	.88	.1	.1	.4
		Pumpernickel bread (⅔ rye flour, ⅓ enr wheat flour):											
6	347	1 lb loaf	1 ea	454	37	1160	41.6	218	18.9	15.6	2.6	3.6	6.4
6	348	Slice, 5x4x⅜ in	1 pce	32	37	80	2.9	15.4	1.33	1.1	.2	.3	.5
6	349	Slice, toasted	1 pce	29	28	80	2.9	15.4	1.33	1.1	.2	.3	.5

(41)926 grams with rind and seeds.

(For purposes of calculations, use "0" for t, <1, <.1, <.01, etc.)

KEY: 1 = BEV 2 = DAIRY 3 = EGGS 4 = FAT/OIL 5 = FRUIT 6 = BAKERY 7 = GRAIN 8 = FISH 9 = BEEF 10 = POULTRY
11 = SAUSAGE 12 = MIXED 13 = NUTS/SEEDS 14 = SWEETS 15 = VEG/LEG 16 = MISC 22 = SOUP/SAUCE

Chol (mg)	Calc (mg)	Iron (mg)	Magn (mg)	Phos (mg)	Pota (mg)	Sodi (mg)	Zinc (mg)	VT-A (RE)	Thia (mg)	Ribo (mg)	Niac (mg)	V-B6 (mg)	Fola (µg)	VT-C (mg)
0	21	.57	16	28	247	2	.19	4	.03	.1	.34	.09	28	85
0	31	1.7	20	37	278	9	.17	7	.05	.14	1.1	.09	47	118
0	28	1.5	18	33	250	8	.15	6	.04	.13	1.02	.08	42	106
0	12	.08	10	8	132	1	.38	77	.09	.02	.13	.06	17	26
0	18	.93	19	25	197	15	.60	212	.13	.11	1.1	.11	34	50
0	45	.5	20	35	443	2	.07	105	.15	.05	.25	.08	8	55
0	38	.82	52	41	560	10	.34	176	.39	.1	.96	.69	10	47
0	13	.27	17	14	186	3	.11	59	.13	.03	.32	.23	3	15
0	29	1.8	14	46	50	245	.35	0	.26	.20	2.4	.03	16	0
t	47	.7	7	36	32	195	.20	3	.08	.08	.8	.01	2	t
t	59	.58	7	129	57	265	.18	4	.12	.11	.85	.01	2	t
1	4	.47	3	79	18	249	.08	0	.08	.05	.67	<.01	1	0
5	122	4.1	31	141	152	736	.50	0	.35	.35	4.8	.02	28	0
3	41	.90	40	72	131	113	.35	0	.06	.04	.7	.06	8	0
0	295	12.1	218	581	608	1966	6.36	0	1.73	1.73	15.3	.42	218	t
0	16	.67	12	32	34	106	.35	0	.1	.1	.84	.02	12	t
0	16	.67	12	32	34	106	.35	0	.07	.1	.84	.02	9	t
0	499	14	91	386	409	2633	2.9	0	2.09	1.59	18.2	.24	168	t
0	39	1.08	7	30	32	203	.22	0	.16	.12	1.4	.02	13	t
0	28	.77	5	21	23	145	.16	0	.12	.09	1	.01	9	t
0	77	12.7	106	350	336	2656	3.1	0	1.86	1.06	15.1	.24	160	0
0	5	.8	7	23	22	176	.2	0	.12	.07	1	.02	11	0
0	472	14.8	222	962	990	1870	5.45	t	1.77	1.73	18.9	.47	295	t
0	27	.8	12	55	56	106	.3	t	.1	.1	1.1	.03	16	t
0	27	.8	12	55	56	106	t	t	.08	.1	1.1	.02	12	t
0	267	12	154	563	707	2231	4.45	0	2.09	1.2	15.4	.07	15	0
0	15	.7	8	31	39	124	.24	0	.12	.07	.85	<.01	<1	0
0	15	.7	8	31	39	124	.24	0	.09	.07	.85	<.01	<1	0
0	49	1.45	16	60	71	339	.47	0	.27	.12	2.21	.02	23	0
0	322	12.4	309	990	1966	2461	5.18	0	1.54	2.36	15	.72	222	0
0	23	.88	22	71	141	277	.4	0	.11	.17	1.06	.05	16	0
0	23	.88	22	71	141	177	.4	0	.09	.17	1.06	.05	12	0

H

(For purposes of calculations, use "0" for t, <1, <.1, <.01, etc.)

TABLE H–1

Food Composition

Grp	Ref	Name	Measure	Wt (g)	H₂O (%)	Ener (kcal)	Prot (g)	Carb (g)	Fiber (g)	Fat (g)	Fat Breakdown (g) Sat	Mono	Poly
		BAKED GOODS—Con.											
		Breads:—continued											
		Raisin bread, enriched:											
6	350	1 lb. loaf	1 ea	454	33	1260	37.3	239	12.3	18	4.1	6.5	6.7
6	351	Slice (18 per loaf)	1 pce	25	33	68	1.9	13.2	.68	1	.23	.36	.37
6	352	Slice, toasted	1 pce	21	24	68	1.9	13	.68	1	.23	.36	.37
		Rye bread, light (⅓ rye flour, ⅔ enr wheat flour):											
6	353	1 lb loaf	1 ea	454	37	1190	38.4	218	30	16.6	3.3	5.2	5.5
6	354	Slice, 4¾x3¾x7⁄16 in	1 pce	25	37	65	2.1	12	1.65	.9	.2	.3	.32
6	355	Slice, toasted	1 pce	22	28	65	2.1	12	1.65	.9	.2	.3	.32
		Wheat bread[45] (blend of enr wheat flour and whole wheat flour):											
6	356	1 lb loaf	1 ea	454	37	1160	43	213	25.3	18.6	3.9	7.3	4.5
6	357	Slice (18 per loaf)	1 pce	25	37	65	2.4	11.8	1.4	1	.21	.4	.28
6	358	Slice, toasted	1 pce	23	28	65	3	12	1.4	1	.21	.4	.28
		White bread, enriched:											
6	359	1 lb loaf	1 ea	454	37	1210	37.6	222	12.3	17.8	5.6	6.5	4.2
6	360	Slice (18 per loaf)	1 pce	25	37	65	2.1	12.2	.68	1	.31	.36	.23
6	361	Slice, toasted	1 pce	22	28	65	2.1	12.2	.68	1	.31	.36	.23
6	362	Slice (22 per loaf)	1 pce	20	37	55	1.7	10	.54	.8	.25	.29	.18
6	363	Slice, toasted	1 pce	17	28	55	1.7	10	.54	.8	.25	.29	.18
		White bread cubes, crumbs:											
6	364	Cubes, soft	1 cup	30	37	80	2.5	14.6	.81	1.2	.4	.4	.3
6	365	Crumbs, soft	1 cup	45	37	120	3.7	22	1.22	1.8	.6	.6	.4
		Whole wheat bread:											
6	366	1 lb loaf	1 ea	454	38	1110	43.7	206	51.4	19.8	5.8	6.8	5.2
6	367	Slice (16 per loaf)	1 pce	28	38	70	3	12.7	3.17	1.2	.36	.42	.33
6	368	Slice, toasted	1 pce	25	29	70	3	12.7	3.17	1.2	.36	.42	.33
		Bread stuffing, prepared from mix:											
6	369	Dry type	1 cup	140	33	500	9.1	49.8	1.3	30.5	6.1	13.3	9.6
6	370	Moist type, with egg	1 cup	203	61	420	8.8	40	1.3	25.6	5.3	11.3	8
		Cakes[46], prepared from mixes:											
		Angel food cake:											
6	371	Whole cake, 9¾ in diam tube	1 ea	635	38	1510	38.3	342	3	2	.4	.2	1
6	372	Piece, 1⁄12 cake	1 pce	53	38	125	3.2	28.5	.25	.2	.03	.02	.08
6	373	Boston cream pie, ⅛ cake	1 pce	120	35	260	2.5	44	.38	8	2.75	3.05	1.5
		Coffee cake:											
6	374	Whole cake, 7¾ x 5⅛ x 1¼ in	1 ea	430	30	1385	27	225	3.25	41	11.8	16.7	9.6
6	375	Piece, ⅙ cake	1 pce	72	30	230	4.5	37.7	.54	6.9	1.98	2.8	1.61
		Devil's food with chocolate frosting:											
6	376	Whole cake, 2 layer, 8 in or 9 in diam	1 ea	1107	24	3755	49	645	5.1	136	55.6	51.4	19.7
6	377	Piece, 1⁄16 of cake	1 pce	69	24	235	3	40.2	.32	8	3.5	3.2	1.2
6	378	Cupcake, 2½ in diam	1 ea	35	24	120	1.6	20.4	.16	4.3	1.76	1.63	.62
		Gingerbread:											
6	379	Whole cake, 8 in square	1 ea	570	37	1575	18	291	3	39	9.6	16.4	10.5
6	380	Piece, ⅑ of cake	1 pce	63	37	174	2	32.2	.34	4.3	1.06	1.81	1.16
		Yellow, with chocolate frosting, 2 layer:											
6	381	Whole cake, 8 in or 9 in diam	1 ea	1108	26	3735	45	638	5	125	47.8	48.8	21.8
6	382	Piece, 1⁄16 of cake	1 pce	69	26	235	2.8	40	.31	7.8	2.99	3.05	1.36

[45] A blend of white and whole wheat flour—no official ratio specified.
[46] Excepting angel food cake, cakes were made from mixes containing vegetable shortening, and frostings were made with margarine. All mixes use enriched flour.

(For purposes of calculations, use "0" for t, <1, <.1, <.01, etc.)

KEY: 1 = BEV 2 = DAIRY 3 = EGGS 4 = FAT/OIL 5 = FRUIT 6 = BAKERY 7 = GRAIN 8 = FISH 9 = BEEF 10 = POULTRY
11 = SAUSAGE 12 = MIXED 13 = NUTS/SEEDS 14 = SWEETS 15 = VEG/LEG 16 = MISC 22 = SOUP/SAUCE

Chol (mg)	Calc (mg)	Iron (mg)	Magn (mg)	Phos (mg)	Pota (mg)	Sodi (mg)	Zinc (mg)	VT-A (RE)	Thia (mg)	Ribo (mg)	Niac (mg)	V-B6 (mg)	Fola (µg)	VT-C (mg)
0	463	14.1	114	395	1058	1657	2.81	1	1.5	2.81	18.6	.15	159	t
0	25	.78	6	22	59	92	.15	t	.08	.15	1.02	<.01	9	t
0	25	.80	6	22	59	92	.15	t	.06	.15	1.02	<.01	8	t
0	363	12.3	109	658	926	3164	5.77	0	1.86	1.45	15	.43	177	0
0	20	.68	6	36	51	175	.38	0	.1	.08	.83	.02	10	0
0	20	.68	6	36	51	175	.38	0	.08	.08	.83	.02	8	0
0	572	15.8	209	835	627	2447	4.77	t	2.09	1.45	20.5	.49	204	t
0	32	.87	12	47	35	135	.26	t	.12	.08	1.13	.03	11	t
0	32	.9	12	47	35	135	.26	t	.10	.08	1.2	.02	8	t
0	572	12.9	95	490	508	2334	2.81	t	2.13	1.41	17	.15	159	t
0	32	.71	5	27	28	129	.15	t	.12	.08	.94	<.01	9	t
0	32	.71	5	27	28	129	.15	t	.09	.08	.94	<.01	9	t
0	25	.57	4	22	22	103	.12	t	.09	.06	.75	<.01	7	t
0	25	.6	4	21	22	103	.12	t	.07	.06	.75	<.01	7	t
0	38	.85	6	32	34	154	.19	t	.14	.09	1.13	.01	10	t
0	57	1.28	9	49	50	231	.28	t	.21	.14	1.69	.01	16	t
0	327	15.5	422	1180	799	2887	7.63	t	1.59	.95	17.4	.85	250	t
0	20	.96	26	74	50	180	.5	t	.1	.06	1.07	.05	16	t
0	20	.96	26	74	50	180	.5	t	.08	.06	1.07	.05	12	t
0	92	2.2	30	136	126	1254	.55	273	.17	.2	2.5	.02	14	0
67	81	2.03	45	134	118	1023	.78	256	.1	.18	1.62	.04	20	t
0	527	2.73	51	1086	845	3226	.81	0	.32	1.27	1.6	.08	51	0
0	44	.23	4	91	71	269	.07	0	.03	.11	.13	<.01	4	0
20	26	.6	11	70	40	225	.23	70	.01	.18	.7	.05	7	0
279	262	7.3	27	748	469	1853	3.7	194	.82	.9	7.7	.12	30	1
47	44	1.22	4	125	78	310	.62	32	.14	.15	1.29	.02	5	t
598	653	22.1	200	1162	1439	2900	7.95	498	1.11	1.66	10	.32	82	1
37	41	1.4	12	72	90	181	.5	31	.07	.1	.6	.02	<1	t
19	21	.7	6	37	46	92	.25	16	.04	.05	.32	.01	3	t
6	513	10.8	41	570	1562	1733	5.52	0	.86	1.03	7.4	.07	36	1
1	57	1.2	4	63	173	192	.61	0	.1	.11	.82	<.01	4	t
576	1008	15.5	72	2017	1208	2515	3.31	465	1.22	1.66	11.1	.45	80	1
36	63	.96	4	126	75	157	.21	29	.08	.1	.69	.03	5	t

H

(For purposes of calculations, use "0" for t, <1, <.1, <.01, etc.)

TABLE H-1

Food Composition

Grp	Ref	Name	Measure	Wt (g)	H$_2$O (%)	Ener (kcal)	Prot (g)	Carb (g)	Fiber (g)	Fat (g)	Fat Breakdown (g) Sat	Mono	Poly
		BAKED GOODS—Con.											
		Cakes from home recipes with enriched flour:											
		Carrot cake, cream cheese frosting:[47]											
6	383	Whole, 9 x 13 in cake	1 ea	1536	23	6175	63	775	11	328	66	135	108
6	384	Piece, ⅟₁₆ of 9 x 13 in sheet cake 2¼ x 3¼ in	1 pce	96	23	385	4.2	48	.69	21	4.1	8.4	6.8
		Fruitcake, dark, 7½ in diam tube-2¼ in high:[47]											
6	385	Whole cake	1 ea	1361	18	5185	74	783	38.1	228	47.6	113	51.7
6	386	Piece, ⅟₃₂ of cake, ⅔ in arc	1 pce	43	18	165	2	25	1.2	7.	1.5	3.6	1.6
		Sheet cake, plain, no frosting:[48]											
6	387	Whole cake, 9 in square	1 ea	777	25	2830	35	434	3	108	29.5	45.1	25.6
6	388	Piece, ⅛ of cake	1 pce	86	25	315	4	48	.34	12	3.3	5	2.83
		Sheet cake, plain, unckd white frosting:[48]											
6	389	Whole cake, 9 in square	1 ea	1096	21	4020	37	694	3	129	41.6	50.4	26.3
6	390	Piece, ⅑ of cake	1 pce	121	21	445	4	77	.34	14	4.6	5.6	2.9
		Pound cake:[49]											
6	391	Loaf, 8½ x 3½ x 3¼ in	1 ea	514	22	2025	33	265	3.75	94	21.1	40.9	26.7
6	392	Piece, ⅟₁₇ of loaf	1 pce	30	22	120	2	15	.22	5	1.2	2.4	1.6
		Cakes, commercial:											
		Pound cake:											
6	393	Loaf, 8½ x 3½ x 3 in	1 ea	500	24	1935	26	257	3.75	94	52	30	4
6	394	Slice, ⅟₁₇ of loaf	1 pce	29	24	110	2	15	.22	5.4	3.02	1.74	.23
		Snack cakes:											
6	395	Chocolate w/creme filling, 2 small cakes per package	1 ea	28	20	105	1	17	.08	4	1.7	1.5	.6
6	396	Sponge cake w/creme filling, 2 small cakes per package	1 ea	42	19	155	1	27	.1	5	2.3	2.1	.5
		White cake with white frosting, 2 layer cake:											
6	397	Whole cake, 8 in or 9 in diam	1 ea	1140	24	4170	43	670	4.5	148	33.1	61.6	42.2
6	398	Piece, ⅟₁₆ of cake	1 pce	71	24	260	3	42	.28	9	2.1	3.84	2.63
		Yellow cake with chocolate frosting, 2 layer cake:											
6	399	Whole cake, 8 in or 9 in diam	1 ea	1108	23	3895	40	620	5	175	92	58.7	10
6	400	Piece, ⅟₁₆ of cake	1 pce	69	23	245	2.5	38.6	.31	10.9	5.73	3.7	.62
		Cheesecake:											
6	401	Whole cake, 9 in diam	1 ea	1110	46	3350	60.2	317	5	213	120	65.5	14.4
6	402	Piece, ⅟₁₂ of cake	1 pce	92	46	278	5	26.3	.41	17.7	9.94	5.43	1.19
		Cookies made with enriched flour:											
		Brownies with nuts:											
6	403	Commercial with frosting, 1½ x 1¾ x ⅞ in	1 ea	25	13	100	1.2	15.9	.22	4.4	1.6	2	.6
6	404	Home recipe[47], 1¾ x 1¾ x ⅞ in	1 ea	20	10	95	1.3	11	.20	6.3	1.4	2.8	1.2
		Chocolate chip cookies:											
6	405	Commercial, 2¼ in diam	4 ea	42	4	180	2.3	28	.17	8.8	2.9	3.1	2.6
6	406	Home recipe, 2⅓ in diam[43]	4 ea	40	3	185	2	25.6	.96	10.7	3.9	4.3	2
6	407	From refrigerated dough, 2¼ in diam	4 ea	48	5	225	2.3	32	.06	11	4	4.4	2

[43]Made with vegetable shortening.
[47]Made with vegetable oil.
[48]Cakes made with vegetable shortening; frosting with margarine.
[49]Made with margarine.

(For purposes of calculations, use "0" for t, <1, <.1, <.01, etc.)

KEY: 1 = BEV 2 = DAIRY 3 = EGGS 4 = FAT/OIL 5 = FRUIT 6 = BAKERY 7 = GRAIN 8 = FISH 9 = BEEF 10 = POULTRY
11 = SAUSAGE 12 = MIXED 13 = NUTS/SEEDS 14 = SWEETS 15 = VEG/LEG 16 = MISC 22 = SOUP/SAUCE

Chol (mg)	Calc (mg)	Iron (mg)	Magn (mg)	Phos (mg)	Pota (mg)	Sodi (mg)	Zinc (mg)	VT-A (RE)	Thia (mg)	Ribo (mg)	Niac (mg)	V-B6 (mg)	Fola (μg)	VT-C (mg)
1183	707	21	197	998	1720	4470	8.15	246	1.83	1.97	14.7	1.38	243	23
74	44	1.3	12	62	108	279	.51	15	.11	.12	.9	.86	15	1
640	1293	37.6	340	1592	6138	2123	6.8	422	2.41	2.55	17	1.72	54	504
20	41	1.2	11	50	194	67	.21	13	.08	.08	.5	.05	2	16
552	497	11.7	56	793	614	2331	2.75	373	1.24	1.4	10.1	.26	54	2
61	55	1.3	6	88	68	258	.31	41	.14	.15	1.1	.03	15	t
636	548	11	56	822	669	2488	2.90	647	1.21	1.42	9.9	.27	110	2
70	61	1.2	6	91	74	275	.32	71	.13	.16	1.1	.03	12	t
555	339	9.3	48	473	483	1645	2.69	1033	.93	1.08	7.8	.39	55	1
32	20	.5	3	28	28	97	.16	60	.05	.06	.5	.02	3	t
1100	146	9.3	48	517	443	1857	1.95	715	.96	1.12	8.1	.38	55	1
64	8	.5	3	30	26	108	.11	41	.06	.06	.5	.02	3	t
15	21	1	2	26	34	105	.17	4	.06	.09	.7	.01	3	0
7	14	.6	3	44	37	155	.21	9	.07	.06	.6	.02	4	0
46	536	15.5	60	1585	832	2827	1.77	194	3.19	2.05	27.6	.16	64	0
3	33	1	4	99	52	176	.11	12	.2	.13	1.7	.01	4	0
609	366	19.9	72	1884	1972	3080	3.3	488	.78	2.22	10	.45	80	0
38	23	1.24	4	117	123	192	.21	30	.05	.14	.62	.03	5	0
2053	622	5.33	111	977	1088	2464	4.66	833	.33	1.44	5.11	.71	200	56
170	52	.44	9	81	90	204	.39	69	.03	.12	.42	.06	17	5
14	13	.6	14	26	50	59	.36	18	.08	.07	.33	.04	5	t
18	9	.4	11	26	35	51	.31	6	.05	.05	.3	.04	4	t
5	16	.8	9	41	56	140	.3	15	.1	.23	.9	.02	4	t
18	13	1	14	34	82	82	.22	5	.06	.06	.58	.03	4	0
22	13	1.04	10	34	62	173	.24	8	.06	.1	.89	<.01	4	0

(For purposes of calculations, use "0" for t, <1, <.1, <.01, etc.)

H

TABLE H–1

Food Composition

Grp	Ref	Name	Measure	Wt (g)	H$_2$O (%)	Ener (kcal)	Prot (g)	Carb (g)	Fiber (g)	Fat (g)	Fat Breakdown (g)		
											Sat	Mono	Poly
		BAKED GOODS—Con.											
		Cookies:—continued											
6	408	Fig bars	4 ea	56	12	210	2	42.3	.80	3.8	1	1.5	1
6	409	Oatmeal raisin cookies, 2⅝ in diam	4 ea	52	4	245	3	36	.21	10	2.5	4.5	2.8
6	410	Peanut butter cookie, home recipe, 2⅝ in diam[43]	4 ea	48	3	245	4	28	1	14	4	5.8	2.8
6	411	Sandwich-type cookies, all	4 ea	40	2	195	2	29	.04	8	2	3.6	2.2
		Shortbread cookies:											
6	412	Commercial, small	4 ea	32	6	155	2	20	.06	8	2.9	3	1.1
6	413	From home recipe, large[49]	2 ea	28	3	145	1.6	17.2	.04	8.3	1.3	2.7	3.4
6	414	Sugar cookies from refrigerated dough, 2½ in diam	4 ea	48	4	235	2	31	.05	12	2.3	5	3.6
6	415	Vanilla wafers	10 ea	40	4	185	2	29	.04	7	1.8	3	1.8
6	416	Corn chips	1 oz	28	1	155	2	16	.3	9	1.4	2.4	3.7
		Crackers:[50]											
6	417	Cheese crackers	10 ea	10	4	50	1	6	.02	3	.9	1.2	.3
6	418	Cheese crackers with peanut butter	4 ea	30	3	150	4.3	18.7	.14	7.5	1.6	3.2	1.2
6	419	Graham crackers	2 ea	14	4	60	1	10.8	1.4	1.5	.4	.6	.4
6	420	Melba toast, plain	1 pce	5	4	20	1	4	.1	.3	.1	.1	.1
6	421	Rye wafers, whole grain	2 ea	14	5	55	1	10	1.45	1	.3	.4	.3
6	422	Saltine crackers[51]	4 ea	12	4	50	1	9	.06	1.1	.5	.4	.2
6	423	Snack-type crackers, Ritz	3 ea	9	3	45	.7	6.4	.24	2.9	.6	1.2	.3
6	424	Wheat cracker, thin	4 ea	8	3	35	1	5	.4	1.4	.5	.5	.4
6	425	Whole wheat wafers	2 ea	8	4	35	1	5	.4	1.5	.5	.6	.4
6	426	Croissant, 4½x4x1¾ in	1 ea	57	22	235	5	27	.47	12	3.5	6.7	1.4
		Danish pastry:											
6	427	Packaged ring, plain, 12 oz	1 ea	340	27	1305	21	152	2.8	71	21.8	28.6	15.6
6	428	Round piece, plain, 4¼ in diam, 1 in high	1 ea	57	27	220	4	26	.47	12	3.6	4.8	2.6
6	429	Ounce, plain	1 oz	28	28	110	2	13	.23	6	1.8	2.4	1.3
6	430	Round piece with fruit	1 pce	65	30	235	4	28	.65	13	3.9	5.2	2.9
		Doughnuts:											
6	431	Cake type, plain, 3¼ in diam	1 ea	50	21	210	2.5	24	.5	12	2.8	5	3
6	432	Yeast-leavened, glazed, 3¾ in diam	1 ea	60	27	235	3.9	26	.48	13	5.2	5.5	.9
		English muffin:											
6	433	Plain, enriched	1 ea	57	42	140	4.5	26.2	1.54	1.1	.3	.2	.3
6	434	Toasted	1 ea	50	29	140	4.5	26.2	1.54	1.1	.3	.2	.3
		Muffins, 2½ in diam, 1½ in high											
		From home recipe:											
6	435	Blueberry[43]	1 ea	45	37	135	3	20	1.32	5	1.5	2.1	1.2
6	436	Bran[47]	1 ea	45	35	125	3	19	2.05	6	1.4	1.6	2.3
6	437	Cornmeal	1 ea	45	33	145	3	21	1.60	5	1.5	2.2	1.4
		From commercial mix:											
6	438	Blueberry	1 ea	45	33	140	2.7	22	1.25	4.9	1.4	2	1.2
6	439	Bran	1 ea	45	28	140	3	24	2.03	4	1.3	1.6	1
6	440	Cornmeal	1 ea	45	30	145	3	22	1.6	6	1.7	2.3	1.4

[43] Made with vegetable shortening.
[47] Made with vegetable oil.
[49] Made with margarine.
[50] Crackers made with enriched flour except for rye wafers and whole wheat wafers.
[51] Made with lard.

H

(For purposes of calculations, use "0" for t, <1, <.1, <.01, etc.)

KEY: 1 = BEV 2 = DAIRY 3 = EGGS 4 = FAT/OIL 5 = FRUIT 6 = BAKERY 7 = GRAIN 8 = FISH 9 = BEEF 10 = POULTRY 11 = SAUSAGE 12 = MIXED 13 = NUTS/SEEDS 14 = SWEETS 15 = VEG/LEG 16 = MISC 22 = SOUP/SAUCE

Chol (mg)	Calc (mg)	Iron (mg)	Magn (mg)	Phos (mg)	Pota (mg)	Sodi (mg)	Zinc (mg)	VT-A (RE)	Thia (mg)	Ribo (mg)	Niac (mg)	V-B6 (mg)	Fola (µg)	VT-C (mg)
27	40	1.36	15	34	162	180	.36	6	.08	.07	.73	.07	4	t
2	18	1.1	26	58	90	148	.53	12	.09	.08	1	.03	6	0
22	21	1.1	19	60	110	142	.36	5	.07	.07	1.9	.04	12	0
0	12	1.4	20	40	66	189	.12	0	.09	.07	.8	.01	1	0
27	13	.8	4	39	38	123	.15	8	.1	.09	.9	.01	3	0
0	6	.55	4	31	18	125	.13	89	.08	.06	.71	<.01	2	t
29	50	.9	8	91	33	261	.24	11	.09	.06	1.1	.02	4	0
25	16	.8	6	36	50	150	.12	14	.07	.1	1	.01	4	0
0	35	.5	19	52	52	233	.42	11	.04	.05	.4	.04[53]	3[54]	1
6	11	.3	2	17	17	112	.1	5	.05	.04	.4	.01	—	0
4	26	1.2	2	94	64	338	.06	2	.16	.12	2.4	.03	—	0
0	6	.37	5	20	36	86	.11	0	.02	.03	.6	.01	2	0
0	6	.1	—	10	11	44	—	0	.01	.01	.1	.01		0
0	7	.5	16	44	65	115	1.6	0	.06	.03	.5	.03	10	0
4	3	.5	3	12	17	165	.07	0	.06	.05	.6	<.01	2	0
0	9	.3	2	18	12	90	.05	t	.03	.03	.3	<.01	1	0
0	3	.3	7[52]	15	17	69	.24[52]	t	.04	.03	.4	.01	3[52]	0
0	3	.2	7[52]	22	31	59	.24	0	.02	.03	.4	.01	3[52]	0
13	20	2.1	6	64	68	452	.32	13	.17	.13	1.3	.03	18	0
292	360	6.5	68	347	316	1302	2.86	99	.95	1.02	8.5	.12	84	t
49	60	1.1	11	58	53	218	.48	17	.16	.17	1.4	.02	14	t
24	30	.55	6	29	27	109	.24	8	.08	.09	.7	.01	7	t
56	17	1.3	13	80	57	233	.55	11	.16	.14	1.4	.02	16	t
20	22	.8	12	111	58	192	.25	5	.12	.12	1.1	.02	4	t
21	17	1.4	12	55	64	222	.3	t	.28	.12	1.8	.28	13	0
0	96	1.7	11	67	331	378	.41	0	.26	.18	2.14	.02	18	0
0	96	1.7	11	67	331	378	.41	0	.23	.18	2.14	.02	15	0
19	54	.9	11	46	47	198	.29	9	.1	.11	.9	<.01	12	1
24	60	1.4	11	125	99	189	.37	30	.11	.13	1.3	.01	9	3
23	66	.9	13	59	57	169	.34	15	.11	.11	.9	.04	5	t
45	15	.9	5	90	54	225	.23	11	.11	.13	1.17	<.01	14	.5
28	27	1.7	4	182	50	385	.95	14	.08	.12	1.9	.12	19	0
42	30	1.3	13	128	31	291	.34	16	.09	.09	.8	.04	5	t

(52)Values derived from whole wheat recipes and retention values.
(53)B₆ values vary from 0 to .04 g between various brands—check label.
(54)Folacin values estimated and derived from values for corn meal and corn tortillas.

H

(For purposes of calculations, use "0" for t, <1, <.1, <.01, etc.)

TABLE H–1

Food Composition

Grp	Ref	Name	Measure	Wt (g)	H₂O (%)	Ener (kcal)	Prot (g)	Carb (g)	Fiber (g)	Fat (g)	Fat Breakdown (g)		
											Sat	Mono	Poly
		BAKED GOODS—Con.											
		Pancakes, 4 in diam:											
6	441	Buckwheat, from mix; egg and milk added	1 ea	27	58	55	2	6	1.3	2	.9	.9	.5
6	442	Plain, from home recipe	1 ea	27	50	60	2	9	.72	2	.5	.8	.5
6	443	Plain, from mix; egg, milk, oil added	1 ea	27	54	60	2	8	.72	2	.5	.9	.5
		Piecrust, with enriched flour, baked:[43]											
6	444	Home recipe, 9 in shell	1 ea	180	15	900	11	79	3.6	60	14.8	25.9	15.7
		From mix:											
6	445	Piecrust for 2 crust pie	1 ea	320	19	1485	20.5	141	6.4	93.1	22.7	41	25
6	446	1 pie shell	1 ea	180	19	835	11.5	79	3.6	52.4	12.8	23.1	14.1
		Pies, 9 in diam; pie crust made with veg shortening, enriched flour:											
		Apple pie[55]:											
6	447	Whole pie	1 ea	945	48	2420	22	360	18.8	105	24.7	45.7	29.1
6	448	Piece, ⅙ of pie	1 pce	158	48	405	3.7	59.5	3.13	17.5	4.12	7.62	4.85
		Banana cream pie[56]:											
6	449	Whole pie	1 ea	1190	66	1917	37.9	283	10.2	77.5	27	29.2	14.9
6	450	⅙ of pie	1 ea	198	66	320	6.3	47.2	1.7	12.9	4.5	4.87	2.48
		Blueberry pie[55]:											
6	451	Whole pie	1 ea	945	51	2285	23	330	22.2	102	24.1	44.8	28.4
6	452	Piece, ⅙ of pie	1 pce	158	51	380	4	55	3.72	17	4.01	7.47	4.73
		Cherry pie[55]:											
6	453	Whole pie	1 ea	945	47	2465	26	363	14.6	107	25.3	47	29.6
6	454	Piece, ⅙ of pie	1 pce	158	47	410	4.3	60.5	2.43	17.8	4.21	7.83	4.93
		Chocolate cream pie[57]:											
6	455	Whole pie	1 ea	1051	63	1864	42.2	255	4.41	76.4	27.2	29.7	14.7
6	456	Piece, ⅙ of pie	1 ea	175	63	311	7	42.5	.73	12.7	4.53	4.95	2.45
		Custard pie:											
6	457	Whole pie	1 ea	910	58	1760	46	204	3.6	85.4	27.9	34.5	16.8
6	458	Piece, ⅙ of pie	1 pce	152	58	293	7.7	34	.6	14.2	.93	5.75	2.8
		Lemon meringue pie[55]:											
6	459	Whole pie	1 ea	840	47	2140	31	317	4.57	86	20.8	37.2	22
6	460	Piece, ⅙ of pie	1 pce	140	47	355	4.7	53	.76	14.3	3.5	6.2	3.67
		Peach pie[55]:											
6	461	Whole pie	1 ea	945	48	2410	24	361	17	105	24.8	46.3	29
6	462	Piece, ⅙ of pie	1 pce	158	48	405	3.5	60.7	2.83	17.5	4.13	7.72	4.83
		Pecan pie[55]:											
6	463	Whole pie	1 ea	825	20	3500	38	551	10.1	142	23.6	75.4	34.3
6	464	Piece, ⅙ of pie	1 pce	138	20	583	6.3	91.8	1.68	23.7	3.93	12.6	5.72
		Pumpkin pie[55]:											
6	465	Whole pie	1 ea	910	59	2250	54	308	15	94.4	34.2	36.5	16.5
6	466	Piece, ⅙ of pie	1 pce	152	59	375	9	51.3	2.5	15.7	5.7	6.08	2.75
		Pies, fried, commercial:											
6	467	Apple	1 ea	85	43	255	2.2	32	1.7	14	5.8	6.6	.6
6	468	Cherry	1 ea	85	43	250	2	32.2	1.31	14.2	5.8	6.7	.6
		Pretzels, made with enriched flour:											
6	469	Thin sticks, 2¼ in long	10 ea	3	2	10	.3	2.4	.07	.1	.02	.04	.04
6	470	Dutch twist, 2¾ x 2⅝ in	1 ea	16	2	65	1.5	12.8	.36	.6	.11	.23	.17
6	471	Thin twists, 3¼ x 2¼ x ¼ in	10 ea	60	3	240	6	48	1.34	2	.4	.8	.60

[43] Made with vegetable shortening.
[55] Recipes updated for latest USDA values for fruits/nuts/fruit juice.
[56] Recipe based on pie crust, cooked vanilla pudding, 2 bananas.
[57] Based on values for pie crust, cooked chocolate pudding with meringue.

(For purposes of calculations, use "0" for t, <1, <.1, <.01, etc.)

KEY: 1 = BEV 2 = DAIRY 3 = EGGS 4 = FAT/OIL 5 = FRUIT 6 = BAKERY 7 = GRAIN 8 = FISH 9 = BEEF 10 = POULTRY
11 = SAUSAGE 12 = MIXED 13 = NUTS/SEEDS 14 = SWEETS 15 = VEG/LEG 16 = MISC 22 = SOUP/SAUCE

Chol (mg)	Calc (mg)	Iron (mg)	Magn (mg)	Phos (mg)	Pota (mg)	Sodi (mg)	Zinc (mg)	VT-A (RE)	Thia (mg)	Ribo (mg)	Niac (mg)	V-B6 (mg)	Fola (µg)	VT-C (mg)
20	59	.4	18	91	66	125	.5	17	.04	.05	.2	.06	6	t
16	27	.5	4	38	33	115	.21	10	.06	.07	.5	.02	4	t
16	36	.7	4	71	43	160	.22	7	.09	.12	.8	.01	3	t
0	25	4.5	31	90	90	1100	1.5	0	.54	.4	5	.17	32	0
0	131	9.3	44	272	179	2600	1.19	0	1.07	.79	9.89	.27	57	0
0	74	5.23	25	153	101	1462	.79	0	.6	.44	5.57	.15	32	0
0	170	10	61	300	600	2844	1.6	177	1.04	.76	9.5	.5	48	2
0	28	1.67	10	50	100	476	.27	30	.17	.13	1.6	.08	8	t
90	880	6.54	186	810	2006	2532	4.05	222	.9	1.75	7.41	1.61	104	20
15	147	1.09	31	135	334	422	.68	37	.15	.29	1.24	.27	17	3
0	155	12.3	60	274	756	2533	1.68	188	1.04	.85	10.4	.43	84	36
0	26	2.1	10	46	126	423	.28	31	.17	.14	1.73	.07	14	6
0	220	19	91	350	920	2873	1.87	685	1.13	.85	9.5	.5	93	5
0	37	3.17	15	58	153	480	.31	114	.19	.14	1.58	.08	16	1
90	958	7.66	176	881	1332	2565	4.34	204	.81	1.83	6.22	.48	73	3
15	160	1.28	29	147	222	428	.72	34	.14	.3	1.04	.08	12	.5
888	742	8.64	110	880	1040	2000	4.75	386	.82	1.6	5.5	.51	91	1
148	124	1.44	18	147	173	333	.79	64	.14	.27	.92	.08	15	t
822	150	8.4	54	412	420	2369	3.06	438	.59	.84	5	.3	78	25
137	25	1.4	9	69	70	395	.51	73	.1	.14	.83	.05	13	4
0	160	11.3	98	332	1408	2533	2.11	555	1.04	.93	13.9	.39	72	28
0	27	1.9	16	55	235	423	.35	93	.17	.15	2.30	.07	12	5
822	210	12	192	777	781	1823	8.8	250	1.63	.99	6.6	.51	110	0
137	35	2	32	130	130	304	1.47	41.7	.27	.17	1.1	.09	18	0
655	1200	15	220	1260	2400	1947	5.75	1116[58]	.82	1.76	7.3	.68	117	6
109	200	2.5	37	210	400	325	.96	186[58]	.14	.29	1.22	.11	20	1
14	12	.94	6	34	42	326	.14	3	.09	.06	1	.03	4	1
13	11	.7	7	41	61	371	.15	19	.06	.06	.6	.04	8	1
0	1	.06	<1	3	3	48	.03	0	<.01	<.01	.13	<.01	<1	0
0	4	.32	4	15	16	258	.17	0	.05	.04	.7	<.01	3	0
0	16	1.2	15	55	61	966	.42	0	.19	.15	2.6	.01	10	0

(58)Latest USDA values of Vitamin A for canned pumpkin are almost 3.5 times greater than previously published values. Canned pumpkin is usually a blend of pumpkin and winter squash.

(For purposes of calculations, use "0" for t, <1, <.1, <.01, etc.)

TABLE H–1

Food Composition

Grp	Ref	Name	Measure	Wt (g)	H₂O (%)	Ener (kcal)	Prot (g)	Carb (g)	Fiber (g)	Fat (g)	Fat Breakdown (g) Sat	Mono	Poly
		BAKED GOODS—Con.											
		Rolls and buns, enriched:											
		Commercial:											
6	472	Cloverleaf rolls, 2½ in diam, 2 in high	1 ea	28	32	85	2	14	.76	2	.5	.8	.6
6	473	Hotdog bun	1 ea	40	34	115	3.3	20	1.08	2.1	.5	.8	.6
6	474	Hamburger bun	1 ea	45	34	129	3.7	22.5	1.21	2.4	.56	.9	.68
6	475	Hard roll, white, 3¾ in diam, 2 in high	1 ea	50	25	155	5	30	.83	2	.4	.5	.6
6	476	Submarine roll or hoagie, 11½ x 3 x 2½ in	1 ea	135	31	400	11	72	2.24	8	1.8	3	2.2
		From home recipe:											
6	477	Dinner roll, 2½ in diam, 2 in high	1 ea	35	26	120	3	20	.94	3	.8	1.2	.9
6	478	Toaster pastry, fortified	1 ea	54	13	210	2.1	38	.6	6	1.7	3.6	.4
		Tortillas:											
6	479	Corn, enriched, 6 in diam	1 ea	30	45	65	2	13	1.23	1	.1	.3	.61
6	480	Flour, 8 in diam	1 ea	35.4	27	105	2.6	19.3	.95	2.7	.4	1.15	1.02
6	481	Taco shell	1 ea	11	4	48	.9	7.6	.71	2.2	.2	.6	1.2
		Waffles, 7 in diam:											
6	482	From home recipe	1 ea	75	37	245	7	26	1.6	13	4	4.9	2.6
6	483	From mix, egg/milk added	1 ea	75	42	205	7	27	1.6	8	2.7	2.9	1.5
		GRAIN PRODUCTS: CEREALS, FLOUR, GRAINS, PASTA and NOODLES, POPCORN											
		Barley, pearled:											
7	484	Dry, uncooked	1 cup	200	11	700	16.4	158	16.4	2	.3	.2	.9
7	485	Cooked	1 cup	200	72	196	4.6	44	4.4	.6	.08	.06	.25
		Breakfast cereals, hot, cooked:											
		Corn grits (hominy) cooked:											
7	486	Yellow, enriched, regular and quick prepared	1 cup	242	85	146	3.5	31.4	.75	.5	t	.1	.2
7	487	White, instant, prepared from packet	1 ea	137	85	80	2.1	17.8	.42	.2	t	.05	.1
		Cream of Wheat®, cooked:											
7	488	Regular, quick, instant	1 cup	244	86	140	3.6	29	.64	.6	.1	.1	.2
7	489	Mix 'n eat, plain, packet	1 ea	142	82	100	3	21	.37	.5	.05	.05	.1
7	490	Malt-O-Meal® cereal, cooked	1 cup	240	88	122	3.6	25.9	.64	.2	t	t	.1
		Oatmeal or rolled oats, cooked:											
7	491	Regular, quick, instant, non-fortified	1 cup	234	85	145	6	25.2	9.23	2.4	.44	.84	1
		Instant, fortified:											
7	492	Plain, from packet	¾ cup	177	86	104	4.4	18.1	6.98	1.7	.3	.6	.7
7	493	Flavored, from packet	¾ cup	164	76	160	4.8	31	6.47	2	.3	.7	.8
7	494	Whole wheat cereal, cooked	1 cup	245	88	110	4.4	23	5.56	.7	.1	.08	.33
		Breakfast cereals; ready to eat:											
7	495	All-Bran®	⅓ cup	28	3	70	4	21	8.4	.5	.1	.1	.3
7	496	Cap'n Crunch®	1 cup	37	2	156	1.9	29.9	.93	3.4	2.23	.44	.54
7	497	Cheerios®	1 cup	23	5	89	3.4	15.7	.92	1.4	.25	.49	.57
7	498	Corn Flakes, Kellogg's®	1¼ cup	28	3	110	2.3	24.4	.49	<.1	.01	.02	.05
7	499	Corn Flakes, Post Toasties®	1¼ cup	28	3	110	2.3	24.4	.49	<.1	.01	.02	.1
7	500	40% Bran Flakes, Kellogg's®	1 cup	39	3	125	4.9	30.5	5.5	.7	.14	.14	.42

(For purposes of calculations, use "0" for t, <1, <.1, <.01, etc.)

KEY: 1 = BEV 2 = DAIRY 3 = EGGS 4 = FAT/OIL 5 = FRUIT 6 = BAKERY 7 = GRAIN 8 = FISH 9 = BEEF 10 = POULTRY 11 = SAUSAGE 12 = MIXED 13 = NUTS/SEEDS 14 = SWEETS 15 = VEG/LEG 16 = MISC 22 = SOUP/SAUCE

Chol (mg)	Calc (mg)	Iron (mg)	Magn (mg)	Phos (mg)	Pota (mg)	Sodi (mg)	Zinc (mg)	VT-A (RE)	Thia (mg)	Ribo (mg)	Niac (mg)	V-B6 (mg)	Fola (µg)	VT-C (mg)
t	33	.81	6	44	36	155	.22	t	.14	.09	1.1	.01	11	t
0	54	1.19	8	44	56	241	.36	t	.2	.13	1.58	.01	15	t
0	61	1.34	9	49	63	271	.41	t	.22	.15	1.78	.02	17	t
0	24	1.4	14	46	49	313	.44	0	.2	.12	1.7	.02	17	0
0	100	3.8	31	115	128	683	1.17	0	.54	.33	4.5	.09	49	0
12	16	1.1	10	36	41	98	.32	8	.12	.12	1.2	.01	12	0
0	104	2.16	10	104	91	248	.31	100[59]	.17	.18	2.27	.2	43	4
0	42	.6	18	55	43	1	.36	8	.05	.03	.4	.09	6	0
0	21	.55	13	59	35	134	.27	0	.13	.08	1.2	.01	16	0
0	21	.21	9	27	20	50	.17	4	<.01	.01	.2	.02	2	0
102	154	1.5	11	135	129	445	.61	39	.18	.24	1.5	.03	13	t
59	179	1.2	11	257	146	515	.52	49	.14	.23	.9	.03	4	t
0	32	4.2	51	378	320	6	4.47	0	.24	.1	7.9	.45	40	0
0	6	1.17	12	112	72	2	1.15	0	.05	.02	1.7	.09	10	0
0	1	1.55[60]	11	29	54	0[62]	.17	15[61]	.24[60]	.15[60]	1.96[60]	.06	2	0
0	7	1[60]	5	16	29	343	.08	0	.18[60]	.08[60]	1.3[60]	.03	1	0
0	54[63]	10.9[63]	12	4[64]	46	564,[65]	.35	0	.24[63]	.07[63]	1.5[63]	.02	9	0
0	20[63]	8.10[63]	7	20[63]	38	241	.20	376[63]	.43[63]	.28[63]	5[63]	.01	5	0
0	5	9.6[63]	14	24[63]	31	2[65]	.17	0	.48[63]	.24[63]	5.8[63]	.02	5	0
0	20	1.59	56	178	132	1[65]	1.15	4	.26	.05	.3	.05	10	0
0	163[60]	6.32[60]	51	133	99	285[60]	1	453[60]	.53[60]	.29[60]	5.49[60]	.74	150	0
0	168[60]	6.7[60]	51	148	137	254[60]	1	460[60]	.53[60]	.38[60]	5.9[60]	.77	150	t
0	17	1.2	33	127	118	3	1.23	0	.15	.05	1.5	.14	25	0
0	23	4.5[60]	106	264	350	320	3.7	375[60]	.37[60]	.43[60]	5[60]	.5	100	15[60]
0	6	9.83[63]	15	47	48	278	4.01	5[60]	.66[63]	.71[63]	8.64[63]	1	238	0
0	38	3.6[60]	31	109	82	246	.63	304[60]	.32[60]	.32[60]	4[60]	.4	5	12[60]
0	1	1.8[60]	3	18	26	351	.08	375[60]	.37[60]	.42[60]	5[60]	.51	100	15[60]
0	1	.7[63]	3	12	33	297	.08	375[60]	.37[60]	.42[60]	5[60]	.51	100	0
0	19	11.2[60]	71	192	248	363	5.15	522[60]	.51[60]	.59[60]	6.86[60]	.7	138	0

[59]Vitamin A values from label declaration varies from 100-150 RE for major brands.
[60]Nutrient added.
[61]Value for yellow corn grits, cooked white corn grits contain 0 RE of Vitamin A.
[62]Cooked without salt. If salt is added according to label recommendation, sodium content is 540 mg.
[63]Nutrient added-value based on label declaration.
[64]For regular and instant cereal. For quick cereal, phosphorus is 102 mg and sodium is 142 mg.
[65]Cooked without salt. If added according to label recommendations, sodium content is: 390 mg for Cream of Wheat; 324 mg for Malt-O-Meal; 374 mg for oatmeal.

(For purposes of calculations, use "0" for t, <1, <.1, <.01, etc.)

TABLE H-1

Food Composition

Grp	Ref	Name	Measure	Wt (g)	H₂O (%)	Ener (kcal)	Prot (g)	Carb (g)	Fiber (g)	Fat (g)	Fat Breakdown (g) Sat	Mono	Poly

Note: H₂O column header is H_2O.

Grp	Ref	Name	Measure	Wt (g)	H_2O (%)	Ener (kcal)	Prot (g)	Carb (g)	Fiber (g)	Fat (g)	Sat	Mono	Poly
		GRAIN PRODUCTS—Con.											
		Breakfast cereals, continued											
7	501	40% Bran Flakes, Post®	1 cup	47	3	152	5.3	37	6.5	.8	.17	.17	.34
7	502	Froot Loops®	1 cup	28	2	111	1.7	25	.3	1	.2	1	1
7	503	Golden Grahams®	1 cup	39	2	150	2.2	33.2	1.4	1.5	1.03	.13	.21
7	504	Granola, homemade	1 cup	122	3	595	15	67.3	8.05	33.1	5.84	9.37	17.2
7	505	Grape Nuts®	½ cup	57	3	202	6.6	26.4	3.31	.2	t	t	.2
7	506	Honey Nut Cheerios®	1 cup	33	3	125	3.6	26.5	.92	.8	.13	.31	.3
7	507	Lucky Charms®	1 cup	32	3	125	2.9	26.1	.7	1.2	.22	.43	.49
7	508	Nature Valley® Granola	1 cup	113	4	503	11.5	75.5	7.46	19.6	13.3	2.82	2.82
7	509	100% Natural cereal, plain	¼ cup	28	2	135	3	18	1.87	6	4.06	1.15	.54
7	510	Product 19®	1 cup	33	3	126	3.2	27.4	.43	.2	t	t	.12
7	511	Raisin Bran, Kellogg's®	1 cup	49	8	211	5.3	52.7	5.8	1.8	.18	.18	.53
7	512	Raisin Bran, Post®	1 cup	56	9	174	5.3	42.9	6.4	1.1	.2	.2	.4
7	513	Rice Krispies, Kellogg's®	1 cup	29	2	112	1.9	24.8	.12	.2	t	t	.1
7	514	Puffed Rice	1 cup	14	3	56	.9	12.6	.11	.1	.03	.03	.04
7	515	Shredded Wheat	¾ cup	32	5	115	3.5	25.4	3.94	.8	.11	.11	.34
7	516	Special K®	1½ cup	32	2	125	6.3	24	.35	.1	t	t	t
7	517	Super Sugar Crisp®	1 cup	33	2	123	2.1	29.8	.62	.3	t	t	.12
7	518	Sugar Frosted Flakes®	1 cup	35	3	133	1.8	31.7	.46	.1	t	t	t
7	519	Sugar Smacks®	¾ cup	28	3	106	2	24.7	.48	.5	.1	.1	.2
7	520	Total®	1 cup	33	4	116	3.3	26	2.4	.7	.12	.12	.35
7	521	Trix®	1 cup	28	2	108	1.5	24.9	.18	.4	.2	.1	.1
7	522	Wheaties®	1 cup	29	5	101	2.8	23.1	3.27	.5	.07	.05	.24
		Buckwheat:											
		Flour:											
7	523	Dark	1 cup	98	12	338	11.5	70.6	8	2.5	.48	.83	.9
7	524	Light	1 cup	98	12	340	6.3	77.9	6	1.1	.2	.4	.4
7	525	Whole grain, dry	1 cup	175	11	586	20.5	128	15.6	4.2	.81	1.4	1.51
		Bulgur:											
7	526	Dry, uncooked	1 cup	170	10	600	19	129	16	2.5	1.2	.3	1.2
7	527	Cooked	1 cup	135	56	246	9.5	44.3	7.07	.9	.43	.11	.43
		Cornmeal:											
7	528	Whole-ground, unbolted, dry	1 cup	122	12	435	11	90	9	5	.5	1.1	2.5
7	529	Bolted, nearly whole, dry	1 cup	122	12	440	11	90.9	7.5	4.2	.5	1.1	2.5
7	530	Degermed, enriched, dry	1 cup	138	12	502	10.9	108	4	1.7	.2	.4	.9
7	531	Degermed, enriched, cooked	1 cup	240	88	120	2.6	25.7	.93	.5	.06	.12	.25
		Macaroni, cooked:											
7	532	Firm stage, hot	1 cup	130	64	190	6.5	39.1	1.04	.7	.09	.08	.27
7	533	Tender stage, cold	1 cup	105	72	115	3.8	24	.84	.4	.06	.05	.18
7	534	Tender stage, hot	1 cup	140	72	155	5	32	1.12	.7	.08	.07	.24
7	535	Millet, cooked	½ cup	95	86	54	1.4	10.8	1.30	.5	.13	.12	.17
		Noodles:											
7	536	Egg noodles, cooked	1 cup	160	70	200	6.6	37.3	.20	2	.5	.6	.6
7	537	Chow mein, dry	1 cup	45	11	220	5.9	26.1	.05	11	2.1	7.3	.4
7	538	Spinach noodles, dry	3½ oz	100	10	380	14	71.3	.90	3.8	.95	1.14	1.14
		Popcorn:											
7	539	Air popped, plain	1 cup	8	4	30	1	6	1.45	.4	t	.1	.2
7	540	Popped in veg oil/salted	1 cup	11	3	55	.9	6	1.45	3.1	.5	1.4	1.2
7	541	Sugar syrup coated	1 cup	35	4	135	2	30	.39	1	.1	.3	.6
		Rice:											
7	542	Brown rice, cooked	1 cup	195	70	232	4.9	49.7	3.90	1.2	.31	.27	.41
		White, enriched, all types:											
7	543	Raw, dry	1 cup	185	12	670	12.4	149	2.59	.7	.2	.2	.27
7	544	Cooked without salt	1 cup	205	73	223	4.1	49.6	.82	.2	.06	.06	.08
7	545	Instant, prepared without salt	1 cup	165	73	180	3.6	39.9	.33	.2	.06	.06	.08

(For purposes of calculations, use "0" for t, <1, <.1, <.01, etc.)

KEY: 1 = BEV 2 = DAIRY 3 = EGGS 4 = FAT/OIL 5 = FRUIT 6 = BAKERY 7 = GRAIN 8 = FISH 9 = BEEF 10 = POULTRY 11 = SAUSAGE 12 = MIXED 13 = NUTS/SEEDS 14 = SWEETS 15 = VEG/LEG 16 = MISC 22 = SOUP/SAUCE

Chol (mg)	Calc (mg)	Iron (mg)	Magn (mg)	Phos (mg)	Pota (mg)	Sodi (mg)	Zinc (mg)	VT-A (RE)	Thia (mg)	Ribo (mg)	Niac (mg)	V-B6 (mg)	Fola (µg)	VT-C (mg)
0	21	7.47[60]	102	296	251	431	2.5	6296[60]	.62[60]	.72[60]	8.36[60]	.85	166	0
0	3	4.5[60]	7	24	26	145	3.7	3756[60]	.4[60]	.4[60]	56[60]	.5	100	15.[60]
0	24	6.2[60]	16	56	86	476	.34	5166[60]	.5[60]	.6[60]	6.9[60]	.7	—	21.[60]
0	76	4.84	141	494	612	12	4.47	4	.73	.31	2.14	.43	99	1
0	22	2.46	38	142	190	394	1.24	7536[60]	.8[60]	.8[60]	10[60]	1	200	0
0	23	5.2[60]	39	122	115	299	.87	4376[60]	.4[60]	.5[60]	5.8[60]	.6	4	17[60]
0	36	5.1[60]	27	88	66	227	.56	4246[60]	.4[60]	.5[60]	5.6[60]	.6	—	17[60]
0	71	3.78	116	354	389	232	2.19	8	.39	.19	.83	.32	85	0
0	49	.83	34	104	138	12	.63	2	.09	.15	.6	.64	8	0
0	4	21[60]	12	47	51	378	.5	17696[60]	1.7[60]	2[60]	23.3[60]	2.3	466	70[60]
0	33	31.6[60]	96	263	404	386	6.6	5006[60]	.66[60]	.76[60]	8.78[60]	.87	140	0
0	27	9.01[60]	96	237	349	370	3.01	7506[60]	.74[60]	.85[60]	10[60]	1.02	200	0
0	4	1.8[60]	10	34	30	340	.48	3886[60]	.4[60]	.4[60]	5[60]	.5	100	15[60]
0	1	.15[60]	4	14	16	.4	.14	0	.01[60]	.01[60]	.42[60]	.01	3	
0	12	1.35	42	112	115	3	1.05	0	.08	.09	1.67	.08	16	0
0	9	5.06[60]	18	62	55	298	4.16	4296[60]	.45[60]	.45[60]	5.63[60]	.56	112	17[60]
0	7	2.1[60]	20	60	123	29	1.7	4376[60]	.4[60]	.5[60]	5.8[60]	.6	116	0
0	1	2.2[60]	3	26	22	284	.05	4636[60]	.5[60]	.5[60]	6.2[60]	.6	124	19[60]
0	3	1.8[60]	13	31	42	75	.28	3756[60]	.37[60]	.43[60]	5[60]	.5	100	15[60]
0	56	21[60]	37	137	123	409	.78	17696[60]	1.7[60]	2[60]	23.3[60]	2.3	466	70[60]
0	6	4.5[60]	6	19	26	179	.13	3756[60]	.4[60]	.4[60]	4.9[60]	.5	—	15[60]
0	44	4.6[60]	32	100	108	363	.65	3886[60]	.4[60]	.4[60]	5.1[60]	.5	9	15[60]
0	32	2.5	135	298	490	1	2.65	0	.58	.15	2.75	.41	125	0
0	11	1	47	86	314	1	2.56	0	.09	.05	.47	.09	100	0
0	200	6.7	315	494	784	4	4.4	0	1.05	.26	7.7	.37	52	0
0	49	9.5	130	575	389	7	3.2	0	.48	.24	7.7	.38	80	0
0	27	2.87	57	263	151	3	2.81	0	.08	.05	4.1	.07	18	0
0	24	2.2	130	312	346	1	2.15	62	.46	.13	2.4	.57	33	0
0	21	2.2	129	272	303	1	2.15	62	.37	.1	2.3	.56	29	0
0	8	5.93	65	137	166	1	1.15	61	.61	.36	4.8	.34	29	0
0	2	1.48	17	34	38	1	.23	14	.14	.1	1.2	.06	6	0
0	14	2.1	17	85	103	1	.61	0	.23	.13	1.82	.1	4	0
0	8	1.31	12	53	64	1	.39	0	.15	.08	1.13	.07	3	0
0	11	1.74	15	70	85	1	.52	0	.2	.11	1.5	.09	4	0
0	3	1.1	38	47	64	1	.42	0	.1	.06	.4	.03	10	0
50	16	2.6	28	94	70	3	.2	34	.22	.13	1.9	.01	7	0
5	14	.4	—	41	33	450	.1	0	.05	.03	.6	.03	10	0
0	41	4.54	38	154	460	35	2.2	18	.98	.47	6.89	.27	73	0
0	1	.2	23	22	20	.5	.22	1	.03	.01	.2	.02	3	0
0	3	.27	25	31	19	86	.28	2	.01	.02	.1	.02	3	0
0	2	.5	29	47	90	.5	.29	3	.13	.02	.4	.03	3	0
0	23	1.17	72	142	137	0	1.05	0	.18	.04	2.73	.29	10	0
0	44	5.4	63	174	170	9	2.41	0	.81	.06	6.48	.3	18	0
0	21	2.87	23	57	57	0	.84	0	.22	.02	2.05	.1	4	0
0	5	1.32	16	31	0	0[66]	.64	0	.21	.02	1.65	.02	7	0

[60] Nutrient added.
[66] If prepared with salt according to label recommendation sodium would = 608 mg.

(For purposes of calculations, use "0" for t, <1, <.1, <.01, etc.)

H

TABLE H-1

Food Composition

Grp	Ref	Name	Measure	Wt (g)	H$_2$O (%)	Ener (kcal)	Prot (g)	Carb (g)	Fiber (g)	Fat (g)	Sat	Mono	Poly
											Fat Breakdown (g)		
		GRAIN PRODUCTS—Con.											
		Rice, continued											
		White, parboiled/converted rice:											
7	546	Raw, dry	1 cup	185	10	683	13.7	150	2.59	1	.2	.2	.4
7	547	Cooked, hot	1 cup	175	73	186	3.7	40.8	.70	.1	.02	.02	.04
7	548	Wild rice, cooked	½ cup	100	76	92	3.6	19	2.56	.2	.05	.05	.07
7	549	Rye flour medium	1 cup	115	11	392	13.2	85.2	8.60	1.9	.35	.53	.89
		Spaghetti, cooked:											
7	550	Firm stage, hot	1 cup	130	64	190	6.5	39.1	1.43	.65	.09	.08	.27
7	551	Tender stage, hot	1 cup	140	72	155	5	32	1.12	.55	.08	.07	.24
7	552	Whole wheat spaghetti, cooked	1 cup	123	67	151	6.6	32.5	4.06	.49	.07	.06	.23
7	553	Wheat bran	½ cup	18	12	38	2.9	11.1	7.92	.83	.12	.1	.39
		Wheat germ:											
7	554	Raw	1 cup	75	12	272	20	35	1.87	8.2	1.39	1.16	4.87
7	555	Toasted	1 cup	113	4	431	32.9	56.1	3.03	12.3	2.09	1.75	7.33
7	556	Rolled wheat, cooked	1 cup	240	80	142	4.2	32.1	4.87	.7	.1	.08	.33
7	557	Whole grain wheat, cooked	⅓ cup	50	86	28	.9	5.7	1.2	.2	.4	.3	1.2
		Wheat flour (unbleached):											
		All purpose, white flour, enriched:											
7	558	Sifted	1 cup	115	12	419	12.1	87.5	3.23	1.1	.18	.09	.51
7	559	Unsifted	1 cup	125	12	455	13.1	95.1	3.51	1.2	.2	.1	.55
7	560	Cake or pastry flour, enriched, sifted	1 cup	96	12	349	7	76	2.5	.96	.15	.08	.4
7	561	Self-rising, enriched, unsifted	1 cup	125	12	440	12	93	3.51	1.2	.2	.1	.55
7	562	Whole wheat, from hard wheats	1 cup	120	12	400	16	85.2	15.2	2.4	.34	.28	1.13
		MEATS: FISH and SHELLFISH											
		Clams:											
8	563	Raw meat only	3 oz	85	82	65	11	.2	.01	1	.3	.3	.3
8	564	Canned, drained	3 oz	85	77	85	13	2	.03	3	.5	.5	.4
		Cod:											
8	565	Baked with butter	3½ oz	100	74	114	23	0	0	6.1	3.2	1.5	.5
8	566	Batter fried	3½ oz	100	61	199	19.6	7.5	0	10.3	2.63	4.4	2.91
8	567	Poached, no added fat	3½ oz	100	78	94	20.9	0	0	1.1	.29	.17	.62
8	568	Crab meat, canned	1 cup	135	77	135	23	1	0	3	.5	.8	1.4
8	569	Fish sticks	2 ea	56	52	140	12	8	.02	6	1.6	2.8	1.6
		Flounder/sole, baked with lemon juice:											
8	570	With butter	3 oz	85	73	120	16	t	0	6	3.2	1.5	.5
8	571	With margarine	3 oz	85	73	120	16	t	0	6	1.2	2.3	1.9
8	572	Without added fat	3 oz	85	78	80	17	t	0	1	.3	.2	.4
8	573	Haddock, breaded/fried[67]	3 oz	85	61	175	17	7	.03	9	2.4	3.9	2.4
8	574	Halibut, broiled with butter and lemon juice	3 oz	85	67	140	20	0	0	6	3.3	1.6	.7
8	575	Herring, pickled	3 oz	85	59	190	17.3	0	0	12.8	4.3	4.6	3.1
8	576	Ocean perch, breaded/fried	3 oz	85	59	185	16	7	.03	11	2.6	4.6	2.8
		Oysters:											
		Raw:											
8	577	Eastern	1 cup	240	85	160	20	8	0	4	1.4	.5	1.4
8	578	Pacific	1 cup	240	85	160	21	8	0	5	1.75	.7	1.75
		Cooked:											
8	579	Eastern, breaded, fried	1 ea	45	65	90	5	5	0	5	1.4	2.1	1.4
8	580	Western, simmered	3½ oz	100	71	135	13.5	7.2	0	3.9	.82	.66	1.48
8	581	Pollock, steamed	3½ oz	100	77	99	23.3	0	0	.9	.1	.1	.5

[67] Dipped in egg, milk and breadcrumbs; fried in vegetable shortening.

(For purposes of calculations, use "0" for t, <1, <.1, <.01, etc.)

KEY: 1 = BEV 2 = DAIRY 3 = EGGS 4 = FAT/OIL 5 = FRUIT 6 = BAKERY 7 = GRAIN 8 = FISH 9 = BEEF 10 = POULTRY 11 = SAUSAGE 12 = MIXED 13 = NUTS/SEEDS 14 = SWEETS 15 = VEG/LEG 16 = MISC 22 = SOUP/SAUCE

Chol (mg)	Calc (mg)	Iron (mg)	Magn (mg)	Phos (mg)	Pota (mg)	Sodi (mg)	Zinc (mg)	VT-A (RE)	Thia (mg)	Ribo (mg)	Niac (mg)	V-B6 (mg)	Fola (µg)	VT-C (mg)
0	111	5.4	34	370	278	17	2.03	0	.81	.07	6.5	.48	22	0
0	33	1.4	11	100	75	9	.56	0	.19	.02	2.1	.17	7	0
0	5	1.1	33	85	55	2	1.17	0	.11	.16	1.6	1.31	35	0
0	36	2.72	90	340	304	1	1.67	0	.36	.15	2.45	.25	91	0
0	14	2.08	17	85	103	1	.61	0	.23	.13	1.82	.1	9	0
0	11	1.74	15	70	85	1	.52	0	.2	.11	1.5	.09	8	0
0	19	1.06	43	106	200	16	.91	0	.21	.09	1.54	.87	25	0
0	21	1.95	91	223	205	3	2.34	0	.14	.06	4.86	.25	46	0
0	54	4.5	252	838	620	2	11	0	1.51	.51	3.15	.69	246	0
0	50	8.71	362	1294	1070	4	18.9	0	1.89	.93	6.32	1.13	474	0
0	19	1.7	58	182	202	2	1.96	0	.17	.07	2.2	.08	27	0
0	3	.3	12	30	29	1	.44	0	.04	.01	.4	.35	6	0
0	18	5.06	24	100	109	2	.76	0	.73	.46	6.08	.05	18	0
0	20	5.5	26	109	119	3	.82	0	.8	.5	6.61	.05	20	0
0	16	4.22	20	70	91	2	.63	0	.6	.38	5.08	.04	15	0
0	331	5.5	26	583	113	1349	.83	0	.8	.5	6.61	.05	20	0
0	49	5.16	168	446	444	4	2.96	0	.66	.14	5.16	.4	58	0
43	59	2.6	31	138	154	102	1.4	26	.09	.15	1.1	.07	13	9
54	47	3.5	8	116	119	102	2.03	26	.01	.09	.9	.07	4	3
60	24	.6	26	220	372	224	.75	30	.07	.08	3	.4	11	t
55	80	.5	24	200	370	100	1	t	.02	.02	1.8	.09	3	t
60	29	.5	26	180	330	110	.75	t	.08	.08	3	.37	14	t
135	61	1.1	50	246	149	1350	5.13	14	.11	.11	2.6	.41	22	0
52	22	.6	32	116	188	106	.5	10	.06	.1	1.2	.12	10	0
68	13	.3	19	187	272	145	.72	54	.05	.08	1.6	.28	10	1
55	14	.3	19	187	273	151	.72	69	.05	.08	1.6	.28	10	1
57	13	.3	19	197	286	101	.72	10	.05	.08	1.7	.28	10	1
75	34	1	26	183	270	123	.85	20	.06	.1	2.9	.13	14	0
62	14	.68	20	206	441	103	.9	174	.06	.07	7.7	.13	6	1
85	29	.9	33	128	85	850	1.75	33	.04	.18	2.8	.11	6	0
66	31	1.2	20	191	241	138	.85	20	.10	.11	2	.22	7	0
120	226	15.6	116	343	290	175	96.7[71]	223	.34	.43	6	.13	24	24
120	202	16.8	54	379	290	185	74.4[71]	223	.29	.43	6	.13	24	72
35	49	3	14	73	64	70	9[71]	44	.07	.1	1.3	.02	2	4
77	75	8.57	31	234	312	165	48[71]	97	.15	.29	2.1	.07	11	15
75	19	.6	31	250	350	97	1	t	.12	.26	4	.62	8	t

[71] Value varies widely.

(For purposes of calculations, use "0" for t, <1, <.1, <.01, etc.)

H

TABLE H-1

Food Composition

Grp	Ref	Name	Measure	Wt (g)	H₂O (%)	Ener (kcal)	Prot (g)	Carb (g)	Fiber (g)	Fat (g)	Fat Breakdown (g)		
											Sat	Mono	Poly
MEATS: FISH and SHELLFISH—Con.													
		Salmon:											
8	582	Canned pink, solids and liquid	3 oz	85	71	120	17	0	0	5	.9	1.5	2.1
8	583	Broiled or baked	3 oz	85	67	140	21	0	0	5	1.2	2.4	1.4
8	584	Smoked	3 oz	85	59	150	18	0	0	8	2.6	3.9	.7
8	585	Atlantic sardines canned, drained	3 oz	85	62	175	20	0	0	9.4	2.1	3.7	2.9
8	586	Scallops, breaded, from frozen	6 ea	90	59	195	15	10	.02	10	2.5	4.1	2.5
		Shrimp:											
8	587	Cooked, boiled	3½ oz	100	62	109	23.8	0	0	1.5	.28	.28	.78
8	588	Canned, drained	3 oz	85	70	100	21	1	0	1	.2	.2	.4
8	589	Fried, 7 medium[69]	3 oz	85	55	200	16	11	.09	10	2.5	4.1	2.6
8	590	Trout, broiled with butter and lemon juice	3 oz	85	63	175	21	.3	0	9	4.1	2.9	1.6
		Tuna, canned, drained solids:											
8	591	Oil pack	3 oz	85	61	165	24	0	0	7	1.4	1.9	3.1
8	592	Water pack	3 oz	85	63	135	30	0	0	1	.3	.2	.3
MEAT and MEAT PRODUCTS													
		Beef, cooked:[70]											
		Braised, simmered, pot roasted:											
		Relatively fat, like chuck blade:											
9	593	Lean and fat, piece 2½x2½x¾ in	3 oz	85	43	325	22	0	0	26	10.8	11.7	.9
9	594	Lean only from item 593	2.2 oz	62	53	170	19	0	0	9	3.9	4.2	.3
		Relatively lean, like round:											
9	595	Lean and fat, piece 4⅛x2¼x¾ in	3 oz	85	54	220	25	0	0	13	4.8	5.7	.5
9	596	Lean only from item 595	2.8 oz	78	57	175	25	0	0	8	2.7	3.4	.3
		Ground beef, broiled, patty 3x⅝ in:											
9	597	Lean	3 oz	85	56	230	21	0	0	16	6.2	6.9	.6
9	598	Regular	3 oz	85	54	245	20	0	0	17.8	6.9	7.7	.7
9	599	Heart, braised	3 oz	85	65	150	24	0	0	5	1.2	.8	1.6
9	600	Liver, fried	3 oz	85	56	185	23	7	0	7	2.5	3.6	1.3
		Roast, oven cooked, no added liquid:											
		Relatively fat, rib:											
9	601	Lean and fat, piece 4⅛x2¼x½ in	3 oz	85	46	315	19	0	0	26	10.8	11.4	.9
9	602	Lean only from item 601	2.2 oz	61	57	150	17	0	0	9	3.6	3.7	.3
		Relatively lean, round:											
9	603	Lean and fat, piece 2½x2½x¾ in	3 oz	85	57	205	23	0	0	12	4.9	5.4	.5
9	604	Lean only from item 603	2.6 oz	75	63	135	22	0	0	5	1.9	2.1	.2
		Steak, broiled, sirloin:											
9	605	Lean and fat, piece 2½x2½x¾ in	3 oz	85	53	240	23	0	0	15	6.4	6.9	.6
9	606	Lean only from item 605	2.5 oz	72	59	150	22	0	0	6	2.6	2.8	.3
9	607	Beef, canned, corned	3 oz	85	59	185	22	0	0	10	4.2	4.9	.4
9	608	Beef, dried, chipped	2.5 oz	72	48	145	24	0	0	4	1.8	2	.2
		Lamb, cooked:											
		Chops (3 per lb with bone):											
		Arm chop, braised:											
9	609	Lean and fat	2.2 oz	63	44	220	20	0	0	15	6.9	6	.9
9	610	Lean part of item 609	1.7 oz	48	49	135	17	0	0	7	2.9	2.6	.4

[69] Dipped in egg, breadcrumbs, and flour; fried in vegetable shortening.
[70] Outer layer of fat removed to about ½ in of the lean. Deposits of fat within the cut remain.

(For purposes of calculations, use "0" for t, <1, <.1, <.01, etc.)

KEY: 1 = BEV 2 = DAIRY 3 = EGGS 4 = FAT/OIL 5 = FRUIT 6 = BAKERY 7 = GRAIN 8 = FISH 9 = BEEF 10 = POULTRY 11 = SAUSAGE 12 = MIXED 13 = NUTS/SEEDS 14 = SWEETS 15 = VEG/LEG 16 = MISC 22 = SOUP/SAUCE

Chol (mg)	Calc (mg)	Iron (mg)	Magn (mg)	Phos (mg)	Pota (mg)	Sodi (mg)	Zinc (mg)	VT-A (RE)	Thia (mg)	Ribo (mg)	Niac (mg)	V-B6 (mg)	Fola (µg)	VT-C (mg)
34	167[68]	.7	23	243	307	443	.77	18	.03	.15	6.8	.38	17	0
60	26	.5	26	269	305	55	.94	87	.18	.14	5.5	.68	17	0
51	12	.8	27	208	327	1700	.34	77	.17	.17	6.8	.59	8	0
85	371[68]	2.6	44	424	349	425	2.21	56	.03	.17	4.6	.28	13	0
70	39	2	62	203	369	298	1.16	21	.11	.11	1.6	.18	11	0
147	320	2.2	110	270	400	180	3.7	18	.03	.03	3.7	.1	15	t
128	98	1.4	31	224	103	1955	1.91	15	.01	.03	1.5	.07	15	0
168	61	2	24	154	189	384	2.21	26	.06	.09	2.8	.05	8	0
71	26	1	30	259	297	122	.22	60	.07	.07	2.3	.41	6	1
55	7	1.6	27	199	298	303	.94	20	.04	.09	10.1	.47	13	0
48	17	.6	26	202	255	468	.94	32	.03	.1	13.2	.42	14	0
87	11	2.5	13	163		53	5.09	t	.06	.19	2	.26	4	0
66	8	2.3	11	146	163	44	3.73	t	.05	.17	1.7	.19	3	0
81	5	2.8	25	217	248	43	4.77	t	.06	.21	3.3	.34	4	0
75	4	2.7	23	212	240	40	4.34	t	.06	.2	3	.32	4	0
74	9	1.8	21	134	256	65	3.74	t	.04	.18	4.4	.39	3	0
76	9	2.1	18	144	248	70	3.88	t	.03	.16	4.9	.39	3	0
164	5	6.4	25	213	198	54	4.92	t	.12	1.31	3.4	.09	5	5
410	9	5.3	16	392	309	90	4.34	9120[71]	.18	3.52	12.3	.31	150	23
72	8	2	17	145	246	54	4.93	t	.06	.16	3.1	.2	4	0
49	5	1.7	17	127	218	45	3.68	t	.05	.13	2.7	.2	3	0
62	5	1.6	23	177	308	50	4.65	t	.07	.14	3	.26	4	0
52	3	1.5	22	170	297	46	4.45	t	.07	.13	2.8	.25	4	0
77	9	2.6	18	186	306	53	4.93	t	.1	.23	3.3	.29	3	0
64	8	2.4	21	176	290	48	4.18	t	.09	.22	3.1	.24	6	0
80	17	3.7	13	90	51	802	3.7	t	.02	.2	2.9	.09	5	0
46	14	2.3	27	287	142	3053	4.11	t	.05	.23	2.7	.14	4	0
77	16	1.5	11	132	195	46	2.9	t	.04	.16	4.4	.11	2	0
59	12	1.3	11	111	162	36	2.26	t	.03	.13	3	.11	2	0

H

(68)If bones are discarded, calcium value greatly reduced.
(71)Value varies widely.

(For purposes of calculations, use "0" for t, <1, <.1, <.01, etc.)

TABLE H–1

Food Composition

Grp	Ref	Name	Measure	Wt (g)	H₂O (%)	Ener (kcal)	Prot (g)	Carb (g)	Fiber (g)	Fat (g)	Sat	Mono	Poly
												Fat Breakdown (g)	

MEAT and MEAT PRODUCTS—Con.
  Lamb, continued
    Loin chop, broiled:

Grp	Ref	Name	Measure	Wt (g)	H₂O (%)	Ener (kcal)	Prot (g)	Carb (g)	Fiber (g)	Fat (g)	Sat	Mono	Poly
9	611	Lean and fat	2.8 oz	80	54	235	22	0	0	16	7.3	6.4	1
9	612	Lean part of item 611	2.3 oz	64	61	140	19	0	0	6	2.6	2.4	.4
		Leg, roasted:											
9	613	Lean and fat, piece 4⅛x2¼x½ in	3 oz	85	59	205	22	0	0	13	5.6	4.9	.8
9	614	Lean only from item 613	3 oz	85	64	163	23.3	0	0	7	2.8	2.56	.47
		Rib, roasted:											
9	615	Lean and fat, piece 2½x2½x¾ in	3 oz	85	47	315	18	0	0	26	12.1	10.6	1.5
9	616	Lean only from item 615	2 oz	57	60	130	15	0	0	7	3.2	3	5
		Pork, cured, cooked (see also items 669-672):											
9	617	Bacon, medium slices	3 pce	19	13	109	5.8	.1	0	9.3	3.33	4.5	1.1
9	618	Canadian-style bacon	2 pce	47	62	86	11.3	.6	0	3.9	1.32	1.88	.37
		Ham, roasted:											
9	619	Lean and fat, 2 pieces 4⅛x2¼x¼ in	3 oz	85	58	207	18.3	0	0	14.2	5.1	6.7	1.54
9	620	Lean only	3 oz	85	66	133	21.3	0	0	4.7	1.56	2.15	.54
9	621	Ham, canned, roasted	3 oz	85	66	140	17.8	.4	0	7.2	2.4	3.5	.8
		Pork, fresh, cooked:											
		Chops, loin (cut 3 per lb with bone):											
		Broiled:											
9	622	Lean and fat	3.1 oz	87	50	275	23.9	0	0	19.2	7	8.83	2.2
9	623	Lean only from item 622	1 ea	72	57	166	23	0	0	7.5	2.6	3.4	.91
		Pan fried:											
9	624	Lean and fat	1 ea	89	45	334	20.7	0	0	27.2	9.8	12.5	3.1
9	625	Lean only from item 624	1 ea	67	54	178	19.3	0	0	10.7	3.66	4.8	1.33
		Leg, roasted:											
9	626	Lean and fat, piece 2½x2½x¾ in	3 oz	85	53	250	21	0	0	18	6.4	8.1	2
9	627	Lean only from item 626	3 oz	85	60	187	24	0	0	9.4	3.23	4.21	1.14
		Rib, roasted:											
9	628	Lean and fat, piece 2½x2½x¾ in	3 oz	85	51	270	21	0	0	20	7.25	9.2	2.3
9	629	Lean only from item 628	2½ oz	71	57	175	20	0	0	9.8	3.4	4.41	1.19
		Shoulder, braised:											
9	630	Lean and fat, 3 pieces, 2½x2½x¼ in	3 pce	85	47	295	22.7	0	0	22	7.9	10	2.4
9	631	Lean only from item 630	2.4 oz	67	54	165	22	0	0	8	2.8	3.7	1
		Veal, medium fat, cooked:											
9	632	Veal cutlet, braised or broiled, 4⅛x2¼x½ in	3 oz	85	60	185	23	0	0	9.4	4.1	4.1	.6
9	633	Veal rib roasted, 2 pieces 4⅛x2¼x¼ in	3 oz	85	55	230	23	0	0	14	6	6	1
9	634	Veal liver, simmered	3 oz	85	53	222	25.1	3.4	0	11.2	4.61	2.62	3.56

(For purposes of calculations, use "0" for t, <1, <.1, <.01, etc.)

KEY: 1 = BEV 2 = DAIRY 3 = EGGS 4 = FAT/OIL 5 = FRUIT 6 = BAKERY 7 = GRAIN 8 = FISH 9 = BEEF 10 = POULTRY
11 = SAUSAGE   12 = MIXED   13 = NUTS/SEEDS   14 = SWEETS   15 = VEG/LEG   16 = MISC   22 = SOUP/SAUCE

Chol (mg)	Calc (mg)	Iron (mg)	Magn (mg)	Phos (mg)	Pota (mg)	Sodi (mg)	Zinc (mg)	VT-A (RE)	Thia (mg)	Ribo (mg)	Niac (mg)	V-B6 (mg)	Fola (μg)	VT-C (mg)
78	16	1.4	21	162	272	62	3.11	t	.09	.21	5.5	.12	18	0
60	12	1.3	18	145	241	54	2.69	t	.08	.18	4.4	.1	16	0
78	8	1.73	20	162	273	57	3.79	t	.09	.25	5.5	.17	3	0
76	7	1.75	20	175	288	58	3.89	t	.09	.23	5.36	.19	3	0
77	19	1.4	15	139	224	60	4	t	.08	.18	5.5	.14	3	0
50	12	1	13	111	179	46	2.26	t	.05	.13	3.50	.09	2	0
16	2	.32	5	64	92	303	.62	0	.13	.05	1.39	.05	1	6[73]
27	5	.38	10	138	181	719	.79	0	.38	.09	3.22	.21	2	10[73]
53	6	.74	16	182	243	1009	1.97	0	.51	.19	3.8	.32	3	0
47	6	.8	19	193	269	1128	2.19	0	.58	.22	4.27	.4	3	0
35	6	.91	16	188	298	908	1.97	0	.82	.21	4.27	.33	4	19[73]
84	4	.7	22	184	312	61	1.68	3	.87	.24	4.35	.35	4	.3
71	4	.66	22	176	302	56	1.61	2	.83	.22	3.99	.34	4	.3
92	4	.75	23	190	323	64	1.74	3	.91	.24	4.58	.35	4	.3
71	3	.67	21	178	305	57	1.61	2	.84	.22	4.03	.34	4	.3
79	5	.85	18	210	280	50	2.43	2	.54	.27	3.89	.33	8	.3
80	6	.95	21	239	317	54	2.77	2	.59	.3	4.2	.38	10	.3
69	9	.76	16	190	313	37	1.67	3	.5	.24	4.17	.3	7	.3
56	8	.71	15	182	300	33	1.58	2	.45	.22	3.8	.28	6	.3
93	6	1.4	12	162	286	75	3.23	3	.46	.26	4.4	.31	4	0
76	5	1.3	15	235	151	68	3.87	2	.4	.24	4	.31	4	0
109	9	.8	15	196	258	56	3.48	t	.06	.21	4.6	.27	3	0
109	10	.7	20	211	259	57	3.48	t	.11	.26	6.6	.27	3	0
280	11	12.1	22	456	385	100	5.23	6464[71]	.21	3.56	14	.62	272	31

[71]Value varies widely.
[73]Values based on products containing added ascorbic acid or sodium ascorbate. If none is added, ascorbic acid content would be negligible.

(For purposes of calculations, use "0" for t, <1, <.1, <.01, etc.)

H

TABLE H–1

Food Composition

Grp	Ref	Name	Measure	Wt (g)	H$_2$O (%)	Ener (kcal)	Prot (g)	Carb (g)	Fiber (g)	Fat (g)	Fat Breakdown (g)		
											Sat	Mono	Poly
MEATS: POULTRY and POULTRY PRODUCTS													
		Chicken, cooked:											
		Fried, batter dipped[72]:											
10	635	Breast (5.6 oz with bones)	1 ea	140	52	364	34.8	12.6	.05	18.5	4.93	7.64	4.31
10	636	Drumstick (3.4 oz with bones)	1 ea	72	53	193	15.8	6	.02	11.3	2.98	4.63	2.73
10	637	Thigh	1 ea	86	52	238	18.6	7.8	.03	14.2	3.79	5.77	3.36
10	638	Wing	1 ea	49	46	159	9.7	5.4	.02	10.7	2.85	4.39	2.48
		Fried, flour coated[72]:											
10	639	Breast (4.2 oz with bones)	1 ea	98	57	218	31.2	1.6	.01	8.7	2.4	3.43	1.92
10	640	Drumstick (2.6 oz with bones)	1 ea	49	57	120	13.2	.8	.01	6.7	1.79	2.66	1.58
10	641	Thigh	1 ea	62	54	162	16.6	2	.01	9.3	2.54	3.64	2.11
10	642	Wing	1 ea	32	49	103	8.4	.8	.01	7.1	1.94	2.84	1.58
		Roasted:											
10	643	All types of meat	1 cup	140	64	266	40.5	0	0	10.4	2.86	3.72	2.37
10	644	Dark meat	1 cup	140	63	286	38.3	0	0	13.6	3.72	4.98	3.17
10	645	Light meat	1 cup	140	65	242	43.3	0	0	6.3	1.78	2.16	1.37
10	646	Breast, without skin	½ ea	86	65	142	26.7	0	0	3	.87	1.07	.66
10	647	Drumstick	1 ea	44	67	76	12.5	0	0	2.5	.65	.82	.6
10	648	Thigh	1 ea	62	59	153	15.5	0	0	9.6	2.86	3.81	2.12
10	649	Chicken meat, stewed, all types	1 cup	140	67	248	38.2	0	0	9.4	2.58	3.34	2.15
10	650	Chicken liver, simmered	1 ea	20	68	30	4.9	1.7	0	1.1	.37	.27	.18
10	651	Duck, meat only, roasted	½ duck	221	64	445	51.9	0	0	24.8	9.22	8.18	3.15
		Turkey, roasted, meat only:											
10	652	Dark meat	3 oz	85	63	159	24.3	0	0	6.1	2.06	1.39	1.84
10	653	Light meat	3 oz	85	66	133	25.4	0	0	2.7	.87	.48	.73
10	654	All types, chopped or diced	1 cup	140	65	240	41	0	0	7	2.29	1.45	2
10	655	All types, slices	3 oz	85	65	145	24.9	0	0	4.2	1.39	.88	1.21
		Poultry food products (see also items 664, 668, 673, 676):											
10	656	Canned, boneless chicken	5 oz	142	69	235	30.9	0	0	11.3	3.12	4.47	2.48
10	657	Chicken frankfurter	1 ea	45	58	115	5.8	3.1	0	8.8	2.49	3.81	1.82
10	658	Chicken roll, light meat	2 pce	57	69	90	11.1	1.4	0	4.2	1.15	1.68	.91
10	659	Gravy and turkey, frozen package	5 oz	142	85	95	8.3	6.5	.43	3.7	1.21	1.4	.7
10	660	Turkey loaf breast meat	2 pce	42	72	46	9.6	0	0	.7	.21	.19	.12
10	661	Turkey patty, breaded, fried	1 ea	64	50	181	9	10	.03	11.5	3	4.8	3
10	662	Turkey, frozen, roasted, seasoned	3 oz	85	68	130	18	3	0	5	1.6	1	1.4
MEATS: SAUSAGES and LUNCHMEATS													
		Bologna:											
11	663	Beef and Pork	1 pce	28	54	89	3.3	.8	0	8	3.03	3.8	.68
11	664	Turkey	2 pce	57	66	113	7.8	.6	0	8.6	2.96	3.71	2.45
11	665	Braunschweiger sausage	2 pce	57	48	205	8	1.8	0	18.3	6.21	8.5	2.12
11	666	Brown and serve sausage links, cooked	1 ea	13	45	50	2	.1	0	5	1.7	2.2	.5
		Frankfurter (see also item 657):											
11	667	Beef and Pork	1 ea	45	54	145	5.1	1.1	0	13.1	4.84	6.15	1.23
11	668	Turkey	1 ea	45	63	102	6.4	.7	0	8.3	2.4	2.73	2.12
		Ham:											
11	669	Ham luncheon meat, canned 3x2x½ in	1 pce	21	52	70	2.6	.4	0	6.4	2.27	3	.75
11	670	Chopped ham, packaged	2 pce	42	61	98	6.7	.1	0	7.9	2.64	3.85	.86
11	671	Ham lunchmeat, regular	2 pce	57	65	103	10	1.8	0	6	1.92	2.81	.69

[72]Fried in vegetable shortening.

(For purposes of calculations, use "0" for t, <1, <.1, <.01, etc.)

KEY: 1 = BEV 2 = DAIRY 3 = EGGS 4 = FAT/OIL 5 = FRUIT 6 = BAKERY 7 = GRAIN 8 = FISH 9 = BEEF 10 = POULTRY
11 = SAUSAGE 12 = MIXED 13 = NUTS/SEEDS 14 = SWEETS 15 = VEG/LEG 16 = MISC 22 = SOUP/SAUCE

Chol (mg)	Calc (mg)	Iron (mg)	Magn (mg)	Phos (mg)	Pota (mg)	Sodi (mg)	Zinc (mg)	VT-A (RE)	Thia (mg)	Ribo (mg)	Niac (mg)	V-B6 (mg)	Fola (µg)	VT-C (mg)
119	28	1.75	34	258	282	385	1.33	28	.16	.2	14.7	.6	8	0
62	12	.97	14	106	134	194	1.67	19	.08	.15	3.67	.2	6	0
80	16	1.24	18	134	165	248	1.75	25	.1	.2	4.92	.23	8	0
39	10	.63	8	59	68	157	.67	17	.05	.07	2.58	.15	3	0
88	16	1.17	29	228	253	74	1.07	15	.08	.13	13.5	.57	4	0
44	6	.66	11	86	112	44	1.42	12	.04	.11	2.96	.17	4	0
60	8	.93	15	116	147	55	1.56	18	.06	.15	4.31	.21	5	0
26	5	.4	6	48	57	25	.56	12	.02	.04	2.14	.13	1	0
125	21	1.69	35	273	340	120	2.94	22	.1	.25	12.8	.65	8	0
130	21	1.86	33	250	336	130	3.92	30	.1	.32	9.17	.5	11	0
118	21	1.49	38	302	345	108	1.73	12	.09	.16	17.4	.84	5	0
73	13	.89	25	196	220	64	.86	5	.06	.1	11.8	.52	3	0
41	5	.57	11	81	108	42	1.4	8	.03	.1	2.67	.17	4	0
58	8	.83	14	108	137	52	1.46	30	.04	.13	3.95	.19	4	0
116	20	1.63	29	210	252	98	2.79	21	.07	.23	8.56	.37	8	0
126	3	1.7	2	62	28	10	.87	983	.03	.35	.89	.12	154	3
198	27	5.97	44	449	557	143	5.75	51	.57	1.04	11.3	.55	22	0
72	27	1.99	21	174	247	67	3.8	0	.05	.21	3.1	.3	8	0
59	16	1.14	24	186	259	54	1.73	0	.05	.11	5.81	.46	5	0
106	35	2.49	37	298	418	99	4.34	0	.09	.26	7.62	.64	10	0
64	21	1.51	22	181	254	60	2.64	0	.05	.15	4.63	.39	6	0
88	20	2.2	17	158	196	714	2.13	48	.02	.18	8.99	.5	4	3
45	43	.9	8	48	38	616	1	17	.03	.05	1.39	.09	2	0
28	24	.55	10	89	129	331	.41	14	.04	.07	3	.31	2	0
26	20	1.32	11	115	87	787	.99	18	.03	.18	2.55	.14	2	0
17	3	.17	8	97	118	608	.48	0	.02	.04	3.54	.15	2	0[74]
40	9	1.41	12	173	176	512	1.5	7	.06	.12	1.47	.13	2	0
45	4	1.4	20	207	253	578	2.37	0	.04	.14	5.3	.24	5	0
16	3	.43	3	26	51	289	.55	0	.05	.04	.73	.05	1	6[73]
56	47	.87	8	74	113	498	.99	0	.03	.09	2.1	.1	3	t
89	6	5.32	6	96	113	652	1.62	2406	.14	.87	4.78	.19	57	5[73]
9	1	.1	2	14	25	105	.15	0	.05	.02	.40	.03	<1	0
23	5	.52	5	39	75	504	.83	0	.09	.05	1.18	.06	2	12[73]
44	53	.77	8	71	84	550	1	17	.11	.12	1.77	.09	2	t
13	1	.15	2	17	45	271	.31	0	.08	.04	.66	.04	1	t
21	3	.4	5	58	119	573	.77	0	.23	.07	1.4	.13	2	.8[73]
32	4	.56	11	140	188	746	1.21	0	.49	.14	2.98	.19	2	16[73]

[73] Values based on products containing added ascorbic acid or sodium ascorbate. If none added, ascorbic acid content would be negligible.
[74] If sodium ascorbate is added, product contains 11 mg ascorbic acid.

(For purposes of calculations, use "0" for t, <1, <.1, <.01, etc.)

TABLE H–1

Food Composition

Grp	Ref	Name	Measure	Wt (g)	H$_2$O (%)	Ener (kcal)	Prot (g)	Carb (g)	Fiber (g)	Fat (g)	Fat Breakdown (g) Sat	Mono	Poly
		MEATS: SAUSAGES and LUNCHMEATS—Con.											
		Ham, continued											
11	672	Ham lunchmeat, extra lean	2 pce	57	70	75	11	.6	0	2.8	.92	1.33	.27
11	673	Turkey ham	2 pce	57	71	75	11	.2	0	3	.95	.75	.75
11	674	Pork sausage link, cooked[75]	1 ea	13	45	50	2.5	.1	0	4	1.4	1.81	.5
		Salami:											
11	675	Pork and beef	2 pce	57	60	145	8	1	0	11.5	4.61	5.23	1.14
11	676	Turkey	2 pce	57	66	111	9.3	.3	0	7.8	2.27	2.58	2
11	677	Dry, beef and pork	2 pce	20	35	85	4.6	.5	0	6.9	2.4	3.42	.64
11	678	Sandwich spread, pork and beef	1 tbsp	15	60	35	1.1	1.8	0	2.6	.9	1.14	.38
11	679	Vienna sausage, canned	1 ea	16	60	45	1.6	.3	0	4	1.48	2.01	.27
		MIXED DISHES and FAST FOODS											
12	680	Beef and vegetable stew, homemade	1 cup	245	82	220	16	15	3.4	11	4.4	4.5	.5
12	681	Beef pot pie, homemade[76]	1 pce	210	55	515	21	39	1.15	30	7.90	12.9	7.4
12	682	Chicken a la king, home recipe	1 cup	245	68	470	27	12	1.33	34	12.9	13.4	6.2
12	683	Chicken and noodles, home recipe	1 cup	240	71	365	22	26	1.2	18	5.1	7.1	3.9
12	684	Chicken chow mein, canned	1 cup	250	89	95	7	18	5	1	.1	.1	.8
12	685	Chicken chow mein, home recipe	1 cup	250	78	255	31	10	4.11	11	3.61	4.31	3.08
12	686	Chicken pot pie, home recipe[76]	1 pce	232	57	545	23	42	1.7	31	10.3	15.5	6.6
12	687	Chili con carne with beans, canned	1 cup	255	72	339	19.1	31.1	5.1	15.6	5.8	7.2	1
12	688	Chop suey with beef and pork	1 cup	250	75	300	26	13	2.4	17	4.3	7.4	4.2
12	689	Corn pudding[77]	1 cup	250	76	271	11	31.9	9.43	13.3	6.34	4.30	1.71
12	690	Cole slaw[78]	1 cup	120	82	84	1.5	14.9	2.4	3.1	.46	.85	1.62
12	691	French toast, home recipe[143]	1 pce	65	53	156	6.4	15.5	.76	7.75	2.37	3.08	1.56
		Macaroni and cheese:											
12	692	Canned[79]	1 cup	240	80	230	9	26	1.4	10	4.7	2.9	1.3
12	693	Home recipe[49]	1 cup	200	58	430	17	40	1.2	22	9.8	7.4	3.6
12	694	Quiche lorraine[76], ⅛ of 8 in quiche	1 pce	176	47	600	13	29	.54	48	23.2	17.8	4.1
		Spaghetti (enriched) in tomato sauce:											
		With cheese:											
12	695	Canned	1 cup	250	80	190	6	39	2.5	2	.4	.4	.5
12	696	Home recipe	1 cup	250	77	260	9	37	2.5	9	3	3.6	1.2
		With meatballs:											
12	697	Canned	1 cup	250	78	260	12	29	2.75	10	2.4	3.9	3.1
12	698	Home recipe	1 cup	248	70	330	19	39	2.75	12	3.9	4.4	2.2
		Burrito[80]:											
12	699	Beef and bean	1 ea	175	54	390	21	40	5	17.5	6.8	6.72	2.29
12	700	Bean	1 ea	174	55	322	13.1	47.1	8.22	9.9	3.76	3.35	2.2
		Cheeseburger:											
12	701	Regular	1 ea	112	46	300	15	28	1.4	15	7.3	5.6	1
12	702	4 oz patty	1 ea	194	46	524	30	39.6	2.32	31.4	15.1	12.2	1.4
12	703	Chicken patty sandwich	1 ea	157	52	436	24.8	33.8	1.35	22.5	6.13	9.5	5.4
12	704	Corn dog	1 ea	111	45	330	10	27.3	.1	20	8.4	10	1.4
12	705	Enchilada[84]	1 ea	230	72	235	20	24	2	16	7.7	6.7	.6
12	706	English muffin with egg, cheese, bacon	1 ea	138	49	360	18	31	1.54	18	8	8	.7

[49] Made with margarine.
[75] One patty (8 per pound) of bulk sausage is equivalent to 2 links.
[76] Crust made with vegetable shortening and enriched flour.
[77] Recipe: 55% yellow corn, 23% whole milk, 14% egg, 4% sugar, 3% salt, and 1% pepper.
[78] Recipe: 41% cabbage, 12% celery, 12% table cream, 12% sugar, 7% green pepper, 6% lemon juice, 4% onion, 3% pimento, 3% vinegar, 2% salt, dry mustard and white pepper.
[79] Made with corn oil.
[80] Made with a 10½ inch diameter flour tortilla.
[84] USDA data was unspecified for type of enchilada.
[143] Recipe: 35% whole milk, 32% white bread, 29% egg and cooked in 4% margarine.

(For purposes of calculations, use "0" for t, <1, <.1, <.01, etc.)

KEY: 1 = BEV 2 = DAIRY 3 = EGGS 4 = FAT/OIL 5 = FRUIT 6 = BAKERY 7 = GRAIN 8 = FISH 9 = BEEF 10 = POULTRY
11 = SAUSAGE 12 = MIXED 13 = NUTS/SEEDS 14 = SWEETS 15 = VEG/LEG 16 = MISC 22 = SOUP/SAUCE

Chol (mg)	Calc (mg)	Iron (mg)	Magn (mg)	Phos (mg)	Pota (mg)	Sodi (mg)	Zinc (mg)	VT-A (RE)	Thia (mg)	Ribo (mg)	Niac (mg)	V-B6 (mg)	Fola (μg)	VT-C (mg)
27	4	.43	10	124	198	810	1.09	0	.53	.13	2.74	.26	2	15[73]
32	6	1.56	12	108	184	565	1.56	0	.04	.15	2.72	.16	4	0
11	4	.16	2	24	47	168	.33	0	.1	.03	.59	.04	<1	t
37	7	1.5	7	66	113	607	1.22	0	.14	.2	2.02	.12	0	7[73]
46	11	.93	9	73	125	535	1.25	0	.06	.15	2.23	.14	5	t
16	2	.3	4	28	76	372	.64	0	.12	.06	.97	.1	0	6[73]
6	2	.12	1	9	16	152	.15	1	.03	.02	.26	.02	<1	0
8	2	.14	1	8	16	152	.26	0	.01	.02	.26	.02	<1	0
71	29	2.9	41	184	613	292	3.9	568	.15	.17	4.7	.28	37	17
42	29	3.8	6	149	334	596	3.17	517	.29	.29	4.8	.24	29	6
221	127	2.5	20	358	404	760	1.8	272	.1	.42	5.4	.23	11	12
103	26	2.2	34	247	149	600	2.07	130	.05	.17	4.3	.16	9	1
8	45	1.3	14	85	418	725	1.3	28	.05	.1	1	.09	12	13
75	58	2.5	28	293	473	718	2.12	50	.08	.23	4.3	.41	19	10
56	70	3	25	232	343	594	2	735	.32	.32	4.9	.46	29	5
28	82	4.3	40	321	594	1354	4.15	15	.08	.18	3.3	.27	41	8
68	60	4.8	32	248	425	1053	3.58	60	.28	.38	5	.32	22	33
230	100	1.4	38	143	402	138	1.26	89	1.03	.32	2.47	.29	63	7.1
10[145]	54	.7	12	38	218	28	.24	98	.08	.07	.33	.17	32	39
140	87	1.34	13	105	112	257	.66	80	.12	.16	1.05	.05	18	t
24	199	1	31	182	139	730	1.34	72	.12	.24	1	.02	8	t
44	362	1.8	37	322	240	1086	1.35	232	.2	.4	1.8	.05	10	1
285	211	1	23	276	283	653	1.95	454	.11	.32	1.2	.15	17	t
3	40	2.8	16	88	303	955	1.12	120	.35	.28	4.5	.13	6	10
8	80	2.3	26	135	408	955	1.3	140	.25	.18	2.3	.2	8	13
23	53	3.3	20	113	245	1220	2.39	100	.15	.18	2.3	.12	5	5
89	124	3.7	40	236	665	1009	2.45	159	.25	.3	.4	.19	7	22
52	165	2.7	61	274	388	516	3.30	58	.26	.29	4.36	.73	48	5
15	181	2.53	76	243	427	1030	2.37	58	.26	.23	2.4	1.01	55	5
44	135	2.3	22	174	219	672	2.53	65	.26	.24	3.7	.11	20	1
104	236	4.45	43	320	407	1224	5.27	128	.33	.48	7.37	.23	23	3
68	44	1.87	30	173	194	2732	1	16	.29	.26	9.21	.37	18	4
37	34	1.94	22	303	164	1252	1.44	t	.28	.17	3.27	.11	2	3
19	322	3.29	76	198	653	1332	1.2	352	.18	.26	t	.25	19	t
213	197	3.1	28	290	201	832	1.86	160	.46	.5	3.71	.15	35	1

[73] Values based on products containing added ascorbic acid or sodium ascorbate. If none added, ascorbic acid content would be negligible.
[145] From dairy cream in recipe.

(For purposes of calculations, use "0" for t, <1, <.1, <.01, etc.)

H

TABLE H–1

Food Composition

Grp	Ref	Name	Measure	Wt (g)	H$_2$O (%)	Ener (kcal)	Prot (g)	Carb (g)	Fiber (g)	Fat (g)	Fat Breakdown (g) Sat	Mono	Poly
		MIXED DISHES and FAST FOODS—Con.											
		Fish sandwich:											
12	707	Regular with cheese	1 ea	140	43	420	16.2	38.5	1.3	22.6	6.3	6.9	7.7
12	708	Large without cheese	1 ea	170	48	470	18	41.1	1.36	26.7	6.3	8.7	9.5
		Hamburger with bun:											
12	709	Regular	1 ea	98	46	245	12	8	1.3	11	4.4	5.3	.5
12	710	4 oz patty	1 ea	174	50	445	25	38	1.35	21	7.1	11.7	.6
12	711	Hotdog/frankfurter and bun	1 ea	85	53	260	8.4	21.1	1.2	15.3	5.3	7	1.8
12	712	Cheese pizza, ⅛ of 15 in round[76]	1 pce	120	46	290	15	39	2.16	9	4.1	2.6	1.3
12	713	Roast beef sandwich	1 ea	150	52	345	22.3	33.8	1.35	13.3	3.5	6.9	1.8
12	714	Beef taco	1 ea	81	55	195	9	15	.91	11	4.1	5.5	.8
12	715	Potato salad with mayonnaise and egg[81]	1 cup	250	76	358	6.7	27.9	3.7	20.5	3.6	6.2	9.34
12	716	Spinach souffle[82]	1 cup	136	74	218	11	2.8	3.81	18.4	7.15	6.84	3.08
12	717	Tuna salad[83]	1 cup	205	63	375	33	19	2.46	19	3.3	4.9	9.2
		NUTS, SEEDS and PRODUCTS											
		Almonds:											
13	718	Slivered, packed	1 cup	135	4	795	26.9	27.5	14.3[85]	70.5	6.68	45.8	14.8
		Whole, dried:											
13	719	Cup	1 cup	142	4	837	28.3	29	15.1[85]	74.1	7.03	48.2	15.6
13	720	Ounce	1 oz	28	4	167	5.7	5.8	3[85]	14.8	1.41	9.63	3.11
13	721	Almond butter	1 tbsp	16	1	101	2.4	3.4	1.44	9.5	.9	6.14	2
13	722	Brazil nuts, dry (about 7)	1 oz	28	3	186	4.1	3.6	2.52	18.8	4.59	6.54	6.85
		Cashew nuts:											
		Dry roasted, salted:											
13	723	Cup	1 cup	137	2	787	21	44.8	8.1	63.5	12.6	37.4	10.7
13	724	Ounce	1 oz	28	2	163	4.3	9.3	1.72	13.2	2.6	7.76	2.23
		Oil roasted, salted:											
13	725	Cup	1 cup	130	4	748	21	37.1	7.9	62.7	12.4	36.9	10.6
13	726	Ounce	1 oz	28	4	163	4.6	8.1	1.72	13.7	2.71	8.07	2.32
13	727	Cashew butter	1 tbsp	16	3	94	2.8	4.4	.97	7.9	1.56	4.66	1.34
13	728	European chestnuts, roasted, 1 cup=approx 17 kernels	1 cup	143	40	350	4.5	75.7	18.5	3.1	.59	1.09	1.24
		Coconut:											
		Raw:											
13	729	Piece 2x2x½ in	1 pce	45	47	159	1.5	6.8	6.12	15.1	13.4	.64	.17
13	730	Shredded/grated[91]	1 cup	80	47	283	2.7	12.2	11.2	26.8	23.8	1.14	.29
		Dried, shredded/grated:											
13	731	Unsweetened	1 cup	78	3	515	5.4	18.5	19.3	50.3	44.6	2.14	.55
13	732	Sweetened	1 cup	93	16	466	2.7	44.3	19.3	33	29.3	1.4	.36
		Filberts (hazelnuts), chopped:											
13	733	Cup	1 cup	115	5	727	15	17.6	7.82	72	5.3	56.5	6.9
13	734	Ounce	1 oz	28	5	179	3.7	4.3	1.93	17.8	1.31	13.9	1.71
		Macadamia nuts, oil roasted, salted:											
13	735	Cup	1 cup	134	2	962	9.7	17.3	5.4	103	15.4	80.9	1.77
13	736	Ounce	1 oz	28	2	204	2.1	3.7	1.14	21.7	3.25	17.1	.38
		Mixed nuts, salted:											
13	737	Dry roasted	1 cup	137	2	814	23.7	34.7	11	70.5	9.45	43	14.8
13	738	Roasted in oil	1 cup	142	2	876	23.8	30.4	11.4	80	12.4	45	18.9

[76] Crust made with vegetable shortening and enriched flour.
[81] Recipe: 62% potatoes, 12% egg, 8% mayonnaise, 7% celery, 6% sweet pickle relish, 2% onion, 1% each for green pepper, pimiento, salt, and dry mustard.
[82] Recipe: 29% whole milk, 26% spinach, 13% egg white, 13% cheddar cheese, 7% egg yolk, 7% butter, 4% flour, 1% salt and pepper.
[83] Made with drained chunk light tuna, celery, onion, pickle relish, and mayonnaise-type salad dressing.
[85] Values reported for dietary fiber in almonds vary from 7.0 to 14.3 per 100 grams.
[91] 1 cup packed = 130 grams.

(For purposes of calculations, use "0" for t, <1, <.1, <.01, etc.)

KEY: 1 = BEV 2 = DAIRY 3 = EGGS 4 = FAT/OIL 5 = FRUIT 6 = BAKERY 7 = GRAIN 8 = FISH 9 = BEEF 10 = POULTRY
11 = SAUSAGE 12 = MIXED 13 = NUTS/SEEDS 14 = SWEETS 15 = VEG/LEG 16 = MISC 22 = SOUP/SAUCE

Chol (mg)	Calc (mg)	Iron (mg)	Magn (mg)	Phos (mg)	Pota (mg)	Sodi (mg)	Zinc (mg)	VT-A (RE)	Thia (mg)	Ribo (mg)	Niac (mg)	V-B6 (mg)	Fola (µg)	VT-C (mg)
56	132	1.85	29	223	274	667	.95	25	.32	.27	3.3	.1	24	3
90	61	2.23	34	246	375	621	.88	15	.35	.24	3.52	.12	42	1
32	56	2.2	19	107	202	463	2	14	.23	.24	3.8	.12	16	1
71	75	4.84	40	225	404	763	5.01	28	.38	.38	7.85	.28	24	2
23	59	1.71	13	83	113	745	1.19	t	.29	.19	2.48	.07	17	12
56	220	1.6	40	216	230	699	1.73	106	.34	.29	4.2	.04	40	2
55	60	4.04	38	222	338	757	3.66	32	.39	.33	6.02	.28	42	2
21	109	1.15	36	134	263	456	1.56	57	.09	.07	1.41	.12	14	1
170	48	1.63	39	130	635	1323	.78	82	.19	.15	2.23	.35	17	25
184	230	1.34	37	231	202	763	1.29	675	.09	.3	.48	.12	62	3
80	31	2.5	42	281	531	877	1.16	53	.06	.14	13.3	.49	41	6
0	359	4.94	400	702	988	15	3.94	0	.28	1.05	4.54	.15	79	1
0	378	5.2	420	738	1034	15[86]	4.15	0	.3	1.11	4.77	.16	83	1
0	75	1.04	84	147	208	3[86]	.83	0	.06	.22	.95	.03	17	t
0	43	.59	48	84	121	2[87]	.49	0	.02	.1	.46	.01	0	t
0	50	.96	64	170	170	0	1.3	t	.28	.04	.46	.07	1	t
0	62	8.22	356	671	774	877[88]	7.67	0	.27	.27	1.92	.35	95	0
0	13	1.7	74	139	160	181[88]	1.59	0	.06	.06	.4	.07	20	0
0	53	5.33	332	554	689	814[89]	6.18	0	.55	.23	2.34	.33	88	0
0	12	1.16	72	121	151	177[89]	1.35	0	.12	.05	.51	.07	19	0
0	7	.09	41	73	87	2[90]	.83	0	.05	.03	.26	.04	11	0
0	42	1.3	47	153	846	3	.81	3	.35	.25	1.92	.71	100	37
0	6	1.09	14	51	160	9	.49	0	.03	<.01	.24	.02	12	1
0	12	1.94	26	90	285	16	.88	0	.05	.02	.43	.04	21	3
0	20	2.59	70	161	423	29	1.57	0	.05	.08	.47	2.34	7	1
0	14	1.79	47	100	313	244	1.69	0	.03	.02	.44	.29	9	1
0	216	3.76	328	359	512	3	2.76	8	.57	.13	1.31	.7	83	1
0	53	.93	81	89	126	1	.68	2	.14	.03	.32	.17	20	t
0	60	2.41	157	268	441	348[92]	1.47	1	.28	.15	2.71	.33	79	0
0	13	.51	33	57	94	74[92]	.31	3	.06	.03	.57	.07	17	0
0	96	5.07	308	596	817	917[93]	5.21	2	.27	.27	6.44	.41	69	1
0	153	4.56	334	659	825	926[93]	7.22	3	.71	.32	7.19	.34	118	1

[86] Salted almonds contain 1108 mg sodium per cup, 221 mg sodium per ounce.
[87] Salted almond butter contains 72 mg sodium per tablespoon.
[88] Dry roasted cashews without salt contain 21 mg of sodium per cup or 4 mg per ounce.
[89] Oil roasted cashews without salt contain 22 mg sodium per cup or 5 mg per ounce.
[90] Salted cashew butter contains 98 mg sodium per tablespoon.
[92] Macadamia nuts without salt contain 9 mg sodium per cup or 2 mg per ounce.
[93] Mixed nuts without salt contain about 15 mg sodium per cup.

(For purposes of calculations, use "0" for t, <1, <.1, <.01, etc.)

H

TABLE H-1

Food Composition

Grp	Ref	Name	Measure	Wt (g)	H₂O (%)	Ener (kcal)	Prot (g)	Carb (g)	Fiber (g)	Fat (g)	Fat Breakdown (g) Sat	Mono	Poly
		NUTS, SEEDS and PRODUCTS—Con.											
		Peanuts:											
		Oil roasted, salted:											
13	739	Cup	1 cup	145	2	841	38.8	26.8	11.7	71.3	9.93	35.5	22.6
13	740	Ounce	1 oz	28	2	165	7.6	5.2	2.2	14.	1.95	7	4.43
		Dried, unsalted:											
13	741	Cup	1 cup	146	7	827	37.5	23.6	13.6	71.8	9.96	35.6	22.7
13	742	Ounce	1 oz	28	7	161	7.3	4.6	2.65	14	1.94	6.93	4.41
13	743	Peanut butter	1 tbsp	16	2	95	4.6	2.5	1.24	8.2	1.4	4	2.5
		Pecans, halves, dried:											
13	744	Cup	1 cup	108	5	720	8.4	19.7	6.54[96]	73.1	5.85	45.6	18.1
13	745	Ounce	1 oz	28	5	190	2.2	5.2	1.72[96]	19.2	1.54	12	4.8
13	746	Pine nuts/pinyon, dried	1 oz	28	6	161	3.3	5.5	1.7	17.3	2.64	6.52	7.3
13	747	Pistachio nuts, dried, shelled	1 oz	28	4	164	5.9	7	1.3	13.7	1.74	9.28	2.08
13	748	Pumpkin kernels, dried, unsalted	1 oz	28	7	154	7	5.1	1.54	13	2.46	4.05	5.94
13	749	Sesame seeds, hulled, dry	¼ cup	38	5	221	9.9	3.5	6	20.6	2.88	7.75	9
		Sunflower seed kernels:											
13	750	Dry	¼ cup	36	5	205	8.2	6.8	2	17.9	1.87	3.4	11.8
13	751	Oil roasted	¼ cup	34	3	208	7.2	5	1.84	19.4	2.03	3.7	12.8
13	752	Tahini (sesame butter)	1 tbsp	15	3	91	2.7	2.7	2.24	8.5	1.19	3.2	3.71
		Black walnuts, chopped:											
13	753	Cup	1 cup	125	4	759	30.4	15.1	10.6	70.7	4.54	15.9	46.9
13	754	Ounce	1 oz	28	4	172	6.9	3.4	2.4	16.1	1.03	3.61	10.7
		English walnuts, chopped:											
13	755	Cup	1 cup	120	4	770	17.2	22	8.4	74.2	6.7	17	47
13	756	Ounce	1 oz	28	4	182	4.1	5.2	1.98	17.6	1.59	4.03	11.1
		SWEETENERS and SWEETS: see also Dairy (milk desserts) and Baked Goods											
14	757	Apple butter	2 tbsp	35	52	66	.1	16.5	.39	.3	.08	.02	.13
14	758	Caramel, plain or chocolate	1 oz	28	8	115	1	22	.06	3	2.2	.3	.1
		Chocolate (see also, items 784, 785 and 971):											
		Milk chocolate:											
14	759	Plain	1 oz	28	1	145	2	16	.31	9	5.4	3	.3
14	760	With almonds	1 oz	28	2	150	2.9	15	.98	10.4	4.4	4.65	1
14	761	With peanuts	1 oz	28	1	155	4.9	10	1.59	11.7	3.5	5.2	2.7
14	762	With rice cereal	1 oz	28	2	140	2	18	.8	7	4.4	2.5	.2
14	763	Semi-sweet chocolate chips	1 cup	170	1	860	7	97	5.4	61	36.2	19.9	1.9
14	764	Sweet dark chocolate	1 oz	28	1	150	1	16	.9	10	5.9	3.3	.3
14	765	Fondant candy, uncoated (mints, candy corn, other)	1 oz	28	3	105	0	27	0	0	0	0	0
14	766	Fudge, chocolate	1 oz	28	8	115	.6	21	.06	2.8	2.1	1	.1
14	767	Gum drops	1 oz	28	12	98	0	24.8	0	.2	t	t	.1
14	768	Hard candy, all flavors	1 oz	28	1	109	0	27.6	0	0	0	0	0
14	769	Jelly beans	1 oz	28	6	104	t	26.4	0	t	t	t	.1 d
14	770	Marshmallows	4 ea	28	17	90	.6	23	0	0	0	0	0
14	771	Gelatin salad/dessert	½ cup	120	84	70	1.8	16.9	.10	0	0	0	0
		Honey:											
14	772	Cup	1 cup	339	17	1030	1	279	0	0	0	0	0
14	773	Tablespoon	1 tbsp	21	17	65	<.1	17.4	0	0	0	0	0
		Jam or preserves:											
14	774	Tablespoon	1 tbsp	20	29	54	.1	14	.12	<.1	0	<.01	<.01
14	775	Packet	1 ea	14	29	38	<.1	9.8	.08	<.1	0	<.01	<.01

[96] Dietary fiber data calculated/derived from data on other nuts.

(For purposes of calculations, use "0" for t, <1, <.1, <.01, etc.)

H

KEY: 1 = BEV 2 = DAIRY 3 = EGGS 4 = FAT/OIL 5 = FRUIT 6 = BAKERY 7 = GRAIN 8 = FISH 9 = BEEF 10 = POULTRY
11 = SAUSAGE 12 = MIXED 13 = NUTS/SEEDS 14 = SWEETS 15 = VEG/LEG 16 = MISC 22 = SOUP/SAUCE

Chol (mg)	Calc (mg)	Iron (mg)	Magn (mg)	Phos (mg)	Pota (mg)	Sodi (mg)	Zinc (mg)	VT-A (RE)	Thia (mg)	Ribo (mg)	Niac (mg)	V-B6 (mg)	Fola (µg)	VT-C (mg)
0	125	2.78	273	734	1020	626[94]	9.6	0	.42	.15	21.5	.58	153	0
0	24	.54	53	144	200	123[94]	1.88	0	.08	.03	4.20	.11	30	0
0	85	4.72	263	559	1047	23	4.78	0	.97	.19	20.7	.43	153	0
0	17	.92	51	109	204	5	.93	0	.19	.04	4.02	.08	30	0
0	5	.29	28	60	110	75[95]	.47	0	.02	.02	2.15	.06	13	0
0	39	2.3	138	314	423	1[97]	5.91	14	.92	.14	.96	.2	42	2
0	10	.6	36	83	111	3[97]	1.55	4	.24	.04	.25	.05	11	1
0	2	.87	67	10	178	20	1.22	1	.35	.06	1.24	.08	19	1
0	38	1.93	45	143	310	2[98]	.38	7	.22	.05	.31	.06	16	t
0	12	4.25	152	333	229	5[99]	2.12	11	.06	.09	.50	.03	26	t
0	49	2.93	130	291	153	15	2.23	t	.27	.03	1.76	.29	38	0
0	42	2.44	128	254	248	1	1.82	2	.82	.09	1.62	.46	85	t
0	19	2.26	43	385	163	205[100]	1.76	2	.11	.1	1.4	.4	79	.5
0	21	.95	53	119	69	5	1.57	1	.24	.02	.85	.06	15	1
0	73	3.84	253	580	655	1	4.28	37	.27	.14	.86	.7	82	1
0	16	.87	57	132	149	0	.97	8	.06	.03	.2	.16	19	t
0	113	2.93	203	380	602	12	3.28	15	.46	.18	1.25	.67	79	4
0	27	.69	48	90	142	3	.78	4	.11	.04	.3	.16	19	1
0	5	.25	2	13	89	1	.01	0	<.01	<.01	.07	<.01	<1	1
1	42	.4	2	35	54	64	.1	t	.01	.05	.1	<.01	0	t
6	50	.4	16	61	96	23	.37	10	.02	.1	.1	.02	<1	t
5	61	.56	33	77	125	23	.48	7	.03	.13	.31	.02	4	t
3	32	.68	35	87	155	19	.68	5	.11	.07	2.2	.05	16	t
6	48	.2	13	57	100	46	.29	8	.01	.08	.1	.01	<1	t
0	51	5.8	230	178	593	24	2.39	3	.1	.14	.9	.04	22	t
0	7	.6	32	41	86	5	.42	1	.01	.04	.1	<.01	4	t
0	2	.1	—	2	1	57	.1	0	<.01	<.01	.01	<.01	0	0
1	22	.3	7	24	42	54	.15	t	.01	.03	.1	<.01	2	t
0	2	.1	—	—	1	10	0	0	0	<.01	.01	0	0	0
0	6	.1	<1	2	1	7	0	0	0	0	0	0	0	0
0	1	.3	—	1	11	7	0	0	0	<.01	.01	—	0	0
0	1	.45	1	2	2	25	<.01	0	0	<.01	.01	<.01	0	0
0	2	.1	<1	23	91	55	.05	0	.01	.01	.2	<.01	0	0
0	17	1.7	8	20	173	17	.27	0	.02	.14	1	.06	34	3
0	1	.11	<1	1	11	1	.02	0	<.01	<.01	.06	<.01	2	t
0	4	.2	1	2	18	2	<.01	t	<.01	.01	.04	<.01	2	.4
0	3	.14	<1	1	13	1	<.01	t	<.01	<.01	.03	<.01	1	t

(94)Peanuts without salt contain 22 mg sodium per cup or 4 mg per ounce.
(95)Peanut butter without added salt contains 3 mg sodium per tablespoon.
(97)Salted pecans contain 816 mg sodium per cup and 214 mg per ounce.
(98)Salted pistachios contain approx 221 mg sodium per ounce.
(99)Salted pumpkin/squash kernels contain approx 163 mg sodium per ounce.
(100)Unsalted sunflower seeds contain 1 mg sodium per ¼ cup.

(For purposes of calculations, use "0" for t, <1, <.1, <.01, etc.)

H

TABLE H–1

Food Composition

Grp	Ref	Name	Measure	Wt (g)	H$_2$O (%)	Ener (kcal)	Prot (g)	Carb (g)	Fiber (g)	Fat (g)	Fat Breakdown (g) Sat	Mono	Poly
		SWEETENERS and SWEETS—Con.											
		Jellies:											
14	776	Tablespoon	1 tbsp	18	28	49	<.1	12.7	0	<.1	<.01	<.01	<.01
14	777	Packet	1 ea	14	28	39	<.1	9.9	0	<.1	<.01	<.01	<.01
14	778	Popsicle, 3oz when fluid	1 ea	95	80	70	0	18	0	0	0	0	0
		Sugars:											
14	779	Brown sugar	1 cup	220	2	820	0	212	0	0	0	0	0
		White sugar, granulated											
14	780	Cup	1 cup	200	1	770	0	199	0	0	0	0	0
14	781	Tablespoon	1 tbsp	12	1	45	0	12	0	0	0	0	0
14	782	Packet	1 ea	6	1	25	0	6	0	0	0	0	0
14	783	White sugar, powdered, sifted	1 cup	100	<1	385	0	99	0	0	0	0	0
		Syrups:											
		Chocolate:											
14	784	Thin type	2 tbsp	38	37	85	1.2	22	.94	.5	.2	.1	.1
14	785	Fudge type	2 tbsp	38	25	125	2	21	.9	5	3.1	1.7	.2
14	786	Molasses, blackstrap[102a]	2 tbsp	40	24	85	0	22	0	0	0	0	0
14	787	Pancake table syrup (corn and maple)	¼ cup	84	25	244	0	64	0	0	0	0	0
		VEGETABLES and LEGUMES											
15	788	Alfalfa seeds, sprouted	1 cup	33	91	10	1.3	1.2	1	.2	.02	.02	.14
15	789	Artichoke, cooked globe (300 g with refuse)	1 ea	120	86	53	2.8	12.4	3.96	.2	.05	<.01	.09
		Asparagus, green, cooked:											
		From raw:											
15	790	Cuts and tips	½ cup	90	92	22	2.3	4	1.62	.3	.06	<.01	.12
15	791	Spears, ½ in diam at base	4 spears	60	92	15	1.6	2.6	1.08	.2	.04	<.01	.08
		From frozen:											
15	792	Cuts and tips	1 cup	180	91	50	5.3	8.8	3.24	.8	.17	.02	.33
15	793	Spears, ½ in diam at base	4 spears	60	91	17	1.8	2.9	1.08	.3	.06	<.01	.11
15	794	Canned, spears, ½ in diam at base	4 spears	80	95	11	1.7	2	1.28	.5	.12	.02	.23
15	795	Bamboo shoots, canned, drained slices	1 cup	131	94	25	2.3	4.2	3.26	.5	.12	.01	.23
		Beans (see also Great Northern item 855; Kidney beans item 860; Navy beans item 876; Pinto beans item 898; Refried beans item 921; Soybeans item 925):											
15	796	Black beans, cooked	1 cup	171	66	225	15	41	15.4	.8	.1	.1	.5
		Lima beans:											
15	797	Thick-seeded (Fordhooks), cooked from frozen	½ cup	85	74	85	5.2	16	4.6	.3	.07	.02	.14
15	798	Thin-seeded (baby), cooked from frozen	½ cup	90	72	94	6	17.5	4.86	.3	.06	.01	.13
15	799	Cooked from dry, drained	1 cup	190	64	260	16.1	49	9.7	.9	.24	.12	.59
		Snap bean/green beans, cuts and french style:											
15	800	Cooked from raw	1 cup	125	89	44	2.4	9.9	3.13	.4	.08	.01	.18
15	801	Cooked from frozen	1 cup	135	92	36	1.8	8.3	3.38	.2	.04	<.01	.09
15	802	Canned, drained	1 cup	136	93	26	1.6	6.1	2.03	.1	.03	<.01	.07

[102a] Light molasses would contain about 66 mg calcium, 2.1 mg iron, 18 mg magnesium, 366 mg of potassium for 2 tbsp.

(For purposes of calculations, use "0" for t, <1, <.1, <.01, etc.)

KEY: 1 = BEV 2 = DAIRY 3 = EGGS 4 = FAT/OIL 5 = FRUIT 6 = BAKERY 7 = GRAIN 8 = FISH 9 = BEEF 10 = POULTRY 11 = SAUSAGE 12 = MIXED 13 = NUTS/SEEDS 14 = SWEETS 15 = VEG/LEG 16 = MISC 22 = SOUP/SAUCE

Chol (mg)	Calc (mg)	Iron (mg)	Magn (mg)	Phos (mg)	Pota (mg)	Sodi (mg)	Zinc (mg)	VT-A (RE)	Thia (mg)	Ribo (mg)	Niac (mg)	V-B6 (mg)	Fola (µg)	VT-C (mg)
0	2	.12	<1	1	16	4	0	t	<.01	<.01	.04	<.01	2	1
0	1	.09	<1	1	12	3	0	t	<.01	<.01	.03	<.01	2	1
0	0	.01	—	0	4	11	0	0	0	0	0	0	0	0
0	187	4.8	135	56	757	97	.08	0	.02	.07	.20	0	0	0
0	3	.1	<1	.1	7	5	.08	0	0	0	0	0	0	0
0	.2	<.01	<1	t	t	t	<.01	0	0	0	0	0	0	0
0	t	<.01	<1	t	t	t	<.01	0	0	0	0	0	0	0
0	0	.08	<1	0	4	2	<.01	0	0	0	0	0	0	0
0	6	.75	26	49	85	36	.39	1	<.01	.02	.11	<.01	3	0
0	38	.5	18	60	82	42	.39	13	.02	.08	.07	<.01	3	0
0	274[102a]	10.1[102a]	103[102a]	34	1171[102a]	38	0	0	.04	.08	.8	.11	6	0
0	2	.06	t	8	14	38	0	0	0	0	0	t	t	0
0	11	.32	9	23	26	2	.30	5	.03	.04	.16	.01	12	3
0	47	1.62	47	72	316	79	.43	17	.07	.06	.71	.1	53	9
0	22	.59	17	55	279	4	.43	75	.09	.11	.95	.13	88	25
0	14	.4	11	37	186	2	.29	50	.06	.07	.63	.09	59	16
0	41	1.15	23	99	392	7	1.01	147	.12	.18	1.87	.16	176	44
0	14	.38	8	33	131	2	.34	49	.04	.06	.62	.06	59	15
0	11	.5	8	30	122	278[101]	.32	38	.05	.07	.7	.04	69	13
0	10	.42	6	33	105	9	.30	1	.03	.03	.18	—	40	1
0	47	2.9	136	239	608	1	1.3	1	.43	.05	.9	.19	84	0
0	19	1.16	29	54	347	45	.37	16	.06	.05	.91	.1	55	11
0	25	1.76	50	101	370	26	.5	15	.06	.05	.69	.1	58	5
0	55	5.9	79	293	1163	4	2.08	0	.25	.11	1.34	.29	170	0
0	58	1.6	32	48	373	4	.45	83[102]	.09	.12	.77	.07	42	12
0	61	1.11	29	33	151	17	.84	71[103]	.07	.1	.56	.08	42	11
0	36	1.22	18	26	148	340[104]	.39	47[105]	.02	.08	.27	.05	40	6

H

(101)Special dietary pack contains 3 mg sodium.
(102)For green varieties; yellow beans contain 10 RE per cup.
(102a)Light molasses would contain about 66 mg calcium, 2.1 mg iron, 18 mg magnesium, 366 mg of potassium for 2 tbsp.
(103)For green varieties; yellow beans contain 15 RE.
(104)Dietary pack contains 3 mg sodium.
(105)For green varieties; yellow beans contain 14 RE.

(For purposes of calculations, use "0" for t, <1, <.1, <.01, etc.)

TABLE H–1

Food Composition

Grp	Ref	Name	Measure	Wt (g)	H$_2$O (%)	Ener (kcal)	Prot (g)	Carb (g)	Fiber (g)	Fat (g)	Fat Breakdown (g) Sat	Mono	Poly
		VEGETABLES and LEGUMES—Con.											
		Beans, continued											
		Navy beans, canned:											
15	803	Pork and beans with tomato sauce	1 cup	255	71	311	15.6	48	18.6	6.6	2.4	2.7	.7
15	804	Pork and beans with sweet sauce	1 cup	255	66	383	15.8	53.8	18	12	4.3	4.9	1.2
15	805	Beans with frankfurters	1 cup	255	71	365	19	32	17.5	18	7.4	8.8	.7
		Bean sprouts (mung):											
15	806	Raw	1 cup	104	90	32	3.2	6.2	1.7	.2	.05	.02	.06
15	807	Cooked, stir fried	1 cup	124	84	62	5.3	13.1	3.4	.3	.05	.07	.08
15	808	Cooked, boiled, drained	1 cup	124	93	26	2.5	5.2	2.5	.1	.03	.01	.04
		Beets:											
		Cooked from fresh:											
15	809	Sliced or diced	½ cup	85	91	26	.9	5.7	1.96	<.1	<.01	<.01	.01
15	810	Whole beets, 2 in diam	2 beets	100	91	31	1.1	6.7	2.3	<.1	<.01	.01	.02
		Canned:											
15	811	Sliced or diced	½ cup	85	91	27	.8	6.1	1.96	.1	.02	.02	.04
15	812	Pickled slices	½ cup	114	82	74	.9	18.6	2.36	.1	.01	.02	.03
15	813	Beet greens, cooked, drained	1 cup	144	89	40	3.7	7.9	2.97	.3	.04	.06	.1
		Blackeyed peas, cooked:											
15	814	From dry with liquid	1 cup	250	80	190	12.8	34.5	10.8	.8	.21	.07	.34
15	815	From fresh, drained	1 cup	165	72	179	13.4	29.9	7.13	1.3	.34	.12	.56
15	816	From frozen, drained	1 cup	170	66	224	14.4	40.4	7.34	1.1	.3	.1	.48
		Broccoli:											
		Raw:											
15	817	Chopped	1 cup	88	91	24	2.6	4.6	3.34	.3	.05	.02	.15
15	818	Spears	1 spear	151	91	42	4.5	7.9	5.74	.5	.08	.04	.25
		Cooked from raw:											
15	819	Spears	1 spear	180	90	53	5.3	10	7.38	.5	.08	.04	.24
15	820	Chopped	1 cup	156	90	46	4.6	8.7	6.4	.4	.07	.03	.21
		Cooked from frozen:											
15	821	Spears	1 spear	30	91	8	.9	1.6	1	<.1	<.01	<.01	.02
15	822	Chopped	1 cup	184	91	51	5.7	9.8	6.07	.2	.03	.01	.1
		Brussels sprouts:											
15	823	Cooked from raw	1 cup	156	87	60	6	13.5	5.62	.8	.16	.06	.41
15	824	Cooked from frozen	1 cup	155	87	65	5.6	12.9	4.96	.6	.13	.05	.31
		Cabbage, common varieties:											
15	825	Raw, shredded or chopped	1 cup	70	92	16	.8	3.8	1.62	.1	.02	.01	.06
15	826	Cooked, drained	1 cup	150	94	32	1.4	7.2	3.95	.4	.05	.03	.18
		Chinese cabbage:											
15	827	Bok choy or Pak-choi, cooked, drained	1 cup	170	96	20	2.6	3	3.4	.3	.04	.02	.13
15	828	Pe-Tsai, raw, chopped	1 cup	76	94	11	.9	2.5	1.67	.1	.03	.02	.06
		Cabbage, red, coarsely chopped:											
15	829	Raw	1 cup	70	92	19	1	4.3	1.82	.2	.02	.01	.09
15	830	Cooked	½ cup	75	94	16	.8	3.5	4	.1	.02	.01	.07
15	831	Savoy cabbage, coarsely chopped, Raw	1 cup	70	91	20	1.4	4.3	1.62	<.1	<.01	<.01	.03
		Carrots:											
		Raw:											
15	832	Whole, 7½ x 1⅛ in	1 carrot	72	88	31	.7	7.3	2.03	.1	.02	<.01	.06
15	833	Grated	½ cup	55	88	24	.6	5.6	1.55	.1	.02	<.01	.04
		Cooked, sliced, drained:											
15	834	Cooked from raw	½ cup	78	87	35	.8	8.2	2.89	.1	.03	<.01	.07
15	835	Cooked from frozen	½ cup	73	90	26	.9	6	2.7	<.1	.01	<.01	.04
15	836	Canned, sliced, drained	½ cup	73	93	17	.5	4	2.04	.1	.03	<.01	.07

H

(For purposes of calculations, use "0" for t, <1, <.1, <.01, etc.)

KEY: 1 = BEV 2 = DAIRY 3 = EGGS 4 = FAT/OIL 5 = FRUIT 6 = BAKERY 7 = GRAIN 8 = FISH 9 = BEEF 10 = POULTRY
11 = SAUSAGE   12 = MIXED   13 = NUTS/SEEDS   14 = SWEETS   15 = VEG/LEG   16 = MISC   22 = SOUP/SAUCE

Chol (mg)	Calc (mg)	Iron (mg)	Magn (mg)	Phos (mg)	Pota (mg)	Sodi (mg)	Zinc (mg)	VT-A (RE)	Thia (mg)	Ribo (mg)	Niac (mg)	V-B6 (mg)	Fola (µg)	VT-C (mg)
10	138	4.6	90	235	536	1181	2.6	33	.2	.08	1.5	.2	61	5
8	161	5.90	90	291	536	969	2.6	33	.15	.1	1.3	.2	61	5
30	94	4.8	90	303	668	1374	2.8	33	.18	.15	3.3	.2	54	.4
0	14	.95	22	56	154	6	.43	2	.09	.13	.78	.09	63	14
0	16	2.4	38	70	200	14	1.12	3	.17	.22	1.49	.1	72	20
0	15	.81	18	34	125	12	.58	2	.06	.13	1.01	.05	35	14
0	9	.53	31	26	266	42	.21	1	.03	.01	.23	.03	49	5
0	11	.62	37	31	312	49	.25	1	.03	.01	.27	.03	86	6
0	13	1.55	13	15	126	233[106]	.18	1	.01	.04	.15	.04	27	4
0	13	.47	17	19	169	301	.3	1	.03	.06	.29	.03	35	3
0	165	2.74	97	58	1308	346	.72	734	.17	.42	.72	.19	47	36
0	43	3.30	117	238	573	20	3.22	3	.40	.1	1	.14	142	0
0	46	2.36	83	197	693	7	1.3	105	.11	.18	1.77	.08	173	3
0	40	3.6	85	208	638	9	2.42	13	.42	.11	1.24	.16	240	4
0	42	.78	22	58	286	24	.36	136[107]	.06	.1	.56	.14	62	82
0	72	1.33	38	99	490	41	.6	233[107]	.1	.18	.96	.24	107	141
0	205	2.16	106	86	293	20	.27	254[107]	.15	.37	1.36	.36	123	113
0	178	1.78	94	74	254	16	.23	220[107]	.13	.32	1.18	.31	107	98
0	15	.18	6	16	54	7	.09	57[107]	.02	.02	.14	.04	26	12
0	94	1.13	37	101	331	44	.56	348[107]	.1	.15	.84	.24	104	74
0	56	1.88	32	87	491	17	.5	112	.17	.12	.95	.31	94	97
0	38	1.15	37	84	504	36	.55	91	.16	.17	.83	.27	157	71
0	32	.4	10	16	172	12	.12	9	.04	.02	.21	.07	40	33
0	50	.58	22	38	308	29	.24	13	.09	.08	.34	.1	31	36
0	158	1.77	18	49	630	57	.43	437	.05	.11	.73	.3	32	44
0	59	.23	10	22	181	7	.17	91	.03	.04	.3	.18	60	21
0	36	.35	11	29	144	8	.15	3	.04	.02	.21	.15	19	40
0	28	.27	8	21	105	6	.11	2	.03	.01	.15	.1	9	26
0	25	.28	20	29	161	20	.26	70	.05	.02	.21	.13	32	22
0	19	.36	11	32	233	25	.14	2025	.07	.04	.67	.11	10	7
0	15	.28	8	24	178	19	.11	1547	.05	.03	.51	.08	8	5
0	24	.48	10	24	177	52	.23	1915	.03	.04	.4	.19	11	2
0	21	.35	7	19	115	43	.17	1292	.02	.03	.32	.09	8	2
0	19	.47	6	17	131	176[108]	.19	1006	.01	.02	.4	.08	7	2

(106)Dietary pack contains 39 mg sodium.
(107)Vitamin A for whole plant: leaves are 1600 RE per 100 grams, raw: flower clusters are 300 per 100 grams, raw; stalks are 40 RE per 100 grams, raw.
(108)Dietary pack contains 31 mg sodium.

(For purposes of calculations, use "0" for t, <1, <.1, <.01, etc.)

TABLE H-1

Food Composition

Grp	Ref	Name	Measure	Wt (g)	H₂O (%)	Ener (kcal)	Prot (g)	Carb (g)	Fiber (g)	Fat (g)	Fat Breakdown (g) Sat	Mono	Poly
		VEGETABLES and LEGUMES—Con.											
15	837	Carrot juice	¾ cup	184	89	73	1.7	17.1	2.5	.3	.05	.01	.13
		Cauliflower:											
15	838	Raw, flowerets	½ cup	50	92	12	1	2.5	1.34	<.1	.01	<.01	.04
		Cooked, drained, flowerets:											
15	839	From raw	½ cup	62	92	15	1.2	2.9	1.67	.1	.02	.01	.07
15	840	From frozen	1 cup	180	94	34	2.9	6.8	3.93	.4	.06	.03	.18
		Celery, pascal-type, raw:											
15	841	Large outer stalk, 8 x 1½ in (at root end)	1 stalk	40	95	6	.3	1.4	.8	<.1	.01	.01	.02
15	842	Diced	½ cup	60	95	10	.4	2.2	1.2	<.1	.02	.01	.04
		Chickpeas (see Garbanzo item 854)											
		Collards, cooked, drained:											
15	843	From raw	1 cup	145	96	20	1.6	3.8	4.08	.2	.06	.03	.12
15	844	From frozen	1 cup	170	88	61	5	12.1	4.76	.7	.1	.1	.4
		Corn:											
		Cooked, drained:											
15	845	From raw, on cob, 5 in long	1 ear	77	70	83	2.6	19.4	3.62	1	.15	.29	.46
15	846	From frozen, on cob, 3½ in long	1 ear	63	73	59	2	14.1	2.96	.5	.07	.14	.22
15	847	Kernels, cooked from frozen	½ cup	82	76	67	2.5	16.8	3.85	<.1	<.01	.02	.03
		Canned:											
15	848	Cream style	½ cup	128	79	93	2.2	23.2	6.27	.5	.08	.16	.25
15	849	Whole kernel, vacuum pack	1 cup	210	77	166	5.1	40.8	10	1.1	.16	.31	.50
		Cowpeas; (see Blackeyed peas items 814-816)											
15	850	Cucumber with peel, ⅛ in thick, 2⅛ in diam	6 slices	28	96	4	.2	.8	.4	<.1	<.01	<.01	.01
		Dandelion greens:											
15	851	Raw	1 cup	55	86	25	1.5	5.1	.94	.4	.05	.04	.23
15	852	Chopped, cooked, drained	1 cup	105	90	35	2.1	6.7	1.4	.6	.15	.04	.35
15	853	Eggplant, cooked	1 cup	160	92	45	1.3	10.6	6	.4	.07	.03	.15
15	854	Garbanzo beans (chickpeas), cooked	1 cup	163	60	270	15	45	8.63	4	.4	.9	1.9
15	855	Great northern beans, cooked	1 cup	180	69	210	14	38.2	12.4	1.1	.14	.14	.64
15	856	Escarole/curly endive, chopped	1 cup	50	94	8	.6	1.7	.75	.1	.02	<.01	.04
15	857	Jerusalem artichoke, raw slices	1 cup	150	78	114	3	26.2	1.95	<.1	—	<.01	<.01
		Kale, cooked, drained:											
15	858	From raw	1 cup	130	91	42	3.5	7.3	3.72	.5	.07	.04	.25
15	859	From frozen	1 cup	130	90	39	3.7	6.8	3.4	.6	.08	.05	.31
15	860	Kidney beans, canned	1 cup	255	76	230	14.5	41.8	20	.9	.1	.1	.6
15	861	Kohlrabi slices, cooked from raw	1 cup	165	90	48	3	11.4	2.3	.2	.02	.01	.09
15	862	Lentils, cooked from dry	1 cup	200	72	215	16	38	10	1	.1	.2	.5
		Lettuce:											
		Butterhead/Boston types:											
15	863	Head, 5 in diam	1 head	163	96	21	2.1	3.8	2.7	.4	.05	.01	.19
15	864	Leaves, 2 inner or outer	2 leaves	15	96	2	.2	.3	.25	<.1	<.01	<.01	.02
		Iceberg/crisphead:											
15	865	Head, 6 in diam	1 head	539	96	70	5.4	11.3	8.95	1	.13	.04	.54
15	866	Wedge, 1/4 of head	1 wedge	135	96	18	1.4	2.8	2.24	.3	.04	.01	.14
15	867	Chopped or shredded	1 cup	56	96	7	.6	1.2	.84	.1	.01	<.01	.06
15	868	Loose leaf, chopped	1 cup	56	94	10	.7	2	.93	.2	.02	<.01	.09

(For purposes of calculations, use "0" for t, <1, <.1, <.01, etc.)

KEY: 1 = BEV 2 = DAIRY 3 = EGGS 4 = FAT/OIL 5 = FRUIT 6 = BAKERY 7 = GRAIN 8 = FISH 9 = BEEF 10 = POULTRY
11 = SAUSAGE 12 = MIXED 13 = NUTS/SEEDS 14 = SWEETS 15 = VEG/LEG 16 = MISC 22 = SOUP/SAUCE

Chol (mg)	Calc (mg)	Iron (mg)	Magn (mg)	Phos (mg)	Pota (mg)	Sodi (mg)	Zinc (mg)	VT-A (RE)	Thia (mg)	Ribo (mg)	Niac (mg)	V-B6 (mg)	Fola (µg)	VT-C (mg)
0	44	.57	26	77	538	54	.33	3167	.17	.1	.71	.4	7	11
0	14	.29	7	23	178	7	.09	t	.04	.03	.32	.12	33	36
0	17	.26	7	22	200	4	.15	t	.04	.04	.34	.12	32	34
0	31	.74	16	43	250	33	.23	4	.07	.1	.56	.16	74	56
0	14	.19	5	10	114	35	.07	5	.01	.01	.12	.01	4	3
0	22	.29	7	16	170	53	.1	8	.02	.02	.18	.02	5	4
0	113	.59	16	15	135	27	.93	322	.03	.06	.34	.06	55	14
0	357	1.9	52	46	427	85	.46	1017	.08	.2	1.08	.19	129	45
0	2	.47	25	79	192	13	.37	17[109]	.17	.06	1.24	.18	36	5
0	2	.38	18	47	158	3	.4	13[109]	.11	.04	.96	.14	19	3
0	2	.25	15	39	114	4	.29	20[109]	.06	.06	1.05	.18	19	2
0	4	.49	22	65	172	365[110]	.68	12[109]	.03	.07	1.23	.08	57	6
0	11	.88	48	134	390	572[111]	.97	51[109]	.09	.15	2.46	.12	104	17
0	4	.08	3	5	42	.6	.07	1	<.01	<.01	.09	.01	4	1
0	103	1.71	20	36	218	42	.62	770	.1	.14	.39	.04	64	19
0	147	1.89	26	44	244	46	.8	1229	.14	.18	.5	.04	82	19
0	10	.56	21	35	397	5	.24	10	.12	.03	.96	.14	23	2
0	80	4.9	115	273	475	11	2.52	3	.18	.1	.9	.39	108	0
0	90	4.9	76	266	749	13	1.72	0	.25	.13	1.3	.4	74	0
0	26	.41	8	14	157	11	.40	103	.04	.04	.2	.01	71	3
0	21	5.1	26	117	644	6	.10	3	.3	.09	1.95	.11	15	6
0	94	1.17	23	36	296	30	.31	962	.07	.09	.70	.18	30	53
0	179	1.22	23	36	417	20	.23	826	.06	.15	.87	.11	31	33
0	74	4.6	75	278	673	968	2	1	.13	.1	1.5	.05	85	0
0	41	.66	31	74	561	34	.32	6	.07	.03	.64	.14	13	89
0	50	4.2	55	238	498	26	1.98	4	.14	.12	1.12	.22	64	0
0	52	.49	18	38	419	8	.42	158	.1	.1	.49	.11	119	13
0	5	.04	2	3	39	t	.04	15	<.01	<.01	.04	.01	11	1
0	102	2.7	48	108	852	48	1.19	178	.25	.16	1.01	.22	302	21
0	26	.68	12	27	213	12	.3	45	.06	.04	.25	.05	76	5
0	11	.28	5	11	89	5	.12	19	.03	.02	.1	.02	31	2
0	38	.78	6	14	148	5	.18	106	.03	.04	.22	.03	60	10

(109)For yellow varieties; white varieties contain only a trace of vitamin A.
(110)Dietary pack contains 4 mg sodium per ½ cup.
(111)Dietary pack contains 6 mg sodium per cup.

H

(For purposes of calculations, use "0" for t, <1, <.1, <.01, etc.)

TABLE H–1

Food Composition

Grp	Ref	Name	Measure	Wt (g)	H$_2$O (%)	Ener (kcal)	Prot (g)	Carb (g)	Fiber (g)	Fat (g)	Fat Breakdown (g) Sat	Mono	Poly
		VEGETABLES and LEGUMES—Con.											
		Lettuce, continued:											
		Romaine:											
15	869	Chopped	1 cup	56	95	9	.9	1.3	.93	.1	.01	<.01	.06
15	870	Inner leaf	1 leaf	10	95	2	.2	.2	.17	<.1	<.01	<.01	.01
		Mushrooms:											
15	871	Raw, sliced	½ cup	35	92	9	.7	1.6	.77	.1	.02	<.01	.06
15	872	Cooked from raw, pieces	½ cup	78	91	21	1.7	4	1.9	.4	.05	<.01	.14
15	873	Canned, drained	½ cup	78	91	19	1.5	3.9	1.83	.2	.03	<.01	.09
		Mustard greens:											
15	874	Cooked from raw	1 cup	140	94	21	3.2	2.9	2.9	.3	.02	.15	.06
15	875	Cooked from frozen	1 cup	150	94	28	3.4	4.7	3.9	.4	.02	.17	.07
15	876	Navy beans, cooked from dry	1 cup	190	69	225	15	40	16.5	1.1	.1	.1	.7
		Okra, cooked:											
15	877	From fresh pods	8 pods	85	90	27	1.6	6.1	2.75	.1	.04	.02	.04
15	878	From frozen slices	½ cup	92	91	34	1.9	7.5	2.98	.3	.07	.05	.07
		Onions:											
		Raw:											
15	879	Chopped	1 cup	160	91	54	1.9	11.7	2.64	.4	.07	.06	.16
15	880	Sliced	1 cup	115	91	39	1.4	8.4	1.9	.3	.05	.04	.12
15	881	Cooked, drained, chopped	½ cup	105	92	30	.8	6.6	1.71	.2	.03	.02	.07
15	882	Dehydrated flakes	¼ cup	14	4	45	1.2	11.7	1.39	<.1	.01	<.01	.03
15	883	Onions, spring, chopped, bulb and top	½ cup	50	91	13	.9	2.8	1.55	<.1	.01	.01	.03
15	884	Onion rings, breaded, prepared from frozen	2 rings	20	29	80	1	8	.2	5	1.7	2.2	1
		Parsley:											
		Raw:											
15	885	Chopped	½ cup	30	88	10	.7	2.1	1.95	<.1	.01	<.01	.04
15	886	Sprigs	10 sprigs	10	88	3	.2	.7	.65	<.1	<.01	<.01	.01
15	887	Freeze dried	¼ cup	1.4	2	4	.4	.6	.56	<.1	<.01	<.01	.03
15	888	Parsnips, sliced, cooked	1 cup	156	78	125	2.1	30.4	4.36	1.4	.1	.2	.1
		Peas:											
		Blackeyed (see Blackeyed peas items 814-816)											
15	889	Edible pods, cooked	1 cup	160	89	67	5.2	11.3	4.8	.4	.07	.04	.16
		Green:											
15	890	Canned, drained	½ cup	85	82	59	3.8	10.7	5.36	.3	.05	.03	.14
15	891	Cooked from frozen	½ cup	80	80	63	4.1	11.4	7.68	.2	.04	.02	.1
15	892	Split, green, cooked from dry	1 cup	200	70	230	16	42	10.2	.6	.1	.1	.3
		Peppers, hot:											
		Hot green chili:											
15	893	Canned	½ cup	68	92	17	.6	4.2	1.22	<.1	<.01	<.01	.04
15	894	Raw	1 pepper	45	88	18	.9	4.3	1.22	<.1	<.01	<.01	.05
15	895	Jalapenos, chopped, canned	½ cup	68	90	17	.5	3.3	2.3	.4	.42	.02	.22
		Peppers, sweet, green:											
15	896	Whole pod (90 g with refuse), raw	1 pod	74	93	18	.6	3.9	1.26	.3	.05	.02	.18
15	897	Cooked, chopped (one pod cooked = 73 g)	½ cup	68	95	12	.4	2.6	1.07	.2	.03	.01	.12
15	898	Pinto beans, cooked from dry	1 cup	180	66	265	15	49	18.9	.8	.1	.1	.5

(For purposes of calculations, use "0" for t, <1, <.1, <.01, etc.)

KEY: 1 = BEV 2 = DAIRY 3 = EGGS 4 = FAT/OIL 5 = FRUIT 6 = BAKERY 7 = GRAIN 8 = FISH 9 = BEEF 10 = POULTRY
11 = SAUSAGE 12 = MIXED 13 = NUTS/SEEDS 14 = SWEETS 15 = VEG/LEG 16 = MISC 22 = SOUP/SAUCE

Chol (mg)	Calc (mg)	Iron (mg)	Magn (mg)	Phos (mg)	Pota (mg)	Sodi (mg)	Zinc (mg)	VT-A (RE)	Thia (mg)	Ribo (mg)	Niac (mg)	V-B6 (mg)	Fola (µg)	VT-C (mg)
0	20	.62	3	25	162	4	.18	146	.06	.06	.28	.03	76	13
0	4	.11	<1	5	29	t	.03	26	.01	.01	.05	.06	14	2
0	2	.43	4	36	130	1	.3	0	.04	.16	1.44	.03	7	1
0	5	1.36	9	68	278	2	.68	0	.06	.23	3.48	.07	14	3
0	9	.62	6	52	101	332	.56	0	.05	.17	1.25	.06	10	0
0	104	1.56	21	57	283	22	.3	424	.06	.09	.61	.18	20	35
0	152	1.68	20	36	209	38	.3	671	.06	.08	.39	.16	20	21
0	95	5.1	89	281	790	13	2.01	0	.27	.13	1.27	.72	108	0
0	54	.38	48	48	274	4	.47	49	.11	.05	.74	.16	39	14
0	88	.62	47	42	215	3	.57	47	.09	.11	.72	.04	134	11
0	40	.59	16	46	248	3	.29	0	.1	.02	.16	.25	32	13
0	29	.43	12	33	178	2	.21	0	.07	.01	.12	.18	23	10
0	29	.21	11	24	159	8	.19	0	.04	<.01	.08	.19	13	6
0	36	.22	13	42	227	3	.26	0	.11	<.01	<.01	.22	23	11
0	30	.94	10	16	128	2	.22	250	.04	.07	.1	.03	8	23
0	6	.3	1	16	26	75	.07	5	.06	.03	.7	.02	1	t
0	39	1.86	13	12	161	12	.22	156	.02	.03	.21	.05	55	27
0	13	.62	4	4	54	4	.07	52	<.01	.01	.07	.02	18	9
0	2	.75	5	8	88	5	.09	89	.01	.03	.15	.02	22	2
0	58	.9	46	108	573	16	.4	0	.13	.08	1.1	.15	91	20[112]
0	67	3.15	42	89	383	6	.6	21	.2	.12	.86	.23	48	77
0	17	.81	15	57	147	186[113]	.6	65	.1	.07	.62	.05	38	8
0	19	1.25	23	72	134	70	.75	53	.23	.14	1.18	.09	47	8
0	23	3.4	70	178	592	26	1.91	8	.28	.18	1.8	.13	16	0
0	5	.34	8	12	143	10	.02	42[114]	.01	.03	.54	.08	35	46
0	8	.54	11	21	153	3	.14	35[115]	.04	.04	.43	.12	10	109
0	18	1.9	8	12	92	995	.13	116	.02	.03	.34	.08	35	9
0	4	.94	10	16	144	2	.13	39[116]	.06	.04	.41	.12	12	95[116]
0	3	.6	7	10	88	1	.08	26[117]	.04	.02	.25	.07	10	76[117]
0	86	5.4	103	296	882	3	2.4	1	.33	.16	.7	.33	137	0

[112]Value for Vitamin C is highest right after harvest and drops after that.
[113]Dietary pack contains 1.7 mg sodium.
[114]For green chili peppers; red varieties contain 809 RE vitamin A.
[115]For green chili peppers; red varieties contain 484 RE vitamin A.
[116]For green sweet peppers; red varieties contain 570 RE vitamin A; 141 mg ascorbic acid.
[117]For green sweet peppers; red varieties contain 256 RE vitamin A; 113 mg ascorbic acid.

H

(For purposes of calculations, use "0" for t, <1, <.1, <.01, etc.)

TABLE H–1

Food Composition

Grp	Ref	Name	Measure	Wt (g)	H₂O (%)	Ener (kcal)	Prot (g)	Carb (g)	Fiber (g)	Fat (g)	Fat Breakdown (g)		
											Sat	Mono	Poly
		VEGETABLES and LEGUMES—Con.											
		Potatoes[118]:											
		Baked in oven, 4¾ x 2⅓ in diam:											
15	899	With skin	1 potato	202	71	220	4.7	51	4.4	.2	.05	<.01	.09
15	900	Flesh only	1 potato	156	75	145	3.1	33.6	3.9	.2	.04	<.01	.07
15	901	Skin	1 ea	58	47	115	2.5	27	1.54	<.1	.01	<.01	.03
		Baked in microwave, 4¾ x 2⅓ in diam:											
15	902	With skin	1 potato	202	72	212	4.9	48.7	4.40	.2	.05	<.01	.09
15	903	Flesh only	1 potato	156	74	156	3.3	36.3	3.9	.2	.04	<.01	.07
15	904	Skin	1 ea	58	64	77	2.5	17.2	1.54	<.1	.01	<.01	.03
		Boiled, about 2½ in diam:											
15	905	Peeled after boiling	1 potato	136	77	119	2.5	27.4	3.2	.1	.04	<.01	.06
15	906	Peeled before boiling	1 ea	135	78	116	2.3	27	1.6	.1	.04	<.01	.06
		French-fried, strips 2-3½ in long, frozen:											
15	907	Oven heated	10 strips	50	53	111	1.7	17	1.6	4.4	2.08	1.78	.33
15	908	Fried in veg oil	10 strips	50	38	158	2	19.8	1.6	8.3	2.50	1.64	3.78
15	909	Hashed brown, from frozen	1 cup	156	56	340	4.9	44	1.6	18	7.01	8.01	2.07
		Mashed:											
15	910	Home recipe with milk[121]	1 cup	210	78	162	4.1	36.9	1.23	1.2	.70	.31	.12
15	911	Home recipe with milk and margarine	1 cup	210	76	222	4	35.1	1.23	8.9	2.17	3.72	2.54
15	912	Prepared from flakes; water, milk, butter, salt added	1 cup	210	76	237	4	31.5	1.2	11.8	7.21	3.32	.52
		Potato products, prepared:											
		Au gratin:											
15	913	From dry mix	1 cup	245	79	228	5.6	31.5	4.21	10.1	6.34	2.88	.33
15	914	From home recipe[119]	1 cup	245	74	322	12.4	27.6	4.41	18.6	11.6	5.27	.68
		Potato salad (see Mixed foods, item 715)											
		Scalloped:											
15	915	From dry mix	1 cup	245	79	228	5.2	31.3	4.55	10.5	6.45	2.97	.47
15	916	Home recipe[124]	1 cup	245	81	210	7	26.4	4.65	9	5.53	2.55	.41
15	917	Potato chips	14 chips	28	2	148	1.8	14.7	.5	10.1	2.58	1.77	5.16
		Pumpkin:											
15	918	Cooked from raw, mashed	1 cup	245	94	50	2	11.9	3.68	.2	.09	.02	.01
15	919	Canned	1 cup	245	90	83	2.7	19.8	5.45	.7	.36	.09	.04
15	920	Red radishes	10 radishes	45	95	7	.3	1.6	.99	.2	.01	<.01	.02
15	921	Refried beans, canned	1 cup	290	72	295	18	51	22	3	.40	.60	1.4
15	922	Sauerkraut, canned with liquid	1 cup	236	92	44	2.1	10.1	4.4	.3	.08	.03	.14
		Seaweed:											
15	923	Kelp, raw	1 oz	28	82	12	.5	2.7	1.4	.2	.07	.03	.01
15	924	Spirulina, dried	1 oz	28	5	82	16.3	6.8	1.03	2.2	.75	.19	.59
15	925	Soybeans, cooked from dry	1 cup	180	71	235	19.8	19.5	4	10.2	1.3	1.9	5.3
		Soybean products:											
15	926	Miso	3 tbsp	52	53	88	5.4	12.2	1[128]	2.5	.34	.49	1.38
15	927	Tofu, piece 2½x2¾x1 in	1 pce	120	85	86	9.4	2.9	2.2[128]	5	.7	1	2.9
		Spinach:											
15	928	Raw, chopped	1 cup	56	92	12	1.6	2	2.28	.2	.03	<.01	.08

[118]Vitamin C varies with length of storage. After 3 months of storage approximately ⅔ of the ascorbic acid remains; after 6-7 months, about ⅓ remains.
[119]Recipe: 55% potatoes; 30% whole milk; 9% cheddar cheese; 3% butter; 2% flour; 1% salt.
[121]Recipe: 84% potatoes; 15% whole milk; 1% salt.
[124]Recipe: 59% potatoes; 36% whole milk; 2% butter; 2% flour; 1% salt.
[128]Estimate based on cooked soybeans.

(For purposes of calculations, use "0" for t, <1, <.1, <.01, etc.)

KEY: 1 = BEV 2 = DAIRY 3 = EGGS 4 = FAT/OIL 5 = FRUIT 6 = BAKERY 7 = GRAIN 8 = FISH 9 = BEEF 10 = POULTRY
11 = SAUSAGE 12 = MIXED 13 = NUTS/SEEDS 14 = SWEETS 15 = VEG/LEG 16 = MISC 22 = SOUP/SAUCE

Chol (mg)	Calc (mg)	Iron (mg)	Magn (mg)	Phos (mg)	Pota (mg)	Sodi (mg)	Zinc (mg)	VT-A (RE)	Thia (mg)	Ribo (mg)	Niac (mg)	V-B6 (mg)	Fola (µg)	VT-C (mg)
0	20	2.75	55	115	844	16	.65	0	.22	.07	3.32	.7	22	26
0	8	.55	39	78	610	8	.45	0	.16	.03	2.18	.47	14	20
0	20	2.2	25	59	332	12	.28	0	.07	.07	1.78	.35	12	8
0	22	2.5	54	212	903	16	.73	0	.24	.07	3.46	.69	24	31
0	8	.64	39	170	641	11	.51	0	.2	.04	2.54	.5	19	24
0	27	3.44	22	48	377	9	.3	0	.04	.04	1.29	.28	10	9
0	7	.42	30	60	515	6	.41	0	.14	.03	1.96	.41	14	18
0	10	.42	26	54	443	7	.37	0	.13	.03	.18	.36	12	10
0	4	.67	11	43	229	15	.21	0	.06	.01	1.15	.12	8	6
0	10	.38	17	47	366	108	.19	0	.09	.01	1.63	.12	14	5
0	24	2.36	26	112	680	53	.5	0	.17	.03	3.78	.2	26	10
4	55	.57	39	100	628	636	.6	12	.18	.08	2.35	.49	17	14
4[123]	54	.55	37	97	607	619	.58	41	.18	.11	2.2	.47	17	13
4[123]	103	.46	37	118	490	697	.37	44	.23	.08	1.41	.02	16	20
12	203	.78	37	233	537	1076	.59	76	.05	.2	2.3	.1	3	8
56[120]	292	1.56	48	277	970	1064	1.69	93	.16	.28	2.43	.43	20	24
27	88	.93	34	137	497	835	.61	51	.05	.14	2.52	.1	3	8
29[125]	140	1.41	46	154	926	821	.98	46	.17	.23	2.58	.44	21	26
0	7	.34	17	43	369	133[126]	.3	0	.04	<.01	1.19	.14	13	12
0	37	1.4	22	74	564	3	.45	265	.08	.19	1.01	.16	33	12
0	64	3.41	56	85	504	12	.42	5404	.06	.13	.9	.14	30	10
0	9	.13	4	8	104	11	.13	t	<.01	.02	.14	.03	12	10
0	141	5.1	171	245	1141	1228	3.43	0	.14	.16	1.40	3.25	106	17
0	72	3.47	31	46	401	1561	.44	4	.05	.05	.34	.31	4	35
0	48	.81	34	12	25	66	.35	3	.01	.04	.13	—	51	—
0	34	8.08	55	33	386	297	—	16	.68	1.04	3.63	.1	—	3
0	132	4.9	1	321	972	4	2.11	5	.39	.15	1.15	.5	76	0
0	35	.89	<1	161	174	1534	3.19	2	.03	.05	.15	—	22	0
0	108	2.23	133	151	50	8	.88	0	.18	.08	.1	.1	55	0
0	55	1.52	44	27	312	44	.3	376	.04	.11	.41	.11	109	16

H

[120]For butter; if margarine is used, cholesterol = 37 mg.
[123]For margarine; if butter is used, cholesterol = 25 mg for 29 total mg.
[125]For butter; if margarine is used cholesterol = 15 mg.
[126]If no salt is added, sodium = 2 mg.

(For purposes of calculations, use "0" for t, <1, <.1, <.01, etc.)

TABLE H–1

Food Composition

Grp	Ref	Name	Measure	Wt (g)	H₂O (%)	Ener (kcal)	Prot (g)	Carb (g)	Fiber (g)	Fat (g)	Fat Breakdown (g)		
											Sat	Mono	Poly
		VEGETABLES and LEGUMES—Con.											
		Spinach, continued:											
		Cooked, drained:											
15	929	From raw	1 cup	180	91	41	5.3	6.8	5.76	.5	.08	.01	.19
15	930	From frozen (leaf)	1 cup	190	90	53	6	10.2	6.27	.4	.06	.01	.16
15	931	Canned, drained solids	1 cup	214	92	50	6	7.3	7.7	1.1	.17	.03	.45
		Spinach souffle (see Mixed foods)											
		Squash, summer varieties, cooked slices:											
15	932	Varieties averaged	1 cup	180	94	36	1.6	7.8	3.24	.6	.12	.04	.24
15	933	Crookneck	1 cup	180	94	36	1.6	7.8	3.24	.6	.12	.04	.24
15	934	Zucchini	1 cup	180	95	29	1.1	7.1	3.20	<.1	.02	<.01	.04
		Squash, winter varieties, cooked:											
		Varieties averaged, baked:											
15	935	Mashed	1 cup	245	89	96	2.2	21.4	5.88	1.5	.32	.12	.65
15	936	Baked cubes	1 cup	205	89	79	1.8	17.9	4.92	1.3	.27	.1	.54
15	937	Acorn, baked, mashed	1 cup	245	90	83	1.6	21.5	5.88	.2	.04	.01	.09
15	938	Butternut, baked cubes	1 cup	205	88	83	1.8	21.5	4.92	.2	.04	.01	.08
		Sweet potatoes:											
		Cooked, 5 x 2 in diam:											
15	939	Baked in skin, peeled	1 potato	114	73	118	2	27.7	2.96	.1	.03	<.01	.06
15	940	Boiled without skin	1 potato	151	73	160	2	37	3.93	.45	.1	.02	.2
15	941	Candied, 2½x2 in	1 pce	105	67	144	.9	29.3	2.11	3.4	1.42	.66	.15
		Canned:											
15	942	Solid pack, mashed	1 cup	265	74	258	5	59.2	6.25	.5	.11	.02	.23
15	943	Vacuum pack, mashed	1 cup	255	76	233	4.2	53.9	6.25	.5	.11	.02	.23
15	944	Vacuum pack, 2¾ x 1 in	1 pce	40	76	36	.7	8.4	.98	<.1	.02	<.01	.04
		Tomatoes:											
		Raw:											
15	945	Whole, 2⅗ diam	1 tomato	123	94	24	1.1	5.3	2.16	.3	.04	.04	.11
15	946	Chopped	1 cup	180	94	35	1.6	7.8	3.17	.4	.05	.06	.16
15	947	Cooked from raw	1 cup	240	92	60	2.7	13.5	5.28	.7	.09	.1	.26
15	948	Canned, solids and liquid	1 cup	240	94	47	2.2	10.3	2.16	.6	.08	.09	.24
15	949	Tomato juice, canned	1 cup	244	94	42	1.9	10.3	1.7	.1	.02	.02	.06
		Tomato products, canned:											
15	950	Paste	1 cup	262	74	220	9.9	49.3	6.2	2.3	.33	.35	.95
15	951	Puree	1 cup	250	87	102	4.2	25.1	4.2	.3	.04	.04	.12
15	952	Sauce	1 cup	245	89	74	3.2	17.6	3.2	.4	.06	.06	.16
15	953	Turnips, cubes, cooked from raw	½ cup	78	94	14	.6	3.8	1.4	<.1	<.01	<.01	.03
		Turnip greens, cooked:											
15	954	From raw (leaves and stems)	1 cup	144	94	29	1.6	6.3	3.8	.3	.08	.02	.13
15	955	From frozen (chopped)	½ cup	82	90	24	2.8	4.1	2.5	.3	.08	.02	.14
15	956	Vegetable juice cocktail, canned	1 cup	242	94	46	1.5	11	1.52	.2	.03	.03	.09
		Vegetables, mixed:											
15	957	Canned, drained	1 cup	163	87	77	4.2	15.1	6.6	.4	.08	.03	.19
15	958	Frozen, cooked, drained	1 cup	182	83	107	5.2	23.8	7.5	.3	.06	.02	.12
		Water chestnuts, canned:											
15	959	Slices	½ cup	70	86	35	.6	8.7	.6	<.1	.01	<.01	.02
15	960	Whole	4 ea	28	86	14	.2	3.5	.24	.1	<.01	<.01	<.01

(For purposes of calculations, use "0" for t, <1, <.1, <.01, etc.)

KEY: 1 = BEV 2 = DAIRY 3 = EGGS 4 = FAT/OIL 5 = FRUIT 6 = BAKERY 7 = GRAIN 8 = FISH 9 = BEEF 10 = POULTRY
11 = SAUSAGE   12 = MIXED   13 = NUTS/SEEDS   14 = SWEETS   15 = VEG/LEG   16 = MISC   22 = SOUP/SAUCE

Chol (mg)	Calc (mg)	Iron (mg)	Magn (mg)	Phos (mg)	Pota (mg)	Sodi (mg)	Zinc (mg)	VT-A (RE)	Thia (mg)	Ribo (mg)	Niac (mg)	V-B6 (mg)	Fola (µg)	VT-C (mg)
0	244	6.42	157	100	838	126	1.37	1474	.17	.42	.88	.44	262	40
0	277	2.89	131	91	566	163	1.33	1479	.11	.32	.8	.28	204	23
0	271	4.92	162	94	740	683[129]	.99	1878	.03	.29	.83	.21	209	31
0	48	.64	44	69	346	2	.71	52[130]	.08	.07	.92	.12	36	9
0	48	.64	44	69	346	2	.71	52[130]	.09	.09	.92	.17	36	10
0	23	.63	40	72	455	5	.32	43[130]	.07	.07	.77	.14	30	8
0	34	.81	20	49	1071	2	.64	872	.21	.06	1.72	.18	69	24
0	28	.67	16	41	895	3	.54	730	.17	.05	1.43	.15	57	20
0	65	1.37	63	67	645	6	.27	63	.24	.02	1.30	.29	28	16
0	84	1.23	59	55	583	7	.27	1435	.15	.04	1.99	.25	39	31
0	32	.52	23	63	397	12	.33	2488	.08	.14	.7	.28	26	28
0	32	.8	15	41	278	20	.4	2575	.08	.21	1	.36	22	26
0[131]	27	1.2	12	27	198	74	.16	440	.02	.04	.41	.17	12	7
0	77	3.4	61	133	536	191	.54	3857	.07	.23	2.4	.48	42	13
0	56	2.27	57	125	796	136	.46	2036	.09	.14	1.89	.48	42	67
0	9	.36	9	20	125	21	.07	319	.01	.02	.3	.08	7	11
0	9	.59	14	28	255	10	.13	139	.07	.06	.74	.09	12	22[132]
0	12	.86	20	42	372	15	.19	204	.11	.09	1.08	.14	17	32[132]
0	20	1.44	33	70	624	25	.32	325	.17	.14	1.72	.15	23	50
0	63[133]	1.45	29	46	529	390[134]	.38	145	.11	.07	1.76	.22	35	36
0	22	1.41	27	47	537	881[135]	.34	136	.12	.08	1.64	.27	49	45
0	92	7.84	134	207	2442	170[136]	2.1	647	.41	.5	8.44	1	40	111
0	37	2.32	60	99	1051	49[137]	.54	340	.18	.14	4.29	.38	39	88
0	34	1.88	46	78	908	1481[138]	.6	240	.16	.14	2.82	.33	39	32
0	18	.17	6	15	106	39	.08	0	.02	.02	.23	.05	7	9
0	198	1.15	32	41	293	41	.29	792	.07	.1	.59	.26	171	40
0	125	1.59	21	27	184	12	.34	654	.04	.06	.38	.06	32	18
0	27	1.02	27	41	467	883	.48	283	.1	.07	1.76	.34	38	67
0	44	1.71	26	68	474	243	.67	1899	.07	.08	.94	.13	38	8
0	46	1.49	40	93	308	64	.89	779	.13	.22	1.55	.14	35	6
0	3	.61	3	14	82	6	.27	t	<.01	.02	.25	—	8	.9
0	1	.25	1	5	33	2	.11	t	<.01	<.01	.1	—	3	.4

H

(129)Dietary pack contains 58 mg sodium.
(130)Applies to squash including skin; flesh has no appreciable vitamin A value.
(131)For recipe using margarine; if butter is used cholesterol = 8 mg.
(132)Year-round average. From June through October, ascorbic acid is approximately 32 mg and 47 mg respectively for one tomato and one cup chopped tomato. From November through May, market samples average around 12 and 18 mg respectively.
(133)Calcium is added as a firming agent.
(134)Dietary Pack contains 31 mg sodium.
(135)If no salt is added, sodium content is 24 mg.
(136)If salt is added, sodium content is 2070 mg.
(137)If salt is added, sodium content is 998 mg.
(138)With salt added.

(For purposes of calculations, use "0" for t, <1, <.1, <.01, etc.)

TABLE H–1

Food Composition

Grp	Ref	Name	Measure	Wt (g)	H$_2$O (%)	Ener (kcal)	Prot (g)	Carb (g)	Fiber (g)	Fat (g)	Fat Breakdown (g)		
											Sat	Mono	Poly
MISCELLANEOUS													
16	961	Carob flour	1 cup	140	3	255	6	126	10.8	.3	—	.1	.10
		Baking powders for home use:											
		Sodium aluminum sulfate:											
16	962	With monocalcium phosphate monohydrate	1 tsp	3	2	5	t	1	0	0	0	0	0
16	963	With monocalcium phosphate monohydrate, calcium sulfate	1 tsp	2.9	1	5	t	1	0	0	0	0	0
16	964	Straight phosphate	1 tsp	3.8	2	5	t	1	0	0	0	0	0
16	965	Low sodium	1 tsp	4.3	1	5	t	1	0	0	0	0	0
16	966	Basil, ground	1 tbsp	5	6	11	.7	2.7	.8	.2	—	—	—
		Catsup:											
16	967	Cup	1 cup	273	69	290	5	69	1.36	1.1	.2	.2	.4
16	968	Tablespoon	1 tbsp	17	69	18	.3	4.3	.09	<.1	.01	.01	.03
16	969	Celery seed	1 tsp	2	6	8	.4	.9	.26	.5	.05	.34	.08
16	970	Chili powder	1 tsp	2.6	8	8	.3	1.4	.58	.4	.1	.1	.2
		Chocolate:											
16	971	Baking	1 oz	28	2	145	3.5	7.5	1.78	15	9	4.5	.5
		Semi-sweet, milk, and dark chocolates (see Sweets and Sweeteners, items 759, 763, 764)												
16	972	Coriander, fresh	¼ cup	4	93	<1	<.1	.1	.03	<.1	—	—	—
16	973	Cinnamon	1 tsp	2.3	10	5	<.1	1.8	.55	<.1	.01	.01	.01
16	974	Curry powder	1 tsp	2	10	5	.2	1.2	.34	.3	127	—	—
		Garlic:											
16	975	Cloves	4 cloves	12	59	18	.8	4	.2	<.1	.01	<.01	.03
16	976	Powder	1 tsp	2.8	6	9	.5	2	.05	<.1	<.01	<.01	.01
16	977	Gelatin, dry, plain	1 envelope	7	13	25	6	0	1	t	t	t	t
16	978	Ginger root, raw, sliced	5 slices	11	87	8	.2	1.7	.11	<.1	.02	.02	.02
16	979	Mustard, prepared, packet (1 packet=1 tsp)	1 tsp	5	80	4	.2	.3	.02	.2	t	.2	t
		Miso (see item 926 under Vegetables, soybean products):												
		Olives:											
16	980	Green	10 olives	39	78	45	.5	.5	1.72	6	.6	3.6	.3
16	981	Ripe, pitted[140]	10 olives	47	81	50	.4	2.9	1.4	4.5	.8	3.4	.32
16	982	Onion powder	1 tsp	2.1	5	5	.2	1.8	.12	<.1	<.01	<.01	.01
16	983	Oregano, ground	1 tsp	1.5	7	5	.2	1	.22	.2	.02	.02	.1
16	984	Paprika	1 tsp	2.1	10	6	.3	1.3	.48	.3	.02	.02	.2
16	985	Pepper, black	1 tsp	2.1	11	5	.2	1.4	.28	<.1	.03	.03	.03
		Pickles:											
16	986	Dill, medium, 3¾ x 1¼ in diam	1 pickle	65	93	5	.5	1.4	.91	.1	.03	<.01	.04
16	987	Fresh pack, slices, 1½ in diam x ¼ in thick	4 slices	30	79	20	.3	5.4	.42	<.1	.01	<.01	.02
16	988	Sweet, small, about 2½ x ¾ in diam	1 pickle	15	61	20	<.1	5.5	.21	<.1	.01	<.01	.02
16	989	Pickle relish, sweet	1 tbsp	15	63	20	<.1	5.2	.28	<.1	.02	<.01	.04
		Popcorn (see Grains, items 539-541)												
16	990	Salt	1 tsp	5.5	0	0	0	0	0	0	0	0	0
16	991	Vinegar, cider	1 tbsp	15	94	2	0	.9	0	0	0	0	0
		Yeast:											
16	992	Bakers, dry, active, package	1 package	7	5	20	2.6	2.6	<.01	.1	t	.1	t
16	993	Brewer's, dry	1 tbsp	8	5	25	3.1	3.1	.14	<.1	t	t	0

(140)This is the most recent tested data from the California Olive industry, October 1986.

(For purposes of calculations, use "0" for t, <1, <.1, <.01, etc.)

Chol (mg)	Calc (mg)	Iron (mg)	Magn (mg)	Phos (mg)	Pota (mg)	Sodi (mg)	Zinc (mg)	VT-A (RE)	Thia (mg)	Ribo (mg)	Niac (mg)	V-B6 (mg)	Fola (μg)	VT-C (mg)
0	390	—	127	102	1275	24	1.12	t	.07	.07	2.2	127	0	t
0	58	0	t	87	5	329	0	0	0	0	0	0	0	0
0	183	0	—	45	4	290	0	0	0	0	0	0	0	0
0	239	0	—	359	6	312	0	0	0	0	0	0	0	0
0	207	0	—	314	891	t	0	0	0	0	0	0	0	0
0	95	1.89	18	22	154	2	.26	42	<.01	.01	.31	—	—	3
0	60	2.2	57	137	991	2845	.64	382	.25	.19	4.4	.29	14	41
0	4	.14	4	9	54	156	.04	24	.02	.01	.27	.02	<1	3
0	38	.97	10	11	30	4	.15	t	.01	.01	.1	—	—	.4
0	7	.37	4	8	50	26	.07	91	<.01	.02	.2	—	1	2
0	22	1.9	82	109	235	1	1.01	1	.01	.1	.38	.01	18	0
0	4	.08	1	1	22	1	—	11	<.01	<.01	.03	—	—	.4
0	28	.87	1	1	12	1	.04	1	<.01	<.01	.03	.02	—	.7
0	10	.62	5	7	31	1	.09	2	<.01	<.01	.07	—	—	.2
0	22	.2	3	18	48	2	1.06	0	.02	.01	.08	.40	<1	4
0	2	.08	2	12	31	1	.07	0	.01	<.01	.02	—	2	t
0	1	0	2	0	2	6	0	0	0	0	0	<.01	0	0
0	2	.05	5	3	46	1	.22	0	<.01	<.01	.08	.02	2	.6
0	4	.1	2	4	7	63	.03	0	<.01	.01	.07	<.01	0	t
0	24	.6	9	6	21	936	.03	12	<.01	<.01	.01	<.01	<1	t
0	42	1.5	10	10	4	410	.14	18	<.01	<.01	0.2	<.01	<1	.5
0	8	.06	3	7	20	1	.05	0	<.01	<.01	.01	.03	3	t
0	24	.66	4	3	25	t	.07	10	<.01	t	.09	—	—	1
0	4	.54	4	7	49	1	.1	127	.01	.04	.35	—	—	1.4
0	9	.49	4	3.67	26.7	1	.03	t	<.01	<.01	.02	0	—	0
0	17	.7	8	14	130	928	.18	7	<.01	.01	.01	<.01	<1	4
0	10	.55	2	8	60	201	0	4	t	<.01	<.01	<.01	0	2
0	2	.25	2	2	30	107	<.01	1	<.01	<.01	<.01	<.01	0	1
0	3	.12	<1	2	30	107	.01	2	t	t	<.01	0	0	1
0	14	<.01	0	3	.3	2132	0	0	0	0	0	0	0	0
0	1	.09	<1	1	15	t	.02	0	0	0	0	0	0	0
0	4	1.1	16	90	140	4	.42	t	.17	.38	2.7	.14	266	t
0	17[139]	1.39	18	140	152	10	.63	t	1.25	.34	3.16	.4	313	t

[139] Value varies from 6-60 mg.

(For purposes of calculations, use "0" for t, <1, <.1, <.01, etc.)

H

TABLE H–1

Food Composition

Grp	Ref	Name	Measure	Wt (g)	H₂O (%)	Ener (kcal)	Prot (g)	Carb (g)	Fiber (g)	Fat (g)	Fat Breakdown (g) Sat	Mono	Poly
		SOUPS, SAUCES, AND GRAVIES											
		Soups, canned, condensed:											
		Prepared with equal volume of whole milk:											
22	994	Clam chowder, New England	1 cup	248	85	163	9.5	16.6	2.5	6.6	2.95	2.26	1.08
22	995	Cream of chicken	1 cup	248	85	191	7.5	15	.13	11.5	4.63	4.45	1.64
22	996	Cream of mushroom	1 cup	248	85	205	6	15	.25	13.6	5.12	2.98	4.61
22	997	Tomato	1 cup	248	85	160	6	22.3	.5	6	2.9	1.6	1.1
		Prepared with equal volume of water:											
22	998	Bean with bacon	1 cup	253	84	173	7.9	22.8	2.55	5.9	1.53	2.18	1.82
22	999	Beef broth, bouillon, consomme	1 cup	240	98	16	2.7	1	0	.5	.26	.22	.02
22	1000	Beef noodle	1 cup	244	92	84	4.8	9	.24	3.1	1.15	1.24	.49
22	1001	Chicken noodle	1 cup	241	92	75	4	9.3	.24	2.5	.65	1.11	.55
22	1002	Chicken rice	1 cup	241	94	60	3.5	7.2	.82	1.9	.5	.9	.4
22	1003	Clam chowder, Manhatten	1 cup	244	90	78	4.2	12.2	1.2	2.3	.44	.41	1.32
22	1004	Cream of chicken	1 cup	244	91	115	3.4	9.3	.61	7.4	2.08	3.28	1.49
22	1005	Cream of mushroom	1 cup	244	90	130	2	9.3	1.48	9	2.4	1.7	4.2
22	1006	Minestrone	1 cup	241	91	80	4.3	11.2	.96	2.5	.54	.69	1.11
22	1007	Split pea with ham	1 cup	253	82	189	10.3	28	.66	4.4	1.8	1.8	.63
22	1008	Tomato	1 cup	244	90	86	2.1	16.6	.49	1.9	.36	.43	.96
22	1009	Vegetable beef	1 cup	244	92	79	5.6	10.2	.81	1.9	.85	.8	.11
22	1010	Vegetarian vegetable	1 cup	241	92	70	2.1	12	1.2	1.9	.29	.83	.73
		Soups, dehydrated:											
		Unprepared, dry products:											
22	1011	Bouillon	1 packet	6	3	15	1	1	0	1	.3	.2	t
22	1012	Onion	1 packet	7	4	20	.8	4	.17	.4	.1	.2	.07
		Prepared with water:											
22	1013	Chicken noodle	¾ cup	188	94	40	2	6	.15	1	.19	.38	.25
22	1014	Onion	¾ cup	184	96	20	.8	3.8	.17	.4	.1	.25	.07
22	1015	Tomato vegetable	¾ cup	189	94	41	1.5	7.6	.4	.7	.3	.25	.06
		Sauces:											
		From dry mixes:											
22	1016	Cheese sauce, prepared with milk	1 cup	279	77	305	16	23	.24	17	9.3	5.3	1.6
22	1017	Hollandaise, prepared with water	1 cup	259	84	240	5	14	—	20	11.6	5.9	.9
22	1018	White sauce, prepared with milk	1 cup	264	81	240	10	21	.33	13	6.4	4.7	1.7
		From home recipe:											
22	1019	White sauce, medium[141]	1 cup	250	73	395	10	24	.41	30	9.1	11.9	7.2
		Ready to serve:											
22	1020	Barbeque sauce	1 tbsp	16	81	10	.2	1.5	.09	.4	.04	.14	.14
22	1021	Soy sauce	1 tbsp	18	68	11	1.5	1.6	0	0	0	0	0
		Gravies:											
		Canned:											
22	1022	Beef	1 cup	233	88	124	8.7	11.2	.4	5.5	2.75	2.3	.21
22	1023	Chicken	1 cup	238	85	189	4.6	12.9	.24	13.6	3.36	6.08	3.58
22	1024	Mushroom	1 cup	238	89	120	3	13	.3	6	1	2.8	2.4
		From dry mix:											
22	1025	Brown	1 cup	261	91	80	3	14	.24	2	.9	.8	.1
22	1026	Chicken	1 cup	260	91	85	3	14	.24	2	.5	.9	.4

(141)Made with enriched flour, margarine, and whole milk.

(For purposes of calculations, use "0" for t, <1, <.1, <.01, etc.)

KEY: 1 = BEV 2 = DAIRY 3 = EGGS 4 = FAT/OIL 5 = FRUIT 6 = BAKERY 7 = GRAIN 8 = FISH 9 = BEEF 10 = POULTRY
11 = SAUSAGE 12 = MIXED 13 = NUTS/SEEDS 14 = SWEETS 15 = VEG/LEG 16 = MISC 22 = SOUP/SAUCE

Chol (mg)	Calc (mg)	Iron (mg)	Magn (mg)	Phos (mg)	Pota (mg)	Sodi (mg)	Zinc (mg)	VT-A (RE)	Thia (mg)	Ribo (mg)	Niac (mg)	V-B6 (mg)	Fola (μg)	VT-C (mg)
22	187	1.48	23	157	300	992	1.3	40	.07	.24	1.03	.13	12	3
27	180	.67	18	152	273	1046	.68	94	.07	.26	.92	.07	8	1
20	178	.59	20	156	270	1076	.64	38	.08	.28	.81	.06	15	2
17	159	1.82	23	148	450	932	.29	109	.13	.25	1.52	.16	21	68
3	81	2.05	44	132	403	952	1.03	89	.09	.03	.57	.04	32	2
.6	15	.41	9	31	130	782	.6	0	<.01	.05	1.87	.07	2	0
5	15	1.1	6	46	100	952	1.54	63	.07	.06	1.07	.04	4	.3
7	17	.78	5	36	55	1106	.4	71	.05	.06	1.39	<.01	2	t
7	17	.75	1	22	101	815	.26	66	.02	.02	1.13	.02	1	t
2	34	1.89	10	58	261	1808	.93	92	.06	.05	1.34	.08	10	3
10	34	.61	3	37	88	986	.63	56	.03	.06	.82	.02	2	t
2	46	.5	5	49	100	1032	.59	0	.05	.09	.7	.01	3	1
2	34	.92	7	56	312	911	.73	234	.05	.04	.94	.10	16	1
0	22	2.3	48	213	399	1008	1.32	44	.15	.08	1.5	.07	2	1
0	13	1.76	8	34	263	872	.24	69	.09	.05	1.42	.11	15	67
5	17	1.11	6	41	173	956	2	189	.04	.05	1.03	.08	11	2
0	21	1.08	7	35	209	823	.46	301	.05	.05	.92	.06	11	1
1	4	.1	4	19	27	1019	.01	t	t	.01	.3	.01	—	0
t	10	.14	3	23	47	627	.06	t	.02	.04	.4	<.01	2	t
2	24	.37	5	24	23	957	.15	5	.05	.04	.66	<.01	1	.2
0	9	.14	6	22	48	635	.06	t	.02	.04	.36	<.01	2	.2
0	6	.47	15	23	78	856	.12	14	.04	.03	.59	.04	2	5
53	569	.3	32	438	552	1565	.95	117	.15	.56	.3	.1	12	2
52	124	.9	—	127	124	1564	—	220	.05	.18	.1	.5	—	t
34	425	.3	35	256	444	797	1.15	92	.08	.45	.5	.08	14	3
32	292	.9	35	238	381	888	1.05	340	.15	.43	.8	.1	12	2
0	3	.12	<1	3	27	128	.03	14	<.01	<.01	.06	.01	<1	t
0	3	.5	8	38	64	1029	.28	0	<.01	.02	.6	.03	4	0
7	14	1.63	3	70	189	117	2.33	0	.07	.08	1.54	.02	7	0
5	48	1.1	5	69	260	1375	1.91	264	.04	.1	1.06	.02	3	0
0	17	1.6	—	36	252	1357	1.66	0	.08	.15	1.6	.05	0	0
2	66	.2	t	47	61	1147	.01	0	.04	.09	.9	<.01	—	0
3	39	.3		47	62	1134	.32	0	.05	.15	.8	.03		3

H

(For purposes of calculations, use "0" for t, <1, <.1, <.01, etc.)

Recommended Nutrient Intakes (RDA, RNI)

Some of the U.S. recommendations appear in the RDA table on the inside front cover. The remaining RDA are here, in Tables I–1 and I–2. The U.S. RDA used on food labels are on the inside back cover. The Canadian recommendations are in Tables I–3 and I–4.

TABLE I–1

Estimated Safe and Adequate Daily Dietary Intakes of Additional Selected Nutrients (United States)[a]

Age (years)	Vitamins			Electrolytes		
	Vitamin K (μg)	Biotin (μg)	Pantothenic acid (mg)	Sodium (mg)	Potassium (mg)	Chloride (mg)
0-0.5	12	35	2	115-350	350-925	275-700
0.5-1	10-20	50	3	250-750	425-1,275	400-1,200
1-3	15-30	65	3	325-975	550-1,650	500-1,500
4-6	20-40	85	3-4	450-1,350	775-2,325	700-2,100
7-10	30-60	120	4-5	600-1,800	1,000-3,000	925-2,775
11+	50-100	100-200	4-7	900-2,700	1,525-4,575	1,400-4,200
Adults	70-140	100-200	4-7	1,100-3,300	1,875-5,625	1,700-5,100

Age (years)	Trace Elements[b]					
	Chromium (mg)	Selenium (mg)	Molybdenum (mg)	Copper (mg)	Manganese (mg)	Fluoride (mg)
0-0.5	0.01-0.04	0.01-0.04	0.03-0.06	0.5-0.7	0.5-0.7	0.1-0.5
0.5-1	0.02-0.06	0.02-0.06	0.04-0.08	0.7-1.0	0.7-1.0	0.2-1.0
1-3	0.02-0.08	0.02-0.08	0.05-0.1	1.0-1.5	1.0-1.5	0.5-1.5
4-6	0.03-0.12	0.03-0.12	0.06-0.15	1.5-2.0	1.5-2.0	1.0-2.5
7-10	0.05-0.2	0.05-0.2	0.1-0.3	2.0-2.5	2.0-3.0	1.5-2.5
11+	0.05-0.2	0.05-0.2	0.15-0.5	2.0-3.0	2.5-5.0	1.5-2.5
Adults	0.05-0.2	0.05-0.2	0.15-0.5	2.0-3.0	2.5-5.0	1.5-4.0

[a]Because there is less information on which to base allowances, these figures are not given in the main table of the RDA and are provided here in the form of ranges of recommended intakes.
[b]Since the toxic levels for many trace elements may be only several times usual intakes, the upper levels for the trace elements given in this table should not habitually be exceeded.

TABLE I-2

Mean Heights and Weights and Recommended Energy Intakes (United States)

Age	Weight		Height		Energy Needs[a]	
(years)	(kg)	(lb)	(cm)	(in)	(kcal)	(MJ)[b]
Infants						
0.0-0.5	6	13	60	24	kg × 115 (95-145)	kg × 0.48
0.5-1.0	9	20	71	28	kg × 105 (80-135)	kg × 0.44
Children						
1-3	13	29	90	35	1,300 (900-1,800)	5.5
4-6	20	44	112	44	1,700 (1,300-2,300)	7.1
7-10	28	62	132	52	2,400 (1,650-3,300)	10.1
Males						
11-14	45	99	157	62	2,700 (2,000-3,700)	11.3
15-18	66	145	176	69	2,800 (2,100-3,900)	11.8
19-22	70	154	177	70	2,900 (2,500-3,300)	12.2
23-50	70	154	178	70	2,700 (2,300-3,100)	11.3
51-75	70	154	178	70	2,400 (2,000-2,800)	10.1
76+	70	154	178	70	2,050 (1,650-2,450)	8.6
Females						
11-14	46	101	157	62	2,200 (1,500-3,000)	9.2
15-18	55	120	163	64	2,100 (1,200-3,000)	8.8
19-22	55	120	163	64	2,100 (1,700-2,500)	8.8
23-50	55	120	163	64	2,000 (1,600-2,400)	8.4
51-75	55	120	163	64	1,800 (1,400-2,200)	7.6
76+	55	120	163	64	1,600 (1,200-2,000)	6.7
Pregnant					+300	
Lactating					+500	

[a]The energy allowances for the young adults are for men and women doing light work. The allowances for the two older age groups represent mean energy needs over these age spans, allowing for a 2 percent decrease in basal (resting) metabolic rate per decade and a reduction in activity of 200 kcal per day for men and women between 51 and 75 years, 500 kcal for men over 75 years, and 400 kcal for women over 75. The customary range of daily energy output, shown in parentheses, is based on a variation in energy needs of ± 400 kcal at any one age, emphasizing the wide range of energy intakes appropriate for any group of people. Energy allowances for children through age 18 are based on median energy intakes of children these ages followed in longitudinal growth studies. The values in parentheses are tenth and ninetieth percentiles of energy intake, to indicate the range of energy consumption among children of these ages.
[b]MJ stands for megajoules (1 MJ = 1,000 kJ).

TABLE I-3

Recommended Nutrient Intakes for Canadians, 1983 (formerly Canadian *Dietary Standard*, 1975)

Age	Sex	Weight (kg)	Protein (g/day)[a]	Vitamin A (RE/day)[b]	Vitamin D (µg/day)[c]	Vitamin E (mg/day)[d]
Months				Fat-Soluble Vitamins		
0-2	Both	4.5	11[f]	400	10	3
3-5	Both	7.0	14[f]	400	10	3
6-8	Both	8.5	17[f]	400	10	3
9-11	Both	9.5	18	400	10	3
Years						
1	Both	11	19	400	10	3
2-3	Both	14	22	400	5	4
4-6	Both	18	26	500	5	5
7-9	M	25	30	700	2.5	7
	F	25	30	700	2.5	6
10-12	M	34	38	800	2.5	8
	F	36	40	800	2.5	7
13-15	M	50	50	900	2.5	9
	F	48	42	800	2.5	7
16-18	M	62	55	1,000	2.5	10
	F	53	43	800	2.5	7
19-24	M	71	58	1,000	2.5	10
	F	58	43	800	2.5	7
25-49	M	74	61	1,000	2.5	9
	F	59	44	800	2.5	6
50-74	M	73	60	1,000	2.5	7
	F	63	47	800	2.5	6
75+	M	69	57	1,000	2.5	6
	F	64	47	800	2.5	5
Pregnancy (additonal)						
1st Trimester			15	100	2.5	2
2nd Trimester			20	100	2.5	2
3rd Trimester			25	100	2.5	2
Lactation (additional)			20	400	2.5	3

Recommended intakes of energy and of certain nutrients are not listed in this table because of the nature of the variables upon which they are based. The figures for energy are estimates of average requirements for expected patterns of activity (see Table I-4). For nutrients not shown, the following amounts are recommended: thiamin, 0.4 mg/1,000 kcal (0.48/5,000 kJ); riboflavin, 0.5 mg/1,000 kcal (0.6 mg/5,000 kJ); niacin, 7.2 NE/1,000 kcal (8.6 NE/5,000 kJ); vitamin B_6, 15 µg, as pyridoxine, per gram of protein; phosphorus, same as calcium. Recommended intakes during periods of growth are taken as appropriate for individuals representative of the mid-point in each age group. All recommended intakes are designed to cover individual variations in essentially all of a healthy population subsisting upon a variety of common foods available in Canada.
Source: *Recommended Nutrient Intakes for Canadians,* Health and Welfare Canada (Ottawa: Canadian Government Publishing Centre, 1984), Table X.1, pp. 179–180.

TABLE I-3

(continued)

Water-Soluble Vitamins			Minerals				
Vitamin C (mg/day)	Folacin (µg/day)[e]	Vitamin B$_{12}$ (µg/day)	Calcium (mg/day)	Magnesium (mg/day)	Iron (mg/day)	Iodine (µg/day)	Zinc (mg/day)
20	50	0.3	350	30	0.4[g]	25	2[h]
20	50	0.3	350	40	5	35	3
20	50	0.3	400	50	7	40	3
20	55	0.3	400	50	7	45	3
20	65	0.3	500	55	6	55	4
20	80	0.4	500	70	6	65	4
25	90	0.5	600	90	6	85	5
35	125	0.8	700	110	7	110	6
30	125	0.8	700	110	7	95	6
40	170	1.0	900	150	10	125	7
40	180	1.0	1,000	160	10	110	7
50	150	1.5	1,100	210	12	160	9
45	145	1.5	800	200	13	160	8
55	185	1.9	900	250	10	160	9
45	160	1.9	700	215	14	160	8
60	210	2.0	800	240	8	160	9
45	175	2.0	700	200	14	160	8
60	220	2.0	800	250	8	160	9
45	175	2.0	700	200	14[i]	160	8
60	220	2.0	800	250	8	160	9
45	190	2.0	800	210	7	160	8
60	205	2.0	800	230	8	160	9
45	190	2.0	800	220	7	160	8
0	305	1.0	500	15	6	25	0
20	305	1.0	500	20	6	25	1
20	305	1.0	500	25	6	25	2
30	120	0.5	500	80	0	50	6

[a]The primary units are expressed per kilogram of body weight. The figures shown here are examples.

[b]One retinol equivalent (RE) corresponds to the biological activity of 1 µg of retinol, 6 µg of β-carotene or 12 µg of other carotenes.

[c]Expressed as cholecalciferol or ergocalciferol.

[d]Expressed as d-α-tocopherol equivalents, relative to which β- and γ-tocopherol and α-tocotrienol have activities of 0.5, 0.1 and 0.3 respectively.

[e]Expressed as total folate.

[f]Assumption that the protein is from breast milk or is of the same biological value as that of breast milk and that between 3 and 9 months adjustment for the quality of the protein is made.

[g]It is assumed that breast milk is the source of iron up to 2 months of age.

[h]Based on the assumption that breast milk is the source of zinc for the first 2 months.

[i]After the menopause the recommended intake is 7 mg/day.

TABLE I–4

Average Energy Requirements (Canada)

Age	Sex	Average Height (cm)	Average Weight (kg)	Requirements[a]					
				kcal/kg[b]	MJ/kg[b]	kcal/day	MJ/day	kcal/cm	MJ/cm
Months									
0-2	Both	55	4.5	120-100	0.50-0.42	500	2.0	9	0.04
3-5	Both	63	7.0	100-95	0.42-0.40	700	2.8	11	0.05
6-8	Both	69	8.5	95-97	0.40-0.41	800	3.4	11.5	0.05
9-11	Both	73	9.5	97-99	0.41	950	3.8	12.5	0.05
Years									
1	Both	82	11	101	0.42	1,100	4.8	13.5	0.06
2-3	Both	95	14	94	0.39	1,300	5.6	13.5	0.06
4-6	Both	107	18	100	0.42	1,800	7.6	17	0.07
7-9	M	126	25	88	0.37	2,200	9.2	17.5	0.07
	F	125	25	76	0.32	1,900	8.0	15	0.06
10-12	M	141	34	73	0.30	2,500	10.4	17.5	0.07
	F	143	36	61	0.25	2,200	9.2	15.5	0.06
13-15	M	159	50	57	0.24	2,800	12.0	17.5	0.07
	F	157	48	46	0.19	2,200	9.2	14	0.06
16-18	M	172	62	51	0.21	3,200	13.2	18.5	0.08
	F	160	53	40	0.17	2,100	8.8	13	0.05
19-24	M	175	71	42	0.18	3,000	12.4		
	F	160	58	36	0.15	2,100	8.8		
25-49	M	172	74	36	0.15	2,700	11.2		
	F	160	59	32	0.13	1,900	8.0		
50-74	M	170	73	31	0.13	2,300	9.6		
	F	158	63	29	0.12	1,800	7.6		
75+	M	168	69	29	0.12	2,000	8.4		
	F	155	64	23	0.10	1,500	6.0		

Source: *Recommended Nutrient Intakes for Canadians,* 1984, Table II.1, pp. 22–23.
[a]Requirements can be expected to vary within a range of ± 30 percent.
[b]First and last figures are averages at the beginning and at the end of the 3-month period.

I

Vitamin/Mineral Supplements Compared

The following tables are useful for comparing the essential vitamin and mineral contents of supplements commonly available in the United States. Notice that blank columns have been provided for the addition of locally available products you may wish to compare with those shown here.

Not all ingredients in vitamin/mineral preparations are of proven benefit. To facilitate meaningful comparison, the table lists only the nutrients known to be needed in supplement form on occasion. Other nutrients and compounds found on the labels of these supplements are listed in the table notes.

When a supplement is needed that supplies certain particular nutrients, this table will ease the task of selecting an appropriate one. Notice, for example, that many preparations marketed for the elderly are composed largely of alcohol, with few vitamins or minerals. These are "tonics," not vitamin/mineral supplements. A tonic may be useful if the only need is for comfort and the benefit of the placebo effect, but if an elderly person needs a balanced assortment of vitamins and minerals and cannot easily take pills, it may be advisable to suggest a liquid preparation designated for infants.

Notice the very low levels of calcium present in some of these preparations. A product that supplies 20 mg of calcium provides only 2 percent of an adult's RDA for calcium and would have no significant impact on a person's calcium nutrition.

TABLE J–1

Supplements for Infants and Children

Company	Lederle	Miles Laboratories	Mead-Johnson	Mead-Johnson	Radiance
Product	Centrum Jr.	Flinstones Plus Iron	Poly-Vi-Sol With Iron (Drops)	Poly-Vi-Sol With Iron (Chewable)	Chewable For Children
Intended Users	Children Over 4	Children 1 to 12	Infants	Children and Adults	Children 2 to 12
Recommended Daily Dose	1 tablet	1 tablet	1 ml	1 tablet	1 tablet
Vitamins					
Vitamin A (IU)	5,000	2,500	1,500	2,500	4,000
Vitamin D (IU)	400	400	400	400	400
Vitamin E (IU)	15	15	5	15	3.4
Vitamin C (mg)	60	60	35	60	60
Thiamin (B_1) (mg)	1.5	1.05	0.5	1.05	2.0
Riboflavin (B_2) (mg)	1.7	1.2	0.6	1.2	2.4
Vitamin B_6 (mg)	2.0	1.05	0.4	1.05	2.0
Vitamin B_{12} (μg)	6.0	4.5	—	4.5	10.0
Niacin (mg)	20.0	13.5	8.0	13.5	10.0
Folacin (mg)	0.4	0.3	—	0.3	—
Minerals					
Calcium (mg)	—	—	—	—	19
Phosphorus (mg)	—	—	—	—	0.0
Iron (mg)	18	15	10	12	12
Potassium (mg)	1.6	—	—	—	4
Magnesium (mg)	25	—	—	—	22
Zinc (mg)	10	—	—	—	—
Copper (mg)	2	—	—	—	0.2
Iodine (μg)	—	—	—	—	—
Manganese (mg)	1	—	—	—	—
Cost per day*					

Radiance Chewables also contain 2 mg pantothenic acid, 10 mg biotin, 2 mg inositol, and 2 mg of a choline compound.

*Since product costs varies so widely by location (and local prices have changed dramatically in the last two years), the computation of cost/ day is left for the reader to complete. To compute this value, divide the total retail price by the number of doses per container. For example: XYZ vitamins are sold in bottles of 100 tablets. The recommended dose is 2 tablets per day, therefore there are 50 doses in the bottle. At $5.00 per bottle, XYZ Vitamins cost $.10 per day.

J

TABLE J–1

(continued)

Chocks	Neolife	J. B. Williams	Upjohn	Amway Nutrilite	Shaklee	Other
Bugs Bunny Plus Iron	Chewable New-Jr.	Chewable Popeye With Mins/Iron	Unicap Chewable	Chewables	Vita-Lea Chewables	
Children 1 to 12	Children 2 and Up	Children	Children	Children	Children	
1 tablet	3 tablets	1 tablet	1 tablet	1 tablet	2 tablets	
2,500	3,000	2,500	5,000	2,500	2,500	
400	300	400	400	400	200	
15	9	15	15	10	15	
60	60	60	60	40	45	
1.05	1.5	1.05	1.5	0.7	1.05	
1.2	1.5	1.2	1.7	0.8	1.2	
1.05	1.2	1.05	2.0	0.7	1.0	
4.5	3.0	4.5	6.0	3.0	4.5	
13.5	10.0	13.5	20.0	9.0	10.0	
0.3	—	0.3	0.4	0.2	0.2	
—	—	—	—	—	160	
—	—	—	—	—	125	
15	3	15	—	5	10	
—	—	40	—	—	100	
—	—	40	—	—	8	
—	—	12	—	—	1	
—	0.002	1.5	—	—	1	
—	75	105	—	—	75	
—	1	—	—	—	—	

Neo-life Chewables also contain 10 mg pantothenic acid, 0.075 mg inositol, and 0.05 mg of a choline compound.
Williams Chewables also contain 2.5 mg pantothenic acid, and 37.5 mg biotin.
Amway Chewables also contain 5 mg pantothenic acid.
Shaklee Chewables also contain 5 mg pantothenic acid, 150 mg biotin, and 0.2 mg inositol.

J

TABLE J–2

Supplements for Adults

Company	Lederle	Lederle	Parke-Davis	Squibb	Miles Lab
Product	Stress Tabs 600	Centrum A To Zinc	Myadec	Theragram M	One-A-Day Plus Iron
Recommended Daily Dose	1 tablet	1 tablet	1 tablet	1 tablet	1 tablet
Vitamins					
Vitamin A (IU)	—	5,000	10,000	10,000	5,000
Vitamin D (IU)	—	400	400	400	400
Vitamin E (IU)	30	30	30	15	15
Vitamin C (mg)	600	90	250	200	60
Thiamin (B_1) (mg)	15.0	2.25	10.0	10.3	1.5
Riboflavin (B_2) (mg)	15.0	2.6	10.0	10.0	1.7
Vitamin B_6 (mg)	5.0	3.0	5.0	4.1	2.0
Vitamin B_{12} (μg)	12	9	6	5	6
Niacin (mg)	100	20	100	100	20
Folacin (mg)	—	0.4	0.4	—	0.4
Minerals					
Calcium (mg)	—	162	—	20	—
Phosphorus (mg)	—	125	—	—	—
Iron (mg)	—	27	20	12	18
Potassium (mg)	—	7.5	—	—	—
Magnesium (mg)	—	100	100	65	—
Zinc (mg)	—	22.5	20	1.5	00
Copper (mg)	—	3	2	2	—
Iodine (μg)	—	150	150	150	—
Manganese (mg)	—	7.5	1.25	1.0	—
Cost per day*					

Lederle Centrum A to Zinc also contains 10 mg pantothenic acid, and 45 μg biotin.
Miles Labs One-A-Day plus Minerals also contains 10 mg pantothenic acid, 10 μg chromium, 10 μg selenium, and 10 μg molybdenum.
Lederle Stress-Tabs 600, Parke-Davis Myadec, and Squibb Theragram M also contain pantothenic acid: 20 mg, 20 mg, 18.4 mg, and 10 mg respectively.
*Since product costs varies so widely by location (and local prices have changed dramatically in the last two years), the computation of cost/day is left for the reader to complete. To compute this value, divide the total retail price by the number of doses per container. For example: XYZ vitamins are sold in bottles of 100 tablets. The recommended dose is 2 tablets per day, therefore there are 50 doses in the bottle. At $5.00 per bottle, XYZ Vitamins cost $.10 per day.

J

TABLE J–2

(continued)

Radiance	Neo-Life	Amway Nutrilite	J. B. Williams	Origin	Miles Lab	Other
Nutri-Mega	Formula IV	Double X	Vitabank	Multi-Vitamin	One-A-Day Plus Minerals	
2 tablets	2 capsules	9 tablets	1 tablet	1 tablet	1 tablet	
10,000	4,000	15,000	5,000	10,000	5,000	
400	400	400	400	400	400	
300	10	30	30	30	30	
300	90	500	90	250	60	
50	10	15	2.25	20	1.5	
50	10	15	2.6	20	1.7	
50	10	15	3.0	5.0	2.0	
50	10	9	9	6	6	
50	50	35	20	150	20	
0.4	0.1	0.4	0.4	0.4	0.4	
200	—	900	170	100	130	
50	—	450	130	—	100	
18	25	18	18	30	18	
30	—	—	7.5	5	5	
50	35	300	100	50	100	
15	—	15	15	7.5	15	
2	2	2	2	1	2	
150	100	150	150	150	150	
30	—	5.0	2.5	1.5	2.5	

Radiance Nutri-Mega also contains 50 mg pantothenic acid, 50 μg biotin, 50 mg inositol, 50 mg PABA, 50 mg choline compound, and 80 mg lecithin.

Neo-Life Formula IV also contains 12 mg pantothenic acid, 65 mg inositol, 30 mg PABA, 30 mg lecithin, 40 mg diastase, 40 mg lipase (pancreatin), and 168 mg linoleic acid.

Origin Multivitamins also contains 20 mg pantothenic acid, 25 μg biotin, 10 mg inositol, and 20 mg of a choline compound.

Amway Nutrilite Double X also contains 10 mg pantothenic acid, 5 μg chromium, and 5 μg selenium.

J. B. Williams Vitabank also contains 18 mg pantothenic acid and 25 μg selenium.

J

TABLE J–3

Supplements and Tonics for the Elderly

Company	Ross Labs	Lederle	J. B. Williams	Upjohn	Other
Product	Vi-Daylin Plus Iron	Gevrabon	Geritol	Unicap Senior	
Recommended Daily Dose	1 tsp	1 oz	1 oz	1 tablet	
Vitamins					
Vitamin A (IU)	2,500	—	—	5,000	
Vitamin D (IU)	400	—	—	—	
Vitamin E (IU)	15	—	—	15	
Vitamin C (mg)	60	—	—	60	
Thiamin (B_1) (mg)	1.05	5.0	5.0	1.2	
Riboflavin (B_2) (mg)	1.2	2.5	5.0	1.7	
Vitamin B_6 (mg)	1.05	1.0	1.0	2.0	
Vitamin B_{12} (μg)	4.5	1.0	1.5	6.0	
Niacin (mg)	13.5	50	100	14.0	
Folacin (mg)	—	—	—	0.4	
Minerals					
Calcium (mg)	—	—	2	—	
Phosphorus (mg)	—	—	—	—	
Iron (mg)	10	15	100	10	
Potassium (mg)	—	—	—	5	
Magnesium (mg)	—	2	—	—	
Zinc (mg)	—	2	—	15	
Copper (mg)	—	—	—	2	
Iodine (μg)	—	100	—	150	
Manganese (mg)	—	2	—	1	
Alcohol (%)	0.5	18	12	—	
Cost per day*					

Lederle Gevrabon also contains 100 mg inositol and 100 mg of a choline compound.
J. B. Williams Geritol also contains 100 mg of a choline compound and 50 mg methionine.
*Since product costs varies so widely by location (and local prices have changed dramatically in the last two years), the computation of cost/day is left for the reader to complete. To compute this value, divide the total retail price by the number of doses per container. For example: XYZ vitamins are sold in bottles of 100 tablets. The recommended dose is 2 tablets per day, therefore there are 50 doses in the bottle. At $5.00 per bottle, XYZ Vitamins cost $.10 per day.

J

Self-Study Forms

This Appendix contains the forms needed to complete the self-study exercises presented throughout the book. For reasons of space, Form 4 appears first, followed by forms 1 through 7.

FORM 4

Percentage of kCalories from Protein, Fat, and Carbohydrate

From Form 3:

Protein: _____ g/day ✕ 4 kcal/g = (P) _____ kcal/day

Fat: _____ g/day ✕ 9 kcal/g = (F) _____ kcal/day

Carbohydrate: _____ g/day ✕ 4 kcal/g = (C) _____ kcal/day

Total kcal/day = (T) _____ kcal/day

Percentage of kcalories from protein:

$$\frac{(P)}{(T)} \times 100 = \underline{\quad\quad} \text{ \% of total kcalories}$$

Percentage of kcalories from fat:

$$\frac{(F)}{(T)} \times 100 = \underline{\quad\quad} \text{ \% of total kcalories}$$

Percentage of kcalories from carbohydrate:

$$\frac{(C)}{(T)} \times 100 = \underline{\quad\quad} \text{ \% of total kcalories}$$

Note: The three percentages can total 99, 100, or 101, depending on the way in which figures were rounded off earlier.

K

FORM 1

Nutrient Intakes (Use One Form for Each Day)

Food	Approximate Measure or Weight	Energy[a] (kcal)	Prot[b] (g)	Carb[b] (g)	Fiber[b] (g)	Fat[b] (g)	Fat Breakdown (g)[b]			Chol[a] (mg)	Calcium[a] (mg)	Iron[c] (mg)	Magn[a] (mg)	Phos[a] (mg)	Potas[a] (mg)	Sodium[a] (mg)	Zinc[b] (mg)	Vit-A[b] (RE)	Thia[c] (mg)	Ribo[c] (mg)	Niac[b] (mg)	V-B$_6$[b] (mg)	Fol[a] (μg)	Vit-C[b] (mg)
							Sat	Mono	Poly															
Total																								

[a]Compute these values to the nearest whole number.
[b]Compute these values to one decimal place.
[c]Compute these values to two decimal places.

K

FORM 2

Average Daily Energy and Nutrient Intakes

Day	Energy (kcal)	Protein (g)	Carb (g)	Fiber (g)	Fat (g)	Fat Breakdown (g) Sat	Mono	Poly	Chol (mg)	Calcium (mg)	Iron (mg)	Magn (mg)	Phos (mg)	Potas (mg)	Sodium (mg)	Zinc (mg)	Vit-A (RE)	Thia (mg)	Ribo (mg)	Niac (mg)	V-B$_6$ (mg)	Fol (µg)	Vit-C (mg)
1																							
2																							
3																							
Total																							
Average daily intake (divide total by 3)																							

FORM 3

Comparison with a Standard Intake

Day	Energy (kcal)	Protein (g)	Fat (g)	Carbo-hydrate (g)	Chol (mg)	Calcium (mg)	Iron (mg)	Magn (mg)	Phos (mg)	Potas (mg)	Sodium (mg)	Zinc (mg)	Vit-A (RE)	Thia (mg)	Ribo (mg)	Niac (mg)	V-B$_6$ (mg)	Fol (µg)	Vit-C (mg)
Average daily intake (from Form 2)																			
Standard[a]																			
Intake as percentage of standard[b]																			

[a] Taken from RDA tables (inside front cover) and Appendix I or *Recommended Nutrient Intakes for Canadians* (Appendix I).
[b] For example, if your intake of protein was 50 g and the standard for a person your age and sex was 46 g, then you consumed (50 ÷ 46) × 100, or 109 percent of the standard.

Food Selection Scorecard

Food Group and Recommended Intake	Your Intake From Group (Specify Food and Amount)	Your Score
Fruits and vegetables—4 or more portions (½ cup cooked edible portion or 3–4 oz, 100 g, raw); at least 1 raw daily		
1 portion vitamin A–rich dark green or deep orange fruit or vegetable (any food with more than your RDA) = 10 points (no more than 10 points allowed)		
1 portion vitamin C–rich fruit or vegetable (any food with more than your RDA) = 10 points (no more than 10 points allowed)		
Other fruits and vegetables, incuding potatoes = 2.5 each		
Subtotal (no more than 25 points allowed)		
Breads and cereals—4 or more portions of whole-grain or enriched (1 oz dry-weight cereal or 1-oz slice bread or equivalent grain product)		
1 portion cereal or 2 bread equivalents = 10 points (no more than 10 points allowed)		
Other bread equivalents = 5 points each		
Subtotal (no more than 25 points allowed)		
Milk and milk products—2 or more portions (8 oz fluid milk; calcium equivalents are 1⅓ oz hard cheese, 1⅓ c cottage cheese, 1 pint ice milk or ice cream)		
One portion = 12.5 points		
Subtotal (no more than 25 points allowed)		
Meat and meat substitutes—2 or more portions of meat (2–3 oz of cooked lean meat, fish, poultry; protein equivalents are 2 eggs, 2 oz hard cheese, or ½ c cottage cheese) and 2 portions legumes or nuts (¾ c cooked legumes, 4 tbsp peanut butter, 1 oz nuts or sunflower seeds); count cheese either in milk group or in meat group, not both		
2 portions meat = 12.5 points		
2 portions legumes = 12.5 points		
Subtotal (no more than 25 points allowed)		
Grand total (no more than 100 points)		

The above are foundation foods. Additional foods are those that do not fit into the above groupings but add flavor, interest, variety, and (often) kcalories. List those eaten:

_____	_____	_____
_____	_____	_____
_____	_____	_____

K

FORM 6

Diet Planning by Exchange Groups

Exchange List	Number of Exchanges[b]	Carbohydrate _____ g	Protein _____ g	Fat _____ g	Energy[c] _____ kcal
		Amounts to be Delivered[a]			
Starch/Bread					
Meat					
Vegetable					
Fruit					
Milk					
Fat					
Total actually delivered					

[a]From step 2.
[b]From steps 4, 5, 6.
[c]From step 7.

FORM 7

Meal Patterns

Exchange List	Total Exchanges to be Consumed Daily[a]	Breakfast	Lunch	Snack	Dinner	Snack
		Exchanges Consumed At Each Meal				
Starch/Bread						
Meat						
Vegetable						
Fruit						
Milk						
Fat						

[a]From Form 6, column 2.

K

Enteral Formulas

As you can see from this appendix, the number of commercially prepared formulas available to meet the nutrient needs of people unable to meet these needs using regular foods is staggering. By the time this appendix has gone to press even more formulas may be on the market. The information presented here can help you see the similarities and differences among formulas, so that you can select the most appropriate one for your client.

Source: Sandoz Nutrition Corporation, Clinical Products Division, Mpls, MN.

TABLE L-1

Enteral Formulas†

Product	Manufacturer	Form	Major Protein Sources	Major Fat Sources	Major Carbohydrate Sources	Protein (g/1000 ml)	Fat (g/1000 ml)	Carbohydrate (g/1000 ml)	kcalories/ml	mOsm/kg
					NUTRIENT SOURCES					
Amin-Aid®1	Kendall McGaw	Powder	Free essential amino acids plus histidine	Partially hydrogenated soybean oil	Maltodextrin, sucrose	19.4	46.2	366	2.0	1095
Citrotein®	SandozNutrition	Powder	Egg white solids	Partially hydrogenated soybean oil	Sucrose, maltodextrin	41	1.6	122	0.66	480 Punch
Compleat® Modified Formula	SandozNutrition	Liquid	Beef, calcium caseinate	Beef, corn oil	Hydrolyzed cereal solids, fruits and vegetables	43	37	141	1.07	300
Compleat® Regular Formula	SandozNutrition	Liquid	Beef, nonfat milk	Beef, corn oil	Hydrolyzed cereal solids, fruits, vegetables, maltodextrin, lactose	43	43	128	1.07	405
Criticare HN®	Mead Johnson	Liquid	Enzymatically hydrolyzed casein, free amino acids	Safflower oil	Maltodextrin, modified corn starch	38	3	222	1.06	650
Enrich™	Ross	Liquid	Sodium and calcium caseinates, soy protein isolate	Corn oil	Hydrolyzed corn starch, sucrose, soy polysaccharide	39.7	37.2	162	1.1	480
Ensure®	Ross	Liquid	Sodium and calcium caseinates, soy protein isolate	Corn oil	Corn syrup, sucrose	37.2	37.2	145	1.06	450
Ensure® HN	Ross	Liquid	Sodium and calcium caseinates, soy protein isolate	Corn oil	Corn syrup, sucrose	44.4	35.5	141	1.06	470
Ensure Plus®	Ross	Liquid	Sodium and calcium caseinates, soy protein isolate	Corn oil	Corn syrup, sucrose	54.9	53.3	200	1.5	600
Ensure Plus® HN	Ross	Liquid	Sodium and calcium caseinates, soy protein isolate	Corn oil	Corn syrup, sucrose	62.6	49.9	200	1.5	650
Entrition®	Biosearch	Liquid	Sodium and calcium caseinates	Corn oil	Maltodextrin	35	35	136	1.0	300
Fortison™	Chesebrough-Pond's	Liquid	Calcium and sodium caseinates	Partially hydrogenated soybean oil	Maltodextrin, sucrose	35	40	125	1.0	300
Hepatic-Aid® II1	Kendall McGaw	Powder	Free amino acids (46% BCAA)	Partially hydrogenated soybean oil	Maltodextrin, sucrose	44.1	36.2	169	1.1	560
Isocal®	Mead Johnson	Liquid	Calcium and sodium caseinates, soy protein isolate	Soybean oil, MCT	Maltodextrin	34	44	133	1.06	300
Isocal® HCN	Mead Johnson	Liquid	Calcium and sodium caseinates	Soybean oil, MCT	Corn syrup	75	91	225	2.0	690
Isotein HN®	SandozNutrition	Powder	Delactosed lactalbumin	Partially hydrogenated soybean oil, MCT	Maltodextrin, monosaccharides	68	34	156	1.2	300
Magnacal®	Chesebrough-Pond's	Liquid	Calcium and sodium caseinates	Partially hydrogenated soybean oil	Maltodextrin, sucrose	70	80	250	2.0	590
Meritene® Liquid	SandozNutrition	Liquid	Concentrated sweet skim milk	Corn oil	Lactose, corn syrup solids, sucrose	57.6	32	110	0.96	505 Van.
Meritene® Powder (Prepared w/whole milk)	SandozNutrition	Powder	Nonfat milk	Milk fat	Lactose, sucrose, corn syrup solids	69	34	119	1.0	690

†Based on Manufacturers' available literature.
*Value not provided in available literature.
+Retinol equivalents
++Tocopherol equivalents
1Does not contain vitamins or electrolytes.
2One packet Sustacal Powder mixed with whole milk to prepare a 40 kcal/fl oz serving.
3At 1.0 kcal/ml dilution.
4Does not contain fat-soluble vitamins or electrolytes.

BCAA: Branched Chain Amino Acids
MCT: Medium chain triglycerides

Volume to meet 100% of U.S. RDA	Vitamin A (IU)	Vitamin D (IU)	Vitamin E (IU)	Vitamin C (mg)	Folacin (µg)	Thiamin (mg)	Riboflavin (mg)	Niacin (mg)	Vitamin B₆ (mg)	Vitamin B₁₂ (µg)	Biotin (mg)	Pantothenic Acid (mg)	Calcium (g)	Phosphorus (g)	Iodine (µg)	Iron (mg)	Magnesium (mg)	Copper (mg)	Zinc (mg)	Vitamin K (µg)	Choline (g)	Potassium g (mEq)	Sodium g (mEq)	Chloride g (mEq)	Manganese (mg)	Selenium (µg)
—	—	—	—	—	—	—	—	—	—	—	—	—	—	—	—	—	—	—	—	—	—	* (<6)	* (<15)	—	—	—
1270	5250	420	31.5	236	830	3.15	3.5	42	4.3	12.6	0.63	20.9	1.06	1.06	158	37.8	420	2.1	16	—	0.35	0.71 (18.2)	0.71 (31)	0.94 (26.5)	5.1	—
1500	3330	267	20	60	270	1.5	1.7	13.3	2.0	4.0	0.20	6.7	0.67	0.93	100	12	267	1.3	10	67	0.20	1.4 (35.9)	0.67 (29.1)	0.47 (13.3)	2.7	67
1500	3330	267	20	60	270	1.5	1.7	13	2.0	4.0	0.20	6.7	0.67	1.3	100	12	267	1.3	10	67	0.20	1.4 (35.9)	1.3 (56.5)	0.87 (24.5)	2.7	67
1892	2642	211	40	159	211	2.0	2.3	26.4	2.6	8.0	0.16	13.2	0.53	0.53	80	9.5	211	1.0	10.6	131	0.26	1.32 (34)	0.63 (27)	1.06 (30)	2.6	*
1391	3593	287	32.5	215	431	1.6	1.9	21.5	2.2	6.7	0.33	10.8	0.719	0.719	108	12.9	287	1.4	16.2	51	0.43	1.564 (40.0)	0.845 (36.8)	1.437 (40.5)	3.6	*
1887	2642	211	23.8	158.5	211	1.6	1.8	21.1	2.1	6.3	0.16	5.3	0.528	0.528	79.5	9.5	211	1.1	11.9	38	0.32	1.564 (40.0)	0.845 (36.8)	1.437 (40.5)	2.6	*
1320	3775	304	34.2	226.6	456	1.7	1.9	22.7	2.28	7.2	0.34	11.3	0.757	0.757	113	13.6	302	1.5	17.0	55	0.45	1.564 (40.0)	0.930 (40.5)	1.437 (40.5)	3.8	*
1600	3525	283	31.7	211	566	2.1	2.4	28.2	2.8	8.5	0.42	14.1	0.706	0.706	106	12.7	283	1.4	15.8	51	0.42	2.113 (54.1)	1.141 (49.6)	1.987 (56)	3.5	*
947	5283	423	47.8	317	845	3.2	3.6	42	4.2	12.7	0.63	21.1	1.056	1.056	159	19.0	423	2.1	23.8	76	0.63	1.818 (46.5)	1.184 (51.5)	1.606 (45.3)	5.3	*
2000	2500	200	30	150	400	1.5	1.7	20	2.0	6.0	0.3	10	0.50	0.50	75	9.0	200	1.0	7.5	100	0.4	1.2 (30.7)	0.70 (30.5)	1.0 (28.2)	2.0	*
2000	2500	200	30	150	200	1.5	1.7	20	2	6	0.15	5	0.5	0.5	75	9	200	1.0	15	150	0.25	1.25 (32)	0.50 (22)	0.85 (24)	2.5	*
—	—	—	—	—	—	—	—	—	—	—	—	—	—	—	—	—	—	—	—	—	—	* (<6)	* (<15)	—	—	—
1892	2638	211	40	158	211	2.0	2.3	26	2.6	8.0	0.16	3	0.634	0.528	80	9.5	211	1.1	10.6	132	0.26	1.32 (34)	0.53 (23)	1.06 (30)	2.6	*
1500	3330	270	50	200	270	2.5	2.9	33	3.3	10	0.20	16.7	0.67	0.67	100	12	270	2.0	20	165	0.33	1.4 (36)	0.80 (35)	1.2 (34)	3.3	*
1770	2820	226	17	51	230	1.27	1.47	11.3	1.7	3.4	0.17	5.7	0.56	0.56	85	10.2	226	1.13	8.5	57	0.06	1.07 (27.4)	0.62 (27)	0.96 (27.1)	2.3	85
1000	5000	400	60	300	400	3	3.4	40	4	12	0.3	10	1.0	1.0	150	18	400	2	30	300	0.50	1.250 (32.1)	1.00 (43.5)	0.950 (26.8)	5	*
1250	4000	320	24	72	320	1.8	2.1	16	2.4	4.8	0.24	8.0	1.2	1.2	120	14.4	320	1.6	12	—	0.08	1.6 (41)	0.88 (38.3)	1.6 (45.1)	3.2	—
1040	4800	385	28.8	57.7	380	1.5	2.6	19.2	1.9	6.9	0.29	9.6	2.2	1.9	146	17.3	385	1.9	14.4	77	0.21	2.8 (71.8)	1.1 (47.8)	2.2 (62.1)	3.8	—

L

TABLE L-1

Enteral Formulas†

Product	Manufacturer	Form	NUTRIENT SOURCES			Protein (g/1000 ml)	Fat (g/1000 ml)	Carbohydrate (g/1000 ml)	kcalories/ml	mOsm/kg
			Major Protein Sources	Major Fat Sources	Major Carbohydrate Sources					
Osmolite®	Ross	Liquid	Sodium and calcium caseinates, soy protein isolate	MCT, corn oil, soybean oil	Hydrolyzed corn starch	37.2	38.5	145	1.06	300
Osmolite® HN	Ross	Liquid	Sodium and calcium caseinates, soy protein isolate	MCT, corn oil, soybean oil	Hydrolyzed corn starch	44.4	36.8	141	1.06	310
Precision High Nitrogen Diet®	SandozNutrition	Powder	Egg white solids	Partially hydrogenated soybean oil	Maltodextrin, sucrose	43.9	1.3	216	1.05	525
Precision Isotonic Diet®	SandozNutrition	Powder	Egg white solids	Partially hydrogenated soybean oil	Glucose, oligosaccharides, sucrose	29	30	144	1.0	300
Precision LR Diet®	SandozNutrition	Powder	Egg white solids	Partially hydrogenated soybean oil	Maltodextrin, sucrose	26	1.6	248	1.1	530 Van.
Pulmocare®	Ross	Liquid	Sodium and calcium caseinates	Corn oil	Sucrose, hydrolyzed corn starch	62.6	92.1	106	1.5	490
Resource® Instant Crystals™	SandozNutrition	Instant Crystals	Sodium and calcium caseinates, soy protein isolate	Hydrogenated soybean oil	Maltodextrin, sucrose	37.2	37.2	145	1.06	450
Ross SLD™	Ross	Powder	Egg white solids	*	Hydrolyzed corn starch, sucrose	37.5	0.5	137	0.82	550
Stresstein®	SandozNutrition	Powder	Free amino acids (44% BCAA)	MCT, soybean oil	Maltodextrin	70	28	170	1.2	910
Sustacal®	Mead Johnson	Liquid	Calcium and sodium caseinates, soy protein isolate	Partially hydrogenated soybean oil	Sucrose, corn syrup	61	23	140	1.0	625
Sustacal® HC	Mead Johnson	Liquid	Calcium and sodium caseinates	Partially hydrogenated soybean oil	Corn syrup solids, sugar	61	58	190	1.5	650
Sustacal® Powder²	Mead Johnson	Powder	Nonfat milk	Milk fat	Lactose, sugar, corn syrup solids	77	34	180	1.33	899
Sustogen®	Mead Johnson	Powder	Nonfat milk, powdered whole milk, calcium caseinate	Milk fat	Corn syrup solids, lactose, dextrose	111.5	16.5	312	1.7	*
Traumacal™ Fulfil™	Mead Johnson	Liquid	Calcium and sodium caseinates	Soybean oil, MCT	Corn syrup, sugar	82.5	68.5	142.5	1.5	550
Traum-Aid® HBC	Kendall McGaw	Powder	Free amino acids (50% BCAA)	Partially hydrogenated soybean oil, MCT	Maltodextrins	56	12.4	166	1.0	675
Travasorb®	Travenol	Liquid	Sodium and calcium caseinates, soy protein isolate	Corn oil, partially hydrogenated soybean oil	Sucrose, corn syrup solids	35	35	136	1.06	488
Travasorb® HN	Travenol	Powder	Enzymatically hydrolyzed lactalbumin	MCT, safflower oil	Glucose oligosaccharides	45	13.4	175	1.0	560
Travasorb® Hepatic	Travenol	Powder	Free amino acids (50% BCAA)	MCT, sunflower oil	Glucose oligosaccharides	28.6	14.3	209	1.1	690
Travasorb® MCT³	Travenol	Powder	Lactalbumin, potassium caseinates	MCT, sunflower oil	Corn syrup solids	49.3	33	123	1.0	312

†Based on Manufacturers' available literature.
*Value not provided in available literature.
+Retinol equivalents
++Tocopherol equivalents
[1]Does not contain vitamins or electrolytes.
[2]One packet Sustacal Powder mixed with whole milk to prepare a 40 kcal/fl oz serving.
[3]At 1.0 kcal/ml dilution.
[4]Does not contain fat-soluble vitamins or electrolytes.

BCAA: Branched Chain Amino Acids
MCT: Medium chain triglycerides

L

Volume to meet 100% of U.S. RDA	Vitamin A (IU)	Vitamin D (IU)	Vitamin E (IU)	Vitamin C (mg)	Folacin (µg)	Thiamin (mg)	Riboflavin (mg)	Niacin (mg)	Vitamin B6 (mg)	Vitamin B12 (µg)	Biotin (mg)	Pantothenic Acid (mg)	Calcium (g)	Phosphorus (g)	Iodine (µg)	Iron (mg)	Magnesium (mg)	Copper (mg)	Zinc (mg)	Vitamin K (µg)	Choline (g)	Potassium g (mEq)	Sodium g (mEq)	Chloride g (mEq)	Manganese (mg)	Selenium (µg)
1887	2642	211	23.8	158.5	423	1.6	1.8	21.1	2.1	6.3	0.32	10.6	0.528	0.528	79.5	9.5	211	1.1	11.9	38	0.32	1.014 (25.9)	0.634 (27.6)	0.845 (23.8)	2.62	*
1320	3804	304	34.2	139	465	1.7	1.9	22.8	2.3	7.2	0.35	11.4	0.76	0.76	114	13.9	304	1.5	17.3	55	0.59	1.564 (40)	0.930 (40.5)	1.437 (40.5)	3.8	*
2850	1760	140	10.5	31.6	140	0.79	0.91	7.0	1.1	2.1	0.11	3.5	0.35	0.35	52.6	6.3	140	0.70	5.3	35.1	0.04	0.91 (23.3)	0.98 (42.6)	1.19 (33.6)	1.4	61
1560	3210	256	19.2	57.7	260	1.44	1.67	12.8	1.92	3.85	0.19	6.41	0.64	0.64	96.2	11.5	256	1.28	9.6	64.1	0.06	0.96 (24.6)	0.77 (19.7)	1.03 (44.8)	2.7	64
1710	2920	235	17.5	52.6	240	1.3	1.5	11.7	1.8	3.5	0.18	5.9	0.58	0.58	88	10.5	234	1.2	8.8	58.5	0.06	0.88 (22.6)	0.70 (30.4)	1.1 (31)	2.4	58.5
960	5283	423	47.8	317	845	3.17	3.59	42	4.2	12.7	0.63	21.1	1.056	1.056	161	19.0	423	2.11	23.7	76	0.63	1.902 (48.8)	1.310 (57.0)	1.691 (47.6)	5.28	*
1896	2642	211	24.1	161	211	1.6	1.8	21.1	2.1	6.3	0.16	5.3	0.55	0.55	80	9.5	211	1.1	15.9	38	0.55	1.56 (40)	0.85 (36.8)	1.4 (40.5)	2.1	—
1200	4167	333	37.5	75	500	1.92	2.17	25	2.5	7.5	0.38	12.5	0.83	0.83	125	15	333	1.67	19.2	30	0.38	0.833 (21)	0.833 (36)	1.00 (28.2)	4.17	*
2000	2500	200	15	30	200	0.75	0.85	10	1.1	3.0	0.15	5.0	0.5	0.5	75	9.0	200	1.0	7.5	35	0.05	1.1 (28.2)	0.65 (28.3)	1.0 (28.2)	2.0	62.5
1080	4690	376	28	56	380	1.4	1.7	20	2.0	5.6	0.28	9.8	1.0	0.93	140	17	380	2	13.7	234	0.23	2.08 (53)	0.94 (41)	1.58 (44)	2.8	*
1200	4220	338	25	76	506	1.9	2.1	25	2.5	7.6	0.38	12.7	0.85	0.85	127	15	338	1.7	12.7	210	0.21	1.48 (38)	0.84 (37)	1.27 (36)	2.5	*
800	6254	498	37.5	75	498	1.9	2.25	26	2.6	7.5	0.38	13	2.2	1.8	187	22	506	2.6	18.8	*	*	3.4 (87)	1.2 (53.5)	1.8 (51)	3.8	*
1030	5275	422	47	316	422	4.0	4.5	52.8	5.3	15.8	0.32	26.4	3.4	2.5	158	19	422	2.1	21	264	0.53	3.38 (86.5)	1.27 (55)	2.85 (80.2)	5.3	*
2000	2500	200	38	150	200	1.9	2.2	25	2.5	7.5	0.15	12.5	0.75	0.75	75	9.0	200	1.5	15	125	0.25	1.4 (36)	1.2 (52)	1.6 (45)	2.5	*
3000	1667	133	20	33	133	0.5	0.57	6.7	0.67	2.0	0.1	3.3	0.40	0.40	50	6.0	133	0.67	6.7	50	0.14	1.167 (30)	0.533 (23)	0.833 (23.4)	1.3	50
1896	2637	211	32	160	211	1.6	1.8	21.1	2.1	6.3	0.16	5.3	0.527	0.527	80	9.5	210	1.05	15.8	1013	0.53	1.266 (32.5)	0.738 (32)	1.055 (29.7)	2.1	*
2000	2500	200	15	45	200	0.75	0.85	10	1.0	3.0	0.15	5.0	0.5	0.5	75	9.0	200	1.0	7.5	75	0.14	1.17 (30)	0.92 (40)	1.37 (38.6)	1.25	*
2100	486 R.E.+	197	4.9 T.E.++	44	195	0.68	0.77	8.7	1.06	1.4	0.07	2.6	0.38	0.47	71	8.6	186	0.95	7.1	50	0.20	1.14 (29)	0.445 (19.3)	0.690 (19.4)	1.21	*
2000	2500	200	30	150	200	1.5	1.7	20	2.0	6.0	0.15	5.0	0.5	0.5	75	9.0	200	1.0	15	75	0.23	1.74 (44.6)	0.350 (15.2)	1.21 (34.1)	2.0	*

L

TABLE L-1

Enteral Formulas[†]

| Product | Manufacturer | Form | NUTRIENT SOURCES | | | Protein (g/1000 ml) | Fat (g/1000 ml) | Carbohydrate (g/1000 ml) | kcalories/ml | mOsm/kg |
			Major Protein Sources	Major Fat Sources	Major Carbohydrate Sources					
Travasorb® MCT Liquid Diet	Travenol	Liquid	Casein, lactalbumin and other whey proteins	MCT, safflower oil	Maltodextrin	74	50	185	1.5	488
Travasorb® Renal[4]	Travenol	Powder	Free amino acids	MCT, sunflower oil	Glucose oligosaccharides, sucrose	22.9	17.7	271	1.35	590
Travasorb® Standard	Travenol	Powder	Hydrolyzed lactalbumin	MCT, sunflower oil	Glucose oligosaccharides	30	13.4	190	1.0	560
TwoCal™ HN	Ross	Liquid	Sodium and calcium caseinates, soy protein isolate	Corn oil, MCT	Hydrolyzed corn starch, sucrose	83.4	90.5	216.4	2.0	740
Vital® HN	Ross	Powder	Protein components, (partially hydrolyzed whey, meat and soy), free amino acids	Safflower oil, MCT	Hydrolyzed corn starch, sucrose	41.7	10.8	185	1.0	460
Vitaneed®	Chesebrough-Pond's	Liquid	Beef, sodium and calcium caseinates	Soybean oil, beef	Maltodextrin, pureed fruit and vegetables	35	40	125	1.0	310
Vivonex® High Nitrogen	Norwich-Eaton	Powder	Free amino acids	Safflower oil	Glucose oligosaccharides	46	0.87	210	1.0	810
Vivonex® Standard	Norwich-Eaton	Powder	Free amino acids	Safflower oil	Glucose oligosaccharides	20.4	1.5	231	1.0	550
Vivonex® T.E.N.	Norwich-Eaton	Powder	Free amino acids (33.1% BCAA)	Safflower oil	Maltodextrins, modified starch	38	3.0	206	1.0	630

[†]Based on Manufacturers' available literature.
[*]Value not provided in available literature.
[+]Retinol equivalents
[++]Tocopherol equivalents
[1]Does not contain vitamins or electrolytes.
[2]One packet Sustacal Powder mixed with whole milk to prepare a 40 kcal/fl oz serving.
[3]At 1.0 kcal/ml dilution.
[4]Does not contain fat-soluble vitamins or electrolytes.

BCAA: Branched Chain Amino Acids
MCT: Medium chain triglycerides

L

Volume to meet 100% of U.S. RDA	Vitamin A (IU)	Vitamin D (IU)	Vitamin E (IU)	Vitamin C (mg)	Folacin (µg)	Thiamin (mg)	Riboflavin (mg)	Niacin (mg)	Vitamin B$_6$ (mg)	Vitamin B$_{12}$ (µg)	Biotin (mg)	Pantothenic Acid (mg)	Calcium (g)	Phosphorus (g)	Iodine (µg)	Iron (mg)	Magnesium (mg)	Copper (mg)	Zinc (mg)	Vitamin K (µg)	Choline (g)	Potassium g (mEq)	Sodium g (mEq)	Chloride g (mEq)	Manganese (mg)	Selenium (µg)
1333	3743	300	45	225	300	2.25	2.5	30	3.0	9.0	0.22	7.5	0.75	0.75	112	13.5	300	1.5	22.5	112	0.34	1.48 (25.6)	0.524 (22.8)	1.81 (51.1)	3.0	*
2100	—	—	—	43	48	0.71	0.81	9.5	4.8	—	0.14	2.6	—	—	—	—	—	—	—	—	0.19	—	—	—	—	—
2000	2500	200	15	45	200	0.75	0.85	10	1.0	3.0	0.15	5.0	0.50	0.50	75	9.0	200	1.0	7.5	75	0.143	1.17 (30)	0.92 (40)	1.5 (42.3)	1.25	*
950	5263	421	48	189.5	674	2.52	2.86	33.6	3.36	10.1	0.506	16.8	1.06	1.06	160	19	422	2.10	24	75.8	0.8	2.316 (59.4)	1.052 (45.7)	1.558 (44.5)	6.32	*
1500	3333	267	30	60	267	1.0	1.1	13.3	1.5	4.0	0.20	6.7	0.667	0.667	100	12.0	267	1.3	10.0	47	0.13	1.333 (34.1)	0.467 (20.3)	0.900 (25.4)	2.5	*
2000	2500	200	30	150	200	1.5	1.7	20	2.0	6.0	0.15	5.0	0.50	0.50	75	9.0	200	1.0	15	150	0.25	1.25 (32)	0.50 (22)	0.85 (24)	2.5	*
3000	1667	133	10.0	20	133	0.5	0.6	6.7	0.7	2.0	0.10	3.3	0.333	0.333	50	6.0	133	0.7	5.0	22	0.02	1.173 (30.0)	0.529 (23.0)	0.815 (23.0)	0.9	50
1800	2778	222	16.7	33	222	0.8	0.9	11.1	1.1	3.3	0.17	5.6	0.556	0.556	83	10.0	222	1.1	8.3	37	0.04	1.172 (30.0)	0.468 (20.4)	0.722 (20.4)	1.6	84
2000	2500	200	15.0	60	400	1.5	1.7	20.0	2.0	6.0	0.30	10.0	0.50	0.50	75	9.0	200	1.0	10.0	22.3	0.07	0.782 (20.0)	0.460 (20.0)	0.819 (23.1)	0.94	50

L

TABLE L-2

Enteral Protein Modules†

Product	Manufacturer	Form	NUTRIENT SOURCE Major Protein Source	g or ml of Product/1000 kcal	NUTRITIONAL PROFILE Protein (g/1000 kcal)	Fat (g/1000 kcal)	Carbohydrate (g/1000 kcal)	% kcal from Protein	% kcal from Fat	% kcal from Carbohydrate	kcalories/ml or g of Product	NUTRIENT ANALYSIS PER 1000 Kcal Calcium (g)	Phosphorus (g)	Potassium g (mEq)	Sodium g (mEq)	Chloride g (mEq)
Casec®	Mead Johnson	Powder	Calcium caseinates	270 g	238	5	0	95	5	0	3.7 kcal/g	4.3	2.2	0.027 (0.7)	0.41 (18)	0.027 (0.8)
Nutrisource® Amino Acids	SandozNutrition	Powder	Free amino acids	256 g	249	0	0	100	0	0	3.9 kcal/g	0	0	0	0	0
Nutrisource® Amino Acids-High Branched Chain	SandozNutrition	Powder	Free amino acids (44% BCAA)	256 g	249	0	0	100	0	0	3.8 kcal/g	0	0	0	0	0
Nutrisource® Protein	SandozNutrition	Powder	Delactosed lactalbumin, egg white solids	248 g	188	21	17	75	19	6	4.0 kcal/g	0.890	0.744	1.414 (36)	0.670 (29)	0.15 (4.3)
ProMod™	Ross	Powder	Whey protein with lecithin	236 g	179	21.4*	24*	71	19	10	4.2 kcal/g	0.82*	0.79*	2.3* (59)	0.46* (20.4)	**
Propac®	Chesebrough-Pond's	Powder	Whey protein	250 g	192	20	13	77	18	5	4.0 kcal/g	1.5	0.77	1.3 (33)	0.58 (25)	0.17 (4.8)
R.D.P.[1]	Navaco	Powder	Whey protein with lecithin	278 g	209	11	14	84	10	6	3.6 kcal/g	1.02	0.89	2.3 (58)	0.64 (28)	0.64 (18)

†Based on manufacturers' available literature.   [1]Also contains trace minerals.   *Does not exceed.
**Value not provided in available literature.

L

TABLE L-3

Enteral Carbohydrate Modules†

Product	Manufacturer	Form	NUTRIENT SOURCE Major Protein Source	NUTRITIONAL PROFILE								NUTRIENT ANALYSIS PER 1000 Kcal				
				g or ml of Product/1000 kcal	Protein (g/1000 kcal)	Fat (g/1000 kcal)	Carbohydrate (g/1000 kcal)	% kcal from Protein	% kcal from Fat	% kcal from Carbohydrate	kcalories/ml or g of Product	Calcium (g)	Phosphorus (g)	Potassium g (mEq)	Sodium g (mEq)	Chloride g (mEq)
Liquid Carbohydrate Supplement	Navaco	Liquid	Glucose polymers	400 ml	0	0	250	0	0	100	2.5 kcal/ml	0.07	0.03	0.07 (2.0)	0.25 (11)	**
Moducal®	Mead Johnson	Powder	Maltodextrins	263 g	0	0	250	0	0	100	3.8 kcal/g	**	**	0.01 (0.3)	0.18 (8)	0.44 (12)
Nutrisource® Carbohydrate	SandozNutrition	Liquid	Deionized corn syrup solids	313 ml	0	0	250	0	0	100	3.2 kcal/ml	0.001	0.006	0.004 (<1)	0.006 (<1)	0.003 (<1)
Polycose® Liquid	Ross	Liquid	Hydrolyzed corn starch	500 ml	0	0	250	0	0	100	2.0 kcal/ml	0.15	0.03	0.10 (2.6)	0.29 (12)	0.54 (15)
Polycose® Powder	Ross	Powder	Hydrolyzed corn starch	263 g	0	0	250	0	0	100	3.8 kcal/g	0.15	0.03	0.10 (2.6)	0.30 (13)	0.56 (16)
Pure Carbohydrate Supplement	Navaco	Powder	Glucose polymers	250 g	0	0	250	0	0	100	4.0 kcal/g	0.02	0.03	Trace	0.04 (1.6)	**
Sumacal®	Chesebrough-Pond's	Powder	Maltodextrins	263 g	0	0	250	0	0	100	3.8 kcal/g	**	**	**	0.26 (11)	0.55 (15)

†Based on manufacturers' available literature.
**Value not provided in available literature.

L

TABLE L-4

Enteral Fat Modules†

Product	Manufacturer	Form	NUTRIENT SOURCE Major Fat Source	g or ml of Product/1000 kcal	Protein (g./1000 kcal)	Fat (g./1000 kcal)	Carbohydrate (g./1000 kcal)	% kcal from Protein	% kcal from Fat	% kcal from Carbohydrate	kcalories/ml or g of Product
High Fat Supplement[1]	Navaco	Powder	Partially hydrogenated coconut oil	163 g	8	77	66[2]	3	70	26	6.12 kcal/g
MCT® Oil	Mead Johnson	Liquid	Coconut oil	130 ml	0	122	0	0	100	0	7.7 kcal/ml
Microlipid®	Chesebrough-Pond's	Liquid	Safflower Oil	222 ml	0	111	0	0	100	0	4.5 kcal/ml
Nutrisource® Lipid-Long Chain Triglycerides	SandozNutrition	Liquid	Soybean oil	455 ml	0	111	0	0	100	0	2.2 kcal/ml
Nutrisource® Lipid-Medium Chain Triglycerides	SandozNutrition	Liquid	Coconut oil	490 ml	0	120	0	0	100	0	2.0 kcal/ml

†Based on manufacturers' available literature.
[1]Contains trace amounts of calcium, phosphorus and sodium.
[2]Contains dried corn syrup as major carbohydrate source.

L

TABLE L-5

Enteral Vitamin Modules†

Product	Manufacturer	Form	NUTRITIONAL PROFILE				NUTRIENT ANALYSIS PER PACKET[1]													
			Protein (g/packet)	Fat (g/packet)	Carbohydrate (g/packet)	kcalories/packet	Vitamin A (IU)	Vitamin D (IU)	Vitamin E (IU)	Vitamin C (mg)	Folacin (μg)	Thiamin (mg)	Riboflavin (mg)	Niacin (mg)	Vitamin B₆ (mg)	Vitamin B₁₂ (μg)	Biotin (mg)	Pantothenic Acid (mg)	Vitamin K (μg)	Choline (g)
Nutrisource® Vitamins	Sandoz Nutrition	Powder	0	0	9	36	5000	200	10	60	400	1.4	1.6	18	2.2	3.0	0.15	5.5	70	0.10

†Based on manufacturers' available literature.
[1]One 10 g packet.

TABLE L-6

Enteral Mineral Modules†

Product	Manufacturer	Form	NUTRITIONAL PROFILE				NUTRIENT ANALYSIS PER PACKET[1]													
			Protein (g/packet)	Fat (g/packet)	Carbohydrate (g/packet)	kcalories/packet	Calcium (g)	Phosphorus (g)	Iodine (μg)	Iron (mg)	Magnesium (mg)	Copper (mg)	Zinc (mg)	Potassium g (mEq)	Sodium g (mEq)	Chloride g (mEq)	Manganese (mg)	Selenium (μg)	Chromium (μg)	Molybdenum (μg)
Nutrisource® Minerals for Amino Acid Formulas	SandozNutrition	Powder	0	0	3	12	0.80	0.80	150	18	350	2	15	2.2 (56.3)	1.3 (56.5)	2.0 (56.4)	4	125	125	325
Nutrisource® Minerals for Amino Acid Formulas-Electrolyte Restricted	SandozNutrition	Powder	0	0	12	48	0.80	0.80	150	18	350	2	15	0.005 (0.2)	0.015 (0.7)	0.025 (0.7)	4	125	125	325
Nutrisource® Minerals for Protein Formulas	SandozNutrition	Powder	0	0	6	24	0.65	0.65	150	18	350	2	15	1.75 (44.8)	1.0 (43.5)	1.8 (50.8)	4	125	125	325
Nutrisource® Minerals for Protein Formulas-Electrolyte Restricted	SandozNutrition	Powder	0	0	13	52	0.65	0.65	150	18	350	2	15	0.005 (0.2)	0.015 (0.7)	0.025 (0.7)	4	125	125	325

†Based on manufacturers' available literature.
[1]One 24 g packet.

L

Index

Nutrient	The RDA for An Adult Man (1968)	The RDA for An Adult Woman (1968)	The U.S. RDA
Nutrients that *must* appear on the label[a]			
protein (g), PER ≥ casein[b]	(45)	—	45
protein (g), PER < casein	(65)	55	65
vitamin A (RE)	(1,000[c])	800[c]	1,000[c]
vitamin C (ascorbic acid) (mg)	(60)	55	60
thiamin (vitamin B_1) (mg)	1.4	1.0	1.5
riboflavin (vitamin B_2) (mg)	(1.7)	1.5	1.7
niacin (mg)	18	13	20
calcium (g)	0.8	0.8	1.0
iron (mg)	10	(18)	18
Nutrients that *may* appear on the label			
vitamin D (IU)	—	—	400
vitamin E (IU)	(30)	25	30
vitamin B_6 (mg)	(2.0)	2.0	2.0
folic acid (folacin) (mg)	(0.4)	0.4	0.4
vitamin B_{12} (μg)	(6)	6	6
phosphorus (g)	0.8	0.8	1.0
iodine (μg)	120	100	150
magnesium (mg)	350	300	400
zinc (mg)	—	—	15
copper (mg)	—	—	2
biotin (mg)	—	—	0.3
pantothenic acid (mg)	—	—	10

Source: Adapted from *Food Technology* 28(7):5, 1974.
[a] whenever nutrition labeling is required.
[b] PER is an index of protein quality explained in Chapter 5.
[c] 1,000 RE was originally expressed as 5,000 IU. 800 RE was originally expressed as 4,000 IU.

As of 1987, the U.S. RDA numbers used on labels were still those taken from the 1968 RDA. There was no great need to update them because they still would be judged generous by any standard, and because the expense of converting labels to a different set of numbers would be too great to warrant the change.

The circled numbers are those chosen for the U.S. RDA from the adult male and female recommendations. In each case, the higher number is chosen.

In the case of thiamin, niacin, iodine, and magnesium the RDA for an adolescent boy is used because this is even higher than the adult RDA.

In the case of calcium and phosphorus, 1 g/day is used, more than the adult RDA. Pregnant and lactating women and rapidly growing teenagers have RDA even higher than this, but 1 g was considered generous enough for use as a standard for labels.

In the case of the last four nutrients—zinc, copper, biotin, and pantothenic acid, RDA had not been set as of 1968 but these nutrients were known to be essential. The agency set "guestimates" for these so that percent-of-U.S.-RDA labels could include them. As of 1980, all four of these nutrients were included in the RDA tables, but the U.S. RDA values were not changed to correspond; they were considered close enough already. For further discussion, see Chapter 2.